Foreword to the student edition

As the new Chief Nurse of the Royal Marsden Hospital, but a contributor and clinical user for many years, it is a special pleasure and honour to be asked to introduce the very first Student Edition of the *The Royal Marsden Hospital Manual of Clinical Nursing Procedures*. The Manual, now in its seventh edition, is internationally renowned and used by student nurses and nurses across the world to help with their clinical practice. When a text is dedicated to clinical practice it is essential that it is regularly updated so that it reflects the most current evidence.

More than ever all nurses need to be able to assure the public, patients and their families that care is based on the best available evidence. As student nurses it is essential that you know the evidence underpinning your clinical skills. For all of us working in the busy day-to-day clinical world it can be challenging to find time to search for the evidence and this is where the *The Royal Marsden Hospital Manual of Clinical Nursing Procedures* can be a real practical help.

At its best, clinical nursing care is an amalgam of a sensitive therapeutic relationship coupled with effective care based on the best evidence that exists. For the first time in the seventh edition reviewing the evidence or sources of knowledge has been made more explicit with each level of evidence graded. This grading provides the reader with an understanding of whether the reference comes from a randomized controlled trial, national or international guidance or from expert opinion.

As you look at the list of contributors to the manual you will see that the seventh edition has continued to ask clinically active nurses to share their practice in their chapters. This has the advantage of ensuring that this manual reflects the reality of practice but also ensures that nurses at the Royal Marsden NHS Foundation Trust are frequently reviewing the evidence and reflecting upon their care.

I commend this Student Edition, an abridged version of *The Royal Marsden Hospital Manual of Clinical Nursing Procedures*, to you. I hope that it will be a valuable resource as you learn the essential skills of professional nursing.

Finally, I would like to pay a warm tribute to the amazing amount of work undertaken by the two editors Lisa Dougherty and Sara Lister and to all the nurses and allied health professionals at the Royal Marsden Hospital who have worked so hard on the seventh edition from which this book has been compiled.

Shelley Dolan
Chief Nurse
The Royal Marsden Hospital
2008

Introduction and guidelines for use

Welcome to this the very first Student Edition of *The Royal Marsden Hospital Manual of Clinical Nursing Procedures*. This edition has been developed after feedback from pre-registration students who tell us how much they use the manual but want a copy they can carry around more easily and focuses on the procedures that they need to learn.

The chapters that have been included have the same content as the full manual and, in addition, multiple choice questions to help you test your knowledge. The chapters that have been included will help you meet the competences of the *Essential Skills Clusters* (NMC 2007):

- Care, Compassion and Communication
- Organizational Aspects of Care
- Infection Prevention and Control
- Nutrition and Fluid Management
- Medicines Management

Ensuring that our care is based on the best available evidence is essential for the safety of our patients and to also ensure that our practice is cost effective. In all the procedures, the evidence underpinning them has been made explicit. The system used to categorize the evidence is broader than that generally used in clinical practice. It has been developed from the types of evidence described by Rycroft-Malone *et al.* (2004) in an attempt to acknowledge that "in reality practitioners draw on multiple sources of knowledge in the course of their practice and interaction with patients" (Rycroft-Malone *et al.* 2004, p.88). The framework still needs to be tested but has been useful in highlighting how little empirical research underpins nursing practice.

The sources of evidence, along with examples, are identified as follows:

1 *Clinical experience (E)*:
- Encompasses expert practical know-how, gained through working with others and reflecting on best practice.

- If there is no written evidence to support clinical experience as a justification for undertaking a procedure the text will be referenced as an E but will not be preceded by an author's name.
- Example: (Dougherty 2008: E). This is drawn from the following article that gives expert clinical opinion: Dougherty, L. (2008) Obtaining peripheral vascular access. In: *Intravenous Therapy in Nursing Practice* (eds L. Dougherty & J. Lamb), 2nd edn. Blackwell Publishing, Oxford.

2 *Patient (P):*
- Gained through expert patient feedback and extensive experience of working with patients.
- Example: (Diamond 1999: P). This has been gained from a personal account of care written by a patient, Diamond, J. (1999) *C Because Cowards Get Cancer Too.* Vermillon, London.

3 *Context (C):*
- Can include Audit and Performance data, Social and Professional Networks, Local and National Policy, guidelines from Professional Bodies (e.g. Royal College of Nursing [RCN]) and manufacturer's recommendations.
- Example: (Department of Health 2001: C). This document gives guidelines for good practice: Department of Health (2001c) *Reference Guide to Consent for Examination or Treatment.* Department of Health, London.

4 *Research (R):*
- Evidence gained through research.
- Example: (Fellowes *et al.* 2004: R 1a). This has been drawn from the following evidence: Fellowes, D., Wilkinson, S. & Moore, P. (2004) Communication skills training for healthcare professionals working with cancer patients, their families and/or carers. *Cochrane Database Syst Rev*, **2**, CD003751. DOI: 10.10002/14651858.CD003571.pub2.

The levels that have been chosen are adapted from Sackett, Strauss and Richardson (2000) as follows:

1 (a) Systematic reviews of randomized controlled trials (RCTs).
  (b) Individual RCTs with narrow confidence limits.
2 (a) Systematic reviews of cohort studies.
  (b) Individual cohort studies and low quality RCTs.
3 (a) Systematic reviews of case-controlled studies.
  (b) Case-controlled studies.
4 Case series and poor quality cohort and case-controlled studies.
5 Expert opinion.

The rationale for the system and further explanation is outlined further in Chapter 1. This chapter also sets out the context of current nursing practice.

Structure of chapters

The structure of each chapter is consistent throughout the book, as outlined below. An explanation of this structure can be found in Chapter 1.

- *Definition*: Each chapter begins with an explanation of the aspect of care, with any technical or difficult concepts explained.
- *Reference material:* This provides background and presents the research and expert opinion in this area. Where appropriate the related anatomy and physiology is explained. Any specific psychological issues that the procedure may raise for the patient have also been included, so the nurse can carry out the procedure with the knowledge and the right attitude.
- *Procedure:* Each chapter includes the current procedures that are used in the acute hospital setting. They have been drawn from the daily nursing practice at The Royal Marsden NHS Foundation Trust. Only procedures where the authors have the knowledge and expertise have been included.
- Each procedure gives detailed step-by-step actions; these are supported by rationale. For the first time where available the known evidence underpinning this rationale has been indicated.
- *Illustrations*: For the first time colour illustrations of the steps of some procedures are included. This will enable the nurse carrying out the procedures to see in more detail such things as the correct position of hands or the angle of a needle.
- *Reference and reading list*: The chapter finishes with a combined reference and reading list. Only recent texts from the last 10 years have been included unless they are seminal texts.

This book is intended as a reference and a resource, not as a replacement for practice-based education. None of the procedures in this book should be undertaken without prior instruction and subsequent supervision from an appropriately qualified and experienced professional. We hope that *The Royal Marsden Hospital Manual of Clinical Nursing Procedures* will be a valuable companion during your training.

References and further reading

NHSE (1999) *Clinical Governance: Quality in the New NHS*. Department of Health, London.

NICE (2005) *Violence. The Short-Term Management of Disturbed/Violent Behaviour in Psychiatric In-Patient Settings and Emergency Departments*. National Institute for Health and Clinical Excellence, London.

NMC (2007) *Essential Skills Cluster for Pre-registration Nursing Programmes.* Annex 2 to NMC Circular 07/2007. http://www.nmc-uk.org/aFrameDisplay.aspx?DocumentID=2690 Accessed 21/09/07.

Rycroft–Malone, J. *et al.* (2004) What counts as evidence in evidence based practice? *J Adv Nurs*, **47**(1), 81–90.

Lisa Dougherty
Sara Lister
Editors

Contents

Foreword to the student edition   *iii*
Introduction and guidelines for use   *v*
Quick reference to the guidelines   *xx*
Acknowledgements   *xxiii*
List of contributors to the student edition   *xxiv*
List of abbreviations   *xxx*

PART ONE

1	The context of nursing	3
	Introduction	3
	What is nursing practice today?	3
	Patients' perspective	3
	What do organizations want from nurses?	12
	Conclusion	21
	References and further reading	22

2	Assessment and the process of care	27
	Introduction	27
	Principles of assessment	28
	Structure of assessment	29
	Methods of assessment	32
	Decision making and nursing diagnosis	36
	Planning and implementing care	39
	Evaluating care	42
	Documenting and communicating care	42
	Summary of recommendations and guidance for practice	44
	References	46
	Multiple choice questions	52

3   **Communication**   54
    Reference material   54
    Procedure guidelines: Provision of information   57
    Conclusion   75
    References   75
    Multiple choice questions   79

PART TWO

4   Aseptic technique   83
    Reference material   84
    Procedure guidelines: Apron: putting on and removing a
        disposable plastic apron   96
    Procedure guidelines: Aseptic technique   99
    Procedure guidelines: Hand washing   102
    Procedure guidelines: Non-sterile gloves use   107
    References and further reading   110
    Multiple choice questions   116

5   Barrier nursing: nursing the infectious or immunosuppressed patient   117
    Barrier nursing   117
    Reference material   118
    Source isolation   124
    Reference material   125
    Procedure guidelines: Isolation of source of infection   135
    Antimicrobial-resistant organisms   142
    Reference material   142
    Clostridium difficile   151
    Reference material   151
    Hepatitis   154
    Hepatitis A   154
    Reference material   154
    Procedure guidelines: Hepatitis A: patient care   157
    Hepatitis B   159
    Reference material   159
    Procedure guidelines: Hepatitis B: patient care   164
    References and further reading   169
    Multiple choice questions   202

6   Cardiopulmonary resuscitation   205
    Reference material   206
    Procedure guidelines: Cardiopulmonary resuscitation (CPR)   221

References and further reading   227
Multiple choice questions   230

7   Discharge planning   232
Reference material   232
Procedure guidelines: Discharge planning   246
References and further reading   252
Multiple choice questions   254

8   Drug administration: general principles   255
Reference material   255
Injections and infusions   275
Summary   289
Procedure guidelines: Self-administration of drugs   290
Procedure guidelines: Oral drug administration   292
Procedure guidelines: Injections: administration   297
Procedure guidelines: Rectal medication administration   307
Procedure guidelines: Vaginal medication administration   307
Procedure guidelines: Topical applications of medication   309
Procedure guidelines: Administration of medication in other forms 310
Procedure guidelines: Continuous infusion of intravenous drugs   313
Procedure guidelines: Intermittent infusion of intravenous drugs   317
Procedure guidelines: Injection (bolus or push) of intravenous drugs 323
Problem solving: Injection and infusion of intravenous fluids
   and drugs   328
References and further reading   338
Multiple choice questions   344

9   Drug administration: delivery (infusion devices)   346
Reference material   347
Infusion devices   359
Gravity infusion devices   359
Infusion pumps   360
Summary   367
Procedure guidelines: Syringe driver: monitoring and infusion   368
Problem solving: Syringe drivers   369
References and further reading   371
Multiple choice questions   374

10 Elimination: bladder lavage and irrigation   375
Reference material   376
Procedure guidelines: Bladder lavage   382

Procedure guidelines: Urinary catheter: maintenance solution
  administration   385
Procedure guidelines: Continuous bladder irrigation   388
Bladder irrigation recording chart   390
Problem solving   392
References and further reading   393
Multiple choice questions   397

11   Elimination: bowel care   **398**
Reference material   398
Procedure guidelines: Bedpan use: assisting a patient   399
Procedure guidelines: Commode use: assisting a patient   401
Enemas   416
Reference material   417
Procedure guidelines: Enema administration   418
Problem solving: Enema administration   421
Suppositories   422
Reference material   423
Procedure guidelines: Suppository administration   424
References and further reading   426
Multiple choice questions   430

12   Elimination: stoma care   **432**
Reference material   432
Procedure guidelines: Stoma care   451
Problem solving: Stoma care   453
Useful addresses   454
References and further reading   454
Multiple choice questions   458

13   Elimination: urinary   **460**
Reference material   461
Procedure guidelines: Urinary catheterization   472
Procedure guidelines: Urine specimen collection: catheter (CSU)   479
Procedure guidelines: Urinary catheter bag: emptying   481
Procedure guidelines: Urinary catheter removal   482
Problem solving: Urinary catheter   483
Penile sheaths   487
Reference material   487
Procedure guidelines: Penile sheath application   488
References and further reading   490
Multiple choice questions   495

14 Intrapleural drainage   497
    Reference material   498
    Procedure guidelines: Intrapleural drain insertion   508
    Procedure guidelines: Intrapleural drain: changing the
      bottle   515
    Procedure guidelines: Intrapleural drain removal   516
    Problem solving: Intrapleural drainage   520
    References and further reading   522
    Multiple choice questions   524

15 Last offices   525
    Reference material   525
    Procedure guidelines: Last offices   527
    Issues specific to critical care   533
    Procedure guidelines: Last offices: additional considerations in
      critical care   534
    Problem solving: Last offices   536
    Procedure guidelines: Last offices: requirements for people of
      different religious faiths   538
    References   544
    Further reading on religious faiths   546
    Multiple choice questions   550

16 Lumbar puncture   551
    Reference material   552
    Procedure guidelines: Lumbar puncture   558
    Problem solving: Lumbar puncture   562
    References and further reading   563
    Multiple choice questions   565

17 Nutritional support   567
    Reference material   568
    Procedure guidelines: Weighing the patient   591
    Procedure guidelines: Feeding an adult   592
    Procedure guidelines: Nasogastric intubation with tubes without
      using an introducer, e.g. a Ryle's tube   594
    Procedure guidelines: Jejunostomy feeding tube care   597
    Procedure guidelines: Enteral feeding tubes: administration
      of medication   598
    Problem solving: Swallowing difficulties   601
    References and further reading   605
    Multiple choice questions   609

18	Observations	611
	Pulse	611
	Reference material	611
	Procedure guidelines: Pulse measurement	618
	Blood pressure	620
	Reference material	620
	Procedure guidelines: Blood pressure (manual)	632
	Respiration	635
	Reference material	635
	Procedure guidelines: Pulse oximetry	650
	Peak flow	652
	Reference material	652
	Procedure guidelines: Peak flow reading using manual peak flow meter	654
	Temperature	656
	Reference material	656
	Procedure guidelines: Temperature measurement	666
	Urinalysis	667
	Reference material	667
	Characteristics of urine	669
	Procedure guidelines: Urinalysis	671
	Blood glucose	673
	Reference material	675
	Procedure guidelines: Blood glucose monitoring	680
	References and further reading	682
	Multiple choice questions	689
19	Observations: neurological	692
	Reference material	692
	Procedure guidelines: Neurological observations and assessment	705
	References and further reading	710
	Multiple choice questions	712
20	Pain management and assessment	714
	Reference material	714
	Procedure guidelines: Pain control: assessment and education of patient prior to surgery	741
	Procedure guidelines: Pain assessment chart: chronic	743
	References and further reading	744
	Multiple choice questions	752

21 Pain management: epidural and intrathecal analgesia 754
    Reference material 756
    Procedure guidelines: Epidural/intrathecal catheter insertion 765
    Procedure guidelines: Epidural/intrathecal catheter for chronic
       pain management: post-insertion management 768
    Procedure guidelines: Epidural/intrathecal exit site dressing change 769
    Procedure guidelines: Epidural/intrathecal catheter removal 771
    Problem solving: Epidural/intrathecal infusions of local
       anaesthetic agents and opioids: management of side-effects 772
    Problem solving: Epidural/intrathecal insertion: complications 774
    Problem solving: Epidural/intrathecal catheter: issues with pump
       and site 776
    References and further reading 778
    Multiple choice questions 782

22 Perioperative care 783
    Preoperative care 783
    Reference material 784
    Procedure guidelines: Antiembolic stockings: fitting
       and wearing 788
    Procedure guidelines: Preoperative care 793
    Intraoperative care 797
    Reference material 797
    Procedure guidelines: Intraoperative care 802
    Postanaesthetic recovery 804
    Reference material 805
    Procedure guidelines: Postanaesthetic recovery 808
    Problem solving: Postanaesthetic recovery 812
    Procedure guidelines: Postoperative recovery 817
    References and further reading 820
    Multiple choice questions 824

23 Personal hygiene: eye care 826
    Reference material 826
    Procedure guidelines: Eye swabbing 839
    Procedure guidelines: Contact lens care 841
    Procedure guidelines: Eye drop instillation 843
    Procedure guidelines: Eye ointment instillation 845
    Procedure guidelines: Eye irrigation 847
    Procedure guidelines: Eyelid closure for comatose patients 849
    References and further reading 850

24   Personal hygiene: mouth care   853
      Reference material   853
      Procedure guidelines: Mouth care   866
      Problem solving: Mouth care   869
      References and further reading   870

25   Personal hygiene: skin care   877
      Reference material   877
      Procedure guidelines: Bed bathing a patient   885
      References and further reading   888
      Multiple choice questions   891

26   Positioning   893
      Reference material   893
      Principles of positioning   894
      Medical considerations   895
      Positioning in bed   896
      Procedure guidelines: Positioning the patient supine   897
      Procedure guidelines: Positioning the patient sitting in bed   898
      Procedure guidelines: Positioning the patient side lying   900
      Guidance for assisting patients to move   901
      Procedure guidelines: Moving from lying to sitting: assisting
        the patient   902
      Procedure guidelines: Positioning the patient in a chair   904
      Procedure guidelines: Moving from sitting to standing: assisting
        the patient   905
      Procedure guidelines: Walking: assisting the patient   912
      Procedure guidelines: Positioning to minimize the work
        of breathing   913
      Procedure guidelines: Positioning to maximize
        ventilation/perfusion (V/Q) matching and oxygenation   914
      Positioning of patients with cardiorespiratory compromise   915
      Positioning to maximize the drainage of respiratory secretions   916
      Positioning the patient with neurological impairment   916
      Procedure guidelines: Positioning the neurological patient with
        tonal problems   920
      Procedure guidelines: Positioning the preoperative and
        postoperative amputee patient   923
      Positioning and amputee management   924
      References and further reading   925
      Multiple choice questions   930

27	Respiratory therapy	932
	Reference material	933
	Continuous positive airway pressure	945
	Reference material	946
	Hazards of oxygen therapy	952
	Procedure guidelines: Humidification for respiratory therapy	953
	Problem solving: Oxygen therapy by nasal cannulae or oxygen mask	954
	References and further reading	955
	Multiple choice questions	958
28	Specimen collection for microbiological analysis	960
	Reference material	960
	Procedure guidelines: Specimen collection: section swabs	969
	Procedure guidelines: Specimen collection: body fluid	973
	References and further reading	976
	Multiple choice questions	980
29	Tracheostomy care and laryngectomy care	982
	Tracheostomy and laryngectomy care	982
	Reference material	982
	Procedure guidelines: Tracheostomy dressing change	1001
	Procedure guidelines: Tracheostomy suction	1002
	Humidification	1005
	Procedure guidelines: Humidification of patient with tracheostomy	1005
	Problem solving: Tracheostomy	1006
	References and further reading	1007
	Multiple choice questions	1011
30	Transfusion of blood and blood products	1013
	Reference material	1013
	Procedure guidelines: Transfusion of blood components	1036
	Problem solving: Transfusion of blood components	1039
	References and further reading	1040
	Multiple choice questions	1043
31	The unconscious patient	1045
	Reference material	1046
	Procedure guidelines: Unconscious patient care	1049

	References and further reading	1052
	Multiple choice questions	1054
32	Venepuncture	1055
	Reference material	1055
	Procedure guidelines: Venepuncture	1065
	Problem solving: Venepuncture	1071
	References and further reading	1075
	Multiple choice questions	1077
33	Violence: prevention and management	1079
	Reference material	1079
	Procedure guidelines: Violence: prevention and management	1090
	References and further reading	1093
	Multiple choice questions	1096
34	Wound management	1097
	Wound healing and management	1097
	Reference material	1097
	Pressure ulcers or decubitus ulcers	1120
	Reference material	1121
	Plastic surgery wounds	1133
	Reference material	1134
	Scarring	1136
	Reference material	1136
	Methods of wound closure	1138
	Procedure guidelines: Wound dressings change for acute and surgical wounds	1140
	Procedure guidelines: Sutures, clips or staples removal	1141
	Procedure guidelines: Wound drain dressing (Redivac: closed drainage systems)	1143
	Procedure guidelines: Change of vacuum drainage system	1144
	Procedure guidelines: Wound drain removal (Yeates vacuum drainage system)	1145
	Procedure guidelines: Wound drain shortening (Penrose: open drainage systems)	1147
	Procedure guidelines: Topical negative pressure (TNP) therapy	1147
	References and further reading	1150
	Multiple choice questions	1161

Appendices
    Appendix 1: The Code: Standards of conduct, performance and
        ethics for nurses and midwives   1163
    Appendix 2: Contributors to previous editions   1171
    Appendix 3: Multiple choice answers   1176

Index   *1187*

Quick reference to the guidelines

Administration of medication in other forms	310
Antiembolic stockings: fitting and wearing	788
Apron: putting on and removing a disposable plastic apron	96
Aseptic technique	99
Bed bathing a patient	885
Bedpan use: assisting a patient	399
Bladder lavage	382
Blood glucose monitoring	680
Blood pressure (manual)	632
Cardiopulmonary resuscitation (CPR)	221
Change of vacuum drainage system	1144
Commode use: assisting a patient	401
Contact lens care	841
Continuous bladder irrigation	388
Continuous infusion of intravenous drugs	313
Discharge planning	246
Enema administration	418
Enteral feeding tubes: administration of medication	598
Epidural/intrathecal catheter for chronic pain management: post-insertion management	768
Epidural/intrathecal catheter removal	771
Epidural/intrathecal catheter insertion	765
Epidural/intrathecal exit site dressing change	769
Eye drop instillation	843
Eye irrigation	847
Eye ointment instillation	845
Eye swabbing	839
Eyelid closure for comatose patients	849
Feeding an adult	592

Hand washing	102
Hepatitis A: patient care	157
Hepatitis B: patient care	164
Humidification for respiratory therapy	953
Humidification of patient with tracheostomy	1005
Injection (bolus or push) of intravenous drugs	323
Injections: administration	297
Intermittent infusion of intravenous drugs	317
Intraoperative care	802
Intrapleural drain insertion	508
Intrapleural drain removal	516
Intrapleural: changing the bottle	515
Isolation of source of infection	135
Jejunostomy feeding tube care	597
Last offices	527
Last offices: additional considerations in critical care	534
Last offices: requirements for people of different religious faiths	538
Lumbar puncture	558
Mouth care	866
Moving from lying to sitting: assisting the patient	902
Moving from sitting to standing: assisting a patient	905
Nasogastric intubation with tubes without using an introducer, e.g. a Ryle's tube	594
Neurological observations and assessment	705
Non-sterile gloves use	107
Oral drug administration	292
Pain assessment chart: chronic	743
Pain control: assessment and education of patient prior to surgery	741
Peak flow reading using manual peak flow meter	654
Penile sheath application	488
Positioning the neurological patient with tonal problems	920
Positioning the patient in a chair	904
Positioning the patient side lying	900
Positioning the patient sitting in bed	898
Positioning the patient supine	897
Positioning the preoperative and postoperative amputee patient	923
Positioning to maximize ventilation/perfusion (V/Q) matching and oxygenation	914
Positioning to minimize the work of breathing	913
Postanaesthetic recovery	808
Postoperative recovery	817
Preoperative care	793

Provision of information   57
Pulse measurement   618
Pulse oximetry   650
Rectal medication administration   307
Self-administration of drugs   290
Specimen collection: body fluid   973
Specimen collection: section swabs   969
Stoma care   451
Suppository administration   424
Sutures, clips or staples removal   1141
Syringe driver: monitoring and infusion   368
Temperature measurement   666
Topical applications of medication   309
Topical negative pressure (TNP) therapy   1147
Tracheostomy dressing change   1001
Tracheostomy suction   1002
Transfusion of blood components   1036
Unconscious patient care   1049
Urinalysis   671
Urinary catheter bag: emptying   481
Urinary catheter removal   482
Urinary catheter: maintenance solution administration   385
Urinary catheterization   472
Urine specimen collection: catheter (CSU)   479
Vaginal medication administration   307
Venepuncture   1065
Violence: prevention and management   1090
Walking: assisting the patient   912
Weighing the patient   591
Wound drain dressing (Redivac: closed drainage systems)   1143
Wound drain removal (Yeates vacuum drainage system)   1145
Wound drain shortening (Penrose: open drainage systems)   1147
Wound dressings change for acute and surgical wounds   1140

Acknowledgements

Since the first edition was conceived by Robert Tiffany, and then published in 1984, *The Royal Marsden Hospital Manual of Clinical Nursing Procedures* has been supported by innovative and enthusiastic editors (including Phylip Pritchard, Jennifer Hunt, Jill David, Valerie Anne Walker, Chris Bailey and Jane Mallett) as well as many previous members of staff. We are continuing their legacy of providing a manual that underpins good nursing practice.

Yet again we have encouraged nursing and allied health professionals at all levels to be involved in contributing to the various chapters, some of whom are contributing for the first time. It has been more challenging for all the authors due to the change in the procedure section and the provision of evidence for each rationale and so the time and effort of all chapter authors should be especially acknowledged in this edition.

We would also like to extend our thanks to some key people who helped in various ways: Sylvie Hampton, Tissue Viability Consultant, for her help in reviewing the wound management chapter; Jo Rycroft-Malone whose work on evidence-based nursing has been invaluable in providing a pragmatic and comprehensive system for grading the source of evidence underpinning the procedures in this manual; Dale Russell and Erika Suchanova of the David Adams Library, The Royal Marsden School of Cancer Nursing and Rehabilitation for their help and support in finding and providing the references required by the authors. In addition, we would also like to thank the student nurses who gave us the idea for the Student Edition in the first place and who gave up their time to help us decide which chapters were relevant for inclusion.

Finally, our thanks go to Beth Knight and Katharine Unwin at Blackwell Publishing for their advice and continual support in all aspects of the publishing process.

Lisa Dougherty
Sara Lister
Editors

List of contributors to the student edition

Karen Allan RN, BSc (Hons)
Senior Staff Nurse, Smithers Ward
(Chapter 25: Personal hygiene: skin care)

Michael Bailey RN, MSc, BSc (Hons), Dip Theo, Dip HE
Senior Staff Nurse, Wilson
(Chapter 18: Observations)

Amanda Baxter RN, RMN, ONC, BSc (Hons), PG Dip
Clinical Nurse Specialist, Pelvic Care
(Chapter 12: Elimination: stoma care)

Jo Bull RN, BN (Hons) Dip ONC
Senior Staff Nurse, Burdet Coutts Ward
(Chapter 10: Elimination: bladder lavage and irrigation)

Suzanne Chapman BSc, MSc
Clinical Nurse Specialist, Pain Management
(Chapter 20: Pain: management and assessment; Chapter 21: Pain: epidural
and intrathecal analgesia)

Maria Crisford RN, BSc (Hons), Dip Nursing, Slice 1 & 2
Colorectal Specialist Sister
(Chapter 11: Elimination: bowel care)

Sharyn Crossen RN, BN, Dip Cancer Nursing
Sister, Wilson Ward
(Chapter 18: Observations)

Nigel Dodds RN, MSc, BSc (Hons), Dip HE, RHV, PG Cert Education
Lead Nurse Hospital and Home Programme
(Chapter 15: Last offices)

Shelley Dolan RN, MSc, BA (Hons)
Chief Nurse
(Chapter 6: Cardiopulmonary resuscitation; Chapter 27: Respiratory therapy)

Lisa Dougherty OBE, RN, MSc
Nurse Consultant Intravenous Therapy
(Chapter 8: Drug administration: general principles)

Ann Farley RN, BA (Hons)
Specialist Sister, Palliative Care
(Chapter 8: Drug administration: general principles)

Jagdesh K. Grewal RN, BA (Hons), PG Dip Nurse Education, DMS
Senior Sister, Theatres
(Chapter 22: Perioperative care)

Diz Hackman Dip Physiotherapy, MCSP, PG Dip Advanced Practice, MSc
Clinical Specialist Physiotherapist in Neurology/Oncology, Physiotherapy
    Department
(Chapter 26: Positioning)

James Neale Hanvey RMN, RN, Dip HE, MSc
Divisional Nurse Director, Rare Cancers Division
(Chapter 30: Transfusion of blood and blood products)

Sarah Hart RN, BSc (Hons), MSc
Clinical Nurse Specialist Infection Control Radiation Protection
(Chapter 4: Aseptic technique; Chapter 5: Barrier nursing: nursing the infectious
    or immunosuppressed patient)

Beverley Henderson RN, PG Dip Counselling & Psychotherapy, BSc (Hons)
Clinical Nurse Specialist, Psychological Care
(Chapter 33: Violence: prevention and management)

Justine Hofland RN, BA (Hons), Dip HE, MSc
Lecturer Practitioner
(Chapter 18: Observations)

Hilary Hollis RN, BSc (Hons), MSc, PG Dip, RNT
Formerly Programme Leader
(Chapter 1: The context of nursing)

Victoria Hollis RN, BN (Hons)
Specialist Sister, Transitional Care Unit
(Chapter 18: Observations)

Lynne Hopwood RN, BSc (Hons)
Assistant Chief Nurse (Operations)
(Chapter 8: Drug administration, general principles)

Sonja Hoy RN, PG Dip, PG Cert, BSc (Hons), Dip Nursing
Lecturer Practitioner
(Chapter 28: Specimen collection for microbiological analysis)

Patricia Hunt RN, MSc, PG Dip
Lecturer Practitioner
(Chapter 31: The unconscious patient)

Kate Jones Dip Physiotherapy, MSc, MCSP
Clinical Specialist Physiotherapist Musculoskeletal/Oncology, Physiotherapy
    Department
(Chapter 26: Positioning)

Jennifer Kelynack RN, BN, Certificate in Intensive Care Nursing Sister,
    Critical Care Unit
(Chapter 31: The unconscious patient)

Sara Lister RN, BSc (Hons), PGDAE, MSc
Assistant Chief Nurse/Head of School
(Chapter 1: The context of nursing)

Chris McNamara RN, BSc (Hons), MSc
Lecturer Practitioner
(Chapter 28: Specimen collection for microbiological analysis)

Neve Mann RN, BSc (Hons), ONC
Formerly Practice Development Facilitator
(Chapter 22: Perioperative care)

David Mathers RN, Dip HE, BSc (Hons)
Deputy Charge Nurse, University Hospitals of Leicester NHS Trust
(Chapter 20: Pain management and assessment)

Carolyn Moore MCSP
Superintendent Physiotherapist, Physiotherapy Department
(Chapter 26: Positioning)

Gillian M. Parker RN, BSc, ONC
Senior Staff Nurse, Burdett Coutts Ward
(Chapter 13: Elimination: urinary)

Sinéad Parry RN, BSc (Hons)
Project Lead, End of Life Care, Learning Disabilities, Trinity Hospice formerly
    Complex Discharge Co-ordinator, Royal Marsden Hospital
(Chapter 7: Discharge planning)

Natalie Pattison BSc (Hons), MSc, N92 Dip Cancer Nursing
Nurse Researcher, Critical Care Nursing
(Chapter 15: Last offices)

Barry Quinn RN, BACC Phil, BD, MSc, PG Cert Teaching
Lecturer Practitioner Haemato-oncology
(Chapter 16: Lumbar puncture; Chapter 32: Personal hygiene: mouth care)

Lara Roskelly RN, Dip General, Psychiatric, Community nursing and midwifery,
    Dip Critical Care Nursing, Cardiothoracics and Trauma
Critical Care Outreach Sister
(Chapter 14: Intrapleural drainage)

Kevin Russell RN, BSc Dip HE, Dip Cancer Nursing, BSc (Hons)
Charge Nurse, Critical Care Unit
(Chapter 19: Observations: neurological; Chapter 23: Personal hygiene: eye care)

Clair Sadler RN, MSc, BSc, PGCE (A), ONC, Dip Couns
Programme Leader
(Multiple choice questions)

Mave Salter RN, NDN (Cert), ONC, Cert Ed, Dip Couns, BSc (Hons), MSc
Complex Discharge Co-ordinator
(Chapter 7: Discharge planning)

Catherine Sandsund Dip Physiotherapy, Advanced Cert Cardiorespiratory
    Physiotherapy, MSc
Senior Physiotherapist, Physiotherapy Department
(Chapter 26: Positioning)

Neelam Sarpal RN, BSc, PG Dip Teaching and Learning
Teaching Sister
(Chapter 8: Drug administration: general principles; Chapter 9: Drug
    administration: infusion devices)

Steve Scholtes RN, BSc, MSc
Charge Nurse, Burdett Coutts Ward
(Chapter 10: Elimination: bladder lavage and irrigation; Chapter 13:
    Elimination: urinary)

Clare Shaw RD (Registered Dietition), BSc (Hons), PhD
Consultant Dietition
(Chapter 17: Nutritional support)

Caroline Soady RN, BSc (Hons), MSc
Clinical Nurse Specialist Head and Neck
(Chapter 29: Tracheostomy care and laryngectomy care)

Catherine South RN, Dip Nursing Studies, BA (Hons)
Specialist Sister, Head and Neck
(Chapter 34: Wound management)

Anna-Marie Stevens RN, RM, ONC, BSc (Hons), MSc
Clinical Nurse Specialist Palliative Care
(Chapter 20: Pain management and assessment; Chapter 31: The unconscious
patient)

Mary Anne Tanay RN, BSc (Hons), Dip Oncology
Research Nurse, Head and Neck
(Chapter 34: Wound management)

Nicola Tinne RN, BSc, Dip Health Studies
Specialist Sister Head, Neck and Thyroid Cancer and Chair Wound
    Management Group
(Chapter 34: Wound management)

Richard Towers RN, Dip Oncology, BSc (Hons), MSc
Lecturer Practitioner Psychological Care
(Chapter 3: Communication)

Caro Watts RN, BSc (Hons), MSc, Dip Oncology, Cert Mgt
Nurse Consultant Transitional Care (Cancer)
(Chapter 2: Assessment and the process of care)

Alexandra Westbrook RN, BSc (Hons), MSc, PG Dip Teaching and Learning
Programmer Leader
(Chapter 2: Assessment and the process of care; Chapter 11: Elimination:
    bowel care)

Barbara Witt RN
Nurse Phlebotomist
(Chapter 32: Venepuncture)

Miriam Wood RN, ONC, BSc (Hons)
Senior Practice Development Facilitator
(Supporting role)

Jacquie Woodcock RN, BEd, MSc, ONC
Programme Leader
(Multiple choice questions)

List of abbreviations

5-FU	5-fluorouracil
A&E	Accident and Emergency
AAMI	Association for the Advancement of Medical Instrumentation
ABG	arterial blood gas
ACoP	Approved Codes of Practice
ADH	antidiuretic hormone
ADL	activities of daily living
AED	automated external defibrillator
AFO	ankle foot orthosis
AHA	American Heart Association
AIDS	acquired immune deficiency syndrome
ALARP	as low as reasonably practicable
ALS	advanced life support
ANH	acute normovolaemic haemodilution
AORN	Association of Perioperative Registered Nurses
AP	alternating pressure
APTR	activated partial thromboplastin ratio
ARDS	acute respiratory distress syndrome/adult respiratory distress syndrome
ARF	acute renal failure
ARSAC	Administration of Radioactive Substances Advisory Committee
ATC	around the clock
AV	atrioventricular
BAL	bronchoscopy with bronchoalveolar lavage
BCC	basal cell carcinoma
BCG	bacille Calmette-Guérin
BCSH	British Committee for Standards in Haematology
BIA	bioelectrical impedance analysis
BLS	basic life support
BMA	British Medical Association

BME	biomedical engineering
BMI	body mass index
BMT	bone marrow transplantation
BOC	British Oxygen Company
BPI	Brief Pain Inventory
Bq	becquerel
BSE	bovine spongiform encephalopathy
BSO	Biological Safety Officer
BUN	blood urea nitrogen
C&R	control and restraint
CAPD	continuous ambulatory peritoneal dialysis
CARES	Cancer Rehabilitation Evaluation System
CAVD	central venous access device
CAVH	continuous arteriovenous haemofiltration
CBE	charting by exception
CCU	coronary care unit
CDC	Centers for Disease Control
CDs	controlled drugs
CE	*Conformité Européene*
cfu	colony-forming units
cGy	centigray
CJD	Creutzfeldt–Jakob disease
CLP	continuous low pressure
CMF	cyclophosphamide, methotrexate and fluorouracil
CMV	cytomegalovirus
CNS	central nervous system
CO	carbon monoxide or cardiac output
CO_2	carbon dioxide
COPD	chronic obstructive pulmonary disease
COSHH	Control of Substances Hazardous to Health
CPAP	continuous positive airway pressure
CPR	cardiopulmonary resuscitation
Cr	creatinine
CRP	C-reactive protein
CRRT	continuous renal replacement therapy
C-SAS	Chemotherapy Symptom Assessment Scale
CSF	cerebrospinal fluid
CSS	Central Sterile Services
CT	computed tomography
CVAD	central venous access device
CVC	central venous catheter
CVP	central venous pressure

CVVHDF	continuous venovenous haemodiafiltration
DBP	diastolic blood pressure
DEFRA	Department of the Environment Food Rural Affairs
DH	Department of Health
DIC	disseminated intravascular coagulation
DMSO	dimethyl sulfoxide
DNA	deoxyribonucleic acid
DNAR	do not attempt resuscitation
DRE	digital rectal examination
DVLA	Driver and Vehicle Licensing Agency
DVT	deep vein thrombosis
EAPC	European Association of Palliative Care
EBV	Epstein–Barr virus
ECG	electrocardiogram
EDTA	ethylenediaminetetra-acetic acid
EGF	epidermal growth factor
ELISA	enzyme-linked immunosorbent assay
EMEA	European Medicines Evaluation Agency
EMRSA	epidemic strains of MRSA
ENT	ears, nose and throat
EPO	erythropoietin
EPP	exposure-prone procedures
ERV	expiratory reserve volume
ESRD	end-stage renal disease
ESRF	end-stage renal failure
EUPAP	European Pressure Ulcer Advisory Panel
FEC	fluorouracil, epirubicin and cyclophosphamide
FFI	fatal familial insomnia
FFP	fresh frozen plasma
FGF	fibroblast growth factor
FNA	fine needle aspirate/fine needle aspiration
FRC	functional residual capacity
FTSG	full-thickness skin graft
FWB	fully weight bearing
G	giga
GCS	Glasgow Coma Scale
G-CSF	granulocyte-colony stimulating factor
GFR	glomerular filtration rate
GI	gastrointestinal
GINA	Global Initiative for Asthma
GISA	glycopeptide intermediate *Staphylococcus aureus*
GM-CSF	granulocyte macrophage-colony stimulating factor

GMM	genetically modified micro-organisms
GP	general practitioner
GRE	glycopeptides-resistant enterococci
GSL	general sales list
GTAC	Gene Therapy Advisory Committee
GVHD	graft-versus-host disease
Gy	gray
HAAg	hepatitis A antigen
HAART	highly active antiretroviral therapy
HACCP	Hazard Analysis Critical Control Points
HCAI	health care-acquired infection
HAV	hepatitis A virus
HBcAg	hepatitis B core antigen
HBIg	hepatitis B immunoglobulin
HBsAg	hepatitis B surface antigen
HBV	hepatitis B virus
HCV	hepatitis C virus
HDN	haemolytic disease of the newborn
HDR	high dose rate
HDV	hepatitis D virus
HEPA	high-efficiency particulate air
HEV	hepatitis E virus
HGV	hepatitis G virus
HIV 1	human immunodeficiency virus 1
HIV 2	human immunodeficiency virus 2
HIV	human immunodeficiency virus
HLA	human leucocyte antigen
HME	heat and moisture exchange(r)
HNIg	human normal immunoglobulin
HPA	Health Protection Agency
HSC	Health Service Circular
HSE	Health and Safety Executive
HSV	herpes simplex virus
HTLV	human T-leukaemia/lymphoma virus
HTLV-1	human T-leukaemia/lymphoma virus type 1
I-131	Iodine-131
IASP	International Association for the Study of Pain
IBCT	Incorrect Blood Component Transfused
IC	inspiratory capacity
ICD	implantable cardioverter defibrillator
ICP	intracranial pressure
ICS	intra-operative cell salvage

ICU	intensive care unit
IDDM	insulin-dependent diabetes mellitus
IGF-1	insulin-like growth factor 1
IgG	immunoglobulin G
IgM	immunoglobulin M
IHD	intermittent haemodialysis
ILCOR	International Liaison Committee on Resuscitation
IMV	intermittent mandatory ventilation
INR	international normalized ratio
IRMER	Ionising Radiation (Medical Exposure) Regulations
IRR	infrared radiation
IRR99	Ionising Radiations Regulations 1999
IRV	inspiratory reserve volume
ISC	intermittent self-catheterization
IV	intravenous
JAPAC	Joint UKBTS/NIBSC Professional Advisory Committee
k	kilo
KGF	keratinocyte growth factor
KVO	keep the vein open
LANSS	Leeds Assessment of Neuropathic Symptoms and Signs
LBC	liquid-based cytology
LCT	long-chain triglycerides
LDR	low dose rate
M	mega
MAC	*Mycobacterium avium intracellulare*
MAP	mean arterial pressure
MBP	mean blood pressure
MBq	megabecquerel
mc	millicuries
MCT	medium-chain triglycerides
MDA	Medical Devices Agency
MDR-TB	multi-drug resistant TB
MeV	megaelectron volts
MHRA	Medicines and Healthcare Products Regulatory Agency
MHSWR	Management of Health and Safety at Work Regulations
MI	myocardial infarction
mIBG	meta-iodobenzylguanidine
MPQ	McGill Pain Questionnaire
MRI	magnetic resonance imaging
MRSA	methicillin-resistant *Staphylococcus aureus*
MSAS	Memorial Symptom Assessment Scale
MSSA	methicillin-sensitive *Staphylococcus aureus*

mSv	millisieverts
MV	minute ventilation
N$_2$O	nitrous oxide
NANB	non-A, non-B (hepatitis)
NANDA	North American Nursing Diagnosis Association
NANDA-I	North American Nursing Diagnosis Association – International
NCI-CTC	National Cancer Institute Common Toxicity Criteria
NGF	nerve growth factor
NHS	National Health Service
NHSE	National Health Service Executive
NICE	National Institute for Health and Clinical Excellence
NIDDM	non-insulin-dependent diabetes mellitus
NINSS	Nosocomial Infection National Surveillance Service
NMC	Nursing and Midwifery Council
NMDA	N-methyl-D-aspartate
NONPF	National Organization of Nurse Practitioner Faculties
NPSA	National Patient Safety Agency
NRPB	National Radiological Protection Board
NRS	Numerical Rating Scales
NSAID	non-steroidal anti-inflammatory drug
NVQ	National Vocational Qualification
NWB	non-weight bearing
O$_2$	oxygen
OAG	Oral Assessment Guide
OMI	Oral Mucositis Index
P	pharmacy medicines
PaCO$_2$	partial pressure of carbon dioxide
PAD	preoperative autologous donation
PASV	pressure-activated safety valve
PBSCs	peripheral blood stem cells
PC	*Pneumocystis carinii*
PCA	patient-controlled analgesia
PCEA	patient-controlled epidural analgesia
PCP	*Pneumocystis carinii* pneumonia
PCR	polymerase chain reaction
PD	peritoneal dialysis
PDGF	platelet derived growth factor
PE	pulmonary embolism/pulmonary embolus
PEA	pulseless electrical activity
PEEP	positive end expiratory pressure
PEFR	peak expiratory flow rate
PEG	percutaneous endoscopically placed gastrostomy

PGD	patient group direction
PHCT	primary health care team
PHN	postherpetic neuralgia
PICC	peripherally inserted central catheter
PN	parenteral nutrition
PNS	peripheral nervous system
POCT	point-of-care testing
POM	prescription only medicine
PPE	personal protective equipment
PSAR	Pain and Assessment Records
psi	pounds per square inch
PTFE	polytetrafluoroethylene
PVC	polyvinylchloride
PWB	partially weight bearing
PWO	partial withdrawal occlusion
RAS	reticular activating system
RCN	Royal College of Nursing
RCS	Royal College of Surgeons for England
RCT	Randomized controlled trial
RCUK	Resuscitation Council UK
Re186 HEDP	rhenium-186 hydroxyethylidene diphosphonate
Rh	rhesus
RIDDOR	Reporting of Incidents, Diseases and Dangerous Occurrences Regulations 1995
RIG	radiologically inserted gastrostomy
RNI	reference nutrient intake
RNIB	Royal National Institute of the Blind
RNID	Royal National Institute of the Deaf
RTO	Resuscitation Training Officer
RV	residual volume
SA	sinoatrial
SABRE	Serious Adverse Blood Reactions and Events
SARS	severe acute respiratory syndrome
SBP	systolic blood pressure
SCC	spinal cord compression
SCNS	Supportive Care Needs Survey
SGA	subjective global assessment
SHOHTS	Safe Handling of Hazardous Therapeutic Substances
SHOT	Serious Hazards of Transfusion
SI	Système International
SIMV	simulated intermittent mandatory ventilation
SIRS	systemic inflammatory response syndrome

SLE	systemic lupus erythematosus
SLT	speech and language therapist
SNBTS	Scottish National Blood Transfusion Service
SPI	Social Problems Inventory
SRHH	Self Report Health History
SSD	sterile supplies department
SSG	split-thickness or split skin graft
SSRI	selective serotonin reuptake inhibitor
SVC	superior vena cava
swg	standard wire gauge
T_3	triiodothyronine
T_4	tetraiodothyronine
TACO	transfusion-associated circulatory overload
TA-GVHD	transfusion-associated graft-versus-host disease
TB	tuberculosis
TCI	target controlled infusion
TEDS	thromboembolic deterrent stockings
TENS	transcutaneous electrical nerve stimulation
TGF	transforming growth factor
TIME	tissue, infection, moisture and edge advancement
TIVA	total intravenous anaesthesia
TLC	total lung capacity
TLD	thermoluminescent
TNP	topical negative pressure therapy
TPI	*Treponema pallidum* immobilization
TRALI	transfusion-related acute lung injury
TRSC	Therapy Related Symptom Checklist
TSEs	transmissible spongiform encephalopathies
TTO	to take out
TV	tidal volume
V/*Q*	ventilation/perfusion
VAC	vacuum-assisted closure
VAD	vascular access device
VC	vital capacity
vCJD	variant Creutzfeldt–Jakob disease
VDRL	venereal disease research laboratory
VDS	Verbal Descriptor Scales
VEGF	vascular endothelial growth factor
VF	ventricular fibrillation
VGF	vascular endothelial growth factor
VISA	vancomycin intermediate *Staphylococcus aureus*
VRI	vancomycin-resistant enterococci

VRSA	vancomycin-resistant *Staphylococcus aureus*
VT	ventricular tachycardia
VTE	venous thromboembolism
VTM	viral transport medium
VZIg	varicella zoster immunoglobulin
VZV	varicella zoster virus
WBP	wound bed preparation
WHO	World Health Organization
WR	Wasserman test

Part one

Chapter 1

The context of nursing

Introduction

> Nursing encompasses autonomous and collaborative care of individuals of all ages, families, groups and communities, sick or well and in all settings. Nursing includes the promotion of health, prevention of illness, and the care of ill, disabled and dying people. Advocacy, promotion of a safe environment, research, participation in shaping health policy and in patient and health systems management, and education are also key nursing roles.
>
> (International Council of Nursing 2007)

Modern nursing practice is explored from two perspectives in this chapter, reminding the reader of the professional context within which any nursing procedure should be undertaken, as well as explaining how the manual can be used by nurses whether at the beginning of their career or in advanced practice roles.

What is nursing practice today?

By nature this book is very procedurally focused, but just carrying out those procedures as tasks without recognizing the humanity of the patient you are caring for is not nursing. If nurses in the UK were asked to describe their job today phrases such as: 'Too much to do too little time . . . too much paper work.' would be heard. With increasing pressure on time nursing can become about performing tasks, but the essence of nursing is not doing but being open in whatever arises in the interaction with the client. It is about being fully present in the moment with unconditional acceptance of the client's experience; with compassion and respect for their choice. Nursing involves the interaction of individuals and is a socially compassionate as well as a scientific profession (Coventry 2006).

Patients' perspective

One of the drivers for nursing practice today is expectations of patients: 'They are more knowledgeable and expect to be treated as partners and equals, and to have choices and options available to them' (DH 2006, p. 6). We know patients want more than just a person who can carry out a series of procedures and interventions dictated by their medical condition. Recent research has explored what patients want from their nurse (Milburn *et al.* 1995; Williams & Iruita 2004). In these two studies the interpersonal aspect of the nurse's role was emphasized as being high on the priority list for patients. From one perspective the time to listen and talk, i.e. performing a social function, helps patients to feel respected and valued as human beings. The social interaction while intimate or difficult procedures are being carried out also provides a valuable distraction. As a patient recently commented, 'Having my chemo was so much better when it was given by a friendly chatty nurse, we talked and gossiped about all sorts'.

Specific therapeutic communication is also highly valued by patients:

> ... I want them to listen to me when I need them. When I get bad news (about this cancer) I need somebody to sit and listen and to know they don't leave you when you get bad news. They take their time ... when you are low, they are there.
>
> (Milburn *et al.* 1995, p. 1096)

Frequently even this therapeutic conversation takes place while the nurse is involved in another procedure or care activity with the patient.

Patients also talk about the importance of the nurse in the 'little things'. Reflecting on an episode of hospital care for the treatment of cancer, K.B. Schwartz wrote in *The Boston Globe* that: 'It is quiet acts of humanity that have felt more healing than the high dose radiation and chemotherapy' (Schwartz 1995). These 'little things' such as changing soiled linen or cleaning up the leaking stoma bag have been described by Darbyshire (1999) as having profound meaning for recovery and, indeed, for cure. He describes this as the essence of nursing, a caring praxis that includes the ability to be with another, sensitively minimizing embarrassing and humiliating experiences.

Practices such as these little yet very complex ones are what helps a patient towards recovery. Giving baths and getting patients to the bathroom are often considered to be the basics of nursing, so are often taken for granted and their complexity and importance are often overlooked. It is when they are carried out by an experienced nurse purposefully and with a patient-centred approach that they make a difference to patients because of the nursing knowledge and skill that is drawn upon (Macleod 1994). The depth of knowledge of the patient and possibilities for recovery influences the timing, pacing and sustainability of action (Benner 1991). Knowledge of the patient is a key component of excellent nursing practice and must be drawn upon when any care activity or procedure is carried out.

Research by Williams and Irurita (2004) found that attention to these interpersonal therapeutic aspects of care provides emotional comfort for patients, which in turn helped patients to feel in control over what was happening to them.

Dignity

When Milburn (Milburn *et al.* 1995, p. 1094) asked patients, 'What care they would like from a nurse?' one of the responses was, 'Being acknowledged and treated as an individual'. They described this as being treated with respect, which meant kind, prompt care and regular contact from the nurses. Patients felt care was dignified not only when they were appropriately dressed or covered but also when there was adequate allocation of time, acknowledgement of their views and feelings and the demonstration of discretion and consideration of their feelings (Walsh & Kowanko 2002).

One of the principles of the revised Nursing and Midwifery Council (NMC) Code is: 'Make the care of people your first concern, treating them as individuals and respecting their dignity' (NMC 2008). There has been much philosophical debate about the concept of dignity, particularly in the provision of care to a diverse population and the challenges of respecting the values, beliefs and practices of different cultures (Willis 1999), age groups and individuals (Coventry 2006). What does this mean in day-to-day nursing practice?

> The most powerful tool a nurse possesses to maintain and promote dignity is herself, to work with feelings, use them constructively to understand patients and to treat them as valid worthy and important at a time when they are vulnerable. In order to promote the dignity of another, feelings need to be clarified and understood, to ensure interactions and interventions are patient focused.
>
> (Haddock 1996, p. 931)

When involved with a physical procedure for a patient, nurses can respect the dignity of the patient by discussing with the patient:

- If they would like the procedure to take place?
- When is the best time for the procedure to take place?
- Where would they like it to take place?
- Who would they like to be there?
- If they need any medication before it begins?
- If they have any questions?
- How much information they would like about the procedure?

(Adapted from Price 2004.)

Patients need to feel that they have an equal and influential role in health care. Communication not only conveys respect but it is also often the only way of assuring patients that we are interested in their experiences, perceptions and needs.

Chapter 3 discusses in more depth the skills of communicating effectively with patients.

Consent

Dignity exists when an individual is capable of exerting control over his or her behaviour, surroundings and the way in which he or she is treated by others. He or she should be capable of understanding information and making decisions. He or she should feel comfortable with his or her physical and psychological status quo (Mairis 1994). Formally and legally this involves ensuring that an individual can give full and appropriate consent for the care and treatment they receive. It would be expected that a nurse would gain a patient's consent for any procedure included in this manual. The NMC (2008) states four over-riding professional responsibilities with regard to obtaining consent:

1   You must ensure that you gain informed consent before you begin any treatment or care.
2   You must be able to demonstrate that you have acted in someone's best interests if you have provided care in an emergency.
3   You must respect and support people's rights to accept or decline treatment and care.
4   You must uphold people's rights to be fully involved in decisions about their care.

'Consent' is a patient's agreement for a nurse and other health professionals to provide care (DH 2001c). The consent process is a partnership between the patient and the nurse involved. It is a two-way process that is dependent upon competence (of the provider and requester of consent) and information. Consent is a core clinical activity and is fundamental to patient care, best practice and clinical governance. Patients may indicate consent non-verbally (for example, by presenting their arm for their pulse to be taken), verbally or in writing (DH 2001c). The Department of Health (DH) guidelines, *Reference Guide to Consent for Examination or Treatment* (DH 2001c), give more details about implementing and having a robust process of consent.

Patients have a fundamental legal and ethical right to determine what happens to their own bodies. Valid consent to treatment is therefore absolutely central in all forms of health care, from providing personal care to undertaking major surgery. Seeking consent is also a matter of common courtesy between health professionals and patients.

While there is no English statute setting out the general principles of consent, case law ('common law') has established that touching a patient without valid consent may constitute the civil or criminal offence of battery. Further, if as a nurse you fail to obtain proper consent and the patient subsequently suffers harm as a result of a procedure or treatment, this may be a factor in a claim of negligence against the health professional involved. Poor handling of the consent process may also result in complaints from patients through the National Health Service (NHS) complaints procedure or to professional bodies (DH 2001c).

English common law identifies three components of a valid consent:

1   Competency.
2   Information.
3   Voluntariness.

This means the nurse has a duty to ensure the person is 'competent' to consent, has adequate information about what is going to take place and is agreeing to it voluntarily (DH 2001c). Adhering to these principles is as important whether you are seeking consent to catheterize a patient or insert a peripheral cannula. If an examination, procedure or treatment is carried out without these requirements being fulfilled then a civil action may be brought in the tort of battery, which protects a person from unwanted touching, or in the tort of negligence, where harm results directly from the procedure.

Documentation

For significant procedures, it is essential for nurses to document clearly both a patient's agreement to the intervention and the discussions that led up to that agreement. Table 1.1 gives examples of procedures that should have written consent and those where informal consent is adequate. This may be done either through the use of a consent form (with further detail recorded in the patient's notes if necessary) or through documenting in the patient's notes that they have given oral consent.

A standard consent form should provide space for a nurse to identify what information they have provided to the patient and to sign confirming that they have done so. The nurse who provides this information must be competent to do so.

Consent is often wrongly equated with a patient's signature on a consent form. A signature on a form is *evidence* that the patient has given consent but is not *proof* of valid consent (DH 2001c). Patients who are rushed into signing a form or are given too little information or too little time may not have given valid consent, despite the signature. Similarly, if a patient has given valid verbal consent, the fact that they are physically unable to sign the form is no bar to treatment (DH 2001c). Patients are entitled to withdraw consent any time after signing a consent form; their signature acts only as evidence of the process of consent giving, it is not a binding contract.

Table 1.1   Examples of patient procedures that may be carried out by a nurse and the type of consent suggested.

Procedures requiring informed written consent by completion of standard consent form	Procedures requiring informed verbal consent and documentation in patient record	Implied consent (procedure discussed with patient but no formal record required)
Therapeutic ■ Chemotherapy (including instillation of chemotherapy via pleural or peritoneal aspiration; oral chemotherapy, e.g. 6 MP, methotrexate, hydroxyurea, and intrathecal chemotherapy) ■ Pleural/abdominal aspiration, drainage ■ IV/sedation for any procedure requiring it ■ Insertion of any indwelling central venous access device ■ Plasma exchange ■ Peripheral blood stem cell harvest (patient or donor) ■ Leucopheresis (therapeutic) ■ Bone marrow harvest (patient or donor) ■ Blood product transfusions *Diagnostic* ■ Breast diagnosis ■ Percutaneous biopsy, e.g. liver, breast, stereotactic wire localization ■ CT-guided biopsies *Other* ■ HIV testing and counselling ■ Photography ■ Genetic testing	■ Female patients undergoing pelvic simulation requiring insertion of vaginal tampon ■ Physio procedures (specific procedures) ■ Complementary therapies	■ Students'/visitors' attendance during treatment procedure ■ Diagnostic tests: – Plain X-ray ■ Clinical examination ■ Breast, rectal, genital examination ■ Urinary catheterization ■ Nasogastric tube insertion ■ Fine-needle aspiration ■ Bone marrow aspiration ■ Bone marrow trephine ■ Skin biopsy ■ Use of patient information ■ Venepuncture

It is rarely a legal requirement to seek written consent, but it is good practice to do so if any of the following circumstances apply:

- The treatment or investigative procedure is complex or involves significant risks (the term 'risk' is used throughout to refer to any adverse outcome, including those which some health professionals would describe as 'sideeffects' or 'complications') (DH 2001c), e.g. breast aspiration.
- The procedure involves a local or general anaesthetic or sedation, e.g. lumbar puncture.
- The clinical care being provided is not the primary purpose of the procedure, e.g. photography (DH 2001c).
- There may be significant consequences for the patient's employment, social or personal life (DH 2001c), e.g. human immunodeficiency virus (HIV) testing.
- For each course of anticancer medical therapy (cytotoxic, radiotherapy, hormonal, biological or other). NB. Course = planned treatments, e.g. one treatment, six treatments or maintenance therapy.
- The treatment is part of a project or programme of research approved by a research ethics committee.

Consent for one procedure or course of treatment does not give any automatic right to undertake any further treatment or procedure.

Once signed, completed consent forms should be filed in the patient's medical notes. If any changes are made to a form after the patient has signed it, these should be initialed and dated by both the patient and health professional. Patients should be given a copy of the consent form that they have signed.

It is generally not necessary to document a patient's consent to routine and low-risk procedures, such as providing personal care or taking a routine blood sample. However, if the nurse has any reason to believe that the consent may be disputed later or if the procedure is of particular concern to the patient (for example, if they have declined, or become very distressed about, similar care in the past), it would be appropriate to do so (DH 2001c). The record should be put in the patient's medical notes and should specify the actual information given to the patient. The health professional carrying out the procedure is ultimately responsible for ensuring that the patient has given valid consent for what is to be done, it is they who will be held responsible in law if this is challenged later (DH 2001c).

Competent staff

Milburn (Milburn *et al.* 1995) probably not unsurprisingly found that patients considered: A good nurse is one who knows what she is doing.

The NMC Code states:

Keep your skills and knowledge up to date.
- You must have the knowledge and skills for safe and effective practice without direct supervision.
- You must keep your knowledge and skills up to date throughout your working life.
- You must recognize and work within the limits of your competence.

(NMC 2008)

As a qualified nurse there is an expectation that you will have the competence on qualifying to carry out fundamental procedures. Competence is defined in the dictionary as having, 'The ability to do something successfully or efficiently' (Pearsall 1998, p. 374). There is considerable debate as to what is needed to achieve this, whether it is just technical ability to perform a skill or whether associated knowledge and the appropriate attitude is also important (Ray 1987; Darbyshire 1999; Arthur *et al.* 2001; Musk 2004). However the NMC states that a registered nurse 'must have the knowledge and skills for safe and effective practice when working without direct supervision'. The manual has been structured to reflect this approach to professional education recognising that competence is not just about knowing how to do something but also about understanding the rationale for doing it and the impact it may have on the patient (see Table 1.2).

Competence develops over time. Benner's (1984) model of skill acquisition offers a framework to define the development from novice through to clinical expert. Based on the Dreyfus model (1982), which distinguishes between the level of skilled performance that can be achieved through principles and theory based in the classroom and context-dependant judgements and skill that can only be acquired in real situations (Dreyfus 1982), the manual is relevant to competence development at all levels.

Stage 1: Novice   As a novice the reference material will give 'objective attributes' (Benner 1984), knowledge of features of the task that can be gained away from the situation, e.g. understanding of venous anatomy of the arm. The procedures will give 'context free rules' (Benner 1984) to guide actions that are not determined by the patient as an indivdual. This is the first step to technical competence (Ray 1987).

Stage 2: Advanced beginner   The advanced beginner who has got some clinical experience and can use the reference material to understand what they have seen in practice and the procedures as a reminder of the steps to follow to undertake

Table 1.2 Structure of chapters.

Definition	Each chapter begins with an explanation of the aspect of care, with any technical or difficult concepts explained
Reference material	This provides background and presents the research and expert opinion in this area. Where appropriate, the related anatomy and physiology is explained. Any specific psychological issues that the procedure may raise for the patient have also been included, so the nurse can carry out the procedure with the knowledge and the right attitude
Procedure	Each chapter includes the current procedures that are used in the acute hospital setting. They have been drawn from the daily nursing practice at The Royal Marsden NHS Foundation Trust. Only procedures where the authors have the knowledge and expertise have been included Each procedure gives detailed step-by-step actions; these are supported by rationale. For the first time, where available, the known evidence underpinning this rationale has been indicated
Illustrations	For the first time colour illustrations of the steps of some procedures are included. This will enable the nurse carrying out the procedures to see in more detail such things as the correct position of hands or the angle of a needle
Reference and reading list	The chapter finishes with a combined reference and reading list. Only recent texts from the last 10 years have been included unless they are seminal texts

a procedure. Chapters such as Assessment (Chapter 2) and Communication (Chapter 3) will also be important at this stage to introduce the nurse to professional aspects of care that are essential in carrying out any procedure holistically as they progress to becoming a competent practitioner.

Stage 3: Competent   At this stage the nurse should be familiar with carrying out core procedures, but they may need to develop problem-solving skills in respect of specific procedures. The problem-solving sections will help them to develop these techniques.

Stage 4: Proficient   Proficient nurses perceive situations as wholes. They will have integrated the knowledge skills and attitudes (Benner 1984). The manual will provide a useful reference to alert them to changes in practice and heighten awareness of the evidence underpinning practice.

Stage 5: Expert The manual will be useful to the expert to highlight areas where further research needs to be done to establish the evidence underpinning practice. It will also be a useful reference to guide them as they learn those procedures that are new to their role.

What do organizations want from nurses?

The expert nurse is frequently being asked to take on new roles and perform procedures to meet the demands of the changing health service. The following factors in the UK are identified as driving the changes needed in nursing (DH 2006, p. 6).

- Society in the UK today is more complex, giving rise to greater social, cultural, racial and geographical diversity.
- There are more people in the older age range so long-term conditions are more prevalent. As a consequence demand for health and social care will continue to rise.
- Major causes of morbidity and mortality such as heart disease and some cancers can respond well to preventative measures, but these frequently require life style changes that can be hard to achieve.
- Health is not distributed equally and inequalities continue to be a major challenge.
- The working population is smaller so fewer people are available to enter the nursing profession.
- Rapid advances in technology mean more effective treatments as well as the ability to provide care in different settings.
- The cost of new treatments, information and communication technology means a greater focus on value for money.

Health care organizations are therefore redefining what they want from their nursing workforce.

Advanced practice

In response to the increasing complexity of health care and the diverse environments in which care takes place, advanced practice nursing roles have developed.

Initially *The New Deal* for doctors (NHSME 1991) began the debate about the areas of medical practice that could be taken over by nurses, with bold statements being made about the potential cost savings (Richardson & Maynard 1995).

With the publication of *The Scope of Professional Practice* (UKCC 1992) procedures previously carried out by doctors became the responsibility of nurses and new advanced practice roles evolved. 'Advanced practice' is an umbrella term relating to the skills, knowledge, expertise and attitude that are firmly grounded in clinical practice, and encompasses aspects of education, research, consultation and case management (Hawkins & Holcombe 1995; NMC 1999; Royal Marsden NHS Trust 2003). The new advanced practice senior clinical roles such as clinical nurse specialists, nurse consultants and nurse practitioners ensure experienced and highly skilled nurses stay close to patient care (DH 2006). The Chief Nursing Officer's '10 key roles' for Nurses in England (DH 2000) provided the legitimacy and authority needed to assume new responsibilities, like the freedom to admit and discharge patients, or order diagnostic investigations. In practice this means that nurses are undertaking procedures that are more numerous, invasive and complex than 20 years ago when the first edition of this manual was published; for example, seroma drainage, the insertion of a peripherally inserted central catheter and removal of a skin-tunnelled catheter. One of the challenges has been assessing competence at this higher level of practice (Lillyman 1998). Benner's (1984) model of skill acquisition offers a framework to define the development from novice through to clinical expert. This and her subsequent work (Benner *et al.* 1996) have been used extensively to articulate the qualities that distinguish an expert nurse and to define expert nursing care. This framework has been used to develop role development profiles, tools that:

> Support competence acquisition in relation to role developments, enabling individuals to take responsibility for planning, managing and evaluating learning and to provide the opportunity for the individual to maintain a record of their own developing competence.
> (Royal Marsden Hospital 2004)

Those activities that have not previously fallen within the scope of nursing practice and for which the nurse has not received education and training may be considered to be role developments. Procedure guidelines are integral to role development and are part of the process of ensuring clinical effectiveness in 'doing the right thing the right way'. Within the UK there are constant challenges for employers to define and manage these roles because currently there is no national legislative statement of what constitutes an advanced practitioner. This also has implications for the general public as any nurse can call themselves an advanced practitioner. The NMC initiated national consultation on this aspect of nursing practice in 2005 with the view of establishing a specific part of the register for nurses who were functioning as advanced practitioners. The competencies required to undertake this role are one aspect of the consultation. These competencies have no legal standing at present but are currently being considered by the Privy Council. For further information see www.nmc.org.uk. These competences are based on those used by Royal College of Nursing Advanced Nursing Practice Programme, that were adapted for use in 2002 from the established work of the National Organization of Nurse Practitioner Faculties (NONPF) in the USA.

Cost effectiveness and patient safety

Developing new roles has obvious risks attached to it and although every individual nurse is accountable for their own actions, every health care organization has to take vicarious liability for the care, treatment and procedures that take place. An organization will have expectations of all its nurses in respect of keeping patients, themselves and the environment safe, for example having knowledge of and complying with the recent publication from the NPSA regarding the standardization of wrist bands in order to improve patient safety, which sets out the details that should be provided and the processes that should be followed on the checking and applying of wrist bands (NPSA 2007). There are the obvious ethical and moral reasons for this: 'Nurses have a moral obligation to protect those we serve and to provide the best care we have available' (Wilson 2005, p. 118).

With increasing emphasis on cost effectiveness the necessity of a registered nurse to carry out all procedures is constantly questioned. A study entitled *Improving the Effectiveness of the Nursing Workforce* (Centre for Health Economics 2003) has highlighted the shift in roles at the other end of the novice-to-expert continuum, with health care assistants taking responsibility for an increasing number of procedures that historically have been the professional domain of nursing (O'Dowd 2003). Although on a day-to-day basis this may look more cost effective, it has been demonstrated that the higher the ratio of registered nurses to patients the lower the mortality rates (Lancaster 1998; Aiken *et al.* 2002). Aiken described nurses as 'the surveillance system' (Lancaster 1998). It is not just the action of taking the vital signs, dressing the wound or starting the intravenous drip. It is the watchfulness that is always part of the nurse's thinking process while activities such as these are completed (Meyer & Lavin 2005). This has been described as vigilance. Vigilance is the search for signals. Signals are events that the individual determines to be indicators of something significant. Vigilance is not seen, it is only an action that occurs as the result of watching out and responding to the signals that others will infer that vigilance has been happening. Meyer and Lavin (2005) propose that vigilance has five components. The manual can help the nurse develop competence in vigilance:

1   Attaching meaning to what is: This is described as the ability to differentiate 'adverse signals' that indicate that there are dangers from the ordinary noise, the normal signs and symptoms. Developing theoretical and professional knowledge is an important part of learning to identify these signals. The reference material in the introductory chapters is essential to developing an understanding of the underlying physiological function or psychological response of the individual so the nurse understands what is normal.

2   Anticipating what might be: Observe, as the normal procedures and responses are described so the abnormal becomes more apparent.
3   Calculating risks: Understanding that there is an inherent risk in every situation. Problem-solving sections help to increase risk awareness and knowledge of the implications of untoward situations associated with procedures.
4   Readiness to act: Developed from a knowledge base, this allows the nurse to know what things might be required in a situation and to make sure interventions can be carried out quickly when necessary. The manual has been written by experts who are sharing years of experience of carrying out the procedures. Therefore they know what equipment is needed, have knowledge of the potential problems that might occur and, over time, they have built up solutions to address them.
5   Monitoring the results of interventions: Experts writing chapters have made explicit the source of rationale for steps in intervention process, i.e. professional knowledge.

If qualified nurses deliver care there is also an increased opportunity for patients to benefit from therapeutic nursing. Evidence demonstrates that this does contribute positively to the patient's experience of care (Spilsbury & Meyer 2001). As well as this often hidden aspect of nursing being essential to organizations, it is also essential for patients as they want to feel secure with the nurses caring for them (Williams & Irurita 2004). They want to be assured that the nurses have the ability to assess their needs as individuals as well as recognize their personal limitations and potential risks.

Clinical governance means that health care providers have a statutory duty for quality improvement to:

Continually improve the overall standard of clinical care, whilst reducing variations in outcomes of, and access to, services as well as ensuring that clinical decisions are based on the most up-to-date evidence of what is known to be effective.

(NHSE 1999a, p. 3)

With this has come an increasing focus on risk management. Risk can be defined as the possibility of incurring misfortune or loss resulting in:

■   Harm to patients.
■   Resources being diverted to provide extra treatment to correct the initial injury.
■   Resources being diverted to the investigation of complaints, adverse incidents and medical negligence.
■   Harm to the reputation of the provider because of poor performance.
■   Reduction in confidence of the public.

(Adapted from Swage 2000.)

Risk management is a means of reducing the risks of adverse events occurring in organizations by systematically assessing, reviewing and then seeking ways to prevent their occurrence (NHSE 1999b).

Having robust evidence-based procedures is a necessary part of the infrastructure of effective risk management and the evidence bases for this edition of the manual will now be considered.

Evidence-based practice

Historically, nursing and specifically clinical procedures have been based upon rituals rather than research (Walsh & Ford 1989; Ford & Walsh 1994). Despite the 1972 Committee on Nursing Report chaired by Briggs identifying that nursing should become a research-based profession (Committee on Nursing 1972), this was slow to happen. Walsh and Ford in 1989 were still challenging some of the rituals that continued in nursing; for example, salt in bath water, nil by mouth from midnight (Walsh & Ford 1989). However, since this time the concept of evidence-based practice or evidence-based nursing has been introduced into health care by the DH through government policy (DH 1997).

Today, evidence-based practice is becoming an integral part of practice, education management and health care strategy and policy, with infrastructures established by the government such as the National Institute for Health and Clinical Excellence (NICE), the Centre for Evidence Based Nursing and the NHS Centre for Reviews and Dissemination at York University. These will increase the likelihood of the care that is delivered to patients being based upon evidence of what works (Rycroft-Malone *et al.* 2004a). With its roots in medicine, questions have been raised as to whether the concept of evidence-based medicine can be transferred to other disciplines within health care including nursing (Freshwater 2004). It is necessary to explore the term evidence-based practice and establish what evidence is used to base practice upon.

What is evidence-based practice?

David Sackett, a leader in the field of evidence-based medicine, defines this as:

> ... the conscientious, explicit and judicious use of current best evidence in making decisions about the care of the individual patients. The practice of evidence-based medicine means integrating individual clinical expertise with the best available external clinical evidence from systematic research.
>
> (Sackett 1996, p. 72)

Consequently it can be seen that from its inception in medicine, with the emphasis on the use of research evidence to underpin evidence-based practice, there is today an increasing emphasis on the limitations of using this alone as a basis for decisions. Rather the ability to use research evidence and clinical expertise together with the preferences and circumstances of the patient to arrive at the best possible decision for that patient is recognized (Guyatt *et al.* 2004). This then opens up challenges as to what can be regarded as evidence to facilitate clinical decision making.

When making clinical decisions clinicians use evidence that relates to the four principal interests of:

1 Feasibility: practical and possible.
2 Appropriateness: fits or is apt for a situation.
3 Meaningfulness: personal experience, opinions, values of the patient.
4 Effectiveness: achieves the intended outcome.

(Pearson *et al.* 2007.)

The leaders of evidence-based practice in the past have focused more upon the evidence of effectiveness through research; however, this is beginning to change. Thus the evidence required today to support all of these principles needs to come from a range of sources, as proposed by Higgs and Jones who consider that evidence should be: 'Knowledge derived from a variety of sources that has been subjected to testing and has found to be credible' (Higgs & Jones 2000, p. 311). Knowledge can be gained that is both propositional, that is from research and generalizable, and non-propositional, that is implicit knowledge derived from practice (Rycroft-Malone *et al.* 2004b). Likewise evidence-bases can be drawn from a number of different sources, and this pluralistic approach needs to be set in the context of the complex clinical environment in which nurses work in today's NHS (Rycroft-Malone *et al.* 2004b; Pearson *et al.* 2007). The evidence-bases that can be drawn upon fall under four main areas:

1 Research.
2 Clinical experience/expertise/tradition.
3 Patient, clients and carers.
4 The local context and environment.

(Rycroft-Malone *et al.* 2004b; Pearson *et al.* 2007.)

In the clinical environment, practitioners will draw upon and integrate these forms of evidence in order to deliver person-centred care.

Of the sources of evidence available, research has been regarded as the best form. However, in some areas of nursing practice there is a lack of evidence available to use to support decisions made in practice (Pearson *et al.* 2007). In addition there is also debate about the types of evidence available to support practice. Within nursing qualitative research is the prevalent design used, whilst within the field of evidence-based practice there is the perception that evidence that is quantitative in nature is superior to that which is qualitative (Rolfe &

Gardner 2006). Whilst there are different opinions on the value of qualitative research to evidence-based practice it is important to consider as Mulhall suggests: 'No single design has precedence over another, rather the design chosen must fit the particular research question' (Mulhall 1998, p. 5). In practice this can be a challenge and currently there will continue to be debate and discussion on the relative merits of different research designs to evidence-based practice. This will be discussed further when considering the grading of evidence.

Clinical experience and expertise play a fundamental role in terms of evidence-based practice. However, there remains some contention in relation to the terminology, role and status within the literature (Rolfe & Gardner 2006; Pearson *et al.* 2007). A clear distinction is apparent between experience as a source of knowledge or evidence and expertise, which is the application of evidence to practice, but these terms are often used interchangeably. So a nurse may have many years of experience, been qualified for 20 years, but may not have developed knowledge as a result of this and thus is not able to apply this to develop expertise when making decisions related to her clinical practice. On the other hand a nurse may have both experience and expertise but these are difficult to capture, make explicit and ensure they are verified for a wider audience (Rycroft-Malone *et al.* 2004b). Expert opinion does have a role within evidence-based practice both within hierarchies of evidence and within the definitions of evidence-based practice, although it is often regarded as poorer evidence compared to research (Rolfe & Gardner 2006). What is perhaps most important is the blending of this knowledge with research and the sharing of this with others to contribute to the evidence-based decision making in practice (Rycroft-Malone *et al.* 2004b).

The involvement of patients in decision making about their own care and wider consultation in relation to the development of services within the NHS is a principle that has been developed and supported by the DH in relation to health care generally and cancer care more specifically (DH 1995; DH 2000). Whilst individual's experiences and preferences should be central to the practice of evidence-based health care, a study by Evans *et al.* (2003) with cancer patients found that the concept of user involvement was an alien one to a significant proportion of cancer service users. The inclusion of patient's values, experiences and preferences into evidence-based practice is complicated and difficult to achieve (Rycroft-Malone *et al.* 2004b). For example, a patient may request a new treatment but the research evidence may not be there to support it, or the patient may decline a treatment for which there is research evidence because from their experience it has unwelcome side-effects. This should not stop us from working towards the patient and carer having a greater role in the decision and care they receive. We must also be mindful that without patient participation the research we use as evidence to underpin our practice would not be possible.

The context within which health care is delivered, whilst not traditionally recognized as a base for evidence, has been suggested to contain sources of evidence that would impact upon evidence-based patient care (Rycroft-Malone *et al.* 2004b). Practitioners will draw upon both local and national sources to underpin their practice and these would include, for example, policies, patient stories, cultural context and professional networks. For some it may include the use of some of the procedures that are contained in this edition. Moreover, in today's NHS in cancer and other specialties it is evident that NICE guidance, the NHS Cancer Plan, published patient stories, patient satisfaction surveys and other sources will influence and impact upon the delivery of patient care. What we have yet to determine is how to appraise and integrate this systematically into the evidence-based agenda in which we work.

Systems and challenges of grading evidence

Within the arena of evidence-based practice today there is requirement for the quality of the evidence to be assessed before it is used to inform practice. To do this hierarchies of evidence have been developed by a range of individuals and organizations in an attempt to identify the 'best' evidence to inform a particular decision that is required to be made in relation to a particular treatment, procedure or area of practice (Sackett 2000; Joanna Briggs Institute, NHS Centre for Reviews and Dissemination). A key underlying assumption of using such a system is that not all evidence is equivalent (Rycroft-Malone 2006) and the quality of the evidence base therefore needs to be judged in some way. Making such judgements about evidence is complex and difficult to achieve. However, the use of an explicit approach as you will find in this edition may help to facilitate critical appraisal of these judgements, provide confidence when applying evidence in practice and improve communication of this information (Grade Working Group 2004).

One of the challenges for nursing is that many of the hierarchies of evidence do not consider some of the evidence-bases discussed in this chapter and put a lower value on research evidence that is not a randomized controlled trial (RCT). To address this problem, some writers such as Rolfe and Gardner (2006) have sought to challenge this and move from an 'exclusive' hierarchy to an 'inclusive' hierarchy that does not only consider evidence from research programmes but considers all sources of evidence together. How this is achieved is under discussion in the literature, so in the interim we have established after much debate a process to grade the procedures in this edition which capture all the evidence-bases not only the research.

Grading evidence in The Royal Marsden Manual of Clinical Nursing Procedures

The evidence underpinning all the procedures has been reviewed and updated. To reflect the current trends in evidence-based practice, the evidence presented to

Table 1.3   Levels of evidence. Adapted from Sackett *et al.* (2000).

1a	Systematic reviews of RCTs
1b	Individual RCTs with narrow confidence limits
2a	Systematic reviews of cohort studies
2b	Individual cohort studies and low quality RCTs
3a	Systematic reviews of case-controlled studies
3b	Case-controlled studies
4	Case series and poor quality cohort and case-controlled studies
5	Expert opinion

RCTs, randomized controlled trials.

support the procedures within the current edition of *The Royal Marsden Manual of Clinical Practice Procedures* have been graded, with this grading made explicit to the reader. The rationale for the system adopted in this edition will now be outlined.

As we have seen there are many sources of evidence and ways of grading evidence, and this has led us to a decision to consider both of these factors when referencing the procedures. You will therefore see that references will identify if the source of the evidence was from:

- Clinical experience (Dougherty 2003: E)
- Patient (Diamond 1999: P)
- Context (DH 2000: C)
- Research (Fellowes *et al.* 2004: R)

If there is no written evidence to support a clinical experience as a justification for undertaking a procedure the text will be referenced as an 'E' but will not be preceded by an author's name.

For the evidence that comes from research this referencing system will be taken one step further and the research will be graded using a hierarchy of evidence. The levels that have been chosen are adapted from Sackett *et al.* (2000) and can be found in Table 1.3.

Taking the example above of Fellowes *et al.* (2004) 'Communication skills training for healthcare professionals working with cancer patients, their families or carer', this is a systematic review of RCTs from the Cochrane Centre and so would be identified in the references as: Fellowes *et al.* (2004: R 1a).

Through this process we hope that you the reader will be able to more clearly identify the nature of the evidence upon which the care of patients is based and that this will assist you when using these procedures in practice. You may also like to consider the evidence-base for other procedures and policies in use in your own organization and consider the evidence-base that underpins these.

Implementing evidence in practice

The implementation of evidence in practice in an organization, be that at a local level in a ward, throughout a hospital or in the community, can be demanding and requires planning, determination and time and the participation of individuals, teams and organization to effect this change. It is beyond the scope of this chapter to consider the process in detail but some key factors to consider in the successful implementation of evidence-based practice are the evidence which has been explored in detail in this chapter, the context and facilitation (Rycroft-Malone *et al.* 2002). Implementation of evidence in practice is most likely to occur when evidence is robust and inclusive, the context is receptive to change and the process is facilitated by someone who has the skills to effect change. Practice development teams in organizations may be best placed to assist with the implementation of evidence in practice.

Conclusion

This chapter has discussed the current context of healthcare, identifying the issues that influence the use and development of nursing procedures in the delivery of patient-centred care. The procedures in this book affect the whole person. They range from those that are observational and physically noninvasive to those involving intrusion into both the physical body and the psychological persona. The intent also varies; some are diagnostic, others therapeutic, and some are supportive with the aim of increasing well-being. This chapter seeks to remind you of the importance of seeing procedures not just as tasks but as part of the whole for the patient.

It is important to remember that even if a procedure is very familiar to us and we are very confident in carrying it out, it may be new to the patient, so time must be taken to explain it and gain consent, even if this is only verbal consent. The diverse range of technical procedures that patients may be subjected to should act as a reminder not to lose sight of the unique person undergoing such procedures and the importance of individualized patient assessment in achieving this:

When a nurse
Encounters another
What occurs is never a neutral event
A pulse taken
Words exchanged
A touch
A healing moment
Two persons
Are never the same

(Anon)
(Dosey Keegan & Guzzetta 2005)

Nurses have a central role to play in helping patients to manage the demands of the procedures described in this manual. It must not be forgotten that for the patient the clinical procedure is part of a larger picture, which encompasses an appreciation of the unique experience of illness. Alongside this we need to be mindful of the evidence upon which we are basing the care we deliver. We hope that through increasing the clarity with which the evidence for the procedures in this edition are presented you will be better able to underpin the care you deliver to your patients in your day-to-day practice.

References and further reading

Aiken, L. *et al.* (2002) Hospital nurse staffing and patient mortality, nurse burnout and job satisfaction. *JAMA*, **288**, 1987–93.

Arthur, D., Pang, S. & Wong, T. (2001) The effect of technology on the caring attributes of an international sample of nurses. *Int J Nurs Stud*, **38**, 37–43.

Benner, P. (1984) *From Novice to Expert*. Addison Wesley, California.

Benner, P. (1991) The role of experience, narrative and community in skilled ethical comportment. *Adv Nurs Sci*, **14**(2), 1–21.

Benner, P., Tanner, C.A. & Chesla, C.A. (1996) *Expertise in Nursing Practice*. Springer, New York.

BMA (1995) *Advance Statements About Medical Treatment*. BMJ Publishing, London.

Briggs, A. (1972) *Report of the Committee on Nursing*. Cmnd 5115. HMSO, London.

Centre for Health Economics (2003) *Improving the Effectiveness of the Nursing Workforce*. University of York, York.

Committee on Nursing (1972) *Report of the Committee on Nursing*. HMSO, London.

Coventry, M. (2006) Care with dignity: a concept analysis. *J Gerontol Nurs*, **32**(5), 42–8.

Cox, C.L. & Reyes-Hughes, A. (2002) Clinical effectiveness, nursing diagnosis and the role of the clinical nurse specialist and nurse practitioner. In: *Clinical Effectiveness in Practice* (eds C.L. Cox & A. Reyes-Hughes). Palgrave, Basingstoke, pp. 1–17.

Darbyshire, P. (1999) Nursing, art and science: revisiting the two cultures. *Int J Nurs Pract*, **5**(3), 123–31.

DH (1995) *Improving the Quality of Cancer Services–A Report by the Expert Advisory Group on Cancer to the Chief Medical Officers of England and Wales*. HMSO, London.

DH (1997) *The New NHS. Modern, Dependable*. HMSO, London.

DH (1998) *A First Class Service*. Department of Health, London.

DH (2000) *The NHS Cancer Plan*. Department of Health, London.

DH (2001a) *National Service Framework for Older People*. Department of Health, London.

DH (2001b) *Essence of Care Benchmarks*. Department of Health, London.

DH (2001c) *Reference Guide to Consent for Examination or Treatment*. Department of Health, London.

DH (2002a) *Chief Nurses. Ten Key Roles*. Department of Health, London.

DH (2002b) *Discharge from Hospital: Pathway, Process and Practice*. Department of Health, London.

DH (2006) *Modernising Nursing Careers*. Department of Health, London.

Dosey, B., Keegan, L. & Guzzetta, C. (2005) *Holistic Nursing Practice*, 4th edn. Jones and Bartlett, Sudbury, MA.

Dreyfus, S.E. (1982) Formal models vs. human situational understanding: inherent limitations on modeling of business expertise. *Office: Technology and People*, **1**, 133–55, cited in Benner, P. (1984) *From Novice to Expert*. Addison Wesley, CA.

Evans, S. *et al.* (2003) User involvement in UK cancer services: bridging the policy gap. *Eur J Cancer Care*, **12**, 331–8.

Fellowes, D., Wilkinson, S. & Moore, P. (2004) Communication skills training for health-care professionals working with cancer patients, their families and/or carers. *Cochrane Database of Syst Rev*, **2**, CD003751.

Ford, P. & Walsh, M. (1994) *New Rituals for Old*. Butterworth Heinemann, Oxford.

Fowell, A. *et al.* (2002) An integrated care pathway for the last two days of life: Wales-wide bench-marking in palliative care. *Int J Palliat Nurs*, **8**(12), 566–73.

Freshwater, D. (2004) Aesthetics and evidence based practice in nursing: an oxymoron. *Int J Human Caring*, **8**(2), 8–12.

GMC (1998) *Seeking Patients' Consent. The Ethical Considerations*. General Medical Council, London.

Goding, L. & Edwards, K. (2002) Evidence-based practice. *Nurse Res*, **9**(4), 45–57.

Grade Working Group (2004) Grading quality of evidence and strength of recommendations. *BMJ*, **328**, 1490–8.

Guyatt, G., Cook, D. & Haynes, B. (2004) Evidence based medicine has come a long way, Editorial. *BMJ*, **29**, 990–1.

Haddock, J. (1996) Towards clarification of the concept 'dignity'. *J Adv Nurs*, **24**(5), 924–31.

Hawkins, J.W. & Holcombe, J.K. (1995) Titling for advanced practice nurses. *Oncol Nurs Forum*, **22**(8), 5–9.

Higgs, J. & Jones, M. (2000) *Clinical Reasoning in the Health Professionals*, 2nd edn. Butterworth Heinemann, Oxford.

International Council of Nursing (2007) www.ICN.ch/definition. Accessed 30/3/07.

Kelson, M. (2001) Patient involvement in clinical governance. In: *Advancing Clinical Governance* (eds M. Lugon & J. Secker-Walker). Royal Society of Medicine Press, London, pp. 5–18.

Kibbe, D.C., Kaluzny, A.D. & McLaughlin, C.P. (1994) Integrating guidelines with continuous quality improvement: doing the right thing the right way to achieve the right goals. *J Quality Improvement*, **20**(4), 181–91.

Kitson, A., Harvey, G. & McCormack, B. (1998) Enabling the implementation of evidence based practice: a conceptual frame-work. *Qual Health Care*, **7**(3), 149–58.

Lancaster, R. (1998) Powerful nurses protecting patients. *Nurs Stand*, **13**(7), 30–1.

Lillyman, S. (1998) Assessing competence. In: *Advanced and Specialist Nursing Practice* (eds G. Castledine & P. McGee). Blackwell Science, Oxford, pp. 119–129.

Ling, J. (1997) Clinical trials, palliative care and the research nurse. *Int J Palliat Nurs*, **3**(4), 192–6.

Macleod, M. (1994) It's the little things that count: the hidden complexity of every day clinical nursing practice. *J Clin Nurs*, **3**, 361–8.

Mairis, E.D. (1994) Concept clarification in professional practice–dignity. *J Adv Nurs*, **19**, 947–53.

Mann, T. (1996) *Clinical Audit in the NHS*. NHSE, Leeds.

Meyer, G. & Lavin, M.A. (2005) Vigilance: the essence of nursing. www.nursing world.org/ojin/topic22/tpc22.6.htm. Accessed 20/4/07.

Milburn, M. *et al.* (1995) Nursing care that patients value. *Br J Nurs*, **4**(18), 1094–8.

Mulhall, A. (1998) Nursing, research, and the evidence. *Evid Based Nurs*, **1**(1), 4–6.

Musk, A. (2004) Proficiency with technology and the expression of caring: can we reconcile these polarized views? *Int J Human Caring*, **8**(2), 13–20.

NHSE (1996) *Achieving Effective Practice: A Clinical Effectiveness and Research Information Pack for Nurses, Midwives and Health Visitors*. Department of Health, Leeds.

NHSE (1997) *The New NHS: Modern, Dependable*. Department of Health, London.

NHSE (1999a) *Clinical Governance: Quality in the New NHS*. Department of Health, London.

NHSE (1999b) *Clinical Governance in London Region, Draft Template of Audit Risk Management Report for a Trust Board*. NHSE London Region, London (www.doh.gov.uk/ntro/risktemp.htm).

NHSE (2000) *The NHS Plan. A Plan for Investment, a Plan for Reform*. Department of Health, London.

NHSME (1991) *Junior Doctors: The New Deal*. NHS Management Executive, London.

NICE (2001) *Pressure Ulcer Risk Assessment and Prevention*. National Institute for Health and Clinical Excellence, London.

NICE/NHS Modernization Agency (2003) *Protocol-Based Care*. Department of Health, London (www.modern.nhs.uk/protocolbasedcare/default.htm).

NMC (1999) *A Higher Level of Practice*. Nursing and Midwifery Council, London.

NMC (2006) A–Z advice sheet: consent. www.nmc-uk.org.

NMC (2008) *The Code: Standards of Conduct, Performance and Ethics for Nurses and Midwives*. Nursing and Midwifery Council, London.

NONPF www.nonpf.org. Accessed 6/8/07.

NPSA (2007) *Standardizing wrist bands improves patient safety*. Safer Practice Notice, 3 July no. 24, National Patient Safety Agency, London.

O'Dowd, A. (2003) Who should perform the caring role? *Nurs Times*, **99**(10), 10–11.

Pearsall, J. (1998) *The New Oxford Dictionary of English*. Oxford University Press, Oxford.

Pearson, A., Field, J. & Jordan, Z. (2007) *Evidence-based Clinical Practice in Nursing and Health Care*. Blackwell Publishing, Oxford.

Price, B. (2004) Demonstrating respect for patient dignity. *Nurs Stan*, **19**(12), 45–51.

Ray, M.A. (1987) Techological caring: a new model in critical care. *Dimens Crit Care Nurs*, **6**(3), 166–73.

Rees, E. (2001) The ethics and practicalities of consent in palliative care research: an overview. *Int J Palliat Nurs*, **7**(10), 489–92.

Resuscitation Council (UK) (2000) *Resuscitation Council Guidelines*. Resuscitation Council (UK), London.

Richardson, G. & Maynard, A. (1995) *Fewer Doctors? More Nurses? A Review of the Knowledge Base of Doctor–Nurse Substitution*. Centre for Health Economics, University of Leeds, Leeds.

Rolfe, G. (2001) *Closing the Theory Practice Gap: A New Paradigm for Nursing*. Butterworth Heinemann, Oxford.

Rolfe, G. & Gardner, L. (2006) Towards a geology of evidence based practice–a discussion paper. *Int J Nurs Stud*, 43, 903–13.

Royal Marsden Hospital (2004) *Developing your role: a guide for nurses*. Royal Marsden NHS Foundation Trust, London (unpublished).

Royal Marsden Hospital Quality Assurance Department (2001) *The Relationship Between Clinical Audit and Clinical Effectiveness*. Royal Marsden NHS Trust, London.

Royal Marsden NHS Trust (2003) *Advanced Nursing Practice at The Royal Marsden NHS Trust 1999–2002*. Royal Marsden NHS Trust, London.

Rycroft-Malone, J. *et al.* (2002) Getting evidence into practice: ingredients for change. *Nurs Stan*, **16**(37), 38–43.

Rycroft-Malone, J. *et al.* (2004a) An exploration of the factors that influence the implementation of evidence into practice. *J Clin Nurs*, **13**, 913–24.

Rycroft-Malone, J. *et al.* (2004b) What counts as evidence in evidence-based practice? *J Adv Nurs*, **47**(1), 81–90.

Rycroft-Malone, J. (2006) The politics of the evidence-based practice movements: legacies and current challenges. *J Res Nurs*, **11**(2), 95–108.

Sackett, D.L. (1996) Evidence based medicine; what it is and what it isn't. *BMJ*, **312**, 71–2.

Sackett, D.L. *et al.* (2000) *Evidence-based Medicine: How to Practice and Teach EBM*, 2nd edn. Churchill Livingstone, New York.

Schwartz, K.B. (1995) 'A patient's story, 16th July'. *The Boston Globe Magazine*. www.thescwartzcentre.org/story/index.html. Accessed 2/4/07.

Smith, R. (1998) Informed consent: edging forwards (and backwards). Informed consent is an unavoidably complicated issue. *BMJ*, **316**(7136), 949–51.

Spilsbury, K. & Meyer, J. (2001) Defining the nursing contribution to patient outcome: lessons from a review of the literature examining nursing outcomes, skill mix and changing roles. *J Clin Nurs*, **10**(1), 3–14.

Swage, T. (2000) *Clinical Governance in Health Care Practice*. Butterworth Heinemann, Oxford.

UKCC (1992) *Scope of Professional Practice*. UKCC, London.

Walsh, K. & Kowanko, I. (2002) Nurses and patients perceptions of dignity. *Int J Nurs Pract*, **8**(3), 143–51.

Walsh, M. & Ford, P. (1989) *Nursing Rituals, Research and Rational Actions*. Heinemann Nursing, Oxford.

Williams, A. & Irurita, V.F. (2004) Therapeutic and non-therapeutic interpersonal interactions: the patients' perspective. *J Clin Nurs*, **13**, 806–15.

Willis, W.O. (1999) Culturally competent nursing care during the perinatal period. *J Perinat Neonatal Nurs*, **13**(3), 45–59.

Wilson, C. (2005) Said another way: my definition of nursing. *Nurs Forum*, **40**(3), 116–18.

Wilson, J.H. (1999) Risk reviews and using a risk management strategy. In: *Clinical Risk Modification, a Route to Clinical Governance?* (eds J. Wilson & J. Tingle). Butterworth Heinemann, Oxford, pp. 39–65.

World Health Alliance (2002) *Factsheet*. www.whpa.org/factptsafety.htm. Accessed 20/8/07.

World Medical Association (2002) *Declaration of Helsinki: Ethical Principles for Medical Research Involving Human Subjects*. World Medical Association General Assembly, Washington, DC.

Chapter 2

Assessment and the process of care

Introduction

For many years, nurses have been expected to demonstrate their contribution to the process of patient care in a structured and comprehensive manner (RCN 2003; NMC 2005; NMC 2008). To achieve this, there is a growing body of evidence underpinning the development of common nursing languages, to enable clearer and more consistent communication and delivery of such care (Muller-Staub *et al.* 2006). In addition to this, there has been an increasing amount of emphasis placed on the importance of critical thinking skills, through thorough assessment, to form accurate clinical judgements and make evidence-based decisions, in order to provide appropriate and individualized care to patients/clients (Daly 1998; Di Vito-Thomas 2000; Seymour *et al.* 2003). Furthermore, as nursing becomes a more autonomous profession in itself, and with continuous developments of new roles and responsibilities it is of utmost importance that we are able to identify what it is that nurses are providing for patients (interventions), for what reason (nursing diagnosis) and with what results (outcomes) (Clark 1999).

Critical thinking is therefore a pivotal skill that underpins clinical judgement and decision making, and culminates in the application of knowledge and experience to clinical practice. However, many authors highlight the lack of a consensus definition around this fundamental, yet complex cognitive process (Daly 1998; Clarke & Holt 2001; Alfaro-Lefevre 2004). Based on some concept analysis work done at The Royal Marsden Hospital in 2004, the following is a definition that integrates many of the key components of critical thinking offered within the nursing literature.

> Critical thinking is a purposeful, reflective and thorough process of reasoning, using cognitive skills including synthesising, interpreting, analysing and evaluating inferences, that enables a clinical issue to be explored from all angles, before arriving at a sound judgement or decision to enhance patient care.
>
> (The Royal Marsden Hospital 2004, unpublished)

The critical thinking approach to nursing care is more than seeking a solution to a problem; it is about challenging assumptions and exploring alternatives in order to most effectively achieve a desired outcome. Critical thinking has arguably the most significant role to play in delivering a consistently high standard of nursing care with demonstrated benefits including improved documentation and enhanced clinical outcomes (Keller *et al.* 2001).

This chapter will consider the role that assessment plays, as an ongoing and central component of everyday care, which nurses achieve by using skills of observation, critical thinking, clinical judgement and communication, and by applying relevant theoretical knowledge (Crow *et al.* 1995; O'Neill & Dluhy 1997; Kennedy 1999; Alfaro-Lefevre 2002). It will then go on to explore the process of identifying nursing diagnoses, as a focus for evidence-based nursing care and identification of measurable and realistic patient outcomes. Some consideration will then be given to how such processes of care can be most effectively communicated and recorded.

Principles of assessment

Assessment is a systematic, deliberate and interactive process that underpins every aspect of nursing care (Heaven & Maguire 1996). It is the process by which the nurse and patient together identify needs and concerns and is seen as the cornerstone of individualized care. It is the only way that the uniqueness of each patient can be recognized and considered in the care process (Holt 1995). Assessment forms an integral part of patient care and should be viewed as a continuous process (Cancer Action Team 2007).

The process of assessment requires nurses to make accurate and relevant observations, to gather, validate and organize data and to make judgements to determine care and treatment needs. A nursing assessment should have physical, psychological, emotional, spiritual, social and cultural dimensions, and it is vital that these are explored with the person being assessed. The patient's perspective of their level of daily activity functioning (Horton 2002) and their educational needs are essential to help maximize their understanding and self-care abilities (Alfaro-Lefevre 2002). It is only after making observations of the person and involving them in the process that the nurse can validate his or her perceptions and make appropriate clinical judgements.

Effective patient assessment is integral to the safety, continuity and quality of patient care and fulfils nurses' legal and professional obligations in practice. The main principles of assessment are outlined below:

1   Patient assessment is patient-focused, being governed by the notion of an individual's actual, potential and perceived needs.
2   It provides baseline information on which to plan the interventions and outcomes of care to be achieved.

3   It facilitates evaluation of the care given and is a dimension of care that influences a patient's outcome and potential survival.
4   It is a dynamic process that starts when problems or symptoms develop, which continues throughout the care process, accommodating continual changes in the patient's condition and circumstances.
5   It is essentially an interactive process in which the patient actively participates.
6   Optimal functioning, quality of life and the promotion of independence should be primary concerns.
7   The process includes observation, data collection, clinical judgement and validation of perceptions.
8   Data used for the assessment process is collected from several sources by a variety of methods, depending on the health care setting.
9   To be effective the process must be structured and clearly documented.
             (Teytelman 2000; Alfaro-Lefevre 2002; White 2003; NMC 2008.)

Structure of assessment

Structuring patient assessment is vital to monitor the success of care and to detect the emergence of new problems. Different conceptual or nursing models, such as Roper *et al.* (2000), provide frameworks for a systematic approach to assessment (such as Roper's Activities of Daily Living) implying that there is a perceived value in the coexistence of a variety of perspectives. There remains, however, much debate about the effectiveness of such models for assessment in practice, some arguing that individualized care can be compromised by fitting patients into a rigid or complex structure (Tierney 1998; Kearney 2001). Nurses therefore need to take a pragmatic approach and utilize assessment frameworks that are useful and appropriate to their particular area of practice. This is particularly relevant in today's rapidly changing health care climate where nurses are taking on increasingly advanced roles, working across boundaries and setting up new services to meet patients' needs (DH 2006).

Nursing models represent a set of concepts and statements integrated into a meaningful conceptual framework (Kozier *et al.* 2003) representing different theoretical approaches to nursing care.

Nursing models can serve as a guide to the overall approach to care within a given health care environment and therefore provide a focus for the clinical judgements and decision-making processes that result from the process of assessment. It has been argued that whilst nursing models have not been widely implemented in clinical practice, nurses do use them as a way to consider the process of nursing (Wimpenny 2001). During any patient assessment, nurses engage in a collection of cognitive, behavioural and practical steps but do not always recognize them as discrete decision-making entities (Ford & McCormack 1999). Nursing models give novice practitioners a structure with which to identify these processes and to reflect on their practice in order to develop analytical, problem-solving and judgement skills needed to provide an effective patient assessment.

Nursing models have been developed according to different ways of perceiving the main focus of nursing. These include adaptation models (e.g. Roy 1984), self-care models (e.g. Orem *et al.* 2001) and activities of daily living models (e.g. Roper *et al.* 2000). Each model represents a different view of the relationship between four key elements of nursing: namely health, person, environment and nursing. It is therefore important that the appropriate model is used to ensure the focus of assessment data collected is effective for particular areas of practice (Murphy *et al.* 2000; Alfaro-Lefevre 2002). Nurses must also be aware of the rationale for implementing a particular model since the choice will determine the nature of patient assessment in their day-to-day work. The approach should be sensitive enough to discriminate between different clinical needs and flexible enough to be updated on a regular basis (Smith & Richardson 1996; Allen 1998).

In the context of cancer care, the Cancer Action Team (2007) have published guidance for an holistic common assessment for assessing the supportive and palliative care needs of adults with cancer. The content of the assessment is divided into five domains including background information and assessment preferences, physical needs, social and occupational needs, psychological well-being and spiritual well-being. The guidance recommends that a structured assessment should be undertaken at key points throughout the person's cancer illness trajectory, recognizing the importance of assessment as an ongoing process (Cancer Action Team 2007).

Incorporating these key dimensions, the framework of choice at The Royal Marsden Hospital is based on Gordon's Functional Health Patterns (Gordon 1994; Box 2.1). The framework facilitates an assessment that focuses on patients'

Box 2.1   Gordon's Functional Health Patterns (Gordon 1994)

- Health perception–health management
- Nutrition–metabolic
- Elimination
- Activity–exercise
- Sleep–rest
- Cognitive–perceptual
- Self-perception–self-concept
- Coping–stress tolerance
- Role–relationship
- Sexuality–reproductivity
- Value–belief

and families' problems and functional status and applies clinical cues to interpret deviations from the patient's usual patterns (Johnson 2000). The model is applicable to all levels of care and allows all problem areas to be identified, and the information derived from the patient's initial functional health patterns is crucial for interpreting both the patient's and their family's pattern of response to the disease and treatment. It is therefore considered particularly applicable for the cancer and palliative care settings where patient's needs and responses vary enormously along their illness trajectory.

The structure of a patient assessment depends not only on the speciality and care setting but also on the purpose of the assessment. A different type of assessment will be required for an acutely ill patient where early recognition of potential or actual deterioration is essential (Ahern & Philpot 2002), from the type of assessment used for a patient with rehabilitation needs. The appropriate type of assessment depends then on the priorities of care and this varies at specific times along the patient's pathway (see Box 2.2 for a summary of the types

---

Box 2.2 Types of patient assessment (Ahern & Philpot 2002; Holmes 2003; White 2003)

Mini assessment

A snapshot view of the patient based on a quick visual and physical assessment. Consider patient's ABC (airway, breathing and circulation), then assess mental status, overall appearance, level of consciousness and vital signs before focusing on the patient's main problem.

Comprehensive assessment

An in-depth assessment of the patient's health status, physical examination, risk factors, psychological and social aspects of the patient's health that usually takes place on admission or transfer to a hospital or health care agency. It will take into account the patient's previous health status prior to admission.

Focused assessment

An assessment of a specific condition, problem, identified risks or assessment of care; for example, continence assessment, nutritional assessment, neurological assessment following a head injury, assessment for day care, outpatient consultation for a specific condition.

Ongoing assessment

Continuous assessment of the patient's health status accompanied by monitoring and observation of specific problems identified in a mini, comprehensive or focused assessment.

of assessment). The single assessment process outlined in *The National Service Framework for Older People* (DH 2001) acknowledges the importance of this and highlights that assessment is a unified process where different professionals are involved in a number of stages. The process utilizes a variety of assessment levels to explore the health and social needs of a particular patient group and facilitates a collaborative, systematic and comprehensive profile of the patient's needs.

Methods of assessment

Assessment information is collected in many different formats and consists of both objective and subjective data. Nurses working in different settings rely on different observational and physical data that may include assessment of vital signs, physical systems, symptoms and laboratory results. Subjective data is based on what the patient perceives and experiences and may include descriptions of their concerns, support network, their awareness and knowledge of their abilities/disabilities, their understanding of their illness and their attitude to and readiness for learning (Coyne *et al.* 2002; White 2003). A variety of methods have been developed to facilitate nurses in eliciting both objective and subjective assessment data on the assumption that if assessment is not accurate, all other nursing activity will also be inaccurate.

Studies of patient assessment by nurses are few but they indicate that discrepancies between nurses' perceptions and those of their patients are common (Lauri *et al.* 1997; McDonald *et al.* 1999; Parsaie *et al.* 2000; Brown *et al.* 2001). Communication is therefore key for as Suhonen *et al.* (2000) suggest, 'there are two actors in individual care, the patient and the nurse' (Suhonen *et al.* 2000, p. 1254). Gaining insight into patients' preferences and individualized needs is facilitated by meaningful interaction and depends both on patients' willingness and capability in participating in the process and in nurses' interviewing skills. The initial assessment interview not only allows the nurse to obtain baseline information about the patient, but also facilitates the establishment of a therapeutic relationship (Crumbie 2006). Patients may find it difficult to disclose some problems and these may only be identified once the nurse–patient relationship develops and the patient trusts that the nurse's assessment reflects concern for his or her well-being.

Assessment interviews

An assessment interview needs structure to progress logically in order to facilitate the nurse's thinking (an example of such a structure can be found in Box 2.3) and to make the patient feel comfortable in telling their story. It can be perceived as being in three phases: the introductory, working and end phases

Box 2.3 Carrying out a patient assessment using Functional Health Patterns (adapted from Gordon 1994)

Pattern	Assessment and data collection is focused on
Health perception–management	■ The person's perceived level of health and well-being, and on practices for maintaining health. ■ Habits that may be detrimental to health are also evaluated. ■ Actual or potential problems related to safety and health management may be identified as well as needs for modifications in the home or needs for continued care in the home.
Nutrition and metabolism	■ The pattern of food and fluid consumption relative to metabolic need. ■ Actual or potential problems related to fluid balance, tissue integrity. ■ Problems with the gastrointestinal system.
Elimination	■ Excretory patterns (bowel, bladder, skin). ■ Excretory problems such as incontinence, constipation, diarrhoea and urinary retention may be identified.
Activity and exercise	■ The activities of daily living requiring energy expenditure, including self-care activities, exercise and leisure activities. ■ The status of major body systems involved with activity and exercise is evaluated, including the respiratory, cardiovascular and musculoskeletal systems.
Sleep and rest	■ The person's sleep, rest and relaxation practices. ■ Dysfunctional sleep patterns, fatigue, and responses to sleep deprivation may be identified.
Cognitive and perceptual ability	■ The ability to comprehend and use information. ■ The sensory functions, neurologic functions.
Perception/ concept of self	■ The person's attitudes toward self, including identity, body image and sense of self-worth. ■ The person's level of self-esteem and response to threats to his or her self-concept may be identified.
Stress and coping	■ The person's perception of stress and on his or her coping strategies. ■ Support systems are evaluated, and symptoms of stress are noted. ■ The effectiveness of a person's coping strategies in terms of stress tolerance may be further evaluated.

Box 2.3 *(cont.)*	
Roles and relationships	■ The person's roles in the world and relationships with others. ■ Satisfaction with roles, role strain or dysfunctional relationships may be further evaluated.
Sexuality and reproduction	■ The person's satisfaction or dissatisfaction with sexuality patterns and reproductive functions. ■ Concerns with sexuality may be identified.
Values and belief	■ The person's values, beliefs (including spiritual beliefs) and goals that guide his or her choices or decisions.

(Crumbie 2006). It is important at the beginning to emphasize the confidential nature of the discussion and to take steps to reduce anxiety and ensure privacy since patients may modify their words and behaviour depending on the environment (Neighbour 1987). In the middle working phase, various techniques can be employed to assist with the flow of information. Open questions are useful to identify broad information that can then be explored more specifically with focused questions to determine the nature and extent of the problem. Other helpful techniques include restating what has been said to clarify certain issues, verbalizing the implied meaning, using silence and summarizing (Morton 1993). It is important to recognize that there may be times when it is not possible to obtain vital information directly from the patient; they may be too distressed, unconscious or unable to speak clearly, if at all. In such situations appropriate details should be taken from relatives or friends and recorded as such. Effort should equally be made to overcome language or cultural barriers by the use of interpreters.

The end phase involves a further summary of the important points and an explanation of any referrals made. In order to gain the patient's perspective on the priorities of care and to emphasize the continuing interest in their needs, a final question asking about their concerns can be used (Alfaro-Lefevre 2002). Examples include: 'Tell me the most important things I can help you with.', 'Is there anything else you would like to tell me?', 'Is there anything that we haven't covered that still concerns you?', or 'If there are any changes or you have any questions do let me know'.

Assessment tools

The use of assessment tools enables a standardized approach to be used to obtain specific patient data. This can facilitate the documentation of change over time and the evaluation of clinical interventions and nursing care (Conner & Eggert

1994). Perhaps more importantly, assessment tools encourage patients to engage in their care and provide a vehicle for communication to allow nurses to follow patients' experiences more effectively. An example of this comes from the European-wide cancer nursing WISECARE project (Kearney 2001). Nurses developed systematic measurements for four chemotherapy treatment-related symptoms and this enhanced care by directly linking nursing interventions to patients' reports of their experience. Improvements in outcomes were demonstrated and patients perceived their feelings and experience had been better considered in their treatment plan (Kearney 2001).

Assessment tools in clinical practice can be used to assess patients' general needs, e.g. the supportive care needs survey (Bonevski *et al.* 2000) or to assess a specific problem, e.g. the oral assessment guide (Eilers *et al.* 1988). The choice of tool depends on the clinical setting although in general the aim of using an assessment tool is to link the assessment of clinical variables with measurement of clinical interventions (Frank-Stromborg & Olsen 1997). To be useful in clinical practice, an assessment tool must be simple, acceptable to patients, have a clear and interpretable scoring system and demonstrate reliability and validity (Brown *et al.* 2001).

Nurse researchers and clinicians have developed a broad spectrum of tools to assess the problems frequently encountered by people with cancer (Box 2.4). More tools are used in practice to assess treatment-related symptoms than other aspects of care, possibly because these symptoms are predictable and of a physical nature and are therefore easier to measure. The most visible symptoms are not always those that cause most distress however (Holmes & Eburn 1989), and acknowledgement of the patient's subjective experience is therefore an important element in the development of assessment tools (McClement *et al.* 1997; Rhodes *et al.* 2000).

Box 2.4   Examples of assessment tools used in cancer care

Generic assessment tools

Cancer Rehabilitation Evaluation System (CARES) (Ganz *et al.* 1992)
Problems checklist (Osse *et al.* 2004)
Supportive Care Needs Survey (SCNS) (Bonevski *et al.* 2000)

Specific assessment tools

Piper Fatigue Scale (Piper 1997)
Oral assessment (Eilers *et al.* 1988)
Chemotherapy Symptom Assessment Scale (C-SAS) (Brown *et al.* 2001)
Pain and Assessment Records (PSAR) (Bouvette *et al.* 2002)

The use of patient self-assessment tools appears to facilitate the process of assessment in a number of ways. It enables patients to indicate their subjective experience more easily, give patients an increased sense of participation (Kearney *et al.* 2000) and prevent patients from being distanced from the process by nurses rating their symptoms and concerns (Brown *et al.* 2001). Many authors have demonstrated the advantages of increasing patient participation in assessment by the use of patient-self-assessment questionnaires (Rhodes *et al.* 2000). A number of patient self-report tools have been developed for cancer patients as a result, and whilst many have been established for research purposes, an increasing number are being used very effectively in everyday clinical practice (Box 2.5).

Box 2.5 Examples of specific patient self-assessment tools used in cancer care

- Self Report Health History (SRHH) (Skinn & Stacey 1994)
- Memorial Symptom Assessment Scale (MSAS) (Portenoy *et al.* 1994)
- Concerns Checklist in Oncology Outpatient Setting (Dennison & Shute 2000)
- Therapy Related Symptom Checklist (TRSC) (Williams *et al.* 2001)
- Social Problems Inventory (SPI) (Wright *et al.* 2001)
- Symptoms and Concerns Checklist (Lidstone *et al.* 2003)

The methods used to facilitate patient assessment are important adjuncts to assessing patients in clinical practice. There is a danger that too much focus can be placed on the framework, system or tool that prevents nurses thinking about the significance of the information that they are gathering from the patient (Harris *et al.* 1998). Rather than following assessment structures and prompts rigidly, it is essential that nurses utilize their critical thinking and clinical judgement throughout the process in order to continually develop their skills in eliciting information about patients' concerns and using this to inform care planning (Edwards & Miller 2001).

Decision making and nursing diagnosis

The purpose of collecting information through the process of assessment is to enable the nurse to make a series of clinical judgements, otherwise known as nursing diagnoses, and subsequently decisions about the nursing care each individual needs. The decision-making process is based upon the cues observed, analysed and interpreted and it has been suggested that expert nurses assess the situation as a whole and make judgements and decisions intuitively (King & Clark 2002;

Peden-McAlpine & Clark 2002; Hedburg & Larsson 2003), reflecting Benner's (1984) renowned novice-to-expert theory. However, others argue that all nurses use a logical process of clinical reasoning in order to identify patients' needs for nursing care and that, while this becomes more automated with experience, and perhaps more subconscious, it should always be possible for a nurse to explain how he or she arrives at a decision about an individual within their care (Putzier & Padrick 1984; Gordon 1994; Rolfe 1999). A further notion is that of a continuum, where our ability to make clinical judgements about our patients lies on a spectrum, with intuition at one end and linear, logical decisions (based on clinical trials, for example) at the other (Thompson 1999; Cader *et al.* 2005). Factors that may influence the process of decision making include time, complexity of the judgement or decision to be made, as well as the knowledge, experience and attitude of the individual nurse.

Nursing diagnosis is a term to describe both a clinical judgement that is made about an individual's response to health or illness, and the process of decision making that leads to that judgement (Box 2.6 illustrates the process of making a nursing diagnosis). The importance of thorough assessment within this process cannot be underestimated. The gathering of comprehensive and appropriate data from patients, including the meanings attributed to events by the patient, is associated with greater diagnostic accuracy and thus more timely and effective intervention (Gordon 1994; Hunter 1998; Alfaro-Lefevre 2002).

Box 2.6 The process of nursing diagnosis (Tanner *et al.* 1987; Gordon 1994)

- Collect information using an appropriate assessment framework.
- Identify clusters of information and consider possible nursing judgements (nursing diagnoses).
- Collect further information to verify these judgements.
- Arrive at an accurate nursing judgement (nursing diagnosis).

The concept of 'nursing diagnosis' has historically generated much debate within British literature, and it is therefore important to clarify the difference between a nursing diagnosis and a patient problem or care need. 'Patient problems' or 'needs' are common terms used within nursing to facilitate communication about nursing care (Hogston 1997). As patient problems/needs may involve solutions or treatments from disciplines other than nursing, the concept of 'patient problem' is similar to but broader than nursing diagnosis. Nursing diagnoses describe problems that may be dealt with by nursing expertise (Leih & Salentijn 1994) (Box 2.7).

Box 2.7 Characteristics of conditions labelled as nursing diagnoses (Gordon 1994)

1 Nurses can identify the condition through a process of diagnostic reasoning (assessment, problem identification).
2 The condition can be resolved primarily by nursing interventions.
3 Nurses assume accountability for patient/outcomes.
4 Nurses assume responsibility for research on the condition and its treatment.

The term nursing diagnosis also refers to a standardized nursing language, to describe patients' needs for nursing care, that originated in America over 30 years ago and has now been developed, adapted and translated for use in numerous other countries. The language of nursing diagnosis provides a classification of over 200 terms (NANDA-I 2007) representing judgements that are commonly made with patients/clients about phenomena of concern to nurses, enabling more consistent communication and documentation of nursing care (see Box 2.8 for an example of a nursing diagnosis). There are different types of nursing diagnoses within the North American Nursing Diagnosis Association–International (NANDA-I) classification system (2007), including actual nursing diagnoses (e.g. acute pain), risk nursing diagnoses (e.g. risk for falls) and wellness diagnoses (e.g. readiness for enhanced nutrition). The different types of diagnoses and the number that already exist have begun to demonstrate the diversity and complexity of nursing practice; however, it should be noted that this language is still under development and is by no means an exhaustive classification of nursing practice. Similar common languages have also been developed for nursing interventions and outcomes, as well as specific languages that have been developed for community nurses and health visitors. Whilst there are claimed to be some disadvantages to using such a standardized system to express nursing care, these are far outweighed by the advantages of having a structured and consistent system to articulate the care that is provided by nurses.

Most significantly, the use of common language enables nurses to clearly and consistently express what they do for patients and why; making the contribution of different nursing roles clearly visible within the multidisciplinary care pathway (Grobe 1996; Moen *et al.* 1999; Payne 2000; Delaney 2001; Elfrink *et al.* 2001). Secondly, an increasingly important reason for trying to structure nursing terms in a systematic way has been the need to create and analyse nursing information in a meaningful way for electronic care records (Clark 1999; Westbrook 2000). The term 'nursing diagnosis' is not commonly used within the UK as no definitive classifications, or common languages, are in general use; however, for the

Box 2.8   An example of a nursing diagnosis (adapted from NANDA-I 2007)

Label	Acute pain
Definition Provides clear meaning of the diagnosis.	An unpleasant sensory and emotional experience associated with actual or potential tissue damage or described in terms of such damage (International Association for the Study of Pain, 2007). Sudden or slow onset of any intensity from mild to severe with an anticipated or predictable end and a duration of < 3 months.
Defining characteristics Cues to determine if the condition or response described by the diagnosis is present for the patient/ client.	For example: ■ The patient states they have pain. ■ Pain assessment: numerical rating scale (0–10) pain score > 2. ■ Evidence of noxious stimuli, e.g surgery, trauma. ■ Guarding of injury. ■ Reduction on patient's normal mobility. Refer to NANDA-I (2007) for a complete list of defining characteristics.
Related factors Factors that contribute to the diagnosis being present. Individualized to each patient or client.	Injury agents (biological, chemical, physical, psychological).

aforementioned reasons, the adaptation and implemention of standard nursing languages within clinical practice in the UK is currently being explored (Chambers 1998; Westbrook 2000; Lyte & Jones 2001).

Planning and implementing care

Nursing diagnoses provide a focus for planning and implementing effective and evidence-based care. This process consists of identifying nursing-sensitive patient outcomes and identifying appropriate interventions that will enable the individual to reach their desired outcome. However, while nurses may gather valuable information through the assessment process, it is often the case that very little of this is translated into the documentation (Ford & Walsh 1994), resulting in the standard of care bearing little relationship to the written documentation (Ford & Walsh 1994; Ballard 2006). Therefore, when planning care it is vital:

40

- To determine the immediate priorities and recognize whether patient problems require nursing care or whether a referral should be made to someone else.
- To identify the anticipated outcome for the patient, noting what the patient will be able to do and in what time frame. The use of 'measurable' verbs that describe patient behaviour or what the patient says facilitates the evaluation of patient outcomes (Box 2.9).
- To determine the nursing interventions, i.e. what nursing actions will prevent or manage the patient's problems so that the patient's outcomes may be achieved.
- To record the care plan for the patient which may be written or individualized from a standardized/core care plan or a computerized care plan.

(Shaw 1998; Alfaro-Lefevre 2002; White 2003.)

Box 2.9 Examples of measurable and non-measurable verbs for use in outcome statements (Alfaro-Lefevre 2002, pp. 134–5)

Measurable verbs (use these to be specific)

- State; verbalize; communicate; list; describe; identify
- Demonstrate; perform
- Will lose; will gain; has an absence of
- Walk; stand; sit

Non-measurable verbs (do not use)

- Know
- Understand
- Think
- Feel

Outcomes should be patient focused and realistic, stating how the outcomes or goals are to be achieved and when the outcomes should be evaluated. Patient-focused outcomes centre on the desired results of nursing care, i.e. the impact of care on the patient, rather than on what the nurse does. Outcomes may be short, intermediate or long term, enabling the nurse to identify the patient's health status and progress (stability, improvement or deterioration) over time. Setting realistic outcomes and interventions requires the nurse to distinguish between nursing diagnoses that are life threatening or are an immediate risk to the patient's safety and those that may be dealt with at a later stage. Identifying which nursing diagnoses/problems contribute to other problems (for example, difficulty breathing will contribute to the patient's ability to mobilize) will make the problem a higher priority. By dealing with the breathing difficulties, the patient's ability to mobilize will be improved.

The nature of the patient outcomes will differ according to the specific patient group or focus of the patient's nursing diagnoses. For example, patient outcomes related to safety, physiological and behavioural responses are defined in the perioperative patient-focused model (Kleinbeck & McKennett 2000). However, in the community setting, patient and family outcomes relate to the knowledge, behaviour and signs and symptoms as described in the Omaha nursing classification system (Martin & Scheet 1992). Health visitors in the UK are now using this framework to demonstrate the effectiveness of care and to facilitate the assessment process and identify clients' progress (Clark *et al.* 2001). Nursing has been shown to influence patient outcomes in the hospital setting according to Lee (1999) in a review of the literature, but more research is necessary to evaluate further the interrelationship. No benefit has been identified from any studies between written care planning, record keeping and patient outcomes (Moloney & Maggs 1999; Currell *et al.* 2003).

The formulation of nursing interventions is dependent on adequate information collection and accurate clinical judgement during patient assessment. As a result specific patient outcomes may be derived and appropriate nursing interventions undertaken to assist the patient to achieve those outcomes (Hardwick 1998). Nursing interventions should be specific to help the patient achieve the outcome and should be evidence based. When determining what interventions may be appropriate in relation to a patient's problem, it may be helpful to clarify the potential benefit to the patient after an intervention has been performed, as this will help to ensure its appropriateness.

It is important to continue to assess the patient on an ongoing basis whilst implementing the care planned. Assessing the patient's current status prior to implementing care will enable the nurse to check whether the patient has developed any new problems that require immediate action. During and after providing any nursing action, the nurse should assess and reassess the patient's response to care. The nurse will then be able to determine whether changes to the patient's care plan should be made immediately or at a later stage. If there are any patient care needs that need immediate action, for example consultation or referral to a doctor, recording the actions taken is essential. Involving the patient and their family or friends will promote the patient's well-being and self-care abilities. The use of clinical documentation in nurse handover will help to ensure that the care plans are up to date and relevant (Alfaro-Lefevre 2002; White 2003).

Evaluating care

42

Effective evaluation of care requires the nurse to critically analyse the patient's health status to determine whether the patient's condition is stable, has deteriorated or improved. Seeking the patient's and family's views in the evaluation process will facilitate decision making. By evaluating the patient's outcomes the nurse is able to decide whether changes need to be made to the care planned. Evaluation of care should take place in a structured manner and on a regular basis by a registered nurse. The frequency of evaluation depends on the clinical environment within which the individual is being cared for as well as the nature of the nursing diagnosis (problem) to which the care relates. Questions such as:

- What are the patient's self-care abilities?
- Is the patient able to do what you expected?
- If not, why not?
- Has something changed?
- Are you missing something?
- Are there new care priorities?

will help to clarify the patient's progress (Alfaro-Lefevre 2002, p. 5; White 2003). It is helpful to consider what is observed and measurable to indicate that the patient has achieved the outcome. There are a variety of different approaches to evaluating care. At The Royal Marsden Hospital a strategy known as 'charting by exception' (CBE) has been implemented, in which only exceptions to the documented care are recorded. This method is reliant on an up-to-date and individualized care plan being maintained and is based on the assumption that, through observation and assessment, the nurse makes a judgement that the care has been provided according to the care plan. If for any reason this is not the case, i.e. if particular interventions have not been provided or if they are now deemed inappropriate, then this would be documented as an exception to the care planned (Murphy 2003).

Documenting and communicating care

Nurses have a professional responsibility to ensure that health care records provide an accurate account of treatment, care planning and delivery, and are viewed as a tool of communication within the team. There should be 'clear evidence of the care planned, the decisions made, the care delivered and the information shared' (NMC 2005, p. 8). The content and quality of record keeping are a measure of standards of practice relating to the skills and judgement of the nurse (NMC 2005). Thus communication and assessment skills are integral to providing quality care.

The ability to develop good practice in record keeping is considered to be an area for improvement by nurses (Frank-Stromborg & Christensen 2001a, b; Rodden & Bell 2002; Wood 2003). Record keeping is an integral part of nursing care (NMC 2005), and the purpose of health records is to ensure that those coming after you can see what has been done, or not done, why and by whom (NHSE 1999). This will ensure not only that patient care is not compromised but also that any decisions made can be justified or reconsidered at a later date (NHSE 1999). Box 2.10 provides some key guidance for documentation.

Box 2.10 Guidelines for nursing documentation (Royal Marsden NHS Trust 2005)

General principles

1 Records should be written legibly in black ink in such a way that they cannot be erased and are readable when photocopied.
2 Entries should be factual, consistent, accurate and not contain jargon, abbreviations or meaningless phrases (e.g. observations fine).
3 Each entry must include the date and the time (using the 24-hour clock).
4 Each entry must be followed by a signature and the name printed as well as:
   - the job role (e.g. Staff Nurse or Clinical Nurse Specialist);
   - if a nurse is a temporary employee (i.e. an agency nurse) the name of the agency must be included under the signature.
5 If an error is made this should be scored out with a single line and the correction written alongside with date, time and initials. Correction fluid should not be used at any time.
6 All assessment and entries made by student nurses must be countersigned by a registered nurse.
7 Health care assistants:
   - can write on fluid balance and food intake charts;
   - who have demonstrated achievement of the learning outcomes for observing and monitoring the patient's condition as defined in *The Royal Marsden Hospital Health Care Assistant Role Assessment and Development Profile* (2001) can write on observation charts;
   - must not write on prescription charts, assessment sheets, care plans or progress notes.

Assessment and care planning

1 The first written assessment and the identification of the patient's immediate needs must begin within 4 hours of admission. This must include any allergies or infection risks of the patient and the contact details of the next of kin.

Box 2.10 *(cont.)*

2 The following must be completed within 24 hours of admission and updated as appropriate:
- completion of nutritional, oral, pressure sore and manual handling risk assessments;
- other relevant assessment tools, e.g. pain and wound assessment.

3 All sections of the Nursing Admission Assessment must be completed at some point during the patient's hospital stay with the identification of the patient's care needs. If it is not relevant or if it is inappropriate to assess certain Functional Health Patterns, e.g. *the patient is unconscious*, then indicate the reasons accordingly.

The ongoing nursing assessment should identify whether the patient's condition is stable, has deteriorated or improved.

4 Care plans should be written wherever possible with the involvement of the patient, in terms that they can understand, and include:
- patient focused, measurable, realistic and achievable goals;
- nursing interventions reflecting best practice;
- relevant core care plans that are individualized, signed, dated and timed.

5 Update the care plan with altered or additional interventions as appropriate.

6 The nursing documentation must be referred to at shift handover so it needs to be kept up to date.

Summary of recommendations and guidance for practice

Principles of assessment

- Assessment should be a systematic, deliberate and interactive process that underpins every aspect of nursing care (Heaven & Maguire 1996: R 5).
- Assessment should be seen as a continuous process (Cancer Action Team 2007: C).

Structure of assessment

- The structure of a patient assessment should take into consideration the speciality and care setting and also the purpose of the assessment (E).
- When caring for individuals with cancer, assessment should be carried out at key points during the cancer pathway and dimensions of assessment should include background information and assessment preferences, physical needs, social and occupational needs, psychological well-being and spiritual well-being (Cancer Action Team 2007: C).
- Functional Health Patterns provide a comprehensive framework for assessment, which can be adapted for use within a variety of clinical specialities and care settings (Gordon 1994: R 5).

Methods of assessment

- Methods of assessment should elicit both subjective and objective assessment data (E).
- An assessment interview must be well structured to progress logically in order to facilitate the nurse's thinking and to make the patient feel comfortable in telling their story (E).
- Specific assessment tools should be used, where appropriate, to enable nurses to monitor particular aspects of care, such as symptom management (e.g. pain, fatigue), over time. This will help to evaluate the effectiveness of nursing interventions whilst often providing an opportunity for patients to become more involved in their care (Conner & Eggert 1994: R 5).

Decision making and nursing diagnosis

- Nurses should be encouraged to provide rationale for their clinical judgements and decision making within their clinical practice (NMC 2005: C; E).
- The language of nursing diagnosis is a tool that can be used to make clinical judgements more explicit and enable more consistent communication and documentation of nursing care (Clark 1999; Westbrook 2000: R 5).

Planning and implementing care

- When planning care it is vital that nurses recognize whether patient problems require nursing care or whether a referral should be made to someone else (E).
- When a nursing diagnosis has been made, the anticipated outcome for the patient must be identified in a manner which is specific, achievable and measurable (NMC 2005: C; E).
- Nursing interventions should be determined in order to address the nursing diagnosis and achieve the desired outcomes (Gordon 1994: R 5).

Evaluating care

- Nursing care should be evaluated using measurable outcomes on a regular basis and interventions adjusted accordingly (The Royal Marsden Hospital; Box 2.10: C).
- Progress towards achieving outcomes should be recorded in a concise and precise manner. Using a method such as charting by exception can facilitate this (Murphy 2003: R 5).

Documenting and communicating care

- The content and quality of record keeping are a measure of standards of practice relating to the skills and judgement of the nurse (NMC 2005: C).
- In addition to the written record of care, the important role that the nursing shift report, or 'handover', plays in the communication and continuation of patient care should be considered, particularly when considering the role of electronic records (Ballard 2006: R 5).

In addition to the written record of care, it is also important to consider the significant role that the nursing shift report, or 'handover', plays in the communication and continuation of patient care, particularly when considering the role of electronic records in enhancing such systems of communication (Ballard 2006). Inter-shift reports can be classified into four different styles, namely the recorded, bedside, written and the verbal (Miller 1998) and each has its benefits and disadvantages. Whilst often seen as a ritual, it is suggested that handover is a ritual that is necessary for team building and continuity of care (Strange 1996; Williams 1998; Lally 1999); however, the question often arises as to what extent such a variety of approaches to handover actually reflect documented care, and vice versa. Rather than referring to the care plan during handover, it has been found that elements such as vital signs, comfort measures and medications are most often referred to (Lally 1999). However if a care plan-orientated style was to be used, it is suggested this can result in improved documentation and the realization that nursing diagnoses (care needs), rather than medical diagnoses, are the primary focus when delivering nursing care (Wallum 1995; Webster 1999). As nursing moves towards electronic methods of documentation, the issue of how such electronic records of nursing care are integrated into shift reports warrants greater attention.

References

Ahern, J. & Philpot, P. (2002) Assessing acutely ill patients on general wards. *Nurs Stand*, **16**(47), 47–52.

Alfaro-Lefevre, R. (2002) *Applying Nursing Process: Promoting Collaborative Care*. Lippincott, Williams & Wilkins, Philadelphia.

Alfaro-Lefevre, R. (2004) *Critical Thinking and Clinical Judgement: a Practical Approach*, 3rd edn. Saunders, MO.

Allen, D. (1998) Record-keeping and routine practice: the view from the wards. *J Adv Nurs*, **27**(6), 1223–30.

Ballard, E. (2006) Improving information management in ward nurses practice. *Nurs Stand*, **20**(50), 43–8.

Benner, P. (1984) *From Novice to Expert: Excellence and Power in Clinical Nursing Practice*. Addison Wesley, Menlo-Park, CA.

Bonevski, B. *et al.* (2000) Evaluation of an instrument to assess the needs of patients with cancer. *Cancer*, **88**, 215–17.

Bouvette, M., Fothergill-Bourbonnais, F. & Perreault, A. (2002) Implementation of the Pain and Symptom Assessment Record (PSAR). *J Adv Nurs*, **40**(6), 685–700.

Brown, V. *et al.* (2001) The development of the Chemotherapy Symptom Assessment Scale (C-SAS): a scale for the routine clinical assessment of the symptom experiences of patients receiving cytotoxic chemotherapy. *Int J Nurs Stud*, **38**(5), 497–510.

Cader, R., Campbell, S. & Watson, D. (2005) Cognitive continuum theory in nursing decision-making. *J Adv Nurs*, **49**(4), 397–405.

Cancer Action Team (2007) *Holistic Common Assessment of Supportive and Palliative Care Needs for Adults with Cancer: Assessment Guidance*. Cancer Action Team, London.

Chambers, S. (1998) Nursing diagnosis in learning disabilities nursing. *Br J Nurs*, **7**(19), 1177–81.

Clark, J. (1999) A language for nursing. *Nurs Stand*, **13**(31), 42–7.

Clark, J. *et al.* (2001) Professional briefing. New methods of documenting health visiting practice. *Community Pract*, **74**(3), 108–12.

Clarke, D.J. & Holt, J. (2001) Philosophy: a key to open the door to critical thinking. *Nurse Educ Today*, **21**, 71–8.

Conner, F.W. & Eggert, L.L. (1994) Psychosocial assessment for treatment planning and evaluation. *J Psychosoc Nurs Ment Health Serv*, **32**(5), 31–42.

Coyne, P.J., Lyne, M.E. & Watson, A.C. (2002) Symptom management in people with AIDS. *Am J Nurs*, **102**(9), 48–57.

Crow, R.A., Chase, J. & Lamond, D. (1995) The cognitive component of nursing assessment: an analysis. *J Adv Nurs*, **22**, 206–12.

Crumbie, A. (2006) Taking a history. In: *Nurse Practitioners Clinical Skills and Professional Issues* (ed. M. Walsh). Butterworth Heinemann, Edinburgh, pp. 14–26.

Currell, R., Wainwright, P. & Urquhart, C. (2003) Nursing record systems: effects on nursing practice and health care outcomes. *Cochrane Database of Systematic Reviews*, Issue 3.

Daly, W.M. (1998) Critical thinking as an outcome of nursing education. What is it? Why is it important to nursing practice? *J Adv Nurs*, **28**(2), 323–31.

Delaney, C. (2001) Health informatics and oncology nursing. *Semin Oncol Nurs*, **17**(1), 2–6.

Dennison, S. & Shute, T. (2000) Identifying patient concerns: improving the quality of patient visits to the oncology outpatient department–a pilot audit. *Eur J Oncol Nurs*, **4**(2), 91–8.

DH (2001) *The National Service Framework for Older People*. Department of Health, London.

DH (2006) *Modernising Nursing Careers: Setting the Direction*. Department of Health, London.

Di Vito-Thomas, P. (2000) Identifying critical thinking behaviours in clinical judgements. *J Nurses Staff Dev*, **16**(4), 174–80.

Edwards, M. & Miller, C. (2001) Improving psychosocial assessment in oncology. *Prof Nurse*, **16**(7), 1223–6.

Eilers, J., Berger, A.M. & Peterson, M.C. (1988) Development, testing and application of the oral assessment guide. *Oncol Nurs Forum*, **15**(3), 325–30.

Elfrink, V. *et al.* (2001) Standardised nursing vocabularies: a foundation for quality care. *Semin Oncol Nurs*, **17**(1), 18–23.

Ford, P. & McCormack, B. (1999) Determining older people's need for registered nursing in continuing health care: the contribution of The Royal College of Nursing's Older People's Assessment Tool. *J Clin Nurs*, **8**(6), 731–42.

Ford, P. & Walsh, M. (1994) *New Rituals for Old. Nursing Through the Looking Glass*. Butterworth Heinemann, Oxford.

Frank-Stromborg, M. & Christensen, A. (2001a) Nurse documentation: not done or worse, done the wrong way–part I. *Oncol Nurs Forum*, **28**(4), 697–702.

Frank-Stromborg, M. & Christensen, A. (2001b) Nurse documentation: not done or worse, done the wrong way–part II. *Oncol Nurs Forum*, **28**(5), 841–6.

Frank-Stromborg, M. & Olsen, S.J. (1997) *Instruments for Clinical Healthcare–Research*, 2nd edn. Jones & Bartlett, London.

Ganz, P.A. *et al.* (1992) The CARES: a generic measure of health-related quality of life for patients with cancer. *Quality of Life Research*, **1**, 19–29.

Gordon, M. (1994) *Nursing Diagnosis, Process and Application*. Mosby, St. Louis.

Grobe, S.J. (1996) The nursing intervention lexicon and taxonomy. Implications for representing nursing care in automated patient records. *Holist Nurs Pract*, **11**(1), 48–63.

Hardwick, S. (1998) Clarification of nursing diagnosis from a British perspective. *Assignment*, **4**(2), 3–9.

Harris, R. *et al.* (1998) Patient assessment: validation of a nursing instrument. *Int J Nurs Stud*, **35**, 303–13.

Heaven, C.M. & Maguire, P. (1996) Training hospice nurses to elicit patient concerns. *J Adv Nurs*, **23**, 280–6.

Hedburg, B. & Larsson, U.S. (2003) Observations, confirmations and strategies–useful tools in decision-making process for nurses in practice. *J Clin Nurs*, **12**(2), 215–22.

Hogston, R. (1997) Nursing diagnosis and classification systems: a position paper. *J Adv Nurs*, **26**, 496–500.

Holmes, H.N. (ed.) (2003) *Three-minute Assessment*. Lippincott, Williams & Wilkins, Philadelphia, pp. 1–32.

Holmes, S. & Eburn, E. (1989) Patients' and nurses' perceptions of symptom distress in cancer. *J Adv Nurs*, **14**(7), 575–81.

Holt, P. (1995) Role of questioning in patient assessment. *Br J Nurs*, **4**, 1145–6.

Horton, R. (2002) Differences in assessment of symptoms and quality of life between patients with advanced cancer and their specialist palliative care nurses in a home care setting. *Palliat Med*, **16**(6), 488–94.

Hunter, M. (1998) Rehabilitation in cancer care: a patient focused approach. *Eur J Cancer Care*, **7**, 85–7.

Johnson, T. (2000) Functional health pattern assessment on-line: lessons learned. *Comput Nurs*, **18**(5), 248–54.

Kearney, N. (2001) Classifying nursing care to improve patient outcomes; the example of WISECARE. *NT Research*, **6**(4), 747–56.

Kearney, N. *et al.* (2000) Collaboration in cancer nursing practice. *J Clin Nurs*, **9**, 429–35.

Keller, C.A., Carolin, K. & Fedoronko, K. (2001) Bone marrow transplant teaching rounds: promoting excellence in nursing care. *Oncol Nurs Forum*, **28**(3), 457–8.

Kennedy, C. (1999) Decision making in palliative nursing practice. *Int J Palliat Nurs*, **5**(3), 142–6.

King, L. & Clark, J.M. (2002) Intuition and the development of expertise in surgical ward and intensive care nurses. *J Adv Nurs*, **37**(4), 322–9.

Kleinbeck, S. & McKennett, M. (2000) Challenges of measuring intraoperative patient outcomes. *AORN J*, **72**(5), 845–50, 853.

Kozier, B. *et al.* (2003) *Fundamentals of Nursing: Concepts, Process and Practice*, 7th edn. Addison Wesley, Menlo Park CA.

Lally, S. (1999) An investigation into the functions of nurses' communication at the intershift handover. *J Nurs Manag*, **7**(1), 29–36.

Lauri, S., Lepisto, M. & Kappeli, S. (1997) Patients' needs in hospital: nurses' and patients' views. *J Adv Nurs*, **25**, 339–46.

Lee, J. (1999) Does what nurses do affect clinical outcomes for hospitalized patients? A review of the literature. *Health Serv Res*, **34**(5), 1011–32.

Leih, P. & Salentijn, C. (1994) Nursing diagnosis: a Dutch perspective. *J Clin Nurs*, **3**, 313–20.

Lidstone, V. *et al.* (2003) Symptoms and concerns amongst cancer outpatients: identifying the need for specialist palliative care. *Palliat Med*, **17**, 588–95.

Lyte, G. & Jones, K. (2001) Developing a unified language for children's nurses, children and their families in the United Kingdom. *J Clin Nurs*, **10**, 79–85.

Martin, K. & Scheet, N. (1992) *The Omaha System: a Pocket Guide for Community Health Nursing*. W.B. Saunders, Philadelphia, pp. 37–41.

McClement, S.E., Woodgate, R.L. & Degner, L. (1997) Symptom distress in adults with cancer. *Cancer Nurs*, **20**(4), 236–43.

McDonald, M.V. *et al.* (1999) Nurses' recognition of depression in their patients with cancer. *Oncol Nurs Forum*, **26**(3), 593–9.

Miller, C. (1998) Ensuring continuing care: styles and efficiency of the handover process. *Aust J Adv Nurs*, **16**(1), 23–7.

Moen, A. *et al.* (1999) Representing nursing judgements in the electronic record. *J Adv Nurs*, **30**(4), 990–7.

Moloney, R. & Maggs, C. (1999) A systematic review of the relationships between written manual nursing care planning, record keeping and patient outcomes. *J Adv Nurs*, **30**(1), 51–7.

Morton, P.G. (1993) *Health Assessment in Nursing*, 2nd edn. Springhouse, Philadelphia.

Muller-Staub, M., Lavin, M. & Needham, I. (2006) Nursing diagnoses, interventions and outcomes: application and impact on nursing practice: systematic review. *J Adv Nurs*, **56**(5), 514–31.

Murphy, E.K. (2003) Charting by exception. *AORN J*, **78**(5), 821–3.

Murphy, K. *et al.* (2000) The Roper, Logan and Tierney (1996) model: perceptions and operationalization of the model in psychiatric nursing within a Health Board in Ireland. *J Adv Nurs*, **31**(6), 1333–41.

NANDA-I (2007) *Nursing Diagnoses: Definitions and Classification 2007–2008*. North American Nursing Diagnosis Association – International, Philadelphia.

Neighbour, R. (1987) *The Inner Consultation*. MTP Press, Lancaster.

NHSE (1999) *For the Records: Managing Records in NHS Trusts and Health Authorities (HSC 199/53 1999)*. NHSE, London.

NMC (2008) *The Code: Standards of Conduct, Performance and Ethics for Nurses and Midwives*. Nursing and Midwifery Council, London.

NMC (2005) *Guidelines for Records and Record Keeping*. Nursing and Midwifery Council, London.

O'Neill, E.S. & Dluhy, N.M. (1997) A longitudinal framework for fostering critical thinking and diagnostic reasoning. *J Adv Nurs*, **26**, 825–32.

Orem, D.E., Taylor, S.G. & Renpenning, K. (2001) *Nursing: Concepts of Practice*, 6th edn. Mosby, St. Louis.

Osse, B.H. *et al.* (2004) Towards a new clinical tool for needs assessment in the palliative care of cancer patients: the PNPC Instrument. *J Pain Symptom Manage*, **28**(4), 329–41.

Parsaie, F.A., Golchin, M. & Asvadi, I. (2000) A comparison of nurse and patient perceptions of chemotherapy treatment stressors. *Cancer Nurs*, **23**(5), 371–4.

Payne, J. (2000) The nursing interventions classification: a language to define nursing. *Oncol Nurs Forum*, **27**(1), 99–103.

Peden-McAlpine, C. & Clark, N. (2002) Early recognition of client status changes: the importance of time. *Dimens Crit Care Nurs*, **21**(4), 144–50.

Piper, B.F. (2004) Measuring fatigue. In: *Instruments for Clinical Health Care Research* (eds M. Frank-Stromborg & S.J. Olsen), 3rd edn. Jones & Bartlett, MA, pp. 538–569.

Portenoy, R.K. *et al.* (1994) The Memorial Symptom Assessment Scale: an instrument for the evaluation of symptom prevalence, characteristics and distress. *Eur J Cancer*, **30**(a), 1326–36.

Price, C.I.M., Han, S.W. & Rutherford, I.A. (2000) Advanced nursing practice; an introduction to physical assessment. *Br J Nurs*, **12**(4), 22–5.

Putzier, D.J. & Padrick, K.P. (1984) Nursing diagnosis: a component of nursing process and decision-making. *Top Clin Nurs*, **5**(1), 21–9.

RCN (2003) *Defining Nursing*. Royal College of Nursing: London.

Rhodes, V.A. *et al.* (2000) An instrument to measure symptom experience: symptom occurrence and symptom distress. *Cancer Nurs*, **23**(1), 49–54.

Rodden, C. & Bell, M. (2002) Record keeping: developing good practice. *Nurs Stand*, **17**(1), 40–2.

Rolfe, G. (1999) Insufficient evidence: the problems of evidence-based nursing. *Nurse Educ Today*, **19**(6), 433–42.

Roper, N., Logan, W. & Tierney, A.J. (2000) *The Roper Logan Tierney Model of Nursing: Based on Activities of Living*. Churchill Livingstone, Edinburgh.

Roy, C. (1984) *Introduction to Nursing: an Adaptation Model*, 2nd edn. Prentice Hall, New Jersey.

Royal Marsden NHS Trust (2001) The Royal Marsden Hospital Health Care Assistant Role Assessment and Development profile. Unpublished.

Royal Marsden NHS Trust (2005) Guidelines for Nursing Documentation. Unpublished.

Seymour, B., Kinn, S. & Sunderland, N. (2003) Valuing both critical and creative thinking in clinical practice: narrowing the research–practice gap. *J Adv Nurs*, **42**(3), 288–96.

Shaw, M. (1998) *Charting Made Incredibly Easy!* Springhouse Corporation, Springhouse PA.

Skinn, B. & Stacey, D. (1994) Establishing an integrated framework for documentation: use of a self-reporting health history and outpatient oncology record. *Oncol Nurs Forum*, **21**(9), 1557–66.

Smith, G. & Richardson, A. (1996) Development of nursing documentation for use in the outpatient oncology setting. *Eur J Cancer Care*, **5**, 225–32.

Strange, F. (1996) Handover: an ethnographic study of ritual in nursing practice. *Intensive Crit Care Nurs*, **12**(2), 106–12.

Suhonen, R., Valimaki, M. & Katajisto, J. (2000) Developing and testing an instrument for the measurement of individual care. *J Adv Nurs*, **32**(5), 1253–63.

Tanner, C.A. *et al.* (1987) Diagnostic reasoning strategies of nurses and nursing students. *Nurs Res*, **36**(6), 358–62.

Teytelman, Y. (2000) Effective nursing documentation and communication. *Semin Oncol Nurs*, **18**(2), 121–7.

Thompson, C. (1999) A conceptual treadmill: the need for 'middle ground' in clinical decision making theory in nursing. *J Adv Nurs*, **30**(5), 1222–9.

Tierney, A.J. (1998) Nursing models; extant or extinct? *J Adv Nurs*, **28**(1), 77–85.

Wallum, R. (1995) Using care plans to replace the handover. *Nurs Stand*, **9**(32), 24–6.

Webster, J. (1999) Practitioner-centred research: an evaluation of the implementation of the bedside hand-over. *J Adv Nurs*, **30**(6), 1375–82.

Wenzel, G. (2002) Creating an interactive interdisciplinary electronic assessment. *Comput Inform Nurs*, **20**(6), 251–60.

Westbrook, A. (2000) Learning curve. Nursing language. *Nurs Times*, **96**(14), 41.

White, L. (2003) *Documentation and the Nursing Process*. Delmar Learning, Clifton Park, NY.

Williams, J. (1998) Managing change in the nursing handover. *Nurs Stand*, **12**(18), 39–42.

Williams, P.D. *et al.* (2001) Treatment type and treatment severity among oncology patients by self-report. *Int J Nurs Stud*, **38**, 359–67.

Wimpenny, P. (2001) The meaning of models of nursing to practising nurses. *J Adv Nurs*, **40**(3), 346–54.

Wood, C. (2003) The importance of good record-keeping for nurses. *Nurs Times*, **99**(2), 26–7.

Wright, E.P. *et al.* (2001) Feasibility and compliance of automated measurement of quality of life in oncology practice. *J Clin Oncol*, **21**(2), 374–82.

Multiple choice questions

1 Nursing assessment should cover which of the following dimensions?

   a Physical, psychological and social
   b Physical, psychological, emotional and cultural
   c Emotional, psychological, spiritual, physical, cultural and social
   d Spiritual, physical, cultural and psychological

2 Nursing assessment should be:

   a Disease focused
   b Process focused
   c Nursing focused
   d Patient focused

3 Nursing models can help nurses to:

   a Reflect on their practice
   b Provide an effective framework for patient assessment
   c Develop analytical problem solving and judgement skills
   d All of the above

4 Assessment tools need to be:

   a Quick and simple
   b Simple, acceptable, reliable and valid with an interpretable scoring system
   c Acceptable, quick and with an interpretable scoring system
   d Quick, reliable and valid

5   Nursing diagnosis can be defined as:

   a   Nurses carrying out a physical assessment
   b   Nurses making clinical judgements about an individual's response to health and illness
   c   Nurses using a nursing model
   d   Nurse using an assessment tool

6   Documentation of care is important in order to:

   a   Record what care has been carried out, when and by whom
   b   Measure nursing care
   c   Provide information to other health care workers
   d   Help nurses think about the care they have delivered

Answers to the multiple choice questions can be found in Appendix 3.

Chapter 3

Communication

Definition

Communication is a reciprocal process that involves the exchange of both verbal and non-verbal messages to convey feelings, information, ideas and knowledge (Wilkinson 1999; Wallace 2001).

Reference material

High quality communication is crucial for the delivery of nursing care and connects the psychological, social and physical domains of patient care.

Good communication involves careful consideration of the patient's perspective. Listening to and supplying patients with the information to understand their illness, treatment and care will support those patients to get what they want from health care services. This will contribute to the efficacy of treatment and result in better care delivery, the promotion of more successful psychological support and consequent patient satisfaction.

It might never be possible to capture a pure and all encompassing description of communication to follow as a procedure; however, it is possible to isolate and define the ingredients of 'communication' and the strategies required to interact well and therefore learn the skills of good communication (Hargie & Dickson 2004; Back *et al.* 2005).

Specific consideration is given to communication in cancer care, although it can be argued that good communication follows similar patterns across a range of situations and disciplines.

Where 'patient' is described this can be extended to include conversations with family members and significant acquired relationships. Extending communication and support to family members (with the consent of the patient) is a crucial way of including personal and social aspects of life, promoting self help, informal support and a genuine understanding of the patient.

People with potentially life-limiting illnesses such as cancer want, among other things:

- Open communication (Heyland *et al.* 2006).
- Clear, honest information (Baile *et al.* 2000; Jenkins *et al.* 2001; Smith *et al.* 2005).
- Emotional support (Smith *et al.* 2005).

Relevant issues in communication

'Psychological distress is common among people affected by cancer' (NICE 2004, p. 9) and effective communication is widely regarded to be a key determinant of patient satisfaction, compliance and recovery (Chant *et al.* 2002), yet poor communication is one of the commonest causes of complaints in health care (Cambell 2006).

It is therefore necessary to have appropriate communication skills and be confident enough to utilize them in our clinical practice.

Numerous issues have been highlighted by the National Institute for Health and Clinical Excellence (NICE) that resonate powerfully when considering how nurses communicate with patients and relatives in cancer care.

Our responsibility lies in ensuring that, 'All patients undergo systematic psychological assessment at key points and have access to appropriate psychological support' (NICE 2004, p. 9).

This means more than referring psychological issues on to appropriate services, it means:

- Recognizing psychological needs on a par with physical needs.
- Being able to maintain a compassionate dialogue.
- Addressing psychological needs with exploratory communication skills.
- Providing emotional support via the skills illustrated in this chapter.
- Understanding the concerns of patients and relatives.

Issues in service provision

Health professionals and nurses especially are considered to be caring. The human suffering generated by illnesses such as cancer might be expected to stimulate an instinctive ability for human connection and empathy.

It might also be sensibly assumed that experience in the field of oncology nursing would have developed communication skills to a level where emotional and psychological support is consistently and skilfully provided to patients and relatives.

The evidence however can contradict these assumptions: 'Research suggests communication skills do not reliably improve with experience' (Cantwell & Ramirez 1997).

Psychological support needs improvement (Maguire *et al.* 1996) and this is highlighted when considering why patients' needs are not always met: 'Professionals are not eliciting the patients' problems or concerns' (NICE 2004, p. 16). 'Patients and carers frequently report the communication skills of health practitioners to be poor' (NICE 2004, p. 8).

Data from the Department of Health (DH) in the UK for the period 2003–04 illustrated that complaints relating to the attitude of staff and communication (written and oral) accounted for nearly 20 000 out of 90 000 complaints (22%) (DH 2005).

The close relationship between good communication and emotional support (NICE 2004, p. 56) should compel our profession to pay greater attention to communication skill development and use.

Reasons for communication problems

A bias towards physical and task related functions in nurse education and problems in the style of communication training may be partly responsible for the evidence seen (Chant *et al.* 2002).

It is still not uncommon to hear qualified nurses outlining the limitations of their education in relation to communication with patients. In practice, confidence is frequently reported to be low in managing commonly occurring emotive situations, e.g. patient's emotional distress.

Evidence also suggests that internal and institutional social barriers can exist within health services that make patient-centred communication difficult and less valued than technical ability (Chant *et al.* 2002; McCabe 2004).

Ward sisters/charge nurses can have a major impact on the style and quality of communication in the workplace (Wilkinson 1991) and therefore have some responsibility for role modelling good communication.

Working in high mortality areas is not without its burdens, and issues like 'death anxiety' are hypothesized to have an impact on our 'comfort level' when talking about serious illness and issues relating to death (Deffner & Bell 2005). End-of-life discussions and high degrees of emotional disclosure are areas that we find difficulty engaging with (Booth *et al.* 1996; Edwards 2005).

Good practice in end-of-life care is, however, not out of reach and is demonstrated by psycho-socially mature staff with well-developed communication skills.

Institutional anxiety about communication and psychological distress/crises is likely to have a negative impact upon the successful management of such issues.

The potential to feel unskilled and inadequately trained to deal with emotional distress and end-of-life issues can be addressed via focused and proven learning of fundamental communication skills. Once applied in the clinical environment these skills are potentially sufficient to provide the necessary emotional support to most patients. These skills are tools by which we can connect more effectively with people, but will only remain effective when coupled with a genuine sense of caring and compassion.

Guidelines for providing information to patients and discussing procedures to be carried out

With any procedure explained within this manual, it is essential that the patient (assuming consciousness and ability to make rational decisions) is psychologically prepared and consented. This requires careful explanation and discussion before a procedure is carried out.

It is easy perhaps for us to become so familiar with procedures that we expect them to be considered 'routine' by our patients. This can prevent us from providing thorough and necessary information and gaining acceptance and cooperation from our patients.

We therefore need to avoid assuming that repetitive or frequent procedures do not require consent, explanation and potential discussion, e.g. taking a temperature.

Procedure guidelines **Provision of information**

Procedure

Action	Rationale
1 Review the changing context of the patient's situation.	
2 Prepare for discussion.	
3 Consider whether the procedure is necessary.	
4 Make use of appropriate patient leaflets.	
5 If possible discuss the procedure some time before it is to be carried out.	Give patients the opportunity to digest information in their own time (Lowry 1995: E). In certain groups it can be demonstrated to improve clinical outcomes; satisfaction; chances of meeting the targeted discharge date; and return to prior functional status sooner (Lookinland & Pool 1998: R 2b).

Procedure guidelines (*cont.*)

6 Introduce yourself.

Ensure patient understands who you are and your role and specific aim. Promote patient satisfaction (Delvaux *et al.* 2004: R 1b).

7 Maintain a warm and approachable demeanour. Do not rush.

Promote patient satisfaction (Delvaux *et al.* 2004: R 1b).

8 Explain that you have a procedure to carry out, considering privacy in giving information.

Promote dignity/preserve confidentiality (NMC 2008: C).

9 Name the procedure. Elicit, clarify and check the information gathered by the patient.

Promote understanding and patient satisfaction.

10 Explain the procedure avoiding the use of medical jargon. Be prepared to repeat information or rephrase until understanding at the patient's desired level is reached.
(If understanding is not achieved, consent has not been achieved.)

Establish mutual understanding. Gain compliance with procedure: minimize risk (NMC 2008: C). Improve outcome and reduce nurses' stress (Fellowes *et al.* 2004: R 1a). Help patients manage side effects and adhere to care and treatment (Chelf *et al.* 2001: R 3a).

11 Confirm consent: ensure that the patient is happy for you to proceed. Allow the patient an opportunity to ask further questions or say no to the procedure. (Full understanding may reveal that the patient is not ready to proceed.)

Respecting the rights of the individual (NMC 2008). Obtaining consent correctly (DH 2001: C; NMC 2006: C).

12 Start the procedure, reiterating the main issues as you go along and keeping the patient updated by progress.

To maintain open dialogue and address issues and questions, as they arise.

13 Make it clear when the procedure has finished and what has been achieved. Offer opportunity for discussion of implications and situation, disclosing information at a level the patient wishes.

So that the patient is aware and has the information they need and want (Jenkins *et al.* 2001: R 2b).

It is important to consider giving information in small amounts and check whether the patient understands what has been said after each part has been explained. Keep language simple and clarify common and complex medical terms, e.g. 'cannula', 'catheter'.

Check frequently whether the patient wishes you to continue to provide them with the same level of information. If confusion is arising, consider whether you are providing too much detail, or using too many medical terms. Be aware whether the patient is paying attention or appears anxious (e.g. fidgety/non-attentive behaviour). Do not ignore these cues: name them. For example: 'I notice you seem a little anxious while I am describing this . . .' or, 'You seem concerned about the procedure, what can I do to help'? This recognition of behaviour will help to fully explore and support the patient's concerns.

Prior to starting, establish how the patient can communicate with you during the procedure, e.g. confirm they can ask questions, request more analgesia or ask for the procedure to stop (if this is realistic).

Information must be presented accurately and calmly and without 'false reassurance', e.g. do not say something 'will not hurt' or it 'will not go wrong', when it might. It is better to explain the risk and likely outcome. Explain that working with the nurse and co-operating with instructions is likely to improve the outcome and that every effort will be made to reduce risk and manage any problems efficiently.

Respect any refusal unconditionally; however, you may wish to explore the reasons for refusal and explain the potential (realistic) consequences. Document carefully and discuss with the multidisciplinary team. If a patient has had a procedure before do not assume they are fully aware of the potential experience or risk involved, which may well have changed.

Attention to good communication, honesty, confidence and calmness will help to reassure the patient, thus gaining their compliance and improving the potential outcome (Maguire & Pitceathly 2002).

Giving the right amount of information is important; for example, it has been shown that getting the level of information wrong (too much or too little) at diagnosis can significantly impact upon the subsequent level of coping (Fallowfield *et al.* 2002). Getting the level right can be achieved by simply asking how much people want to know and frequent checking if the level of information is satisfactory for the individual.

Recognizing our own agenda

When meeting and caring for patients we do so with our role and purpose clearly identified. Information needs to be gathered in order to provide safe and efficient care. This occurs in a time-pressured environment with practical and technical issues requiring dedicated and simultaneous attention for several patients. In summary, nurses are required to manage a lot and therefore there may be a tendency to impose a structure of control upon the working environment to facilitate organization and safety. Although this is clearly necessary to get the job done, it controls the environment to an extent where it may be difficult to hand control over to the patient to lead their own care, or initiate a discussion involving psychological and emotional needs. In addition, factors like the wearing of uniform and the physical environment are likely to influence the type of dialogue that occurs (Hargie & Dickson 2004; Edwards 2005).

Patients may expect that the principal reason for communication is the physical problem: this is frequently confirmed by the questioning and communication bias that nurses can use.

Combine this with a tendency for patients to withhold or delay the disclosure of psycho-social concerns until later in a conversation (Silverman *et al.* 2005) and we can partly understand why a patient's psycho-social needs may not be being met.

Resolving demands upon time and meeting psychological support needs

Part of the answer lies in a change of emphasis and a shift in the culture of health care (Smith *et al.* 2005). Psychological care issues need to be considered on a par with physical and technical care. Psychological support can be integrated with everyday nursing activity and may take a lot less time than anticipated. Investing time in listening and managing psychological care issues (like anxiety) early in a patient's journey might significantly reduce the overall demands made upon the nursing team over a longer period (Carlson & Bultz 2004): consider how much an anxious patient seeks frequent attention, often disrupting the flow of work. Early recognition and appropriate management of psychological issues will promote understanding and compliance, demanding less nursing time and crucially improve the patient's experience.

Investing time in psychological care is essential for the patient's experience to improve and this time will develop empathy and promote a less technological and more human bias to delivering care with nurses getting more reward from their working environment.

If we can adopt a position where the patient is allowed to take the lead in dialogue, all the required information can still be gathered but the patient's priorities will have been acknowledged and we can contextualize this information within a broader bio-psycho-social framework. This offers a better understanding of the patient's experience and will enable us to care for patients more holistically.

Communication skills

Listening

Listening is ask ill often assumed to be natural. Rarely would we consider we were physically unable to listen and perhaps this makes us pay little attention to this crucial skill area.

How to let someone know you are listening to them

- Non-verbal encouragement
- Verbal characteristics
- Questioning
- Paraphrasing
- Clarifying
- Summarizing
- Empathy

The physical act of hearing is distinct from that of 'listening'.

Hearing can be seen to be passive, but listening requires active processing and the attachment of meaning.

It might be difficult for us to answer the question 'How do we listen?' and perhaps a procedure of 'How to listen' wouldn't do justice to the sophistication and success of good listeners. However there are ways of describing the constituent parts of listening which, if followed, would make the person speaking appreciate that they were being listened to.

Problems can emerge as two people may interpret the meaning of the same dialogue differently. For example if you have asked the question, 'How are you?' and the patient replies 'Getting by', do you assume they are doing well and coping or do you assume that this means they are struggling and 'Putting on a brave face'?

Hopefully we will be attending to numerous non-verbal cues to decipher what the patient actually means. If there is a suggestion of 'incongruence' where the patient says, 'Getting by' with a low and sad sounding voice, coupled with a simultaneous lowering of the head, we might consider the latter assumption. Alternatively if the patient sounds upbeat and looks you in the face with a smile you might be reassured they mean the former (for further information see the Non-verbal communication section below).

One thing is certain: an amount of concentration is required to make sure we are getting the right message. In a difficult working environment for intimate and in-depth discussion (Edwards 2005) we need to make the best use of available space, minimize potential distractions, setting time aside by confidently letting your colleagues know you are going to 'talk'. Challenge any indication that this isn't a legitimate use of nursing time.

There are strategies to promote successful listening, e.g. 'summarizing' and 'clarifying' (at suitable moments) what the patient is saying (see sections below). Listening remains the fundamental skill in communication and is the way that we are most likely to show care and provide support.

Verbal responses

The way things are said makes a big difference, so attention needs to be paid to the tone, rate and depth of speech. This means sounding alert, interested and caring, but not patronizing. Speech should be delivered at an even rate: not too fast or too slow (unless presenting difficult or complex information).

Non-verbal characteristics of speech should naturally correspond with the verbal message.

Non-verbal responses

Non-verbal communication generally indicates information transmitted without speaking. Included in this would be the way you sit or stand, facial expression, gestures and posture, whether you nod or smile, the clothes worn: all will have an impact on the total communication taking place (Hargie & Dickson 2004).

Egan (2002) usefully describes the acronym SOLER to summarize the constituent elements of non-verbal communication. The acronym indicates: facing the patient **Squarely**; maintaining an **Open** posture; **Leaning** slightly towards the patient to convey interest; having appropriate Eye contact, not staring, nor avoiding (a cultural dimension needs to be considered); and being **Relaxed**. By learning an awareness of these factors and making this behaviour part of your normal demeanour, patients will be encouraged to talk more openly, facilitating emotional disclosure.

Saying nothing says something, so there is always communication however reluctant you or the patient are.

It can be argued that non-verbal information is more powerful than verbal information, e.g. in the case of 'incongruence' where the verbal message indicates one thing and the non-verbal suggests another (see above). There is a tendency to believe the non-verbal message over the verbal in these instances.

This highlights the need to communicate with genuine compassion. Without this, communication can be severely reduced in its effectiveness.

Non-verbal communication becomes even more important in the case of people whose verbal communication is impaired, e.g. by stroke, trauma or surgery. Patients need to be supported, ensuring, for example, they have constant access to pen and paper; the use of communication boards can be used to good effect and it is worth considering the use of information technology and communication software, if available. The experience of losing the ability to speak can be very isolating and frustrating and preparation of the patient and practice with communication aids is important to maximize the success of communication. It is essential that people with a speech deficit are given more time to communicate their needs, and we must be patient and persist with interaction until a satisfactory level of understanding is gained.

We can use non-verbal behaviour to encourage patients to talk by nodding/making affirming noises, e.g. 'Hmmm'. This 'affirming' is mostly done naturally, e.g. at points of eye contact, as specific points are made and during slight pauses in dialogue. It can be especially important to affirm when the patient is talking about psychological or emotional issues as they will need you to validate that this is an acceptable topic of conversation.

Paying attention to and tailoring the environment facilitates good communication, e.g. promoting privacy, removing distractions and sitting at the same level as the patient to talk are the minimum necessary considerations.

Questioning

One skill that needs to be used in close collaboration with listening is that of questioning. When specific information is required, e.g. in a crisis, closed questions are indicated. Closed questions narrow the potential answer (Silverman *et al.* 2005) and allow the gathering of specific information for a purpose. Closed questions therefore are ones which are likely to generate a short yes or no answer, e.g. 'Are you alright'?

In cancer care however a broader assessment of the patient's perspective is required and there is a need to show compassion and support psycho-social issues. Open questions and listening are therefore required. Open questions do the opposite of closed questions; they broaden the potential answer (Silverman *et al.* 2005) and hand the initiative and agenda over to the patient. So instead of asking, 'Are you alright?' ask, 'How are you today?' or, 'What has your experience of treatment been like'?

It is good to include a psychological focus to make it clear that this is part of what you are interested in; for example, 'How did that make you feel?' or, 'What are your main concerns'?

Open questions cannot be used in isolation as the opportunity for open discussion can easily be blocked by failing to ensure that the rest of the fundamental communication elements are in place. Attention therefore must be paid to providing sufficient time, verbal space (not interrupting) and encouragement (in the form of non-verbal cues, paraphrasing, clarifying and summarizing), so that the patient and/or relative can express their feelings and concerns.

Open questions may not be appropriate with people who have a communication problem: perhaps following head and neck surgery, or where complex communication is going to be difficult, as with a difficulty talking in the English language.

Try to use one question at a time: it is easy to ask more than one question in a sentence and this can make it unclear where your focus is and lead the patient to answer only one part of your question.

Reflecting back

You can repeat the same words back to the patient: this signals that their focus is a legitimate topic for discussion (Perry & Burgess 2002), but if this technique is overused it can sound unnatural (Silverman *et al.* 2005).

When it is used it needs to be done with thought and include, 'Something of you in your response' (Egan 2002, p. 97), meaning that you remain alert and caring.

Paraphrasing

This technique involves telling the patient what they have told you but using different words that retain the same meaning; for example:

Patient: I need to talk to them but whenever they start to talk to me about the future, I just start to get wound up and shut down.
Nurse: So when your family try to talk, you get tense and you stop talking . . . .

Clarifying

The aim of this technique is to reduce ambiguity and help the patient define and explore the central or pivotal aspect of issues raised. Many of us may be reluctant to explore emotional or psychological issues too much; just in case issues are raised that are emotional and hard to deal with (Perry & Burgess 2002). However, if the principles of good communication are applied and a focus on the patient's agenda is maintained, distressing and difficult situations can be moved forward positively.

Once open questions have opened dialogue, it is likely that certain issues will be raised that would benefit from further exploration. Clarification encourages the expression of detail and context to situations and may help to draw out pertinent matters, perhaps not previously considered by either patient or health professional. A mixture of open or closed questions can be used in clarification; for example:

- 'Are you feeling like that now'?
- 'You say that you've not had enough information: can you tell what you do know'?

- 'You mention that you are struggling: what kinds of things do you struggle with'?
- 'You say it's been hard getting this far: what has been the hardest thing to cope with'?
- 'You seem to be down today, am I right'?
- 'Can you describe how the experience made you feel'?

It might be necessary for you to clarify your own position too: perhaps acknowledge that you don't know something and cannot answer certain questions, e.g. 'Will the treatment work'?

Sometimes not knowing can be a valuable position, enabling you to seek out the patient's experience and not just imagine it. Our imagination and experience might be relevant but each patient and relative will require the opportunity to tell it in their words and need to feel 'heard'.

Summarizing

This intervention can usefully be used as a way of opening or closing dialogue. An opening can be facilitated by recapping over a previous discussion or outlining your understanding of the patient's position. Summarizing can be used to punctuate a longer conversation and highlight specific issues raised.

This serves several purposes:

- It informs your patient that you have listened and understood their position.
- It allows the patient to correct any mistakes or misconceptions generated.
- It brings the conversation from the specific to the general (which can help in recontextualizing issues within a bigger picture).
- It gives an opportunity for agreement to be made about what may need to happen.

An example of summarizing:

It sounds like you are tired and are struggling to manage the treatment schedule: it also sounds like you don't have enough information and we could support you more with that . . . .

Summarizing can be a useful opportunity to plan and agree what actions are necessary. Avoid getting caught up with planning though: the important issue is that you have listened and understood. In our nursing role we are familiar with 'doing' and correcting problematic situations, and although interventions can be helpful in psycho-social issues, sometimes it is necessary not to act and to just 'be' with the patient, accepting their experience as it is, however emotionally painful.

Recognizing when to act and when to sit with distress can be difficult but it is important for us to develop this awareness and accept that sometimes there are no solutions to difficult situations and the temptation to always correct problems might only serve to negate the patient's experience.

Empathy

Sharing time and physical space with other people demands the development of a relationship. In nursing, the relationship with patients is defined by many factors, e.g. physical and medical care. In clinical roles it might be possible to be emotionally detached and to exist behind a 'professional mask' (Taylor 1998, p. 74), but to work in a supportive role a shared experience and bond is generated, inclusive of feelings.

Recognizing our own feelings is important to allow us to understand and to 'tolerate another person's pain' (McKenzie 2002, p. 34).

As nurses we demonstrate empathy when there is a 'desire to understand the client (patient) as fully as possible and to communicate this understanding' (Egan 2002, p. 97).

This means attempting to understand what the patient might be going through, taking into consideration their physical, social and psychological environment. This inferred information can be used to 'connect' with the patient, all the time checking that our interpretation of their experience is accurate (we can be wrong even if we have experienced similar things).

As the patient's environment can change considerably in short spaces of time it is essential to remain alert to the consequent change and interdependency of bio-psycho-social elements.

Rogers seminally described the skill of empathy as: 'The ability to experience another person's world as if it were one's own, without losing the "as if" quality' (Rogers 1975, p. 2). That means allowing ourselves to get into the patient's shoes and experience some of what they might be experiencing, without allowing ourselves to enter the experience wholly (it isn't our experience to own). Empathy allows for an opportunity to 'taste' and therefore to attempt to understand the patient's perspective. Understanding emotions and behaviours in this way encourages an acceptance and positive negotiation of them. Maintaining the 'as if' quality protects us from adopting too great an emotional load. Having too much of a sense of loss or sorrow may prevent us from offering effective support, as we are drawn to focus on our own feelings more than is necessary or helpful (for ourselves or the patient).

Empathy may not always come easily, especially if a patient is angry. What can be very useful in the development and use of empathy is the ability to step back from the situation and reflect upon what it is that you, as the nurse feel and how this relates to what is happening for the patient.

Supporting ourselves

Sharing a patient's distress is difficult and we can help ourselves by sharing and reflecting upon these experiences.

If you communicate well and allow patients to talk, you will be exposed to weighty emotional experiences, e.g. fear, loss and profound sadness. This emotional experience is part of working as a nurse in oncology and arguably health services in general.

Sitting with emotional pain is not without its consequence or burden (Dunne 2003) and it is therefore essential that our own needs are recognized and nurses learn ways of processing this burden.

Historically the nursing culture is more synonymous with 'getting on with it' than with the idea of self care. However 'getting on with it' means disowning the feelings that emotive situations generate within us (Johns & Freshwater 1998). If we do this then weare failing to empathize and may deprive patients and relatives of supportive and good quality care. To facilitate empathy and the subsequent management of psycho-social issues there needs to be an equivalent commitment to 'self care'.

The first challenge is to recognize this need and develop the emotional maturity to accept that a person cannot support without being 'supported' themselves.

Secondarily it will require institutions and the senior staff within them to place psychological care on a par with physical care and to do more than pay lip service to a holistic concept of care. This also means making a commitment to communication training that follows a proven approach (for examples of these see Razavi *et al.* 2000a, b; Wilkinson *et al.* 2002, 2003; Delvaux *et al.* 2004; Boyd 2005).

Thirdly there must be action on the part of the institution and individual to take on the responsibility for safe and effective clinical supervision to allow people to reflecton issues in a non-threatening environment (Dunne 2003).

The more developed our communication skills are, the more effectively we can manage situations. This can provide greater job satisfaction and reduce stress (Fellowes *et al.* 2004).

Everyone needs to be able to reflect upon their skills of communication and everyone can develop their skills via appropriate training (Jenkins & Fallowfield 2002; Wilkinson *et al.* 2002; Delvaux *et al.* 2004; Fellowes *et al.* 2004).

Specific issues

Blocking

Blocking means avoiding addressing the patient's agenda by:

- Failing to pick up on cues (ignoring).
  e.g. Not responding to a patient's disclosure of concern.
- Selectively focusing on the physical aspects of care.
  e.g. Making it clear that your priority is physical care.

- Premature or false reassurance.
  e.g. Where someone is worried, telling them it will be okay.
- Inappropriate encouragement or trivializing.
  e.g. Telling someone they look fine when they have expressed altered body image.

- Passing the buck.
  e.g. Suggesting it is another professional's responsibility to answer questions or sort out the problem.
- Changing the subject.
- Jollying along.
  e.g. 'Don't worry, the sun is still shining (!)'
- Using closed questions.

(Faulkner & Maguire 1994.)

The greater the emotional disclosure, the more nurses use blocking behaviours (Booth *et al.* 1996) and the highest blocking behaviour by health professionals occurs with patients with recurrent cancer (Wilkinson 1991). Interestingly nurses who felt supported practically and emotionally by supervisors decreased their blocking behaviours (Booth *et al.* 1996).

For further discussion about blocking and how nurses and health professionals lack (or perceive a lack of) necessary skills to communicate and support people effectively, readers are directed to Wilkinson 1991; Booth *et al.* 1996; Wilkinson *et al.* 1998 and Fallowfield 2002.

Recognizing blocking tactics and honestly considering how much this occurs in our own practice can help us to reduce this behaviour and support our patients better.

Language and cultural issues

Illness and medical environments are not culturally neutral (Moore & Spiegel 2004, p. 17). We work with and need to care for people from different cultures who may have a primary language other than English. Beliefs and values may be very different from our own and lead to misunderstanding. Consideration must be given to patients speaking a different language and, 'Suitably trained and skilled interpreters and advocates should be available for patients' (NICE 2004, p. 57).

It is not possible to list all the cultural considerations required when communicating with people from different cultural backgrounds; however, it is vital that we remain aware that our assumptions about good communication may not span all cultures. Offence can easily be caused by inappropriate eye contact or touch and an open attitude, and sensitivity to these issues will serve us well in practice.

Including a cultural dimension to nursing care involves addressing these issues by observing acceptable interaction between family members and simply asking patients from different cultural backgrounds about specific considerations, preferences and things to avoid.

Depression and anxiety

Depression in cancer patients is a frequently occurring phenomenon, with the type of cancer and stage of progression influencing the prevalence (Fallowfield *et al.* 2002; Massie 2004). In our daily work with cancer patients we need to be able to assess low mood and the level of coping amongst patients in our care. At diagnosis a good proportion of patients and families are understandably in a state of shock and have anxiety and low mood as part of a stress reaction. Importantly, 'A substantial minority go on to develop persistent psychological disorders' (Moorey & Greer 2002, p. 5).

Where persistent and unrealistic negative predictions and expressions of hopelessness are apparent we need to recognize them and act. Concern about a patient's behaviour, e.g. significant lethargy that isn't accounted for by treatment side effects, should be sensitively explored and further support offered.

Frequently depression can present with anxiety. Anxiety occurs frequently and to some extent can be seen as 'normal' given the threats and stresses inherent in treatment and potentially life-threatening disease (Stark *et al.* 2002).

It is important to avoid labelling and pathologizing normal anxiety reactions to stressful experiences. When patients are anxious they require support and realistic reassurance, not a psychological diagnosis.

Significant and prolonged anxiety can lead to 'panic attacks' which require calm management. Various symptoms can be experienced by the person, e.g. abdominal discomfort, dizziness, tingling in fingers and toes, mostly caused by changes in breathing. This is a very distressing state for the patient, who may attribute the sensations to more serious causes.

Anxiety can be avoided by making time for patients to talk things through, eliciting and addressing concerns realistically and giving accurate information. Where fears are realistic, work with the patient to explore and focus upon their strengths and what will help them get through difficult situations. 'Ignorance is the parent of fear' (Melville 1994, p. 40).

Supporting patients with severe anxiety/suffering panic attacks

- Stay with the patient, remain calm. Ensure the patient is suffering anxiety and not something more serious.
- Reassure the patient that they will feel better shortly if they follow your advice. Gain eye contact, speak confidently and calmly. Offer to hold their hand but be aware that some people may not want this.
- Encourage the person to breathe deeply and slow their breathing down (it might help to demonstrate). Get them to breathe with you: count slowly one, two, three to breathe in, pause, and one, two, three to breathe out.
- As their breathing slows, encourage them with positive affirmation that they are controlling the situation.

- Once the crisis has passed it is important to reflect upon what prompted the anxiety in that situation, how it builds up, and for the person to raise their awareness of their breathing. The patient needs to recognize how shallow or rapid breathing can cause many of the symptoms they have experienced and are afraid of, e.g. light-headedness, tingling in fingers and toes, abdominal discomfort.
- Refer for further exploration and psychological support if occurring frequently or there is a history of anxiety.
- Use of prescribed benzodiazepines may help if the above strategy is not immediately helpful.

Denial and collusion

Denial is a coping mechanism to enable people to deal with shocking, painful or distressing information (Goldbeck 1997) and for this reason many patients with cancer use it functionally. Denial frequently generates discomfort and uncertainty for the health professional. There is a potential risk of using the term to explain away certain patient behaviours, or to avoid tackling difficult issues with people. Careful management of denial is required, but is within the scope of someone with good communication skills.

Denial and collusion: key points

- Denial is a coping mechanism.
- We need to consider carefully when to respect it and when to challenge it, sharing this with colleagues.
- Collusion needs to be understood and recognized in staff and or in families. It is best addressed and worked through as early as possible to avoid the situation becoming too complicated.

The degree of denial varies considerably and has different implications for the health professional.

It is often inappropriate to challenge functional denial; however, this can become complex when trying to ensure whether someone has understood his or her diagnosis and the implications of treatment.

If the process of information giving and the delivery of bad news is handled professionally and the process is clearly documented it can be easier to assess whether denial or ignorance is represented by certain behaviours.

Once the duty to disclose information has been met, the degree to which the patient accepts the information is variable and needs to be respected.

It can generally be assumed that where denial does not affect the treatment regime or damage family relationships then it need not be confronted.

Breaking denial down and forcing someone to confront their reality can be particularly harmful. An individual's ability to cope with further information can change, so it can be useful to 'test' denial from time to time; for example: 'How do you feel things are going for you?' or, 'Do you require any further information or clarification of information'?

Exploring what and how much a patient wants to know can indicate whether they want to retain their denial as a coping mechanism or are ready to confront their situation further. Remember that 'most patients want as much information as possible about treatment and illness' (Jenkins *et al.* 2001, p. 49).

Working in oncology we may feel pressured to provide and maintain hope for patients (Houldin 2000). The maintenance of hope is very valuable for patients when they are confronting and going through tough physical and psychological times. Maintaining inappropriate hope however is similar to providing premature or inappropriate encouragement (see Blocking section above), and may say more about our own difficulty in tackling difficult emotional issues than the patient's ability to deal with the consequences of reality.

At the point where hopes for a cure or significantly prolonged life become unrealistic, we need to recognize the issue and make it explicit, i.e. share information with the patient and their family (with consent) as well as other professional colleagues involved in care. If this doesn't occur then collusive relationships may develop and health professionals might attempt to conceal reality from the patient.

Poor professional communication can lead to the patient receiving mixed messages about their situation, which is potentially far more distressing than confronting reality.

Collusion can leave health professionals feeling confused, deceitful and disturbed. There can be a feeling that nurses should not challenge the information giving of medical staff and it certainly offers no advantage to be contradicting one another in the health setting. In a nursing role however we should acknowledge our ability to recognize collusion where it occurs and face up to the situation with colleagues. With good planning, honest information can be given to the patient and family, to allow them to make decisions about their care, treatment and future, however short that time may be.

Collusion within families can also occur with family members expressing a desire to protect the patient from bad news, or alternatively the patient wishes to do the same for their family. The motive in these situations is frequently one of protection and arises from love.

Managing collusion with professionals and patients and their families requires an exploration of the consequences of maintaining the silence. If delicately managed, this exploration will often lead to some acceptance that the truth is less harmful, e.g. by the realization that people will not be able to say things they wish to say, or organize things they wish to happen. If agreement cannot be gained, then it must be pointed out that there is a duty to be truthful if the party lacking information 'wants to know'. A statement can be made that if the patient or relative states clearly that they do not wish to know bad news then this wish will be respected.

Breaking bad news

Bad news is: 'Any information that produces a negative alteration to the person's expectations about their present and future' (Buckman 1992, p. 15). Being involved with breaking bad news is an unavoidable part of oncology nursing. Bad news is often formally given by doctors; however, nurses often clarify and confirm the information given either immediately or in the following hours and days.

The use of a breaking bad news model is indispensable, e.g. SPIKES (a six-step approach). Models provide a valuable framework to ensure that we meet the individual information needs of our patients. The SPIKES model involves:

- Setting up the interview.
- Assessing the patient's Perception (of their current situation).
- Obtaining the patient's Invitation (to disclose information).
- Giving Knowledge and information.
- Addressing the Emotions with Empathy.
- Strategy and Summary (making a plan for the future/avoiding abandoning the patient). (Baile *et al.* 2000.)

A poorly planned and insensitive approach to breaking bad news has been shown to increase patient distress with a possible lasting impact on coping ability, potentially even influencing psychological pathology, e.g. anxiety and depression (Maguire 1998; Fallowfield & Jenkins 2004).

Communicating with the blind or partially sighted

Sight loss can be very variable, ranging from mild to complete. Any sight disturbance is a significant issue in caring for patients. It might simply mean ensuring glasses are kept safely, within reach and clean, or providing large print documents, braille or audio information.

Blind people will rely more heavily on other senses, especially their hearing and it might therefore be necessary to read things carefully for them. Be open about the visual impairment: ask what helps and what doesn't.

Good communication practice becomes more important, e.g. introducing yourself even when the person may have met you on numerous occasions (as your voice may not always be distinguishable). A lack of non-verbal information can compromise verbal meaning. Consider describing something complex on the phone: it takes a lot more verbal information. Careful explanation and repetitive checking of understanding is a key technique. To some extent you may be the eyes of the patient and you need to relay information that they will not be aware of, e.g. the patient's relative has arrived on the ward but is waiting.

There will be an increased demand for empathic skills.

Make it clear when you are leaving to avoid confusion (visual cues are not always available to the blind or partially sighted).

In situations where confusion may occur as to whom is being spoken to, use the patient's name or a light touch when addressing them.

- Blind and partially sighted people have the same information needs as everyone else and need accessible information in a suitable format.
- Access to information facilitates informed decisions and promotes independence.
- No single method will suit all. Even the same person might use different methods at different times and under different circumstances. It is important to identify the preferred method(s) for each person.
- It is also important to remember the blind or partially sighted person does not necessarily have a hearing loss.

There is now a legal duty to meet the information needs of blind and partially sighted people (Disability Discrimination Act 1999).

Ethnic minorities
There is very little material available in large print, Braille or on tape in ethnic languages.

Resources
Royal National Institute of the Blind (RNIB): See It Right, 105 Judd Street, London, WC1H 9NE. Tel. 020 7391 2397. Email: www.seeitright@rnib.org. Helpful website of the RNIB: www.rnib.org.uk.

Communicating with the deaf or hard of hearing

As with blindness, the extent of the impairment varies significantly. Mild hearing loss might simply require more care with clarity of speech and ensuring the patient is able to see your face clearly. If a hearing aid is used, make sure it is in use and working. Reduce noise in the environment: hearing aids amplify everything, even background noise. More severe hearing problems will not benefit from a hearing aid and these patients reply more on lip reading and/or signing.

Lip reading is a difficult skill and requires a lot of concentration. Not all sounds/words produce a shape on the lips and so the lip-reader has to piece together

74

meaning from what they do distinguish. What information you do convey via your facial expression and lip movement needs to be accentuated, hence pay attention to the direction of light (not behind you) and ensure the patient is ready to begin. Contextualize your discussion by giving the topic for conversation first. Try to relax and allow your body language and gesture to flow normally. Speak normally: not too fast or too slow (although slightly slower speech may be beneficial).

Keep your hands away from your face, avoid using complex words and be prepared to repeat yourself as many times as it takes. If you cannot make yourself understood, write things down. Use sentences not single word answers: this again helps to contextualize information.

Suggestions when communicating with someone who is deaf or hard of hearing

- Find a suitable place to talk, with good lighting and no noise or distractions.
- Be patient and allow extra time for the consultation/ conversation.
- If the person is wearing a hearing aid, do not assume they can hear you. Ask if it is on and if they still need to lip read.
- If an interpreter is required always remember to talk directly to the person you are communicating with, not the interpreter.
- Make sure you have the listener's attention before you start to speak.
- Talk clearly, but not too slowly, and do not exaggerate your lip movements.
- Use natural facial expressions and gestures.
- Use plain language; avoid waffling, jargon and unfamiliar abbreviations.
- Check the person understands you.
- Depending on the purpose of the consultation, writing down a summary of the key points made might be helpful.

Resources

Royal National Institute of the Deaf (RNID): 19–23 Featherstone Street, London, EC1Y 8SL. Tel. 0207296 8264. Text-phone 020 7296 8246. Fax 020 7196 8199. Email: support-erservices@rnid.org.uk. Website: www.rnid.org.uk.

Communicating with a person with aphasia (complex disorder of language processing)

- Make an early referral to a speech and language therapist (SLT).
- Be aware of where the aphasic patient is within their disease trajectory.
- Be aware if the patient has impaired attention, concentration and/or memory.
- Minimize distractions, both visual and auditory.
- Allow enough time, with a calm, friendly, encouraging approach.
- Make sure the aphasic patient understands the purpose of the conversation.

- Talk directly to the aphasic patient and ask them what is/isn't helpful.
- Have a pen and paper for both people to use: writing or drawing can support what is being said.
- Speech should be clear, slightly slower and of normal volume.
- Use straightforward language and avoid jargon (medical terminology).
- Say one thing at a time and pause between 'chunks' of information.
- Structure questions carefully and check the patient understands.
- Make it clear when there is a change of topic.
- Support the spoken language with appropriate non-verbal communication.
- Abilities may fluctuate, so what helps one moment might not work another.
- Be prepared for their and your frustration. You might have to come back to a topic at another time.
- Confusion or miscommunication can be avoided by using a notebook to record salient/key information, especially when the information is new and/or complex, anxiety is present or memory function is impaired.

Conclusion

As nurses we have a profound responsibility to include good communication and psychological support as part of our role. These skills need to be incorporated as a priority, alongside technological advances and extended roles. We cannot afford to forget that people have emotions and psychological needs that require as much, if not more, attention than the physical and technical care delivered. Without this consideration the processes of successful treatment and recovery can be seriously impaired and undermined. Everyone can develop and improve their communication skills, and by paying attention to this crucial aspect of the nursing role, may be pleased to discover how rewarding and valuable this investment is for both nurse and patient.

References

Back, A.L. *et al.* (2005) Approaching difficult communication tasks in oncology. *CA Cancer J Clin*, **55**, 164–77.

Baile, W.F. *et al.* (2000) SPIKES – a six-step protocol for delivering bad news: application to the patient with cancer. *Oncologist*, 5(4), 302–11.

Booth, K. *et al.* (1996) Perceived professional support and the use of blocking behaviours by hospice nurses. *J Adv Nurs*, **24**, 522–7.

Booth, K., Maguire, P. & Hillier, V.F. (1999) Measurement of communication skills in cancer care: myth or reality? *J Adv Nurs*, **30**(5), 1073–97.

Boyd, K. J. (2005) *Enhancing clinical communication: developing an education programme for consultants in SE Scotland*. MMedSci Clinical Education Thesis, University of Nottingham (unpublished).

Buckman, R. (1992) *Breaking Bad News: A Guide for Health Care Professionals.* Johns Hopkins University Press, Baltimore, p. 15.

Cambell,S. (2006) A project to promote better communication with patients. *Nurs Times,* **102**(19), 28–30.

Cantwell, B.M. & Ramirez, A.J. (1997) Doctor–patient communication: a study of junior house officers. *Med Educ,* **31**(1), 17–21. In: Fellowes, D., Wilkinson, S. & Moore, P. (2004) Communication skills for health care professionals working with cancer patients, their families and/or carers. *Cochrane Database Syst Rev,* **2**, CD003751.

Carlson, L.E. & Bultz, B.D. (2004) Efficacy and medical cost offset of psychosocial interventions in cancer care: making the case for economic analyses. *Psychooncology,* **13**, 837–49.

Chant, S. *et al.* (2002) Communication skills: some problems in nurse education and practice. *J Clin Nurs,* **11**, 12–21.

Chelf, J.H. *et al.* (2001) Cancer-related patient education: an overview of the last decade of evaluation and research. *Oncol Nurs Forum,* **28**(7), 1139–47.

Cooley, C.M. (2005) Communication skills in palliativecare. In: *Handbook of Palliative Care* (eds C. Faull, Y. Carter & L. Daniels), 2nd edn. Blackwell Publishing, Oxford, pp. 86–97.

Deffner, J.M. & Bell, S.K. (2005) Nurses' death anxiety, comfort level during communication with patients and families regarding death, and exposure to communication education: a quantitative study. *J Nurses Staff Dev,* **21**(1), 19–23.

Delvaux, N. *et al.* (2004) Effects of a 105 hours psychological training program on attitudes, communication skills and occupational stress in oncology: a randomised study. *Br J Cancer,* **90**, 106–14.

DH (2005) www.performance.doh.gov.uk/hospitalactivity/data_requests/download/nhs_complaints/complaint_04_summary.xls. Accessed 11/5/05.

DH (2001) *Consent: What You Have a Right to Expect (A Guide for Adults).* Department of Health, London.

DH (2000) *The NHS Cancer Plan.* Department of Health, London.

Disability Discrimination Act Section 21 (1999) www.opsi.gov.uk/acts/acts2005/200513.htm, DDA 2005. Accessed 10/05.

Drew, A. & Fawcett, T.N. (2002) Responding to the information needs of patients with cancer. *Prof Nurse,* **17**(7), 443–6.

Dunne, K. (2003) The personal cost of caring. Guest editorial. *Int J Palliat Nurs,* **9**(6), 232.

Edwards, P. (2005) An overview of the end-of-life discussion. *Int J Palliat Nurs,* **11**(1), 21–27.

Egan, G. (2002) *The Skilled Helper. A Problem–Management and Opportunity–Development Approach to Helping,* 7th edn. Brooks/Cole, Pacific Grove, CA.

Fallowfield, L. & Jenkins, V. (2004) Communicating sad, bad, and difficult news in medicine. *Lancet,* **363**, 312–19.

Fallowfield, L., Jenkins, V.A. & Beveridge, H.A. (2002) Truth may hurt but deceit hurts more: communication in palliative care. *Palliat Med,* **16**, 297–303.

Faulkner, A. & Maguire, P. (1994) *Talking to Cancer Patients and their Relatives.* Oxford University Press, Oxford.

Fellowes, D., Wilkinson, S. & Moore, P. (2004) Communication skills for health care professionals working with cancer patients, their families and/or carers. *Cochrane Database Syst Rev*, **2**, CD003751.

Goldbeck, R. (1997) Denial in physical illness. *J Psychosom Res*, **43**(6), 575–93.

Hargie, O. (2006) *The Handbook of Communication Skills*, 3rd edn. Routledge, London.

Hargie, O. & Dickson, D. (2004) *Skilled Interpersonal Communication: Research Theory and Practice*, 4th edn. Routledge, London.

Heyland, D.K. *et al.* (2006) What matters most in end-of-life care: perceptions of seriously ill patients and their family members. *CMAJ*, **174**(5), 627–33.

Houldin, A.D. (2000) *Patients with Cancer: Understanding the Psychological Pain*. Lippincott, Philadelphia.

Jenkins, V.A. & Fallowfield, L.J. (2002) Can communication skills training alter physicians' beliefs and behaviour in clinics? *J Clin Oncol*, **20**, 765–9.

Jenkins, V.A., Fallowfield, L.J. & Saul, J. (2001) Information needs of patients with cancer: results from a large study in UK cancer centres. *Br J Cancer*, **84**(1), 48–51.

Johns, C. & Freshwater, D. (1998) *Transforming Nursing through Reflective Practice*. Blackwell Science, London.

Lookinland, S. & Pool, M. (1998) Study on effect of methods of pre-operative education in women. *AORN J*, **67**(1), 203–13.

Lowry, M. (1995) Knowledge that reduces anxiety: creating patient information leaflets. *Prof Nurse*, **10**(5), 318–20.

McCabe, C. (2004) Nurse–patient communication: an exploration of patients' experiences. *J Clin Nurs*, **13**, 41–9.

McKenzie, R. (2002) The importance of philosophical congruence for therapeutic use of self in practice. In: *Therapeutic Nursing. Improving Patient Care through Self-awareness and Reflection* (ed. D. Freshwater). Sage Publications, London, pp. 22–38.

Maguire, P., Faulkner, A., Booth, K., Elliott, C. & Hillier, V. (1996) Helping cancer patients disclose their concerns. *Eur J Cancer*, 32 A, No. 1 78–81.

Maguire, P. (1998) Breaking bad news. *Eur J Surg Oncol*, **24**(3), 188–91.

Maguire, P. & Pitceathly, C. (2002) Key communication skills and how to acquire them. *Br Med J*, **325**, 697–700.

Massie, M.J. (2004) Prevalence of depression in patients with cancer. *J Natl Cancer Inst*, **32**, 57–71.

Melville, H. (1994) *Moby Dick*. Penguin Classics, London.

Moore, R.J. & Spiegel, D. (2004) *Cancer, Culture and Communication*. Kluwer Academic/Plenum Publishers, New York.

Moorey, S. & Greer, S. (2002) *Cognitive Behaviour Therapy for People with Cancer*. Oxford University Press, Oxford.

NICE (2004) *Improving Supportive and Palliative Care for Adults with Cancer*. National Institute for Health and Clinical Excellence, London.

NMC (2006) *A–Z Advice Sheet Consent*. www.nmc.org.

NMC (2008) *The Code: Standards of Conduct, Performance and Ethics for Nurses and Midwives*. Nursing and Midwifery Council, London.

Perry, K.N. & Burgess, M. (2002) *Communication in Cancer Care*. Blackwell Publishing, Oxford.

Razavi, D. *et al.* (2000a) Testing health care professionals' communication skills: the usefulness of highly emotional standardized role-playing sessions with simulators. *Psychooncology*, 9(4), 293–302.

Razavi D. *et al.* (2000b) Does training increase the use of more emotionally laden words by nurses when talking with cancer patients? A randomized study. *Br J Cancer*, 87, 1–7.

Rogers, C.R. (1975) Empathic: An Unappreciated Way of Being. *Counselling Psychologist*, 5, 2–10.

Scott, T. (2004) *Integrative Psychotherapy in Healthcare. A Humanistic Approach*. Palgrave, Basingstoke.

Silverman, J., Kurtz, S. & Draper, J. (2005) *Skills for Communicating with Patients*, 2nd edn. Radcliffe Publishing, Abingdon.

Smith, C., Dickens, C. & Edwards, S. (2005) Provision of information for cancer patients: an appraisal and review. *Eur J Cancer Care*, 14, 282–8.

Stark, D. *et al.* (2002) Anxiety disorders in cancer patients: their nature, associations and relation to quality of life. *J Clin Oncol*, 20(14), 3137–48.

Street, R. (2003) Interpersonal communication skills in health care contexts. In: *Handbook of Communication and Social Interaction Skills* (eds J. Greene & B. Burleson). Lawrence Erlbaum Associates, Mahwah, NJ, pp. 909–35.

Taylor, B. (1998) Ordinariness in nursing as therapy. In: *Nursing as Therapy* (eds R. McMahon & A. Pearson). Stanley Thornes, Cheltenham, pp. 64–75.

Van de Molen, B. (1999) Relating information needs to the cancer experience, part 1: information as a key coping strategy. *Eur J Cancer Care*, 8(4), 238–44.

Wallace, P.R. (2001) Improving palliative care through effective communication. *Int J Palliat Nurs*, 7(2), 86–90.

Wilkinson, S. (1999) Communication: it makes a difference. *Cancer Nurs*, 22(1), 17–20.

Wilkinson, S., Roberts, A. & Aldridge, A. (1998) Nurse–patient communication in palliative care: an evaluation of a communication skills programme. *Palliat Med*, 12(1), 13–22.

Wilkinson, S.M. (1991) Factors which influence how nurses communicate with cancer patients. *J Adv Nurs*, 16, 677–88.

Wilkinson, S.M., Gambles, M. & Roberts, A. (2002) The essence of cancer care: the impact of training on nurses' ability to communicate effectively. *J Adv Nurs*, 40(6), 731–8.

Wilkinson, S.M. *et al.* (2003) Can intensive 3-day programmes improve nurses' communication skills in cancer care? *Psychooncology*, 12(8), 747–59.

Multiple choice questions

1 Non-verbal communication makes up an important part of any interaction. Egan (2002) offers a useful acronym to summarize the significant parts. What does SOLER stand for?

   a Squarely, Open posture, Leaning slightly forward, Eye contact, Relaxed
   b Squarely, Open posture, Limit time, Eye contact, Relaxed
   c Squarely, Open posture, Leaning slightly forward, Eye contact, Respectful
   d Sitting, Open posture, Leaning slightly forward, Eye contact, Relaxed

2 'The ability to experience another person's world as if it were one's own, without losing the "as if" quality'. This definition by Rogers (1975) is of which communication skill?

   a Sympathy
   b Pity
   c Reflection
   d Empathy

3 'You say it has been hard getting this far: what has been the hardest thing to cope with?' What skill of communication is demonstrated in this quote?

   a Empathy
   b Clarifying
   c Summarizing
   d Paraphrasing

4 Bad news is 'any information that produces a negative alteration in the person's expectations about their present and future' (Buckman 1992) and is an unavoidable part of many nursing roles. Which of these is essential when breaking bad news?

a Assess patient's perception of the situation
b Obtain patient's invitation to disclose information
c Address emotions with empathy
d All of the above

Answers to the multiple choice questions can be found in Appendix 3.

Part two

Chapter 4

Aseptic technique

Definition

Aseptic means 'without micro-organisms'. Aseptic technique refers to the practice used to prevent the risk of infection. There are two aims of an aseptic technique: first, to protect the patient from contamination by pathogenic organisms during medical and nursing procedures; secondly, to protect the health care worker during nursing and medical procedures from being exposed to potentially infectious blood and body fluids. This can be achieved by ensuring that only sterile equipment and fluids are used during invasive medical and nursing procedures. The aseptic technique procedure has continually developed and is a skill-based procedure evolved from ritualistic and evidence-based practice (Preston 2005).

Ayliffe *et al.* (2000) suggest that there are two types of asepsis: medical and surgical asepsis. Medical or clean asepsis reduces the number of organisms and prevents their spread; surgical or sterile asepsis includes procedures to eliminate micro-organisms from an area and is practised by nurses in operating theatres and treatment areas.

A randomized prospective study has been undertaken to evaluate whether some procedures should be included in the medical or surgical category. Using a medical aseptic non-touch technique compared to a surgical technique when changing central venous devices, fluids or lines caused no difference in infection rates, indicating that it was safe to use the simpler non-touch medical aseptic technique (Larwood *et al.* 2000). However, limiting entry to sterile sites by adopting a closed system for intravascular devices (Rosenthal & Maki 2004) and urinary catheterization (Stephan *et al.* 2006) reduces the incidence of intravenous (IV) and urinary catheter-associated infection.

Indications

Patients have a right to be protected from preventable infection and nurses have a duty to safeguard the well-being of their patients, as health care-acquired infection is recognized as a major and increasing problem for our patients (Chalmers & Straub 2006). An aseptic technique should be implemented during any invasive procedure that bypasses the body's natural defences, e.g. the skin and mucous membranes, or when handling equipment such as IV cannulae and urinary catheters that have been used during these procedures.

Whilst it is difficult to maintain sterility, it is important to prevent contamination of sterile equipment. Poor aseptic techniques can lead to contamination. A 22% syringe contamination rate was observed for syringes prepared by intensive care unit nurses, compared to a 1% rate for the syringes prepared by pharmaceutical technicians (Van Grafhorst et al. 2002).

A study to establish nurses' actions whilst carrying out aseptic techniques suggested that not all nurses followed the same actions and that the rationale for the practice of aseptic techniques is not always research based (Preston 2005). Similar discrepancies were found amongst medical staff (Stein et al. 2003). Nurses can feel uncertain about how to undertake an aseptic technique (Hallett 2000). Unfortunately some infection control practices routinely used cannot be rigorously studied for ethical or logistical reasons; for example, wearing versus not wearing gloves (Mangram et al. 1999). Other problems relate to nurses not always understanding that research is an important part of a nurse's role (Kuuppelomaki & Tuomi 2005).

Chalmers and Straub (2006) suggest that incorporating risk management strategies during health care can help to prevent and control health care-associated infection. By predicting and planning for potential problems asepsis can be maintained.

Reference material

Health care-acquired infection (HCAI) (also called nosocomial infection) is defined as infection occurring in patients after admission to any health care facility that was neither present nor incubating at the time of admission. Infections acquired in hospital but not manifest until after the patient is discharged are included in the definition (Ayliffe et al. 2000). Crowe and Cooke (1998) reviewed the case definition for nosocomial infections, finding areas of consensus and variation which made comparisons of infection rates difficult.

No single factor explains why patients acquire an infection, but it is estimated that one in 10 National Health Service (NHS) hospital patients will acquire a HCAI, which is costing at least £1 billion a year. The commonest sites of infection are:

- urinary (23%) (80% of urinary tract infections are associated with indwelling urinary catheters);
- lung (22%);

- wound (9%);
- blood (6%) (the UK has one of the highest rates of meticillin-resistant *Staphylococcus aureus* blood isolates in Europe. Sixty per cent of blood infections are associated with intravascular devices).

(DH 2003)

Immunocompromised patients have an increased risk of HCAI. Risk factors include underlying disease, invasive procedures, medical devices and length of hospital stay. Prevention of infection for those immunocompromised patients with multiple risk factors cannot always be achieved (DH 2003). Infections acquired by neutropenic patients differ from those of general hospitalized patients. Bloodstream infections are the most common infections for neutropenic patients with haematological malignancies (Glauser & Calandra 2000) and recovery from these is often poor (Garrouste-Orgeas *et al.* 2000).

Risk factors associated with HCAI include invasive procedures, indwelling devices, malignancy, a stay in intensive care or surgical department and length of hospital stay (DH 2003).

The cost of infection is high, to both the patient and the hospital. HCAI increases mortality and morbidity (DH 2003) and causes an increase in pain and suffering, slower recovery, longer hospital stay, loss of earnings and disability experienced by the patients (Chalmers & Straub 2006). The hospital will have increased waiting lists and increased hospital costs. Breaks in aseptic techniques have been implicated in post-operative wound infections (Michalopoulos & Sparos 2003). It is essential when aseptic techniques are used as a method of preventing infection that these procedures are sound in theory and are carried out correctly.

Hospitals recognize the significance of nosocomial infections and employ infection control teams to:

- Reduce the likelihood of patients being exposed to infectious micro-organisms while in hospital.
- Provide adequate care for patients with communicable infections.
- Minimize the likelihood of employees, visitors and communicable contacts being exposed to infectious micro-organisms.
- Develop policies for appropriate management of patients with communicable infections.
- Provide surveillance systems which give adequate feedback to appropriate staff.
- Provide education in techniques to prevent the emergence and spread of infection.

Prevention of HCAI requires specific expertise (Gordts 2005). Analysis has demonstrated that infection control programmes are not only clinically effective but also cost effective (Scheckler *et al.* 1998).

Table 4.1   Surgical site infections can be further divided by surgical category.

Surgical category	Infection risk
Clean (non-traumatic wound where respiratory, alimentary and genitourinary tracts were not entered)	1.5–4.2%
Clean/contaminated (non-traumatic wound in which respiratory, alimentary and genitourinary tracts were entered without significant spillage)	<10%
Contaminated (fresh traumatic wound from a relatively clean source or an operative wound with gross spillage from the gastrointestinal tract or entrance into genitourinary or biliary tract in the presence of infected urine or bile)	10–20%
Dirty or infected (traumatic wound from a dirty source or delayed treatment, faecal contamination, foreign bodies, a devitalized viscus or pus)	20–30%

Factors that influence compliance with infection control procedures included lack of knowledge, lack of time, shortage of staff, lack of facilities such as hand wash basins, lack of isolation rooms (Wilcox 2005) and bed occupancy and turnover intervals (Cunningham *et al.* 2005) as relevant indicators. It was suggested that greater emphasis and knowledge may motivate staff to make time for correct compliance with infection-control procedures.

All staff involved in patient care must receive education and training in the prevention of HCAI (DH 2001a). Creativity is required when facilitating learning related to infection control (Ford & Koehler 2001). Feedback of infection rates can achieve changes in practice (Reilly 2002).

When cross-infection does occur, the cost of investigating and controlling even a small outbreak is high. It has been estimated that an infection increases the costs of health care by more than 300% (Whitehouse *et al.* 2002), emphasizing how important it is to prevent infection. The Infection Control Standards Working Party has prepared standards for practice to make prevention, detection and control of infection in hospitals as effective as possible (Infection Control Standards Working Party 1993). Surgical wound infections are the third most common nosocomial infection in England and Wales (DH 2003) (see Table 4.1). Between October 1997 and June 2001, 140 English hospitals participated in the Nosocomial Infection National Surveillance Service (NINSS) of surgical site infection. One of the findings found that mortality rates were significantly higher following hip prostheses if the patient developed a wound infection (Coello *et al.* 2005). This data emphasizes the need for flawless aseptic technique principles in the operating theatre and the wards.

The diagnosis of infection relies on classic signs of inflammation such as local redness, swelling and pain, although decreased numbers of neutrophils produce minimal or atypical clinical signs of infection (van der Meer & Kuijpers 2000). These local signs and symptoms can precede a further sequence of events, which can be lymphangitis, lymphadenitis, bacteraemia and septicaemia, which, if not promptly recognized and treated, can result in death.

Some patients die each year as a result of HCAI. Whilst many of these fatalities occur in patients already dying from other causes and/or in patients whose infections were not preventable, a proportion of these deaths are avoidable (DH 1995; Taylor *et al.* 2001). The risk of death increases with the severity of the patient's underlying disease.

A survey completed by nurses working on wards assessed adherence to aspects of aseptic technique, and revealed an enormous level of variability, with 3% not washing their hands when delivering medication via a peripherally inserted central line (Galway *et al.* 2003). Nurses' heavy workload has been reported as a contributing factor in poor compliance with hygiene measures (Cunningham *et al.* 2005), which suggests that unnecessary time-consuming aspects of an aseptic technique should be avoided. This view is supported by Bree-Williams and Waterman's (1996) study, which highlighted that the practice of aseptic technique has become ritualistic and complex, and simpler practices are easier, cheaper and not detrimental to the patients.

Continuous education in basic infection control procedures and policies is essential, followed by audits to measure improvements (Michalopoulos & Sparos 2003). Reviews of the literature suggest that the majority of nurses have an incomplete knowledge on how to prevent cross-infection. This should be provided during pre-registration as well as in-service training (Roberts 2000). Bissett (2006) suggests that it is impossible to completely remove the risk of infection. But the National Audit Office estimates that if infection control guidelines were adhered to, HCAI could be reduced by 15% (Taylor *et al.* 2001). One multiple education approach targeted at central venous catheters was found to reduce infection rates and improve compliance to catheter care policies (Lobo *et al.* 2005). A different educational approach using local incidents of non-compliance to standard precautions may also enhance training (Ferguson *et al.* 2004) as a creative approach to training is often needed when undertaking in-service training for a large number of staff (Ford & Koehler 2001).

Principles of asepsis

Infection is caused by organisms which invade the host's immunological defence mechanisms, although susceptibility to infection may vary from person to person (Chalmers & Straub 2006). The risk of infection is increased if the patient is immunocompromised by:

- Age. Neonates and the elderly are more at risk because their immune systems are less efficient.
- Underlying disease. For example, those patients with severe debilitating or malignant disease.
- Prior drug therapy, such as the use of immunosuppressive drugs or the use of broad-spectrum antimicrobials.
- Patients undergoing surgery.

(Calandra 2000.)

The following factors must be considered when nursing immunocompromised patients:

- Classic signs and symptoms of infection are often absent.
- Untreated infection may disseminate rapidly.
- Infections may be caused by unusual organisms or organisms which, in most circumstances, are non-pathogenic.
- Some antibiotics are less effective in immunocompromised patients.
- Repeated infections may be caused by the same organism.
- Superinfections, where a patient acquires a more pathogenic organism (of the same or different species) than the one already causing infection (Laurence & May 2003), require nursing care of the highest standard, including strict adherence to aseptic technique to prevent such infections.

Chalmers and Straub (2006) suggest that a basic principle of infection control for all patients is to assess the risk of the transmission of infection from one patient to another and to plan nursing care accordingly before action is taken. Ryan *et al.* (2006) discusses how an awareness of risk amongst anaesthetists contributes to compliance to infection control guidelines. A prospective study investigating whether a risk asessment programme was effective, found that infections could be prevented which increased patients' safety (Segers *et al.* 2005). This suggests that if each patient is evaluated individually it is possible to focus more closely on those patients who are most susceptible to infection. The most usual means for spread of infection include:

- Hands of the staff involved.
- Inanimate objects, e.g. instruments and clothes.
- Dust particles or droplet nuclei suspended in the atmosphere.

Hand washing

Hand washing is well researched and uncontroversial, having been found to be the single most important procedure for preventing nosocomial infection as hands have been shown to be an important route of transmission of infection (DH 2001a). The type and amount of micro-organisms colonizing health care workers

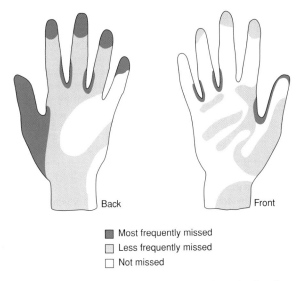

Back   Front

■ Most frequently missed
□ Less frequently missed
□ Not missed

Figure 4.1 Areas most commonly missed following hand washing. (Reproduced by kind permission of *Nursing Times*, where this article first appeared in 1978.)

and patients' intact skin can vary from 102 to 106/cm^2 (Akyol *et al.* 2006). Contamination of hands can easily occur: one study evaluating contamination of gloves during a surgical aseptic technique found that contamination occurred in 55% of gloved hands (Kocent *et al.* 2002). Unfortunately, recent studies (McArdle *et al.* 2006) support those done earlier showing that hand washing is rarely carried out in a satisfactory manner. Studies have shown that up to 89% of staff miss some part of the hand surface during hand washing (Taylor 1978) (Figure 4.1), with the most important factor inhibiting hand washing being busyness (Blatnik & Lesnicar 2005) or inaccessible sinks (Harris *et al.* 2000), with compliance improving when hand washing facilities were installed close to each patient's bed (Cam 2004). Compliance can improve and be sustained when new products are introduced accompanied by an associated behavioral modification programme (Whitby *et al.* 2006).

Hands must be cleaned before and after every patient contact (DH 2001a). Hand washing can be achieved by three methods:

■ Soap and water are effective in removing physical dirt or soiling and transient micro-organisms (Grinbaums *et al.* 1995). Bars of soap can become slimy and be heavily contaminated during use and should not be used in patient areas.

Therefore liquid soap in closed containers that do not come into contact with the user's hands should be used (Subbannayya *et al.* 2006).

■ Antimicrobial detergent is effective in removing physical dirt and soiling and more effective in removing resident micro-organisms than soap and water.

■ Alcohol-based handrub, whilst not effective in removing physical dirt or soiling, is more effective in destroying transient bacteria than more time-consuming hand wash methods. Therefore, hands that are visibly soiled or potentially contaminated with dirt or organic matter must be washed first with liquid soap and running water before using alcohol-based handrub (DH 2001a).

Hand washing must include the following:

1 Roll up sleeves, remove rings and wristwatches.
2 Use continuously running water.
3 Use soap.
4 Position hands to avoid contaminating arms.
5 Avoid splashing clothing or floor.
6 Rub hands together vigorously.
7 Use friction on all surfaces.
8 Rinse hands thoroughly with hand held down to rinse.
9 Dry hands thoroughly.

Hand washing should be undertaken after patient contact and before an aseptic technique is performed (DH 2001a). The use of 'glow and tell' hand washing inspection cabinets to assess the effectiveness of hand washing has been seen to improve hand washing technique (Bissett & Craig 2005).

A dispenser of alcoholic handrub should be placed on the lower shelf of all trolleys used for aseptic techniques to allow hands to be cleaned during the aseptic procedure. A nurse with 'socially clean' hands will not need to wash them during the aseptic procedure, but should use a bactericidal alcoholic handrub whenever disinfection is required, e.g. after opening the outer wrappers of dressings. The use of a handrub will also remove the need for the nurse to leave the patient during the procedure to wash the hands at the nearest basin, during which time contamination may occur.

Compliance with hand washing can be improved through multifaceted approach to training (Aragon *et al.* 2005). Ward-based infection-control link nurses can increase infection-control awareness and motivate staff to improve practice (Dawson 2003). It has been suggested that successful campaigns to improve hand washing will reduce infection rates but hospital management support is required (Pittet 2003). The wearing of rings increases the number of bacteria under the ring compared to adjacent skin or the opposite hand (Kelsall *et al.* 2006). Effective hand washing is difficult to achieve if watches and rings are not removed;

rings can also cause micro-tears around the base of the finger which could expose patients to bacterial contamination (Kelsall *et al.* 2006). Artificial nails harbour microbes and cannot be cleaned as effectively as short, natural nails and must not be worn by those undertaking aseptic techniques (Porteous 2002).

Washed, wet and poorly dried hands can more easily transfer micro-organisms to other surfaces than dry hands (Gould 2000): the damper the hands, the greater the number of micro-organisms (Taylor *et al.* 2000). Thorough drying of hands after hand washing is essential but lapses in hand drying do occur (Chandra & Milind 2001). Electric air drying or disposable paper towels are the usual method of hand drying; the choice depends on the area where the hand washing is being undertaken and on issues such as noise and heat generation, waste disposal and the availability of a regular supply of paper towels. Research indicates that bacteria counts on palms and hands can increase after being dried using warm air, whilst paper towels were the most useful for removing bacteria from fingertips (Yamamoto *et al.* 2005). This suggests that the preferred method is the drying of hands with a good-quality paper towel (DH 2001a). Towel holder type and position must be considered, to ensure they are in the correct position for ease of use and that a paper towel can be removed without contaminating the remaining towels and the holder does not jam or allow the towels to fall out (Harrison *et al.* 2003). Care must be taken not to contaminate the hand wash area. Taps and the paper towel dispenser exit are the most likely areas to be contaminated, which can lead to contamination of the hands of the next user of the hand wash area (Griffith *et al.* 2003).

Non-touch technique

A non-touch technique is essential to ensure that hands, even though they have been washed, do not contaminate the sterile equipment or the patient. This can be achieved by the use of either forceps or sterile gloves (DH 2001a). However, it must be remembered that forceps may damage tissue (David 1991) and gloves can become damaged during use (Kelsall *et al.* 2006). There is no direct evidence that gloves that leak result in transmission of infection (DH 2001a). However, gloves can become contaminated during use with firm touching of the skin rather than light touching, leading to increased contamination (Kocent *et al.* 2002). Gloves must be removed carefully to prevent hands becoming contaminated during removal. Hands must be washed following removal of gloves (DH 2001a). Gloves are single-use items and must not be washed during use (Chalmers & Straub 2006).

Inanimate objects

All instruments, fluids and materials that come into contact with the wound must be sterile if the risk of contamination is to be reduced. Crow (1994) suggests four principles of asepsis, which are: (i) know what is sterile; (ii) know what is not sterile; (iii) keep these two types of items separate; and (iv) replace contaminated items immediately. There will be times when wounds will be in contact with tap water, maybe to remove dressings or during routine showering/bathing (Heal *et al.* 2006). A small double-blind randomized controlled trial comparing tap water and normal saline found no difference in healing or infection rates (Griffiths *et al.* 2001). Once the exposure to tap water is finished, the wound should be redressed using aseptic technique.

The sterile supplies department should normally provide all sterile instruments. The Department of Health (DH) (NHSE 2000) requires that all surgical instruments are traceable to the process that washed, packed and autoclaved the pack, and on whom the pack has been used. A traceability system means that the cleaning, packing and sterilization process can be checked. This ensures that the correct procedure had been undertaken at all stages of the process. If a problem occurs either with the pack or with the patient on whom the pack has been used, the instruments can be traced. These systems involve the instrument pack being labelled to prove it has gone through a sterile process. Prior to the pack being released from the autoclave, a trained person inspects the autoclave cycle responsible for the sterilization of the pack, to ensure the autoclave cycle was completed satisfactorily (NHSE 2000). When using the pack it must be checked for conformance; this includes whether the steam indicator has changed colour, the product is in date and it is undamaged. Once the pack has been used, the label has to be removed from the pack and put in the patient's notes.

All medical devices must carry the *Conformité Europèene* (CE) marking which allows patients, clinicians and other users to be confident that the medical device will perform as the manufacturer intends and is safe when used as instructed (MHRA 2006). Any faults or incidents with medical devices must be reported (MHRA 2005).

The manufacturer's recommendations for all clinical supplies must be followed at all times. The reuse of single-use items must not occur and could result in legal, economic and ethical consequences (Medical Devices Agency 2000).

Forceps can be used to arrange the dressing pack, and then to remove the used dressing before being discarded. Alternatively the washed hands can be inserted into the polythene waste bag to arrange the pack before removing the used dressing. The bag which contains the used dressing is then inverted, before the bag is attached to the dressing trolley. Any equipment that becomes contaminated during a procedure must be discarded. On *no* account should it be returned to the sterile field. Care must also be taken to ensure that equipment and lotions are sterile and that packaging is undamaged before use (Ayliffe *et al.* 2000).

While following aseptic technique, it is important to evaluate the whole procedure to ensure that the principles are followed throughout the whole process. Potential problems such as reusing left-over dressings or taking tape from a contaminated roll (Oldman 1991) will therefore be avoided.

The dressing trolley

Most disinfectants are not sporicidal, have a limited antimicrobial spectrum and must be used only on clean surfaces or equipment, e.g. instruments, as they may fail to penetrate blood or pus (Ayliffe *et al.* 2000). Therefore it is essential that equipment such as a trolley is cleaned daily and, when it becomes contaminated, with a detergent solution and dried carefully with paper towels. This will remove a high proportion of micro-organisms, including bacterial spores (Ayliffe *et al.* 2000). Prior to use for aseptic technique, trolleys should be wiped over with chlorhexidine in 70% ethanol alcohol using a clean paper towel (Ayliffe *et al.* 2000). Trolleys used for aseptic procedures must not be used for any other purpose.

93

Personal protective equipment

Personal protective equipment (PPE) means all equipment that is intended to be worn to protect a person against risks to their health and that which may compromise their safety. The *Personal Protective Equipment at Work Regulations* (HSE 1992) requires employers to carry out a formal assessment of the PPE needs of their employees. The aim of the assessment is to identify any foreseeable risks that cannot be controlled by other means and the suitable PPE available to reduce risk (Masterson & Teare 2001). All PPE must have an appropriate British Standard kitemark or European Community CE mark. Staff required to wear PPE must be provided with information, instruction and training on the hazards from which the PPE does or does not protect the wearer, and the purpose, correct use, limitations, maintenance and storage information related to the PPE (HSE 1992). If an individual is carrying out any task that involves blood or body fluids they require PPE for the following reasons:

- To prevent the user's clothing becoming contaminated with pathogenic micro-organisms, which may subsequently be transferred to other patients in their care.
- To prevent the user's clothing becoming soiled, wet or stained during the course of their duties.
- To prevent transfer of potentially pathogenic micro-organisms from user to patient.
- To prevent the user acquiring infection from the patient (DH 2001a).

Uniform and other protective clothing should not be taken home for laundering. Changing facilities should be provided for staff to encourage them to change out of their uniform in the workplace (NHSE 2002). Nurses' uniforms can become contaminated with pathogenic micro-organisms (Perry *et al.* 2001). It is therefore recommended that a disposable plastic apron, which is impermeable to bacteria, is worn during aseptic procedures. Plastic aprons are single-use items and are worn for one procedure or episode of patient care and then removed (DH

2001a). Gowns must be worn when undertaking invasive surgical procedures; for example, when inserting central venous catheters (DH 2001b). Surgical masks are an integral part of theatre clothing. However, it has never been shown that wearing a surgical mask decreases post-operative wound infections (Lipp & Edwards 2005). Masks must be worn as part of routine universal precautions when there is a risk of airborne aerosol of blood or body fluids, administration of toxic drugs or contact with patients who are smear positive with drug-resistant tuberculosis (DH 2001a; NICE 2006). These masks must comply with the Control of Substances Hazardous to Health (COSHH) (DH 2002) regulations. For surgical procedures undertaken on the wards, masks are generally not required. There is no evidence that wearing a face mask is important in preventing catheter-related infection during central catheter insertion (DH 2001b).

Gloves

Disposable gloves are available in latex and synthetic materials, in sterile and non-sterile form, with and without powder. Gloves must conform to European Community (CE) standards, must not be powdered nor made from polythene. Alternatives to latex gloves must be available because of the increase in sensitivity to latex amongst patients and health care workers (DH 2001a).

Latex allergy guidelines pertaining to the safety of patients and staff must be available. All health care workers must be knowledgeable about latex allergy and its related issues (Wright *et al.* 2001). Problems related to latex allergies must be reported to the Occupational Health Department immediately for early diagnosis and treatment (Medical Devices Agency 1996). Incidences of latex sensitivity are reportable to the Health and Safety Executive under the Reporting of Injuries, Diseases and Dangerous Occurrences Regulations (1985) (RIDDOR) (HSE 1995; NHSE 1999).

Boxed, clean, non-sterile, powder-free gloves made from materials other than latex are safe for routine use (Rossoff *et al.* 1993), in particular to protect hands from contamination with organic matter and micro-organisms (DH 2001a). However, boxed, clean, non-sterile gloves should not be used for aseptic techniques as there is insufficient evidence to justify a practice change to non-sterile gloves for aseptic techniques (St. Clair & Larrabee 2002). Efforts must be made when wearing gloves to avoid glove contamination (Kocent *et al.* 2002) and glove damage (Cork *et al.* 1995).

Failure to change gloves after each patient contact does occur particularly when handling food (Blenkharn 2006). Generally compliance with correct glove use is poor (Girou *et al.* 2004).

Protective footwear

Micro-organisms can be found on the bottom of footwear (Haigh 1993). However, the risk of acquiring infection from floors (Ayliffe *et al.* 2000) and the bottom of health care workers' footwear is low (Haigh 1993). Whilst washable shoes must be kept for those entering the operating theatre (Ayliffe *et al*. 2000), footwear worn elsewhere in the hospital is chosen to comply with risk management rather than infection control.

Environmental cleanliness

The NHS requires that patients are nursed in a clean, comfortable and safe environment (DH 2003). The NHS Performance Assessment Framework (NHSE 2001) includes a cleanliness standard. The standard can be used to monitor and improve cleaning services. The standard has five key objectives: (i) take cleaning seriously; (ii) listen to patients; (iii) infection control; (iv) education; (v) development and monitoring. Included in the standard are lists of elements and their cleaning requirements. These include odour control and a tidy, uncluttered, well-maintained environment (NHSE 2001).

Good hospital hygiene is an integral and important component for preventing HCAI. Unfortunately extensive contamination of the hospital environment is known to occur (Oie *et al*. 2002). Cleaning and disinfecting programmes and protocols for patient care areas must be clearly defined and carefully monitored to ensure high standards of cleanliness are achieved (DH 2003), to ensure that the patient area must be visibly clean, free of dust and soilage before an aseptic technique is commenced. Therefore thorough cleaning, clean laundry, safe collection of waste and food hygiene and pest control are essential (DH 2001a).

Routine cleaning of the environment is the responsibility of the hospital domestic staff. Cleaning must be suspended during aseptic techniques (Ayliffe *et al*. 2000).

Patient hygiene

The majority of infections in susceptible patients are caused by the patient's own endogenous flora (Glauser & Calandra 2000). Preoperative bathing or showering is a well-accepted procedure for reducing skin micro-organisms (Webster & Osborne 2006). Bathing and showering using an antiseptic detergent to eliminate meticillin-resistant *Staphylococcus aureus* (MRSA) colonization of skin is well documented (Rohr *et al*. 2003), although a study comparing routine skin cleaning with soap and water to chlorhexidine solution found no difference in wound infections (Kalantar-Hormozi & Davami 2005). The general population's showering habits vary considerably (Wilkes *et al*. 2005). It is well documented that illness affects patients' well-being which may influence their energy levels (Munch *et al*. 2005); therefore, nurses must be prepared to assist patients with their daily bath or shower.

Studies have established that it is not detrimental for stitches of surgical wounds to get wet (Heal *et al*. 2006). After showering any non-waterproof dressing should be changed immediately. The use of a transparent film dressing allows continuous inspection and more secure anchorage as well as being comfortable and protecting against wetting during showering (Cosker *et al.* 2005).

Airborne contamination

The spread of airborne infection is most likely to occur following procedures such as bed making (Shiomori *et al.* 2002) and cleaning, which can disperse organisms into the air. Airborne contamination of sterile goods can occur (Dietze *et al.* 2001). Ideally such activities should cease 30 minutes before a dressing is to be undertaken. To reduce further the risk of airborne contamination of open wounds, the wound should be exposed for as short a time as possible (Ayliffe *et al.* 2000). Dirty dressings should be placed carefully in a yellow clinical waste bag, which is sealed before disposal (DH 2006a). Clean wounds should be dressed before contaminated wounds. Colostomies and infected wounds should be dressed last of all to minimize environmental contamination and cross-infection.

Air movement should be kept to a minimum during the dressing. This means that adjacent windows should be closed and the movement of personnel within the area discouraged.

Procedure guidelines **Apron: putting on and removing a disposable plastic apron**

Action	Rationale
1 Adequate supply of disposable aprons in a dispenser made for this purpose to be available.	Staff are more likely to put on an apron if they are readily available (E).
2 Dispenser to be positioned away from any source of contamination, but near enough to the point of use to be readily available. For example outside a barrier nursing room.	Plastic aprons generally are in rolls or packs of 100 or 200. Micro-organisms such as MRSA and VRE will survive on contaminated equipment (Dietze *et al.* 2001: R 1b).
3 Colour-coded aprons to be in areas of high risk, for example in Critical Care Units, where each bed has a different colour apron designated for that bed space.	By colour coding aprons it is possible to see if the correct colour apron is being used for the correct task or environment (E).
4 Plastic aprons are single-use items and must be only worn for one procedure or episode of patient care.	Single patient-use items only and cannot be cleaned and reused for another patient (MHRA 2002: E).

5 Used aprons must be discarded and disposed of in a yellow clinical waste bag.

All waste contaminated with blood, body fluids, excretions, secretions and micro-organisms disposed as clinical waste. Yellow is the recognized colour for clinical waste (DH 2005: C; DH 2006a: C).

6 Plastic aprons must be worn during close contact with a patient, patient equipment or the environment when contamination with pathogenic micro-organisms or blood and body fluids is expected. Perspiration is an exception (Pratt *et al.* 2007).

To protect the clothing that is covered by the plastic apron from contamination (Pratt *et al.* 2007: R 1a).

97

7 Remove a plastic apron from the dispenser making sure no other aprons are dislodged at the same time. If this does occur the dislodged unwanted apron should be disposed of as domestic waste in a black polythene bag.

Dislodged aprons can become contaminated; as this apron has not been used and therefore is not contaminated it can be disposed of as domestic waste (DH 2005: C; DH 2006a: C).

8 Pull the apron over your head, avoid touching your hair and uniform (see Action figure 8).

Hands may become contaminated when touching hair and skin as hair and skin can be colonized with micro-organisms such as *Staphylococcus aureus* and *epidemidis*, which can cause infections (Mims *et al.* 2004: R 1a).

9 Tie the apron loosely at the back.

Tightly tied aprons can cause the wearer to become hot and uncomfortable, as well as make the apron more difficult to remove (E).

10 Cleanse hands, using an alcoholic handrub.

Hands must be cleansed before and after every contact with patients and their equipment. As hands would have been cleansed after the previous patient's contact, hands would have been clean before putting on the apron (Pratt *et al.* 2007: R 1a).

Procedure guidelines *(cont.)*

11   If required put on single-use disposable gloves. Gloves should be put on after the apron is put on and removed before the apron is removed.

Sterile gloves to be worn for invasive procedures, contact with sterile sites, non-intact skin or mucous membranes. Clean gloves to be worn when exposure to blood, body fluids, secretions and excretions is likely to occur (Pratt *et al.* 2007: R 1a).

12   Undertake procedure. On completion of the procedure remove the apron. This is achieved by pulling on the apron to break the loop around the neck and the ties behind the back. This is achieved by pulling on the part of the apron that is clean for example the neck and sides (see Action figures 12a–c).

Hands may become contaminated during the procedure by removing the apron, unhooking the neck loop or untying the apron's ties, which could contaminate the wearer's neck, hair and the back of their clothing (E).

13   Clean hands using a liquid soap and warm running water and carefully dry with a paper towel.

Alcoholic handrub is only suitable for clean hands, whilst liquid soap and water removes contamination (Pratt *et al.* 2007: R 1a).

14   If extensive splashing of blood, body fluids, secretions and excretions are expected a full body fluid-repellent gown must be worn as a single-use item.

A gown offers more protection than a plastic apron which only covers the front of the wearer's uniform (Pratt *et al.* 2007: R 1a).

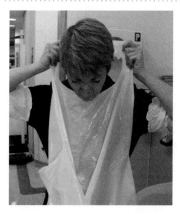

Action 8   Pull the apron over your head, avoiding touching your hair and uniform.

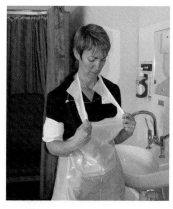

Action 12a   To remove apron, pull apron to break loop around neck and ties behind the back.

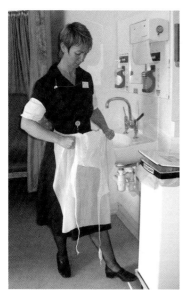

Action 12b Avoid touching uniform whilst removing apron.

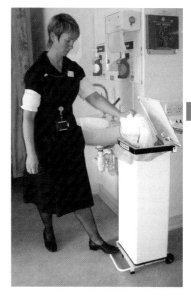

Action 12c Dispose of used plastic apron as clinical waste.

Procedure guidelines Aseptic technique

Equipment

1 Sterile dressing pack* containing gallipots or an indented plastic tray, low-linting swabs and/or medical foam, disposable forceps, gloves, sterile field, disposable bag.
2 Fluids for cleaning and/or irrigation.
3 Hypo-allergenic tape.
4 Appropriate dressing (see Chapter 34).
5 Appropriate hand hygiene preparation.
6 Any other material will be determined by the nature of the dressing: special features of a dressing should be referred to in the patient's nursing care plan.

7 Any extra equipment that may be needed during procedure, e.g. sterile scissors.
8 Chlorhexidine in 70% spirit and paper towels for cleaning trolley.
9 Total traceability system for surgical instruments and patient record form.

Procedure guidelines *(cont.)*

Procedure

Action	Rationale
1 Explain and discuss the procedure with the patient.	To ensure that the patient understands the procedure and gives his or her valid consent (NMC 2006: C; Wilson 2006: E).
2 Clean hands with bactericidal alcohol rub.	Hands must be cleaned before and after every patient contact and before commencing the preparations for aseptic technique, to prevent cross-infection (DH 2005: C).
3 Clean trolley with chlorhexidine in 70% spirit with a paper towel.	To provide a clean working surface (Ayliffe *et al.* 2000: C).
4 Place all the equipment required for the procedure on the bottom shelf of the clean dressing trolley.	To maintain the top shelf as a clean working surface (E).
5 Take the patient to the treatment room or screen the bed. Position the patient comfortably so that the area to be dealt with is easily accessible without exposing the patient unduly.	To allow any airborne organisms to settle before the sterile field (and in the case of a dressing, the wound) is exposed (Ayliffe *et al.* 2000 C). Maintain the patient's dignity and comfort (E).
6 If the procedure is a dressing and the wound is infected or producing copious amounts of exudate, put on a disposable plastic apron.	To reduce the risk of cross-infection (DH 2005: C).
7 Take the trolley to the treatment room or patient's bedside, disturbing the screens as little as possible.	To minimize airborne contamination (Ayliffe *et al.* 2000: C).
8 Loosen the dressing tape.	To make it easier to remove the dressing (E).
9 Clean hands with a bactericidal alcohol handrub.	To reduce the risk of wound infection (DH 2005: C).

10 Check the pack is sterile (i.e. the pack is undamaged, intact and dry. If autoclave tape is present, check that it has changed colour from beige to beige and brown lines), open the outer cover of the sterile pack and slide the contents onto the top shelf of the trolley.

To ensure that only sterile products are used (MHRA 2005: E).

11 Open the sterile field using only the corners of the paper.

So that areas of potential contamination are kept to a minimum (E).

12 Check any other packs for sterility and open, tipping their contents gently onto the centre of the sterile field.

To prepare the equipment and, in the case of a wound dressing, reduce the amount of time that the wound is uncovered. This reduces the risk of infection and a drop in temperature of the wound which will delay wound healing (Naylor et al. 2001: R 1a).

13 Clean hands with a bactericidal alcohol rub.

Hands may become contaminated by handling outer packets, etc. (DH 2005: C).

14 Place hand in disposable bag, arrange contents of dressing pack.

To maintain sterility of pack (E).

15 Remove used dressing with hand covered with the disposable bag, invert bag and stick to trolley.

To minimize risk of contamination, by containing dressing in bag (E).

16 Where appropriate, swab along the 'tear area' of lotion sachet with chlorhexidine in 70% spirit/swab saturated with 70% isopropyl alcohol. Tear open sachet and pour lotion into gallipots or on indented plastic tray.

To minimize risk of contamination of lotion (E).

17 Put on sterile gloves, touching only the inside wrist end.

To reduce the risk of infection. Gloves provide greater sensitivity than forceps and are less likely to cause trauma to the patient (David 1991: E).

Carry out procedure
18 Make sure the patient is comfortable.

19 Dispose of waste in yellow plastic clinical waste bags. Remove gloves.

To prevent environmental contamination. Yellow is the recognized colour for clinical waste (DH 2006a: C).

Procedure guidelines *(cont.)*

20 If necessary, draw back curtains or, if appropriate, help the patient back to the bed area and ensure the patient is comfortable.

21 Check that the trolley remains dry and physically clean. If necessary, wash with liquid detergent and water and dry throughly with a paper towel.

To reduce the risk of spreading infection (Ayliffe *et al.* 2000: C).

22 Clean hands with bactericidal alcohol handrub.

To reduce the risk of spreading infection (DH 2005: C).

23 Place sterility label from the outside of any surgical instrument packs used during the procedure on the patient record form which is to be placed in the patient's notes.

Provides a record, as the sterility label proves the pack has gone through a sterile process and that prior to release has been inspected by a trained person In the Sterile Services Department (NHSE 2000).

NB. Please note that for some procedures it may be more appropriate to use different types of sterile packs (e.g. IV packs). Since usage of these will vary locally reference is generally made to 'sterile dressing pack'.

Procedure guidelines   Hand washing

Hands must be cleaned before and after each patient contact, and after any task that may have resulted in the hands becoming contaminated. There is substantial evidence to indicate that hand washing is the single most important action to reduce the incident of hospital-acquired infection (DH 2001a).

Equipment and facilities

Wrist/knee/elbow or automatic taps should be used in all clinical areas in order to prevent dirty hands contaminating the taps, which could lead to cross-contamination of the next person who uses the taps. Hand basins should be located conveniently near to where they are required. They must be maintained in good working order and always kept stocked with a plentiful supply of paper towels and liquid soap in disposable containers. This ensures the soap containers are not topped up from a larger container. Soap containers can become contaminated (Ayliffe *et al.* 2000) and by renewing them on a regular basis, a potential source of infection is removed. It is important that the design of the paper towel dispenser allows for easy removal of the paper towel without contaminating the remaining towels. Contaminated paper towels could lead to cross-infection.

Procedure

Action	Rationale
1 Remove rings, bracelets and wristwatch.	Jewellery inhibits good hand washing. Dirt and bacteria can remain beneath jewellery after hand washing (DH 2001a: C).
2 Roll up sleeves.	Long sleeves prevent washing of wrists (E).
3 Cover cuts and abrasions on hands with waterproof dressing.	Cuts and abrasions can become contaminated with bacteria and cannot be easily cleaned. Repeated hand washing can increase the injury (DH 2001a: C).
4 Remove nail varnish and artificial nails. Nails must also be short and clean.	Long nails and false nails may be a source of infection by harbouring dirt and bacteria. Nail varnish can become cracked, which could lead to contamination if the nail polish fell into a patient's wound. Nail polish can also inhibit effective hand washing by potentially harbouring bacteria in microscopic imperfections of nail varnish (DH 2001a: C).
5 Hands that are visibly or potentially soiled or contaminated with dirt or organic material should be washed with liquid soap from a dispenser and running hand-hot water.	Liquid soap is very effective in removing dirt, organic material and any loosely adherent transient flora, but has little antimicrobial activity. Liquid soap must be used, as tablets of soap can become contaminated (DH 2001a: C).
(a) Turn on the taps using wrist/elbow or foot and direct the water flow away from the plughole. Run the water at a flow rate that prevents splashing.	Plugholes are often contaminated with micro-organisms that could be transferred to the environment or the user if splashing occurs (NHSE 2002: C).
(b) Run the water until hand hot.	Hand-hot water to be used to ensure that the skin of hands is not damaged by cold water. Water that is too hot could cause scalding. Soap is more effective in breaking down dirt and organic matter when used with hand-hot water (DH 2001a: C).

Procedure guidelines *(cont.)*

(c) Wet the surface of hands and wrists.

Soap applied directly onto dry hands may damage the skin. The water will also quickly mix with the soap to speed up hand washing (DH 2001a: C).

(d) Apply liquid soap and water to all surfaces of the hands.

To ensure all surfaces of the hands are cleaned (DH 2001a: C).

(e) Rub hands together for a minimum of 10–15 seconds, with particular attention to between the fingers and the tips of fingers and thumbs.

To ensure all surfaces of the hands are cleaned. Areas that are missed can be a source of cross-infection (DH 2001a: C).

(f) Nail brushes should not be used.

Nail brushes may damage the skin and result in increased shedding of bacteria from the hands (Winnefeld *et al.* 2000: C).

(g) Rinse soap thoroughly off hands.

A residue of soap can lead to irritation and damage to the skin. Damaged skin does not provide a barrier to infection for the health care worker and can become colonized with potentially pathogenic bacteria, leading to cross-infection (DH 2001a: C).

(h) Care must be taken not to contaminate the taps, sink or nozzle of the soap dispenser with dirt or organic material that is washed off hands.

Contamination of the nozzle of the soap dispenser can result in contamination of the liquid soap, leading to cross-infection (E).

(i) Dry hands thoroughly with a good-quality disposable paper towel from a towel dispenser.

Damp hands encourage the multiplication of bacteria and can potentially become sore (DH 2001a: C).

(j) Dispose of used paper towels in a black bag on a foot-operated stand.

Black is the colour coding for paper waste. Using a foot-operated waste bag stand prevents contamination of the hands (E).

6 Hands that are visibly clean and not soiled or contaminated with dirt, organic material or toxic substances can be cleaned using an alcoholic handrub.

The antimicrobial activity of alcohol is due to its ability to denature proteins. Alcoholic handrub solutions are a quick convenient method of cleansing clean hands of Gram-negative, Gram-positive vegetative bacteria, tuberculosis and a variety of fungi, but have poor activity against bacterial spores and cannot remove dirt, organic material or toxic substances such as drugs or radioactivity. Alcoholic handrub comes in a variety of solutions, gels and foams with an emollient (which reduces the drying effect of the alcohol) (DH 2001a: C).

(a) Follow the manufacturer's instructions for the amount of handrub to be used.

The instructions must be followed so that the correct amount of handrub is used to ensure effective hand cleaning. Too much will cause delays and leave hands sticky, too little will not clean hands adequately (E).

(b) Rub an alcoholic handrub into **all** areas of the hands, until the hands are dry.

To ensure all areas of the hands are cleaned. Alcohol is a rapid-acting disinfectant, with the added advantage that it evaporates, leaving the hands dry. This prevents contamination of equipment, whilst facilitating the application of unpowdered gloves (DH 2001a: C).

7 Hand washing using a bacterial detergent for surgical procedures to be undertaken outside the operating theatre:

Rapid multiplication of bacteria occurs under surgical gloves if hands are washed with a non-bactericidal soap. The use of bactericidal soap reduces the resident skin flora. Bactericidal detergents have a persistent activity, which means that following use the bacteria appear to reproduce slowly on hands.

(a) Turn on the taps using wrist/elbow or foot and direct the water flow away from the plughole. Run the water at a flow rate that prevents splashing.

Plugholes are often contaminated with micro-organisms that could be transferred to the environment or the user if splashing occurs (DH 2001a: C).

(b) Run the water until hand hot.

Hand-hot water to be used to ensure that the skin of hands is not damaged by cold water. Water that is too hot could cause scalding. Soap is more effective in breaking down dirt and organic matter when used with hand-hot water (DH 2001a: C).

(c) Wet hands with hand-hot water.

Applying bactericidal detergent directly onto dry hands increases the risk of skin damage/irritation (E).

(d) Apply the amount of bactericidal detergent advised by the manufacturer.

The correct amount of detergent must be used to ensure effective hand cleaning (E).

Procedure guidelines *(cont.)*

(e) The following washing/rubbing actions should be undertaken five times:
  - Rotational rubbing of wrists.
  - Palm to palm.
  - Right palm to back of left hand.
  - Left palm to back of right hand.
  - Palm to palm, fingers interlaced.
  - Back of fingers of one hand to palm of other hand with fingers interlaced.
  - Rotational rubbing of right thumb in left palm and left thumb in right palm.
  - Rotational rubbing of fingers in clasped palm of opposite hand.

All surfaces of hands must be thoroughly washed for effective hand washing to have taken place (DH 2001a: C).

(f) Holding hands upright, rinse them and wrists under hand-hot running water to remove soap.

Soap residue can cause skin damage. Hands must be held upright to ensure water splashes from unwashed areas of arm do not run down onto clean hands (E).

(g) Dry hands carefully using a good-quality paper towel.

Wet hands can encourage the growth of bacteria and may lead to sore hands (Gould & Chamberlain 1994: R 1a).

- -

Hand washing for surgical procedures in theatre

8 The routine is the same as above but the forearms are included. The hand washing is extended to 2 minutes during which time repeated applications of the bactericidal detergent are required. Hands are dried using a sterile disposable paper towel.

The optimal length of the hand washing is unknown. The important factor is that all areas have been effectively cleaned and rinsed (E).

To prevent contamination from unsterile paper towels (E).

Procedure guidelines Non-sterile gloves use

Equipment

Gloves are single-use items. Single-use items cannot be cleaned and reused for the same or another patient (MHRA 2002: E). Clean boxed gloves are suitable for non-touch aseptic techniques and when there is a risk of exposure to blood, body fluids, excretions, secretions and micro-organisms. Gloves provide a barrier to the hands from contamination from blood, body fluids, excretions, secretions and micro-organisms (Pratt *et al*. 2007: C). Gloves that are CE marked must be available in all clinical areas. CE marking denotes the standard and suitability of the product (Pratt *et al*. 2007: C). Gloves should be stored safely to ensure they are protected from contamination. Powdered and polythene gloves should not be used. Alternatives to natural rubber latex gloves must be available for all staff who have a history of latex sensitivity. Emphasis should be placed on providing alternatives to latex for all staff.

A full range of small, medium and large gloves must be accessible to ensure a correctly fitting glove is available for all staff. Incorrectly fitting gloves decreases dexterity of the wearer and could lead to accidents or poor care (E).

Action	Rationale
1 Hands to be cleaned prior to putting on gloves.	Hands must be cleansed before and after every patient contact or contact with patient's equipment (Pratt *et al*. 2007: C).
2 Gloves should be removed from the box singly, to prevent contamination of the lower down gloves.	To prevent cross-infection (E).
3 Holding the cuff of the gloves, pull the glove into position taking care not to contaminate the glove from the wearer's skin. This is particularly important when the second glove is being put on, as the gloved hand of the first glove can touch the skin of the ungloved second hand if care is not taken.	To prevent cross-infection (E).
4 During the procedure or when undertaking two procedures with the same patient, it may be necessary to change gloves. Gloves are single-use items and must not be cleansed and reused.	Gloves are single patient-use items only and cannot be cleaned and reused for the same or another patient (MHRA 2002: C).

Procedure guidelines *(cont.)*

5 Similarly if gloves become damaged during use they must be replaced.	Damaged gloves do not provide protection (E).
6 When the procedure is completed and the gloves are to be removed, care must be taken to ensure contamination of the wearer does not occur.	The outside of the glove may be contaminated (E).
7 The first glove can be removed by firmly holding the glove wrist and pulling off the glove in such a way as to turn it inside out.	Whilst removing the first glove the second gloved hand continues to be protected. By turning the glove inside out during removal the contamination is contained inside the glove (E).
8 The second glove is removed by slipping the fingers of the other ungloved hand inside the wrist of the glove and pulling it off whilst at the same time turning it inside out.	By putting the fingers inside the glove, the fingers will not be in contact with the potentially contaminated outer surface of the glove (E).
9 Used gloves are to be disposed of in the yellow clinical waste bag.	All waste contaminated with blood, body fluids, excretions, secretions and micro-organisms should be disposed of as clinical waste. Yellow is the recognized colour for clinical waste (DH 2005: C; DH 2006a: C).
10 Hands to be cleansed after taking off gloves, ideally by washing with liquid soap and running water.	Hands may have become contaminated. Alcoholic handrub is only suitable for clean hands whilst liquid soap and water removes contamination (Pratt *et al.* 2007 C).
11 If an apron is being worn at the same time as the gloves, the gloves are to be removed first followed by the apron and then the hands should be washed.	The gloves are more likely to be contaminated than the apron and therefore should be removed first to prevent cross-infection (E).

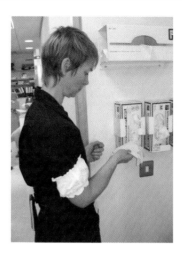

Action 2   Carefully remove gloves to prevent contamination of remaining gloves.

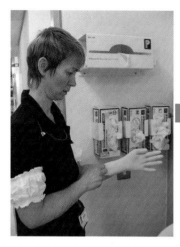

Action 3   Holding the cuff of the glove, pull the glove into position.

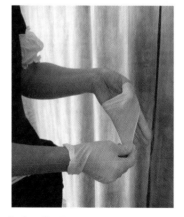

Action 7   Holding the cuff, remove the first glove, turning it inside out.

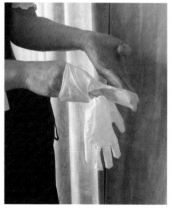

Action 8   Remove second glove by inserting fingers inside the wrist of the glove; pull it off whilst turning it inside out.

References and further reading

Akyol, A., Ulusoy, H. & Ozen, I. (2006) Handwashing: a simple, economical and effective method for preventing nosocomial infections in intensive care units. *J Hosp Infect*, **62**(4), 395–405.

Aragon, D., Sole, M.L. & Brown, S. (2005) Outcomes of an infection prevention project focusing on hand hygiene and isolation practices. *AACN Clin Issues*, **16**(2), 121–32.

Ayliffe, G.A.J. *et al.* (2000) *Control of Hospital Infection. A Practical Handbook*, 4th edn. Arnold, London.

Bissett, L. (2006) Reducing the risk of acquiring antimicrobial-resistant bacteria. *Br J Nurs*, **15**(2), 68–71.

Bissett, L. & Craig, K. (2005) Hand inspection cabinets as an aid to washing technique. *Nurs Times*, **1001**(31), 38–40.

Blatnik, J. & Lesnicar, G. (2005) Propagation of Methicillin-resistant *Staphylococcus aureus* due to the overloading of medical nurses in intensive care units. *J Hosp Infect*, **63**(2), 162–6.

Blenkharn, J.I. (2006) Glove use by ancillary and support staff: a paradox of prevention? *J Hosp Infect*, **62**(4), 519–20.

Bree-Williams, E.J. & Waterman, H. (1996) An examination of nurses' practices when performing aseptic technique for wound dressing. *J Adv Nurs*, **23**, 48–54.

Calandra, T. (2000) Practical guide to host mechanisms and the predominant infections encountered in immunocompromised patients. In: *Management of Infections in Immuno-compromised Patients*, Part I (Section 1) (eds M.P. Glauser & P.A. Pizzo). W.B. Saunders, London, pp. 3–17.

Cam, J. (2004) What does it take to ensure effective hand decontamination by nurses? *Prof Nurse*, **19**(12), 26–8.

Chalmers, C. & Straub, M. (2006) Standard principles for preventing and controlling infection. *Nurs Stand*, **20**(23), 57–65.

Chandra, P.N. & Milind, K. (2001) Lapses in measures recommended for preventing hospital-acquired infection. *J Hosp Infect*, **47**(3), 218–22.

Coello, R. *et al.* (2005) Adverse impact of surgical site infections in English hospitals. *J Hosp Infect*, **60**(2), 93–103.

Cork, R.C. *et al.* (1995) Leak rate of latex gloves after tearing adhesive tape. *Am J Anesthesiol*, **22**(3), 133–7.

Cosker, T. *et al.* (2005) Choice of dressing has a major impact on blistering and healing outcomes in orthopaedic patients. *Wound Care*, **14**(1), 27–9.

Crow, S. (1994) Asepsis: a prophylactic technique. *Semin Perioper Nurs*, **3**(2), 93–100.

Crowe, M.J. & Cooke, E.M. (1998) Review of case definition for nosocomial infection – towards a consensus. Presentation by nosocomial infection surveillance unit to hospital infection liaison group, subcommittee of Federation of Infection Societies. *J Hosp Infect*, **39**(1), 3–11.

Cunningham, J.B., Kernohan, W.G. & Sowney, R. (2005) Bed occupancy and turnover interval as determinant factors in MRSA infections in acute settings in Northern Ireland: 1 April 2001 to 31 March 2003. *J Hosp Infect*, **61**(3), 189–93.

David, J. (1991) Letters. *Wound Manage*, **1**(2), 15.

Dawson, S.J. (2003) The role of the infection control link nurse. *J Hosp Infect*, **54**(4), 251–7.

DH (1995) *Hospital Infection Control: Guidance on the Control of Infection in Hospitals.* Department of Health, London.

DH (1998) *Prevention and Control of Tuberculosis in the United Kingdom* (HSC 1998/196). Department of Health, London.

DH (2001a) Standard principles for preventing hospital-acquired infection. *J Hosp Infect*, **47**(Suppl), S21–37.

DH (2001b) Guidelines for preventing infections associated with the insertion and maintenance of central venous catheters. *J Hosp Infect*, **47**(Suppl), S49–67.

DH (2002) *Control of Substances Hazardous to Health Regulations.* COSSH, Department of Health, London.

DH (2003) *Winning Ways.* Department of Health, London.

DH (2005) *Hazardous Waste (England) Regulations.* Department of Health, London.

DH (2006a) *Health Technical Memorandum 07-01: Safe management of healthcare waste.* Department of Health, London.

DH (2006b) *Saving Lives: A Delivery Programme to Reduce Healthcare Associated Infection including MRSA.* Department of Health, London.

Dietze, B. *et al.* (2001) Survival of MRSA on sterile goods packaging. *J Hosp Infect*, **49**(4), 255–61.

Ferguson, K.J. *et al.* (2004) Critical incidents of nonadherence with standard precautions guidelines among community hospital-based health care workers. *J Gen Intern Med*, **19**(7), 808–9.

Ford, D.A. & Koehler, S.H. (2001) A creative process for reinforcing aseptic technique practices. *AORN J*, **73**(2), 446–50.

Galway, R. *et al.* (2003) Central venous access and handwashing: variability in policies and practice. *Paediatr Nurs*, **15**(10), 14–18.

Garrouste-Orgeas, M. *et al.* (2000) A one-year prospective study of nosocomial bacteraemia in ICU and non-ICU patients and its impact on patients' outcome. *J Hosp Infect*, **44**(3), 206–13.

Girou, E., Chai, S.H. & Oppein, F. (2004) Misuse of gloves: the foundation for poor compliance with hand hygiene and potential for microbial transmission. *J Hosp Infect*, **57**(2), 162–9.

Glauser, M.P. & Calandra, T. (2000) Infections in patients with hematologic malignancies. In: *Management of Infections in Immunocompromised Patients*, Part II (Section 4) (eds M.P. Glauser & P.A. Pizzo). W.B. Saunders, London, pp. 141–88.

Gordts, B. (2005) Models for the organisation of hospital infection control and prevention programmes. *Clin Microbiol Infect*, Suppl **1**, 19–23.

Gould, D. (2000) Innovations in hand hygiene: manual from SSL International. *Br J Nurs*, **9**(20), 2175–80.

Gould, D. & Chamberlain, A. (1994) Gram-negative bacteria. The challenge of preventing cross-infection in hospital wards: a review of the literature. *J Clin Nurs*, **3**(6), 339–45.

Griffith, C.J. *et al.* (2003) Environmental surface cleanliness and the potential for contamination during handwashing. *Am J Infect Control*, **31**(2), 93–6.

Griffiths, R.D., Fernandez R.S. & Ussia, C.A. (2001) Is tap water a safe alternative to normal saline for wound irrigation in the community setting. *J Wound Care*, **10**(10), 407–11.

Grinbaums, R.S., de Mendonca, J.S. & Cardo, D.M. (1995) An outbreak of handscrubbing-related surgical site infections in vascular surgical procedures. *Infect Control Hosp Epidemiol*, **16**(4), 198–202.

Haigh, C. (1993) A study of micro-organism levels on nurses' footwear. *Br J Nurs*, **2**(22), 1109–12.

Haley, R.W. *et al.* (1985a) The efficiency of infection surveillance and control programmes in preventing nosocomial infections in US hospitals. *Am J Epidemiol*, **121**, 182–205.

Hallett, C.E. (2000) Infection control in wound care: a study of fatalism in community nursing. *J Clin Nurs*, **9**(1), 103–9.

Hambraeus, A. (1973) Transfer of *Staphylococcus aureus* via nurses' uniform. *J Hyg*, **71**, 799–814.

Hampton, S. (2002) The appropriate use of gloves to reduce allergies and infection. *Br J Nur*, **11**(17), 1120–4.

Harris, A.D. *et al.* (2000) A survey on handwashing practices and opinions of health care workers. *J Hosp Infect*, **45**(4), 318–21.

Harrison, W.A. *et al.* (2003) Techniques to determine contamination exposure routes and the economic efficiency of folded paper-towel dispensing. *Am J Infect Control*, **31**(2), 104–8.

Heal, C. *et al.* (2006) Can sutures get wet? Prospective randomised controlled trial of wound management in general practice. *BMJ*, **332**(7549), 1053–4.

HSE (1992) *Personal Protective Equipment at Work Regulations*. Department of Health, London.

HSE (1995) *Reporting of Injuries, Diseases and Dangerous Occurrences Regulations (RIDDOR)*. Department of Health, London.

Infection Control Standards Working Party (1993) *Standards in Infection Control in Hospitals*. HMSO, London.

Kalantar-Hormozi, A.J. & Davami, B. (2005) No need for preoperative antiseptics in elective outpatients plastic surgical operations: a prospective study. *Plast Reconstr Surg*, **116**(2), 529–31.

Kelsall, N.K.R. *et al.* (2006) Should finger rings be removed prior to scrubbing for theatre? *J Hosp Infect*, **62**(4), 450–2.

Kocent, H. *et al.* (2002) Washing of gloved hands in antiseptic solution prior to central line insertion reduces contamination. *Anaesth Intensive Care*, **30** (3), 338–40.

Kuuppelomaki, M. & Tuomi, J. (2005) Finnish nurses' attitudes towards nursing research and related factors. *Int J Nurs Stud*, **42**(2), 187–96.

Larwood, K.A., Anstey, C.M. & Dunn, S.V. (2000) Managing central venous catheters: a prospective randomised trial of two methods. *Aust Crit Care*, **13**(2), 44–50.

Lawrence J. & May D. (2003) *Infection Control in the Community*. Churchill Livingstone, Edinburgh.

Lipp, A. & Edwards, P. (2005) Disposable surgical face masks: a systematic review. *Can Oper Room Nurs J*, **23**(3), 20–1.

Lobo, R.D. *et al.* (2005) Impact of an educational program and policy changes on decreasing catheter-associated bloodstream infections in a medical intensive care unit in Brazil. *Am J Infect Control*, **33**(2), 83–7.

Mangram, A.J. *et al.* (1999) Guideline for prevention of surgical site infection, 1999. Centers for Disease Control and Prevention [CDC] Hospital Infection Practices Advisory Committee. *Am J Infect Control*, **27**(2), 97–132.

Masterson, R.G. & Teare, E.L. (2001) Clinical governance and infection control in the United Kingdom. *J Hosp Infect*, **47**(1), 25–31.

McArdle, F.I. *et al.* (2006) How much time is needed for hand hygiene in intensive care? A prospective trained observer study of rates of contact between healthcare workers and intensive care patients. *J Hosp Infect*, **62**(3), 304–10.

Medical Devices Agency (1996) *Latex Sensitivities in Health Care Setting (Use of Latex Gloves)*. MDA DB 9601. Medical Devices Agency, London.

Medical Devices Agency (2000) *Equipped to Care. The Safe Use of Medical Devices in the 21st Century*. Medical Devices Agency, London.

MHRA (2005) *Safeguarding Public Health. Guidance for Manufacturers on Clinical Investigations to be Carried out in the UK*. Medicines and Healthcare Products Regulatory Agency. Department of Health, London.

MHRA (2006) *The CE Mark*. Bulletin No 2. Medicines and Healthcare Products Regulatory Agency. Department of Health, London.

MHRA (2002) Devices labeled single use only. *One Liners*, **19**. Department of Health, London.

Michalopoulos, A. & Sparos, L. (2003) Post-operative wound infections. *Nurs Stand*, **17**(44), 53–6, 58, 60.

Mims, C. *et al.* (2004) Infection of the skin, soft tissue, muscle and associated systems. In: *Medical Microbiology Updated*, Vol. 4(26), 3rd edn, pp. 350–77. Mosby, Edinburgh.

Munch, T.N. *et al.* (2005). The association between anaemia and fatigue in patients with advanced cancer receiving palliative care. *J Palliat Med*, **8**(6), 1144–9.

Naylor, W. *et al.* (2001) *The Royal Marsden Hospital Handbook of Wound Management in Cancer Care*. Blackwell Science, Oxford.

NHSE (1999) *Latex Medical Gloves and Powdered Latex Medical Gloves*. Department of Health, London.

NHSE (2000) *Decontamination of Medical Devices*. Department of Health, London.

NHSE (2001) *National Standards of Cleanliness for the NHS*. Department of Health, London.

NHSE (2002) *Infection Control in the Built Environment*. Department of Health, London.

NICE (2006) *Tuberculosis*. National Institute for Health and Clinical Excellence, London.

NMC (2006) *A–Z Advice Sheet Consent*. www.nmc.org.

North Thames Audit and Clinical Effectiveness in Occupational Health (2000) *Report on Latex Gloves Policies and Procedures*. Royal Free Hampstead Centre, London.

Oie, S., Hosokawa, I. & Kamiya, A. (2002) Contamination of room handles by Methicillin-sensitive/Methicillin-resistant *Staphylococcus aureus*. *J Hosp Infect*, **51**(2), 140–3.

Oldman, P. (1991) A sticky situation – microbiological study of adhesive tape used to secure IV cannulae. *Prof Nurse*, **6**(5), 265–9.

Pereira, L.J., Lee, G.M. & Wade, K.J. (1997) An evaluation of five protocols for surgical handwashing in relation to skin condition and microbial counts. *J Hosp Infect*, **36**, 49–65.

Perry, C., Marshall, R. & Jones, E. (2001) Bacterial contamination of uniforms. *J Hosp Infect*, **48**(3), 238–41.

Pittet, M.W. (2003) Hand hygiene: improve standards and practice for hospital care. *Curr Opinion Infect Dis*, **16**(4), 327–35.

Porteous, J. (2002) Artificial nails: very real risk. *Can Oper Room Nurs*, **20**(3), 16–17, 20–1.

Pratt, R.J. *et al.* (2007) Epic 2 national evidence-based guidelines for preventing healthcare-associated infection in NHS hospitals in England. *J Hosp Infect*, **65**(Suppl 1), S2–12.

Preston, R.M. (2005) Aseptic technique: evidence-based approach for patients' safety. *Br J Nurs*, **14**(10), 540–2, 544–6.

Reilly, J. (2002) Changing surgical practice through feedback of performance data. *J Adv Nurs*, **38**(6), 607–14.

Roberts, C. (2000) Universal precautions: improving knowledge of trained nurses. *Br J Nurs*, **9**(1), 43–7.

Rohr, U. *et al.* (2003) Methicillin-resistant *Staphylococcus aureus* whole body decolonization among hospitalized patients with variable site colonization by using mupirocin in combination with octenidine dihydrochloride. *J Hosp Infect*, **54**(4), 305–9.

Rosenthal, V.D. & Maki, D.G. (2004) Prospective study of the impact of open and closed infusion stems on rates of central venous catheter-associated bacteraemia. *Am J Infect Control*, **32**(3), 135–41.

Rossoff, L.J. *et al.* (1993) Is the use of boxed gloves in an intensive care unit safe? *Am J Med*, **94**(6), 602–7.

Ryan, A.J. *et al.* (2006) A national survey of infection control practices by New Zealand anaesthetists. *Anaesth Intensive Care*, **34**(1), 68–74.

Scheckler, W.E. *et al.* (1998) Requirements for infrastructure and essential activities of infection control and epidemiology in hospitals: a consensus panel report. Society for Healthcare Epidemiology of America. *Infect Control Hosp Epidemiol*, **19**(2), 114–24.

Segers, P. *et al.* (2005) Risk control of surgical site infection after cardiothoracic surgery. *J Hosp Infect*, **62**(4), 437–45.

Shiomori, T. *et al.* (2002) Evaluation of bed making-related airborne and surface Methicillin resistant *Staphylococcus aureus* contamination. *J Hosp Infect*, **50**(1), 30–5.

St. Clair, K. & Larrabee, J.H. (2002) Clean versus sterile gloves; which to use for postoperative dressing changes? *Outcomes Manag*, **6**(1), 17–21.

Stein, A.D., Makarawo, T.P. & Ahmad, M.F.R. (2003) A survey of doctors' and nurses' knowledge, attitude and compliance with infection control guidelines in Birmingham teaching hospitals. *J Hosp Infect*, **54**(1), 68–73.

Stephan, F. *et al.* (2006) Reduction of urinary tract infection and antibiotic use after surgery: a controlled, prospective, before–after intervention study. *Clin Infect Dis*, **42**(11), 1544–51.

Subbannayya, K. *et al.* (2006) Can soap act as fomites in hospitals? *J Hosp Infect*, **62**(2), 244–5.

Taylor, J.H. *et al.* (2000) A microbiological evaluation of warm air hand driers with respect to hand hygiene and the washroom environment. *J Appl Microbiol*, **89**(6), 910–19.

Taylor, K., Plowman, R. & Roberts, J.A. (2001) *The Challenge of Hospital Acquired Infection*. National Audit Office, London.

Taylor, L. (1978) An evaluation of handwashing techniques 1. *Nurs Times*, **74**(2), 54–5.

van der Meer, J.W.M. & Kuijpers, T.W. (2000) Infections in patients with primary (congenital) immunodeficiences. In: *Management of Infections in Immmunocompromised Patients*, Part II (Section 1) (eds M.P. Glauser & P.A. Pizzo). W.B. Saunders, London, pp. 47–78.

Van Grafhorst, J.P. *et al.* (2002) Unexpected high risk of contamination with Staphylo-cocci species attributable to standard preparation of syringes for continuous intravenous drug administration in a simulation model in intensive care units. *Crit Care Med*, **30**(4), 833–6.

Ward, V. *et al.* (1997) *Preventing hospital acquired infection. Clinical guidelines*. Public Health Laboratory Service, London.

Webster, J. & Osborne, S. (2006) Preoperative bathing or showering with skin antiseptics to prevent surgical site infection. *Cochrane Database Syst Rev*, **19**(2), CD004985.

Whitby, M., McLaws, M.L. & Ross, M. (2006) Why healthcare workers don't wash their hands: a behavioral explanation. *Infect Control Hosp Epidemiol*, **27**(5), 484–92.

Whitehouse, J.D. *et al.* (2002) The impact of surgical-site infections following orthopaedic surgery at a community hospital and a university hospital: adverse quality of life, excess length of stay and extra cost. *Infect Control Hosp Epidemiol*, **23**(4), 183–9.

Wilcox, A. (2005) Preventing healthcare-associated infection in primary care. *Primary Health Care*, **15**(8), 43–50.

Wilkes, C.R., Mason, A.D. & Hern, S.C. (2005) Probability distribution for showering and bathing water-use behavior for various US subpopulations. *Risk Anal*, **25**(2), 317–37.

Wilson, J. (2006) *Infection Control in Clinical Practice*, 3rd edn. Bailliere Tindall, London.

Winnefeld, M. *et al.* (2000) Skin tolerance and effectiveness of two hand decontamination procedures in everyday hospital use. *Br J Dermatol*, **14**(393), 546–50.

Wright, L., Spickett, G. & Stoker, S. (2001) Latex allergy awareness among hospital staff. *Nurs Times*, **97**(38), 49–52.

Yamamoto, Y., Ugai, K. & Takahashi, Y. (2005) Efficiency of hand drying for removing bacteria from washed hands: comparison of paper towel drying with warm air drying. *Infect Control Hosp Epidemiol*, **26**(3), 316–20.

Multiple choice questions

1 Which is the commonest type of hospital acquired infection?

    a   Urinary
    b   Lung
    c   Wound
    d   Blood

2 Studies suggest that up to 89% of staff miss some or part of their hands when hand washing. What are the most commonly missed sites?

    a   Palms and wrists
    b   Backs of hands
    c   Backs of thumbs and fingertips
    d   Index fingers

3 All waste contaminated with blood, body fluids, excretions and secretions should be disposed of in what colour waste bags?

    a   Red
    b   Black
    c   Clear
    d   Yellow

4 In order to ensure a clean work surface to perform aseptic technique, trolleys should be cleaned with what percentage of chlorhexidine?

    a   50% in spirit
    b   100% in spirit
    c   35% in spirit
    d   70% in spirit

Answers to the multiple choice questions can be found in Appendix 3.

Chapter 5

Barrier nursing: nursing the infectious or immunosuppressed patient

Barrier nursing

Definition

Barrier nursing is the use of infection control practices aimed at controlling the spread of, and eradicating, pathogenic organisms (Garner 1996a, b). These practices may require the setting up of mechanical barriers to contain pathogenic organisms within a specified area.

Indications

Barrier nursing includes:

- Source isolation to segregate infected patients in single rooms to prevent the spread of infection.
- Cohort source isolation to segregate a number of patients with the same infection in one ward when there are inadequate number of single rooms, to prevent the spread of infection (NHS Estates 2002).
- Protective isolation (reverse barrier nursing) to segregate immunosuppressed patients (individuals with impaired immunity due to disease or treatment) to protect them from acquiring an exogenous infection.
- Strict source isolation to segregate patients infected with a serious contagious disease, e.g. viral haemorrhagic fever, in isolation units to prevent the spread of infection (DH 1998a).

Reference material

It is estimated that health care-associated infection (HCAI) affects one in 10 NHS patients each year, and costs the National Health Service (NHS) one billion pounds annually (DH 2003a). This means there are at least 100 000 infections a year, which results in about 5000 deaths where infection is the primary cause of death and a further 15 000 where infection is a substantial contributory factor in the death (DH 2002a). The indiscriminate and inappropriate use of antibiotics to treat infection promotes the emergence of antibiotic resistant micro-organisms (DH 2003a). Infection with a resistant micro-organism increases the risk of death from infection (Coia *et al.* 2006).

The main sites of infection are:

- Urinary (23%) (80% of these are related to urinary catheterization).
- Lung (22%) (with pneumonia occurring most frequently among patients who had been ventilated).
- Wound (9%).
- Blood (6%) (60% of blood infections were related to intravenous feeding devices, urinary catheters or similar devices (DH 2003a). In one matched cohort study of adult patients being cared for in intensive care units, it was found that blood stream infections increased the risk of death (42% with blood stream infection dying compared with 26% who did not; Laupland *et al.* 2006).

Those patients with a more serious illness, such as cancer, are particularly vulnerable and susceptible to infection (DH 2003a). Neutropenic patients with haematological malignancies are at increased risk of infectious morbidity and mortality. One USA study found a 6.8% inpatient mortality rate for neutropenia hospitalization (Caggiano *et al.* 2005), whilst another more recent study put the rate at 9.5% (Kuderer *et al.* 2006). A further prospective surveillance study of hematology–oncology patients found that the incidence of HCAI in neutropenic patients is significantly higher (up to 25.3%) than in immune-competent patients, with length of neutropenia a marker for risk of infection (Engelhart *et al.* 2002). The incidence of infection is directly related to the neutrophil count, with the probability that 25% of patients with a neutrophil count less than $100/mm^3$ for 1 week will develop an infection. Bloodstream infections are the most common type of infection (Glauser & Calandra 2000).

The risk of infection also depends on the patient's ability to respond to infection, rather than the number of neutrophils in the peripheral blood (Dale & Liles 1998). A careful patient medical history and physical examination provides an initial risk assessment of the patient's susceptibility to infection.

Risk assessment includes establishing the known or suspected risk, establishing what preventative measures are already in place and then producing an action plan, which should include specific precautions for the patient (HSE 2003a). Using this approach, inappropriate and unnecessary precautions are not adopted (Garner 1996a, b). An oncology centre in the USA has developed a risk assessment complication tool using risk factors from published studies and national guidelines. A retrospective survey of records found that the tool was effective in helping to determine which patients were at high risk of developing an infection (Donohue 2006).

Most precautions against transferring infection demand more effort, take more time and cost more when neutropenic patients are cared for, than the comparable procedures in normal circumstances. However, the cost of an outbreak of infection can be far more (Wilcox & Dane 2000).

For the infected patient the consequences can be considerable and may include:

- Delayed or prevented recovery.
- Increased pain, discomfort and anxiety.
- Extended hospitalization, which has implications for the patient, the family and the hospital:
  - If isolated the patient may receive less care (Evans *et al.* 2003).
  - Psychological stress as a result of loneliness and boredom from periods spent in isolation (Maunder *et al.* 2003). A study of the psychological and occupational impact of a severe acute respiratory syndrome (SARS) outbreak, found that isolated patients reported fear, loneliness, boredom, anger and worries about the risk to family and friends. Staff, however, were affected by fear of contagion and of infecting their family, friends and work colleagues (Maunder *et al.* 2003).

Sources of infection

Self-infection (endogenous infection)

Self-infection results when tissues become infected from other sites in the patient's body. The normal microbial flora of the human body consists largely of the organisms in the alimentary tract, upper respiratory tract, female genital tract and on the skin. This flora may include versatile pathogens (e.g. *Staphylococcus aureus*) that may cause disease in almost any tissue, as well as others (e.g. *Micrococcus* species and diphtheroids), which are usually of very low pathogenicity and rarely cause infection. Many organisms exist with capabilities between these extremes. Many infections acquired by immunosuppressed patients are caused by the patient's own microbial flora (Glauser & Calandra 2000). For example, septicaemia in neutropenic patients is often due to translocation of micro-organisms from the gut (Paulus *et al.* 2005).

Cross-infection (exogenous infection)

Cross-infection may be caused by infection from patients, hospital staff or visitors who are suffering from the relevant disease (cases) or who are symptomless carriers. Food and the environment may also be factors in cross-infection (Ayliffe *et al*. 2000). For example, blood stream infections in neutropenic patients can be due to contamination of a central venous catheter by micro-organisms not carried by the patient but acquired exogenously from the environment, other patients or staff (Paulus *et al*. 2005).

Transmission of infection is directly related to the environment and management, with insufficient working space, overcrowding of patients and understaffing predisposing to cross-infection (NHS Estates 2002).

Routes and reservoirs of infection

A reservoir of infection is anywhere where organisms can survive and multiply. For infection to occur there has to be a route of transmission between the reservoir and the susceptible host (Ayliffe *et al*. 2000).

The health care environment is a secondary reservoir for organisms with the potential for infecting patients. It is essential that all plans for new or renovated health care buildings are designed to ensure that HAI is reduced (NHS Estates 2002). Routes of spread include the following.

Direct contact

Organisms can be transmitted directly to susceptible people by the hands of health care workers and by contaminated equipment. Therefore it is essential that all equipment is cleaned following each and every episode of use (MDA 2002). Hand washing has been shown to reduce the spread of infection, so hands must be washed before and after every patient contact and contact with contaminated equipment (DH 2001a). However, studies of hand washing by nurses and others have shown that this procedure is generally not carried out efficiently (Creedon 2005), although compliance does seem to improve during dirty high-risk situations (Kuzu *et al*. 2005). Teaching interventions, belief in the benefits of the activity, peer pressure of senior physicians, administrators' role modelling (Whitby *et al*. 2006) and feedback on performance (Kuzu *et al*. 2005) may all improve compliance with hand-washing requirements. Patient education programmes that enable the patient to ask the health care workers providing direct care to them, 'Did you wash your hands?' have also been seen to increase compliance with hand washing (McGuckin *et al*. 2004).

Hand washing with soap removes transient micro-organisms, whilst the use of bactericidal soap removes both transient and resident skin micro-organisms

(DH 2001a). In clinical areas washing in running water is essential. Basins should be deep enough to contain any splashing water and should be plugless. Taps should not be operated by hand but by remote control, elbow, knee or foot, as appropriate (Chapter 4).

A quick, convenient and effective disinfectant for clean hands, without the use of soap and water, is an alcoholic handrub, which can remove organisms and reduce nosocomial infections (Johnson *et al.* 2005). This handrub is less drying to hands (Creedon 2005) and well liked if introduced following educational initiatives. Alcoholic handrubs are not effective on hands that are visibly soiled or potentially contaminated with dirt or organic matter. In such circumstances washing with soap and running water, followed by careful drying with a good-quality paper towel, is required (DH 2001a).

Any item or equipment used near or in a patient area may be a reservoir of micro-organisms. This can range from obvious items such as stethoscopes (Hill *et al.* 2006), commodes (Vardhan *et al.* 2000), children's toys (Fleming & Randle 2006), cot mattresses (Jenkins & Sherburn 2005), fabrics (Neely & Maley 2000) and blood pressure cuffs (Walker *et al.* 2006) to patients' files (Panhotra *et al.* 2005), computer keyboards (Wilson *et al.* 2006) and doctors' ties (Ditchburn 2006). This research emphasizes the importance of cleaning items after patient use.

Airborne

Organisms can be transmitted in dust or skin scales carried by air. This is likely to occur during procedures such as bed making (Sexton *et al.* 2006), when particles may land directly on open wounds or puncture sites. Doors of isolation rooms must be kept closed to minimize airborne spread of micro-organisms (Sexton *et al.* 2006). The hospital ward environment must be visibly clean, free from dust and soilage and acceptable to patients, their visitors and staff. The Secretary for State has stated that: 'Patients rightly expect hospitals to be clean.' The message it gives spreads far beyond infection to say to patients, 'You are in safe hands' (DH 2004a, p. 1). Sites most likely to fail a ward cleaning inspection are the toilets and kitchen (Griffith *et al.* 2000).

Airborne infection may also occur through droplets. Water from nebulizers or humidifiers may be contaminated by *Pseudomonas* species (Ayliffe *et al.* 2000). Fine droplet spray from ventilation cooling towers or showers contaminated with *Legionella pneumophila* correlates with the incidence of nosocomial Legionnaires' disease (Declerck *et al.* 2006).

Positive pressure air conditioning protects immunosuppressed patients by reducing the entry of outside air into the room. Negative pressure air conditioning reduces the amount of air leaving the room therefore keeping pathogenic micro-organisms within the barrier nursing room. When negative pressure air conditioning is being used, for example with a patient with tuberculosis, the air changes should be 12 per hour with the pressure regularly monitored (CDC 2003).

Food borne

Food poisoning occurs when contaminated foods are ingested, with *Campylobacter* species being one of the most common causes (Gillespie *et al.* 2006). *Salmonella* species continues to be a problem and is particularly associated with contaminated eggs (Gillespie *et al.* 2005) and chicken (Meldrum *et al.* 2005), and contamination was linked to cross-contamination and inadequate heat treatment (Gillespie *et al.* 2005). Prevention includes good infection control practices (Maguire *et al.* 2001). New food hygiene legislation (Food Standards Agency 2006) applies to all food businesses in the UK. An internationally recognized and recommended system for food hygiene, called Hazard Analysis Critical Control Points (HACCP), focuses on identifying the critical points in the entire food chain where problems could occur and then putting in steps to prevent the problems occurring (Food Standards Agency 2006). Hand washing, thorough cooking, storage, segregation of cooked and uncooked food, clean environment and equipment are essential. Hot food must be kept hot and cold food must be kept chilled. As some organisms such as *Listeria* can survive in low temperatures (Flessa *et al.* 2005), ideally ward refrigerators should be kept below 5°C. Food products must also be obtained from reputable suppliers (Ejidokun *et al.* 2000) (Table 5.1).

Blood borne

Blood, or bloodstained material, is potentially hazardous, transmitting infection through inoculation accidents, existing breaks in the skin, gross contamination of mucous membranes, sexual activity or, prenatally, from mother to baby (UK Health Department 2002a).

Vector borne (an insect or animal carrier/transmitter of disease)

International movement of people and products is associated with the emergence of infectious diseases (Mangili & Gendreau 2005) by introducing infectious agents into areas in which they had previously been absent (Gezairy 2003). Research on vaccines, environmentally safe insecticides, vector control and training programmes for health care workers can assist in disease control (Gezairy 2003). Although disease transmitted by biting insects is not a major problem in the UK, insects such as cockroaches can carry pathogenic organisms on their bodies and in their digestive tracts. This may infect the hospital environment, which includes food and sterile supplies (Lemos *et al.* 2006). Storage of supplies in dry, clean,

Table 5.1 Temperature required to prevent food infections.

Refrigeration	A food temperature of 8°C or below is effective in controlling the multiplication of most micro-organisms. It is recommended that the temperature of refrigerators holding perishable food, i.e. milk, is at 5°C or below. Ward refrigerators must have their temperature checked and recorded regularly through the day. Any problems in maintaining the low temperature must be reported and repaired immediately. Food in refrigerators at a temperature above 8°C should not be used
Freezers	Freezing food at temperatures below −18°C will prevent micro-organisms multiplying
Cooking	Temperatures of 75°C or above are effective in destroying most bacteria
Hot food holding	Food should be delivered to the patient as soon as it is cooked and served. Temperatures above 63°C will control the multiplication of bacteria in correctly prepared and cooked food
Cooling	Cooked food that is served cold must be cooled as quickly as possible and then refrigerated
Reheating of cooked food	This must only be undertaken by staff with catering/food hygiene qualifications (Food Standards Agency 2006)

123

well-ventilated areas is therefore essential. Statutory requirements related to pest control must also be met (DH 2001a).

Types of barrier nursing

1 Source isolation also termed 'transmission based precautions' (Garner 1996a, b).
2 Protective isolation.

Source isolation is designed to prevent the spread of pathogenic micro-organisms from an infected patient to other patients, hospital personnel and visitors. The need for isolation is determined by the ease with which the disease can be transmitted in hospital and, if it is transmittable, by its severity. As infectious diseases are transmitted by different routes, isolation procedures must, in order to be effective, provide appropriate barriers to the route of transmission. In addition, the procedures imposing these barriers must be adhered to universally by all hospital staff entering the isolation unit. Risk assessment of the patient to evaluate the risk of cross-infection to other patients must be undertaken, to ensure the most appropriate restrictions are implemented (HSE 2003a).

Protective isolation protects the patient from the hospital environment. Protective isolation techniques have also been referred to as reverse barrier nursing and reverse isolation, and include the use of high-efficiency particulate air (HEPA) filters (Cacciari *et al.* 2004; Wilson 2006).

Source isolation

Definition

Source isolation or transmission based precautions is a process of care whereby an infectious patient and any material that has been in contact with them or eliminated by them are isolated from others to prevent the spread of infection. This is achieved by achieving standard precautions for all patients, and adding airborne, droplet or contact precautions depending on the patient's causative organism (Garner 1996a, b).

Indications

The decision to isolate a patient will be influenced by the availability of facilities as well as by the physical condition of the area where the isolation is to take place. In determining the most suitable area, a number of criteria need to be met. Among these are the relative cleanliness of the ward, the standard of domestic services support, the infected patient's causative pathogen, the immune status of the other patients and the anticipated length of the isolation. A review of the effectiveness of different isolation polices and practices in the UK, suggests that a concerted effort that includes isolation of meticillin-resistant *Staphylococcus aureus* (MRSA) -positive patients, can reduce the incidence of MRSA, even when MRSA is endemic (Cooper *et al.* 2003).

Unfortunately facilities for the isolation of infected patients are not always available. The NHS Estates highlights that the NHS rarely provides more than 20% of single rooms in NHS hospitals (NHS Estates 2005). A 12-month prospective observational study of the demand and availability of single rooms carried out in a large UK teaching hospital found that there were 845 patients requiring isolation facilities, of whom 185 (22%) did not have this need met (Wigglesworth & Wilcox 2006).

The NHS Estates suggests that with the increase in antibiotic-resistant bacteria and immunocompromised inpatients, there is an increasing need for en-suite single rooms and negative as well as positive pressure isolation rooms (NHS Estates 2002).

Reference material

Source isolation may be achieved by:

1   Purpose-built infectious disease wards.
    Advantages:
    (a) decreased risk of cross-infection;
    (b) less disruption to general wards;
    (c) nurses often more informed and motivated;
    (d) improved, supervised cleaning;
    (e) improves decolonization of patients with MRSA (Fitzpatrick *et al.* 2000).

    Disadvantages:
    (a) increased costs;
    (b) when full, similar patients have to remain on general wards;
    (c) when there are no infectious patients requiring admission, beds are closed to the admission of patients without a contagious infection;
    (d) inadvisable to admit immunosuppressed patients who would be at significant risk of morbidity and mortality if cross-infection were to occur with virulent infections such as drug-resistant tuberculosis, although this can be prevented by ventilation systems. These are capable of being switched to negative pressure for infected patients and positive pressure for immunosuppressed patients (Cacciari *et al.* 2004);
    (e) problem of staff recruitment;
    (f) staff may not be conversant with patients' underlying clinical conditions (Chattopadhyay 2001);
    (g) isolation on general wards can result in isolated patients being seen less often than non-isolated patients (Evans *et al.* 2003).

2   Negative pressure plastic isolator used for dealing with patients who have highly contagious infections such as Ebola virus infection (Bruce & Brysiewicz 2002).
    Advantages:
    (a) provides a high degree of protection to those in contact with patient;
    (b) said to be comfortable and acceptable to patients (Trexler *et al.* 1977).
    Disadvantages:
    (a) not freely available;
    (b) expensive to obtain and maintain;
    (c) limited experienced health care workers to provide required care.

3   Single rooms on general wards.
    Advantages:
    (a) allows patients to remain on ward, which provides continuity of care;
    (b) will reduce cross-infection (Eveillard *et al.* 2001);
    (c) en-suite single rooms provide greater privacy and are preferred by many patients (NHS Estates 2002);

(d) some patients suggest barrier nursing in a single room allows greater freedom for visitors and from routine (Newton *et al.* 2001).

Disadvantages:

(a) some patients report a negative experience of barrier nursing, with feelings of being 'a leper' (Newton *et al.* 2001);

(b) shortage of suitable single rooms, resulting in patients with known infections being cared for in open wards. Hospitals with 10% of their beds as single rooms often find these inadequate to cope with every infected patient (NHS Estates 2002).

4 Cohort barrier nursing: when a group of patients have the same infection, it may be necessary to cohort barrier nurse these patients in a small bay.

Advantage:

(a) undertaken correctly can successfully control and contain infection (Zafar *et al.* 1998).

Disadvantage:

(a) restrictions on admissions to these beds.

One small case-controlled study found that nursing catheterized patients in single rooms reduced the transmission rate of micro-organisms compared to those catheterized patients in shared rooms, as standard precautions were more likely to be adopted in single rooms (Fryklund *et al.* 1997). This supports the use of single rooms for infected patients as the bed around infected patients can often be contaminated with the infecting organism (Widdowson *et al.* 2002).

Effective source barrier nursing practice is achieved most easily by isolating the patient in a single room with the following:

- An anteroom area for protective clothing.
- Hand-washing facilities.
- Toilet facilities.

However, with good technique, an area in the ward away from especially vulnerable patients can be used. In some instances where cross-infection has occurred it may be more appropriate to cohort nurse these patients together in a small ward with designated staff, so containing the infection to one area, rather than using side rooms on different wards (NHS Estates 2002). Uninfected patients must not be admitted into this area until all the infected patients have been discharged and the area has been thoroughly cleaned.

General principles of source isolation

The main emphasis for successful source isolation nursing procedures is on hand washing and protection of clothes; both have been seen to reduce cross-infection

---

Box 5.1   Standard barrier nursing precautions

Standard precautions include:
- Hospital environment clean, free from dust and soilage.
- Hands must be decontaminated immediately before and after every patient contact.
- Personal protective equipment worn when exposed to blood or body fluids, These include gloves, masks, eye protection, face shield, aprons and gowns.
- Safe use and disposal of waste in particular sharps (DH 2001a).
- Safe handling of used, foul or infected linen.
- All reusable shared equipment cleaned, disinfected or sterilized after each patient use.
- Health care workers fit and free from infection.

(Lucet *et al.* 2005). Several general principles need to be adhered to if effective barrier nursing is to occur. Every effort must be made to ensure that instructions are kept simple and realistic. Regular assessment and evaluation of the situation must take place to ascertain whether barrier nursing continues to remain the most appropriate form of care.

Standard precautions should be adopted for all patients (Box 5.1). When a patient has been found to have an infection that required source isolation, besides using standard precautions, additional precautions should be adopted based on transmission-based precautions. These included: droplet, airborne and contact precautions (Garner 1996a, b) (Box 5.2).

Protective clothing

Uniforms

Microbiological sampling of nurses' uniforms detected *Staphylococcus aureus*, *Clostridium difficile* and vancomycin-resistant enterococci (VRE) on uniforms both before and after wear (Perry *et al.* 2001). This study was supported by a laboratory study that tested the survival of micro-organisms on various hospital fabrics and plastics and found that *Staphylococcus aureus* survived on polyester material for up to 56 days (Neely & Maley 2000). These studies reiterate the need for uniforms to be changed daily and when soiled (Perry *et al.* 2001). Changing and laundry facilities must be provided to all staff (NHS Estates 2002). If health care workers take their uniforms home to wash, the uniforms must be washed, tumbled dry and ironed to ensure the effectiveness of home laundering (Patel 2005).

128

Box 5.2   Routes of transmission of infection and extra precautions used with standard precautions to prevent cross-infection

Airborne transmission

Passage of micro-organisms from a source person through aerosols spread.

Airborne precautions

Designed to reduce the transmission of micro-organisms in droplets and evaporated droplets that remain suspended in the air or dust particles containing infectious agents. Examples: tuberculosis and varicella.

Droplet transmission

Passage of airborne residue of a potentially infectious micro-organism aerosol from which most of the liquid has evaporated.

Droplet precautions

Designed to reduce the risk of transmission of infectious micro-organisms by air. This achieved by the use of masks, aprons and gloves. Examples: influenza, meningococcal meningitis.

Contact transmission

Passage of micro-organisms by direct or indirect contact.

Contact precautions

Designed to reduce the risk of transmission of micro-organisms by direct or indirect contact. This is achieved by wearing gloves and apron. Examples: MRSA, *Clostridium difficile*.

Plastic apron

The wearing of a plastic apron is an accepted part of barrier-nursing technique. Uniforms can become contaminated during close contact with infected patients (DH 2001a). The wearing of an apron can protect the uniform and prevent the spread of micro-organisms from one patient to the next (Callaghan 1998). Disposable plastic aprons are cheap, impermeable to bacteria and water, are easy to put on, protect the probable area of maximum contamination and are preferable to cotton gowns, which provide increased cover but are readily penetrated by moisture and bacteria (Belkin 2002).

Gowns

When there is a risk of extensive splashing of blood and body fluids, secretions and excretions, a full body, fluid-repellent gown should be worn to protect the wearer (DH 2001a), as well as patients, as wearing a gown and gloves has been shown to reduce the transmission of micro-organisms such as VRE (Srinivasan *et al.* 2002). However, another study found that wearing gowns and overshoes routinely did not prevent infection in patients undergoing bone marrow transplantation (BMT), and by eliminating the unnecessary use of gowns and overshoes saved nursing time and hospital resources (Duquette-Petersen *et al.* 1999). Belkin (2002) suggests that staff and visitors should select a gown that is appropriate for the task and degree of exposure anticipated, to prevent contamination of blood and body fluids to the wearer of the gown.

Doctors' white coats

Doctors should also be encouraged to change their white coats regularly as it has been shown that a white coat can easily be contaminated and that the design should be modified in order to facilitate hand washing (Loh *et al.* 2000).

Caps

Although the wearing of disposable head covering while nursing infected patients is still practised, hair that is clean and tidy has not been implicated in cross-infection. Therefore, unless heavy contamination or splashing is present or expected, the wearing of caps is not justified. However, head covering continues to be required in the operating theatre, as its use has been shown to reduce wound infections (Friberg *et al.* 2001).

Masks

Masks are worn to protect the wearer from infection, for example from severe respiratory infection (SARS), which requires a FFP 3 mask (Chia *et al.* 2005), or aerosol-generating procedures, when a PPF 2 mask is generally worn (Aisien & Ujah 2006). Masks are also worn by a person undertaking an aseptic technique to reduce the risk of airborne contamination during the surgical procedure (Friberg *et al.* 2001). A small randomized controlled trial showed a trend towards masks being associated with fewer infections, whilst a larger study found no difference in infection rates between masked and unmasked persons undertaking clean surgery (Lipp & Edwards 2002). Masks suitable to be worn as personal protective equipment (PPE) must meet the European standard EN 149 (2001) that is approved for use in the UK. Masks are graded depending on total inward leakage. FF 1 is the lowest level of protection and FFP 3 is the highest level of protection. If a mask needs to be worn it must be a filter type and fit the face closely (Ayliffe *et al.* 2000). Masks are single-use items and manufacturer's instructions must always be followed (Lipp & Edwards 2005).

Eye protection

Eye protection must be worn to prevent contamination by micro-organisms, blood and body fluids (DH 2001a), for example in the operating theatre (Keogh *et al.* 2001), when barrier nursing (Parker & Goldman 2006) or when a patient is bleeding (Ho *et al.* 2005).

Overshoes

The floors of hospital wards become easily contaminated by large numbers of bacteria (Ayliffe *et al.* 2000). Shoe coverings should be used when contamination of the environment occurs, as part of the Control of Substances Hazardous to Health (COSHH) requirements for PPE (HSE 2002). However, there is no evidence that shoe coverings reduce contamination of clean floors (Santos *et al.* 2005).

Gloves

Gloves reduce hand contamination by transient pathogens (Kac *et al.* 2005). Gloves must conform to *Conformité Européene* (CE) standards, be of acceptable quality and available in all clinical areas (DH 2001a). Gloves should be unpowdered (MDA 1998) and not made of latex (MDA 1996; NHS Executive 1999a), as latex allergies have serious implications for patients and health care workers (Wright *et al.* 2001). A 1-year longitudinal study of operating room personnel reported a significant decrease in natural rubber latex sensitivity after changing to powder-free low-protein gloves (Korniewicz *et al.* 2005).

Boxed, clean non-sterile gloves (termed examination gloves: DH 2005a) are adequate for routine non-invasive nursing care (Rossoff *et al.* 1993). Clean gloves must be worn when handling blood or body fluids, or cleaning (DH 2001a). Gloves must be changed between patients, and hands must be washed with bactericidal soap and water or bactericidal alcohol handrub after removing gloves.

The practice of double gloving is an option that can be adopted during surgical procedures when gloves may become damaged. It is suggested that double gloving can cause loss of tactile sensitivity and increased costs. However, it is a necessary and sensible practice when there is a risk of gloves being damaged during use (Twomey 2003).

Incorrect use of gloves has been found to be common, poor practice exposing patients to the risk of cross-infection (Girou *et al.* 2004). Examination gloves must be worn if there is a risk of exposure to body fluids. Sterile gloves must be worn for surgical aseptic techniques, for example for the insertion of medical devices (DH 2005a). Gloves are single-use items and must not be cleaned and reused for the same or another patient (NICE 2003).

Cleaning

Some bacteria can survive in the environment for long periods of time, for example *Enterococcus faecium* can survive for 60 days (Gastmeier *et al.* 2006). Thorough cleaning of the environment is essential, as dust from floors and surfaces contain organisms that, if transferred to patients, can cause infection (Dancer *et al.* 2006). All furniture must be damp dusted to remove organisms dispersed into the air from bed making. The floor must be vacuum cleaned with a machine fitted with a filter followed by damp mopping with hot, soapy water (the mop head must be laundered daily) and then the washed area must be dried carefully (De Lorenzi *et al.* 2006). Dry dusting or the use of a broom should be forbidden as studies have shown this method of cleaning simply redisperses the organisms into the air (Ayliffe *et al.* 2000). Cleaning equipment must be washed and dried after each use.

Ensuring a clean patient environment is every health care worker's responsibility; included in this objective is ensuring that maintenance of the environment is achieved. The Department of Health's (DH) Matron Charter, an action plan for cleaner hospitals (DH 2004b), has placed the responsibility for ensuring the patient environment is clean and well maintained within the remit of the Moden Matron (Gamble 2005).

Antibacterial surfaces and materials have been developed that will inhibit colonization and growth of micro-organisms. These surfaces may be designed to gradually diffuse agents into the surrounding area that prevent contamination of micro-organisms, or the surface is bonded with the agent that destroys micro-organisms on contact. Silver, for example, has been shown to have disinfectant activity against *Staphylococcus aureus* and *Pseudomonas* (Brady *et al.* 2003). However, the use of these products does not provide a substitute for careful cleaning of the environment and equipment.

Patient hygiene

Essence of care is a patient-focused benchmark for clinical governance. Included in the 10 bench marks is a benchmark for patients' personal and oral hygiene. All patients must be individually assessed to identify advice or care required to maintain and promote personal hygiene. Patients must be provided with hygiene information, education and assistance when required, as well as toiletries for their own personal use (DH 2003a). Maintaining patient hygiene is a fundamental part of nursing care and should not be delegated to unqualified staff (Whiting 1999). It is essential patients wash their hands and they should be encouraged to use alcoholic handrub to improve their compliance with hand washing (Banfield & Kerr 2005).

Patients should be encouraged, and when necessary helped, to shower or bath daily and more frequently, for example, if incontinent. Analysis of showering and bathing showed that age and level of education significantly influenced showering/bathing frequency. This information can be used to establish patient current hygiene practices, to establish where changes need to be made (Wilkes *et al.* 2005). As cancer is known to cause fatigue it is essential that nurses play a key role in identifying and managing unwillingness to maintain personal hygiene for what ever reason (Mock & Olsen 2003).

A study evaluating:

(a) daily soap and water baths;
(b) cleansing with cloths saturated with 2% chlorhexidine gluconate;
(c) cloths without chlorhexidine;

found that the incidence of VRE acquisition was reduced with all three methods but cleansing with chlorhexidine-saturated cloths was a simple and statistically effective strategy to reduce VRE contamination of patients' skin. It has led to a reduction of VRE in the environment and on health care workers' skin (Vernon *et al.* 2006).

It is essential that baths are cleaned and dried between patients with a non-abrasive cleaning agent, ideally incorporating a hypochlorite, as viable organisms can survive in bath scum (Ayliffe *et al.* 2000). If bed bathing is unavoidable, the patient should be supplied with their own bowl, which is washed and dried after use and stored at the bedside to prevent cross-infection.

Waste

Collection, transportation and disposal of hazardous and non-hazardous waste is regulated by the following: Environment Protection Act 1990; The Safe Management of Healthcare Waste 2006 (DH 2006a); The Carriage of Dangerous Goods (Classification, Packaging and Labelling) and Use of Transportable Pressure Receptacles Regulations 2004 (DH 2004d); and The Control of Substances Hazardous to Health Regulations (COSHH) (HSE 2002).

Domestic waste, which includes all waste not contaminated with blood, body fluids and toxic chemicals is disposed of in black polythene bags. From July 2005, Hazardous Waste (England and Wales) Regulations 2005 replaced The Special Waste Regulations 1996. Under the new regulations hazardous and non-hazardous waste must be separated.

Within a source barrier nursing room all waste other than sharps or unused drugs must be put into the appropriate waste bag, sealed securely in the room, labelled with ward, hospital and date and sent for incineration.

Sharps and unused drugs must be placed in disposal boxes (that conform to UN3291 and BS7320) at the point of use. These boxes must not be overfilled. When full, the container must be shut, labelled with ward, hospital and date and sent for incineration. Containers must not be left on the floor in public areas (DH 2001a).

Linen

Infected linen must be placed in a red alginate polythene bag. The bag is tied shut and then placed in a red linen bag to be sent in a safe manner to the laundry for barrier washing. This entails placing the full alginate bag in the washing machine where it dissolves, allowing the hot water to wash and disinfect the linen. In this way staff and the environment are protected from contamination (DH 1995a).

Cutlery and crockery

Crockery and cutlery can become contaminated with pathogenic organisms. Hands must be washed after handling utensils used by patients (NHS Executive 1995).

All crockery should have excess food removed (Stahl Wernersson *et al.* 2004) and must be machine washed in a dishwasher with a final rinse of 80°C for 1 minute to disinfect it (Ayliffe *et al.* 2000). Disposable crockery and cutlery are needed only when gross contamination has occurred or if a dishwasher is not available (Redpath & Farrington 1997).

133

Urine, faeces and vomit

These must be disposed of immediately and carefully to prevent contamination of the environment. This may be by using a bedpan washer or macerator. Gloves must be worn when handling and disposing of urine, faeces and vomit. Hands must be washed following removal of the gloves (DH 2001a).

Notification of infection

If a patient develops signs and symptoms of infection, or if bacteriological analysis identifies an organism that necessitates barrier nursing, swift communication and action are needed to instigate this. Any problems may be discussed with the infection control team.

Informing the patient and visitors

Giving careful explanation to the patient is essential so that they can co-operate fully with the restrictions (Ayliffe *et al.* 2000). This will include the provison of written information (Ward 2000). The nurse should have a full understanding of the epidemiology and transmission of the micro-organism that has necessitated the patient being barrier nursed (Stirling *et al.* 2004) and be sensitive to the psychological implications of being labelled 'infectious' and of being confined in isolation (Gammon 1999). It is important that nurses are aware of strategies for dealing with and preventing the effects of isolation (Madeo 2003).

The emergence of resistant micro-organisms has led to an increase in barrier nursing. A US study (Catalano *et al.* 2003) compared two groups of seriously ill patients, one of which required isolation because of resistant micro-organism infections. This study, using the Hamilton Depression Anxiety Rating Scale, found that the isolated group had significantly higher scores on both anxiety and depression at the time of follow up. A cross-sectional matched controlled UK study found that hospitalized patients with MRSA had higher levels of depression and anxiety symptoms than the MRSA negative group of patients (Tarzi *et al.* 2001). Tarzi and colleagues recommend that further studies are needed to examine the best ways of managing the detrimental effects of barrier nursing (Tarzi *et al.* 2001). Fortunately, many patients in fact preferred a single room, and adapted well to any subsequent loneliness and boredom. A review of the literature of nurses' perceptions of single rooms compared with shared rooms, found that nurses believed that a single room impacts positively on the patient's hospital experience, by increasing privacy, improving the interaction with staff and the patients' families and by reducing noise and anxiety (Chaudhury *et al.* 2006). The patient's visitors must also be told why the barrier nursing restrictions are necessary. Visitors will generally be allowed into the room at the discretion of the infection control team. They must be taught to observe the correct procedures for entering and leaving the room. As children are more susceptible to infection than adults, any visit by a child should be discussed with the infection control team.

Domestic staff

The domestic manager must be informed as soon as barrier nursing is commenced. He or she will then provide the ward domestic with written instructions.

The ward domestic staff must understand clearly why barrier nursing is required and should be instructed on the correct procedure. The nursing staff must check that the ward domestics understand and are following their instructions correctly. If the patient is in a single room, a mop (laundered daily), bucket (washed and dried after use), cleaning fluid and disposable cloths should be used solely for this patient's use. If the patient is in a general ward, special care must be taken with the cleaning so that potentially infectious material is not transferred from the area around the infected patient to other patient areas. The infected patient's area must be cleaned last and separately.

Staff allocation

A minimum number of staff should be involved in caring for an infected patient. The nurse concerned with the infected patient should not also attend to other susceptible patients. If barrier nursing is for an infectious disease such as chickenpox, it is important that only personnel who have already had the disease should attend this patient.

The protection of staff against the risk of infection is one of the main functions of the occupational health department. This department offers an immunization and counselling service.

Procedure guidelines   Isolation of source of infection

Equipment

1 Isolation suite if possible. A single room with en-suite facilities will prevent cross-infection (NHS Estates 2002).
2 All items required to meet the patient's nursing needs during the period of isolation, e.g. instruments to assess vital signs.

3 Protective clothing.
4 Alcoholic handrub.

Procedure

Isolation room preparation

Action	Rationale
1 Place a barrier nursing sign outside the door.	To inform anyone intending to enter the room of the situation (Dhaliwal & McGeer 2005: R 1b).
2 List requirements for personnel before entering and after leaving the isolation area.	To decrease entries to and exits from the room (E).
3 Remove all non-essential furniture. The remaining furniture should be easy to clean and should not conceal or retain dirt or moisture either within or around it.	To minimize the risk of furniture harbouring microbial spores or growth colonies (NHS Estates 2002: C).
4 Stock the hand basin with a suitable bactericidal soap preparation and paper towels for staff use.	Facilities for hand washing within the infected area are essential for effective barrier nursing (NHS Estates 2002: C).
5 Place yellow clinical waste bag in the room on a foot operated stand. The bag must be sealed before it is removed from the room.	For containing contaminated rubbish within the room. Yellow is the recognized colour for clinical waste (DH 2006a: C).
6 Place a container for sharps in the room.	To contain contaminated sharps within the infected area (DH 1996a: C).
7 When the sharps container is two-thirds full it must be firmly shut and sent for incineration.	To minimize the risk of leakage from the sharps container (DH 2006a: C).

Procedure guidelines *(cont.)*

8 Keep the patient's personal property to a minimum. Advise him/her to wear hospital clothing. All belongings taken into the room should be washable, cleanable or disposable.

The patient's belongings may become contaminated and cannot be taken home unless they are washable or cleanable (E).

9 Provide the patient with his/her own thermometer and sphygmomanometer, and all items necessary for attending to personal hygiene.

Equipment used regularly by the patient should be kept within the infected area to prevent the spread of infection (Walker *et al.* 2006: R 1b).

10 Keep dressing solutions, creams and lotions, etc., to a minimum and store them within the room.

All partially used materials must be discarded when barrier nursing ends (sterilization is not possible), therefore unnecessary waste should be avoided (Dietze *et al.* 2001: R 1h)

11 Set up a trolley outside the door to hold plastic aprons and bactericidal alcoholic handrub (this is contraindicated if the trolley causes an obstruction or is a hazard to staff and others).

Staff are more likely to use the equipment if it is readily available (E).

Entering the isolation room
Action

Rationale

1 Collect all equipment needed.

To avoid entering and leaving the infected area unnecessarily.

2 Roll up long sleeves to the elbow.

To allow hand washing to take place (E).

3 Put on a disposable plastic apron.

A plastic apron is inexpensive, quick to put on and protects the front of the uniform, which is the most likely area to come in contact with the patient (DH 2005a: R 1a).

4 Put on a disposable, impermeable gown when heavy contamination is anticipated.

To fully protect clothing from contamination to shoulders, arms and back, as permeable cotton gowns are an ineffective barrier against bacteria, particularly when wet (DH 2005a: R 1a).

5 Put on a disposable well-fitting mask if there is a risk of airborne contamination, i.e.: (a) Meningococcus meningitis. (b) Blood and body fluids. (c) Tuberculosis.	To reduce the risk of inhaling organisms and to comply with safe techniques and practices (DH 2005a: R 1a).
6 Safety glasses, visors and goggles should be put on when it is likely that aerosolized droplets of blood or body fluids are present in the air.	To give protection to the conjunctiva from blood and body fluid splashes (DH 2005a: R 1a).
7 Rinse hands with bactericidal alcoholic handrub.	Hands must be cleaned before and after patient contact to reduce the risk of cross-infection (DH 2005a: R 1a).
8 Put on disposable gloves only if you are intending to deal with blood, excreta or contaminated material.	To reduce the risk of hand contamination (DH 2005a: R 1a).
9 Enter the room, shutting the door behind you.	To reduce the risk of airborne organisms leaving the room (Kao & Yang 2006: R 1b).

137

Attending to the patient in isolation

Action	Rationale
1 *Meals.* Meals only need to be served on disposable crockery and eaten with disposable cutlery if deemed necessary by the infection control team. Disposables and uneaten food should be discarded in the appropriate bag.	Contaminated crockery is a potential disease vector (Ayliffe *et al.* 2000: E).
2 *Non-disposable crockery and cutlery* must be washed in a dishwasher with a hot disinfecting cycle.	Water at 80°C for 1 minute in a dishwasher will disinfect crockery and cutlery (Ayliffe *et al.* 2000: E).
3 *Excreta.* A toilet should be kept solely for the patient's use. If neither this nor disposable items are available, a separate bedpan or urinal and commode should be left in the patient's room. Gloves must be worn by staff when dealing with excreta. Bedpans and urinals should be bagged in the isolation room, emptied and then washed in a bedpan washer.	To minimize the risk of infection being spread from excreta, e.g. via a toilet seat or a bedpan (Hota 2004: R 1a).

Procedure guidelines *(cont.)*

4 *Accidental spills*. Any suspected contaminated fluids must be mopped up immediately and the area cleaned with disinfectant.

Surfaces must be left as dry as possible after cleaning (Ayliffe *et al*. 2000: E) as damp areas encourage microbial growth and increase the risk of spread of infection.

5 *Bathing*. If an en-suite bathroom is not available, an infected patient must be bathed last on the ward. Clean and dry the bath after the previous patient and after the infected patient.

Surfaces must be left as dry as possible after cleaning (Ayliffe *et al*. 2000: E). Leaving the bath dry after disinfection reduces the risk of microbes surviving and infecting others. Bacteria will not easily grow on clean, dry surfaces.

6 *Dressings*. Aseptic technique must be used for changing all dressings. Waste materials and dirty dressings should be discarded in the appropriate yellow clinical waste bag. Used lotions, creams, etc., must be kept in the room and not used for other patients. Sterile packs must be stored safely to protect them from contamination and damage.

Aseptic procedure minimizes the risk of cross-infection. Lotions and creams can become easily contaminated. Micro-organisms can survive on unopened sterile packs (Dietze *et al*. 2001: R 1a).

7 *Linen*. Place infected linen in a red alginate polythene bag, which must be secured tightly before it leaves the room. Just outside the room, place this bag into a red linen bag which must be secured tightly and not used for other patients. These bags should await the laundry collection in a safe area.

Placing infected linen in a red alginate polythene bag confines the organisms and allows staff handling the linen to recognize the potential hazard (DH 1995a: C).

8 *Waste*. Yellow clinical waste bags should be kept in the room for disposal of all the patient's rubbish. The top of the bag should be sealed and labelled with the name of the ward or department before it is removed from the room.

Yellow is the international colour for clinical waste (DH 2006 a: C).

Leaving the isolation room

Action	Rationale
1 If wearing gloves, remove and discard them in the yellow clinical waste bag. Clean hands with bactericidal alcoholic handrub.	To remove pathogenic organisms acquired during contact with patient before removing gown, so preventing contamination of uniform (DH 2005a: R 1a).
2 Remove apron and discard it in the appropriate bag. Clean hands with bactericidal alcoholic handrub.	Hands may be contaminated by a used plastic apron (DH 2005a: R 1a).
3 Reusable gowns must be worn once and then sent to the laundry.	To reduce the risk of cross-infection by contaminated uniforms, as staff find it hard to distinguish the inside/outside of a gown. If the gown is worn inside out, uniforms can be contaminated (E).
4 Leave the room, shutting the door behind you.	To reduce the risk of airborne spread of infection (Kao & Yang 2006: R 1a).
5 Rub hands with a bactericidal alcoholic handrub.	To remove pathogenic organisms acquired from such items as the door handle (Oie *et al*. 2002: R 1a).

Cleaning the isolation room

Action	Rationale
1 Domestic staff must be educated and trained to understand why barrier nursing is required to prevent a health care-acquired infection and should be instructed on the correct procedure when cleaning an isolation room.	To reduce the risk of mistakes and to ensure that barrier nursing is maintained (DH 2001a: R 1b).
2 The area where barrier nursing is being carried out must be cleaned last.	To reduce the risk of the transmission of organisms (Gould 2005: E).
3 Separate cleaning equipment must be kept for this area.	Cleaning equipment can easily become infected. Cross-infection may result from shared cleaning equipment (Wilson 2006: E).
4 Members of the domestic services staff must wear gloves and plastic aprons.	To reduce the risk of cross-infection (DH 2005a: R 1b).

Procedure guidelines *(cont.)*

5 Floor (hard surface). This must be washed daily with a disinfectant as appropriate. All excess water must be removed.

Daily cleaning will keep bacterial count reduced. Organisms, especially Gram-negative bacteria, multiply quickly in the presence of moisture and on equipment (Wilson 2006: E).

6 Cleaning solutions must be freshly diluted and the spray container emptied, cleaned and dried daily.

Cleaning fluid can easily become contaminated (Dharan *et al.* 1999: R 1b).

140

7 After use, the bucket must be cleaned and dried.

Bacteria will not easily survive on clean, dry surfaces (Ayliffe *et al.* 2000: E).

8 Mop heads should be laundered in a hot wash daily.

Mop heads become contaminated easily (Wilson 2006 E).

9 Floor (carpet). The use of carpets in clinical areas must be avoided (DH 2002b). If an infected patient has been admitted into a room with a carpet, a vacuum cleaner should be used which is fitted with an efficient filter. After use the dust bag must be changed and the brush head washed and dried.

Vacuum cleaning reduces the dust, thus reducing organisms (Trakumas *et al.* 2001: R 1b).

10 On discharge, the carpet must be carefully cleaned.

Micro-organisms can easily survive in carpet fibres (Malik *et al.* 2006: R 1b).

11 Furniture and fittings should be damp dusted using a disposable cloth and a detergent solution or a disinfectant if appropriate.

To remove any organisms (Wilson 2006: E).

12 The toilet, shower and bathroom area must be cleaned at least once a day using a non-abrasive hypochlorite powder or cream. A disinfectant will only be required if soiling of the area has occurred.

Non-abrasive powders or creams preserve the integrity of the surfaces. These areas recontaminate rapidly after cleaning and routine chemical disinfection is of little value and should be saved for terminal cleaning following discharge of the patient (Ayliffe *et al.* 2000: E).

Transporting infected patients outside the source isolation area

Action	Rationale
1 Inform the department concerned about the diagnosis.	To allow other departments time to make their own arrangements (E).
2 Arrange for the patient to have the last appointment of the day.	The department concerned, the hospital corridors, lifts, etc., will be less busy and will allow more time for special cleaning and disinfecting (E).
3 Any porters involved must be instructed carefully. The trolley or chair should be cleaned after use.	Protection and reassurance of porters are necessary to allay fear and to minimize the risk of the infection being spread to them (Ayliffe *et al.* 2000: E).
4 It may be necessary for the nurse to escort the patient.	To ensure the necessary precautions are maintained (E).
5 In some circumstances, for example meningococcus meningitis and tuberculosis, the patient should wear a mask when leaving the room.	To prevent airborne cross-infection (E).

Discharging the patient from isolation

Action	Rationale
1 Inform the infection control team when the patient is due for discharge.	The infection control team may need to provide advice on any special precautions (E).
2 The room should be stripped. All textiles must be changed and curtains sent to the laundry.	Curtains readily become colonized with bacteria (Patel 2005: E).
3 Impervious surfaces, e.g. lockers, stools and blinds, should be washed with soap and water.	Wiping of surfaces is the most effective way of removing contaminants. Relatively inaccessible places, e.g. ceilings, may be omitted; these are not generally relevant to any infection risk (Wilson 2006: E).
4 The floor must be washed and dried thoroughly.	To remove any organisms present (Ayliffe *et al.* 2000: E).
5 The room can be reused as soon as it has been correctly and thoroughly cleaned.	Most organisms will survive in the environment for long periods of time. Effective cleaning will remove these organisms. Once cleaning has been completed correctly, the room is ready to admit another patient (Samuelsson *et al.* 2003: R 1a).

Antimicrobial-resistant organisms

Definition

The term *antimicrobial resistance* denotes a strain of organism not killed or inhibited by antimicrobial agents to which the species is generally sensitive, leading to an increase in length of hospital stay and severity of illness (DH 2000a).

Reference material

The increase in antimicrobial-resistant organisms is the inevitable consequence of the widespread use of antibiotics (Chen *et al.* 2004). The importance cannot be overemphasized. The increasing resistance of organisms to antibiotics brings the prospect of a return to the pre-antibiotic era (Bissett 2006). The DH (2000a) UK Antimicrobial Resistance Strategy and Action plan aims to minimize the morbidity and mortality due to antibiotic-resistant infections and to maintain the effectiveness of antimicrobials for the treatment and prevention of infection in humans and animals. Key interrelated elements of this strategy include surveillance, prudent antimicrobial use and infection control. The Standing Medical Advisory Committee (1998) points out that micro-organisms are getting ahead in the development of new antibiotics and therapeutic options are narrowing (DH 1998b).

Some new antimicrobial drugs have been developed that are effective against some antimicrobial-resistant micro-organisms (Leuthner *et al.* 2006). Unfortunately the introduction of new antimicrobial drugs into clinical practice eventually leads to the emergence of strains of bacteria resistant to the new drugs (Potoski *et al.* 2006).

Emphasis on antibiotic resistance has shifted from recognition to prevention (DH 2003a). In addition, research has been aimed at improving understanding of resistance and transmissibility of resistant organisms (Coia *et al.* 2006). The widespread and often indiscriminate use of antibiotics for prophylactic and veterinary purposes, as well as the inappropriate selection of these antibiotics, is believed to be an important factor in the development of resistant forms of bacteria (Lefebvre *et al.* 2006).

The transmission of genetic material between bacteria by conjugation has been well documented. Conjugation accounts in part for the rapid spread of resistance, with mutation, transformation and transduction also being involved (Corkill *et al.* 2005; Tenover 2006). The possibility of VRE transferring the vancomycin resistance gene to MRSA is a growing concern. It is also important that the relevant national surveillance network is notified (Health Protection Agency) to ensure that accurate information about the epidemiology and spread of these organisms is gathered (Coia *et al.* 2006).

Patient risk factors for developing an infection with an antimicrobial-resistant organism include: advanced age, underlying disease, severity of illness, interinstitutional transfer of patient, especially from a nursing home, prolonged hospitalization, surgery or transplantation, invasive devices and antibiotic therapy (Safdar & Maki 2002). The consequences of a patient being infected with a resistant form of bacteria are demanding in terms of increased length of stay in hospital, costs of care and treatment (Coia *et al.* 2006). Resistance to antiviral drugs has also been seen (Longerich *et al.* 2005; Jabs *et al.* 2006).

The DH (2003a) states that compliance with infection control measures and restrictive use of antibiotics are the key measures to prevent epidemics of multiresistant bacterial infection. When an outbreak of infection does occur, the control of contamination of the environment can control the outbreak without requiring ward closure (Wilks *et al.* 2006). Infection control includes establishing best practice, education and training, establishing and monitoring standards and organizational support (DH 2000b).

Theoretically any organism can develop antimicrobial resistance. In practice, MRSA, *Staphylococcus epidermidis*, VRE and Gram-negative micro-organisms are of particular concern (Jones 2001).

Gram-negative bacteria

Gram-negative bacteria normally inhabit the gut, but can cause infections in the urinary tract, respiratory tract and wounds. Antimicrobial resistant strains have emerged, which have caused significant mortality and morbidity (Wu *et al.* 2006) and pose a significant risk due to limited treatment options (Navon-Venezia *et al.* 2005). This may be the consequence of excessive use of broad-spectrum antibiotics (Rolston 2005). Important resistant Gram-negative bacteria include *Klebsiella pneumoniae, Escherichia coli, Proteus mirabilis, Pseudomonas aeruginosa, Acinetobacter* and *Stenotrophomonas maltophilia* (Picazo 2005). *Pseudomonas* species, *E. coli* and *Klebsiella* (Babay *et al.* 2005) cause particular problems, being ubiquitous in the hospital environment (Vianelli *et al.* 2006). Resistant strains spread easily in hospitals and communities (Landman *et al.* 2002). Resistance in many Gram-negative bacteria is caused by the β-lactamase production enzyme, which can inactivate antibacterial agents (McGowan 2006). These organisms can multiply in warm, moist conditions and have been identified in eye drops, soap solutions, lotions, tubing used for ventilators and incubators, and the environment (Dancer *et al.* 2002). Risk factors for spread include overcrowded wards, lapses in hygiene and poor infection control practices. Spread is primarily by direct or indirect person-to-person contact (Casolari *et al.* 2005). However, contamination of equipment such as humidifiers and nebulizers has also been implicated in spread (Rae 1998).

Gram-negative bacteraemia is associated with septic shock (Candel *et al.* 2005), which occurs primarily in debilitated, hospitalized patients, who are the group that also develop the resistant form of Gram-negative bacteraemia (Lin *et al.* 2006). The major problem regarding Gram-negative-resistant organisms is that shock progresses before antibiotic sensitivities are known, producing increased clinical manifestations of infection, which can result in death (Blot *et al.* 2005). Therefore, timely initiation of antibiotic therapy is crucial for severe infection.

Prevention of Gram-negative resistant micro-organisms relies on improved antibiotic usage and infection control (Paterson 2006), along with appropriate investigations to allow accurate and speedy diagnosis, so that effective treatment can be achieved (Anderson *et al.* 2006). One measure that has reduced the incidence of *Pseudomonas* infection is the use of filters on water outlets (Trautmann *et al.* 2005).

Gram-positive bacteria

Meticillin-resistant *Staphylococcus aureus* (MRSA)
(coagulase-positive *Staphylococcus aureus*)

Staphylococcus aureus is part of the normal human flora, with large numbers of the organism being found on the skin and mucosa. Colonization or infection by MRSA is therefore more likely to occur in the nose, lesions and sites of abnormal skin, and in indwelling devices such as catheters and tracheostomies (Ayliffe *et al.* 2000). MRSA bacteraemia is associated with an increased risk of death compared with meticillin-sensitive *Staphylococcus aureus* (MSSA) (Gastmeier *et al.* 2005). Soon after the introduction of benzyl penicillin in the 1940s incidences of resistance were seen. With penicillin usage, the prevalence of resistant strains increased. In the 1960s meticillin was introduced and MRSA was soon reported (Jevons 1961). *Staphylococcus aureus* resistance to meticillin results from the expression of cell wall synthesizing enzyme, which has a low affinity for all β-lactams (Fuda *et al.* 2004). In 1981 the first epidemic strains of MRSA (EMRSA) were reported. Since this time MRSA has become endemic in some hospitals, with some senior nurses suggesting it is out of control (Lines 2006). There are increased rates of MRSA in the UK compared to most other European countries. It is difficult to establish reasons for this, but it has been suggested that facilities and resources provided, coupled with senior management support in controlling infection is important (Humphreys 2006). The media has labelled MRSA 'the super bug'. A study to measure MRSA awareness among health care workers, patients and their visitors, found increased levels of awareness amongst all patients, visitors and staff, and concerns about their own safety (Gill *et al.* 2006).

Resistance to other antibiotics have emerged: vancomycin intermediate *Staphylococcus aureus* (VISA); glycopeptide intermediate *Staphylococcus aureus* (GISA);

and vancomycin-resistant *Staphylococcus aureus* (VRSA). Inappropriate or unnecessary use of antibiotics will further increase this resistance (Coia *et al*. 2006). New drugs have been developed that are effective against MRSA (Leuthner *et al*. 2006), but resistance (Potoski *et al*. 2006) and toxicity have already been seen (Bishop *et al*. 2006). The patient with increased resistance may become a reservoir for further dissemination of difficult-to-treat resistant strains of MRSA (Gales *et al*. 2006).

The use of mupirocin nose cream and chlorhexidine baths or showers has been seen to irradicate colonization of MRSA and decrease the incidence of MRSA cross-infection (Sandri *et al*. 2006). However, resistance to mupirocin cream is also occurring (Fawley *et al*. 2006). Other products such as fusidic acid continue to be effective for irradication of MRSA colonization (Nishijima & Kurikawa 2002). Fortunately, disinfectant agents used for hand washing and cleaning remain equally effective against sensitive and resistant antibiotic strains of bacteria if manufacturers' recommendations are followed (Payne *et al*. 1998). Revised guidelines for the control of MRSA in hospitals have been compiled (Coia *et al*. 2006). The guidelines include recommendations that emphasize the need for active and timely interventions in reducing the numbers of patients colonized and infected with MRSA (Coia *et al*. 2006).

While rates of patients colonized with MRSA appear to be greater than those infected with MRSA, these infections are significant due to the difficulties in treating systemic infection and the ability of the organism to spread and colonize debilitated patients. Deaths from MRSA infection have increased (Crowcroft & Catchpole 2002).

Risk factors for MRSA include previous hospitalization, particularly in high-dependency units, presence of intravenous catheters, tracheotomies, wounds and pressure ulcers, underlying disease and recent antibiotics. Colonization with MRSA has been seen to be a risk factor for acquiring a hospital infection (Coia *et al*. 2006). Actively seeking and treating carriers has been seen to lead to a reduction in MRSA (McNeil *et al*. 2002). Screening specimens include nose, throat, axilla, groin and wounds. Delay in initiation of effective therapy has been shown to be a significant morbidity factor (Coia *et al*. 2006).

MRSA infection results in increased workload (Farrington *et al*. 2000) and increased length of stay in hospital with associated costs, in particular intravenous antibiotics. In addition, the detrimental effects on patients, their family and friends, such as pain, anxiety and depression, are a vital consideration. In one study, five patients being barrier nursed due to MRSA infection expressed feelings of loneliness, stigma, monotony and issues of control (Oldman 1998).

Screening

Until recently microbiological testing of specimens for MRSA took 2–3 days. However, rapid polymerase chain reaction (PCR) tests are now available where

145

same day results can be achieved (Davidson *et al.* 2006). This is important as it enables the diagnosis of MRSA more rapidly, which in turn allows appropriate treatment to be started earlier and the risk of MRSA cross-infection reduced.

Active screening of patients for MRSA should be performed. The 2006 MRSA guidelines suggest that certain high-risk patients should be screened routinely. These groups should be determined locally, based on local experience. Generally those included in screening would be frequent readmissions to any health care facility, direct interhospital transfers and persons known to have been infected or colonized with MRSA in the past (Coia *et al.* 2006).

Patients transferred from all hospitals where MRSA infection/colonization is common should be screened on admission, and treated as suspect until the results of screening specimens are known. These restrictions may be minimal, with nursing care involving good hand washing following patient contact. However, if the patient is obviously ill, for example with a discharging wound, then this would necessitate source isolation nursing (see Source isolation section, above). Any patients in contact with infected patients must be screened to detect cross-infection. This would include nose swabs and swabs from skin lesions and urinary and intravenous catheters. If cross-infection occurs, it may be necessary to close a ward to new admissions, particularly to surgical or intensive care patients.

Screening of health care workers is not recommended routinely, but if MRSA cross infection occurs in wards, screening of staff should be considered as health care workers have been seen to acquire and transmit MRSA to patients. MRSA eradication and treatment for health care workers should be the same as for a patient (Coia *et al.* 2006).

In patients known to be colonized with MRSA, signs of infection must be treated as significant, with MRSA considered to be the possible cause. Early investigations, appropriate specimen collection and treatment are essential (see Chapter 28). Relapses may occur, especially in debilitated patients and particularly in sites such as tracheotomies (MacKinnon & Allen 2000). This means that source isolation must be maintained even after three negative cultures have been obtained. The presence of MRSA should be documented in the patient's records in order to alert staff should readmission be necessary (Coia *et al.* 2006).

Transmission

MRSA is mainly spread by hands; therefore, hand hygiene is the most important factor in controlling an outbreak of MRSA (Coia *et al.* 2006). Environmental cleanliness is also important, as MRSA can survive for a long period in the environment. Microbiological sampling of MRSA-positive patients' rooms in a hospital in Ireland found that the mattress, linen and furniture were all positive for MRSA. Increased contamination was found in patients infected with MRSA compared to those colonized with MRSA (Sexton *et al.* 2006). This study emphasized the importance of cleaning and keeping the door of the room closed to prevent the airborne spread of MRSA. Similarly it has been found that there is a correlation between increased rates of MRSA and bed occupancy, particularly with the rapid turnover of patients in acute hospitals (Cunningham *et al.* 2005).

Once patients have been discharged, the ward must be cleaned thoroughly before new patients are admitted (Coia *et al.* 2006). A prospective microbiological study of MRSA contamination of isolation rooms following the discharge of a MRSA-positive patient, found that daily routine cleaning over a 4-week period did not remove MRSA contamination. Inadequate cleaning and therefore the removal of exogenous MRSA predisposes to cross-infection with MRSA (Sexton *et al.* 2006).

147

A 3-year prospective study monitoring MRSA infection and daily workload of nurses, found a correlation between nurses with a very high workload and MRSA cross-infection (Blatnik & Lesnicar 2006). A year-long intensive care study found that segregation of MRSA-positive patients did not prevent the spread of MRSA, but did produce a potential risk to the patient by being segregated (Cepeda *et al.* 2005). Other studies emphasize the importance of hand washing but continue to advocate segregation of MRSA colonized or infected patients (Henderson 2006).

Patients with large wounds, eczema or respiratory tract infection with a productive cough will be heavy dispersers of MRSA and are often responsible for spread. Faulty ventilation systems (Cotterill *et al.* 1996) and crowded conditions have also been implicated in the spread of MRSA (Kibbler *et al.* 1998). Source isolation in a single room with the door closed and limiting the movement of MRSA-positive patients will minimize spread (Coia *et al.* 2006). Studies comparing isolation strategies found that when using single rooms there was a decrease in the risk of cross-infection due to the correct use of PPE on entry, signage and encouraging/reminding of the importance of hand washing (Dhaliwal & McGeer 2005).

When there are large numbers of MRSA-infected/colonized patients, cohort nursing in one ward is an effective means of controlling outbreaks. Other measures include:

- Correctly performed hand washing before and after patient contact. A bactericidal alcoholic handrub can be used when hands are clean.
- High standard of ward cleaning, as inanimate surfaces near affected patients are commonly contaminated with MRSA.
- Careful containment and disposal of waste.
- Careful segregation, containment and laundering of used linen.
- Careful education of the patient and their visitors to ensure compliance to policy, as familial carriage and subsequent infection have been reported.
- Planned cleaning of the ward, including difficult-to-clean areas such as blinds.
- Appropriate investigation and treatment of health care workers. While MRSA rarely causes infection in healthy persons, health care workers can become

colonized with MRSA and go on to transmit MRSA to their patients. Staff screening is indicated if transmission of MRSA continues in spite of control measures being undertaken. Investigation and treatment of health care workers is the responsibility of the occupational health department, with the help of the infection control team.

■ Wearing of masks during some procedures, e.g. suctioning, can reduce the risk of health care workers acquiring MRSA (Coia *et al.* 2006).

In areas where MRSA is endemic a risk assessment may need to be undertaken. The 2006 MRSA guidelines suggest there are some patients at increased risk of MRSA. These include:

1 Frequent readmissions to any health care facility.
2 Direct interhospital transfers.
3 Recent inpatient at hospitals abroad or hospitals in the UK which are known or likely to have high prevalence of MRSA.
4 Residents of residential care facilities where there is known or likely high prevalence of MRSA carriage (Coia *et al.* 2006).

Some patients are at increased risk of serious MRSA infection. These include: HIV-positive persons; patients with eczema, dermatitis, psoriasis; patients in intensive care; neonatal, burns, transplantation, cardiothoracic, orthopaedic, trauma, vascular surgery and renal patients (Coia *et al.* 2006). Attempts to control MRSA require a comprehensive approach to reduce the associated morbidity and mortality (Fairclough 2006).

Community care

Interhospital movement should be restricted to the absolute minimum. If the patient must be transferred to another hospital the receiving hospital must be informed in plenty of time for the necessary arrangements to be made. The ambulance service should be notified if it is being used to transfer an MRSA patient, mainly to prevent another patient being placed in the same vehicle before it is cleaned. Hand washing by the ambulance service staff and cleaning of local areas of patient contact, i.e. chair or stretcher, are all that is required after transport of an affected patient.

People colonized with MRSA do not present a risk to healthy people in the community, and should live their lives without restrictions. However, in care of the elderly wards and residential homes where other residents may have postoperative wounds, strict attention to hand washing, environmental cleanliness and compliance with aseptic technique is important, which generally makes segregation unnecessary (Coia *et al.* 2006).

Staphylococcus epidermidis (coagulase-negative staphylococci)

Staphylococcus epidermidis is part of the body's normal commensal flora (Ziebuhr *et al.* 2006) and an important cause of infection as well as a significant cause of morbidity and mortality (Yang *et al.* 2006). This is particularly problematic in immunosuppressed patients (Falcone *et al.* 2004) or in those with invasive devices such as intravenous catheters, particularly for those patients with cancer who are hospitalized for several days (Knauer *et al.* 2004). Significant levels of resistance are seen, reflecting antibiotic usage (Trueba *et al.* 2006), and are associated with a poor prognosis (Rabaud & Mauuary 2001). Cross-infection may occur, which can become endemic in hospitals (Monsen *et al.* 2005).

Staphylococcus epidermidis can organize into a complex multi-layer of cells covered with polysaccharide, called a biofilm. This biofilm allows the organism to adhere to foreign objects such as catheters and become less susceptible to antibiotics (Rohde *et al.* 2005). Research and technology continue to produce devices such as tracheostomy tubes that will inhibit the formation of biofilms (Jarrett *et al.* 2002).

Streptococcus pneumoniae

There are over 30 species of *Streptococcus pneumoniae*, some of which can cause programme cell death or apoptosis during pneumococcal meningitis and pneumonia (Marriott & Dockrell 2006). Different species have differing pathogenicity (Aricha *et al.* 2004). *Streptococcus pneumoniae* is the major cause of community-acquired pneumonia (File 2006) and can also be the cause of bacteraemia, otitis media, meningitis, peritonitis and sinusitis. Most patients who develop this infection have other risk factors that predispose them to infection, for example malignancy, splenectomy, AIDS, malnutrition, age (very young and elderly) and, in particular, alcohol consumption (de Roux *et al.* 2006).

Streptococcus pneumoniae is carried asymptomatically in the nose and throat of healthy persons and can be easily transmitted by person-to-person spread (Serrano *et al.* 2006).

Resistant *S.pneumoniae* was recognized in the 1960s, but was not seen in the UK until 1976 in a patient with a history of foreign travel (Meers & Matthews 1978). Since this time, resistance to penicillin has been increasing with a marked ability to cause cross-infection (File 2006). The increased incidence of *S.pneumoniae* infection has led to the increased use of vaccine. These vaccines are based on the serotype antigen of the *pneumoniae*; therefore, the serotype of the organism needs to be known to ensure the appropriate vaccine is given. Currently there are multi-valent vaccines available that contain the antibiotic-resistant serotypes (Berg *et al.* 2006).

Vancomycin-resistant enterococci

Vancomycin-resistant enterococci (VRE) are also referred to as glycopeptide-resistant enterococci (GRE) (Cookson *et al.* 2006). Enterococcus species were once considered normal bacterial flora which occasionally acted as opportunistic pathogens. The genus *Enterococcus* includes 21 species with *Enterococcus faecalis* and *faecium* an important cause of nosocomial infection (Cookson *et al.* 2006). The origin of VRE may be due to selection of VRE by the use of vancomycin, or introduced into the hospital by patients already colonized with VRE due to acquisition from animals or via the food chain. VRE infections are associated with greater rates of clinical treatment failures and mortality compared to vancomycin-sensitive enterococci infections (Brown *et al.* 2006a).

VRE infection and colonization are associated with previous vancomycin use and/or broad-spectrum antibiotic therapy, severe underlying disease, immunosuppression, intra-abdominal surgery and prolonged hospitalization, with the risk of acquisition of VRE directly proportional to the length of stay in hospital (McEvoy *et al.* 2006). Most VRE infections are endogenous, with the colonization of the human bowel prolonged often for months, sometimes years (Brown *et al.* 2006a). Cross-infection does occur (Samuelsson *et al.* 2003); however, transmission from patient to patient or by direct contact, particularly by unwashed hands or contamination of equipment or the environment, frequently occurs (Cookson *et al.* 2006). The food chain, especially raw minced meat, is thought to be responsible for the increased incidence of VRE in humans, due to use of the glycopeptide avoparcin as a food additive. However, a large German study of raw minced meat and pork failed to demonstrate a connection between 8% of meat samples positive for VRE and patients' clinical isolates, which were of different resistance patterns (Klein *et al.* 1998). A great cause of concern is the appearance of transferable high-level glycopeptide resistance in enterococci, producing some strains that are now resistant to all available antibiotics. Enterococci readily colonize the bowel, spread rapidly among hospital patients and transfer their antibiotic resistance widely among themselves and other Gram-positive species (French 1998). Patients with diarrhoea or incontinence pose a significant risk of cross-infection to others and should be segregated in a single room with an en-suite toilet (Mayer *et al.* 2003).

Contamination of the environment readily occurs (Wendt *et al.* 1998). Reducing environmental contamination will control spread (Hayden *et al.* 2006). VRE can survive temperatures of 71°C for 10 minutes or 80°C for 3 minutes (Bradley & Fraise 1996); it can survive in 150 parts per million available chlorine for 5 minutes (Kearnes *et al.* 1995) and in the environment for longer than 11 days (Neely & Maley 2000). Inoculation studies found that VRE can survive on stethoscopes and telephones for 30 minutes and on fingertips for 60 minutes (Noskin *et al.* 1995). Thorough cleaning of the environment and equipment both during the patient admission and on discharge of the patients is important in preventing cross-infection of VRE (Martinez *et al.* 2003). Strict attention to hand washing before and after patient contact is essential. Patients must wash their hands after visiting the toilet and before meals. While universal precautions are generally adequate for caring for VRE-positive patients, when patients have diarrhoea or cannot comply with infection control policies barrier nursing is required, particularly if other patients in the area are immunocompromised (Mayer *et al.* 2003).

From September 2003 it became compulsory for all Trusts in England to monitor VRE bacteraemia as part of the Healthcare Associated Infection Development Strategy to combat infectious diseases (Brown *et al.* 2006a).

151

Clostridium difficile

Definition

Clostridium difficile is a slender, Gram-positive anaerobic rod which is spore forming, motile and widely distributed in soil and the intestinal tract of animals (DH 2003a). Approximately 3% of healthly adults are carriers of *C. difficile*. This increases to 7% in residents of long-term care facilities, 14% of hospitalized elderly on acute medical wards and 20% of elderly patients in chronic care wards (DH 2003b). *Clostridium difficile* is capable of surviving in the environment for prolonged periods (Cunha 1998). Bacteria of this type may be a normal component of gut flora and flourish when other gut organisms are eradicated by antibiotics (Mohan *et al.* 2006).

The typing system for *C. difficile* uses a test called ribatyping. Over 100 types have been identified. Type 027 has been identified as producing 16 times more toxin A and 23 times more toxin B and has been implicated in outbreaks associated with severe disease. Type 027, whilst rare in the UK, has been found in isolates obtained from the National Public Health Service for Wales that were tested as part of a research study with specimens from the USA and Canada (Warny *et al.* 2005). Recently multi-drug resistant strains with increased virulence have been found (Sebaihia *et al.* 2006), in particular the strain called Ribotype 1 (Hawkyard & Bignardi 2006) has caused outbreaks of infection in North America and Europe (McDonald *et al.* 2005; Warny *et al.* 2005). Typing of *C. difficile* isolates allows for investigation of outbreaks of infection (DH 2003b).

Reference material

Clostridium difficile causes gastrointestinal infection ranging from symptomless colonization to severe foul smelling diarrhoea, abdominal pain and fever, with toxin-producing strains causing pseudomembranous colitis (Mohan *et al.* 2006). It is now one of the most commonly detected enteric pathogens, an important cause of nosocomial infection in nursing homes and hospitals, and a common cause of mortality and morbidity in hospitalized patients. The incidence and severity has increased in the past several years (Oldfield 2006).

Diarrhoea can be caused by disruption of the normal flora of the gut by antibiotics which allow *C. difficile* to multiply. The colonic mucosa becomes covered with a characteristic fibrinous pseudomembrane. Signs and symptoms can be relatively mild, resolving when antibiotics are discontinued, or more severe, as in cases of pseudomembranous colitis, which may require surgical resection of parts of the colon and is associated with a significant mortality rate (Koss *et al.* 2006).

Since April 2003 NHS Trusts in England are required to report cases of *C. difficile* to their regional Communicable Disease Surveillance Centre as part of CoSurv (a systematic national alert organisms laboratory reporting system) (DH 2003b).

Diagnosis

Diagnosis is based on clinical findings, endoscopy and laboratory evaluation. Clinical findings range from profuse, watery, green, foul smelling or bloody diarrhoea, with cramping abdominal pains, tenderness and high fever, to hypovolaemic shock and overwhelming sepsis. Endoscopy may reveal effects similar to those seen in non-specific colitis, or may show the yellow–white raised plaques which go on to form a membrane on the inflamed intestinal mucosa (DH 2003b).

Laboratory diagnosis

All patients with diarrhoea should have a stool sample sent to microbiology. *Clostridium difficile* is difficult to isolate in ordinary culture because of overgrowth by other organisms. To overcome this, a selective culture medium is used. The presence of *C. difficile* in culture is not by itself an indication of infection, it simply marks the organism's presence. Infection or disease is indicated by the presence of toxins produced by the organism, which can be identified using screening tests such as commercially available neutralized cell cytotoxicity assay or an immunoassay that will detect both toxin A and toxin B (DH 2003b). Pathogenic strains of *C. difficile* produce two protein exotoxins, toxin A (enterotoxin) and toxin B (cytotoxin). *Clostridium difficile* toxin A induces detachment of human epithelial cells from the basement membrane and subsequent death by apoptosis. This process may be asymptomatic or cause mild diarrhoea or it can lead to pseudomembranous colitis (Voth & Ballard 2005). Recurrence is common (DH 2003b).

Treatment

Initial treatment involves discontinuing antibiotics and providing supportive care, which includes hydration to compensate for loss of electrolytes (Wiesen *et al.* 2006) and antidiarrhoeal oral medication (Aslam & Musher 2006). However, significant infection can be treated with antibiotics (DH 2003b). In extreme cases of pseudomembranous colitis, surgery will be required, which may include resectional or diversion procedures (Koss *et al.* 2006), but death can occur even when diagnosis is made early and appropriate therapy is given (Mohan *et al.* 2006).

Studies using probiotics, which are live organisms that improve the microbial balance of the host, are ongoing (Novak & Katz 2006), as well as intravenous immunoglobulin, which has been given for severe refractory or recurrent *C. difficile* diarrhoea after failed conventional treatment (McPherson *et al.* 2006).

153

Transmission

Pseudomembranous colitis develops from overgrowth of *C. difficile* already present in the gut, or from exogenous organisms acquired via person-to-person contact or the faecal–oral route following contamination of the environment or poor hand washing by patients, visitors or health care workers. *Clostridium difficile* leads to increased costs associated with increased length of hospital stay (DH 2003b), and outbreaks in hospital have resulted in deaths (Sunenshine & McDonald 2006). Bignardi (1998) identified nine risk factors that appear to influence the chance of acquiring *C. difficile*; these were increasing age, severity of underlying disease, non-surgical gastrointestinal procedures, presence of nasogastric tube, antiulcer medication, stay in Intensive Care Unit (ITU), duration of hospital stay, duration of antibiotic therapy and administration of multiple antibiotics.

Antibiotic use was shown to be statistically significantly associated with both diarrhoea and carriage of *C. difficile*. Risks include type of antibiotic, route of administration and dose (Dial *et al.* 2004). Accurate identification of risk factors allows for appropriate decisions to be made to reduce risk and thereby reduce incidence. High-risk patients can be monitored closely to facilitate early detection of infection, commencement of treatment and infection control precautions.

Prevention of spread and management of infection

Reservoirs of *C. difficile* have been found, which included carpets, blood pressure cuffs, thermometers, nurses' uniforms (DH 2003b), radiators, curtain rails, commodes, floors and toilets (Verity *et al.* 2001). *Clostridium difficile* spores are capable of being transferred during periods of air disturbances by, for example, air conditioning, open windows and floor buffing (Fawley *et al.* 2005).

Reducing the risk of cross-infection by *C. difficile* relies on the adoption of several factors, which include the restriction of the use of those antibiotics that encourage the growth of *C. difficile*, reducing the duration of antibiotic courses and the length of stay in hospital, careful hand washing, environmental decontamination and isolation of symptomatic patients (DH 2003b). Hands may become contaminated following contact with a patient with *C. difficile* who is incontinent or has diarrhoea, therefore they should be washed with detergent and water, dried carefully and have a final cleanse with alcoholic handrub (Boyce *et al.* 2006). Cross-infection has been seen to be reduced by thorough cleaning of the environment and the use of clean equipment for each patient. Cleaning with a hypochlorite has been seen to reduce the incidence of *C. difficile* (Wilcox *et al.* 2003).

Nursing care

Careful barrier nursing is required for all patients with toxin-producing *C. difficile* or unexplained diarrhoea. Segregation from other patients must continue until signs and symptoms of infection have ceased. Healthy staff and visitors who are not receiving antibiotics are not at risk (Sanderson 1999).

Hepatitis

Hepatitis may be caused by a variety of agents including viruses and certain chemicals, and it may be secondary to other illnesses. Nurses need to be aware of the epidemiology, modes of transmission and prevention of hepatitis (Table 5.2).

Hepatitis A

Definition

Hepatitis A virus (HAV) is an enterically transmitted positive strand RNA virus classified as a hepavirus, a member of the Picornaviridae family (Mims *et al.* 2004). It was first identified 35 years ago, and causes an acute, self-limiting infection of the liver (Martin & Lemon 2006). It can also cause significant infection in vulnerable people, for example pregnant women (Elinav *et al.* 2006).

Reference material

HAV is a small, symmetrical RNA virus (enterovirus type 72). The virus is unusually stable, resisting heat at 60°C for 1 hour, at 25°C for 3 months, indefinite cold storage (5°C), acidic conditions (pH 3) and non-ionic detergents. It can survive

Table 5.2 Types and infection routes of hepatitis viruses.

Subtypes	A	B	C	D	E	F	G
Infection route	Oral–faecal, sexual	Sexual, contact with blood and body fluids	Contact with blood and body fluids; sexual	As hepatitis B	Oral–faecal	As hepatitis B	As hepatitis C
Vaccine	Yes	Yes	No	No/ indirect from hepatitis B vaccine	No	No	No
Natural history	Acute	Acute–chronic	Acute–chronic	Acute–chronic	Acute–chronic	Not clear	Not clear
Long-term prognosis	Recovery	Carrier, cirrhosis, cancer	Carrier, cirrhosis, cancer	Carrier, cirrhosis, cancer	Unknown	Unknown	Unknown

for several months in sewage and the environment (Brundage & Fitzpatrick 2006). One study found HAV in mussels following marinating in an acid marinade with a pH of 3.75 for 4 weeks (Hewitt & Greening 2004). However, HAV can be inactivated after 4 minutes at 70°C, after 5 seconds at 80°C and instantly at 85°C (Battegay *et al.* 1995).

HAV is spread predominantly by the faecal–oral route, which can lead to large outbreaks of infection (Perrett *et al.* 2003). Following infection, the virus enters the bloodstream from unknown sites in the gastrointestinal tract. It can then infect liver cells when passing via the biliary tract to the intestine and into the faeces. Viral replication probably occurs in the jejunum before transmission via the portal vein to the liver. HAV has been associated with the following:

■ Contaminated water, milk and food. Any uncooked food and drink could be responsible for infection. However, particular problems are due to contamination at the time of harvesting and packaging of uncooked frozen foods, which are then thawed and used (Fiore 2004). Large outbreaks of hepatitis A can be due to contamination of uncooked or cooked food, by an infected food handler or infected food source (Koopmans & Duizer 2004).

■ Poor general hygiene and low economic status, contact with children in day care centres and intensive care units. Outbreaks of HAV at school, as well as among health care workers, have been associated with lack of toilet paper, soap and hand towels, and poor hygiene in school toilets (Chodick *et al.* 2006).

- Foreign travel to countries where HAV is endemic (Wasley *et al.* 2006).
- Blood transfusions (Gowland *et al.* 2004).
- Contact with a case of hepatitis A in the home (Sonder *et al.* 2004), during social activities (Sundkvist *et al.* 2000) or in hospital due to breaches in infection control measures (Chodick *et al.* 2006).
- Sexual contact. HAV can be reduced among homosexual men by HAV vaccination (Franco *et al.* 2003).
- Perinatal transmission of hepatitis A is uncommon (Duff 1998).
- Intravenous drug misusers. Needle-sharing practices contribute to the spread of HAV (Wells *et al.* 2006).

Following ingestion of HAV, multiplication occurs as the virus moves through the stomach, small intestine and large intestine. The virus eventually reaches the liver after leaving the alimentary system via the blood. Further replication occurs in the liver before being released into bile (Cuthbert 2001).

Diagnosis of acute HAV infection is usually confirmed serologically, by detecting immunoglobulin M (IgM) antibodies to hepatitis A antigen (HAAg), which appear in serum 2–7 weeks after oral inoculation, and may persist for some time, occasionally for more than a year. Evidence of past infection, and therefore immunity which can persist for life, is obtained by detecting serologically the presence of IgG antibody to HAAg. HAV can be detected by a variety of immunological and molecular techniques (Mims *et al.* 2004).

HAV has an incubation period of 2–7 weeks. HAV usually causes a minor illness in children and young adults, with a few cases being symptomatic. The illness often presents as an upper respiratory infection with the following signs and symptoms: anorexia, malaise, weight loss, pyrexia, diarrhoea, vomiting and jaundice (Mims *et al.* 2004). Complications of HAV can occur, which can lead to fulminant hepatitis (Beyazit *et al.* 2006).

A population based seroprevalence study in England and Wales indicated a low incidence of hepatitis A infection (Morris-Cunnington *et al.* 2004). Control and prevention of HAV rely on provision of good sanitation facilities, clean drinking water and supervision of food handlers. Careful personal hygiene and the use of condoms will limit person-to-person spread (Leung *et al.* 2005). Passive immunization with intramuscular normal pooled immunoglobulin (human normal immunoglobulin [HNIg]) gives protection against clinical hepatitis for about 3 months in most people. Post-exposure prophylaxis is advisable for household contacts during outbreaks of HAV infection (DH 2006b).

Hepatitis A vaccine is available and immunization has been seen to be effective (Brundage & Fitzpatrick 2006). The vaccine should be administered to those travelling in developing countries (Dick 1998), in areas of moderate or high HAV endemicity, particularly where sanitation and food hygiene are poor, but it is not an alternative to preventive behaviours. The DH (2006b) has recommended that sewage workers, military personnel and foreign diplomats should be considered for vaccination. In institutions for the care of the mentally ill, and in children's centres where the children are not toilet trained, vaccination policy should be formulated according to local circumstances (DH 2006b).

A combined hepatitis A and B vaccine is also available, which increases convenience and compliance, and reduces costs whilst providing prolonged dual protection (Van der Wielen *et al.* 2006). HNIg offers short-term protection for up to 4 months and can be given to people who have been in close contact with infected cases and to those travelling to areas where the disease is endemic (DH 2006b; Fiore *et al.* 2006).

HAV infection does not generally require hospital treatment. If admitted, strict barrier nursing in a single room with en-suite toilet would be required. Outbreaks of HVA among health care workers have been attributed to inadequate hand washing and then eating on the ward (Chodick *et al.* 2006).

Procedure guidelines   Hepatitis A: patient care

Hepatitis A: outpatient care

Action	Rationale
1 It is not usually necessary to admit the individual to hospital.	Usually a self-limiting disease (Kyrlagkitsis *et al.* 2002: R 1b; Lewis & Martin 2006: R 1b).
2 Patient education is essential and must include advice on good personal hygiene and careful hand washing.	Limits the spread of the virus. Careful hand washing removes contamination from hands (Banfield & Kerr 2005: R 1b).
3 Separate soap, flannel and towel must be provided.	To minimize the risk of infection being spread via equipment used for hygiene purposes (E).
4 Meticulous cleaning of bath, wash basin and toilet with a cream cleaner and hot water.	To remove contamination (Ayliffe *et al.* 2000: 5).
5 Bath and wash basin must be allowed to dry after use.	Viruses will not live on clean dry surfaces (Weaving 2006: 5).
6 Soiled bed linen and underclothing should be washed.	To remove contamination (DH 1995a: C).

Procedure guidelines *(cont.)*

7 Patient should refrain from intimate kissing and sexual intercourse while symptoms are present.	To reduce risk of cross-infection (Sonder *et al.* 2004: 5).
8 People with hepatitis A should avoid contact with susceptible people, i.e. the very young or old or those with debilitating illness.	To reduce the likelihood of infection (Sonder *et al.* 2004: 5).
9 Crockery and cutlery must be washed and rinsed in hot water.	Heat destroys the virus (Ayliffe *et al.* 2000: C).
10 Close contacts of the infected person should seek medical advice from their general practitioner.	To enable the general practitioner to assess whether the contact person should receive human normal immunoglobulin (HNIg) prophylaxis (DH 2006b: C).

Hepatitis A: inpatient care

Action	Rationale
1 Whenever possible, the patient should have medical or surgical treatment postponed until he/she is symptom free.	Medical and surgical treatment will debilitate the patient further and recovery will be slower (E).
2 Ideally, the patient should be discharged.	Cross-infection is less likely to occur at home (E).
3 A single room with separate toilet should be made available for the patient.	To prevent cross-infection (Chodick *et al.* 2006: 5).
4 Blood, secretions and excreta (particularly faeces) must be disposed of immediately in a heat-disinfecting bedpan washer.	To prevent cross-infection (Ayliffe *et al.* 2000: 5).
5 Careful hand washing after patient contact.	To prevent cross-infection (Chodick *et al.* 2006: 5).

Hepatitis B

Definition

Hepatitis B is a serious infectious disease caused by the hepatitis B virus (HBV), which produces an inflammatory condition of the liver leading to acute and in some cases chronic infection (Mims *et al.* 2004).

Reference material

HBV is a 42 nm double-shelled particle, inside which is a 27 nm inner core particle that contains the viral nucleic acid and represents the intact infectious virion (Mims *et al.* 2004).

HBV infection is a serious global health problem with 2 billion people infected world-wide, with 350 million of these suffering from chronic HBV infection. HBV infection is the 10th leading cause of death world-wide, with 500 000 to 1.2 million deaths per year caused by chronic HBV infection, cirrhosis and hepatocellular carcinoma (Lavanchy 2004). The incidence of HBV in the UK is low. An analysis of routine laboratory surveillance data between 1995–2000 in England and Wales suggests the incidence is 7.4 per 100 000 of the population. Intravenous drug use was the most frequent route of transmission, with numbers due to heterosexual contact transmission remaining stable, and a reduction in the number of cases related to men having sex with men. Whilst transmission during childhood remains rare, it is more frequently reported among South Asians, where their risk factors were medical treatment overseas and heterosexual contact (Hahne *et al.* 2004).

Prevention of HBV includes vaccination, prophylaxis, improved infection control and safer sex practices (Aggarwal & Ranjan 2004).

Epidemiology

HBV may be found in virtually all body secretions and excreta of patients with acute hepatitis B and carriers of the virus. Blood, semen and vaginal fluids are mainly implicated in the transmission of infection, which occurs by:

- Sexual transmission, both vaginal and anal.
- Accidental inoculation of blood following, for example, a sharps injury, or by drug addicts sharing used needles and syringes.
- Contamination of mucous membranes, eye, nose or mouth.
- Contamination of non-intact skin.

- Perinatal route at or about the time of birth.
- Blood transfusion. The estimated frequency of HBV-positive blood donations entering the blood supply during 1996–2003 was 1.66 per million donations (Soldan *et al.* 2005).

HBV infection acquired during infancy and early childhood has a high likelihood of progressing to chronic infection, which can lead to chronic hepatitis, cirrhosis and primary hepatocellular carcinoma. Vaccination would reduce this risk (Hahne *et al.* 2003).

Clinical response

HBV infection is clinically extremely variable, with the incubation period varying from 4 weeks to as long as 6 months.

Symptoms of acute HBV infection include jaundice of skin and eyes, dark urine, fatigue, nausea, vomiting and abdominal pain. Recovery can take several months to a year. Chronic infection can predispose the infected person to develop cirrhosis or cancer of the liver. HBV reactivation can occur in patients following allogeneic BMT (Kempinska *et al.* 2005).

Infectivity

The progress of HBV can be monitored by serological testing. Hepatitis B surface antigen (HBsAg) is detected in the blood approximately 3–4 weeks after exposure, with antibodies to hepatitis B core antigen (HBcAg) developing about 2 weeks after HBsAg occurs. Anti-HBc will eventually be replaced by anti-HBs, the antibody to HBsAg, which marks the end of high infectivity and the development of immunity to subsequent HBV infection. The antigen HBeAg is an internal component of the core of HBs and is an indicator of high infectivity; it will be replaced eventually by anti-HBe, which correlates with loss of viral replication (Mims *et al.* 2004). HBV is capable of surviving outside the body (Thompson *et al.* 2003), but will not multiply in the environment (Weaving 2006).

Diagnosis

Diagnosis is confirmed by a virological blood test with regular monitoring of antigen and antibody status to evaluate progress (Burek 2005). The diagnosis of chronic HBV infection is made using a combination of serological, virological, biochemical and histological markers (Park & Keeffe 2004).

Screening policy for HBsAg

Screening of the entire hospital patient population would be an effective way to identify hepatitis B infection, but this would be costly and time consuming in terms of the benefits derived.

In general, the best compromise is to test those patients belonging to groups in which there is a high prevalence of hepatitis B. These include the following people:

- All new admissions who currently live or were born in countries where there is a high prevalence of hepatitis B.
- Drug addicts.
- Institutionalized people with learning difficulties.
- All patients acutely or recently jaundiced.

HBV is not transmitted by normal daily contact including coughing, sneezing, hugging, holding hands or sharing bathrooms and toilets, cups and crockery with an HBV-positive person (DH 2003c).

Transmission of HBV in the health care setting

Transmission of HBV to health care workers can be substantially reduced by vaccination and adoption of universal safe precautions (Talaat *et al.* 2003).

Following all accidents involving inoculation or exposure to mucous membranes or non-intact skin, the patient should be tested for HBV, with the incident fully evaluated by the Occupational Health Unit and appropriate care provided. Health care workers who are involved in an incident can experience considerable distress and anxiety. Transmission of HBV from infected health care workers to their patients has occurred (Puro *et al.* 2003). The DH (2003a) requires that HBeAg-positive staff are not to undertake EPP. Those staff who are HBeAg negative must have additional testing to establish viral load. Those persons with HBV DNA levels exceeding 10^3 genome equivalents per millilitre cannot undertake EPP. Those whose viral load is below this figure have to be retested yearly (DH 2003a).

Immunization and vaccination

Passive protection against hepatitis B

Specific hepatitis B immunoglobulin (HBIg), prepared from pooled plasma with a high titre of hepatitis B surface antibody, is available for passive protection and is usually used in combination with hepatitis B vaccine to confer passive/active immunity under certain defined conditions (DH 2006b), including:

- Persons who have an inoculation, ingestion or splashing accident with HBsAg-infected blood.
- Babies of mothers with hepatitis B. In these cases babies should receive HBIg no later than 48 hours after birth. All pregnant women should be offered HBV testing at the beginning of antenatal care (DH 2004c).
- Sexual partners and, in some cases, family contacts judged to be high risk, or individuals suffering from acute hepatitis B and who are seen within 1 week of onset of jaundice.

162 Active immunization

Active immunization is by hepatitis B vaccine. Hepatitis B vaccine is a genetically engineered vaccine. The basic regimen consists of three doses of vaccine over 6 months, with a booster dose every 5 years. An accelerated schedule of three doses over 3 months with a booster at 12 months and then every 5 years can be given when rapid acquisition of immunity is required.

Health care workers involved in EPP, including theatre nurses, are required to be immunized against HBV. This means theatre nurses will have to provide evidence of HBV vaccination prior to employment. Those who fail to respond to vaccine have to be tested for HBV every 6 months to prove their continuing non-carrier status (DH 2003c).

Indications for immunization include:

- Personnel including teaching, training and nursing staff directly involved over a period of time in patient care where there is a high prevalence of HBV or where blood and blood products are handled regularly.
- Laboratory workers.
- Dentists and dental personnel.
- Medical and surgical personnel.
- Health care personnel on secondment to work in areas of the world where there is a high prevalence of HBV.
- Patients on entry to residential institutions where there is a high prevalence of HBV.
- Patients treated by maintenance haemodialysis.
- Sexual contacts of patients with acute HBV or carriers of HBV.
- Infants born to mothers who are HBsAg positive.
- Health care workers who receive an inoculation accident from a needle used on a patient who is HBsAg positive, either used alone or in combination with HBIg.

In addition, HBV vaccine is offered to selected high-risk populations; this includes homosexual men attending genitourinary clinics, as studies indicate they are at the greatest risk of acquiring HBV (McMillan 2005). A combined HBV and

HAV vaccine is now available, which has been seen to be safe and well tolerated (Van der Wielen *et al*. 2006).

Prevention of hepatitis B in health care workers

It is important that health care workers adopt safe techniques when in contact with blood and body fluids of all patients, regardless of their hepatitis status.

Avoiding inoculation accidents and contamination of mucous membranes and skin is an essential component of safe techniques (DH 2001a).

Death of patients with hepatitis B

When infected patients die, their bodies are no more hazardous than when they were alive, providing that appropriate precautions against contamination with blood and body fluids are maintained (Sa *et al*. 2006). Guidelines recommend that bodies of patients known to be infected with hepatitis should be placed in a body bag. Relatives and significant others should be permitted to view, touch and spend time with the deceased person. However, embalming should not be undertaken (Healing *et al*. 1995).

Patient education

The DH (2006b) recommends that individuals found to be HBsAg carriers should be educated about the ways in which hepatitis B may spread and the precautions that can be taken to reduce the risk to others. It is stressed that unnecessary restrictions and precautions may cause distress and should be avoided.

Antiviral therapy

Treatment is aimed at preventing the progression of infection to hepatocellular cancer and cirrhosis. Treatments to decrease viral replication and improve the immune response include interferon-α administered three times a week for 4–6 months, lamidivudine and adefovir dipivoxil, which blocks viral replication. Long-term therapy is required, which can lead to the development of resistance to treatment (Aggarwal & Ranjan 2004). Combinations of antiviral drugs have been tried in patients failing to respond to mono-therapy, which has been seen to reduce the levels of HBV in blood (Santos *et al*. 2006; Sokucu *et al*. 2006).

Excellent long-term results have been achieved following liver transplantation for chronic liver disease (Bruix *et al*. 2006). Prophylactic therapy is necessary following bone or stem cell transplantation to prevent reactivation of HBV (Kempinska *et al*. 2005).

Procedure guidelines   Hepatitis B: patient care

Procedure

Action	Rationale
1 The patient may be nursed on an open ward using all the patients' facilities as normal unless there is a high risk of blood contamination of the ward environment.	If adequate precautions can be adhered to on an open ward, there is no need to isolate the patient (HSE 2005: E).
2 The patient must be assessed daily to establish accurately any sites of bleeding. Changes in the patient's condition should be recorded in the care plan.	Sites of bleeding must be identified in order that the appropriate precautions can be taken (E).
3 Used sharps must be correctly disposed of in a sharps bin.	Contaminated sharps are a potential Inoculation hazard to others, so particular caution must be taken in handling them. Overloaded sharps containers may cause needles to pierce the walls of the container or even protrude through the top (DH 2001a: C).
4 A yellow clinical waste bag should be kept on a regular holder with a lid for the patient's disposable waste. When full this should be securely closed, and sent for incineration.	To confine potentially contaminated material, e.g. bloodstained tissues. Yellow is the internationally recognized colour for clinical waste (DH 2006a: C).
5 The patient's personal hygiene equipment must be kept at the bedside.	To prevent accidental use of equipment by others (E).
6 Used linen that is not bloodstained is placed in the white linen bags in the usual way.	Linen free from blood stains is not contaminated and may be dealt with in the normal manner (DH 1995a: C).
7 During venepuncture or other procedures likely to cause bleeding, furniture, bedding and clothing in the adjacent area should be protected with polythene sheeting.	To prevent contamination of the environment with spilled blood (E).

8 All staff involved with the patient should cover any cuts or grazes on their hands with waterproof dressings.

Broken skin provides a portal of entry for the hepatitis virus in the event of contact with the patient's blood (E).

9 Routine daily cleaning procedures may be carried out as normal. As part of universal safe technique and practices, domestic staff will be aware of the potential hazard associated with any blood contamination.

Education is necessary so the domestic staff can understand the hazards involved (E).

Accidental inoculation or spillage of blood from patient with hepatitis B

Action	Rationale
1 Any accident involving skin penetration or heavy contamination of abraded skin or mucosal surfaces of staff should be recorded on an accident form and this taken to bacteriology immediately. Occupational health must be informed, who will make an assessment for the need of HBV vaccine or HBV IgG.	To protect personnel. To comply with legal and/or hospital requirements (HSE 2005: C).
2 Blood spillage onto unbroken skin should be washed off with soap and running water. A scrubbing brush should not be used as this could break the skin. Complete an accident form, as above, and inform occupational health.	To remove the source of potential contamination. To comply with legal and/or hospital requirements (HSE 2005: C).
3 Accidental inoculation sites should be cleaned under running water, encouraged to bleed freely and then covered with waterproof plaster. Complete an accident form, as above.	Bleeding helps to expel the inoculated virus from the site. To comply with legal and/or hospital requirements (HSE 2005: C).
4 Blood spilled on hard surfaces must be wiped up immediately with paper towels and the area washed well with a solution such as hypochlorite.	To prevent viral spread. Dried blood remains infectious for several days (Wilson 2006: E).
5 Linen stained with blood should be treated as infected linen and placed in a red alginate polythene bag before being placed in a red linen bag.	Bloodstained linen is highly infectious. All linen in red alginate polythene bags will be washed in a barrier wash at the laundry (DH 1995a: C).

Procedure guidelines *(cont.)*

Precautions if patient with hepatitis B is bleeding

Action	Rationale
1 If significant bleeding is present in the mouth:	
(a) Consider the use of disposable crockery and cutlery and, with any contaminated food, dispose of as clinical waste.	Significant amounts of blood contamination on crockery and cutlery may contaminate the ward kitchen and lead to cross-infection (E).
(b) Keep a personal food tray and water jug at the bedside.	Significant blood can be removed from jug and tray before it leaves the room to be thoroughly cleaned in a dish washer, so preventing cross-contamination (E).
(c) Disposable mouth-care equipment, sputum pot and tissues should be kept at the bedside.	The sputum may be contaminated with blood from the mouth, therefore precautions must include avoiding contact with the patient's sputum (E).
2 If haematuria or melaena is present:	
(a) Wear plastic gowns and gloves when handling excreta.	Blood present in the urine or faeces makes the patient's excreta a potential source of hepatitis B contamination (HSE 2005: E).
(b) Keep a toilet and handbasin for the patient's sole use, if practicable.	Blood present in the urine or faeces makes the patient's excreta a potential source of hepatitis B contamination (HSE 2005: E).
(c) If a toilet is not available for the patient's sole use, bedpans or urinals must be used. These should be washed in the usual manner in the bedpan washer. Disposable bedpans are dealt with in the routine manner.	Blood present in the urine or faeces makes the patient's excrete a potential source of hepatitis B contamination (HSE 2005: E).
3 If the patient has a wound or a break in the skin:	
(a) Cover the area adequately so that there is no seepage.	To prevent the spread of the virus from dried or fresh blood. Dried blood can remain infectious for several days (HSE 2005: C).
(b) Used dressings should be sealed securely in a plastic bag before being disposed of as clinical waste.	To prevent the spread of the virus (HSE 2005: C).

(c) All tapes, lotions and creams are kept solely for the patient's use.	To prevent contamination and therefore the spread of the virus (E).
(d) The dressing trolley must be cleaned carefully before reuse.	To prevent contamination and therefore the spread of the virus (E).
(e) Non-disposable equipment should be emptied and wiped clean, placed in a central sterile supplies department bag, securely stapled shut and sent to the sterile supplies department in a safe manner, to be resterilized.	To remove any contamination and therefore reduce the risk of cross-infection (E).

Invasive procedures, specimens and transport for patient with hepatitis B

Action	Rationale
1 All departments and staff who will be undertaking invasive procedures to the patient must be made aware of the patient's hepatitis B diagnosis.	To allow them to make their own precautionary arrangements (E).
2 All request cards to be labelled appropriately.	To alert the receiving department of the diagnosis (HSE 2003b: C).
3 All specimens to be labelled appropriately and correctly bagged. (For further information on specimen collection see Chapter 28.)	To alert the receiving department of the diagnosis and prevent contamination of the environment (HSE 2003b: C).
4 If a patient who is bleeding has to be transported elsewhere, a nurse must accompany the patient and the porter involved should be provided with the following:	To prevent the contamination of the porter or other patients (E).
(a) Disposable gloves and aprons.	To prevent the contamination of the porter (E).
(b) Cleaning equipment for the trolley or chair before use by the next patient.	To remove any contamination and therefore reduce the risk of cross-infection (E).

Discharging the patient with hepatitis B

Action	Rationale
1 The majority of precautions can cease.	Discharge normally implies that the risk of cross-infection is no longer present (E).

Procedure guidelines *(cont.)*

2 The patient should be advised not to share razors, toothbrushes or similar personal property likely to be contaminated by blood.	To reduce the risk of cross-infection (E).
3 If bleeding occurs, the patient clears up the blood himself/herself and disposes safely of such items as contaminated tissues by burning or flushing down the toilet. If regular persistent bloodstained waste is generated, the health authority must be requested to make special collections.	To reduce the risk of cross-infection (E).
4 If emergency treatment or dental care is required, the patient must inform the health care worker of the fact that he/she has a recent history of hepatitis B infection.	To allow the correct precautions to be taken (E).

Death of a patient with hepatitis B

Action	Rationale
1 There should be minimal handling of the body. However, routine last offices can be undertaken (see Chapter 15).	To reduce the risk of infecting the nursing staff (E).
2 Nurses should wear disposable plastic aprons and gloves when handling the body.	
3 The body should be totally enclosed in a body bag specifically designed for infected patients.	To reduce the risk of infecting the nursing staff (E).
4 The mortuary staff should be informed of the diagnosis.	To ensure that all staff are aware of the infection risk.
5 If the relatives want to view the body, they must be supervised. The body bag can be opened by a nurse to allow viewing.	To prevent contamination (E).

References and further reading

Abdel-Haq, N. *et al.* (2006) New antiviral agents. *Indian J Pediatr*, **73**(4), 313–21.

Abdulmalik, A. *et al.* (2006) Varicella-associated purpura fulminans: chickenpox is not always benign. *Med Princ Pract*, **15**(3), 232–4.

Abe, K. *et al.* (2004) Molecular epidemiology of hepatitis B, C, D and E viruses among children in Moscow, Russia. *J Clin Virol*, **30**(1), 57–61.

Afessa, B. & Peters, S.G. (2006) Major complications following hematopoietic stem cell transplantation. *Semin Respir Crit Care Med*, **27**(3), 297–309.

Aggarwal, R. & Ranjan, P. (2004) Preventing and treating hepatitis B infection. *BMJ*, **329**, 1080–6.

Aisenberg, G.M. *et al.* (2005) Extrapulmonary tuberculosis active infection misdiagnosed as cancer: *Mycobacterium tuberculosis* disease in patients at a Comprehensive Cancer Centre (2001–2005). *Cancer*, **104**(12), 2882–7.

Aisien, A.O. & Ujah, I.A. (2006) Risk of blood splashes to masks and goggles during cesarean section. *Med Sci Monit*, **12**(2), CR94–97.

Albert, J. *et al.* (1990) Replicative capacity of HIV-2 like HIV-1, correlates with severity of immunosuppression. *AIDS*, **4**(4), 291–5.

Ali, R. *et al.* (2006) Invasive pulmonary aspergillosis: role of early diagnosis and surgical treatment in patients with acute leukemia. *Ann Clin Microbiol Antimicrob*, **5**(1), 17–23.

Amin, Z. (2006) Clinical tuberculosis problems and management. *Acta Med Indones*, **38**(2), 109–16.

Anaya, I. *et al.* (2006) Survivability of *Salmonella* cells in popcorn after microwave oven and conventional cooking. *Microbiol Res,* [Epub ahead of print].

Anderson, D.J. *et al.* (2006) Predictors of mortality in patients with blood stream infection due to ceftazidime-resistant *Klebsiella pneumoniae*. *Antimicrob Agents Chemother*, **50**(5), 1715–20.

Andrei, G. *et al.* (2005) Susceptabilities of several clinical varicella-zoster virus (VZV) isolates and drug-resistant VZV strains to bicyclic furano pyrimidine nucleosides. *Antimicrob Agents Chemother* **49**(3), 1081–6.

Arduino, P.G. & Porter, S.R. (2006) Oral and perioral herpes simplex type 1(HSV-1) infection: review of management. *Oral Dis*, **12**(3), 254–70.

Aricha, B., Fishov, I. & Cohen, Z. (2004) Differences in membrane fluidity and fatty acid composition between phenotypic variants of *Streptococcus pneumoniae*. *J Bacteriol*, **186**(14), 4638–44.

Aslam, S. & Musher, D.M. (2006) An update on diagnosis, treatment and prevention of *Clostridium difficile*-associated disease. *Gastroenterol Clin North Am*, **35**(2), 315–35.

Avery, R.K. *et al.* (2004) Use of leflunomide in an allogeneic bone marrow transplant recipient with refractory cytomegalovirus infection. *Bone Marrow Transplant*, **34**(12), 1071–5.

Aveyard, H. (2002) The requirement for informed consent prior to nursing care procedures. *J Adv Nurs*, **37**(3), 243–9.

Ayliffe, G.A.J. *et al.* (2000) *Control of Hospital Infection. A Practical Handbook*, 4th edn. Arnold, London.

Babay, H.A. *et al.* (2005) Bloodstream infections in pediatric patients. *Saudi Med J*, **26**(10), 1555–61.

Bakardjiev, A.I., Theriot, J.A. & Portnoy, D.A. (2006) *Listeria monocytogenes* traffics from maternal organs to the placenta and back. *PLoS Pathog*, **2**(6), e66.

Baker, S.A. (1994) Hepatitis: protecting BMETs and CEs. *J Clin Eng*, **19**(6), 446–51.

Ball, J. *et al.* (1991) Long lasting viability of HIV after patient's death. *Lancet*, **338**(8758), 63.

Banfield, K.R. & Kerr, K.G. (2005) Could hospital patients' hands constitute a missing link? *J Hosp Infect*, **61**(3), 183–8.

Baqai, R., Anwar, S. & Kazmi, S.U. (2005) Detection of *Cryptosporidium* in immunosuppressed patients. *J Ayub Med Coll Abbottabad*, 17(3), 38–40.

Barber, F.D. (2001) Management of fever in neutropenic patients with cancer. *Nurs Clin North Am*, **36**(4), 631–44.

Barin, F. *et al.* (1985) Serological evidence for virus related to Simian T-lymphotropic retrovirus III in residents of West Africa. *Lancet*, **ii**, 1387–9.

Battegay, M., Gust, I.D. & Feinstone, S.M. (1995) Hepatitis A virus. In: *Principles and Practice of Infectious Diseases*, Vol. 2, 4th edn (eds G.L. Mandell, J.E. Bennett & R. Dolin). Churchill Livingstone, New York, pp. 1636–66.

BCSH (1995) Guidelines on the provision of facilities for the care of adult patients with haematological malignancies (including leukaemia and lymphoma and severe bone marrow failure). *Clin Lab Haematol*, **17**, 3–10.

Belkin, N.L. (2002) A historical review of barrier materials. *AORN J*, **76**(4), 648–53.

Berg, S. *et al.* (2006) Serotypes of *Streptococcus pneumoniae* isolated from blood and cerebrospinal fluid related to vaccine serotypes and to clinical characteristics. *Scand J Infect Dis*, **38**(6), 427–32.

Bernardi, M., Catania, G. & Marceca, F. (2005) The world of nursing burn out. A literature review. *Prof Inferm*, **58**(2), 75–9.

Bernstein, W.B. *et al.* (2006) Acquired immunodeficiency syndrome-related malignancies in the era of highly active antiretroviral therapy. *Int J Hematol*, **84**(1), 3–11.

Berrington, J.E. *et al.* (2000) Unsuspected *Pneumocystis carinii* pneumonia at presentation of severe primary immunodeficiency. *Arch Dis Child*, **82**(2), 144–7.

Beyazit, Y. *et al.* (2006) Acute pericarditis and renal failure complicating acute hepatitis A infection. *South Med J*, **99**(1), 82–4.

Bignardi, G.E. (1998) Risk factors for *Clostridium difficile* infection. *J Hosp Infect*, **40**, 1–15.

Bishop, E. *et al.* (2006) Good clinical outcomes but high rates of adverse reactions during linezolid therapy for serious infection: a proposed protocol for monitoring therapy in complex patients. *Antimicrob Agents Chemother*, **50**(4), 1599–602.

Bissett, L. (2006) Reducing the risk of acquiring antimicrobial-resistant bacteria. *Br J Nurs*, **15**(2), 68–71.

Blajchman, M.A. (2006) The clinical benefits of the leukoreduction of blood products. *J Trauma*, **60**(6)(Suppl), S83–90.

Blatnik, J. & Lesnicar, G. (2006) Propagation of methicillin-resistant *Staphylococcus aureus* due to the overloading of medical nurses in intensive care units. *J Hosp Infect*, **63**(2), 162–6.

Bloomfield, S.F. & Scott, E.A. (2003a) Developing an effective policy for home hygiene: a risk-based approach. *Int J Environ Health Res*, **13**(Suppl 1), S57–66.

Bloomfield, S.F. (2003b) Home hygiene: a risk approach. *Int J Hyg Environ Health*, **206**(1), 1–8.

Blot, S. *et al*. (2005) Colonization status and appropriate antibiotic therapy for nosocomial bacteria caused by antibiotic-resistant gram-negative bacteria in intensive care unit. *Infect Control Hosp Epidemiol*, **26**(6), 575–9.

Boden, M. (1999) Contamination in moving and handling equipment. *Prof Nurse* **14**(7), 484–7.

Bodey, G.P. (2005) Managing infections in the immunocompromised patient. *Clin Infect Dis*, **40**(Suppl 4), S239.

Boeckh, M. *et al*. (2002) Late cytomegalovirus disease and mortality in allogeneic hematopoietic stem cell transplant recipients: importance of viral load and T-cell immunity. *Blood*, **101**(2), 407–14.

Boeckh, M. *et al*. (2006) Long term acyclocir for prevention of varicella zoster virus disease after allogeneic hematopoietic cell transplantation – a randomized double-blind placebo-controlled study. *Blood*, **107**(5), 1800–5.

Borella, P. *et al*. (2005) *Legionella* contamination in hot water of Italian hotels. *Appl Environ Microbiol*, **71**(10), 5805–13.

Boussemart, T. *et al*. (1998) Cytomegalovirus, pregnancy and occupational risk. *Arch Pediatr*, **5**(1), 24–6.

Bowden, R.A. (2000) Infection in blood and bone marrow transplant patients: allogeneic and autologous transplantation. In: *Management of Infections in Immunocompromised Patients*, Part II, Chapter 5 (eds M.P. Glauser & P.A. Pizzo). W.B. Saunders, London, pp. 189–218.

Bower, M. *et al*. (2004) HIV-associated anal cancer: has highly active antiretroviral therapy reduced the incidence or improved the outcome? *J Acquir Immune Defic Syndr*, **37**(5), 1563–5.

Boxall, E.H. & Smith, N. (2004) Antenatal screening for HIV; are those who refuse testing at higher risk than those who accept testing? *J Public Health (Oxf)*, **26**(3), 285–7.

Boxall, E. *et al*. (2006) Transfusion-transmitted hepatitis E in a 'nonhyperendemic' country. *Transfus Med*, **16**(2), 79–83.

Boyce, J.M. *et al*. (2006) Lack of association between the increased incidence of *Clostridium difficile* associated disease and the increasing use of alcoholic-based handrub. *Infect Control Hosp Epidemiol*, **27**(5), 479–83.

Bradley, C.R. & Fraise, A.P. (1996) Heat and chemical resistance of enterococci. *J Hosp Infect*, **34**, 191–6.

Brady, M.J. *et al*. (2003) Persistent silver disinfectant for the environment control of pathogenic bacteria. *Am J Infect Control*, **31**(4), 208–14.

Braitstein, P. *et al*. (2006) Mortality of HIV-1 infected patients in the first year of antiretroviral therapy: comparison between low-income and high-income countries. *Lancet*, **11**(367; 9513), 817–24.

Brant, L. *et al*. (2005) Pathways of care and resource utilization in a national cohort of patients with transfusion-acquired hepatitis C. *J Viral Hepat*, **12**(6), 618–26.

Brisson, M. & Edmunds, W.J. (2003) Epidemiology of varicella-zoster virus in England and Wales. *J Med Virol*, **70**(Suppl 1), S9–14.

Brown, D.F.J. *et al.* (2006a) National glycopeptide-resistant enterococcal bacteraemia surveillance working group report to the Department of Health, August 2004. *J Hosp Infect*, **62**(Suppl 1), 1–27.

Brown, E.L. *et al.* (2006b) Maternal herpes simplex virus antibody avidity and risk of neonatal herpes. *Am J Obstet Gynecol*, **195**(1), 115–20.

Bruce, J. & Brysiewicz, P. (2002) Ebola fever: the African emergency. *Int J Trauma Nurs*, **8**(2), 36–41.

Bruix, J. *et al.* (2006) New aspects of diagnosis and therapy of hepatocellular carcinoma. *Oncogene*, **25**(27), 3848–56.

Brundage, S.C. & Fitzpatrick, A.N. (2006) Hepatitis A. *Am Fam Physician*, **73**(12), 2162–8.

Burek, V. (2005) Laboratory diagnosis of viral hepatitis B and C. *Acta Med Croatica*, **59**(5), 405–12.

Burnard, P. (1992) Nurse training needs in AIDS counselling. *Nurs Stand*, **6**(34), 34–39.

Cacciari, P. *et al.* (2004) Consideration on isolation rooms and alternative pressure ventilation systems. *Ann Ig*, **16**(6), 777–801.

Caccio, S.M. (2005) Molecular epidemiology of human cryptosporidiosis. *Parassitologia*, **47**(2), 185–92.

Caccio, S.M. & Pozio, E. (2006) Advances in the epidemiology, diagnosis and treatment of cryptosporidiosis. *Expert Rev Anti Infect Ther*, **4**(3), 429–43.

Caggiano, V. *et al.* (2005) Incidence, cost, and mortality of neutropenia hospitalization with chemotherapy. *Cancer*, **103**(9), 1916–24.

Calandra, T. (2000) Practical guide to host defence mechanisms and the predominant infections encountered in immunocompromised patients. In: *Management of Infections in Immmunocompromised Patients*, Part I, Chapter 1 (eds M.P. Glauser & P.A. Pizzo). W.B. Saunders, London, pp. 3–16.

Callaghan, I. (1998) Bacterial contamination of nurse's uniform: a study. *Nurs Stand*, **13**(1), 37–42.

Campana, S. *et al.* (2004) Molecular epidemiology of *Pseudomonas aerginosa*, *Burkholderia cepacia* complex and methicillin-resistant *Staphyloccocus aureus* in a cystic fibrosis centre. *J Cyst Fibros*, **3**(30), 159–63.

Candel, F.J. *et al.* (2005) Bacteremia and septic shock after solid-organ transplantation. *Transplant Proc*, **37**(99), 4097–9.

Carmona, E.M. *et al.* (2006) Pneumocystis cell wall beta-glucans induce dentritic cell costimulatory molecule expression and inflammatory activation through a Fas-Fas ligand mechanism. *J Immunol*, **177**(1), 459–67.

Casemore, D.P. (1998) *Cryptosporidium* and the safety of our water supplies. *Commun Dis Public Health*, **1**(4), 218–19.

Casolari, C. *et al.* (2005) A simultaneous outbreak of *Serratia marcescens* and *Klebsiella pneumoniae* in a neonatal intensive care unit. *J Hosp Infect*, **61**(4), 312–20.

Casper, C. & Wald, A. (2002) Condom use and the prevention of genital herpes acquisition. *Herpes*, **9**(1), 10–14.

Castognola, E. *et al.* (2006) Fungal infections in children with cancer: a prospective, multicenter surveillance study. *Pediatr Infect Dis J*, **25**(7), 634–9.

Catalano, G. *et al.* (2003) Anxiety and depression in hospitalized patients in resistant organism isolation. *South Med J*, **96**(2), 141–5.

CDC (1992) Revised classification system for HIV infection and expanded surveillance case definition for AIDS among adolescents and adults. *MMWR Morb Mortal Wkly Rep*, **41**, 1–19.

CDC (2003) Guidelines for environmental infection control health-care facilities. *MMWR Morb Mortal Wkly Rep*, **52**(RR10), 1–42.

CDC (2005) Guidelines for preventing the transmission of *Mycobacterium tuberculosis* in health care setting. *MMWR Morb Mortal Wkly Rep*, **54**(RR17), 1–141.

CDC (2006) Rapid HIV test distribution – United States, 2003–2005. *MMWR Morb Mortal Wkly Rep*, **55**(24), 673–6.

Cepeda, J.A. *et al.* (2005) Isolation of patients in single rooms or cohorts to reduce spread of MRSA in intensive-care units: prospective two-centre study. *Lancet*, **365**(9456), 295–304.

Chang, B. *et al.* (2004) Quality of life in tuberculosis: a review of the English language literature. *Qual Life Res*, **10**, 1633–42.

Chattopadhyay, B. (2001) Control of infection wards: are they worthwhile? *J Hosp Infect*, **47**(2), 88–90.

Chaudhury, H., Mahmood, A. & Valente, M. (2006) Nurses perception of single-occupancy versus multioccupancy rooms in a city care environment: an exploratory comparative assessment. *Appl Nurs Res*, **19**(3), 118–25.

Chen, C.Y. *et al.* (2004) Trends and antimicrobial resistance of pathogens causing blood-stream infection among febrile neutropenic adults with hematological malignancy. *J Formos Med Assoc*, **103**(7), 526–632.

Chen, L. & Lee, C. (2006) Distinguishing HIV-1 drug resistance, accessory, and viral fitness mutations using conditional selection pressure analysis of treated versus untreated patients' samples. *Biol Direct*, **1**(1), 14–30.

Chia, S.E. *et al.* (2005) Appropriate use of personal protective equipment among healthcare workers in public sector hospitals and primary healthcare polyclinics during the SARS outbreak in Singapore. *Occup Environ Med*, **62**(7), 473–7.

Chodick, G., Ashkenazi, S. & Lerman, Y. (2006) The risk of hepatitis A infection among healthcare workers: a review of reported outbreaks and sero-epidemiologic studies. *J Hosp Infect*, **62**(4), 414–20.

Clavel, F. *et al.* (1986) Isolation of a new human retrovirus from West African patients with AIDS. *Science*, **233**, 343–6.

Coaquette, A. *et al.* (2004) Mixed cytomegalovirus glycoproteins B genotypes in immuno-compromised patients. *Clin Infect Dis*, **39**(2), 155–61.

Codeluppi, M. *et al.* (2005) Rituximab as treatment of posttransplant lymphoproliferative disorder in patients who underwent small bowel/multivisceral transplantation: report of three cases. *Transplant Proc*, **37**(6), 2634–5.

Coia, J.E. *et al.* (2006) Guidelines for the control and prevention of methicillin-resistant *Staphylococcus aureus* (MRSA) in healthcare facilities by the joint BSAC/HIS/ICNA working party on MRSA. *J Hosp Infect*, **63**(Suppl 1), S1–44.

Communicable Disease Surveillance Centre (2002a) *HIV and AIDS in the UK in 2001.* Public Health Laboratory Service, London.

Communicable Disease Report (CDR) (2002b) First report of the Department of Health's mandatory MRSA Bacteremia Surveillance Scheme in acute NHS Trusts in England April to September 2001. *CDC Weekly* Public Health Laboratory Service, London., **12**(6), 1–15.

Conaty, S.J. *et al.* (2005) Women who decline antenatal screening for HIV infection in the era of universal testing: results of an audit of uptake in three London Hospitals. *J Public Health (Oxf)*, **27**(1), 114–7.

Cookson, B.D. *et al.* (2006) Guidelines for the control of glycopeptide-resistant enterococci in hospital. *J Hosp Infect*, **62**(1), 6–21.

Cooper, E.E. *et al.* (2003) Influence of building construction work on *Aspergillus* infection in a hospital setting. *Infect Control Hosp Epidemiol*, **24**(7), 472–6.

Corkill, J.E., Anson, J.J. & Hart, C.A. (2005) High prevalence of the plasmid-mediated quinolone resistance determinant qnrA in multi-drug resistant Enterobacteriaceae from blood cultures in Liverpool, UK. *J Antimicrob Chemother*, **56**(6), 1115–17.

Cotterill S. *et al.* (1996) An unusual source for the outbreak of methicillin resistant *Staphylococcus aureus* on an intensive therapy unit. *J Hosp Infect*, **329**(3), 207–16.

Coupe, S. *et al.* (2006) Detection of *Cryptosporidium*, *Giardia* and *Enterocytozoon bieneusi* in surface water, including recreational areas: a 1-year prospective study. *FEMS Immunol Med Microbiol*, **47**(3), 351–9.

Creedon, S.A. (2005) Healthcare workers hand decontamination practices: compliance with recommended guidelines. *J Adv Nurs*, **51**(3), 208–16.

Creeson, S.A. (2006) Health care workers hand decontamination practices: an Irish study. *Clin Nurs Res*, **15**(1), 6–26.

Crimi, P. *et al.* (2006) Correlation between *Legionella* contamination in water and surrounding air. *Infect Control Hosp Epidemiol*, **27**(7), 771–3.

Croner (1998) *Health Service Risk Management and Practice Special Report*. www.croner.co.uk

Crowcroft, N.S. & Catchpole, M. (2002) Mortality from methicillin resistant *Staphylococcus aureus* in England and Wales: analysis of death certificates. *Br Med J*, **325**(7377), 1390–1.

Cunha, B.A. (1998) Nosocomial diarrhoea. *Crit Care Clin*, **14**(2), 329–38.

Cunha, B.A. (2006) The atypical pneumonias: clinical diagnosis and importance. *Clin Microbiol Infect*, **12**(Suppl 3), 12–24.

Cunningham, J.B., Kernohan, W.G. & Rush, T. (2005) Bed occupancy, turnover intervals and MRSA rates in English hospitals. *Br J Nurs*, **15**(12), 656–60.

Custovic, A. *et al.* (1998) Domestic allergens in public places. *Clin Exp Allergy*, **28**(1), 53–9.

Cuthbert, J.A. (2001) Hepatitis A: old and new. *Clin Microbiol Rev*, **14**(1), 38–58.

Dadd, G., McMinn, P. & Monterosso, L. (2003) Protective isolation in hemopoietic stem cell transplants: a review of the literature and single institution experience. *J Pediatr Oncol Nurs*, **20**(6), 293–300.

Dale, D.C. & Liles, C. (1998) How many neutrophils are enough? *Lancet*, **351**(9118), 1752–3.

Dale, J.W. *et al.* (2005) Origins and properties of *Mycobacterium tuberculosis* isolates in London. *J Med Microbiol*, **54**, 575–82.

Danaher, E.H. *et al.* (2006) Fatigue and physical activity in patients undergoing hematopoietic stem cell transplant. *Oncol Nurs Forum*, **33**(3), 614–24.

Dancer, S., Raeside, J. & Boothman, M. (2002) Environmental organisms from different hospital wards. *Br J Infect Control*, **3**(94), 10–14.

Dancer, S.J. *et al.* (2006) Antibiotic use is associated with resistance of environmental organisms in a teaching hospital. *J Hosp Infect*, **62**(2), 200–6.

Davidson, M.M., Evans, R. & Hay, A.J. (2006) Same day detection of methicillin-resistant *Staphylococcus aureus* from screening swabs by real time polymerase chain reaction. *J Hosp Infect*, **62** (4), 484–5.

Davis, M.M. (2006) Successes and remaining challenges after 10 years of varicella vaccination in the USA. *Expert Rev Vaccines*, **5**(2), 295–302.

Dawson, D. (2005) Foodborne protozoan parasites. *Int J Food Microbiol*, **103**(2), 207–27.

Dawson, S. *et al.* (2006) *Listeria* outbreak associated with sandwich consumption from a hospital retail shop, United Kingdom. *Euro Surveill*, **11**(6), 89–91.

De la Rua-Domenech, R. (2006) Human *Mycobacterium bovis* infection in the United Kingdom: incidence, risks, control measures and review of the zoonotic aspects of bovine tuberculosis. *Tuberculosis (Edinb)*, **86**(2):77–109.

De Lorenzi, S. *et al.* (2006) Comparison of floor sanitation methods. *J Hosp Infect*, **62**(3), 346–8.

De Schryver, A. *et al.* (1999) Risk of cytomegalovirus infection among educators and health care personnel serving mentally disabled children. *J Infect*, **38**(1), 36–40.

De Souza, W. & Benchimol, M. (2005) Basic biology of *Pneumocystis carinii*: a mini review. *Mem Inst Oswaldo Cruz*, **100**(8), 903–8.

De Vries, G., Sebek, M.M. & Lambregts-van Weezenbeek, C.S. (2006) Health care workers with tuberculosis infected during work in the Netherlands. *Eur Respir J*, **28**(6), 1216–21.

Declerck, P. *et al.* (2006) Detection and quantification of *Legionella pneumophila* in water samples using competitive PCR. *Can J Microbiol*, **52**(6), 584–90.

Deeks, S.G. (2006) Antiretroviral treatment of HIV infected adults *BMJ*, **332**, 1489.

DeMille, D. *et al.* (2006) The effect of the neutropenic diet in the outpatient setting: a pilot study. *Oncol Nurs Forum*, **33**(2), 337–43.

de Roux, A. *et al.* (2006) Impact of alcohol abuse in the etiology and severity of community-acquired pneumonia. *Chest*, **129**(5), 1219–25.

DH (1995a) *Hospital Laundry Arrangements for Used and Infected Linen*. Department of Health, London.

DH (1995b) *Hepatitis C and Blood Transfusion Look Back*. PL CMO (95)1. HMSO, London.

DH (1995c) *Hospital Infection Control, Guidance on the Control of Infection in Hospitals*. 2383 IP 25K. Health Publications Unit, Heywood, Lancashire.

DH (1996a) *Guidelines for Pre-Test Discussion on HIV Testing*. HMSO, London.

DH (1998a) *Management and Control of Viral Haemorrhagic Fevers. Summary of Guidance from the Advisory Committee on Dangerous Pathogens*. 12491 HP 14k 1P Mar 98 (MUL). HMSO, London.

DH (1998b) *Standing Medical Advisory Committee, Sub Group on Antimicrobial Resistance. The Path of Least Resistance*. HMSO, London.

DH (1998c) Third Report of the Group of Experts (1998) *Cryptosporidium in Water Supplies*. Department of the Environment, Transport and the Regions, and Department of Health, London.

DH (1998d) *The Prevention and Control of Tuberculosis in the United Kingdom*. HSC 1998/196. HMSO, London.

DH (2000a) *HIV Post Exposure Prophylaxis: Guidance from the UK Chief Medical Officer' Expert Advisory Group on AIDS*. Department of Health, London.

DH (2000b) *United Kingdom Antimicrobial Resistance Strategy and Action Plan.* Department of Health, London.

DH (2001a) Standard principles for preventing hospital-acquired infections. *J Hosp Infect,* **47**(Suppl), S21–37.

DH (2001b) *The Essence of Care: Patients Focused Benchmarking for Health Care Practitioners.* Department of Health, London.

DH (2002a) *Hepatitis C for England Strategy.* HMSO, London.

DH (2002b) *Getting Ahead of the Curve. A Strategy for Combating Infectious Diseases (Including Other Aspects of Health Promotion).* HMSO, London.

DH (2003a) *Winning Ways. Working Together to Reduce Healthcare Associated Infection in England.* Department of Health, London.

DH (2003b) *National Clostridium difficile Standards Group. Report to the Department of Health, February 2003.* Department of Health, London.

DH (2003c) *Health Clearance for Serious Communicable Diseases: New Health Care Workers.* Department of Health, London.

DH (2003d) *Transmissible Spongiform Encephalopathy Agents: Safe Working and Prevention of Infection.* Department of Health, London.

DH (2004a) *Towards Cleaner Hospitals and Lower Rates of Infection.* Department of Health, London.

DH (2004b) *Matrons Charter, an Action Plan for Cleaner Hospitals.* Department of Health, London.

DH (2004c) *Children in Need and Blood-borne Viruses: HIV and Hepatitis.* Department of Health, London.

DH (2004d) *The Carriage of Dangerous Goods (Classification, Packaging and Labelling) and Use of Transportable Pressure Receptacles Regulations.* SI 2004, No. 568. Department of Health, London.

DH (2005a) *Saving Lives: A Delivery Programme to Reduce Healthcare Associated Infection including MRSA.* Department of Health, London.

DH (2005b) *HIV-infected Healthcare Workers: Guidance on Management and Patient Notification.* Department of Health, London.

DH (2005c) *Hazardous waste (England) regulations.* Department of Health, London.

DH (2006a) *Environment and sustainability Health Technical Memorandum 07-01: Safe management of healthcare waste.* Department of Health, London.

DH (2006b) *Immunisation Against Infectious Disease.* HMSO, London.

DH (2006c) *Water systems Health technical memorandum 04-01: The control of legionella, hygiene, "safe" hot water, cold water and drinking water systems.* Department of Health, Leeds

DH (2006d) *Infection Control Guidance for Care Homes.* Department of Health, London.

Dhaliwal, J. & McGeer, A. (2005) *Does Isolation Prevent the Spread of Methicillin-resistant Staphylococcus aureus? CMAJ,* **172**(7), 875.

Dharan S. *et al.* (1999) Routine disinfection of patients' environmental surfaces. Myth or reality. *J Hosp Infect,* **42**(2), 113–7.

Dial, S. *et al.* (2004) Risk of *Clostridium difficile* diarrhea among hospital patients prescribed proton pump inhibitors: cohort and case-control studies. *CMAJ,* **171**(1), 3–38.

Diamond, C. *et al.* (2005) Increased incidence of squamous cell anal cancer among men with AIDS in the era of highly active antiretroviral therapy. *Sex Transm Dis,* **32**(5), 314–20.

Diamond, C. *et al.* (2006a) Changes in acquired immunodeficiency syndrome-related non-Hodgkin lymphoma in the era of highly active antiretroviral therapy: incidence, presentation, treatment and survival. *Cancer*, **106**(1), 128–35.

Diamond, C. *et al.* (2006b) Highly active antiretroviral therapy is associated with improved survival among patients with IDS-related primary central nervous system non-Hodgkin's lymphoma. *Curr HIV Res*, **4**(3), 375–8.

Diaz-Pedroche, C. *et al.* (2006) Valganciclovir preemptive therapy for the prevention of cytomegalovirus disease in high-risk seropositive solid-organ transplant recipients. *Transplantation*, **82**(1), 30–5.

Dick, L. (1998) Travel medicine: helping patients prepare for trips abroad. *Am Fam Physician*, **58**(2), 383–98.

Diederen, B.M. & Peeters, M.F. (2006) Evaluation of two new immunochromatographic assays (rapid U *Legionella* antigen test and SD Bioline *Legionella* antigen test) for detection of *Legionella pneumophila* serogroup 1 antigen in urine. *J Clin Microbiol*, **44**(8), 2991–3.

Dietze, B. *et al.* (2001) Survival of MRSA on sterile goods packaging. *J Hosp Infect*, **49**(4), 255–61.

Ditchburn, I. (2006) Should doctors wear ties? *J Hosp Infect*, **63**(2), 227–8.

Donohue, R. (2006) Development and implementation of a risk assessment tool for chemotherapy-induced neutropenia. *Oncol Nurs Forum*, **33**(2), 347–52.

Duff, P. (1998) Hepatitis in pregnancy. *Semin Perinatol*, **22**(4), 277–83.

Duquette-Petersen L. *et al.* (1999) The role of protective clothing in infection prevention in patients undergoing autologous bone marrow transplantation. *Oncol Nurs Forum*, **26**(8), 1319–24.

Dyer, C. (2004) Payments announced for patients infected with hepatitis C. *BMJ*, **328**, 246.

Dykewicz, C.A. (2001) Hospital infection control in hematopoietic stem cell transplant recipients. *Emerg Infect Dis*, **7**(2), 263–7.

Editorial (2002) Transfusion transmission of HCV infection before anti-HCV testing of blood donations in England: results of the national HCV Lookback program. *Transfusion*, **42**(9), 1146– 53.

Ehlert, K. *et al.* (2006) Treatment of refractory CMV-infection following hematopoietic stem cell transplantation with the combination of foscarnet and leflunomide. *Klin Padiatr*, **218**(3), 180–4.

Ejidokun, O.O. *et al.* (2000) Four linked outbreaks of *Salmonella enteritidis* phage type 4 infection: the continuing egg threat. *Commun Dis Public Health*, **3**(2), 95–100.

Elinav, E. *et al.* (2006) Acute hepatitis A infection in pregnancy is associated with high rates of gestational complications and preterm labor. *Gastroenterology*, **130**(4), 1129–34.

Ellett, M.L. (1999) Hepatitis A, B, and D. *Gastroenterol Nurs*, **22**(6), 236–44.

Elliott, S.K., Keeton, A. & Holt, A. (2005) Medical students' knowledge of sharps injuries. *J Hosp Infect*, **60**(4), 374–7.

El-Mahallawy, H.A. *et al.* (2004) Epidemiologic profile of symptomatic gastroenteritis in pediatric oncology patients receiving chemotherapy. *Pediatr Blood Cancer*, **42**(4), 338–42.

Emerson, S.U., Arankalle, V.A. & Purcell, R.H. (2005) Thermal stability of hepatitis E virus. *J Infect Dis*, **1**(295), 930–3.

Engelhart, S. *et al*. (2002) Surveillance for nosocomial infections and fever of unknown origin among adult hematology–oncology patients. *Infect Control Hosp Epidemiol*, **23**(5), 244–8.

Errico, A. *et al*. (1999) Survey of measures for the prevention of infection in bone marrow transplantation centers. *Assist Inferm Ric*, **18**(2), 80–6.

European Standard EN 149 (2001) *Respiratory protective devices, filtering half masks to protect against particles. Requirements, testing, marking.* www.bsi-global.com/en/

Evans, B.G. *et al*. (1991) HIV 2 in the United Kingdom. A review. *Commun Dis Rep*, **1**(2), R19–32.

Evans, H.L. *et al*. (2003) Contact isolation in surgical patients: a barrier to care? *Surgery*, **134**(2), 180–8.

Evans, H.S. *et al*. (1998) General outbreaks of infectious intestinal disease in England and Wales, 1995–1996. *Commun Dis Public Health*, **1**(3), 165–71.

Eveillard, M. *et al*. (2001) Evaluation of the contribution of isolation precautions in prevention and control of multi-resistant bacteria in a teaching hospital. *J Hosp Infect*, **47**(2), 116–24.

Eveillard, M. *et al*. (2002) Prevalence of methicillin resistant *Staphylococcus aureus* carriage at the time of admission in two acute geriatric wards. *J Hosp Infect*, **50**(?), 122 6.

Fafi-Kremer, S. *et al* (2005a) A prospective follow-up of Epstein–Barr virus LMP1 genotypes in saliva and blood during infectious mononucleosis. *J Infect Dis*, **192**(12), 2108–11.

Fafi-Kremer, S. *et al*. (2005b) Long-term shedding of infectious Epstein–Barr virus after infectious mononucleosis. *J Infect Dis*, **191**(6), 985–9.

Fairclough, S.J. (2006) Why tackling MRSA needs a comprehensive approach. *Br J Nurs*, **15**(2), 72–5.

Falcone, M. *et al*. (2004) Methicillin-resistant *Staphylococcus* bacteremia in patients with hematologic malignancies: clinical and microbiological retrospective comparative analysis of *S. haemolyticus*, *S epidermidis* and *S Aureus*. *J Chemother*, **16**(6), 540–8.

Farrington M. & Pascoe G. (2001) Risk management and infection control-time to get our priorities right in the United Kingdom. *J Hosp Infect*, **47**(1), 19–24.

Farrington M. *et al*. (2000) Effects on nursing workload of different methicillin-resistant *Staphylococcus aureus* (MRSA) control measures. *J Hosp Infect*, **46**(2), 118–22.

Fawley, W.N. *et al*. (2005) Molecular epidemiology of endemic *Clostridium difficile* significance of subtypes of the United Kingdom Epidemic (Ribotype 1). *J Clin Microbiol*, **43**(6), 2685–96.

Fawley, W.N. *et al*. (2006) Surveillance for mupirocin resistance following introduction of routine peri-operative prophylaxis with nasal mupirocin. *J Hosp Infect*, **62**(3), 327–32.

Felmingham, D. (2004) Comparative antimicrobial susceptibility of respiratory tract. *Chemotherapy*, **50**(Suppl 1), 3–10.

Fields, B.S., Benson, R.F. & Besser, R.E. (2002) *Legionella* and Legionnaires' disease: 25 years of investigation. *Clin Microbiol Rev*, **15**(3), 506–26.

File, T.M. (2006) Clinical implications and treatment of multiresistant *Streptococcus pneumoniae* pneumonia. *Clin Microbiol Infect*, **12**(Suppl 3), 31–41.

Fillet, A.M. (2002) Prophylaxis of herpesvirus infections in immunocompetent and immunocompromised older patients. *Drugs Aging*, **19**(5), 343–54.

Fiore, A.E. (2004) Hepatitis A transmitted by food. *Clin Infect Dis*, **1**(38; 5), 705–15.

Fiore, A.E., Wasley, A. & Bell, B.P. (2006) Prevention of hepatitis A through active or passive immunization: recommendations of the advisory committee on immunization practices (ACIP). *MMWR Recomm Rep*, **55**, RR-701–23.

Fitzpatrick, F. *et al.* (2000) A purpose built MRSA cohort unit. *J Hosp Infect*, **46**(4), 271–9.

Flandre, P. *et al.* (2006) Analyzing plasma HIV-1 RNA measurements as multiple recurrent events in clinical trials. *HIV Clin Trials*, **7**(3), 116–24.

Fleming, K. & Randle, J. (2006) Toys – friend or foe? A study of infection risk in a paediatric intensive care unit. *Paediatr Nurs*, **18**(4), 14–18.

Flessa, S., Lusk, D.M. & Harris, L.J. (2005) Survival of *Listeria monocytogenes* on fresh and frozen strawberries. *Int J Food Microbiol*, **101**(3), 255–62.

Food Standards Agency (2006) *Food Hygiene Legislation*. www.foodstandards.gov.uk

Forns, X. & Bukh, J. (1998) Methods for determining the hepatitis C virus genotype. *Viral Hep Rev*, **4**(1), 1–19.

Fowler, K.B. & Pass, R.F. (2006) Risk factors for congenital cytomegalovirus infection in the offspring of young women: exposure to young children and recent onset of sexual activity. *Pediatrics*, **118**(2), 286–92.

Franca, P.H. *et al.* (2004) Strong association between Genotype F and hepatitis B antigen-negative variants among HBV-infected Argentinians. *J Clin Microbiol*, **42**(11), 5015–21.

Franco, E. *et al.* (2003) Risk groups for hepatitis A virus infection. *Vaccine*, **21**(19–20), 2224–33.

Fraser, D.W. *et al.* (1977) Legionnaires' disease: description of an epidemic of pneumonia. *N Engl J Med*, **297**, 1189–97.

Freije, M.R. (2004) The word of water: new CDC guidelines recommend a proactive approach to *Legionella*. *Health Facil Manage*, **17**(10), 33–4.

French, G.L. (1998) Enterococci and vancomycin resistance. *Clin Infect Dis*, **27**(Suppl 1), S75–83.

Friberg, B. *et al.* (2001) Surgical area contamination comparable bacterial counts using disposable head and mask and helmet aspirator system, but dramatic increase upon omission of head-gear: an experimental study in horizontal laminar air-flow. *J Hosp Infect*, **47**(2), 110–15.

Fryklund, B. *et al.* (1997) Transmission of urinary bacterial strains between patients with indwelling catheters nursing in the same room and in separate rooms compared. *J Hosp Infect*, **36**, 147–53.

Fuda, C. *et al.* (2004) The basis for resistance to beta-lactam antibiotics by penicillin-binding protein 2 a of methicillin-resistant *Staphylococcus aureus*. *J Biol Chem*, **279**(39), 40802–6.

Gaber, K.A. *et al.* (2005) An outbreak of tuberculosis in the South West of England related to a public house. *Prim Care Respir J*, **14**(1), 51–5.

Gal, A.A. *et al.* (2002) Granulomatous *Pneumocystis carnii* pneumonia complicating hematopoietic cell transplantation. *Pathol Res Pract*, **198**(8), 553–8.

Galadari, I. & Fowzan, A.W. (2006) A comparative study between viral isolates and indirect immunofluorescence in diagnosis of herpes simplex virus. *Allerg Immunol*, **38**(2), 62–4.

Gales, C. *et al.* (2006) Emergence of linezolid-resistant *Staphylococcus aureus* during treatment of pulmonary infection in a patient with cystic fibrosis. *Int J Antimicrob Agents*, **27**(4), 300–2.

Gamble, M.J. (2005) Using the modern charter to improve hospital cleaning. *Nurs Times*, **101**(15), 26–7.

Gammon, J. (1999) The psychological consequences of source isolation: a review of the literature. *J Clin Nurs*, **8**(1), 13–21.

Garner, J.S. (1996a) Guidelines for isolation precautions in hospitals. Part 1: evaluation of isolation practices. Hospital Infection Control Practices Advisory Committee. *Am J Infect Control*, **24**(1), 24–31.

Garner, J.S. (1996b) Guidelines for isolation precautions in hospitals. Hospital Infection Control Practices Advisory Committee. *Am J Infect Control*, **17**(1), 53–80.

Garner, J.S. & Simmons, B.P. (1983) CDC guidelines for isolation precautions in hospital. *Infect Control*, **4**(4), 245–325.

Garrouste-Orgeas, M. *et al.* (2000) A 1 year prospective study of nosocomial bacteraemia in ICU and non ICU patients and its impact on patient outcome. *J Hosp Infect*, **44**(3), 206–13.

Gastmeier, P. *et al.* (2005) Mortality risk factors with nosocomial *Staphylococcus aureus* infections in intensive care units: results from the German Nosocomial Infection Surveillance System (KISS). *Infection*, **33**(2), 50–5.

Gastmeier, P. *et al.* (2006) Correlation between genetic diversity of nosocomial pathogens and their survival time in intensive care units. *J Hosp Infect*, **62**(2), 181–6.

Gellaitry, G. *et al.* (2005) Patients' perception of information about HAART: impact on treatment decisions. *AIDS Care*, **17**(3), 367–76.

Gerberding, J.L. (1998) Nosocomial transmission of opportunistic infections. *Infect Control Hosp Epidemiol*, **19**(8), 574–7.

Gezairy, H.A. (2003) Travel epidemiology: WHO perspective. *Int J Antimicrob Agents*, **21**(2), 86–8.

Gheorghe, L. *et al.* (2005) Natural history of compensated viral B and D cirrhosis. *Rom J Gastroenterol*, **14**(4), 329–35.

Gianfranceschi, M. *et al.* (2006) Listeriosis associated with gorgonzola (Italian blue-veined cheese). *Foodborne Pathog Dis*, **3**(2), 105–9.

Gibb, A.P., Fleck, B.W. & Kepton-Smith, L. (2006) A cluster of deep bacterial infections following eye surgery associated with construction dust. *J Hosp Infect*, **63**(2), 197–200.

Gigliotti, F. & Wright, T.W. (2005) Immunopathogenesis of *Pneumocystis carinii* pneumonia. *Exper Rev Mol Med*, **7**(26), 1–16.

Gill, J. *et al.* (2006) Methicillin resistant *Staphylococcus aureus*: awareness and perceptions. *J Hosp Infect*, **62**(3), 333–7.

Gillespie, I.A. *et al.* (2001) General outbreak of infectious intestinal disease associated with fish and shell fish, England and Wales, 1992–1999. *Commun Dis Public Health*, **4**(2), 117–23.

Gillespie, I.A. *et al.* (2005) Foodborne general outbreaks of *Salmonella enteritidis* phage type 4 infection, England and Wales, 1992–2002: where are the risks? *Epidemiol Infect*, **133**(5), 795–801.

Gillespie, I.A. *et al.* (2006) Investigating vomiting and/or bloody diarrhoea in *Campylobacter jejuni* infection. *J Med Microbiol*, **55**(6), 741–6.

Girou, E. *et al.* (2004) Misuse of gloves: the foundation for poor compliance with hand hygiene and potential for microbial transmission. *J Hosp Infect*, **57**(2), 162–9.

Glasmacher, A. & Prentice, A.G. (2005) Evidence-based review of antifungal prophylaxis in neutropenic patients with haematological malignancies. *J Antimicrob Chemother*, 56(Suppl 1), 123–32.

Glauser, M.P. & Calandra, T. (2000) Infections on patients with hematologic malignancies. In: *Management of Infections in Immunocompromised Patients*, Part II, Chapter 4 (eds M.P. Glauser & P.A. Pizzo). W.B. Saunders, London, pp. 141–88.

Goldie, S.J. *et al.* (2002) Prophylaxis for human immunodeficiency virus-related Pneumocystis cariniii pneumonia: using simulation modelling to inform clinical guidelines. *Arch Intern Med*, 162(8), 921–8.

Golec, M. *et al.* (2004) Immunologic reactivity to work-related airborne allergens in people occupationally exposed to dust from herbs. *Ann Agric Environ Med*, 11(1), 121–7.

Gomes, S.A. *et al.* (2004) Uncommon mutation pattern of a hepatitis B virus isolate from genotype F infection a patient with AIDS. *J Infect*, 48(1), 102–8.

Gona, P. *et al.* (2006) Incidence of opportunistic and other infections in HIV-infected children in the HAART era. *JAMA*, 296(3), 292–300.

Gottschalk, S., Roomey, C.M. & Heslop, H.E. (2005) Post-transplant lymphoproliferative disorders. *Annu Rev Med*, 56, 29–44.

Gould, D. (2005) Infection control: the environment and service organisation. *Nurs Stand*, 20(5), 57–65.

Gowland, P. *et al.* (2004) Molecular and serologic tracing of a transfusion-transmitted hepatitis A virus. *Transfusion*, 44(11), 1555–61.

Graczyk, T.K. *et al.* (2004) Mechanical transmission of *Cryptosporidium parvum* oocysts by flies. *Wiad Parazytol*, 50(2), 243–7.

Greub, G., Koh, A. & Calandra, T. (2000) Practical guide to antimicrobial agents commonly used in the immunocompromised patients. In: *Management of Infections in Immunocompromised Patients*, Vol. 2(3), (eds M.P. Glauser & P.A. Pizzo). W.B. Saunders, London, pp. 33–42.

Griffith, C.J. *et al.* (2000) An evaluation of hospital cleaning regimes and standards. *J Hosp Infect*, 45(1), 19–28.

Griffiths, P.D. (2006) CMV as a cofactor enhancing progression of AIDS. *J Clin Virol*, 35(4), 489–92.

Grunfeld, E. *et al.* (2005) Job stress and job satisfaction of cancer care workers. *Psychooncology*, 14(1), 61–9.

Gunsar, F. *et al.* (2005) Two-year interferon therapy with or without ribavirin in chronic delta hepatitis. *Antivir Ther*, 10(6), 721–6.

Hadziyannis, S.J. (1997) Review: hepatitis delta. *J Gastroenterol Hepatol*, 12(4), 289–98.

Hahn, T. *et al.* (2002) Efficacy of high-efficiency particulate air filtration in preventing aspergillosis in immunocompromised patients with hematologic malignancies. *Infection Control Hosp Epidemiol*, 23(9), 525–31.

Hahne, S. *et al.* (2003) Hepatitis B incidence among South Asian children in England and Wales: implications for immunisation policy. *Arch Dis Child*, 88, 1082–3.

Hahne, S. *et al.* (2004) Incidence and routes of transmission of hepatitis B virus in England and Wales, 1995–2000: implications for immunisation policy. *J Clin Virol*, 29(4), 211–20.

Hall, J. & Sutton, A. (2002) Non-HIV nurses knowledge of HIV therapy. *Nurs Stand*, 16(43), 33–6.

Hamid, S.S. *et al.* (2002) Heptitis E virus super infection in patients with chronic liver disease. *Hepatology*, **36**(2), 474–8.

Hansel, N.N. *et al.* (2004) Quality of life in tuberculosis: patient and provider perspectives. *Qual Life Res*, **13**(3), 639–52.

Haque, T. *et al.* (1997) A prospective study in heart and lung transplant recipients correlating persistent Epstein–Barr virus infection with clinical events. *Transplantation*, **64**(7), 1028–34.

Harris, H.E. *et al.* (2000) The HCV national register: towards informing the natural history of hepatitis C infection in the UK. *J Viral Hepat*, **7**(6), 420–7.

Hauggaard, A., Ellis, M. & Ekelund, L. (2002) Early chest radiography and CT in the diagnosis management and outcome of invasive pulmonary aspergillosis. *Acta Radiol*, **43**(3), 292–8.

Hawkyard, C. & Bignardi, G.E. (2006) Has the severity of *Clostridium difficile* infection increased? *J Hosp Infect*, **63**(1), 111–12.

Hayden, M.K. *et al.* (2006) Reduction in acquisition of vancomycin-resistant enterococcus after enforcement of routine environmental cleaning measures. *Clin Infect Dis*, **42**(11), 1552–60.

Hayes-Lattin, B., Leis, J.F. & Maziarz, R.T. (2005) Isolation in the allogeneic transplant environment: how protective is it? *Bone Marrow Transplant*, **36**(5), 373–81.

Haynes, B.F. & Montefiori, D.C. (2006) Aiming to induce broadly reactive neutralizing antibody responses with HIV-1 vaccine candidates. *Expert Rev Vaccines*, **5**(3), 347–63.

He, Z. *et al.* (2003) Retrospective analysis of non-A–E hepatitis: possible role of hepatitis B and C virus infection. *J Med Virol*, **69**(1), 59–65.

Healing, T.D. *et al.* (1995) The infection hazards of human cadavers. *Commun Dis Rep*, **5**, R61–9.

Health Protection Agency (2006) www.hpa.org.uk. Accessed 26/11/06.

Heinonen, H. *et al.* (2005) Stress among allogeneic bone marrow transplantation patients. *Patient Educ Couns*, **56**(1), 62–71.

Heldal, E. *et al.* (2003) Risk factors for recent transmission of *Mycobacterium tuberculosis*. *Eur Respir J*, **22**(4), 637–42.

Hemsworth, S. & Pizer, B. (2006) Pet ownership in immunocompromised children – a review of the literature and survey of existing guidelines. *Eur J Oncol Nurs*, **10**(2), 117–27.

Henderson, D.K. (2006) Managing methicillin-resistant staphylococci: a paradigm for preventing nosocomial transmission of resistant organisms. *Am J Infect Control*, **34**(5 Suppl), S46–54.

Henry, L. (1997) Immunocompromised patients and nutrition. *Prof Nurse*, **12**(9), 655–9.

Hewitt, J. & Greening, G.E. (2004) Survival and persistence of norovirus, hepatitis A virus, and feline calicivirus in marinated mussels. *J Food Prot*, **67**(8), 1743–50.

Highleyman, L. (2006) Nutrition and HIV. *BETA*, **18**(2), 18–32.

Hill, C., King, T. & Day, R. (2006) A strategy to reduce MRSA colonization of stethoscopes. *J Hosp Infect*, **62**(1), 122–3.

Hill, G. *et al.* (2005) Recent steroid therapy increases severity of varicella infections in children with acute lymphoblastic leukemia. *Pediatrics*, **116**(4), 525–9.

Ho, E.C., Patriar, S. & Corbridge, R. (2005) How we do it: blood contamination during management of epistaxis-awareness, utilization and availability of barrier protection. *Clin Otolaryngol*, **30**(1), 71–2.

182

Hodgson, I. (2006) Empathy, inclusion and enclaves: the culture of care of people with HIV/AIDS and nursing implications. *J Adv Nurs*, **55**(3), 283–90.

Hogg, R.S. *et al.* (2006) Emergence of drug resistance is associated with an increase risk of death among patients first starting HAART. *PLoS Med*, **3**(19), 1–18.

Hohenthal, U. *et al.* (2005) Bronchoalveolar lavage in immunocompromised patients with haematological malignancy-value of new microbiological methods. *Eur J Haematol*, **74**(3), 203–11.

Holmes, R.D. & Sokol, R.J. (2002) Epstein–Barr virus and post-transplant lymphoproliferative disease. *Pediatr Transplant*, **6**(6), 456–64.

Horng, Y.T. *et al.* (2006) Development of an improved PCR–ICT hybrid assay for direct detection of *Legionellae* and *Legionella pneumophila* from cooling tower water specimens. *Water Res*, **40**(11), 2219–21.

Hota, B. (2004) Contamination, disinfection and cross-colonization: are hospital surfaces reservoirs for nosocomial infection. *Clin Infect Dis*, **39**(8), 1182–9.

HSE (2000) *Legionnaires' Disease*. Health and Safety Executive, London.

HSE (2002) *Control of Substances Hazardous to Health (COSHH) Approved Code of Practice*. Health and Safety Executive, London.

HSE (2003a) *Five Steps to Risk Assessment*. Health and Safety Executive, London.

HSE (2003b) *Safe Working and the Prevention of Infection in Clinical laboratories and Similar Facilities*. Health and Safety Executive, London.

HSE (2005a) *Blood-borne Viruses in the Workplace. Guidance for Employers and Employees*. Health and Safety Executive, London.

HSE (2005b) *European Working Party for Legionella Infection*. Health and Safety Executive, London.

Hsu, Y.S. *et al.* (2002) Long term outcome after spontaneous HbeAg seroconversion in patients with chronic hepatitis B. *Hepatology*, **35**(6), 1522–57.

Huber, M.A. (2003) Herpes simplex type-1 virus infection. *Quintessence Int*, **34**(6), 453–67.

Humphreys, H. (2004) Positive-pressure isolation and the prevention of invasive aspergillosis. What is the evidence? *J Hosp Infect*, **56**(2), 93–100.

Humphreys, H. (2005) On the wrong scent: banning fresh flowers from hospitals. *J Hosp Infect*, **62**(94), 527–8.

Humphreys, H. (2006) Implementing guidelines for the control of methicillin-resistant *Staphylococcus aureus* and vancomycin-resistant enterococci: how valid are international comparisons of success? *J Hosp Infect*, **62**(2), 133–5.

Hunter, P.R. & Syed, Q. (2002) A community survey of self-reported gastroenteritis undertaken during an outbreak of cryptosporidiosis strongly associated with drinking water after much press interest. *Epidemiol Infect*, **128**(3), 433–8.

Hunter, P.R. & Thompson, R.C. (2005) The zoonotic transmission of *Giardia* and *Cryptosporidium*. *Int J Parasitol*, **35**(11–12), 1181–90.

Husa, P. *et al.* (2005) Hepatitis D. *Acta Viron*, **49**(4), 219–25.

ILSI Research Foundation; Risk Science Institute (2005) Achieving continuous improvement in reductions in foodborne listeriosis – a risk-based approach. *J Food Prot*, **68**(9), 1032–94.

Insulander, M. *et al.* (2005) An outbreak of cryptosporidiosis associated with exposure to swimming pool water. *Scand J Infect Dis*, **37**(5), 354–60.

183

Irshad, M. (1997) Hepatitis E virus: a global view of its seroepidemiology and transmission pattern. *Trop Gastroenterol*, **18**(2), 45–9.

Irshad, M. *et al.* (2006) Transfusion-transmitted virus in associated with hepatitis A–E viral infections in various forms of liver diseases in India. *World J Gastroenterol*, **12**(15), 2432–6.

Jabs, D.A. *et al.* (2006) Detection of ganciclovir resistance in patients with AIDS and cytomegalovirus retinitis: correlation of genotypic methods and viral phenotypes and clinical outcome. *J Infect Dis*, **193**(12), 1728–37.

Jardi, R. *et al.* (2001) Quantitative detection of hepatitis B virus DNA in serum by a new rapid real-time fluorescence PCR assay. *J Viral Hepat*, **8**(6), 465–71.

Jarrett, R.F. (2006) Viruses and lymphoma/leukaemia. *J Pathol*, **208**(2), 176–86.

Jarrett, W.A., Ribes, J. & Manaligot, J.M. (2002) Biofilm formation on tracheostomy tubes. *Ear Nose Throat J*, **81**(9), 659–61.

Jarvis, L.M. *et al.* (2006) Detection of HCV and HIV-1 antibody negative infections in Scottish and Northern Ireland blood donations by nucleic acid amplification testing. *Vox Sang*, **89**(3), 128–34.

Jayshree, R.S. *et al.* (2006) Microscopic, cultural and molecular evidence of disseminated invasive aspergillosis involving the lungs and the gastrointestinal tract. *J Med Microbiol*, **55**(Pt 7), 961–4.

Jenkins, R.O. & Sherburn, R.E. (2005) Growth and survival of bacteria implemented in sudden infant death syndrome on cot mattress material. *J Appl Microbiol*, **99**(3), 573–9.

Jevons, M.P. (1961) Celberin resistant staphylococci. *Br Med J*, **1**, 124–5.

Jindal, N. *et al.* (2005) HIV-1 infection in early seroconversion stage missed by rapid or ELISA tests – two case reports. *Indian J Pathol Microbiol*, **48**(3), 395–6.

Johnson, E. *et al.* (2000) Preventing fungal infections in immunocompromised patients. *Br J Nurs*, **9**(17), 1154–64.

Johnson, P.D. *et al.* (2005) Efficacy of an alcoholic/chlorhexidine hand hygiene program in a hospital with high rates of nosocomial methicillin resistant *Staphylococcus aureus* (MRSA) infection. *Med J Aust*, **183**(10), 509–14.

Jones, R.N. (2001) Resistance patterns among nosocomial pathogens: trends over the past few years. *Chest*, **119**(2 Suppl), S397–404.

Kac, G. *et al.* (2005) Microbiological evaluation of two hand hygiene procedures achieved by healthcare workers during routine patients care: a randomized study. *J Hosp Infect*, **60**(1), 32–9.

Kao, P.H. & Yang, R.J. (2006) Virus diffusion in isolation rooms. *H Hosp Infect*, **62**(3), 338–45.

Kawamura, M. *et al.* (1989) HIV 2 in West Africa in 1966. *Lancet*, **i**, (8634), 385.

Kato, H. *et al.* (2001) Determination of hepatitis B virus genotype G by polymerase chain reaction with hemi-nested primers. *J Virol Methods*, **98**(2), 153–9.

Kato, H. *et al.* (2002) Hepatitis B e antigen in sera from individuals infected with hepatitis B virus of genotype G. *Hepatology*, **35**(4), 922–9.

Kato, H. *et al.* (2005) Classifying genotype F of hepataitis B virus into F1 and F2 subtypes. *World J Gastroenterol*, **11**(40), 6295–304.

Kearnes, A.M., Freeman, R. & Lightfoot, N.F. (1995) Nosocomial enterococci; resistance to heat and sodium hypochlorite. *J Hosp Infect*, **30**, 193–9.

Kedzierski, M. (1991) Understanding virology. *Prof Nurse*, **7**(2), 99–102.

Kemp, C. & Stepp, L. (1995) Palliative care for patients with acquired immunodeficiency syndrome. *Am J Hosp Palliat Care*, **12**(6), **14**, 17–27.

Kempinska, A.M., Kwak, E.J. & Angel, J.B. (2005) Reactivation of hepatitis B infection following allogeneic bone marrow transplantation in a hepatitis B-immune patient: case report and review of the literature. *Clin Infect Dis*, **41**(9), 1277–82.

Keogh, I.J. *et al.* (2001) Blood splash and tonsillectomy: an underestimated hazard to the otolaryngologist. *J Laryngol Otol*, **115**(6), 455–6.

Kiang, K.M. *et al.* (2006) Recurrent outbreaks of cryptosporidiosis associated with calves among students at an educational farm programme in Minnesota. *Epidemiol Infect*, **134**(4), 878–86.

Kibbler, C.C., Quick, A. & O'Neil, A.M. (1998) The effect of increased bed numbers on MRSA transmission in acute medical wards. *J Hosp Infect*, **39**, 213–19.

Kim, P.W. *et al.* (2003) Rates of hand disinfection associated with glove use, patient isolation and changes between exposure to various body sites. *Am J Infect Control*, **31**(2), 97–103.

Kimberlin, D.W. (2005) Herpes simplex virus infections in neonates and early childhood. *Semin Pediatr Infect Dis*, **16**(4), 271–81.

King, D. (2001) Ice machines – an audit of their use in clinical practice. *Commun Dis Public Health*, **4**(1), 49–52.

Kirkup, B. (2002) Incident arising in October 2002 from a patient with Creutzfeldt–Jakob disease in Middlesbrough. Report of incident review. www.dh.gov.uk. Accessed 25/11/06.

Klassen, T.P. *et al.* (2005) Acyclovir for treating varicella in otherwise healthy children and adolescents. *Cochrane Database Syst Rev*, **4**, CD002980.

Klein, G., Pack, A. & Reuter, G. (1998) Antibiotic resistance patterns of enterococci and occurrence of vancomycin-resistant enterococci in raw minced beef and pork in Germany. *Appl Environ Microbiol*, **64**(5), 1825–30.

Klastersky, J. (2004) Management of fever in neutropenic patients with different risks of complications. *Clin Infect Dis*, **39**(Suppl 1), S32–7.

Kleymann, G. (2003) Novel agents and strategies to treat herpes simplex virus infections. *Expert Opin Investig Drugs*, **12**(2), 165–83.

Klont, R.R. *et al.* (2006) *Legionella pneumophilia* in commercial bottles water. *FEMS Immunol Med Microbiol*, **47**(1), 42–4.

Knauer, A. *et al.* (2004) Effect of hospitalization and antimicrobial therapy on antimicrobial resistance of colonizing *Staphylococcus epidermidis*. *Wien Klin Wochenschr*, **116**(14), 489–94.

Knysz, B. *et al.* (2005) Hepatitis D virus superinfection – a rare cause of occupational disease. *Med Pr*, **56**(4), 317–18.

Koopmans, M. & Duizer, E. (2004) Food borne viruses: an emerging problem. *Int J Food Microbiol*, **90**(1), 23–41.

Korniewicz, D.M. *et al.* (2005) Impact of converting to powder-free gloves. Decreasing the symptoms of latex exposure in operating room personnel. *AAOHN J*, **53**(3), 111–16.

Koss, K. *et al.* (2006) The outcome of surgery in fulminant *Clostridium difficile* colitis. *Colorectal Dis*, **8**(2), 149–54.

Krasuska, M.E. & Stanislawek, A. (2003) Communication with patients and their families, who undergo bone marrow transplantation. *Ann Univ Mariae Curie Sklodowska*, **58**(2), 168–73.

Krasuska, M.E. *et al.* (2002) Information needs of the patients undergoing bone marrow transplantation. *Ann Univ Mariae Curie Sklodowska*, **57**(2), 178–85.

Kriesel J.D. *et al.* (2005) Recurrent antiviral-resistant genital herpes in an immunocompetent patient. *J Infect Dis*, **192**(1), 156–61.

Kruger, W.H. *et al.* (2001) Practices of infectious disease prevention and management during hematopoietic stem cell transplantation: a survey from the European group for blood and marrow transplantation. *J Hematother Stem Cell Res*, **10**(60), 895–903.

Kuderer, N.M. *et al.* (2006) Mortality, morbidity, and cost associated with febrile neutropenia in adult cancer patients. *Cancer*, **106**(10), 2258–66.

Kuehn, B.M. (2006) UNAIDS report. AIDS epidemic slowing but huge challenges remain. *JAMA*, **296**(1), 29–30.

Kumar, R.M. *et al.* 2001. Sero-prevalence and mother-to-infant transmission of hepatitis E virus among pregnant women in the United Arab Emirates. *Eur J Obstet Gynecol Reprod Biol*, **100**(1), 9–15.

Kusne, S. & Krystofiak, S. (2001) Infection control issues after bone marrow transplantation. *Curr Opin Infect Dis*, **14**(4), 427– 31.

Kuzu, N. *et al.* (2005) Compliance with hand hygiene and glove use in university-affiliated hospital. *Infect Control Hosp Epidemiol*, **26**(3), 312–15.

Kyrlagkitsis, I, *et al.* (2002) Acute hepatitis A virus infection: a review of prognostic factors from 25 years experience in a tertiary referral center. *Hepatogastroenterology*, **49**(44), 524–8.

Lam, P.K. *et al.* (2006) Factors related to response to intermittent treatment of *Mycobacterium avium* complex lung disease. *Am J Respir Crit Care Med*, **173**(11), 1283–9.

Lanari, M. *et al.* (2006) Neonatal cytomegalovirus blood load and risk of sequelae in symptomatic and asymptomatic congenitally infected newborns. *Pediatrics*, **117**(1), 76–83.

Landman, Q. *et al.* (2002) City-wide clonal outbreak of multiresistant *Acinetobacter baumannii* and *Pseudomonas aerginosa* in Brooklyn NY. *Arch Intern Med*, **162**(13), 1515–20.

Larson, E. & Nirenberg, A. (2004) Evidence-based nursing practice to prevent infection in hospitalized neutropenic patients with cancer. *Oncol Nurs Forum*, **31**(4), 717–24.

Larson, J.L. *et al.* (2003) Potential nosocomial exposure to *Mycobacterium tuberculosis* from a bronchoscope. *Infect Control Hosp Epidemiol*, **24**(11), 825–30.

Laupland, K.B. *et al.* (2006) Cost of intensive care unit-acquired bloodstream infections. *J Hosp Infect*, **63**(2), 124–32.

Lavanchy, D. (2004) Hepatitis B virus epidemiology, disease burden, treatment, and current and emerging prevention and control measures. *J Viral Hepat*, **11**(2), 97–107.

Laws, H.J. *et al.* (2006) Surveillance of nosocomial infections in paediatric recipients of bone marrow or peripheral blood stem cell transplantation during neutropenia, compared with adult recipients. *J Hosp Infect*, **62**(1), 80–8.

Lee, J.V. *et al.* (2002) Guidelines for investigating single cases of Legionnaires' disease. *Commun Dis Public Health*, **5**(2), 157–62.

Lefebvre, B. *et al.* (2006) Growth performance and shedding of some pathogenic bacteria in feedlot cattle treated with different growth-promoting agents. *J Food Prot*, **69**(6), 1256–64.

Lefebvre, S.L. *et al.* (2006) Prevalence of zoonotic agents in dogs visiting hospitalized people in Ontario: implications for infection control. *J Hosp Infect*, **62**(3), 458–66.

Lehto, J.T. *et al.* (2005) Bronchoscopy in the diagnosis and surveillance of respiratory infections in lung and heart–lung transplant recipients. *Transpl Int*, **18**(5), 562–71.

Lemos, A.A. *et al.* (2006) Cockroaches as carriers of fungi of medical importance. *Mycoses*, **49**(1), 23–5.

Lettinga, K.D. *et al.* (2002) Legionnaires disease at a Dutch flower show: prognostic factors and impact of therapy. *Emerg Infect Dis*, **8**(12), 1448–54.

Leung, A.K., Kellner, J.D. & Davies, H.D. (2005) Hepatitis A: a preventable threat. *Adv Ther*, **22**(6), 578–86.

Leuthner, K.D., Cheung, C.M. & Rybak, M.J. (2006) Comparative activity of the new lipoglycopeptide telavancin in the presence and absence of serum against 50 glycopeptide non-susceptible staphylococci and three vancomycin-resistant *Staphylococcus aureus*. *J Antimicrob Chemother*, **58**(2), 338–43.

Levine, A.S., Siegal, S.E. & Schrieber, A.D. (1973) Protected environment and prophylactic antibiotics. A perspective controlled study of their utility in the therapy of acute leukaemia. *N Engl J Med*, **288**, 477–83.

Lewis, A.M. & Martin, R.C. (2006) The treatment of hepatic metastases in colorectal carcinoma. *Am Surg*, **72**(6), 466–73.

Lewis, H. *et al.* (2006) Indigenous hepatitis E virus infection in England and Wales. *BMJ*, **332**, 1509–10.

Li, J. *et al.* (2006a) Epidemiology of hepatitis B, C, D and G viruses and cytokine levels among intravenous drug users. *J Huazhong Univ Sci Technolog Med Sci*, **26**(2), 221–4.

Li, J. *et al.* (2006b) *Pneumocystis carinii* pneumonia in patients with connective tissue disease. *Clin Rheumatol*, **12**(3), 114–17.

Li, Y. *et al.* (2002) Mild heat treatment of lettuce enhances growth of *Listeria monocytogenes* during subsequent storage at 5°C or 15°C. *J Appl Microbiol*, **92**(2), 269–75.

Liljestrand, P. (2004) HIV care: continuing medical education and consultation needs of nurses, physicians and pharmacists. *J Assoc Nurses AIDS Care*, **15**(2), 38–50.

Limaye, A.P. *et al.* (2006) Impact of cytomegalovirus in organ transplant recipients in the era of antiviral prophylaxis. *Transplantation*, **81**(12), 1645–52.

Lin, C.C. *et al.* (2000) Diagnostic value of immunoglobulin G (IgG) and IgM anti-hepatitis E virus (HEV) tests based on HEV RNA in an area where hepatitis E is not endemic. *J Clin Microbiol*, **38**(11), 3915–18.

Lin, Y.C. *et al.* (2006) Clinical characteristics and risk factors for attributable mortality in *Enterobacter cloacae* bacteremia. *J Microbiol Immunol Infect*, **39**(1), 67–72.

Lines, L. (2006) A study of senior nurses perception about MRSA. *Nurs Times*, **102**(15), 32–5.

Lionakis, M.S. *et al.* (2005) *Aspergillus* susceptibility testing in patients with cancer and invasive aspergillosis: difficulties in establishing correlation between *in vitro* susceptibility data and the outcome of initial amphotericin B therapy. *Pharmacotherapy*, **25**(9), 1174–80.

Lipp, A. & Edwards, P. (2002) Disposable surgical face masks for preventing surgical wound infection in clean surgery. *Cochrane Database Syst Rev*, **1**, CD002929.

Lipp, A. & Edwards, P. (2005) Disposable surgical masks: a systematic review. *Can Oper Room Nurs J*, **23**(3), 20–1.

Loach, L. (1997) Blue days. *Nurs Times*, **93**(32), 31–2.

Loens, K. *et al.* (2006) Development of conventional and real-time NASBA® for the detection of *Legionella* species in respiratory specimens. *J Microbiol Methods*, **67**(3), 408–15.

Loh, W., Ng, V.V. & Holton, J. (2000) Bacterial flora on the white coats of medical students. *J Hosp Infect*, **45**(1), 65–8.

Longerich, T. *et al.* (2005) Recurrent herpes simplex virus hepatitis after liver retransplantation despite acyclovir therapy. *Liver Transpl*, **11**(10), 1289–94.

Lucet, J.C. *et al.* (2005) Successsful long term program for controlling methicillin-resistant *Staphylococcus aureus* in intensive care units. *Intensive Care Med*, **31**(8), 1051–7.

Lugauskas, A., Repeckiene, J. & Novosinskas, H. (2005) Micromycetes, producers of toxins, detected on stored vegetables. *Ann Agric Environ Med*, **12**(2), 253–60.

Luzuriaga, K. *et al.* (2006) Vaccines to prevent transmission of HIV-1 via breast milk: scientific and logistical priorities. *Lancet*, **368**(9534), 511–21.

MacKellar, D.A. *et al.* (2005) Unrecognized HIV infection, risk behaviors, and perceptions of risk among young men who have sex with men: opportunities for advancing HIV prevention in the third decade of HIV/AIDS. *J Acquir Immune Defic Syndr*, **38**(5), 603–14.

MacKinnon, M.M. & Allen, K.D. (2000) Long-term MRSA carriage in hospital patients. *J Infect Control*, **46**(3), 216–21.

Madeo, M (2003) The psychological impact of isolation. *Nurs Times*, **99**(7), 54–5.

Maertens, J. & Boogaerts, M. (2005) The place for itraconazole in treatment. *J Antimicrob Chemother*, **56**(Suppl 1), i33–8.

Maertens, J., Vrebos, M. & Boogaerts, M. (2001) Assessing risk factors for systemic fungal infections. *Eur J Cancer Care (Engl)*, **10**(1), 56–62.

Maguire, H. *et al.* (2001) Hospital outbreak of *Salmonella virchow* possibly associated with a food handler. *J Hosp Infect*, **44**(4), 261–6.

Mahan, S.S. *et al.* (2006) Lack of value of repeat stool testing for *Clostridium difficile* toxin. *Am J Med*, **119**(4), 356–8.

Malik, Y.S. *et al.* (2006) Disinfection of fabrics and carpets artificially contaminated with calicivirus: relevance in institutional and healthcare centres. *J Hosp Infect*, **63**(2), 205–10.

Maloney, B.J. *et al.* (2005) Challenges in creating a vaccine to prevent hepatitis E. *Vaccine*, **23**(15), 1870–4.

Manfredi, R., Calza, L. & Chiodo, F. (2006) Primary cytomegalovirius infection in otherwise healthy adults with fever of unknown origin: a 3-year prospective survey. *Infection*, **34**(2), 87–90.

Mangili, A. & Gendreau, M.A. (2005) Transmission of infectious diseases during commercial air travel. *Lancet*, **365**(9463), 989–96.

Manian, F.A. (2003) Vascular and cardiac infections in end-stage renal disease. *Am J Med Sci*, **325**(4), 243–50.

Mank, A. *et al.* (2003) Is there still an indication for nursing patients with prolonged neutropenia in protective isolation? An evidence based nursing and medical study of 4 years experience for nursing patients with neutropenia without isolation. *Eur J Oncol Nurs*, **7**(1), 17–23.

Marr, K.A. *et al.* (2002) Invasive aspergillosis in allogenic stem cell transplant recipients: change in epidemiology and risk factors. *Blood*, **100**(13), 4358–66.

Marra, C.A. *et al.* (2004) Factors influencing quality of life in patients with active tuberculosis. *Health Qual Life Outcomes*, **2**, 58.

Marras, T.K. *et al.* (2002) Aerosolized pentamindine prophylaxis for *Pneumocystis carinii* pneumonia after allogeneic marrow transplantation. *Transpl Infect Dis*, **4**(2), 66–74.

Marriott, H.M. & Dockrell, D.H. (2006) *Streptococcus pneumoniae*: the role of apoptosis in host defense and pathogenesis. *Int J Biochem Cell Biol*, **38**(11), 1848–54.

Marrs, J.A. (2006) Care of patients with neutropenia. *Clin J Oncol Nurs*, **10**(2), 164–6.

Martin, A. & Lemon, S.M. (2006) Hepatitis A virus: from discovery to vaccines. *Hepatology*, **43**(2 Suppl 1), S164–72.

Martinez, J.A. *et al.* (2003) Role of environmental contamination as a risk factor for acquisition of vancomycin-resistant enterococci in patients treated in a medical intensive care unit. *Arch Intern Med*, **163**(16), 1905–12.

Marx, P.A. *et al.* (2004) AIDS as a zoonosis? Confusion over the origin of the virus and the origin of the epidemics. *J Med Primatol*, **33**(5-6), 220–6.

Masterton, R.G. & Teare, E.L. (2001) Clinical governance and infection control in the United Kingdom. *J Hosp Infect*, **47**(1), 25–31.

Maunder, R. *et al.* (2003) The immediate psychological and occupational impact of the 2003 SARS outbreak in a teaching hospital. *CMAJ*, **168**(10), 1245–51.

May, M.T. *et al.* (2006) HIV treatment response and prognosis in Europe and North America in the first decade of highly active antiretroviral therapy: a collaborative analysis. *Lancet*, **368**(9534), 451–8.

Mayer, R.A. *et al.* (2003) Role of fecal incontinence in contamination of the environment with vancomycin-resistant enterococci. *Am J Infect Control*, **31**(4), 221–5.

McCarthy, G.M. *et al.* (2002) Transmission of HIV in the dental clinic and elsewhere. *Oral Dis*, **8**(Suppl 2), 126–35.

McDonald, L.C. *et al.* (2005) An epidemic toxic gene variant strain of *Clostridium difficile*. *N Eng J Med*, **353**(23), 2433–41.

McEvoy, S.P. *et al.* (2006) Risk factors for the acquisition of vancomycin-resistant enterococci during a single-strain outbreak at a major Australian teaching hospital. *J Hosp Infect*, **62**(2), 256–8.

McGowan, J.E. (2006) Resistance in nonfermenting gram-negative bacteria: multidrug resistance to the maximum. *Am J Infect Control*, **34**(5)(Suppl 1), S29–37.

McGuckin, M. *et al.* (2004) Evaluation of a patient education model for increasing hand hygiene compliance in an inpatient rehabilitation unit. *Am J Infect Control*, **32**(4), 235–8.

McMichael, A.J. (2006) HIV vaccines. *Annu Rev Immunol*, **24**, 227–55.

McMillan, A. (2005) Hepatitis B vaccination of men who have sex with men: experience with an accelerated course of vaccination in a genitourinary medicine clinic. *Int J STD AIDS*, **16**(9), 633–5.

McNeil, S.A., Mody, L. & Bradley, S.F. (2002) Methicillin-resistant *Staphylococcus aureus*. Management of asymptomatic colonization and outbreaks of infection in long-term care. *Geriatrics*, **57**(6), 16–27.

McPherson, S. *et al.* (2006) Intravenous immunoglobulin for the treatment of severe refractory and recurrent *Clostridium difficile* diarrhea. *Dis Colon Rectum*, **49**(5), 640–5.

MDA (1996) *Latex Sensitisation in the Health Care Setting*. Department of Health, London.

MDA (1998) *Latex Medical Gloves*. Department of Health, London.

MDA (2002) *Sterilization, Disinfection and Cleaning of Medical Equipment*. Department of Health, London.

Medland, J., Howard-Ruben, J. & Whitaker, E. (2004) Fostering psychosocial wellness in oncology nurses. Addressing burnout and social support in the workplace. *Oncol Nurs Forum*, **31**(1), 47–54.

Meers, P.D. & Matthews, R.B. (1978) Multiple-resistant pneumococcus. *Lancet*, **2**(8082), 219.

Meier, J. & Lopez, L. (2001) Listeriosis: an emerging food-borne disease. *Clin Lab Sci*, **14**(3), 187–92.

Meldrum, R.J. *et al.* (2005) Survey of *Salmonella* and *Campylobacter* of whole raw poultry in sales in Wales in 2003. *J Food Prot*, **68**(7), 1447–9.

Meyer, I.D. (1986) Infection in bone marrow transplant recipients. *Am J Med*, **81**, 27–8.

Miguez-Burbano, M.J. *et al.* (2006) Non-tuberculous mycobacteria disease as a cause of hospitalization in HIV-infected subjects. *Int J Infect Dis*, **10**(1), 47–55.

Mims, C.A. *et al.* (2004) *Medical Microbiology*, 3rd edn. Mosby, London.

Miyakoshi, K. *et al.* (1998) Prenatal ultrasound diagnosis of small bowel torsion. *Obstet Gynecol*, **91**(5, Part 2), 802–3.

Mock, V. & Olsen, M. (2003) Current management of fatigue and anemia in patients with cancer. *Semin Oncol Nurs*, **19**(4 Suppl 2), 36–41.

Mohamed, M.K. *et al.* (2006) Transmission of hepatitis C virus between parents and children. *Am J Trop Med Hyg*, **75**(1), 16–20.

Mohan, S.S. *et al.* (2006) Lack of value of repeat stool testing for *Clostridium difficile*. *Am J Med*, **119**(4), 356–8.

Monsen, T., Karisson, C. & Wistrom, J. (2005) Spread of clones of multidrug-resistant coagulase negative staphylococcus within a university hospital. *Infect Control Hosp Epidemiol*, **26**(1), 76–80.

Monso, E. (2004) Occupational asthma in greenhouse workers. *Curr Opin Pulm Med*, **10**(2), 147–50.

Moody, K. *et al.* (2006) Feasibility and safety of a pilot randomized trial of infection rate: neutropenic diet versus standard food safety guidelines. *J Pediatr Hematol Oncol*, **28**(3), 126–33.

Morris, K. *et al.* (2005) First HIV 'window period' donation in a UK blood donor. *Transfus Med*, **15**(3), 249–50.

Morris-Cunnington, M.C. *et al.* (2004) A population-based seroprevalence study of hepatitis A virus using oral fluid in England and Wales. *Am J Epidemiol*, **159**(8), 786–94.

Navon-Venezia, S., Ben-Ami, R. & Carmeli, Y. (2005) Update on *Pseudomonas aerginosa* and *Acinetobacter baumannii* infection in the healthcare setting. *Curr Opin Infect Dis*, **18**(4), 306–13.

Nazzaro, A.M. *et al.* (2006) Knowledge, attitudes, and behaviours of youths in the US hemophilia population: results of a national survey. *Am J Public Health*, **96**(9), 1618–22.

Neely, A.N. & Maley, M.P. (2000) Survival of enterococci and staphylococci on hospital fabrics and plastic. *J Clin Microbiol*, **38**(1), 724–6.

Neuberger, P. *et al.* (2006) Case-control study of symptoms and neonatal outcome of human milk-transmitted cytomegalovirus infection in premature infants. *J Pediatr*, **148**(3), 326–31.

Neville, K., Renbarger, J. & Dreyer, Z. (2002) Pneumonia in the immunocompromised pediatric cancer patient. *Semin Respir Infect*, **17**(1), 21–32.

Newman, K., Maylor, U. & Chansarkar, B. (2002) The nurse satisfaction, service quality and nurse retention chain: implications for management of recruitment and retention. *J Manage Med*, 16(4–5), 271–91.

Newton, J.T., Constable, D. & Senior, V. (2001) Patients perceptions of methicillin-resistant *Staphylococcus aureus* and source isolation: a qualitative analysis of source-isolated patients. *J Hosp Infect*, 48(4), 275–80.

Nguyen, D.M., Mascola, L. & Brancoft, E. (2005) Recurring methicillin-resistant *Staphylococcus aureus* in a football team. *Emerg Infect Dis*, 11(4), 526–32.

NHS Estates (2002) *Infection Control in the Built Environment. Design and Planning.* HMSO, Norwich.

NHS Estates (2005) *Ward Layouts with Single Rooms and Space for Flexibility.* National Health Service Estates, Leeds.

NHS Executive (NHSE) (1994) *The control of Legionellae in Health Care Premises*, Health Technical Memorandum 2040, Code of Practice NHS Estates. HMSO, London.

NHS Executive (NHSE) (1995) *Hospital Infection Control: Guidance on the Control of Infection in Hospitals.* HSG (95) 10 1995. HMSO, London.

NHS Executive (NHSE) (1999a) *Latex Medical Gloves and Powdered Latex Medical Gloves.* Department of Health, London.

NHS Executive (NHSE) (1999b) *Variant Creutzfeldt–Jakob Disease (vCJD). Minimising the Risk of Transmission.* Department of Health, London.

NICE (2003) *Infection control. Prevention of healthcare-associated infection in primary and community care.* National Institute for Health and Clinical Excellence, London.

NICE (2006) *Tuberculosis.* National Institute for Health and Clinical Excellence, London.

Niro, G.A. *et al.* (2005) Lamivudine therapy in chronic delta hepatitis: a multicentre randomized-controlled pilot study. *Aliment Pharmacol Ther*, 22(3), 227–32.

Nishijima, S. & Kurikawa, I. (2002) Antimicrobial resistance of *Staphylococcus aureus* isolated from skin infections. *Int J Antimicrob Agents*, 19(3), 241–3.

NMC (2005) *Guidelines for Records and Record Keeping.* Nursing and Midwifery Council, London.

NMC (2006) *A–Z Advice Sheet Consent.* www.nmc.org.

Norgard, B. *et al.* (2006) Maternal herpes labialis in pregnancy and neural tube defects. *Dev Med Child Neurol*, 48(8), 674–6.

Nosari, A. *et al.* (2001) Invasive aspergillosis in haematological malignancies: clinical findings and management for intensive chemotherapy completion. *Am J Hematol*, 68(4), 231–6.

Noskin, G.A. *et al.* (1995) Recovery of vancomycin-resistant enterococci on fingertips and environmental surfaces. *Infect Control Hosp Epidemiol*, 16(10), 577–81.

Novak, J. & Katz, J.A. (2006) Probiotics and prebiotics for gastrointestinal infections. *Curr Infect Dis Rep*, 8(2), 103–9.

Nozzoli, C. *et al.* (2006) Epstein–Barr virus-associated post-transplant lymphoproliferative disease with central nervous system involvement after unrelated allogeneic hematopoietic stem cell transplantation. *Leuk Lymphoma*, 47(1), 167–9.

Nyiri, P. *et al.* (2004) Sharps discarded in inner city parks and play grounds—risk of blood-borne virus exposure. *Commun Dis Public Health*, 7(4), 287–8.

Oie, S., Hosokawa, I. & Kamiya, A. (2002) Contamination of room door handles by methicillin resistant *Staphylococcus aureus*. *J Hosp Infect*, 51(2), 140–3.

Oldfield, E.C. (2006) *Clostridium difficile*-associated diarrhea: resurgence with a vengeance. *Rev Gastroenterol Disord*, **6**(2), 79–96.

Oldman, T. (1998) Isolated cases. *Nurs Times*, **94**(11), 67–71.

Oncu, S. *et al.* (2006) Prevalence and risk factors for HEV infection in pregnant women. *Med Sci Monit*, **12**(1), CR36–9.

O'Neill, E. & Humphreys, H. (2005) Surveillance of hospital water and primary prevention of nosocomial legionellosis: what is the evidence? *J Hosp Infect*, **59**(4), 273–9.

O'Neill, J. & Buttery, J. (2003) Varicella and paediatric staff: current practice and vaccine cost-effectiveness. *J Hosp Infect*, **53**(2), 117–19.

Ormerod, L.D. *et al.* (1998) Rapidly progressive herpetic retinal necrosis: a blinding disease characteristic of advanced AIDS. *Clin Infect Dis*, **26**(1), 34–45.

Ormerod, L.P. (1996) Tuberculosis and immigration. *Br J Hosp Med*, **56**(5), 209–12.

Ornoy, A. & Diav-Citrin, O. (2006) Fetal effects of primary and secondary cytomegalovirus infection in pregnancy. *Reprod Toxicol*, **21**(4), 399–409.

Ozerol, I.H. *et al.* (2006) Legionnaires' disease: a nosocomial outbreak in Turkey. *J Hosp Infect*, **62**(1), 50–7.

Pancham, S. *et al.* (2005) Caspofungin for invasive fungal infections: combination treatment with liposomal amphotericin B in children undergoing hemopoietic stem cell transplantation. *Pediatr Transplant*, **9**(2), 254–7.

Panhotra, B.R., Saxena, A.K. & Al-Mulhim, A.S. (2005) Contamination of patients' files in intensive care units: an indication of strict hand washing after entering case notes. *Am J Infect Control*, **33**(7), 398–401.

Parise, E.R. *et al.* (2006) Response to treatment with interferon-α and ribavirin in patients with chronic hepatitis C virus genotypes 2 and 3 depends on the degree of hepatic fibrosis. *Braz J Infect Dis*, **10**(2), 78–81.

Park, S.H. *et al.* (2006) Current trends of infectious complications following hematopoietic stem cell transplantation in a single center. *J Korean Med Sci*, **21**(2), 199–207.

Park, W. & Keeffe, E.B. (2004) Diagnosis and treatment of hepatitis B. *Minerva Gastroenterol Dietol*, **50**(4), 289–303.

Parker, M.J. & Goldman, R.D. (2006) Paediatric emergency department staff perceptions of infection control measures against server acute respiratory syndrome. *Emerg Med J*, **23**(5), 349–53.

Patel, S. (2005) Minimising cross-infection risks associated with beds and mattresses. *Nurs Times*, **101**(8), 52–3.

Patel, S.N., Murray-Leonard, J. & Wilson, A.P.R. (2006) Laundering of hospital staff uniforms at home. *J Hosp Infect*, **62**(1), 89–93.

Paterson, D.L. (2006) Resistance in gram-negative bacteria: Enterobacteriaceae. *Am J Infect Control*, **34**(5 Suppl 1), S20–8.

Paterson, P.J. *et al.* (2003) Treatment failure in invasive aspergillosis: susceptibility of deep tissue isolates following treatment with amphotericin B. *J Antimicrob Chemother*, **52**(5), 873–6.

Patterson, A.J. (1993) Review of current practices in clean diets in the UK. *J Hum Nutr Diet*, **6**, 3–11.

Patterson, W.J. *et al.* (1997) Colonization of transplant unit water supplies with *Legionella* and protozoa: precautions required to reduce the risk of legionellosis. *J Hosp Infect*, **37**(1), 7–17.

Paul, N. & Jacob, M.E. (2006) An outbreak of cadaver-acquired chickenpox in a health care setting. *Clin Infect Dis*, **43**(5), 599–601.

Paulus, S.C. *et al.* (2005) A prospective study of septicaemia on a paediatric oncology unit: a 3-year experience at the Royal Liverpool Children's Hospital, Alder Hey UK. *Eur J Cancer*, **41**(14), 2132–40.

Payne, D.N., Gibson, S.A. & Lewis, R. (1998) Antiseptics: a forgotten weapon in the control of antibiotic resistant bacteria in hospital and community setting. *J R Soc Health*, **118**(i), 18–22.

Pedro-Botet, L. & Yu, V.L. (2006) *Legionella*: macrolides or quinolones? *Clin Microbiol Infect*, **12**(Suppl 3), 25–30.

Peron, J.M. *et al.* (2006) Hepatitis E is an autochthonous disease in industrialized countries. Analysis of 23 patients in South-West France over a 13-month period and comparison with hepatitis A. *Gastroenterol Clin Biol*, **30**(5), 757–62.

Perrett, K. *et al.* (2003) Changing epidemiology of hepatitis A: should we be doing more to vaccinate injecting drug users? *Commun Dis Public Health*, **6**(2), 97–100.

Perry, C., Marshall, R. & Jones, E. (2001) Bacterial contamination of uniforms. *J Hosp Infect*, **48**(3), 238–41.

Petchey, R. *et al.* (2000) The last resort would be to go to the GP. Understanding the perceptions and use of general practitioner services among people with HIV/AIDS. *Soc Sci Med*, **50**(2), 233–45.

Petchey, R., Farnsworth, W. & Heron, T. (2001) The maintenance of confidentiality in primary care: a survey of policies and procedures. *AIDS Care*, **13**(2), 251–6.

Petersen, F.B. *et al.* (1987) Infectious complications in patients undergoing marrow transplantation: a prospective randomized study of the additional effects of contamination and laminar air flow isolation among patients receiving prophylactic systemic antibiotics. *Scand J Infect Dis*, **19**(5), 559–67.

Picazo, J.J. (2005) Management of febrile neutropenic patients. *Int J Antimicrob Agents*, **2**(Suppl), S12–22.

Pinna, A.D. *et al.* (2002) Five cases of fulminant hepatitis due to herpes simplex virus in adults. *Dig Dis Sci*, **47**(4), 750–4.

Pinot de Moira, A., Edmunds, W.J. & Breuer, J. (2006) The cost-effectiveness of antenatal varicella screening with post-partum vaccination of susceptibles. *Vaccine*, **24**(9), 1298–307.

Poe, S.S *et al.* (1994) A national survey of infection prevention practices on bone marrow transplant units. *Oncol Nurs Forum*, **21**(10), 1687–93.

Potoski, B.A. *et al.* (2006) Epidemiology profile of linezolid-resistant coagulase-negative staphylococci. *Clin Infect Dis*, **43**(2), 165–71.

Preiss, J.C. *et al.* (2006) Autochthonous hepatitis E virus infection in Germany with sequence similarities to other European isolates. *Infection*, **34**(3), 173–5.

Puro, V., Scognamiglio, P. & Ippolito, G. (2003) HIV, HBV, or HDV transmission from infected health care workers to patients. *Med Lav*, **94**(6), 556–68.

Quinn, B. (2003) Exploring nurses experiences of supporting a cancer patient in their search for meaning. *Eur J Oncol Nurs*, **7**(3), 164–71.

Quinn, B. (2005) Cancer and the treatment: does it make sense to patients. *Hematology*, **10**(Suppl 1), 325–8.

Rabaud, C. & Mauuary, G. (2001) Infection and/or colonization by methicillin-resistant *Staphylococcus epidermidis* (MRSE). *Pathol Biol (Paris)*, **49**(10), 812–14.

Radwin, L. (2000) Oncology patients' perception of quality nursing care. *Res Nurs Health*, **23**(3), 179–90.

Rae, G.G. (1998) Risk factors for the spread of antibiotic-resistant bacteria. *Drugs*, **55**(3), 323–30.

Redpath, C. & Farrington, M. (1997) Dispose of disposables. *J Hosp Infect*, **35**(4), 313–17.

Reglier-Poupet, H. *et al.* (2005) Evaluation of the quality of hospital food from the kitchen to the patients. *J Hosp Infect*, **59**(2), 131–7.

Respaldiza, N. *et al.* (2004) High seroprevalence in *Pneumocystis* infection in Spanish children. *Clin Microbiol Infect*, **10**(11), 1029–31.

Ribas-Mundom, M., Granena, A. & Rozman, C. (1981) Evaluation of a protective environment in the management of granulocytopenic patients. A comparative study. *Cancer*, **48**, 419–24.

Ricketts, K.D. & Joseph, C.A. (2006) The impact of new guidelines in Europe for the control and prevention of travel-associated Legionnaires' disease. *Int J Hyg Environ Health*, **209**(6), 547– 52.

Robertson, C.B. *et al.* (2006) Effect of X-ray irradiation on reducing the risk of listeriosis in ready-to-eat vacuum-packaged smoked mullet. *J Food Prot*, **69**(7), 1561–4.

Robinson, L. *et al.* (2006) Palliative home nursing interventions for people with HIV/AIDS: a pilot study. *J Assoc Nurses AIDS Care.* **17**(3), 37–46.

Rohde, H. *et al.* (2005) Induction of *Staphylococcus epidermidis* biofilm formation via proteolytic processing of the accumulation associated protein by *Staphylococcus* and host proteases. *Mol Microbiol*, **55**(6), 1883–995.

Rolston, K.V. (2001) The spectrum of pulmonary infections in cancer patients. *Curr Opin Oncol*, **13**(4), 218–23.

Rolston, K.V. (2005) Challenges in the treatment of infections caused by gram-positive and gram-negative bacteria in patients with cancer and neutropenia. *Clin Infect Dis*, **40**(Suppl 4), S246–52.

Ronning, C.M. *et al.* (2005) Genomics of *Aspergillus fumigatus*. *Rev Iberoam Micro*, **22**(4), 223–8.

Ross, D.S. *et al.* (2006) The epidemiology and prevention of congenital cytomegalovirus infection and disease: activities of the Centers for Disease Control and Prevention Workgroup. *J Womens Health (Larchmt)*, **15**(3), 224–9.

Rossoff, L.J. *et al.* (1993) Is the use of boxed gloves in an intensive care unit safe? *Am J Med*, **94**, 602–7.

Roxas, M. (2006) Herpes zoster and postherpetic neuralgia: diagnosis and therapeutic considerations. *Altern Med Rev*, **11**(2), 102–13.

Russell, J.A. *et al.* (2000) Early outcomes after allogeneic stem cell transplantation for leukaemia and myelodysplasia without protective isolation: a 10 year study. *Biol Blood Marrow Transplant*, **6**(2), 109–14

Russian, D.A. & Levine, S.J. (2001) *Pneumocystis carinii* pneumonia in patients with HIV infection. *Am J Med Sci*, **321**(1), 56–65.

Sa, D.H. *et al.* (2006) Practice of universal precautions among healthcare workers. *J Natl Med Assoc*, **98**(5), 722–6.

Sabria, M. & Yu, V.L. (2002) Hospital acquired legionellosis: solutions for a preventable infection. *Lancet Infect Dis*, **ii**(6), 368–73.

Sabria, M. *et al.* (2006) A community outbreak of Legionnaires' disease: evidence of a cooling tower as the source. *Clin Microbiol Infect*, **12**(7), 642–7.

Sadler, G.J. *et al.* (2006) UK acquired hepatitis E – an emerging problem? *J Med Virol*, **78**(4), 473–5.

Safdar, N. & Maki, D.G. (2002) The commonality of risk factors for nosocomial colonization and infection with antimicrobial-resistant *Staphylococcus aureus*, enterococcus, Gram negative bacilli, *Clostridium difficile* and *Candida*. *Ann Intern Med*, **136**(11), 834–44.

Sambatakou, H. *et al.* (2006) Voriconazole treatment for subacute invasive and chronic pulmonary aspergillosis. *Am J Med*, **119**(6), 527.e17–24.

Samuelsson, A. *et al.* (2003) Clustering of enterococcal infections in a general intensive care unit. *J Hosp Infect*, **54**(3), 188–95.

Sanderson, P.J. (1999) What should we do about patients with *Clostridium difficile*? *J Hosp Infect*, **43**(4), 251–3.

Sandri, A.M. *et al.* (2006) Reduction in incidence of nosocomial methicillin-resistant *Staphylococcus aureus* (MRSA) infection in an intensive care unit: role of treatment with mupirocin ointment and chlorhexidine baths for nasal carriers of MRSA. *Infect Control Hosp Epidemiol*, **27**(2), 185–7.

Santamauro, J.T., Aurora, R.N. & Stover, D.E. (2002) *Pneumocystis carinii* pneumonia in patients with and without HIV infection. *Compr Ther*, **28**(2), 96–108.

Santos, A.M., Lacerda, R.A. & Graziano, K.U. (2005) Evidence of control and prevention of surgical site infection by shoe cover and private shoes: a systematic literature review. *Rev Lat Am Enfermagem*, **13**(1), 86–92.

Santos, S.A. *et al.* (2006) Effect of switching to tenofovir with emtricitabine in patients with chronic hepatitis B failing to respond to an adefovir containing regimen. *Eur J Gastroenterol Hepatol*, **18**(12), 1253–7.

Sarrazin, U. *et al.* (2004) Postexposure prophylaxis after occupational exposure to HBV, HCV and HIV. *Radiologe*, **44**(2), 181–94.

Sasaki, T. *et al.* (2000) Mental disturbance during isolation in bone marrow transplant patients with leukemia. *Bone Marrow Transplant*, **25**(3), 315–18.

Saville, R.D. *et al.* (2001) Fourth-generation enzyme linked immunosorbent detection of human immunodeficiency virus antigen and antibody. *J Clin Microbiol*, **39**(7), 2518–24.

Saxena, A.K. & Panhotra, B.R. (2004) The impact of nurse understaffing on the transmission of hepatitis C virus in a hospital-based hemodialysis unit. *Med Princ Pract*, **13**(3), 129–35.

Saxena, A.K. *et al.* (2003) Impact of dedicated space, dialysis equipment, and nursing staff on the transmission of hepatitis C virus in a hemodialysis unit of the middle east. *Am J Infect Control*, **31**(1), 26–33.

Schim van der Loeff, M.F. *et al.* (2001) HIV-2 does not protect against HIV-1 infection in a rural community in Guinea-Bissau. *AIDS*, **15**(17), 2303–10.

Schlundt, J. *et al.* (2004) Emerging food-borne zoonoses. *Rev Sci Tech*, **23**(2), 513–33.

Schraub, S. & Marx, E. (2004) Burn out syndrome in oncology. *Bull Cancer*, **91**(9), 673–6.

Schulmeister, L., Quiett, K. & Mayer, K. (2005) Quality of life, quality of care, and patient satisfaction: perception of patients undergoing outpatient autologous stem cell transplantation. *Oncol Nurs Forum*, **32**(1), 57–67.

Sebaihia, M. *et al.* (2006) The multidrug-resistant human pathogen *Clostridium difficile* has a highly mobile, mosaic genome. *Nat Genet*, **38**(7), 779–86.

Sepkowitz, K.A. (2005) Treatment of patients with hematologic neoplasm, fever and neutropenia. *Clin Infect Dis*, **40**(Suppl 4), S253–6.

Serrano, I., Melo-Cristino, J. & Ramirez, M. (2006) Heterogeneity of pneumococcal phase variants in invasive human disease. *BMC Microbiol*, **6**(1), 67.

Sexton, T., Clarke, P. & O'Neill, E. (2006) Environmental reservoirs of methicillin-resistant *Staphylococcus aureus* in isolation rooms: correlation with patient isolates and implications for hospital hygiene. *J Hosp Infect*, **62**(2), 187–94.

Sharma, A. & Lokeshwar, N. (2005) Febrile neutropenia in haematological malignancies. *J Postgrad Med*, **51**(Suppl 1), S42–8.

Sheffer, P.J. *et al.* (2005) Efficacy of new point-of-use water filter for preventing exposure to *Legionella* and waterborne bacteria. *Am J Infect Control*, **33**(5 Suppl 1), S20–5.

Sheffield, J.S. *et al.* (2006) Valacyclovir prophylaxis to prevent recurrent herpes at delivery: a randomized clinical trial. *Obstet Gynecol*, **108**(1), 141–7.

Shelton, B.K. (2003) Evidence-based care for the neutropenic patients with leukaemia. *Semin Oncol Nurs*, **19**(2), 133–41.

Shinjo, K. *et al.* (2002) Efficacy of the Shinki bioclean room for preventing infection in neutropenic patients. *J Adv Nurs*, **37**(3), 227–33.

Sinclair, J. & Sissons, P. (2006) Latency and reactivation of human cytomegalovirus. *J Gen Virol*, **87**(Pt 7), 1763–79.

Singhal, R., Mirdha, B.R. & Guieria, R. (2005) Human pneumocystosis. *Indian J Chest Dis Allied Sci*, **47**(4), 273–83.

Sixbey, J.W. *et al.* (1984) Epstein–Barr virus replication in oropharyneal epithelial cells. *N Engl J Med*, **310**(19), 1225–30.

Slota, M. *et al.* (2001) The role of gown and glove isolation and strict handwashing in the reduction of nosocomial infection in children with solid organ transplantation. *Crit Care Med*, **29**(2), 405–12.

Smith, A. *et al.* (2006) Outbreaks of waterborne infectious intestinal disease in England and Wales, 1992–2003. *Epidemiol Infect*, **134**(6), 1141–9.

Smith, H.V. *et al.* (2006) Tools for investigating the environmental transmission of *Cryptosporidium* and *Giardia* infections in humans. *Trends Parasitol*, **22**(4), 160–7.

Smith, T.L. & Nathan, B.R. (2002) Central nervous system infections in the immune-competent adult. *Curr Treat Options Neurol*, **4**(4), 323–32.

Snoeck, R. & De Clercq, E. (2002) Role of cidofovir in the treatment of DNA virus infections, other than CMV infections, in immunocompromised patients. *Curr Opin Investig Drugs*, **3**(11), 1561–6.

Sobaszek, A. *et al.* (2000) Prevalence of cytomegalovirus infection among health care workers in pediatric and immunosuppressed adult units. *J Occup Environ Med*, **42**(11), 1109–14.

Sokucu, S. *et al.* (2006) Comparison of interferon monotherapy with interferon-lamivudine combination treatment in children with chronic hepatitis B. *Indian J Gastroenterol*, **25**(3), 136–9.

Soldan, K., Davison, K. & Dow, B. (2005) Estimates of the frequency of HBV, HCV, and HIV infectious donations entering the blood supply in the United Kingdom, 1996 to 2003. *Euro Surveill*, **10**(2), 17–19.

Sonder, G.J. *et al.* (2004) Hepatitis A virus immunity and seroconversion among contacts of acute hepatitis A patients in Amsterdam, 1996–2000: an evaluation of current prevention policy. *Am J Public Health*, **94**(9), 1620–6.

Special Waste Regulations (1996) HMSO, London.

Srinivasan, A. *et al.* (2002) A prospective study to determine whether cover gowns in addition to gloves decrease nosocomial transmission of vancomycin-resistant enterococci in the intensive care unit. *Infect Control Hosp Epidemiol*, 23(8), 424–8.

Sritangratanakul, S., Nuchprayoon, S. & Nuchprayoon, I. (2004) Pneumocystis pneumonia: an update. *J Med Assoc Thai*, 87(2), S309–17.

Staat, M.A. *et al.* (2006) Varicella-related hospitalization and emergency department visit rates, before and after introduction of varicella vaccine, among white and black children in Hamilton County, Ohio. *Pediatrics* 117 (5), e833–9.

Stahl Wernersson, S., Johansson, E. & Hakanson, H. (2004) Cross contamination in dishwashers. *J Hosp Infect*, 56(4), 312–17.

Stebbing, J. *et al.* (2006) A prognostic index for AIDS-associated Kaposi's sarcoma in the era of highly active antiretroviral therapy. *Lancet*, 367(9521), 1495–502.

Stirling, B., Littlejohn, P. & Willbond, M.L. (2004) Nurses and the control of infectious disease. Understanding epidemiology and disease transmission is vital to nursing care. *Can Nurse*, 100(9), 16–20.

Storb, R. *et al.* (1983) GVHD and survival in patients with aplastic anaemia treated by bone marrow grafts with HLA identifiable siblings. *N Engl J Med*, 308, 302–7.

Su, C.W. *et al.* (2006a) Genotypes and viremia of hepatitis B and D viruses are associated with outcomes of chronic hepatitis D patients. *Gastroenterology*, 130(6), 1625–35.

Su, H.P. *et al.* (2006b) A legionellosis case due to contaminated spa water and confirmed by genomic identification in Taiwan. *Microbiol Immunol*, 50(5), 371–7.

Sundkvist, T. *et al.* (2000) Outbreak of hepatitis A spread by contaminated drinking glasses in a public house. *Commun Did Public Health*, 3(1), 60–2.

Sunenshine, R.H. & McDonald, L.C. (2006) *Clostridium difficile*-associated disease: new challenges from an established pathogen. *Cleve Clin J Med*, 73(2), 187–97.

Sunnotel, O. *et al.* (2006) *Cryptosporidium*. *Lett Appl Microbiol*, 43(1), 7–16.

Takada, Y. *et al.* (2006) Clinical outcomes of living donor living transplantation for hepatitis C virus (HCV)-positive patients. *Transplantation*, 81(3), 350–4.

Takahashi, M. *et al.* (2004) High prevalence of antibodies to hepatitis A and E viruses and viremia of hepatitis B, C and D viruses among apparently healthy populations in Mongolia. *Chin Diag Lab Immunol*, 11(2), 392–98.

Takemoto, K. *et al.* (2006) Comparative study on the efficacy of AmBisome and Fungizone in a mouse model of pulmonary aspergillosis. *J Antimicrob Chemother*, 57(4), 724–31.

Talaat, M. *et al.* (2003) Occupational exposure to needlestick injuries and hepatitis B vaccination coverage among health care workers in Egypt. *Am J Infect Control*, 31(8), 469–74.

Tan, H.H. & Goh, C.L. (2006a) Viral infections affecting the skin in organ transplant recipients: epidemiology and current management strategies. *Am J Clin Dermatol*, 7(1), 13–29.

Tan, M.P. & Koren, G. (2006b) Chickenpox in pregnancy: revisited. *Reprod Toxicol*, 21(4), 410–20.

Tao, Q. *et al.* (2006) Epstein–Barr virus (EBV) and its associated human cancers – genetics, epigenetics, pathobiology and novel therapeutics. *Front Biosci*, 11, 2672–713.

Taormina, P.J. & Beuchat, L.R. (2001) Survival and heat resistance of *Listeria monocytogenes* after exposure to alkali and chlorine. *Appl Environ Microbiol*, 67(6), 2555–63.

Tarantino, G. *et al.* (2006) Metabolic factors involved in the therapeutic response of patients with hepatitis C virus-related chronic hepatitis. *Gastroenterol Hepatol*, **21**(8), 1266–8.

Tarzi, S. *et al.* (2001) Methicillin resistant *Staphylococcus aureus*: psychological impact of hospitalization and isolation in the older adult. *J Hosp Infect*, **49**(4), 250–4.

Tattevin, P. *et al.* (2006) Increasing incidence of severe Epstein–Barr virus-related infectious mononucleosis: surveillance study. *J Clin Microbiol*, **44**(5), 1873–4.

Taylor, J.M. (2006) Hepatitis delta virus. *Virology*, **344**(1), 71–6.

Taylor, K., Plowman, R. & Roberts, J.A. (2001) *The Challenge of Hospital Acquired Infection*. National Audit Office, London.

Tenover, F.C. (2006) Mechanisms of antimicrobial resistance in bacteria. *Am J Med*, **119**(6 Suppl 1), S3–10.

Thevenot, D., Dernburg, A.M. & Vernozy-Rozand, C. (2006) An updated review of *Listeria monocytogenes* in the pork meat industry and its products. *J Appl Microbiol*, **101**(1), 7–17.

Thoen, C., Lobue, P. & De Kantor, I. (2006) The importance of *Mycobacterium bovis* as a zoonosis. *Vet Microbiol*, **112**(2–4), 339–45.

Thompson, S.C., Boughton, C.R. & Dore, G.J. (2003) Blood-borne viruses and their survival in the environment: is public concern about community needlestick exposures justified? *Aust N Z J Public Health*, **27**(6), 602–7.

Toivgoogin, A. *et al.* (2005) Validity of using tuberculin skin test erythema measurement for contact investigation during a tuberculosis outbreak in schoolchildren previously vaccinated with BCG. *J Epidemiol*, **15**(2), 56–64.

Tormom Molina, R. *et al.* (2002) Pollen and spores in the air of a hospital out-patient ward. *Allergol Immunopathol (Madr)*, **30**(4), 232–8.

Torres, H.A. *et al.* (2006) Cytomegalovirus infection in patients with lymphoma: an important cause of morbidity and mortality. *Clin Lymphoma Myeloma*, **6**(5), 393–8.

Trad, O. *et al.* (2003) Eradication of *Cryptosporidium* in four children with acute lymphoblastic leukemia. *J Trop Pediatr*, **49**(2), 128–30.

Trakumas, S. *et al.* (2001) Particle emission characteristics of filter-equipped vacuum cleaners. *Am Ind Hyg Assoc J*, **62**(4), 482–93.

Trautmann, M., Lepper, P.M. & Haller, M. (2005) Ecology of *Pseudomonas aeruginosa* in the intensive care unit and the evolving role of water outlets as a reservoir of the organism. *Am J Infect Control*, **33**(5 Suppl 1), S41–9.

Trexler, P.C. (1975) Microbial isolators for use in the hospital. *Biomed Eng*, **10**(2), 63–7.

Trexler, P.C., Emond, R.T. & Evans, B. (1977) Negative pressure plastic isolator for patients with dangerous infections. *Br Med J*, **ii**(6086), 559–61.

Trim, J.C., Adams, D. & Elliott, T.S. (2003) Healthcare workers' knowledge of inoculation injuries and glove use. *Br J Nurs*, **12**(4), 215–21.

Trueba, F. *et al.* (2006) High prevalence of teicoplanine resistance among *Staphylococcus epidermidis* strains in a 5 year study. *J Clin Microbiol*, **44**(5), 1922–3.

Tsatsralt-Od, B. *et al.* (2005) High prevalence of dual or triple infection of hepatitis B, C and delta viruses among patients with chronic liver disease in Mongolia. *J Med Virol*, **77**(4), 491–9.

Tsiodras, S. *et al.* (2000) Infection and immunity in chronic lymphocytic leukemia. *Mayo Clin Proc*, **75**(10), 1039–54.

Turner, J.M. *et al.* (2006) Behavioural predictors of subsequent hepatitis C diagnosis in a UK clinic sample of HIV positive men who have sex with men. *Sex Transm Infect*, **82**(4), 298–300.

Twomey, C.L. (2003) Double gloving: a risk reduction strategy. *Jt Comm J Qual Saf*, **29**(7), 369–78.

UK Health Department (2002a) *AIDS/HIV Infected Health Care Workers: Guidance on the Management of Infected Health Care Workers and Patient Notification*. UK Health Department, Wetherby.

UK Health Department (2002b) *Guidance for Clinical Health Care Workers. Protection against Infection with Blood Borne Viruses*. UK Health Department, Wetherby.

Ungar, B.L.P. (1995) *Cryptosporidium*. In: *Principles and Practices of Infectious Disease*, 4th edn, Vol. 2 (eds G.L. Mandell, J.E. Bennett & R. Dolan). Churchill Livingstone, New York, pp. 2500–10.

Urrea, M. *et al.* (2004) Nosocomial infections among pediatric hematology/oncology patients: results of a prospective incidence study. *Am J Infect Control*, **32**(4|), 205–8.

Vamvakas, E.C. (2005) Is white blood cell reduction equivalent to antibody screening in preventing transmission of cytomegalovirus by transfusion? A review of the literature and meta-analysis. *Transfus Med Rev*, **19**(3), 181–99.

van der Kooij, D., Veenendaal, H.R. & Scheffer, W.J. (2005) Biofilm formation and multiplication of *Legionella* in a model warm water system with pipes of copper, stainless steel and cross-linked polyethylene. *Water Res*, **39**(13), 2789–98.

van der Wielen, M. *et al.* (2006) Hepatitis A/B vaccination of adults over 40 years old: comparison of three vaccine regimens and effect of influencing factors. *Vaccine*, **24**(26), 5509–15.

Vardhan, M.S., Allen, K.D. & DeRuiter, G. (2000) Commodes: a health hazard. *J Hosp Infect*, **44**(4), 320–1.

Vaughn, T.E. *et al.* (2004) Factors promoting consistent adherence to safe needle precautions among hospital workers. *Infect Control Hosp Epidemiol*, **25**(7), 548–55.

Vento, S., Cainelli, F. & Longhi, M.S. (2002) Reactivation of replication of hepatitis B and C viruses after immunosuppressive therapy: an unresolved issue. *Lancet Oncol*, **3**(6), 333–40.

Verity, P. *et al.* (2001) Prospective evaluation of environmental contamination by *Clostridium difficile* in isolation side rooms. *J Hosp Infect*, **49**(3), 204–9.

Vernon, M.O. *et al.* (2006) Chlorhexidine gluconate to cleanse patients in medical intensive care units: the effectiveness of source control to reduce the bioburden of vancomycin-resistant enterococci. *Arch Intern Med*, **166**(3), 306–12.

Vianelli, N. *et al.* (2006) Resolution of a *Pseudomonas aerginosa* outbreak in a hematology unit with the use of disposable sterile water filters. *Haematologica*, **91**(7), 983–5.

Vonberg, R.P. & Gastmeier, P. (2006) Nosocomial aspergillosis in outbreak settings. *J Hosp Infect*, **63**(3), 246–54.

Vonberg, R.P. *et al.* (2005a) Reusable terminal tap water filters for nosocomial legionellosis prevention. *Ann Hematol*, **84**(6), 403–5.

Vonberg, R.P. *et al.* (2005b) Use of terminal tap water filter systems for prevention of nosocomial legionellosis. *J Hosp Infect*, **60**(2), 159–62.

Voth, D.E. & Ballard, J.D. (2005) *Clostridium difficile* toxins: mechanism of action and role in disease. *Clin Microbiol Rev*, **18**(2), 247–63.

Walch, S.E., Roetzer, L.M. & Minnett, T.A. (2006) Suppport group participation among persons with HIV: demographic characteristics and perceived barriers. *AIDS Care*, **18**(4), 284–9.

Walker, N., Gupta, R. & Cheesbrough, J. (2006) Blood pressure cuffs, friend or foe? *J Hosp Infect*, **63**(2), 167–9.

Ward, D. (2000) Infection control: reducing the psychological effects of isolation. *Br J Nurs*, **9**(3), 162–70.

Warny, M. *et al.* (2005) Toxin production by an emerging strain of *Clostridium difficile* associated with outbreaks of severe disease in North America and Europe. *Lancet*, **366**(9491), 1079–84.

Wasley, A., Fiore, A. & Bell, B.P. (2006) Hepatitis A in the era of vaccination. *Epidemiol Rev*, **28**(1), 101–11.

Wazir, J.F. & Ansari, N.A. (2004) *Pneumocystis carnii* infection. Update and review. *Arch Pathol Lab Med*, **128**(9), 1023–7.

Weaving, P. (2006) Treatment strategies for bacteria and viruses. Why clinical management must be different. *Nurs Times*, **102**(24), 42–3.

Weitzel, T. *et al.* (2006) Evaluation of seven commercial antigen detection tests for *Giardia* and *Cryptosporidium* in stool samples. *Clin Microbiol Infect*, **12**(7), 656–9.

Wells, R. *et al.* (2006) Hepatitis A prevalence among injection drug users. *Clin Lab Sci*, **19**(1), 12–17.

Welsby, P.D. (2006) Chickenpox, chickenpox vaccination, and shingles. *Postgrad Med J*, **82**(967), 351–2.

Wendt, C. *et al.* (1998) Survival of vancomycin-resistant and vancomycin-susceptible enterococci on dry surfaces. *J Clin Microbiol*, **36**(12), 3734–6.

Whitby, M., McLaws, M.L. & Ross, M.W. (2006) Why healthcare workers don't wash their hands: a behavioral explanation. *Infect Control Hosp Epidemiol*, **27**(5), 484–92.

Whiting, L.S. (1999) Maintaining patients' personal hygiene. *Prof Nurse*, **14**(5), 338–40.

Whitley, R. (2006) New approach to the therapy of HSV infections. *Herpes*, **13**(2), 53–5.

Whitley, R.J. (2002) Herpes simplex virus in children. *Curr Treat Options Neurol*, **4**(3), 231–7.

Widdowson, M.A. *et al.* (2002) An outbreak of diarrhea in a neonatal medium care unit caused by a novel strain of rotavirus: investigation using both epidemiologic and microbiological methods. *Infect Control Hosp Epidemiol*, **23**(11), 665–70.

Wiesen, P., Van Gossum, A. & Preiser, J.C. (2006) Diarrhoea in the critically ill. *Curr Opin Crit Care*, **12**(2), 149–54.

Wigglesworth, N. & Wilcox, M.H. (2006) Prospective evaluation of hospital isolation room capacity. *J Hosp Infect*, **63**(2), 156– 61.

Wilcox, M.H. & Dane, J. (2000) The cost of hospital-acquired infection and the value of infection control. *J Hosp Infect*, **45**(2), 81–4.

Wilcox, M.H. *et al.* (2003) Comparison of the effect of detergent versus hypochlorite cleaning on environmental contamination and incidence of *Clostridium difficile* infection. *J Hosp Infect*, **54**(2), 109–14.

Wilkes, C.R., Mason, A.D. & Hern, S.C. (2005) Probability distribution for showering and bathing water-use behavior for various US subpopulations. *Risk Anal*, **25**(2), 317–37.

Wilks, M. *et al.* (2006) Control of an outbreak of multidrug-resistant *Acinetobacter baumannii-calcoaceticus* colonization and infection in an intensive care unit without closing the ICU or placing patients in isolation. *Infect Control Hosp Epidemiol*, 27(7), 654–8.

Willocks, L.J. *et al.* (2000) Compliance with advice to boil drinking water during an outbreak of cryptosporidiosis. *Commun Dis Public Health*, 3(2), 137–8.

Wilson, A.P. *et al.* (2006) Computer keyboards and the spread of MRSA. *J Hosp Infect*, 62(3), 390–2.

Wilson, B.J. (2002) Dietary recommendations for neutropenic patients. *Semin Oncol Nurs*, 81(1), 44–9.

Wilson, J. (2006) *Infection Control in Clinical Practice*, 3rd edn. Bailliere Tindall, London.

Wilson, L.E. *et al.* (2006) Progression of liver fibrosis among injection drug users with chronic hepatitis C. *Hepatology*, 43(4), 788–95.

Wolosin, R.J. (2005) HIV/AIDS patient satisfaction with hospitalization in the era of highly active antiretroviral therapy. *J Assoc Nurses AIDS Care*, 16(5), 16–25.

Wood, E. *et al.* (2006) Impact of baseline viral load and adherence on survival of HIV-infected adults with baseline CD4 cell counts $\geq$200 cells/μL. *AIDS*, 20(8), 1117–23.

Woodman, C.B. *et al.* (2005) Role of sexual behaviour in the acquisition of asymptomatic Epstein–Barr virus infection: a longitudinal study. *Pediatr Infect Dis J*, 24(6), 498–502.

Working Group (2000) Guidelines for preventing opportunistic infections among hematopoietic stem cell transplant recipients. *Biol Blood Marrow Transplant*, 6(6A), 7–83.

WHO (2002) *Framework for Effective Tuberculosis Control*. World Health Organization, Geneva.

Wright, D. (2005) Hepatitis C nightmare. Interview by Charlotte Alderman. *Nurs Stand*, 20(5), 26–7.

Wright, L., Spickett, G. & Stoker, S. (2001) Latex allergy awareness among hospital staff. *Nursing Times Plus*, 97(38), 4–8.

Wu, C.J. *et al.* (2006) Predominance of gram-negative bacilli and increasing antimicrobial resistance in nosocomial blood stream infections at a university hospital in southern Taiwan 1996–2003. *J Microbiol Immunol Infect*, 39(2), 135–43.

Wyles, D.L. *et al.* (2005) Development of herpes simplex virus disease in patients who are receiving cidofovir. *Clin Infect Dis*, 41(5), 676–80.

Yang, X.M. *et al.* (2006) Comparative proteomic analysis between invasive and commensal strains of *Staphylococcus epidermidis*. *FEMS Microbiol Lett*, 261(1), 32–40.

Yates, J.W. *et al.* (1973) A controlled study of isolation and endogenous microbial suppression in acute myelocytic leukaemia patients. *Cancer*, 32, 1490–8.

Yu, J. *et al.* (2005) *Aspergillus flavus* genomics: gateway to human and animal health, food safety, and crop resistance to diseases. *Rev Iberoam Micol*, 22(4), 194–202.

Zafar, A.B. *et al.* (1998) Effectiveness of infection control program in controlling nosocomial *Clostridium difficile*. *Am J Infect Control*, 26(6), 588–93.

Ziebuhr, W. *et al.* (2006) Nosocomial infections by *Staphylococcus epidermidis*: how a commensal bacterium turns into a pathogen. *Int J Antimicrob Agents*, Suppl 1: S14-20.

Ziyaeyan, M. *et al.* (2006) Diagnosis and monitoring of human cytomegalovirus infection in bone marrow transplant recipients by quantitative competitive PCR. *Exp Clin Transplant*, 4(1), 470–4.

Multiple choice questions

1 **The term 'barrier nursing' includes:**

   a Source isolation
   b Protective isolation
   c Protective isolation, source isolation, cohort source isolation
   d Strict source isolation, cohort source isolation, protective isolation, source isolation

2 **Endogenous infection is infection caused by:**

   a Other patients
   b Self-infection
   c Staff
   d Visitors

3 **Exogenous infection is caused by:**

   a Self-infection
   b Visitors, staff, other patients
   c Food, environment, hospital staff, patients, visitors
   d Staff not washing their hands correctly

4 **Microbiological sampling of nurses uniform detected the following:**

   a *Clostridium difficile*
   b *Staphylococcus aureus, Clostridium difficile*
   c *Clostridium difficile, Staphylococcus aureus,* Vancomycin-resistant enterococci
   d Vancomycin-resistant enterococci, *Staphylococcus aureus*

5 Hospital cleaning is of high importance. Some bacteria can live for up to:

   a   16 days
   b   60 weeks
   c   60 hours
   d   60 days

6 Infected linen should be placed in:

   a   Black alginate bag with a hazard label
   b   Red alginate bag tied shut and put in a red linen bag
   c   Clear alginate bag tied shut and put in a red linen bag
   d   Red linen bag and tied up

7 The increase in antimicrobial resistant organisms is a consequence of:

   a   Poor hygiene
   b   Widespread use of antibiotics
   c   New bacteria
   d   None of the above

8 Gram-negative bacteria can normally be found in the:

   a   Respiratory tract
   b   Urinary tract
   c   Gut
   d   All of the above

9 *Staphylococcus aureus* is part of the normal human flora with large numbers usually found on:

   a   Wounds
   b   Skin and mucous
   c   Skin
   d   Hair

10 **Transmission of hepatitis B virus to health workers can be substantially reduced by:**

  a   Use of universal precautions
  b   Vaccination
  c   Vaccination and use of universal precautions
  d   None of the above

Answers to the multiple choice questions can be found in Appendix 3.

Chapter 6

Cardiopulmonary resuscitation

Definition

Sudden death as a result of cardiac arrest is responsible for 60% ischaemic heart disease deaths across Europe (RCUK 2005). Survival to hospital discharge is cited as 10.7% of all types of cardiac arrest with survival being higher (21.2%) in ventricular fibrillation arrests (RCUK 2005).

The term cardiac arrest implies a sudden interruption of cardiac output. It may be reversible with appropriate treatment (Handley 2004). The patient will collapse, lose consciousness, stop breathing and will be pulseless (Jevon 2001).

The four arrhythmias that cause cardiac arrest are:

■ Asystole.
■ Ventricular fibrillation (VF).
■ Pulseless ventricular tachycardia (VT).
■ Pulseless electrical activity (PEA).

For the purposes of resuscitation guidelines these rhythms are divided into two groups by their treatment.

■ VF and pulseless VT, which require defibrillation.
■ Non-VF/VT, which do not require defibrillation (RCUK 2005).

Indications

The patient is unconscious, has absent or agonal (gasping) respirations and has no pulse (Perkins *et al.* 2005). Other clinical features such as pupil size, cyanosis and pallor are unreliable and so the practitioner should not waste time looking for them (Skinner & Vincent 1997).

Reference material

Principles

Failure of the circulation for 3–4 minutes will lead to irreversible cerebral damage (Docherty & Hall 2002). Basic life support (BLS) acts to slow down the deterioration of the brain and the heart until defibrillation and/or advanced life support (ALS) can be provided (RCUK 2005).

Resuscitation is the emergency treatment of any condition in which the brain fails to receive enough oxygen. The basic technique involves a rapid simple assessment of the patient followed by the BLS resuscitation. The first international consensus evidence based guidelines on resuscitation were published in 2000 (AHA/ILCOR 2000). These guidelines were reviewed in 2004/05 by the International Liaison Committee on Resuscitation and published in 2005 (International Liaison Committee on Resuscitation 2005). These internationally agreed guidelines based on research and audit now form the basis for the European Resuscitation Guidelines (European Resuscitation Council 2005) as well as the UK Resuscitation Guidelines (RCUK 2005).

Assessment

There are two stages of assessment.

1   An immediate assessment by the rescuer to ensure that cardiopulmonary resuscitation (CPR) may safely proceed (i.e. checking there is no immediate danger to the rescuer from any hazard, for example electrical power supply).
2   Assessment by the rescuer of the likelihood of injury sustained by the patient, particularly injury to the cervical spine. Although there may be no external evidence of injury, the immediate situation may provide the necessary evidence. For example, trauma to the cervical spine should be suspected in an accelerating/decelerating injury such as a road traffic accident with a motorbike travelling at speed. Once these two aspects have been assessed, the patient's level of consciousness should be checked by gently shaking his shoulders and asking loudly if he is alright (Figure 6.1). If there is no response the rescuer should commence the BLS assessment (Figure 6.2) immediately.

Note: if the arrest is witnessed or monitored, and a defibrillator is not immediately to hand, a single precordial thump should be administered. If delivered within 30 seconds after cardiac arrest, a sharp blow with a closed fist on the patient's sternum may convert VF back to a perfusing rhythm (RCUK 2005).

Basic life support

Basic life support (BLS) is sometimes known as the 'ABC'.

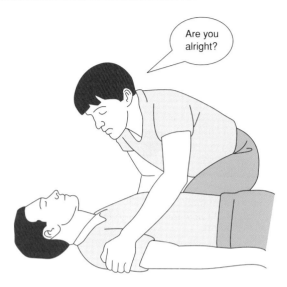

Figure 6.1   Initial verbal assessment.

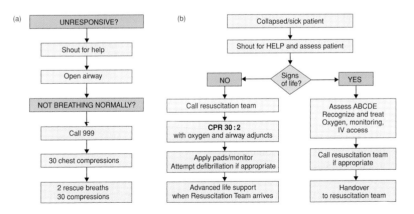

Figure 6.2   (a) Basic life support algorithm. (b) In-hospital resuscitation algorithm. CPR, cardiopulmonary resuscitation; IV, intravenous. Courtesy of RCUK (2005).

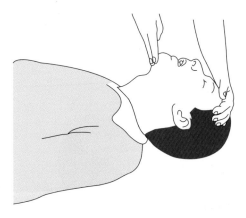

208

Figure 6.3 Head tilt/chin lift manoeuvre.

Airway

The rescuer should look in the mouth and remove any visible obstruction (leave well-fitting dentures in place). The most likely obstruction in an unconscious person is the tongue. The head tilt/chin lift manoeuvre (Figure 6.3), which removes the tongue from occluding the oropharynx, is an effective method of opening an airway and relieving obstruction in 80% of patients (Simmons 2002).

Note: if there is any suspicion of cervical spine injury (see above) try to avoid head tilt.

Breathing

Keeping the airway open, the rescuer should look, listen and feel for breathing (more than an occasional gasp or weak attempts at breathing) for up to 10 seconds. If the patient is breathing they should be turned into the recovery position (Figure 6.4). If the adult patient is not breathing and there is no suspicion of trauma or drowning, an immediate call for the cardiac arrest team should be made. It should be noted that in 40% of cases a person who has arrested still has agonal (gasping) respirations and these can be mistaken for normal breaths (Hauff *et al.* 2003). Artificial ventilation must then be commenced and maintained. If there are no aids to ventilation available then direct mouth-to-mouth ventilation should be used (Figure 6.5). The recommended length for each breath is now 1 second (RCUK 2005). When cardiac arrest occurs in hospital, the RCUK (2005) recommend the use of adjuncts such as the pocket mask or the bag mask unit. They can be used to avoid direct person-to-person contact and some devices may reduce the risk of cross-infection between patient and rescuer (RCUK 2005).

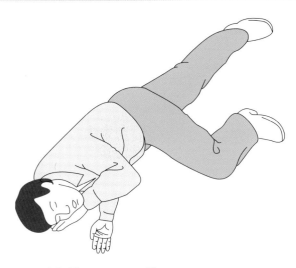

Figure 6.4   The recovery position.

In 2005 in recognition of the concern in providing mouth-to-mouth resuscitation, the guidelines changed and the BLS algorithm now starts with chest compressions and then proceeds to two breaths (RCUK 2005).

One of the most easily learnt aids is the 'mouth-to-face mask' method. This is where a valved exhaled air ventilation mask with an oxygen attachment valve is used. The mask directs the patient's exhaled air and any fluid away from the rescuer and the oxygen port allows attachment of oxygen with enrichment up to 45%.

If the operator is skilled in airway management, an Ambu bag and mask may be used. When the bag is attached to oxygen, high levels, of up to 85%, can be obtained. However, it should be emphasized that to manipulate the head tilt, and hold on a face mask while squeezing a bag is a procedure that requires practice and is most safely achieved by two people, one holding the mask and one squeezing the bag (Hodgetts & Castle 1999).

The most effective method of airway management is to use an endotracheal tube, thus enabling the application of 100% oxygen (Bossaert *et al.* 1998). This method of airway management is included in the advanced life support algorithm (Figure 6.6).

Circulation

Circulation is assessed by looking for any signs of movement, including swallowing or breathing. If trained to do so, a check should also be made for the carotid

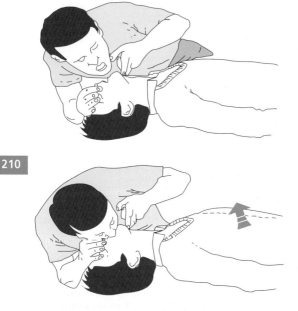

210

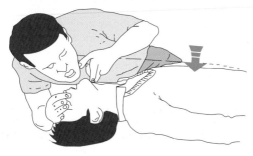

Figure 6.5 If patient is not breathing, expired air resuscitation must be started immediately. Courtesy of Colqhoun *et al.* (1999).

pulse (Figure 6.7) for up to 10 seconds. If no circulation is detected it must be maintained by compressions. The correct place to compress is in the centre of the lower half of the sternum (Figure 6.8). The rescuer should position themselves vertically above the patient with arms straight and elbows locked. The sternum should be pressed down to depress it by 4–5 cm. This should be repeated at a rate

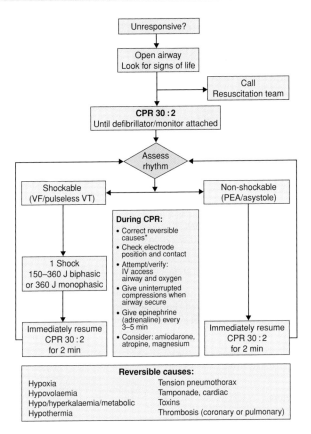

211

Figure 6.6 The advanced life support algorithm for the management of cardiac arrest in adults. CPR, cardiopulmonary resuscitation; IV, intravenous; PEA, pulseless electrical activity; VF, ventricular fibrillation; VT, ventricular tachycardia. Courtesy of RCUK (2005).

of about 100 times a minute. After 30 compressions two rescue breaths are given, continuing compressions and rescue breaths in a ratio of 30:2 (RCUK 2005). There is evidence that chest compressions are often interrupted and that this is associated with a reduction in the chance of survival, it is therefore imperative that interruptions to chest compressions are minimized by effective coordination between rescuers (Eftestol *et al.* 2002; Van Alem *et al.* 2003).

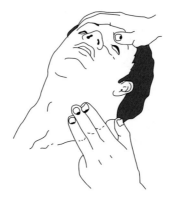

Figure 6.7 If patient does not have a pulse in a major artery (carotid), or if there is a neck injury, the femoral artery may be felt. Circulation must then be established with compression. Courtesy of Colqhoun *et al.* (2004).

Potentially reversible causes of a cardiopulmonary arrest

During cardiac arrest, potential causes or aggravating factors for which specific treatment exists should be considered. For ease of memory there are eight common causes of arrest, four of which begin with the letter H and four with the letter T:

- Hypoxia.
- Hypovolaemia.
- Hypothermia.
- Hypo/hyperkalaemia.
- Thromboembolism.
- Tension pneumothorax.
- Tamponade.
- Toxicity (metabolic or drug induced) (RCUK 2005).

Hypoxia

There are many reasons why a patient may become severely hypoxic (see Chapters 18 & 27), the most common being the following:

- Acute respiratory failure.
- Airway difficulties.
- Acute lung injury.
- Severe anaemia.
- Neuromuscular disorders.

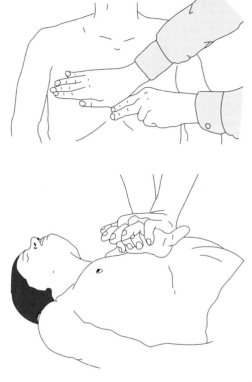

Figure 6.8   Establishing circulation with compression. Note fingers are clear of chest wall. Courtesy of Colqhoun *et al.* (1999).

For healthy cell metabolism the body requires a constant supply of oxygen. When this is interrupted for more than 3 minutes in most situations (except when there is severe hypothermia) cell death occurs, followed by lactic acidosis and very rapidly a cardiorespiratory arrest. The risk of hypoxia is minimized by ensuring that the patient's lungs are ventilated adequately with 100% oxygen (RCUK 2005).

Hypovolaemia

Hypovolaemia in adults that results in PEA is usually due to severe blood loss. While it is not the nurse's role to make a medical diagnosis, they may be aware of significant factors in the history of a patient that may have led to PEA.

The most common causes of severe blood loss are:

- Trauma.
- Surgical procedure.
- Gastrointestinal mucosa erosion.
- Oesophageal varices.
- Peripheral vessel erosion (by tumour usually).
- Clotting abnormality.

Note: blood loss, although usually overt, can be covert such as a gastrointestinal bleed which may only become apparent when the patient collapses.

The treatment for hypovolaemia is identifying and stopping the source of fluid or blood loss, and replacing the circulating volume with the appropriate fluid. Fluid resuscitation is normally started with a crystalloid, e.g. 0.9% sodium chloride, and/or colloid, e.g. Gelofusin (depending on local protocols). Blood is likely to be required rapidly if the blood loss exceeds 1500–2000 ml in an adult (RCUK 2005).

Hypothermia

Hypothermia should be suspected in any submersion or immersion injury. During a prolonged resuscitation attempt, a patient who was normothermic at the onset of cardiac arrest may become hypothermic (RCUK 2005). A low reading thermometer should be used if available. Resuscitation in the presence of hypothermia may be prolonged.

Hypo/hyperkalaemia and other metabolic disorders

Because potassium is so closely linked with muscle and nerve excitation, any imbalance will affect both the nervous conduction and the muscular working of the heart. Therefore a severe rise or fall in potassium can cause arrest arrhythmias. The causes of hypokalaemia are:

- Gastrointestinal fluid losses.
- Urinary fluid loss.
- Drugs that affect cellular potassium, e.g. antifungal agents such as amphotericin.

The immediate treatment for hypokalaemia that has resulted in an arrest is to give concentrated infusions of potassium while carefully monitoring the serial potassium measurements. Most intensive care unit (ICU)/Accident and Emergency (A&E) departments and coronary care units (CCUs) will have an arterial blood gas analyser that enables the potassium to be measured in 1 minute.

The patients who are most at risk of hyperkalaemia are those with renal failure or Addison's disease. The immediate treatment for hyperkalaemia is to give intravenous calcium. This has the effect of protecting the myocardium during the cardiac arrest. If the patient is successfully resuscitated it will be essential to monitor their serum potassium and if it remains high to commence therapy to lower or remove the potassium (RCUK 2006).

Thromboembolism

The commonest cause of thromboembolic or mechanical circulatory obstruction is a massive pulmonary embolus. Options for definitive treatment include thrombolysis or, if available, cardiopulmonary bypass and operative removal of the clot (RCUK 2005).

Tension pneumothorax

A tension pneumothorax is the sudden collapse of a lung, usually under pressure, which results in a severe change in intrathoracic pressure and cessation of the heart as a pump (Bersten & Soni 2003). The most common causes are:

- Trauma.
- Acute lung injury.
- Mechanical ventilation of the newborn.

The immediate treatment is the insertion of a large-bore cannula into the second intercostal space at the mid-clavicular line of the affected side (RCUK 2005). Arrangements should be made for the insertion of a formal chest tube and underwater seal drain (see Chapter 14).

Tamponade

This is where there is an acute effusion of fluid in the pericardial space and as it enlarges, the heart is splinted and finally cannot beat. The fluid is usually blood but can be malignant or infected fluid (Dolan & Preston 2006). The most common cause for a sudden tamponade is trauma. The immediate treatment is the insertion of a catheter or surgical drainage of the fluid. After drainage, the cause of the tamponade should be sought and corrected where possible, for example with appropriate antibiotic therapy for a bacterial aetiology or surgical repair of a myocardial laceration (Shoemaker 2000).

Toxicity: poisoning and drug intoxication

Poisoning rarely leads to cardiac arrest but it is a leading cause of death in patients less than 40 years old. Self-poisoning with therapeutic or recreational drugs is the main reason for hospital admission (RCUK 2005). There are few specific therapeutic measures for poisons that are useful in the immediate situation. The emphasis must be on intensive supportive therapy, with correction of hypoxia, acid/base balance and electrolyte disorders. Specialist help can be obtained by telephoning one of the regional National Poisons Information Service Centres (RCUK 2005).

Drugs

Only a few drugs are indicated during the immediate management of a cardiac arrest and there is only limited scientific evidence supporting their use. Drugs should be considered only after a sequence of shocks has been delivered (if indicated) and chest compressions and ventilation started (RCUK 2005). Central venous access is optimum as it allows for drugs to be delivered rapidly. However, this is dependent on the skills available. If a peripheral intravenous cannula is already in place it should be used first (RCUK 2005). Selected drugs (epinephrine, atropine, naloxone and lidocaine) can be administered down the endotracheal tube but the dose of the drug should be increased to 2–3 times the intravenous dose (AHA/ILCOR 2000). It is also possible to administer drugs using the intraosseous route, which is used commonly in the resuscitation of children.

The drugs used in the treatment of cardiac arrest are:

1 Epinephrine (adrenaline) 1 mg (10 ml of a 1 : 10 000 solution) given intravenously. The main purpose of adrenaline is to utilize its inotropic effect to maintain coronary and cerebral perfusion during a prolonged resuscitation attempt. It is the first drug used in cardiac arrest of any aetiology. Epinephrine is included in the ALS universal algorithm (see Figure 6.6), 1 mg to be given every 3–5 minutes (RCUK 2005).

2 Atropine 3 mg given intravenously once only reduces cardiac vagal tone, increases the rate of discharge of the sinoatrial node and increases the speed of conduction through the atrioventricular node. Its use is advocated in asystolic cardiac arrest and bradycardic PEA of less than 60 beats per minute. Note: although there is no conclusive evidence that atropine is of value in asystole during a cardiac arrest, there are anecdotal accounts of success following its administration (RCUK 2005).

3 Amiodarone (300 mg in 20 ml) should be considered in VF or pulseless VT. It increases the duration of the action potential in the atrial and ventricular myocardium; thus the QT interval is prolonged. In refractory VT or VF following recovery from cardiac arrest a further 300 mg may be given followed by an infusion of 900 mg over 24 hours (RCUK 2005). Note: lidocaine can still be considered if amiodarone is not available (RCUK 2005).

4 Calcium chloride (10 ml of 10%) is only given during resuscitation when specifically indicated, i.e. for the treatment of PEA caused by hyperkalaemia, hypocalcaemia or overdose of calcium channel blocking drugs (RCUK 2005).

Although it plays a vital role in the cellular mechanisms underlying myocardial contraction there are very few data supporting any beneficial action for calcium following most cases of cardiac arrest (RCUK 2005).

5   Sodium bicarbonate 8.4% is only used in prolonged cardiac arrest or according to serial blood gas analyses. Potential adverse effects of excessive sodium bicarbonate administration include hypokalaemia, exacerbation of respiratory acidosis and increased affinity of haemoglobin for oxygen. The high concentration of sodium can also exacerbate cerebral oedema. Other adverse effects are increased cardiac irritability and impaired myocardial performance. Sodium bicarbonate is usually given in 25–50 mmol aliquots and repeated as necessary. It can also be given in the special circumstances of tricyclic overdose or hyperkalaemia (Winser 2001).

6   Magnesium sulphate. Magnesium (4–8 mmol of 50%) should be given in cardiac arrest where there is a suspicion of hypomagnesaemia as this may precipitate refractory VF/VT (Winser 2001). The normal value for magnesium is 0.8–1.2 mmol/l (Wakeling & Mythen 2000).

217

Defibrillation

Defibrillation causes a simultaneous depolarization of the myocardium and aims to restore normal rhythm to the heart. This is the definitive treatment for VF/pulseless VT. It has been suggested that 80–90% of adults who collapse because of non-traumatic cardiac arrest are found to be in VF when first attached to a monitor (Varon *et al.* 1998). In hospital cardiac arrest is more likely to present as non-VF/VT. Early defibrillation is a vital link in the chain of survival and developments in public access defibrillation and first responder defibrillation by ward nurses in hospitals are focusing firmly on this link. Delay in defibrillation decreases the chances of success by 7–10% each minute (Bossaert *et al.* 1998). Nurses are often first on the scene at a cardiac arrest, highlighting the obvious need for nurse-led defibrillation at ward level. While not all nurses are trained in defibrillation, they should understand why it is necessary and how it is done and be able to assist in an emergency (Austin & Snow 2000).

Safe defibrillation practice

Defibrillation in an environment where high flows of oxygen are present could represent a danger to patients and rescuers. It is essential therefore to ensure that oxygen tubing and equipment is moved away from the chest when defibrillation is performed. Using adhesive electrodes to deliver the shock as opposed to paddles may also minimize the danger (RCUK 2005).

Placement of paddles or self-adhesive electrodes

The right paddle or electrode should be placed to the right of the sternum below the clavicle and the left vertically in the mid-axillary line approximately level with the position V6 used in electrocardiogram (ECG) monitoring (see Figure 6.6 for the universal ALS algorithm for the management of cardiac arrest in adults).

Cardiopulmonary resuscitation standards and training

The Resuscitation Council UK (RCUK), formed in 1981, aims to promote the education of lay and professional personnel in the most effective methods of resuscitation appropriate to their needs. In its report *CPR Guidance for Clinical Practice and Training in Hospitals* (RCUK 2004), the Council made a number of recommendations relating to the provision of a resuscitation service in hospital:

- A resuscitation committee. This should comprise of medical and nursing staff who advise on the role and composition of the cardiac arrest team, resuscitation equipment and resuscitation training equipment.
- A Resuscitation Training Officer (RTO), who should be responsible for training in resuscitation, equipment maintenance and the auditing of resuscitation/clinical trials.
- Resuscitation training. Hospital staff should receive at least annual resuscitation training appropriate to their level and role. Medical and nursing staff should receive basic resuscitation training and should be encouraged to recognize patients who are at risk of having a cardiac arrest and call for appropriate help early. This is the most effective method of improving outcome (Jevon 2002). All medical staff should have advanced resuscitation training and senior nurses and doctors working in acute specialities (CCU, ITU, A&E) should hold a valid RCUK ALS certificate.
- A cardiac arrest team. Each hospital should have a team of about five people including a minimum of two doctors (physician and anaesthetist), an ALS trained nurse, the RTO and a porter when possible. Clear procedures should be available for calling the cardiac arrest team. The Resuscitation Council has recommended the development of a medical emergency team who recognize patients who are at risk of having a cardiac arrest and initiate the most appropriate clinical intervention to prevent it (Jevon 2002).
- Resuscitation equipment. Ideally this should be standardized throughout the hospital (see Procedure guidelines: Cardiopulmonary resuscitation, below). Defibrillators should also be standardized. The widespread deployment of automated or shock advisory defibrillators is a realistic strategy to reduce mortality from cardiac arrests related to ischaemic heart disease (Jevon 2002). Bossaert (1997) believes that defibrillation should be a basic skills requirement of all nurses. With the advent of automated external defibrillators (AEDs) this may become a possibility in the near future.

- Audit and reporting of standards. All resuscitation attempts should be audited, ideally using a nationally recognized template such as Utstein template (recommended for use by the RCUK).
- Decisions relating to CPR. Every hospital should have a 'Do not attempt resuscitation' (DNAR) policy based on national guidelines (Jevon 2001; BMA, RCN, RCUK 2001).

If these recommendations are implemented, the standards in resuscitation and resuscitation training should improve (Jevon 2002).

Ethics

The increase in skills, knowledge, technology and pharmacological support has proved effective in prolonging quality of life for many patients. Many patients have good reason to be thankful for CPR and the numbers rise daily (RCUK 2005). Resuscitation attempts in the mortally ill, however, do not enhance the dignity that most people hope for in death. Ideally, resuscitation should only be attempted in patients who have a high chance of successful revival for a good quality of life (i.e. as deemed acceptable by the individual patient). There are many important factors that need to be considered when deciding whether or not to resuscitate a patient:

- The patient's own wishes.
- The views of relatives or close friends, who may be aware of the wishes of a patient who cannot communicate.
- The patient's disease and prognosis.
- The quality of life of the patient and expected quality should resuscitation be 'successful'.

Decision making: do not attempt resuscitation

In an attempt to reduce the number of futile resuscitation attempts many hospitals have introduced formal DNAR policies, which can be applied to individual patients in specific circumstances. Health care professionals must be able to show that their decisions relating to CPR are compatible with the human rights set out in the Human Rights Act 1998 implemented on 2 October 2000 (e.g. the right to life, the right to be free from inhuman or degrading treatment and freedom of expression) (BMA 2000). The following guidelines are based on those provided in a joint statement by the British Medical Association (BMA), the Royal College of Nursing (RCN) and the RCUK (BMA, RCN, RCUK 2001). (Note: where no decision has been made and the express wishes of the patient are unknown, CPR should be performed without delay.)

- Sensitive advance discussion between experienced medical/nursing staff and patients regarding attempting CPR should be encouraged but not forced. Where patients lack competence to participate, people close to them can be helpful in reflecting their views. (Note: in England, Wales and Northern Ireland, no person is legally entitled to give consent to medical treatment on behalf of another adult.) Information about CPR needs to be realistic. Written information explaining CPR should be available for patients and those close to them to read. The BMA, in liaison with the RCUK, has published an information leaflet that may help patients and families discuss DNAR with medical and nursing staff (BMA 2002).
- Patients are entitled to refuse CPR even when there is a reasonable chance of success.

- Some patients may ask that no DNAR order be made. Patients cannot demand treatment which the health care team judges to be inappropriate, but all efforts should be made to accommodate their wishes and preferences.
- An advance DNAR order should only be made after consideration of the likely clinical outcome, the patient's wishes and the patient's human rights. It should be considered on an individual patient basis where:

  1 Attempting CPR will not start the patient's heart and breathing.
  2 There is no benefit in restarting the patient's heart and breathing.
  3 The expected benefit is outweighed by the burdens (RCUK 2005).

- The overall responsibility for decisions about CPR and DNAR orders rests with the consultant in charge of the patient's care. Issues should, however, be discussed with other members of the health care team, the patient and people close to the patient where appropriate.
- There are exceptional cases where resuscitation discussions with a patient may be inappropriate, e.g. where senior members of the medical and nursing team consider that CPR would be futile and that such a discussion would cause the patient unnecessary distress and anguish. This could apply to patients in the terminal phase of their illness.
- The most senior members of the medical and nursing team available should clearly document any decisions made about CPR in the patient's medical and nursing notes. The decision should be dated and the reasons for it given. This information must be communicated to all other relevant health care professionals. Unless it is against the wishes of the patient, their family should also be informed.
- The DNAR order should be reviewed on each admission or in light of changes in the patient's condition (BMA, RCN, RCUK 2001).

Finally, it should be noted that a DNAR order applies only to CPR and should not reduce the standard of medical or nursing care.

Procedure guidelines   Cardiopulmonary resuscitation (CPR)

Equipment

All hospital wards and appropriate departments, e.g. theatre, computed tomography (CT) scanning, should have a standardized cardiac arrest trolley or box. Resuscitation equipment should be checked on a daily basis (RCUK 2005) by the staff on the wards or clinical areas responsible for it, and a record of this check should be maintained. Below is a list of the minimum equipment recommended by the Resuscitation Council for the management of an adult cardiac arrest.

Airway management

- Pocket masks with oxygen port.
- Self-inflating resuscitation bag with oxygen reservoir and tubing.
- Clear face masks in sizes 4, 5 and 6.
- Oropharyngeal airways in sizes 2, 3 and 4.
- Yankauer suckers × 2.
- Endotracheal suction catheters × 10.
- Laryngeal mask airway (size 4) or Combitube (small).
- McGill forceps.
- Endotracheal tubes: oral, cuffed, sizes 6, 7 and 8.
- Gum elastic bougie.
- Lubricating jelly.
- Laryngoscopes × 2: normal and long blades.
- Spare laryngoscope bulbs and batteries.
- 1 inch ribbon gauze/tape.
- Scissors.
- Syringe: 20 ml.
- Clear oxygen mask with reservoir bag.
- Oxygen cylinders × 2 (if no wall oxygen).
- Cylinder key.

Circulation equipment

- Intravenous cannulae: 18 gauge × 3, 14 gauge × 3.
- Hypodermic needles: 21 gauge × 10.
- Syringes: 2 ml × 6, 5 ml × 6, 10 ml × 6, 20 ml × 6.
- Cannula fixing dressings and tapes × 4.

Additional items

- ECG electrodes.
- Defibrillation gel pads/unless using fast patch electrodes.
- Clock.
- Gloves/goggles/aprons.
- A sliding sheet or similar device should be available for safe handling.

Drugs

Immediately available prefilled syringes of:

- Atropine: 3 mg × 1.
- Amiodarone: 300 mg × 1.
- Epinephrine/adrenaline: 1 mg (1 : 10 000) × 4.

Other readily available drugs

- Epinephrine (adrenaline): 1 mg (1 : 10 000) × 4.
- Sodium bicarbonate 8.4%: 50 ml × 1.
- Calcium chloride 10%: 10 ml × 2.
- Lidocaine/lignocaine: 100 mg × 2.
- Atropine: 1 mg × 2.
- 0.9% sodium chloride: 10 ml ampoules × 10.
- Naloxone: 400 g × 2.
- Epinephrine/adrenaline 1 : 1000 × 2.
- Amiodarone: 150 mg × 4.
- Magnesium sulphate 50% solution: 2 g (4 ml) × 1.
- Potassium chloride 40 mmol × 1.
- Adenosine: 6 mg × 10.
- Hydrocortisone: 200 mg × 1.
- Glucose 10%: 500 ml × 1.

Procedure guidelines *(cont.)*

- Seldinger wire central venous catheter kits × 2.
- 12 gauge non-Seldinger central venous catheter × 2.
- Intravenous administration sets × 3.
- 0.9% sodium chloride: 1000 ml bags × 2.

Procedure

Action	Rationale
1 Note time of arrest, if witnessed.	Lack of cerebral perfusion for approximately 3–4 minutes can lead to irreversible brain damage (E).
2 Give patient precordial thump.	This may restore cardiac rhythm, which will give a cardiac output (E).
3 Summon help. If a second nurse is available, he/she can call for the cardiac arrest team, bring emergency equipment and screen off the area.	Maintain patient's privacy and dignity. CPR is more effective with two rescuers. One is responsible for inflating the lungs, and the other for chest compressions. Continue until medical help arrives (RCUK 2005: C).
4 Lie patient flat on a firm surface/bed. If on a chair, lower the patient to the floor, ensuring that the head is supported.	Effective external cardiac massage can be performed only on a hard surface (E; RCUK 2005: C).
5 If patient is in bed, remove bed head, and ensure adequate space between back of bed and wall.	To allow easy access to patient's head in order to facilitate intubation (E).
6 Ensure a clear airway. If cervical spine injury is excluded, extend, not hyperextend, the neck (thus lifting the tongue off the posterior wall of the pharynx). This is best achieved by lifting the chin forwards with the finger and thumb of one hand while pressing the forehead backwards with the heel of the other hand (see Figure 6.3). If this fails to establish an airway, there may be obstruction by a foreign body. Try to remove the obstruction if visible.	To establish and maintain airway, thus facilitating ventilation (RCUK 2005: C).

Do not remove well-fitted dentures.

They help to create a mouth to mask seal during ventilation (E).

7 Place the heel of one hand in the centre of the sternum and place the other on top, ensuring that the hands are located between the middle and the lower half of the sternum. Ensure that only the heel of the dominant hand is touching the sternum.

To ensure accuracy of external cardiac compression and reduced delay in commencing cardiac compressions (RCUK 2005: C).

Place the other hand on top, straighten the elbows and make sure shoulders are directly over the patient's chest.

The sternum should be depressed sharply by 4–5 cm. The cardiac compressions should be forceful, and sustained at a rate of 100 per minute.

This produces a cardiac output by applying direct downward force and compression (Smith 2000: R3).

8 Compress the Ambu bag in a rhythmical fashion: the bag should be attached to an oxygen source. In order to deliver 85% oxygen, a reservoir may be attached to the Ambu bag. If, however, oxygen is not immediately available, the Ambu bag will deliver ambient air.

Room air contains only 21% oxygen. In shock, a low cardiac output, together with ventilation–perfusion mismatch, results in severe hypoxaemia. The importance of providing a high oxygen gradient from mouth to vital cells cannot be exaggerated and so oxygen should be added during CPR as soon as it is available (80–100% is desirable) (Simmons 2002. R3).

9 Maintain cardiac compression and ventilation at a ratio of 30 : 2. This rate can be achieved effectively by counting out loud 'one and two', etc. There should be a slight pause to ensure that the delivered breath is sufficient to cause the patient's chest to rise. This must continue until cardiac output returns and the patient has a palpable blood pressure.

Counting aloud will ensure co-ordination of ventilation and compression ratio. To maintain circulation and oxygenation, thus reducing risk of damage to vital organs (E).

10 When the cardiac arrest team arrives, it will assume responsibility for the arrest in liaison with the ward staff.

To ensure an effective expert team co-ordinates the resuscitation (E; RCUK 2005: C).

Procedure guidelines *(cont.)*

11 Attach patient to ECG monitor using three electrodes or defibrillation patches/paddles.	To obtain adequate ECG signal. Accurate recording of cardiac rhythm will determine the appropriate treatment to be initiated (E).

Intubation in CPR

Action	Rationale
12 Continue to ventilate and oxygenate the patient before intubation.	The risks of cardiac arrhythmias due to hypoxia are decreased (RCUK 2005: C).

224

13 Equipment for intubation should be checked before handing to appropriate medical/nursing staff: (a) Suction equipment is operational. (b) The cuff of the endotracheal tube inflates and deflates. (c) The endotracheal tube is well lubricated. (d) That catheter mount with swivel connector is ready for use.	
14 During intubation, the anaesthetist may request cricoid pressure. This involves compressing the oesophagus between the cricoid ring and the sixth cervical vertebra.	To prevent the risk of regurgitation of gastric contents and the consequent risk of pulmonary aspiration (RCUK 2006: C).
15 Recommence ventilation and oxygenation once intubation is completed.	Intubation should interrupt resuscitation only for a maximum of 16 seconds to prevent the occurrence of cerebral anoxia (Handley *et al*. 1997: R 3).
16 Once the patient's trachea has been intubated, chest compressions, at a rate of 100 per minute, should continue uninterrupted (except for defibrillation and pulse check when indicated) and ventilation should continue at approximately 12 breaths per minute.	Uninterrupted compression results in a substantially higher mean coronary perfusion pressure. A pause in chest compressions allows the coronary perfusion pressure to fall. On resuming compressions, there is some delay before the original coronary perfusion pressure is restored (RCUK 2005: C).

Intravenous access in CPR

Action	Rationale
17 Venous access must be established through a large vein as soon as possible.	To administer emergency cardiac drugs and fluid replacement (RCUK 2005: C).
18 Asepsis should be maintained throughout.	To prevent local and/or systemic infection (DH 2005:C).
19 The correct rate of infusion is required.	To ensure maximum drug and/or solution effectiveness (E).
20 Accurate recording of the administration of solutions infused and drugs added is essential.	To maintain accurate records, provide a point of reference in the event of queries and prevent any duplication of treatment (NMC 2005: C).

Defibrillation

Used to terminate VF or VT.

Post-resuscitation care

After cardiac arrest, return of spontaneous circulation is just the first phase in a continuum of resuscitation. To return the patient to a state of normal cerebral function with no neurological deficit, a stable cardiac rhythm and normal haemodynamic function requires further resuscitation tailored to each patient's individual needs (RCUK 2005).

Action	Rationale
1 Check patient by assessing airway, breathing, circulation, blood pressure and urine output.	To ensure a clear airway, adequate oxygenation and ventilation and aim to maintain normal sinus rhythm and a cardiac output adequate for perfusion of vital organs. To ensure adequacy of ventilation and oxygenation (E).
2 Check arterial blood gases.	To ensure correction of acid/base balance (RCUK 2005: C).

Procedure guidelines *(cont.)*

3 Check full blood count, clotting and biochemistry.

To exclude anaemia as a contributor to myocardial ischaemia. A clotting disorder may have contributed to a major haemorrhage. Replacement stored blood for transfusion has less clotting factors and the patient may require replacement of clotting factors usually in the form of fresh frozen plasma (E). To assess renal function and electrolyte balance (K+, Mg^{2+} and Ca^{2+}). To ensure normoglycaemia. To commence serial cardiac enzyme assay (RCUK 2006: C).

226

4 Monitor patient's cardiac rhythm and record 12-lead ECG.

Normal sinus rhythm is required for optimum cardiac function (RCUK 2006: C). An assessment of whether cardiac arrest has been associated with a myocardial infarction should be made, as the patient may be suitable for coronary angioplasty or thrombolytic therapy.

5 A chest X-ray should be taken.

To establish correct siting of tracheal tube, gastric tube and central venous catheter. To exclude left ventricular failure, pulmonary aspiration and pneumothorax. To establish size and shape of heart (E).

6 Continue respiratory therapy.

Hypoxia and hypercarbia both increase the likelihood of a further cardiac arrest (RCUK 2006: C).

7 Assess patient's level of consciousness. This can be done by use of the Glasgow Coma Scale. Although this is intended primarily for head injury, it is clinically relevant. It contains five levels of consciousness:
  (a) Conscious and alert.
  (b) Drowsy but responsive to verbal commands.
  (c) Unconscious but responsive to minimal painful stimuli.
  (d) Unconscious and responsive to deep painful stimuli.
  (e) Unconscious and unresponsive.
  (See Chapter 19).

Once a heart has been resuscitated to a stable rhythm and cardiac output, the organ that influences an individual's survival most significantly is the brain (RCUK 2006: C). Initial assessment and regular monitoring will alert the nurse to any changes in function.

8 The patient should be made comfortable and nursed in the appropriate position, i.e. upright or in the recovery position. Avoid nursing supine as this physiologically hinders cardiac output and respiration. Careful explanation and reassurance is vital at all times, particularly if the patient is conscious and aware.

9 Following stabilization of the patient's condition, consideration should be given to moving them to an appropriate critical care environment. All established monitoring should continue during transfer.

To facilitate a safe transfer of the patient between the site of resuscitation and an appropriate place of definitive care (E).

A critical care outreach service, if available, may contribute to the care of the patient during stabilization and transfer.

To export the expertise of critical care to the patient and enhance the skills and understanding of ward staff in the delivery of critical care (Ridley 2002: E; RCUK 2006: C).

Please note: whether the resuscitation attempt was successful or not, the patient's relatives will require considerable support. Equally, the pastoral needs of all those associated with the arrest should not be forgotten (RCUK 2005: C).

References and further reading

AHA/ILCOR (2000) Guidelines 2000 for CPR and emergency care: an international consensus on science. *Resuscitation*, **46**(1), 73–92, 109–14.

Austin, R. & Snow, A. (2000) Defibrillation. In: *Resuscitation: A Guide for Nurses* (ed. A. Cheller). Harcourt, London, pp. 141–57.

Baskett, P.J.F., Steen, P.A. & Bossaert, L. (2005) European Resuscitation Council Guidelines for Resuscitation 2005. Section 8: The ethics of resuscitation and end of life decisions. *Resuscitation*, **67**(Suppl 1), S171–80.

Bersten, A.D. & Soni, N. (2003) *Oh's Intensive Care Manual*, 5th edn. Butterworth Heinemann, Edinburgh.

BMA (2000) *The Impact of the Human Rights Act on Medical Decision-Making*. British Medical Association, London.

BMA (2002) *Decisions Relating to Cardiopulmonary Resuscitation: Model Information Leaflet*. British Medical Association, London.

BMA, RCN, RCUK (2001) *Decisions Relating to Cardiopulmonary Resuscitation: A Joint Statement*. Resuscitation Council UK, London.

Bossaert, L. (1997) Fibrillation and defibrillation of the heart. *Br J Anaesth*, **79**(2), 203–13.

Bossaert, L. *et al.* (1998) European Resuscitation Council Guidelines for adult advanced life support. *Resuscitation*, **37**(1), 81–94.

Colqhoun, M., Handley, A.J. & Evans, T.R. (2004) *ABC of Resuscitation*, 5th edn. BMJ Publishing Group, London.

DH (2005) *Saving Lives: A Delivery Programme to Reduce Healthcare Associated Infection including MRSA*. Department of Health, London.

Docherty, B. & Hall, S. (2002) Basic life support and AED. *Prof Nurse*, **17**(12), 705–6.

Dolan, S. & Preston, N.J. (2006) Malignant effusions. In: *Nursing Patients with Cancer* (eds N. Kearney & A. Richardson). Elsevier, Churchill Livingstone, Edinburgh, pp. 619–33.

Eftestol, T., Sunde, K. & Steen, P.A. (2002) Effects of interrupting precordial compressions on the calculated probability of defibrillation success during out-of-hospital cardiac arrest. *Circulation*, **105**, 2270–3.

European Resuscitation Council (2005) *European Resuscitation Council Guidelines for Resuscitation*, **67**(Suppl 1), S1–190.

Gabbott, D. *et al.* (2005) Cardiopulmonary resuscitation standards for clinical practice and training in the UK. *Resuscitation*, **64**, 13–19.

Handley, A.J. (2004) Basic life support. In: *ABC of Resuscitation* (eds M. Colqhoun, A. Handley & T. Evans), 4th edn. BMJ Books, London, pp. 1–4.

Handley, A.J. *et al.* (1997) Single rescuer adult basic life support: an advisory statement by the Basic Life Support Working Group of the International Liaison Committee on Resuscitation. *Resuscitation*, **34**, 101–7.

Hauff, S.R. *et al.* (2003) Factors impeding dispatcher-assisted telephone cardiopulmonary resuscitation. *Ann Emerg Med*, **42**, 731–7.

Hodgetts, T. & Castle, N. (1999) *Resuscitation Rules*. BMJ Books, London.

International Liaison Committee on Resuscitation (2005) International consensus on cardiopulmonary resuscitation and emergency cardiovascular care science with treatment recommendations. *Resuscitation*, **67**, 157–341.

Jevon, P. (2001) Cardiopulmonary resuscitation. Initial assessment. *Nurs Times*, **97**(42), 41–2.

Jevon, P. (2002) Resuscitation in hospital: Resuscitation Council (UK) recommendations. *Nurs Stand*, **16**(33), 41–4.

NMC (2005) *Guidelines for Records and Record Keeping*. Nursing and Midwifery Council, London.

Perbedy, M.A. *et al.* (2003) Cardiopulmonary resuscitation of adults in the hospital: a report of 14 720 cardiac arrests from the National Registry of Cardiopulmonary Resuscitation. *Resuscitation*, **58**, 297–308.

Perkins, G.D. *et al.* (2005) Birmingham assessment of breathing study (BABS). *Resuscitation*, **53**, 29–36.

RCUK (2001) *Decisions Relating to Cardiopulmonary Resuscitation: A Joint Statement from the British Medical Association, the Resuscitation Council (UK) and the Royal College of Nursing*. Resuscitation Council, UK, London.

RCUK (2004) *CPR Guidance for Clinical Practice and Training in Hospitals*. Resuscitation Council UK, London.

RCUK (2005) *Adult Basic Life Support: Resuscitation Guidelines*. Resuscitation Council UK, London.

RCUK (2006) *Advanced Life Support*, 5th edition. Resuscitation Council UK, London.

Ridley, S. (2002) Critical care – modality, metamorphosis and measurement. In: (ed S.A. Ridley) *Outcomes in Critical Care*. Butterworth Heinemann, Oxford, pp. 1–21.

Shoemaker, W.C. (2000) Pericardial tamponade. In: *Oxford Textbook of Critical Care* (eds A. Webb *et al.*). Oxford University Press, London, pp. 276–9.

Simmons, R. (2002) The airway at risk. In: *ABC of Resuscitation* (eds M. Colqhoun, A. Handley & T. Evans), 5th edn. BMJ Books, London, pp. 25–31.

Skinner, D. & Vincent, R. (1997) *Cardiopulmonary Resuscitation*. Oxford University Press, London.

Smith, D. (2000) Basic life support. In: *Resuscitation: A Guide for Nurses* (ed. A. Cheller). Harcourt, London, pp. 65–80.

Van Alem, A., Sanou, B. & Koster, R. (2003) Interruption of CPR with the use of the AED in out of hospital cardiac arrest. *Ann Emerg Med*, **42**, 449–57.

Varon, J., Marik, P.E. & Fromm, R.E. Jr (1998) Cardiopulmonary resuscitation: a review for clinicians. *Resuscitation* **36**(2), 133–45.

Wakeling, H.G. & Mythen, M.C. (2000) Hypomagnesemia. In: *Oxford Textbook of Critical Care* (eds A. Webb *et al.*). Oxford University Press, London pp. 561–4.

Winser, H. (2001) An evidence base for adult resuscitation. *Prof Nurse*, **16**(7), 1210–13.

Multiple choice questions

1 Irreversible brain damage will occur if there is a failure of circulation for:

    a   34 minutes
    b   3–4 minutes
    c   58 minutes
    d   6–7 minutes

2 The arrhythmias caused by cardiac arrest are:

    a   Flat line, pulseless ventricular tachycardia
    b   Asystole, ventricular fibrillation, pulseless electrical activity
    c   Pulseless electrical activity, asystole, ventricular fibrillation
    d   Asystole, pulseless electrical activity, ventricular tachycardia, ventricular fibrillation

3 What is the most likely cause of airway obstruction in the unconscious person?

    a   Food
    b   Dentures
    c   Tongue
    d   Foreign body

4 Which manoeuvre will open the airway and relieve obstruction in 80% of patients?

    a   Head lift
    b   Head tilt
    c   Chin tilt
    d   Head tilt/chin lift

5 How many compressions of the sternum should be made before two breaths are given?

   a   15
   b   13
   c   30
   d   25

6 What is the first drug used in a cardiac arrest, whatever the cause?

   a   Magnesium sulphate 4–8 mmol of 50%
   b   Sodium bicarbonate 8.4%
   c   Calcium chloride 10 m of 10%
   d   Epinephrine 1 mg

Answers to the multiple choice questions can be found in Appendix 3.

Chapter 7

Discharge planning

Definition

Discharge planning is a process and not an isolated event. It should involve the development and implementation of a plan to facilitate the transfer of an individual from hospital to an appropriate setting and include the multidisciplinary team, the patient and their carers. Furthermore, it involves building on, or adding to, any assessments undertaken prior to admission (DH 2003a).

Reference material

One of the key elements of the Clinical Governance agenda is improved quality and effectiveness (DH 1998a). Good quality discharge should reduce delayed discharges (Tarling & Jauffur 2006) and facilitate meeting the targets set by The NHS Plan (DH 2000a), National Service Framework for Older People (DH 2002) and commissioning a patient-led National Health Service (NHS) (DH 2004a).

Therefore all hospitals should have a discharge policy which is developed, agreed and ideally jointly published with all the relevant local health and social service agencies. Standards should be applicable to the planning and delivery of care at all stages: preadmission and admission; the period as an inpatient; predischarge; the discharge process and postdischarge (Health Services Accreditation 1996). Patient preadmission clinics are an ideal opportunity to assess care required on discharge (DH 2003a).

Your Guide to the National Health Service (NHSE 2001) states that from the moment a patient arrives:

> Arrangements for discharging you from hospital will begin, and your discharge plan will be agreed with you, taking account of your needs. When you are ready to leave hospital, the nurses and doctors will talk to you about what will happen to you during your recovery and you will be told who to contact in an emergency.
>
> If you need ongoing care at home, your GP, midwife, health visitor, community nurse or social services department will be there to help you.

> **Box 7.1   Patients who may have particular care needs on discharge***
>
> The following patients were identified as having particular care needs:
> - Live alone.
> - Are frail and/or elderly.
> - Have care needs which place a high demand on carers.
> - Have a limited prognosis.
> - Have serious illnesses and will be returning to hospital for further treatments.
> - Have continuing disability.
> - Have learning difficulties.
> - Have mental illness or dementia.
> - Have dependents.
> - Have limited financial resources.
> - Are homeless or live in poor housing.
> - Do not have English as their first language.
> - Have been in hospital for an 'extended stay'.
> - Require aids/equipment at home.
>
> *DH 1989; DH 2004b.

If you need any medical equipment for your return home, the NHS and your social services department will aim to provide it promptly. If you need your home to be adapted in any way, your social services department will assess your needs.

(NHSE 2001, p. 30)

All patients, whether short- or long-stay, those with few needs or those with complex needs, should receive comprehensive discharge planning. Some patients may have particular care needs on discharge; examples are listed in Box 7.1.

Aims of discharge planning

- To ensure patients have a safe discharge from hospital to the community.
- To ensure patients and carers are involved throughout the discharge planning process.
- To provide patients and carers with written and verbal information to meet their needs on discharge.
- To provide continuity of care between the hospital and the agreed environment by facilitating effective communication. (Adapted from DH 2004b.)

Principles of discharge planning

The key principles for effective discharge planning are that:

- Unnecessary admissions are avoided and discharge is facilitated by a whole system approach to care planning.

- Patients and carers should be actively involved in the process (DH 1995; DH 2004c).
- Discharge planning should commence on the initial contact with patients.
- Discharge should be co-ordinated by a named person.
- Discharge planning should be a multidisciplinary process by which resources to meet the needs of patients and carers are put in place (Salter 1996).
- Effective use is made of transitional and intermediate care services, so that patients achieve their optimal outcome and acute hospital beds are used appropriately.
- Patients and carers understand the discharge planning process, their rights and receive appropriate information to enable them to make informed decisions about their future care. (Adapted from DH 2003a.)

234 The discharge planning process and the primary/secondary care interface

The discharge planning process can be initiated by a member of the primary health care team (PHCT) or social services staff in the patient's home, prior to admission, in preadmission clinics or on hospital admission (Health Services Accreditation 1996). Importance is attached to developing a primary care-led NHS, reinforced by the government's white paper, 'The New NHS: Modern, Dependable' (DH 1998b). The focus on quality, patient-centred care and services closer to where people live will be dependent on primary, secondary and tertiary professionals working together (Davis 1998).

However, it is important to note that the Community Care (Delayed Discharges) Act (DH 2003b) introduced a system of reimbursement to NHS bodies from social services departments for delays caused by the failure of social services departments to provide timely assessment and/or services for a patient being discharged from an acute hospital bed.

The discharge planning process takes into account a patient's physical, psychological, social, cultural and economic needs. It involves not only patients but can involve families, friends, carers, the hospital multidisciplinary team and the community health/social services teams (Nixon *et al.* 1998), with the emphasis on health and social services departments working jointly.

In recent years the reduction in hospital beds has resulted in an increasing emphasis on shorter inpatient stays (Stewart 2000). However, the notion of a seamless service may be idealistic because of increasing time constraints and the complex care needs of high-dependency patients (Smith 1996).

Occasionally the discharge process may not proceed as planned; a discharge may be delayed for a number of reasons and a system should be in place to record this (for example see Figure 7.1). Patients may take their own discharge against medical advice and this should be documented accordingly (for example see

DISCHARGE DELAY MONITORING FORM
Please refer to accompanying guidelines

Ward
Week commencing

Were there any delayed discharges this week (please tick)   YES ☐   NO ☐

If yes please complete form fully.

Please complete this form for patients who no longer need clinical care in a comprehensive cancer centre, but who stay in the hospital because of 'delayed or lack of appropriate Community/Social Services or internal failures to plan the discharge properly'

Patient's Details: (Give full address inc. postcode)   **Hospital No:** _____

Name: _____   **Consultant:** _____

Address: _____

_____

_____ **Postcode:** _____

Expected Date of Discharge: _____ | **Actual Date of Discharge:** _____

Reason for Delay in Discharge: (Please tick the appropriate boxes)

Royal Marsden NHS Trust Failure	☐	Other Hospital Failure	☐
Hospice Failure	☐	Transport failure	☐
		Internal Social Services failure	☐
Community Health Service Failure e.g. D/N, Macmillan	☐	External Social Services failure	☐
Identify Health Authority _____		*Identify Social Services Dept.* _____	
Patient/Relative choice	☐	Other	☐
(Don't count if 24 hour's notice given to relatives)		Please specify _____	

Full details of delay: Please complete

_____

_____

_____

_____

Signature: _____ **Print Name:** _____

Please send completed forms to Complex Discharge Co–Ordinator / Tracking Officer

Figure 7.1 Example of discharge delay monitoring form. Source: Royal Marsden NHS Foundation Trust (2006).

Box 7.2 Patients taking discharge against medical advice*

Nursing staff responsibility

If a patient wishes to take his/her own discharge the ward sister/co-ordinator should contact:

1 A member of the medical team.
2 The manager on call.
3 The Complex Discharge Co-ordinator.

The Complex Discharge Co-ordinator will inform social services if appropriate. Out of hours, following a risk assessment, the manager on call will contact the local social services department, if felt appropriate, and inform the hospital social services department the following day.

Medical staff responsibility

The doctor, following consultation with the patient, should complete the appropriate form prior to the patient leaving the hospital. The form must be signed by the patient and the doctor and filed in the medical notes. The doctor must immediately contact the patient's general practitioner (GP).

*Source: Royal Marsden NHS Foundation Trust 2006.

Box 7.2). Some patients receiving news of a poor prognosis may prefer to go home to die and plans would need to be set up at short notice (Figure 7.2).

The role of informal carers

Engaging and involving patients and carers as equal partners is central to successful discharge planning (DH 2003a). The hospital discharge process is a critical time for carers. It may be the first time they are confronted with the reality of their role, the effect it may have on their relationship with the person needing care, their family and their employment (Hill & Macgregor 2001). Research suggests that if carers are unsupported it can result in early readmission of the patient (Holzhausen 2001). Recent government policy (DH 2004c) builds on existing legislation to support carers in a practical way by providing information, helping carers to remain at work and by helping carers to care for themselves. Throughout discharge planning, carers' needs should be acknowledged. Carers may have different needs from patients and they are entitled to a separate assessment (DH 2004c). Health care professionals should allow carers sufficient time and information to make decisions, provide written information on the discharge plan and ensure adequate support is in place before discharge (Hill & Macgregor 2001). This will promote a successful and seamless transfer from hospital to home.

Name:	Hospital No:

Checklist for Discharge

This form should be used to assist with planning an urgent discharge home for a patient with terminal care needs. It should be used in conjunction with the discharge policy.

Sign and date to confirm when arranged and equipment given. Document relevant information in the discharge planning section of the nursing documentation. Document if item or care is not applicable.

Appoint a designated ward based discharge lead:

Name:.. Designation:.. Contact No:............

	Date & Time	Signature, Print Name & Job Title
Patient / Family issues		
Meeting with patient/family to discuss: patient's condition and prognosis		
Plan agreed and discussed with patient and carers. Explain the level of care that will be provided in the community. Ensure an understanding that there will not be 24-hour nursing presence.		

	Date & Time	Signature, Print Name & Job Title
Communication with District Nurse and Community Palliative Care Team		
Discuss • Patient and family needs • The role of each service and the timing and frequency of visits • Community Service cover at night (to support family) e.g. Marie Curie or other local services • The need to complete the Continuing Care Application Form, if necessary		
Agreed planned date and time of district nurses first visit..		
Agreed planned date and time of community palliative care team first visit..		
Night nursing service Start date....................................		
Communication with GP and Community Palliative Care Medical Team - Medical Responsibilities **(Hospital medical team to organize – the nurse to confirm when arranged)**		
Registrar to discuss with GP the patient needs and their prognosis, medication and the need to review the patient in the community for death certification purposes.		
Oxygen cylinder/ concentrator (delete as appropriate) ordered through GP and delivery date organized for.................................		
Medical summary faxed to GP ☐ copy with patient ☐		
Registrar to discuss with the Palliative Care Medical team the patient's needs and proposed plan of care		
Adequate supply of drugs prescribed for discharge (TTOs) including crisis drugs, i.e. Midazolam and morphine sulphate		
Medical letter or authorization for drugs to be administered by community nurses.		
'Do Not Attempt Resuscitation' letter for Community Staff		
'Do Not Attempt Resuscitation' letter for Ambulance Crew		

237

Figure 7.2 Checklist for patients being discharged home for urgent palliative care (*continued on p. 238*).

	Date & Time	Signature, Print Name & Job Title
Equipment – confirm delivery of equipment		
Hospital bed (electric/manual – please circle)		
Pressure relieving equipment		
Commode/urinal		
Hoist		
Backrest/mattress variator		
Other, please state......................................		
Provide 7 days supply of:		
Dressings		
If patient is being discharged with a syringe driver in situ then complete the syringe driver discharge checklist		
Sharps bin		
Continence aids		
Transport (confirm by ticking appropriate boxes) CHECK OTHER DISCHARGE DOCUMENTATION		
Transport booked: Date and Time.. Oxygen/suction ☐ Stretcher ☐ Paramedic crew ☐		
Escort (family/nurse)		
'Do Not Attempt Resuscitation' letter given to ambulance crew		
Family informed and aware that the patient may not survive the transfer journey and that the ambulance crew will not attempt resuscitation		
Written Information and Documentation		
Community Care Referral form completed and faxed for the attention of..		
Community Care Referral form and medical summary given to patient or relative (specify)		
Community Palliative Care Team form completed and faxed for the attention of..		
Patient/carer given list of contact numbers of community services **(including night service)**		
Medication list, stating reasons for drugs, given and explained to patient/relative		
Confirm with the Hospital Consultant whether a bed should be held for this patient for 24/48 hrs (delete as appropriate)		

Signature/print name of designated ward based discharge lead:...

Date/Time...

File this form in the patient's records on discharge.

Figure 7.2 (*cont.*)

Communication and discharge planning

Effective, safe discharge planning needs to be patient and carer focused. Therefore it is dependent on a multidisciplinary approach and the sharing of good practice (Martin 2001). There is consistent evidence to suggest that best practice in hospital discharge involves multidisciplinary teamwork throughout the process (Borill *et al.* 2001). The multidisciplinary approach, where all staff have a clear understanding of their roles and responsibilities (for example see Box 7.3), will

Box 7.3   Guide to discharge planning for nursing staff

YOUR RESPONSIBILITIES:

The aim of this guide is to make discharge planning more effective. It should be used in conjunction with the Royal Marsden's *Discharge Policy and Procedure* (Royal Marsden NHS Foundation Trust 2006).

- Within 24 hours of each admission, make every effort to complete the full nursing assessment and discharge planning section of the care plan.
- On admission a provisional discharge date should be discussed with patients, carers and the medical team and documented. This must be reviewed daily.
- Be aware: if patients require a care package on discharge, social services require a minimum of 3 days to assess their needs under the Community Care (Delayed Discharges) Act 2003 (DH 2003b).
- Discharge date should be set in negotiation with the multidisciplinary team and discussed with the patient and carers.
- Please ensure that all complex discharges are discussed at ward multidisciplinary meetings.

AS APPROPRIATE:

- Refer to other members of the multidisciplinary team.
- If a social services care package is essential on discharge, forward Section 2/Section 5 Notification Forms to the Tracking Officer.
- For information regarding social services or carers support please complete a Trigger Form only and forward to the social services department.
- Refer to district nursing/specialist community services (try to give 48 hours notice). Complete the Community Care Referral Form and fax.
- Request nursing equipment for use in the community (it can take a week to obtain).
- Complete the NHS Continuing Healthcare assessment form if the patient may meet the criteria for NHS funded care, due to prognosis or complexity of need.
- Refer to Community Palliative Care Team and specify if urgent. Document all referrals made to community services with **DATE, CONTACT NAME, TELEPHONE AND FAX NUMBERS.**
- Give written details of services arranged to patient and/or carer.

DISCHARGE DELAYS:

For a definition of a delayed discharge at the Royal Marsden, please refer to the Discharge Policy.

- All delayed discharges must be discussed at ward multidisciplinary meetings and highlighted to the Complex Discharge Co-ordinators.
- Discharge Delay Monitoring Form to be completed for every delay by the ward manager or designated deputy and forwarded to the site-specific Tracking Office, Chelsea or Sutton.

For further information or advice on discharge planning please contact the Complex Discharge Co-ordinator or social services department.

239

also help to prevent inappropriate readmissions and delayed discharges (Stewart 2000). This approach also promotes the highest possible level of independence for the patient, their partner and family by encouraging appropriate self-care activities.

Ineffective discharge planning has been shown to have detrimental effects on a patient's psychological and physical well being and their illness experience (Smith 1996; Nazarko 1998). Planning care, providing adequate information and involving patients, families and health care professionals will keep disruption to a minimum.

Discharge Co-ordinators are health or social care professionals who have both hospital and community experience. Their role is to advise and help with planning the care patients may need when leaving hospital, particularly when the nursing and care needs are complex. McKenna *et al.* (2000) cite poor communication between hospital and community, and to this end Nixon *et al.* (1998) have endorsed the value of co-ordination in a climate of shorter hospital stays and timely patient discharge.

For complex discharges, it is helpful if a key worker is appointed to manage the discharge (DH 2003a), the Discharge Co-ordinator for example, and, where appropriate, for family meetings/case conferences to take place and include the patient/carer, multidisciplinary team and PHCT and representatives (Health Services Accreditation 1996; Salter 1996). Additionally a guide to planning a complex discharge (Box 7.4) can highlight the communication required by the multidisciplinary team.

Nurse-led discharge

In The NHS Plan (DH 2000a) the Chief Nursing Officer identified 10 key roles for nurses, one being admitting and discharging patients with specific conditions using agreed protocols. Nurse discharge protocols can assist hospitals in reducing length of stay, reducing delays associated in waiting for a doctor to review a patient for discharge or to prescribe medication to take home, and also avoids unnecessary delays at weekends and evenings (NHS Modernisation Agency 2003).

Single Assessment Process

Referred to in The NHS Plan (DH 2000a) and reinforced in The National Service Framework for Older People (DH 2001a), the Single Assessment Process is designed to replace fragmented assessments carried out by different agencies with one seamless procedure (Hunter 2001). The aim is to produce a single, centrally held, electronic summary/tool containing all the information needed to assess, and in turn provide for, an older person's health and social care needs. The end result

Box 7.4   Guide to arranging a complex discharge home

Helpful hints on arranging a complex discharge home

NB: This is not an exhaustive list and MUST BE DISCUSSED with the Complex Discharge Co-ordinator/ Specialist Sister, Discharge Planning, Palliative Care.

Complex discharge definition:

- A large package of care involving different agencies.
- The patient's needs have changed since admission, with different services requiring co-ordination.
- The family/carer requires intensive input into discharge planning considerations (e.g. psychological interventions):
  - Patients who are entitled to Continuing NHS Funded Care and who require a package of care on discharge.
  - Patients for repatriation.

1 **Comprehensive assessment by nurse on admission and document care accordingly.**

(a) Provisional discharge date set.

- This will only be an approximate date, depending on care needs, equipment, etc.
- It should be reviewed regularly with multidisciplinary team.
- Discharge should **not** be arranged for a Friday or weekend.

(b) Referrals to relevant members of multidisciplinary team.

e.g. Occupational therapist, physiotherapist, social services.

(c) Referral to Community Health Services (in liaison with multidisciplinary team).

e.g. District nurse (who may be able to arrange for night sitters), Community Palliative Care Team.

(d) Request equipment from district nurse and discuss with family.

e.g. Hoist, hospital bed, pressure-relieving mattress/cushion, commode, nebulizer.

- **If oxygen is required,** medical team to complete Home Oxygen Ordering Form (HOOF) and Home Oxygen Consent Form (HOCF) forms for oxygen cylinders and concentrators at home. Fax to relevant oxygen supplier.

Box 7.4   *(cont.)*

2 **Discuss at ward multidisciplinary meeting, arrange family meeting/case conference as required**, and invite all appropriate health care professionals, including community staff.

(a) Appoint discharge co-ordinator at the multidisciplinary meeting.	▪ To act as co-ordinator for referrals and point of contact for any discharge concerns.
	▪ To plan and prepare the family meeting/case conference and to arrange a chairperson and minute-taker for the meeting.
	▪ Primary Team Nurse to liaise with discharge co-ordinator.
(b) Formulate a discharge plan at meeting.	▪ At the meeting, formulate a discharge plan in conjunction with patient, carers, and all hospital and community personnel involved and agree a discharge date: an occupational therapist home visit may be required.
(c) Ascertain discharge address.	▪ Liaise with services accordingly.
	▪ It is important to agree who will care for patient/where the patient will be cared for, e.g. ground/first floor.
	▪ Ascertain type of accommodation patient lives in so that the equipment ordered will fit in appropriately.
	▪ NB. IF NOT RETURNING TO OWN HOME, A GP WILL BE REQUIRED TO TAKE PATIENT ON AS A TEMPORARY RESIDENT.
(d) Confirm PROVISIONAL discharge date.	▪ This will depend on when community services and equipment can be arranged.
	▪ This must be agreed with the patient and family/informal carer/s.

3 **Ascertain whether district nurse is able to undertake any necessary clinical procedures** in accordance with their Primary Care Trust policy, e.g. care of skin-tunnelled catheters. Consider alternative arrangements if necessary.

Box 7.4 *(cont.)*

(a) Confirm equipment agreed and delivery date.

NB. Family must be informed of delivery date and also requested to contact ward to inform that this has been received.

(b) Confirm **start date** for care.

e.g. Social services/district nurse/community palliative care.

(c) Confirm with patient/family agreed discharge date.

- Liaise with Complex Discharge Co-ordinator for 'Community Services Arrangements' Form
- Check community services able to enter patient home as necessary.

4 **Forty-eight hours prior to discharge,** Fax and telephone district nurse with Community Care Referral Form and discuss any special needs of patient, e.g. syringe driver, oxygen, wound care, intravenous therapy, methicillin-resistant *Staphylococcus aureus* (MRSA) or other infection status. Give written information and instructions.

(a) Arrange transport and assess need for escort/oxygen during transport.

(b) Ongoing review.

- Should be in place for any change in patient's condition/treatment plan.
- IF THERE IS A CHANGE, notify/liaise with Multidisciplinary Team and Community Services

(c) If NO change within 24 hours of discharge, confirm that:

- Patient is medically fit for discharge
- All Community Services are in place as agreed above

Patient has drugs to take out (TTO) and next appointment.

- Ensure patient has drugs TTO with written and verbal instructions.
- Next in/out-patient appointment as required.

Access to home, heating and food are checked.

- Check arrangements for patient to get into home (front door key), heating, food and someone there to welcome them home, as appropriate.

5 **Hospital equipment:** e.g. syringe drivers: ensure clearly marked and arrangements made for return.

6 **After discharge,** follow-up phone call to patient by ward nurse/Complex Discharge Co-ordinator as agreed to ensure all services in place.

will be a comprehensive 'individual care plan' that will lay out their full needs and entitlements (Hunter 2001). Examples of health care professionals who may be involved in contributing to the Single Assessment Process are nurses and doctors, occupational therapists, physiotherapists, dietitians and speech therapists.

Although there has been a high level of commitment to the Single Assessment Process from both health and social care professionals, implementation has occurred at different rates. It appears that more progress has been made in the community rather than hospitals and general practitioner practices (NHS Connecting for Health 2005).

Intermediate care

The National Bed Enquiry (DH 2000b), The NHS Plan (DH 2000a) and The National Service Framework for Older People (DH 2001a) signalled the development of intermediate care as one of the major initiatives for services in the future. It is recognized that older people are best cared for at home if at all possible. To aid the transition period from hospital to home, intermediate care teams may provide a period of intensive care/rehabilitation following a hospital stay. It may be provided in a care home or in the individual's own home. It is likely to be limited to a maximum of 6 weeks; however, there are local variations in practice. Intermediate care needs to have a person centred approach involving patients and carers in all aspects of assessment, goal setting and discharge planning. Its success depends on local knowledge of the service and interagency collaboration (Hancock 2003). There is growing evidence that supports intermediate care initiatives reducing admissions to acute hospitals and reducing residential/nursing home placements (DH 2002).

Discharge to a care home

Discharge to a care home (whether it be in the form of a residential or nursing home) requires careful thought as for many patients the concept and planning of giving up their own home is one of the most traumatic events that a person has to consider. A thorough multidisciplinary assessment is essential, taking into account the individual needs of the patient and carer and exploring all the options before agreeing on a care home. Placements can be delayed while waiting for a vacancy and it may be necessary to consider an interim placement (DH 2003a).

In 2001 there were important changes in the funding arrangement for adults requiring registered nursing care in nursing homes in England (DH 2001b). All adults needing the skills and knowledge of a registered nurse to meet all or certain elements of their care needs have that care paid for by the NHS. The amount of funding, paid directly to the nursing home, is dependent on a comprehensive assessment of the patient's care needs by a registered nurse, who will usually be employed by the local Primary Care Trust. NHS-funded nursing care was provided via payment 'bands', which relate to the level of nursing care required. However, the National Framework (DH 2006), which came into effect in October 2007, replaced the banding system with a weekly rate for NHS-funded nursing care.

NHS Continuing Healthcare

NHS Continuing Healthcare is a general term that describes the care that people need over an extended period of time as the result of disability, accident or illness to address both physical and mental health needs. It may require services from the NHS and/or social care. It can be provided in a range of settings, for example, from a care home to care in people's own homes. NHS Continuing Healthcare describes a package of care arranged and funded solely by the NHS. NHS Continuing Healthcare should be awarded when it is established (through multidisciplinary assessment) that an individual's overall care needs are such that their primary need is a health need. There has been inconsistency in applying the criteria nationally (House of Commons Health Committee 2005) resulting in the Department of Health producing a National Framework for NHS Continuing Healthcare (DH 2006). This aims to establish a single policy on who should receive NHS funding and a standard process for assessing eligibility.

245

Discharge delays

A discharge delay is when a patient remains in hospital beyond the date agreed by the multidisciplinary team and beyond the time they are medically fit to leave (DH 2003a). For every patient who is 'delayed' the ward nurse should complete a form, similar to that in Figure 7.1, highlighting the reasons for the delay. It is the responsibility of health authorities, in collaboration with social services departments, to monitor the way in which discharges from hospitals are being undertaken and, if problems occur, to establish the reasons, so that any necessary changes are made to address the local needs (DH 1989). Each hospital should have at least a basic system of audit and quality control of discharge practice and procedures.

Conclusion

From the patient's and carer's perspective, discharge may be one of the most important events of the hospital stay (Holzhausen 2001). Planning for hospital discharge is an integral part of care and an ongoing process that should start prior to admission for planned admissions and as soon as possible for all other admissions (DH 2003a). It should involve the assessment and implementation of a multidisciplinary plan to facilitate the transfer of the patient from hospital to an appropriate setting and patients and carers should be involved at all stages.

Procedure guidelines   Discharge planning

Procedure

Action   Rationale

Initial assessment (at preadmission clinic or within first 24–48 hours of admission)

1 The admitting nurse is responsible for ensuring that an initial assessment is completed when the patient is admitted and is documented in the patient's care plan. Assessment should be ongoing and regularly reviewed with the multidisciplinary team.

To enable the physical, psychological and social care needs of the patient and carers to be identified at an early stage (Biddington 2000: C; DH 2000c: C).

2 An expected date of discharge should be established.

To ensure planning for discharge commences (Biddington 2000: C).

3 Clarify whether the patient has dependants, e.g. elderly relatives, children or a disabled partner who is unwell. If so, establish who is looking after them and whether they receive any services.

Arrangements may need to be made for alternative carer or an increase in services. Notification may need to be made, e.g. to school nurse/teacher if patient has children at school (E).

4 Establish who else is involved in giving care/support and the type of help given, e.g. local support group, voluntary agency, church.

To assess the support that the patient and carers may require at home so that appropriate services can be mobilized. To establish social network in order to co-ordinate care between voluntary and statutory agencies (E).

5 Ascertain the type of accommodation the patient is living in, e.g. house, bungalow (council or privately owned), residential or nursing home, sheltered housing.

To identify any potential accommodation needs which may entail social work intervention (E).

6 Ensure that the home address and telephone number of the patient are documented accurately in the care plan. Establish where the patient will be going on discharge and document the discharge address if different from the permanent address.

Personal information may not have been updated on previous nursing or medical records. It is crucial that this information is accurate when making referrals to community services, to ensure appropriate service provision (E).

7 Ensure that the patient is registered permanently with a GP, and with a GP on a temporary basis if going to a different address on discharge. Check the names, addresses and telephone numbers with the patient.

Community nursing services are unable to accept the patient without medical support. Accurate information is required to establish which district nurse will have responsibility for patient care. It is important for the patient that medical care can be provided at home (E).

8 Establish whether any statutory community health or social services have been involved before the patient's admission. Include the health visitor when the patient has children under the age of 5 years.

To enable contact for exchange of information. Valuable information can be obtained from community services to assist in assessing potential needs on discharge (DH 2003a: C).

247

Referrals for discharge planning

9 Assess the patient's ability to carry out activities of daily living at home prior to admission, e.g. was she/he able to climb stairs? Consider patient's current level of functioning and whether this will change as a result of treatment and/or rehabilitation.

To establish at an early stage whether an occupational therapy/physiotherapist assessment is required. Home assessment may be required by occupational therapy prior to discharge, which may involve complex planning and preparation (Kumar 2000; DH 2001c: C).

10 Refer to other hospital personnel as soon as potential needs are recognized, e.g. occupational therapist, physiotherapists, dietitian. Referral as soon as possible after admission is essential: do not wait until treatment is completed and discharge is imminent.

To ensure multidisciplinary planning and co-ordination. Considerable time may be needed to arrange community services and early referral helps to prevent discharge delays (E).

11 Patients identified as requiring local authority social services support are referred to the social services department. Some hospitals use a 'trigger' form as an aid to assessment, an example of which can be found in Box 7.1.

To ensure early and appropriate referral to the social services department for assessment (E).

Procedure guidelines *(cont.)*

12 A discharge planning care plan should be commenced. All members of the multidisciplinary team should document in the care plan their assessment, plans and action taken.

To facilitate multidisciplinary planning, co-ordination and communication (E).

13 Where there is a designated discharge co-ordinator s/he can act as a resource offering support and education to the ward team in the preparation of discharge plans, especially for those patients requiring a complex package of care.

To facilitate effective discharge planning and utilize expertise appropriately (E).

14 Formulate a discharge plan in conjunction with patient and carers and all involved hospital and community personnel and agree a discharge date.

To collate information and co-ordinate planning (DH 2004h· C).

15 For complex discharges a discharge planning meeting should be held.

To co-ordinate continuity of care planning (E).

16 The ward-based nurse is responsible for arranging and co-ordinating community nursing services (including the Community Palliative Care Team) in consultation with the discharge co-ordinator, if applicable.

To facilitate continuity of care between hospital and community (E).

17 Refer to the community nursing services with a minimum of 48 hours' notice. If a complex package of care is being organized more notice will be required. Invite community nurses to visit the ward where appropriate.

Community nurses may wish to assess the patient's nursing care needs and ensure preparation of the home prior to discharge. They need time to liaise with other agencies to co-ordinate care and to obtain any equipment required (E).

18 Ascertain whether district nurses are able to carry out necessary clinical procedures in accordance with their Trust policy, e.g. care of skin-tunnelled catheters. Consider alternative arrangements if necessary. Give written information and instructions.

District nurses may not have been trained in certain procedures or may be unfamiliar with particular equipment (E).

248

19 Details of patient's MRSA status (or other infections) must be given to community personnel and written in requirements.	To reduce risk of cross-infection. Community staff require full knowledge of the patient's history and nursing referral details (Halm *et al.* 2003: E; Smith 2003: E, C).
20 Complete the community care referral form or update letter. The form/letter should be completed and signed and a copy provided for all community services.	Provide information for community staff to ensure that they have accurate information (Halm *et al.* 2003: E).
21 Ensure any essential medical/nursing aids or equipment have been obtained before discharge by community services, e.g. oxygen, nebulizers, commode, pressure-relieving mattress, hoist. Home assessment may be required by occupational therapy prior to discharge.	Some equipment may not be available or may take some time to obtain. Equipment may be loaned from the community and appropriate legislation procedures must be followed for safety reasons (DH 2001c: C).
22 Patients requiring community nursing, physiotherapy, occupational therapy, stoma care, speech therapy and/or dietetic support on discharge will be referred by the appropriate hospital-based health care professional to their equivalent in the community.	To ensure continuity of specialist care (E).

Leaving the hospital on discharge

23 Medical staff are responsible for assessing the patient's medical fitness for discharge and for liaising with other members of the multidisciplinary team regarding arrangements for meeting the patient's care needs in the community.	To ensure that both health and social care needs are taken into consideration when formulating discharge plans (DH 2003a: C).

249

Procedure guidelines *(cont.)*

24 Ensure that patient and, with his/her agreement, carers have full information regarding the patient's medical condition and care required.	To prepare carers and to enable patient/carer support (E).
25 Teach the patient and carers any necessary skills, allowing sufficient time to practise before discharge. This should include information on the safe use of equipment, e.g. a hoist.	To enable the patient to be as independent as possible and promote an understanding of self-care techniques (E).
26 Ensure that the patient has a door key and can gain entrance to their residence. Wherever possible, ensure that someone is at home to receive the patient.	The patient may have left their key with a neighbour. It is helpful for someone to be available to welcome the patient and attend to any immediate needs (E).
27 Book transport if required with 48 hours' notice, using relevant form. Specify if patient needs a stretcher or chair, or requires escort. Ensure that transport is also booked for return clinic appointment if necessary.	The patient may not have private transport facilities and may be too weak to use public transport (E).
Cancel transport if discharge date or out-patients department appointment is altered.	To prevent a waste of resources (E).
28 Patients should be given an appropriate supply of medication and, where necessary, a supply of wound dressings or medical equipment.	To ensure the safe and continuous administration of medication and use of equipment at home. Time is needed to obtain supplies in the community (E).
29 Discharge plans should not be altered without consultation with all the hospital personnel who have been involved in the planning, e.g. occupational therapist, social worker, Discharge Co-ordinator and also patient/family carers.	If there is no consultation this causes considerable confusion and stress for the patient/carers, and all involved services. It may result in the patient being unsupported at home (E).

30 If discharge is cancelled or postponed, or if the patient dies, ensure that all relevant community services are informed.

To avoid distress to relatives. To avoid wasted visits and promote good community relations (E).

31 Weekend discharge: patients who require a high level of health and social services support should not be discharged home on a Friday or Saturday or a public holiday. This applies particularly to patients who were previously unknown to community services. (NB. it may be appropriate, under the Community Care (Delayed Discharges) Act, 2003, to discharge patients if agreement has been obtained with Local Authority social services.) *Note*: assessment and planning for weekend leave are as important as for final discharge.

All community services will be operating at a reduced level and emergency medical back-up may be difficult to obtain (E).

Patient information on hospital discharge

32 Inform the patient and carers of potential side-effects of treatment and management.

To alleviate anxiety and to promote patient comfort, knowledge and safety (E).

33 Ensure that patient and carers have information on local support groups or national specialist organizations as appropriate.

Some patients may benefit from the kind of support offered by the organizations (E).

34 Reinforce any special instructions with written information or by giving an approved patient education booklet, e.g. one of the Royal Marsden Hospital series.

To promote an understanding of disease and treatment. To confirm arrangements made. To enable the patient to contact the appropriate services (E).

35 Information on community services arranged, including names and telephone numbers and expected date of first visit, should be given to the patient and carers prior to discharge. This information should also be documented in the patient's care plan.

To confirm arrangements made. To enable the patient to contact the appropriate services (E).

Procedure guidelines *(cont.)*

36 Ensure that arrangements have been made to provide patient with food at home on discharge and that there will be adequate heating.	To supply immediate needs (E).
37 Ensure that the patient and carers are given verbal and written information on the dosage, route, frequency and side-effects of any medication and how to obtain further supplies.	Lack of information makes it difficult for the GP to provide the medical care required (DH 2003a: C).

After discharge from hospital

38 A follow-up phone call should be made to establish how the patient is managing.	To ensure services are in place (E).

References and further reading

Biddington, W. (2000) Reviewing discharge planning processes and promoting good practice. *JCN*, **14**(5), 4–6.

Borill, C. *et al.* (2001) *Team Working and Effectiveness in Health Care.* Aston Centre for Health Service Organisation Research, Aston, Yorkshire.

Davis, S. (1998) *Primary Secondary Care Interface.* Proceedings of conference, 25 March. NHS Executive, June, Issue 2.

DH (1989) *Discharge of Patients from Hospital.* Health Circular (89) 5. HMSO, London.

DH (1995) *Carer's (Recognition and Services) Act.* HMSO, London.

DH (1998a) *A First Class Service: Quality in the New NHS.* NHSE, London.

DH (1998b) *The New NHS: Modern, Dependable.* HMSO, London.

DH (2000a) *The NHS Plan. A Plan for Investment, a Plan for Reform.* HMSO, London.

DH (2000b) *Shaping the Future NHS: Long Term Planning for Hospitals and Related Services. Consultation Document on the Findings of the National Bed Enquiry.* HMSO, London.

DH (2000c) *Patient and Public Involvement in the NHS.* HMSO, London.

DH (2001a) *The National Service Framework for Older People.* HMSO, London.

DH (2001b) *NHS Funded Nursing Care in Nursing Homes: What It Means for You.* HMSO, London.

DH (2001c) *Guide to Integrating Community Equipment Services.* HMSO, London.

DH (2002) *National Service Framework for Older People – Intermediate Care: Moving Forward.* HMSO, London.

DH (2003a) *Discharge from Hospital: Pathway, Process and Practice.* HMSO, London.

DH (2003b) *Delayed Transfers of Care: Planning for Implementation of Reimbursement and Improving Hospital Discharge Practice.* HMSO, London.

DH (2004a) *The NHS Improvement Plan: Putting People at the Heart of Public Services.* HMSO, London.

DH (2004b) *Achieving Timely 'Simple' Discharge from Hospital – a Toolkit for the Multi-disciplinary Team*. HMSO, London.

DH (2004c) *Carers and Disabled Children Act 2000 and Carers (Equal Opportunities) Act 2004. Combined Policy Guidance*. HMSO, London.

DH (2004d) *National Standards, Local Action: Health and Social Care Standards and Planning Framework*. Department of Health Publications, London (www.dh.gov.uk).

DH (2005/6–2007/8) *National Standards, Local Action; Health and Social Care Standards and Planning Framework*. Department of Health Publications, London (www.dh.gov.uk).

DH (2006) *National Framework for NHS Continuing Healthcare and NHS-funded Nursing Care in England. Consultation Document*. HMSO, London.

Halm, J. *et al.* (2003) Interdisciplinary rounds: impact on patients, family and staff. *Clin Nurse Spec*, **17**(3), 133–42.

Hancock, S. (2003) Intermediate care and older people. *Nurs Stand*, **17**(48), 45–51.

Health Services Accreditation (1996) *Service Standards for Discharge Care*. NHS, East Sussex.

Hill, M. & Macgregor, G. (2001) *Health's Forgotten Partners? How Carers are Supported Through Hospital Discharge*. Carers UK, London (www.carershealthmatters.org.uk).

Holzhausen, F. (2001) *'You Can Take Him Home Now'. Carers' Experiences of Hospital Discharge*. Carers National Association, London.

House of Commons Health Committee (2005) *NHS Continuing Care, Sixth Report of Session 2004–2005*, Vol. 1. House of Commons, Norwich, pp. 399–1.

Hunter, M. (2001) Will social services suffer in new regime? *Commun Care*, **13**(87), 10–11.

Kumar, S. (2000) *Multidisciplinary Approach to Rehabilitation*. Butterworth Heinemann, London.

Martin, J. (2001) Benchmarking – how do you do it? *Nurs Times*, **97**(42), 30–1.

McKenna, H. *et al.* (2000) Discharge planning: an exploratory study. *J Adv Nurs*, 9, 594–601.

Nazarko, L. (1998) Improving discharge: the role of the discharge co-ordinator. *Nurs Stand*, **12**(49), 35–7.

NHS Connecting for Health (2005) *CRDB SAP Action Team Output V1.0*. Crown Copyright.

NHSE (2001) *Your Guide to the National Health Service*. HMSO, London.

NHS Modernisation Agency (2003) *National Institute for Clinical Excellence: Protocol Based Care*. Department of Health, London.

Nixon, A., Whitter, M. & Stitt, P. (1998) Audit in practice: planning for discharge from hospital. *Nurs Stand*, **12**(26), 35–8.

Royal Marsden NHS Foundation Trust (2006) *Discharge Policy and Procedure*, Internal Document, The Royal Marsden NHS Foundation Trust, London.

Salter, M. (1996) Nursing the patient in the community. In: *Nursing the Patient with Cancer* (ed. V. Tschudin). Prentice Hall, Hemel Hempstead, pp. 438–51.

Smith, A. (2003) Antibiotic resistance. In: *Infection Control in the Community* (eds J. Lawrence & D. May). Churchill Livingstone, London, pp. 319–32.

Smith, S. (1996) Discharge planning: the need for effective communication. *Nurs Stand*, **10**(38), 39–41.

Stewart, W. (2000) Development of discharge skills: a project report. *Nurs Times*, **96**(41), 37.

Tarling, M. & Jauffur, H. (2006) Improving team meetings to support discharge planning. *Nurs Times*, **26**, 32–5.

Multiple choice questions

1 On discharge from hospital, who is responsible for ensuring a patient's fitness for discharge?

    a   Hospital medical staff
    b   General practitioner
    c   Nurse
    d   Any of the above

2 If a patient wishes to take their own discharge against medical advice, who should the nurse in charge of the ward contact?

    a   A member of the medical team
    b   The manager on call
    c   Complex discharge coordinator
    d   All of the above

3 When discharging a patient from hospital to community nursing services, how much notice should be given?

    a   Minimum 24 hours
    b   Minimum 48 hours
    c   Once transport has been arranged
    d   Once the doctor in charge of the patient's care has said the patient is fit to leave

4 The Single Assessment Process for Older People was introduced in 2001. What is it?

    a   An assessment to ensure that people who live alone are discharged safely and appropriately
    b   The discharge of patients with no comorbidities
    c   Production of a centrally held summary of care resulting in an individual care plan
    d   A government initiative to reduce the numbers of health care professionals necessary to coordinate a discharge effectively

Answers to the multiple choice questions can be found in Appendix 3.

Chapter 8

Drug administration:
general principles

Definition

Drug administration can be defined as the way medicines are selected, procured, delivered, prescribed, administered and reviewed to optimize the contributions that medicines make to producing informed and desired outcomes of patient care (Audit Commission 2001). The professional role of the nurse in medicines management is the safe handling and administration of medicines, including a responsibility for making sure that patients understand what medicines they are taking and why, including the likely side-effects (Luker & Wolfson 1999). Medicinal products are defined, according to the Medicines Act 1968, as, 'substances sold or supplied for administration to humans (or animals) for medicinal purposes' (HMSO 1968).

Indications

Drugs can be administered for the following purposes.

- Diagnostic purposes, e.g. assessment of liver function or diagnosis of myasthenia gravis.
- Prophylaxis, e.g. heparin to prevent thrombosis or antibiotics to prevent infection.
- Therapeutic purposes, e.g. replacement of fluids or vitamins, supportive purposes (to enable other treatments, such as anaesthesia), palliation of pain and cure (as in the case of antibiotics).

Reference material

Drug administration has been one of the most common clinical procedures a nurse has undertaken for at least the past 50 years (Shepherd 2002a). With changes in legal, professional and cultural boundaries in health care, the role of the nurse has broadened to one of medicines management.

The legal and professional context

Medicines management and specifically drug administration require thought and professional judgement (Luker & Wolfson 1999; NMC 2008a). All aspects of a medicine's use must be managed with a multidisciplinary approach to ensure it is supported by a strong evidence base and that the safety and well being of the patient remain paramount (Shepherd 2002a; NMC 2008b).

Legislation

Legislative frameworks, government guidelines and professional regulations govern medicines management in the UK. The two pieces of primary legislation of importance are the Medicines Act 1968 and the Misuse of Drugs Act 1971 (HMSO 1971).

The Medicines Act 1968

The Medicines Act 1968 (HMSO 1968) establishes a licensing system for medicines for human use, controlling the manufacture and distribution, regulating who can lawfully supply and be in possession of medicines and how they should be packaged and labelled. The Medicines and Health Care Products Regulatory Agency (MHRA) in the UK and the European Medicines Evaluation Agency (EMEA) are responsible for issuing the product licences. The availability of products is restricted by defining which of the following legal categories they are in:

- Prescription-only medicines (POM).
- Pharmacy only medicines (P).
- General sales list medicines (GSL).

Different requirements apply to the sale, supply and labelling of medicines in each category. In National Health Service (NHS) hospitals, adherence to the Act means that a pharmacist supervises the purchasing and supply of medicines, and that supply or administration to a patient is only on a doctor's prescription. Sections 9, 10 and 11 of the Act exempt doctors, dentists, pharmacists and nurses, respectively, from many restrictions otherwise imposed by the Act on the general public, and thus allow them to supply and use drugs in the practice of their respective professions.

Unlicensed medicines

An unlicensed medicine is a term used to refer to a medicine with no product licence. 'Off label' medicines refer to drugs which are licensed but used outside of the licensed indications. If a medicine is unlicensed, it should only be administered to a patient/client with their informed consent against a patient-specific direction not against a patient group direction (PGD) (NMC 2008a). However, 'off label' medicines, 'may be administered under a PGD if such use is exceptional, justified by best practice and the staus of the product clearly described' (NMC 2008a). The use of unlicensed and 'off label' medicines is common in hospitals, particularly in oncology and palliative care for clinical trials and symptom control. If an unlicensed medicine is administered to a patient/client, the manufacturer has no liability for any harm which may ensue (NMC 2008a). Therefore, it is very important that all prescribers, dispensing pharmacists and administering nurses are aware of their responsibilities with these medicines, and that the associated medico-legal implications are encompassed within organizations' clinical governance arrangements.

The Misuse of Drugs Act 1971

For reasons of public safety the Misuse of Drugs Act (1971) controls the import, export, production, supply, possession and manufacture of controlled drugs to prevent abuse as most are potentially addictive or habit forming. Other regulations of the Act govern safe storage, destruction and supply to known addicts.

The level of control to be exercised is related to the potential for abuse or misuse of the substances concerned. Under the current 2001 Misuse of Drugs regulations, controlled drugs are classified into five schedules, each representing a different level of control (HMSO 2001). The requirements of the Act as they apply to nurses working in a hospital with a pharmacy department are described in Table 8.1.

Implications of the Act for nursing practice

Hospital wards and departments are authorized to hold a stock of controlled drugs. These should be stored in a suitably secure cupboard, which is kept locked and to which access is restricted to registered nurses and pharmacy staff. Controlled drugs are obtained by the use of a special duplicate order form signed by the nurse in charge who is then responsible for them. The order forms must be stored in a locked cupboard when not in use.

Controlled drugs may be administered only to a patient in that ward or department when prescribed by an authorized medical or non-medical prescriber. A prescription must be written in the prescriber's handwriting. To write a prescription for a controlled drug, a prescriber must be resident in the UK and the pharmacist must know and have a record of his/her signature. In the hospital setting this excludes locum doctors from writing prescriptions for controlled drugs. The Aitken report (Central Health Services Council 1958) recommends that two nurses check all controlled drug entries. Appropriate records of their use must

Table 8.1 Summary of legal requirements for handling of controlled drugs (CDs) as they apply to nurses in hospitals with a pharmacy.

	Schedule 1: CDs Home Office Licence	Schedule 2: CDs subject to full controls	Schedule 3: CDs with no register entry	Schedule 4: CDs anabolic steroids/ benzodiazepines	Schedule 5: CDs needing invoice retention
Drugs in the schedule	Cannabis + derivatives but excluding nabilone, LSD (lysergic acid diethylamide)	Most opioids in common use including: alfentanyl; amphetamines; cocaine; diamorphine; methadone; morphine papaveretum; fentanyl; phenoperidine. Pethidine; codeine; Dihydrocodeine injections; Pentazocine	Minor stimulants Barbiturates (but excluding hexobarbitone, thiopentone) Diethylpropion Buprenorphine Temazepam†	Part 1: anabolic steroids Part 2: benzodiazepines	Some preparations containing very low strengths of: cocaine; codeine; morphine; pholcodine; and some other opioids
Ordering	Possession and supply permitted only by special licence from the Secretary of State issued (to a doctor only) for scientific or research purposes	A requisition must be signed in duplicate by the nurse in charge. The requisition must be endorsed to indicate that the drugs have been supplied. Copies should be kept for 2 years	As Schedule 2	No requirement*	No requirement*
Storage	Must be kept in a suitable locked cupboard to which access is restricted	As Schedule 1	Buprenorphine and diethylpropion: as Schedule ' drugs All other drugs no requirement	No requirement*	No requirement*
Record keeping	Controlled drug register must be used	As Schedule 1	No requirement	No requirement*	No requirement*

Prescription	Prescription must include: ■ the name and address of patient ■ the drug, the dose, the form of preparation ■ the total quantity of drug or the total number of dosage units to be supplied. This quantity must be stated in words and figures The prescription must be written indelibly in the prescriber's own handwriting	As Schedule 1	As Schedule 1 Except for phenobarbitone (this includes all preparations of phenobarbitone and phenobarbitone sodium). Because of its use as an antiepileptic, it does not need to be written in the prescriber's own handwriting	No requirement*	No requirement*
Administration to patients	Under special licence only A doctor or dentist or anyone acting on their instructions may administer these drugs to anyone for whom they have been prescribed	A doctor or dentist or anyone acting on their instructions may administer these drugs to anyone for whom they have been prescribed	A doctor or dentist or anyone acting on their instructions may administer these drugs to anyone for whom they have been prescribed	No requirement*	No requirement*

* 'No requirement' indicates that the Misuse of Drugs Act 1971 imposes no legal requirements additional to those imposed by the Medicines Act 1968 (HMSO 1968).

† Temazepam preparations are exempt from record keeping and prescription requirements, but are subject to storage requirements.

259

be maintained. There is no legal requirement for the nurse in charge or acting in charge of a ward or department to keep a record of Schedule 1 or 2 controlled drugs obtained or supplied. However, the Aitken report (Central Health Services Council 1958) recommended that this should be done and in practice a controlled drug register is usually kept according to the following guidelines:

- Each page should be clearly headed to indicate the drug and preparation to which it refers.
- Entries should be made as soon as possible after the relevant transaction has occurred and always within 24 hours.
- No cancellations or obliteration of an entry should be made. Corrections should be made by means of a note in the margin or at the foot of the page and this should be signed, dated and cross-referenced to the relevant entry.
- All entries should be indelible.
- The register should be used for controlled drugs only and for no other purposes and be stored in a locked cupboard when not in use.
- Completed registers and copies of orders should be kept for 2 years.

Unwanted drugs should normally be destroyed in the pharmacy but may, under some circumstances, be disposed of on the ward under the supervision of a pharmacist. An appropriate entry should then be made in the ward register.

In response to seven case reports, published between 2000 and 2005, regarding deaths due to the administration of high-dose (30 mg or greater) morphine or diamorphine to patients who had not previously received doses of opiates, the National Patient Safety Agency (NPSA) released a safer practice notice in 2006, *Ensuring Safer Practice with High Dose Ampoules of Morphine and Diamorphine* (NPSA 2006). In line with this safer practice notice the following guidance should be adhered to:

- High-strength preparations of morphine or diamorphine (30 mg or above) should be stored in a separate location from lower-strength preparations (10 mg) within the controlled drugs cupboard.
- Awareness should be raised of the similarities of drug packaging, and consider use of alert stickers being attached to high-strength preparations by pharmacy.
- A review of stock levels should be taken in all clinical areas where morphine and diamorphine are stored to assess if high-strength preparations need to be kept on a permanent basis or whether they could be ordered according to specific patient requirements.
- Clear guidance should be provided to ensure the correct doses of diamorphine and morphine are prepared in the appropriate clinical situation. For example, diamorphine 5-mg and 10-mg ampoules could be used for both bolus administration and patients newly commenced on diamorphine infusions;

diamorphine 30-mg ampoules could be reserved for patients already receiving diamorphine infusions and who require higher daily doses.
■ Patients should be observed for the 1st hour after receiving their first dose of diamorphine or morphine injection.
■ Naloxone injections should be available in all clinical areas where morphine and diamorphine is stored.

Storage of medicines

The Duthie Report (DH 1988) requires NHS Trusts to establish, document and maintain procedures to ensure and demonstrate that medicines are stored and handled in a safe and secure manner. Under the Duthie Report the nurse in charge of a ward or clinical area is responsible for the safe storage of all medicines. Some of these duties may be delegated, such as the ordering of additional medicines, but the responsibility remains with the nurse in charge. He/she is also responsible for controlling access (by keys or other means) to the medicines cupboards even if he/she decides to delegate this duty.

The storage of medicines is governed by the following principles.

Security

All drugs should be stored in locked cupboards with separate storage for internal medicines, external medicines, controlled drugs and medicines needing refrigeration or storage in a freezer.

Diagnostic reagents, intravenous and topical agents should also be kept separately.

Stability

No medicinal preparation should be stored where it may be subject to substantial variations in temperature, e.g. not in direct sunlight. The normal temperature ranges for storage are 'a cool place', normally interpreted as meaning between 1 and 15°C; 'refrigerated' at a temperature between 2 and 8°C; 'room temperature' between 15 and 25°C. Refrigerators must have their temperatures monitored and recorded daily and appropriate action taken if the recordings are not within 2 and 8°C.

Labelling

The wording of labels is chosen carefully to convey clearly all essential information. Printed labels should always be used.

Containers

The type of container used may have been chosen for specific reasons. Therefore all medicines should be stored in the containers in which they were supplied by pharmacy. Medicinal preparations should never be transferred (in bulk) from one container to another except in the pharmacy.

Stock control

A system of stock rotation must be operated (e.g. first in, first out) to ensure that there is no accumulation of old stocks. Only one pack/container of a named medicine should be in use at any one time.

Storage requirements of specific preparations

- *Aerosol containers* should not be stored in direct sunlight or over radiators: there is a risk of explosion if they are heated.
- *Creams* may deteriorate rapidly if subjected to extremes of temperature.
- *Eye drops and ointments* may become contaminated with micro-organisms during use and thus pose a danger to the recipient. Therefore in hospitals, eye preparations should be discarded 7 days after they are first opened. For use at home this limit is extended to 28 days.
- *Mixtures* may have a relatively short shelf-life. Most antibiotic mixtures require refrigerated storage and even then have a shelf-life of only 7–14 days. Always check the label for details.
- *Tablets and capsules* are relatively stable but are susceptible to moisture unless correctly packed. They should be stored only in the containers in which they were supplied by the pharmacy.
- *Vaccines* and similar preparations usually require refrigerated storage and may deteriorate rapidly if exposed to heat.

Patient's own drugs

Patients are encouraged to bring their medication into hospital with them to facilitate the collection of a comprehensive and accurate medication history. These medicines remain the patient's property and should either be stored securely in the ward's drug cupboard until discharge or sent home with a relative or carer. These medicines should neither be disposed of without the patient's consent nor used for other patients.

Types of medicinal preparations of drugs

Preparations for oral administration

Tablets
These come in a great variety of shapes, sizes, colours and types. The formulation may be very simple and result for instance in a plain, white, uncoated tablet, or complex and designed with specific therapeutic aims. Sugar coatings are used to improve appearances and palatability. In cases where the drug is a gastric irritant

or is broken down by gastric acid, an enteric coating may be used. This is designed to allow the tablet to remain intact in the stomach and to pass unchanged into the small bowel where the coating dissolves and hence the drug is released and absorbed. Tablets may be formulated specifically to achieve control of the rate of release of drug from the tablet as it passes through the alimentary tract. Terms such as 'sustained-release', 'controlled-release' and 'modified-release' are used by manufacturers to describe these preparations. Tablets may also be formulated specifically to dissolve readily ('soluble' or 'effervescent'), to be chewed or to be held under the tongue ('sublingual') or placed between the gum and inside of the mouth ('buccal'). Unscored or coated tablets should not be crushed or broken, nor should most 'slow-release' or 'sustained action' tablets, since this can alter the rate of release of drug from the tablet.

Capsules

These offer a useful method of formulating drugs which are difficult to make into a tablet or are particularly unpalatable.

The capsule shells are usually made of gelatin and the contents of the capsules may be solid, liquid or of a paste-like consistency. The contents do not cause deterioration of the shell. The shell, however, is attacked by the digestive fluids and the contents are then released. Delayed-release capsule formulations also exist. Gastro-resistant capsules are delayed-release capsules that are intended to resist the gastric fluid and to release their active substance or substances in the intestinal fluid (British Pharmacopoeia 2007). If for any reason the capsule is unsuitable, the contents should not routinely be removed from the shell without first seeking advice from a pharmacist. Removing contents from the capsule could destroy their properties and cause gastric irritation or premature release of the drug into an incompatible pH (Downie *et al.* 2000).

Lozenges and pastilles

Lozenges and pastilles are solid, single-dose preparations intended to be sucked to obtain a local or systemic effect to the mouth and/or throat (British Pharmacopoeia 2007).

Elixirs, linctuses and syrups

Elixirs   These are clear, flavoured oral liquids containing one or more active ingredients dissolved in a vehicle that usually contains a high proportion of sucrose.

Linctuses   These are viscous oral liquids that may contain one or more active ingredients; the solution usually contains a high proportion of sucrose. Linctuses are intended for use in the treatment or relief of cough (British Pharmacopoeia 2007).

Syrups   These do not contain active ingredients and many are used as vehicle ingredients for their flavouring and sweetening.

Mixtures

These are flavoured solutions or suspensions of drugs used mainly when patients cannot swallow a tablet or the drug is not available as a tablet. It is particularly important that suspensions are thoroughly mixed by shaking before each dose is measured. This ensures that the measured volume always contains the correct amount of drug.

Rectal and vaginal preparations

Enemas

These are solutions which are instilled into the rectum as laxatives or to obtain other localized therapeutic effects, or for diagnostic purposes.

Suppositories

These are solid wax pellets for rectal administration. They may either melt at body temperature or dissolve or disperse in the mucous secretions of the rectum. They may be used to obtain local effect (e.g. as laxatives) or for systemic therapy. Many drugs, such as the opioids; are well absorbed when administered this way. Suppositories sometimes offer a useful alternative to injections for very sick patients unable to take drugs orally. They must be administered according to the manufacturer's recommendations.

Pessaries

These are solid pellets for vaginal administration and are usually designed to have a local therapeutic action.

Topical preparations

Creams

Creams are emulsions of oil and water and are generally well absorbed into the skin. They are usually more cosmetically acceptable than ointments because they are less greasy and easy to apply (BNF 2008). They may be used as a 'base' in which a variety of drugs may be applied for local therapy (BNF 2008).

Ointments

Ointments are greasy preparations, which are normally anhydrous and insoluble in water, and are more occlusive than creams (BNF 2008). They are absorbed more slowly into the skin and leave a greasy residue. They have similar uses to creams, and are particularly suitable for dry, scaly lesions (BNF 2008).

Transdermal patches

A number of drugs such as hyoscine to prevent motion sickness, oestrogens for hormone replacement therapy and fentanyl for pain control are now available in 'transdermal patches'. A very small volume of drug solution is contained in a reservoir which is stuck on the skin. Drug molecules diffuse at a constant rate through a semipermeable membrane which is in direct contact with the skin when the patch is applied. The drug is absorbed through the skin and into the capillary blood supply from where it enters the systemic circulation. Advantages include a constant rate of drug administration over several days which may reduce the incidence of side-effects and improve patient compliance.

Wound products

See Chapter 34.

Injections

Injections are sterile solutions, emulsions or suspensions. They are prepared by dissolving, emulsifying or suspending the active ingredient and any added substances in water for injections, in a suitable non-aqueous liquid or in a mixture of these vehicles (British Pharmacopoeia 2007).

Single-dose preparations

The volume of the injection in a single-dose container is sufficient to permit the withdrawal and administration of the nominal dose using a normal technique.

Multidose preparations

Multidose aqueous injections contain a suitable antimicrobial preservative at an appropriate concentration except when the preparation itself has adequate antimicrobial properties. When it is necessary to present a preparation for parenteral use in a multidose container, the precautions to be taken for its administration and more particularly for its storage between successive withdrawals are given.

Parenteral infusions

Parenteral infusions are sterile, aqueous solutions or emulsions with water; they are free from pyrogens and are usually made isotonic with blood. They are principally intended for administration in large volume. Parenteral infusions do not contain any added antimicrobial preservative (British Pharmacopoeia 2007).

Inhalations

Two techniques, nebulization and aerosolization, permit the inhalation of a range of drugs with the aim of a localized therapeutic effect.

265

Nebulization involves the passage of air or oxygen driven through a solution of a drug. The resulting fine mist is then inhaled via a face mask (Trounce & Gould 2000). Some antibiotics and bronchodilators may be given in this way.

Aerosolization involves the use of a solution of drug in an inert diluent. Passing a metred volume of this solution through a valve under pressure allows the delivery to the patient of a measured dose of drug in a very fine spray of controlled particle size. Bronchodilators and steroids are administered commonly in this way. Although a very small total dose of drug is administered, the concentration achieved at the site of action is high. Rapid and effective control of symptoms is achieved but without the side-effects commonly associated with an equivalent systemic (oral or parenteral) dose of the drug(s).

Many patients can be taught to use aerosol inhalers effectively but some patients, particularly the elderly and small children, may find it difficult to use them. Spacer devices can help such patients because they remove the need to co-ordinate actuation with inhalation (BNF 2008). For those who cannot co-ordinate aerosol inhalation, alternative methods of administration include breath-actuated inhalers or dry powder inhalers which merely require the patient to breathe in. No co-ordination of hand movement and breathing is required. Some dry powder inhalers occasionally cause coughing due to irritation of the throat and trachea by the dry powder (Downie *et al.* 2000).

Administration

The effective and safe administration of drugs to patients demands a partnership between the various health professionals concerned, i.e. doctors, pharmacists and nurses. A medicine is an active chemical or biological substance with diagnostic, curative or preventive purposes. The manner in which it is administered determines the extent to which a patient gains any clinical benefit and whether any adverse effect is experienced. One of the main factors that determine whether or not a medicine will reach its intended site of action in the body is how it is given (Shepherd 2002a). Nurses are responsible for the correct administration of prescribed drugs to patients in their care at all times, being guided by the Nursing and Midwifery Council (NMC) *Standards for Medicines Management* (NMC 2008a).

All medicines administered in hospital must be considered prescription only. This is because administration, whether by a nurse or by a patient to themselves, may only take place in accordance with one or more of the following processes:

- Patient specific direction (PSD).
- Patient medicines administration chart (MAR).
- Patient group direction (PGD).
- Medicines Act exemption.

- Standing orders.
- Homely remedy protocol.
- Prescription form.

(NMC 2008a, pp. 13–16).

'Verbal orders'

The NMC clearly states that the instruction by telephone to administer a previously unprescribed medicine is unacceptable. In exceptional circumstances, where the medication has been previously prescribed and the prescriber is unable to issue a new prescription, but where changes to the dose are considered necessary, the use of information technology (such as fax or e-mail) is the preferred method. This should be followed up by a new prescription confirming the changes . . . within a maximum of 24 hours. In any event the changes must be authorized before the new dosage is administered (NMC 2008a).

Medicine administration should ensure that the correct patient receives:

267

- the appropriate medicine;
- in the appropriate formulation;
- by the appropriate route;
- at the appropriate dose;
- at the appropriate time;
- at the appropriate rate;
- for the appropriate duration of therapy;
- with the appropriate monitoring to ensure safety and efficacy of therapy;
- with the appropriate reporting of adverse drug reactions (Sexton 1999, p. 240).

To achieve this, the nurse must have a sound knowledge of the use, action, usual dose and side-effects of the drugs being administered. Institutional policies and procedures also assist the nurse to administer drugs safely and a sound knowledge of local procedures is essential. The importance of reporting errors to the appropriate authority should never be underestimated as research suggests that many undeclared medication errors are made by nurses. The immediate and honest disclosure that an error has occurred results in the patient receiving the required emergency treatment. Organizational policies therefore need to reflect a culture that encourages disclosure and in which the management of medication errors is viewed as a learning process as opposed to a punitive act (Martin 1994; Gladstone 1995). The NMC states that all errors and incidents require a thorough and careful investigation at a local level, taking full account of the context, circumstances and position of the practitioner involved. Such incidents require a sensitive management and a comprehensive assessment of all the circumstances before a professional and managerial decision is reached on the appropriate way to proceed (NMC 2008a).

It must be recognized, however, that errors in drug administration can have traumatic consequences for the individual nurse involved and that disciplinary procedures invoke fear in most nurses (Arndt 1994).

Single nurse administration of medicines

In the majority of hospitals it is policy that medicines administration is carried out by a single qualified nurse. It is thought that single nurse administration of medicines will result in greater care being given since the nurse will be aware that she or he is solely responsible and accountable.

Those nurses who wish or need to have their administration supervised will retain the right to do so until such time as all parties agree that the requested level of proficiency has been achieved. The nurse checking the medicine must be able to justify any action taken and be accountable for the action taken. This is in keeping with the principles of *The Code* (NMC 2008b).

Self-administration of medicines

With evidence that between 30 and 70% of patients are non-compliant with taking prescribed medication (Royal Pharmaceutical Society 1997), the self-administration of medicines in hospitals is encouraged. Non-adherence to medication regimens is a significant problem in older patients (McGraw & Drennan 2001). Self administration of medicines is recommended by the *National Service Framework for Older People* (Pratt *et al.* 2007) as a strategy to address this major issue. All patients benefit significantly from the opportunity to adjust to the responsibility of self-administration while still having access to professional support (NMC 2008a). It has also been found that patients who had administered their own medications in hospital were more likely to report that their overall care was excellent and that they were satisfied with the discharge process than patients who had not (Deeks & Byatt 2000). Bird (1990) suggests that for the majority of hospital patients, self-administration of drugs would appear to be a more appropriate method than the conventional system. Self-administration is not merely the process of patients taking their own drugs; it can also help clients retain or regain control over their health.

The safety and success of a self-administration system in hospital are based upon the nursing assessment of the patient and the subsequent teaching (Shepherd 2002b). The nursing assessment should include a measure of the patient's ability to interpret and participate in the prescribed treatment regimen and seek to determine whether the patient already takes prescribed treatment at home and how they manage that and whether they can understand the medicine labels and the dosage instructions (Shepherd 2002b). Teaching patients to take their own medication correctly forms part of their programme of rehabilitation, which should begin with the first multidisciplinary assessment on their arrival in hospital. Patients taught to self-administer their drugs in hospital are encouraged to regain independence and to participate in their own care. Self-administration also provides an opportunity to identify additional education needs and improve compliance. Importantly, it also raises awareness of those patients who are unable to self-administer and will need additional support on discharge (Shepherd 2002b).

Although, by definition, self-administration of medicines shifts the balance of responsibility for this part of care towards the patient, it in no way diminishes the fundamental professional duty of care. It is therefore essential that local policies, procedures and records are adequate to ensure that this duty is, and can be shown to be, discharged.

Even if a patient is self-administering their medication, continual assessment of this aspect of their care while they are in hospital is important. The nurse must continually be aware of the patient's capability to self-administer and the action of the drugs the patient is taking. No drug produces a single effect. The combined effect of two or more drugs taken together may be different from the effects when taken separately. The effectiveness of any drug should be noted and any signs of resistance or dependence reported.

Provision must be made for the patients to have access to their own lockable cupboard, usually at the bedside, for the specific purpose of allowing the safe storage of medicines.

Covert drug administration

The NMC recognizes that 'this a complex issue', as covert drug administration 'involves the fundamental principles of patient and client autonomy and consent to treatment, which are set out in common law and statute and underpinned by the Human Rights Act 1998' (NMC 2008a). The covert administration of medicines 'should not be confused with the administration of medicines against someone's will, which in itself may not be deceptive, but may be unlawful' (NMC 2008a).

Some vulnerable groups of patients, for example those who are confused, may refuse to take medication. Traditionally, in some places, medication has therefore been hidden or disguised in food. The NMC (2001a, b; 2008a) offered the following position statement:

> As a general principle, by disguising medication in food or drink, the patient or client is being led to believe that they are not receiving medication when in fact they are. The registered nurse, midwife or health visitor will need to be sure that what they are doing is in the best interests of the patient or client and be accountable for this decision.
> (NMC 2001a; NMC 2008a.)

Disguising medication in food and drink is acceptable under exceptional circumstances in which covert administration may be considered to prevent a patient, who is incapable of informed consent, from missing out on essential treatment (NMC 2001b; NMC 2008a). The following principles should be followed when making such a decision.

- The medication must be considered essential for the patient's health and well-being.
- The decision to administer medication covertly should be considered only as a contingency in an emergency, not as regular practice.
- The registered practitioner must make the decision only after discussion and with the support of the multiprofessional team and, if appropriate, the patient's relatives, carers or advocates.
- The pharmacist must be involved in these decisions as adding medication to food or drink can alter its pharmacological properties and thereby affect its performance.
- The decision and action taken must be fully documented in the patient's care plan and regularly reviewed.
- Regular attempts should continue to be made to encourage the patient to take the medication voluntarily (Treloar *et al.* 2000; NMC 2001b; NMC 2008a).

Nurse prescribing and Patient Group Directions

As nurses have undertaken increasingly specialized roles the need for them to have powers to prescribe has become more apparent. The Report of the Advisory Committee on Nurse Prescribing (DH 1989) initially recommended a limited nurses' formulary for District Nurses and Health Visitors. The Medicinal Products: Prescription by Nurse etc. Act (1992) granted the statutory authority for this to occur. The Crown Report (DH 1989) also recommended that doctors and nurses collaborate in drawing up local protocols for the administration of medicines in situations that would benefit specific groups of patients, for example those requiring vaccinations.

The practice of prescribing under group protocols became widespread across the NHS, and they were used to support initiatives such as nurse-led clinics (Laverty *et al.* 1997; Mallett *et al.* 1997). The legality of this practice was then questioned. Section 58 of the Medicines Act (1968) states that no one should administer any medication (other than to himself) unless he is the appropriate practitioner or a person who is acting according to directions from an appropriate practitioner. The terms *direction* and *administration* were open to interpretation and how they were used varied across the country (McHale 2002).

Nurse prescribing was therefore reviewed and two further reports were published:

- *Review of Prescribing, Supply and Administration of Medicines. A Report on the Supply and Administration of Medicines under Group Protocols* (DH 1998).
- *Review of Prescribing, Supply and Administration of Medicines. Final Report* (DH 1999).

The first specifically offered guidance about group protocols, including changing the name to patient group directions (PGDs).

- *Patient Group Directions.* This is defined as a specific written instruction for the supply or administration by nurses, pharmacists or other authorized named professionals of named medicines in an identified clinical situation, in the absence of a prescription. It is drawn up locally by doctors, pharmacists and other appropriate professionals and must be approved by the employer, advised by the relevant professional advisory committee. It applies to groups of patients or other service users who may not be individually identified before presentation for treatment (DH 2004). The Health and Safety Commission (HSC) advised that the majority of medication 'should be prescribed and administered on an individual patient specific basis', but that it is appropriate to use PGDs for the supply and administration of medicines in situations where this offers an advantage for patient care (DH 2000). Shepherd suggests that this means, 'where medical staff are either inaccessible or unavailable' (Shepherd 2002b, p. 44). The flowchart in Figure 8.1 aims to assist practitioners in deciding the appropriate system for the prescription, supply or administration of medicines.

271

The second report looked at the existing arrangements for prescribing, supply and administration of medicines and suggested the introduction of a new form of prescribing to be undertaken by non-medical health professionals (DH 2003a). Independent nurse prescribing was initially allowed from an extremely limited formulary (Shuttleworth 2005). It was then extended a number of times until finally appropriately qualified nurses were allowed to prescribe from the whole *British National Formulary.*

There are now two categories of prescriber:

1. *Independent prescribing:* This allows nurses who are registered as independent prescribers to prescibe any licensed medicine for any medical condition (this also includes some controlled drugs) but only within their own level of experience and competence, and acting in accordance with of the NMC's Code (NMC 2008b). Only those who have undergone appropriate training and are registered with the NMC as an independent prescriber can prescribe (NMC 2006). It must also be judged that it is part of the nurse's role.

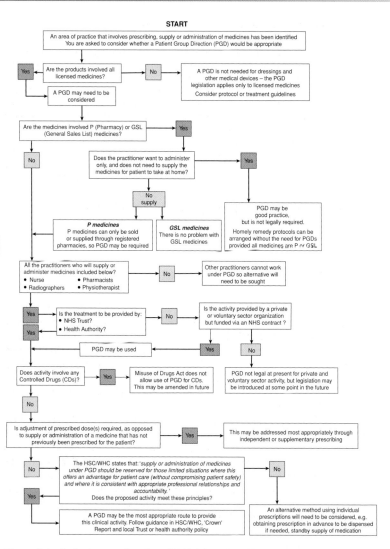

START

An area of practice that involves prescribing, supply or administration of medicines has been identified
You are asked to consider whether a Patient Group Direction (PGD) would be appropriate

Yes — Are the products involved all licensed medicines? — No — A PGD is not needed for dressings and other medical devices – the PGD legislation applies only to licensed medicines. Consider protocol or treatment guidelines

A PGD may need to be considered

Are the medicines involved P (Pharmacy) or GSL (General Sales List) medicines? — Yes

No

Does the practitioner want to administer only, and does not need to supply the medicines for patient to take at home? — Yes

No supply

PGD may be good practice, but is not legally required. Homely remedy protocols can be arranged without the need for PGDs provided all medicines are P or GSL

P medicines
P medicines can only be sold or supplied through registered pharmacies, so PGD may be required

GSL medicines
There is no problem with GSL medicines

All the practitioners who will supply or administer medicines included below?
• Nurse   • Pharmacists
• Radiographers   • Physiotherapist
— No — Other practitioners cannot work under PGD so alternative will need to be sought

Yes — Is the treatment to be provided by:
• NHS Trust?
• Health Authority?
— No — Is the activity provided by a private or voluntary sector organization but funded via an NHS contract ?

Yes

PGD may be used — Yes

No

Does activity involve any Controlled Drugs (CDs)? — Yes — Misuse of Drugs Act does not allow use of PGD for CDs. This may be amended in future

PGD not legal at present for private and voluntary sector activity, but legislation may be introduced at some point in the future

No

Is adjustment of prescribed dose(s) required, as opposed to supply or administration of a medicine that has not previously been prescribed for the patient? — Yes — This may be addressed most appropriately through independent or supplementary prescribing

No

The HSC/WHC states that: 'supply or administration of medicines under PGD should be reserved for those limited situations where this offers an advantage for patient care (without compromising patient safety) and where it is consistent with appropriate professional relationships and accountability.'
Does the proposed activity meet these principles?
— No

Yes

A PGD may be the most appropriate route to provide this clinical activity. Follow guidance in HSC/WHC, 'Crown' Report and local Trust or health authority policy

An alternative method using individual prescriptions will need to be considered, e.g. obtaining prescription in advance to be dispensed if needed, standby supply of medication

272

Figure 8.1   Patient group directions (PGDs) flowchart. The diagram above takes the practitioner through a logical process that aims to assist decision making. **The majority of clinical care should still be provided on an individual, patient-specific basis.**

2 *Supplementary prescribing* has been defined as:

> A voluntary prescribing partnership between an independent prescriber and a supplementary prescriber to implement an agreed patient specific clinical management plan with the patient's agreement' (DH 2003b). Amendments to the Prescription Only Medicines Order and the NHS regulations allowed supplementary prescribing by suitably trained nurses from April 2003. Supplementary prescribers prescribe in partnership with a doctor or dentist (the independent prescriber) and are able to prescribe any medicine including controlled drugs and unlicensed medicines that are listed in an agreed Clinical Management Plan. The plan is drawn up with the patient's agreement, following diagnosis of the patient by an independent prescriber and following consultation and agreement between the independent and supplementary prescribers.
> (DH 2003b, p. 6 and 7)

The key principles that underpin supplementary prescribing are:

- The importance of communication between prescribing partners.
- The need for access to shared patient records.
- The patient is treated as a partner in their care and is involved at all stages in decision making, including whether part of their care is delivered via supplementary prescribing (NPC 2003a).

273

Preparation for both independent nurse prescribing and supplementary prescribing is at least 26 days in length and must follow the standards set out in NMC's *Circular 25/2002* (NMC 2001c). Any preparation must enable independent and supplementary non-medical prescribers to reach the competencies outlined in *Maintaining Competency in Prescribing: An Outline Framework to Help Nurse Prescribers* (NPC 2001) and the additional guidance in *Maintaining Competency in Prescribing: An Outline Framework to Help Nurse Supplementary Prescribers* (NPC 2003b).

The addition of prescriptive authority to the nurse role has been a positive way of making a service not only more responsive for service users, but also has helped to resource increasing demands on health services (Bridge *et al.* 2005). In 2005 it was estimated that there were 28 000 nurses who were able to prescribe from the limited formulary and 4000 extended prescribers (MHRA 2005). In a national survey of 246 nurse prescribers they concluded that nurse prescribing is largely successful in both practice and policy terms (Latter *et al.* 2005): this is discussed in more detail in Table 8.2.

Intravenous administration

Intravenous therapy is now an integral part of the majority of nurses' professional practice (RCN 2005). The nurse's role has progressed considerably from being able to add drugs to infusion bags (DHSS 1976) to now assessing patients and

Table 8.2 An evaluation of nurse prescribing. Source: Latter *et al.* 2005 (cited in Shuttleworth 2005).

- Most nurse prescribers were confident in their prescribing practice
- Most felt extended prescribing had a positive impact on patient care and enabled them to make better use of their skills
- Most felt that the limited nurse formulary imposed unhelpful limitation on their practice
- Nurses were satisfied with the support received from their medical practitioner
- Patients are positive about their experience of nurse prescribing
- Doctors were positive about the development of nurse prescribers in their teams

inserting the appropriate vascular access devices (VAD) prior to drug administration (Gabriel 2005).

Any nurse administering intravenous drugs must be competent in all aspects of intravenous therapy and act in accordance with the NMC Code (2008b), i.e. to maintain knowledge and skills (RCN 2005; Hyde 2008). Training and assessment should comprise both a theoretical and practical component and include legal and professional issues, fluid balance, pharmacology, drug administration, local and systemic complications, infection control issues, use of equipment and risk management (RCN 2005; Hyde 2008).

The nurse's responsibilities in relation to intravenous drug administration include:

1 Knowing the therapeutic use of the drug or solution, its normal dosage, side-effects, precautions and contraindications.
2 Preparing the drug aseptically and safely, checking the container and drug for faults, using the correct diluent and only preparing it immediately prior to administration.
3 Identifying the patient and checking allergy status.
4 Checking the prescription chart.
5 Checking and maintaining patency of the VAD.
6 Inspecting the site of the VAD and managing/reporting complications where appropriate.
7 Controlling the flow rate of infusion and/or speed of injection.
8 Monitoring the condition of the patient and reporting changes.
9 Make clear and immediate records of all drugs administered (RCN 2005; Finlay 2008; NMC 2008a, 2008b).

The NMC Standards for Medicines Management states that 'wherever possible two registrants should check medication to be administered intravenously, one of whom should also be the registrant who then administers the intravenous medication (NMC 2008a, p. 31).

274

Injections and infusions

Injections can be described as the act of giving medication by use of a syringe and needle, and an infusion is defined as an amount of fluid in excess of 100 ml designated for parenteral infusion because the volume must be administered over a long period of time. However, medications may be given in small volumes (50–100 ml) or over a shorter period (30–60 minutes) (Weinstein 2007).

There are a number of routes for injection or infusion. The selection may be predetermined, e.g. intra-arterial, intracardiac or intrathecal injections. The choice of other routes will normally depend on the desired therapeutic effect and the patient's safety and comfort.

The NMC clearly states that:

> It is unacceptable to prepare substances for injection in advance of their immediate use or to administer medication drawn into a syringe or container by another registrant when not in their presence. An exception of this is an already established infusion which has been instigated by another registrant following the principles set out above, or medication prepared under the direction of a pharmacist from a central intravenous additive service and clearly labelled for that patient/client.

> (NMC 2008a.)

275

However, the NMC acknowledges that a registrant 'may be required in an emergency to prepare substances for other professionals' (NMC 2008a).

Intra-arterial

This special technique allows the delivery of a high concentration of drug to the tissues supplied by a particular artery. This route can be used for the administration of chemotherapy and vasodilators and for diagnostic purposes. Injection of drugs into an artery is a rare and hazardous procedure. The introduction of the cannula or catheter must be performed with care as the vessel may go into spasm, causing pain and occlusion. This could result in necrosis of an organ or part of a limb. Injection of irritant chemicals increases the risk of spasm and its sequelae (see Chapter 45, Professional edition); however, arterial catheterization is occasionally performed when it is desirable to deliver a high concentration of a drug to a tumour mass (see Chapter 12, Professional edition). The most common procedures are catheterization of the hepatic artery and isolated limb perfusion.

Intra-articular

In inflammatory conditions of the joints, corticosteroids are given by intra-articular injection to relieve inflammation and increase joint mobility (Downie et al. 2000).

Intrathecal

It may be necessary to administer some drugs intrathecally if they have poor lipid solubility and, as a result, do not pass the blood–brain barrier (Downie *et al.* 2000). A drug specially prepared for the intrathecal route should be used; doses should be carefully calculated and are usually much smaller than would be given by intramuscular or intravenous injection. In the treatment of meningitis, water-soluble antibiotics are administered by the intrathecal route to achieve adequate concentrations in the cerebrospinal fluid (CSF). In addition, antifungal agents, opioids, cytotoxic therapy and radio-opaque substances (used in the diagnosis of spinal lesions) are sometimes administered by this route (Downie *et al.* 2000) (see Chapter 12, Professional edition).

Intradermal

The intradermal route provides a local, rather than systemic effect, and is used primarily for diagnostic purposes such as allergy or tuberculin testing. It can also be used for the administration of local anaesthetics (Workman 1999). Observation of an inflammatory reaction is a priority, so the best sites are those that are lowly pigmented, thinly keratinized and hairless. Chosen sites are the inner forearms and the scapulae. The injection site most commonly used is the medial forearm area. The injections are best performed using a 25 G needle inserted at a 10–15° angle, bevel up, just under the epidermis. Volumes of 0.5 ml or less should be used (Workman 1999).

Subcutaneous

Subcutaneous injections

These are given beneath the epidermis into the fat and connective tissue underlying the dermis. Injections are usually given using a 25 G needle, at a 45° angle. With the introduction of shorter length needles it is recommended that insulin injections be given at an angle of 90° (King 2003). The skin should be gently pinched into a fold to elevate the subcutaneous tissue which lifts the adipose tissue away from the underlying muscle (Workman 1999). The practice of aspirating to ensure a blood vessel has not been pierced is no longer recommended as it has been shown that this is unlikely to occur (Peragallo-Dittko 1997). The maximum volume tolerable using this route for injection is 2 ml and drugs should be highly soluble to prevent irritation (Workman 1999). Administration of infusions of drugs or fluids requires the insertion of a 25 G winged infusion set or a 24 G cannula. These should be inserted at an angle of 45° and secured with a transparent dressing to enable inspection of the site. This may also be appropriate for patients not receiving a continuous infusion but requiring frequent subcutaneous injections; this is common practice in palliative care in order to reduce the number of needlesticks injuries.

Injection sites

Sites recommended are the abdomen in the umbilical region, the lateral or posterior aspect of the lower part of the upper arm, the thighs (under the greater trochanter rather than mid-thigh) and the buttocks. It has been found that the amount of subcutaneous tissue at sites varies more than was previously thought; this is particularly significant for administration of insulin as inadvertent intramuscular administration can result in rapid absorption and hypoglycaemic episodes (King 2003). Rotation of sites can decrease the likelihood of irritation and ensure improved absorption.

Subcutaneous infusions of fluids (hypodermoclysis)

Subcutaneous fluids can be given to maintain adequate hydration in patients with mild or moderate dehydration (Sasson & Shvartzman 2001). The use of this route is generally limited to palliative care or elderly patients. It is not recommended for patients needing rapid administration of fluids, it is also contraindicated in patients with clotting disorders or who have problems with fluid overload (such as patients with cardiac failure).

A volume of 1000–2000 ml can be given over 24 hours; this can be given as a continuous infusion, over a number of hours (such as overnight) or as intermittent boluses (Moriarty & Hudson 2001). It is recommended that electrolyte containing fluids such as sodium chloride 0.9% or dextrose saline be used although 5% glucose has also been used (Noble-Adams 1995). More than one site can be used to allow administration of a greater volume of fluid.

Advantages of this route include:

- Side effects are few and not generally significant.
- As it is a relatively easy procedure it can be carried out at home, reducing the need for hospitalization.
- Intravenous access can be problematic in elderly or debilitated patients; avoidance of this can reduce anxiety and distress (Noble-Adams 1995).

Research has shown that the use of peripheral cannulae rather than steel winged infusion devices results in sites remaining viable for longer (Torre 2002). Incidence of needlestick injuries may also be reduced (Dawkins *et al.* 2000). It is now recommended that subcutaneous infusion be given via a plastic cannula (e.g. Insyte 24 G; 0.7 × 19 mm).

Side-effects of subcutaneous fluid administration include pain, bruising, local oedema, erythema and local infection.

Hyaluronidase is an enzyme which increases the rate of subcutaneous absorption of fluids. It can be given as a subcutaneous injection before commencing fluids. A randomized study compared absorption and side effects of administration of subcutaneous fluids with or without hyaluronidase. No significant differences were found although patients not receiving hyaluronidase showed an increase in size of the limb in which the fluid had been administered, but no differences in pain or local discomfort were found; so no clear benefit to use of hyaluronidase was demonstrated (Constans *et al.* 1991). It is currently unclear from the evidence available whether hyaluronidase should routinely be used (Rochon *et al.* 1997). Rarely severe allergic reactions have been reported.

There is a lack of clear evidence regarding the use of hydration in dying patients. It has been suggested that incidence of delirium may be reduced. It has also been suggested that administration of fluids can reduce feelings of thirst; studies have shown that this is not the case and it may be that a variety of factors play a part, for example certain drugs can cause a dry mouth (Viola *et al.* 1997). Currently practice varies but the risks and benefits for each patient should be carefully considered before a decision is made bearing in mind that issues of nutrition and hydration are particularly sensitive when the patient is dying.

Subcutaneous infusions of drugs

This may be the route of choice in patients with problems such as vomiting, diarrhoea or dysphagia and who are unable to tolerate drugs by the oral route; patients in bowel obstruction whose gut absorption may be impaired may also benefit. It is also commonly used for patients who are dying and no longer able to manage medication orally. Continuous subcutaneous infusion of insulin is used in a small number of diabetic patients; this may be used when adequate control cannot be achieved with multiple daily insulin doses. Such patients need to be under the care of a multidisciplinary team familiar with the use of such infusions (NICE 2003).

Infusions of a single drug, such as an antiemetic or analgesic, do not generally cause problems with stability. The drug should be diluted with a suitable diluent, sodium chloride is recommended for most drugs, and given over 12–24 hours (Dickman *et al.* 2005). The use of a combination of drugs can be problematic; there is anecdotal evidence regarding combinations of drugs but not many pharmaceutical studies confirming compatibility. Combinations of up to four drugs have been reported, but if compatibility is uncertain it may be best to use a second syringe pump. It is also important to ensure that the diluent used is compatible with all the drugs in the infusion. It is recommended that infusions are not exposed to direct sunlight or to increased temperatures as drug instability may result (Dickman *et al.* 2005).

Infusion sites

Choice of site should be based both on thickness of subcutaneous tissue and patient convenience. Sites recommended for subcutaneous infusion of drugs or fluids are the lateral aspects of the upper arms and thighs, the abdomen, the chest and the scapula (Mitten 2001). The following areas should not be used:

- Lymphoedematous areas, as absorption may be impaired and infection may be introduced.
- Sites over bony prominences, as there may be insufficient subcutaneous tissue.
- Previously irradiated skin areas, as absorption may be impaired.
- Sites near a joint, as movement may cause the cannula to become dislodged.
- Any areas of inflamed, infected or broken skin (Mitten 2001).

Care of the site

The site should be assessed regularly for patency; redness, leakage of fluid, bleeding, pain or swelling at the site can be signs of irritation and poor absorption. The time a site can be used for can vary from 1 to 14 days (Kain *et al.* 2006). The syringe should also be inspected for precipitation or cloudiness which may indicate imcompatibility. Some drugs are particularly likely to cause irritation and may need to be diluted in a greater volume of diluent; cyclizine and levomepromazine are among these.

279

If skin sites break down rapidly, suggestions include:

- Check compatibility of drugs and diluents.
- Consider increasing the amount of diluent or changing the diluent.
- Change the infusion device.
- Use a different site cleanser.
- Change the dressing used.
- Consider adding dexamethasone 1 mg to the driver; this may be helpful but is not currently recommended for routine use, care should also be taken as dexamethasone is incompatible with a number of drug combinations (Dickman *et al.* 2005).

Intramuscular

Intramuscular injections should be given into the densest part of the muscle. The injectable volume will depend on the muscle bed. In children, injectable volumes should be halved because muscle mass is less (Workman 1999). Current research evidence suggests that there are five sites that can be utilized for the administration of intramuscular injections (Workman 1999; Rodger & King 2000). These sites (Figure 8.2) are described below.

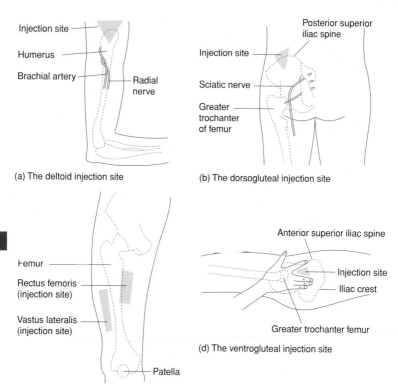

(a) The deltoid injection site

(b) The dorsogluteal injection site

(c) The rectus femoris and vastus lateralis injection sites

(d) The ventrogluteal injection site

Figure 8.2   Intramuscular injection sites. From Rodger and King (2000).

1 The mid-deltoid site (Figure 8.2a). This site has the advantage of being easily accessible whether the patient is standing, sitting or lying down. Owing to the small area of this site, the number and volume of injections which can be given into it are limited. Drugs such as narcotics, sedatives and vaccines, which are usually small in volume, tend to be administered into the deltoid site (Workman 1999). Rodger and King (2000) state that the maximum volume that should be administered at this site is 1 ml.

2 The dorsogluteal site (Figure 8.2b) is used for deep intramuscular and Z-track injections. The gluteus muscle has the lowest drug absorption rate. The muscle mass is also likely to have atrophied in elderly, non-ambulant and emaciated patients. This site carries with it the danger of the needle hitting the sciatic

nerve and the superior gluteal arteries (Workman 1999). The Z-track method involves pulling the skin downwards or to one side of the injection site and inserting the needle at a right angle to the skin, which moves the cutaneous and subcutaneous tissues by approximately 1–2 cm (Workman 1999). The injection is given and the needle withdrawn, while releasing the retracted skin at the same time. This manoeuvre seals off the puncture tract. In adults up to 4 ml can be safely injected into this site (Rodger & King 2000).

3   The rectus femoris site (Figure 8.2c) is used for antiemetics, narcotics, sedatives, injections in oil, deep intramuscular and Z-track injections. The rectus femoris is the anterior quadriceps muscle, which is rarely used by nurses, but is easily accessed for self-administration of injections or for infants (Workman 1999).

4   The vastus lateralis site (Figure 8.2c) is used for deep intramuscular and Z-track injections. One of the advantages of the vastus lateralis site is its ease of access but more importantly, there are no major blood vessels or significant nerve structures associated with this site. Up to 5 ml can be safely injected (Rodger & King 2000).

5   The ventrogluteal site (Figure 8.2d) is used for antibiotics, antiemetics, deep intramuscular and Z-track injections in oil, narcotics and sedatives. This is the site of choice for intramuscular injections (Rodger & King 2000). Up to 2.5 ml can be safely injected into the ventrogluteal site (Rodger & King 2000).

Skin preparation

There are many inconsistencies regarding skin cleaning prior to subcutaneous or intramuscular injections. Previous studies have suggested that cleaning with an alcohol swab is not always necessary, does not result in infections and may predispose the skin to hardening (Dann 1969; Koivistov & Felig 1978; Workman 1999).

Dann (1969), in a study over a period of 6 years involving more than 5000 injections, found no single case of local and/or systemic infection. Koivistov and Felig (1978) concluded that whilst skin preparations did reduce skin bacterial count, they are not necessary to prevent infections at the injection site. Some trusts accept that if the patient is physically clean and the nurse maintains a high standard of hand hygiene and asepsis during the procedure, skin disinfection is not necessary (Workman 1999).

In the immunosuppressed patient, the skin should be cleaned as such patients may become infected by inoculation of a relatively small number of pathogens (Downie *et al.* 2000). The practice at The Royal Marsden Hospital is to continue to clean the skin prior to injection in order to reduce the risk of contamination from the patient's skin flora. The skin should be cleaned using an 'alcohol swab' (containing 70% isopropyl alcohol) for 30 seconds and then allowed to dry. If the skin is not dry before proceeding, skin cleaning is ineffective and the antiseptic may cause irritation by being injected into the tissues (Downie *et al.* 2000).

Needle bevel

Three categories of needle bevel are available:

1 *Regular*: for all intramuscular and subcutaneous injections.
2 *Intradermal*: for diagnostic injections and other injections into the epidermis.
3 *Short*: rarely used.

Intramuscular needle gauge size and length

Needles should be long enough to penetrate the muscle and still allow a quarter of the needle to remain external to the skin (Workman 1999). The most common sizes are 21 or 23 G and 2.5–5.0 cm long. Lenz (1983) states that when choosing the correct needle length for intramuscular injections it is important to assess the muscle mass of the injection site, the amount of subcutaneous fat and the weight of the patient. Without such an assessment, most injections intended for gluteal muscle are deposited in the gluteal fat. The following are suggested by the author as ways of determining the most suitable size of needle to use.

Deltoid and vastus lateralis muscles

The muscle to be used should be grasped between the thumb and forefinger to determine the depth of the muscle mass or the amount of subcutaneous fat at the injection site.

Gluteal muscles

The layer of fat and skin above the muscle should be gently lifted with the thumb and forefinger for the same reasons as before. Use the patient's weight to calculate the needle length required. Lenz (1983) recommends the following guide:

31.5–40.0 kg:	2.5 cm needle.
40.5–90.0 kg:	5.0–7.5 cm needle.
90 kg:	10–15 cm needle.

Intramuscular injections and pain

Patients are often afraid of receiving injections because they perceive the injection will be painful (Workman 1999). Torrence (1989) listed a number of factors that cause pain:

- The needle.
- The chemical composition of the drug/solution.
- The technique.

- The speed of the injection.
- The volume of drug.

Workman (1999) listed a number of techniques that could be utilized to reduce pain and discomfort experienced by the patient such as adequate preparation of the patient, using ice or freezing spray to numb the skin, correct choice of site and technique and positioning of the patient so that the muscles are relaxed. Field (1981) attempts to answer the question of what it is like to give an injection, and goes on to explore the meaning and use of language relating to injections, the feelings involved in preparing and administering injections, and the meaning of the patient's response to the nurse.

Intravenous

Advantages of using the intravenous route

1. An immediate, therapeutic effect is achieved owing to rapid delivery of the drug to its target site, which allows a more precise dose calculation and there-fore more reliable treatment.
2. Pain and irritation caused by some substances when given intramuscularly or subcutaneously are avoided.
3. The vascular route affords a route of administration for the patient who can-not tolerate fluids or drugs by the gastrointestinal route or is unable to take them by mouth.
4. Some drugs cannot be absorbed by any other route; the large molecular size of some drugs prevents absorption by the gastrointestinal route, while other drugs, unstable in the presence of gastric juices, are destroyed.
5. The intravenous route offers the facility for control over the rate of adminis-tration of drugs; prolonged action can be provided by administering a dilute infusion intermittently or over a prolonged period of time (Weinstein 2007; Whittington 2008).

283

Disadvantages of using the intravenous route

1. There is an inability to recall the drug and reverse its action. This may lead to increased toxicity or a sensitivity reaction.
2. Insufficient control of administration may lead to speed shock or circulatory overload.
3. Additional complications may occur, such as the following:
   (a) microbial contamination (extrinsic or intrinsic);
   (b) vascular irritation, e.g. chemical phlebitis;
   (c) drug incompatibilities and interactions if multiple additives are prescribed (Weinstein 2007).
4. Needle phobia.

5 Altered body image, especially with central vascular access devices (Dougherty 2008).

6 Time taken for administration (Hockley *et al.* 1995).

Principles to be applied throughout preparation and administration

Asepsis and reducing the risk of infection

Microbes on the hands of health care personnel contribute to hospital-associated infection (Weinstein 2007). Therefore aseptic technique must be adhered to throughout all intravenous procedures (see Chapter 4). The nurse must employ good hand washing and drying techniques using a bactericidal soap or a bactericidal alcohol handrub. If asepsis is not maintained, local infection, septic phlebitis or septicaemia may result (RCN 2005; Hart 2008; Pratt *et al.* 2007).

The insertion site should be inspected at least once a day for complications such as infiltration, phlebitis or any indication of infection, e.g. redness at the insertion site of the device or pyrexia (RCN 2005). These problems may necessitate the removal of the device and/or further investigation (Finlay 2008).

It is desirable that a closed system of infusion is maintained wherever possible, with as few connections as is necessary for its purpose (Finlay 2008; Hart 2008). This reduces the risk of bacterial contamination. Any extra connections within the administration system increase the risk of infection. Three-way taps have been shown to encourage the growth of micro-organisms. They are difficult to clean due to their design, as micro-organisms can become lodged and are then able to multiply in the warm, moist environment (Finlay 2008; Hart 2008). This reservoir for micro-organisms may then be released into the circulation.

The injection sites on administration sets or injection caps should be cleaned using an alcohol-based antiseptic, allowing time for it to dry (Pratt *et al.* 2007). Connections should be cleaned before changing administration sets and manipulations kept to a minimum. Administration sets should be changed according to use (intermittent/continuous therapy), type of device and type of solution, and the set must be labelled with the date and time of change (RCN 2005; NPSA 2007).

To ensure safe delivery of intravenous fluids and medication:

- Replace all tubing when the vascular device is replaced (Pratt *et al.* 2007).
- Replace solution administration sets and stopcocks used for continuous infusions every 72 hours unless clinically indicated, e.g. if drug stability data indicate otherwise (RCN 2005; Pratt *et al.* 2007). Research has indicated that routine changing of administration sets (used for infusing solutions) every 48–72 hours instead of every 24 hours is not associated with an increase in infection and could result in considerable savings for hospitals (RCN 2005; Pratt *et al.* 2007).

- Replace solution administration sets used for lipid emulsions and parenteral nutrition at the end of the infusion or within 24 hours of initiating the infusion (RCN 2005; Pratt *et al.* 2007). Certain intravenous fluids including lipid emulsions, blood and blood products are more likely than other parenteral fluids to support microbial growth if contaminated and therefore replacement of the intravenous tubing is required more frequently than 48–72 hours (Pratt *et al.* 2007).
- Replace blood administration sets at least every 12 hours and after every second unit of blood (McClelland 2007; RCN 2005; Pratt *et al.* 2007).
- All solution sets used for intermittent infusions, e.g. antibiotics, should be discarded immediately after use and not allowed to hang for reuse (RCN 2005).

Inspection of fluids, drugs, equipment and their packaging must be undertaken to detect any points where contamination may have occurred during manufacture and/or transport. This intrinsic contamination may be detected as cloudiness, discoloration or the presence of particles (Perucca 2001; Weinstein 2007; BMA & RPS 2008). Infusion bags should not be left hanging for longer than 24 hours. In the case of blood and blood products this is reduced to 5 hours (McClelland 2007; RCN 2005).

Safety
All details of the prescription and all calculations must be checked carefully in accordance with hospital policy in order to ensure safe preparation and administration of the drug(s).

Drug calculations
The following formulas can be applied to calculate dose, volume or rate of infusion, as illustrated in Higgins (2005).

The drug volume required from stock strength

$$\frac{\text{Strength required}}{\text{Stock strength}} \times \text{Volume of stock solution} = \text{Volume required}$$

What you want/What you have got × Volume of stock solution

Infusion rates   *Gravitational flow administration:*

Volume required/Duration (hour)

× Set value (drops/ml)/Minutes (60) = Drops per minute

Volumetric infusion pumps:

Volume to be infused/Duration of infusion = Volume per hour

Weight-related doses

Prescribed volume × Body weight = volume, e.g. ml per weight, e.g. kg

Prescribed dose × Body weight = dose, e.g. mg per weight, e.g. kg

It is important to note that the 'use of calculators to determine the volume or quantity of medication should not act as a substitute for arithmatical knowledge and skill' (NMC 2008a).

The nurse must also check the compatibility of the drug with the diluent or infusion fluid. The nurse should be aware of the types of incompatibilities, and the factors which could influence them. These include pH, concentration, time, temperature, light and the brand of the drug. If insufficient information is available, a reference book (e.g. *British National Formulary* [BMA & RPS 2008]) or the product data sheet must be consulted (NPSA 2007; Whittington 2008). If the nurse is unsure about any aspect of the preparation and/or administration of a drug, they should not proceed and should consult with a senior member of staff (NMC 2008a). Constant monitoring of both the mixture and the patient is important. The preferred method and rate of intravenous administration must be determined.

Drugs should never be added to the following: blood; blood products, i.e. plasma or platelet concentrate; mannitol solutions; sodium bicarbonate solution, etc. Only specially prepared additives should be used with fat emulsions or amino acid preparations.

Accurate labelling of additives and records of administration are essential (RCN 2005; NPSA 2007).

Any protective clothing which is advised should be worn, and vinyl gloves should be used to reduce the risk of latex allergy (Hart 2008). Health care professionals who use gloves frequently or for long periods face a high risk of allergy from latex products. All health care facilities should develop policies and procedures that determine measures to protect staff and patients from latex exposure and outline a treatment plan for latex reactions (Dougherty 2002).

It has been suggested that needle-free systems can increase the risk of bloodstream infections (Danzig *et al.* 1995). However, most studies have found no difference in microbial contamination when comparing conventional and needle-free systems (Brown *et al.* 1997; Luebke *et al.* 1998; Mendelson *et al.* 1998). It appears that an increased risk is only associated where there is lack of compliance with cleaning protocols or changing of equipment (Pratt *et al.* 2007).

Preventing needlestick injuries should be key in any health and safety programme and organizations should introduce safety devices and needle-free systems wherever possible (NHS Employers 2005). Basic rules of safety include not resheathing needles, disposal of needles immediately after use into a recognized sharps bin and convenient location of sharps bins in all areas where needles and sharps are used (MHRA 2004; RCN 2005; Hart 2008).

Comfort

Both the physical and psychological comfort of the patient must be considered. Comprehensive explanation of the practical aspects of the procedure together with information about the effects of treatment will contribute to reducing anxiety and will need to be tailored to each patient's individual needs.

Methods of administering intravenous drugs

There are three methods of administering intravenous drugs: continuous infusion, intermittent infusion and intermittent injection.

Continuous infusion

Continuous infusion may be defined as the intravenous delivery of a medication or fluid at a constant rate over a prescribed time period, ranging from 24 hours to days to achieve a controlled therapeutic response. The greater dilution also helps to reduce venous irritation (Weinstein 2007; Whittington 2008).

A continuous infusion may be used when:

- The drugs to be administered must be highly diluted.
- A maintenance of steady blood levels of the drug is required.

Preprepared infusion fluids with additives such as those containing potassium chloride should be used whenever possible. This reduces the risk of extrinsic contamination, which can occur during the mixing of drugs (Weinstein 2007). Only one addition should be made to each bottle or bag of fluid after the compatibility has been ascertained. More additions can increase the risk of incompatibility occurring, e.g. precipitation (Weinstein 2007; Whittington 2008). The additive and fluid must be mixed well to prevent a layering effect which can occur with some drugs (Whittington 2008). The danger is that a bolus injection of the drug may be delivered. To safeguard against this, any additions should be made to the infusion fluid and the container inverted a number of times to ensure mixing of the drug and prevent a bolus of the drug being infused, before the fluid is hung on the infusion stand (NPSA 2007). The infusion container should be labelled clearly after the addition has been made. Constant monitoring of the infusion fluid mixture (Weinstein 2007; Whittington 2008) for cloudiness or presence of particles should occur, as well as checking the patient's condition and intravenous site for patency, extravasation or infiltration.

Intermittent infusion

Intermittent infusion is the administration of a small-volume infusion, i.e. 50–250 ml, over a period of between 20 minutes and 2 hours. This may be given as a specific dose at one time or at repeated intervals during 24 hours (Pickstone 1999).

An intermittent infusion may be used when:

- A peak plasma level is required therapeutically.
- The pharmacology of the drug dictates this specific dilution.
- The drug will not remain stable for the time required to administer a more dilute volume.
- The patient is on a restricted intake of fluids (Whittington 2008).

Delivery of the drug by intermittent infusion may utilize a system such as a 'Y' set, if the primary infusion is of a compatible fluid, or a burette set with a chamber capacity of 100 or 150 ml. This is when the drug can be added to the burette and infused while the primary infusion is switched off. A small-volume infusion may also be connected to a cannula specifically to keep the vein open, and maintain patency.

All the points considered when preparing for a continuous infusion should be taken into account here, e.g. preprepared fluids, single additions of drugs, adequate mixing, labelling and monitoring.

Direct intermittent injection

Direct intermittent injection (also known as intravenous push or bolus) involves the injection of a drug from a syringe into the injection port of the administration set or directly into a vascular access device. Most are administered anywhere from 3 to 10 minutes depending upon the drug (Weinstein 2007; Whittington 2008).

A direct injection may be used when:

- A maximum concentration of the drug is required to vital organs. This is a 'bolus' injection which is given rapidly over seconds, as in an emergency, e.g. adrenaline.
- The drug cannot be further diluted for pharmacological or therapeutic reasons or does not require dilution. This is given as a controlled 'push' injection over a few minutes.
- A peak blood level is required and cannot be achieved by small-volume infusion.

Rapid administration could result in toxic levels and an anaphylactic-type reaction. Manufacturers' recommendations of rates of administration (i.e. millilitres or milligrams per minute) should be adhered to. In the absence of such recommendations, administration should proceed slowly, over 5–10 minutes (Dougherty 2002).

Delivery of the drug by direct injection may be via the cannula through a resealable needleless injection cap, extension set or via the injection site of an administration set.

- If a peripheral device is in situ the bandage and dressing must be removed to inspect the insertion of the cannula, unless a transparent dressing is in place (Finlay 2008).
- Patency of the vein must be confirmed prior to administration and the vein's ability to accept an extra flow of fluid or irritant chemical must also be checked (Dougherty 2008).

Administration into the injection site of a fast-running drip may be advised if the infusion in progress is compatible in order to dilute the drug further and reduce local chemical irritation (Dougherty 2002). Alternatively, a stop–start procedure may be employed if there is doubt about venous patency. This allows the nurse to constantly check the patency of the vein and detect early signs of extravasation. If the infusion fluid is incompatible with the drug, the administration set may be switched off and a compatible solution may be used as a flush (NPSA 2007).

If a number of drugs are being administered, 0.9% sodium chloride must be used to flush in between each drug to prevent interactions. In addition, 0.9% sodium chloride should be used at the end of the administration to ensure that all of the drug has been delivered. The device should then be flushed to ensure patency is maintained (see Chapter 45, Main edition) (Dougherty 2008).

Summary

The nurse is responsible for the administration of drugs by a variety of methods. The NMC's *Standards for Medicines Management* emphasizes that this 'is not solely a mechanistic task to be performed in strict compliance with the written prescription of a medical practitioner (now independent supplementary prescriber)' (NMC 2008a, p. 6). Shepherd (2002b) maintains that the administration of a medicine is arguably the most common clinical procedure that a nurse will undertake. He goes on to state that it is the manner in which a medicine is administered that determines to some extent whether or not the patient gains any clinical benefit and whether any adverse effect is experienced.

The nurse is accountable for the safe administration of drugs. In order to do this the nurse requires a thorough knowledge of the principles and their application, and a responsible attitude, which ensures that medications are not given without full knowledge of immediate and late effects, toxicities and nursing implications. The nurse must also be able to justify any actions taken and be accountable for the action taken (NMC 2008b).

Procedure guidelines Self-administration of drugs

Equipment

1 Drugs to be administered.
2 Recording sheet or book as required by law or hospital policy.
3 Patient's prescription chart, to check dose, route, etc.

4 Any protective clothing required by hospital policy for specified drugs, such as antibiotics or cytotoxic drugs (see Chapter 12, Professional edition).

Procedure

Action

1 Discuss medication history with the patient on his/her admission. This should include an assessment of the patient's ability to self-administer medication using the following criteria.

■ Is the patient willing to participate in self-administration?
■ Is the patient confused or forgetful?
■ Does the patient have a history of drug/alcohol abuse/self-harm?
■ Does the patient self-administer medicines at home?
■ Can the patient read the labels on the medicines?
■ Can the patient open the medicine containers?
■ Can the patient open the locker where the medicines are stored while they are in hospital?
■ Does the patient know what his/her medicines are for, their dosage, instructions and potential side-effects (Shepherd 2002b)?

Document this assessment in the patient's nursing records.

Rationale

To ensure an accurate record of: all medicines being taken (prescribed or otherwise); dietary supplements, e.g. multivitamins, herbal remedies, complementary therapies; allergies or hypersensitivities; understanding of current medicines; possible problems with self-administration (Shepherd 2002b: E; Jordan *et al.* 2003: E; NMC 2005: C; NMC 2008a: C).

If frequent changes of drug or dose are expected, immediate self-administration may be undesirable and/or impractical.

Appropriate medicines already in the patient's possession may be used, subject to local policy and agreement with the pharmacist (Shepherd 2002b: E; NMC 2007: C).

2 Review proposed (inpatient) prescription in liaison with pharmacist and compare with details given by patient and medicines in his/her possession.

290

3 Consider whether there are any constraints on self-administration, and if so, how they might be overcome. Discuss this with appropriate members of the multidisciplinary team.	To promote successful and safe self-administration and ensure that medicines are dispensed and labelled appropriately for the patient's needs (Shepherd 2002a: E; DH 2003d: C; NMC 2008a: C). Constraints such as physical or visual handicap must be addressed. Changes in performance status may result from the underlying condition or its treatment, and must be allowed for (Shepherd 2002a: E; NMC 2008a: C). If a compliance aid such as a 'dosette' box is to be used, responsibility for filling and labelling the aid, especially whilst used on the ward, must be agreed and documented in local policies (Shepherd 2002a: E; NMC 2008a: C).

4 Regularly discuss with the patient his/her medication and any problems they may be having with the regimen. Document discussions in the care plan. Teach any special skills required, e.g. correct use of aerosol inhalers.	To promote the informed commitment and involvement of patients in their own care, where appropriate. To ensure that treatment is received as intended (Shepherd 2002b: E; NMC 2008a: C).
5 Check that drugs are taken as intended, and that the necessary records are kept.	To discharge the nurse's overall responsibility for patient care and well being. To maintain a record of responsibilities undertaken (NMC 2005: C; NMC 2008a: C; NMC 2008b: C). Particular care with record keeping is needed in the period of gradual transition from nurse administration to self-administration. Any problems encountered must be addressed (NMC 2005: C; NMC 2008a: C; NMC 2008b: C). The detail and format of the record may vary according to: the patient's needs and performance status; the complexity of treatment; and local circumstances and policy (NMC 2005: C; NMC 2008a: C; NMC 2008b: C).

Procedure guidelines *(cont.)*

6 Monitor changes in the patient's prescription.	To ensure that: changes are put into effect promptly; drugs are properly relabelled or redispensed; any discontinued drugs are retrieved from the patient (Shepherd 2002b: E; DH 2003d: C; NMC 2008a: C).
7 Check when drug supplies are expected to run out and make arrangements for resupply. Order drugs to take out (TTO) as far in advance as possible.	To ensure that drugs are represcribed and dispensed in time to allow uninterrupted treatment and to facilitate planned discharge (Shepherd 2002b: E; DH 2003d: C; NMC 2008a: C).
8 Evaluate the effectiveness of the self-administration teaching programme and record any difficulties encountered and interventions made.	To identify further learning and teaching needs and modify care plan accordingly (Shepherd 2002b: E; NMC 2005: C; NMC 2008a: C; NMC 2008b: C).

292

Procedure guidelines Oral drug administration

Equipment

1 Refer to Procedure guidelines: Self-administration of drugs.

2 Medicine container (disposable if possible).

Procedure

Action	Rationale
1 Wash hands with bactericidal soap and water or bactericidal alcohol handrub.	To minimize the risk of cross-infection (DH 2007: C).
2 Before administering any prescribed drug, check that it is due and has not already been given. Check that the information contained in the prescription chart is complete, correct and legible.	To protect the patient from harm (DH 2003d: C; NMC 2008a: C).

3 Before administering any prescribed
   drug, consult the patient's prescription
   chart and ascertain the following:

   (a) Drug.

   (b) Dose.

   (c) Date and time of administration.

   (d) Route and method of
       administration.

   (e) Diluent as appropriate.

   (f) Validity of prescription.

   (g) Signature of doctor.

   (h) The prescription is legible.

To ensure that the patient is given the
correct drug in the prescribed dose using
the appropriate diluent and by the correct
route (DH 2003d: C; NMC 2008a:C).
To protect the patient from harm (DH
2003d: C; NMC 2008a: C).
To protect the patient from harm (DH
2003d: C; NMC 2008a: C).
To protect the patient from harm (DH
2003d: C; NMC 2008a: C).
To protect the patient from harm (DH
2003d: C; NMC 2008a: C).

4 Select the required medication and
  check the expiry date.

Treatment with medication that is outside
the expiry date is dangerous. Drugs
deteriorate with storage. The expiry date
indicates when a particular drug is no
longer pharmacologically efficacious (DH
2003d: C; NMC 2008a: C).

293

5 Empty the required dose into a
  medicine container. Avoid touching the
  preparation.

To minimize the risk of cross-infection.
To minimize the risk of harm to the nurse
(DH 2007: C).

6 Take the medication and the
  prescription chart to the patient. Check
  the patient's identity by asking the
  patient to state their full name and date
  of birth. If patient unable to confirm
  details then check patient identity band
  against prescription chart.

To ensure that the medication is
administered to the correct patient
(NPSA 2005: C).

7 Evaluate the patient's knowledge of
  the medication being offered. If this
  knowledge appears to be faulty or
  incorrect, offer an explanation of the
  use, action, dose and potential
  side-effects of the drug or drugs
  involved.

A patient has a right to information about
treatment (NMC 2008a: C; NMC 2008b:
C).

Procedure guidelines *(cont.)*

8 Administer the drug as prescribed.	To meet legal requirements and hospital policy (DH 2003d: C; NMC 2005: C; NMC 2008a: C; NMC 2008b: C).
9 Offer a glass of water, if allowed.	To facilitate swallowing the medication (Jordan *et al.* 2003: E).
10 Record the dose given in the prescription chart and in any other place made necessary by legal requirement or hospital policy.	To meet legal requirements and hospital policy (DH 2003d: C; NMC 2005: C; NMC 2008a: C; NMC 2008b: C).
11 Administer irritant drugs with meals or snacks.	To minimize their effect on the gastric mucosa (Shepherd 2002a: E; Jordan *et al.* 2003: E).
12 Administer drugs that interact with food, or that are destroyed in significant proportions by digestive enzymes, between meals or on an empty stomach.	To prevent interference with the absorption of the drug (Shepherd 2002a: E; Jordan *et al.* 2003: E).
13 Do not break a tablet unless it is scored and appropriate to do so. Break scored tablets with a file or a tablet cutter. Wash after use.	Breaking may cause incorrect dosage, gastrointestinal irritation or destruction of a drug in an incompatible pH. To reduce risk of contamination between tablets (Shepherd 2002a: E; Jordan *et al.* 2003: E; DH 2003d: C; NMC 2008a: C).
14 Do not interfere with time-release capsules and enteric coated tablets. Ask patients to swallow these whole and not to chew them.	The absorption rate of the drug will be altered (Shepherd 2002a: E; Jordan *et al.* 2003: E).
15 Sublingual tablets must be placed under the tongue and buccal tablets between gum and cheek.	To allow for correct absorption (Shepherd 2002a: E).

16 When administering liquids to babies and young children, or when an accurately measured dose in multiples of 1 ml is needed for an adult, an oral syringe should be used in preference to a medicine spoon or measure.

An oral syringe is much more accurate than a measure or a 5 ml spoon.

Use of a syringe makes administration of the correct dose much easier in an uncooperative child.

Oral syringes are available and are designed to be washable and reused for the same patient. However, in the immunocompromised patient single use only is recommended. Oral syringes must be clearly labelled for oral or enteral use only (DH 2003d: C).

17 In babies and children especially, correct use of the syringe is very important. The tip should be gently pushed into and towards the side of the mouth. The contents are then *slowly* discharged towards the inside of the cheek, pausing if necessary to allow the liquid to be swallowed. If children are uncooperative it may help to place the end of the barrel between the teeth.

To prevent injury to the mouth and eliminate the danger of choking the patient (Watt 2003: E).

To get the dose in and to prevent the patient spitting it out (Watt 2003: E).

295

Controlled drug administration
Equipment

1 Refer to Procedure guidelines: Self-administration of drugs or Procedure guidelines: Injections: administration.

Action

1 Consult the patient's prescription chart, and ascertain the following:
  (a) Drug.
  (b) Dose.
  (c) Date and time of administration.
  (d) Route and method of administration.
  (e) Diluent as appropriate.
  (f) Validity of prescription.
  (g) Signature of doctor.

Rationale

To ensure that the patient is given the correct drug in the prescribed dose using the appropriate diluent and by the correct route (DH 2003d: C; NMC 2008a: C).

Procedure guidelines *(cont.)*

2 Select the correct drug from the
controlled drug cupboard.

3 Check the stock against the last entry
in the ward record book. (At The
Royal Marsden Hospital, a second
person is required to check the
stock level and both nurses are
required to sign the controlled drugs
book.)

To comply with hospital policy (DH
2003d: C; NMC 2008a: C; NPSA 2006:
C).

4 Check the appropriate dose against
the prescription chart.

5 Return the remaining stock to
the cupboard and lock the
cupboard.

6 Enter the date, dose and the patient's
name in the ward record book.

7 Take the prepared dose to the patient,
whose identity is checked.

To prevent error and confirm patient's
identity (NPSA 2005: C).

8 Administer the drug after checking the
prescription chart again. Once the
drug has been administered, the
prescription chart is signed by the
nurse responsible for administering the
medication.

9 Record the administration on
appropriate charts.

To maintain accurate records, provide a
point of reference in the event of any
queries and prevent any duplication of
treatment (DH 2003d: C; NMC 2005: C;
NMC 2008a: C; NMC 2008b: C).

Procedure guidelines   Injections: administration

Equipment

1 Clean tray or receiver in which to place drug and equipment.
2 21 G needle(s) to ease reconstitution and drawing up, 23 G if from a glass ampoule.
3 21, 23 or 25 G needle, size dependent on route of administration.
4 Syringe(s) of appropriate size for amount of drug to be given.
5 Swabs saturated with isopropyl alcohol 70%.
6 Sterile topical swab, if drug is presented in ampoule form.
7 Drug(s) to be administered.
8 Patient's prescription chart, to check dose, route, etc.
9 Recording sheet or book as required by law or hospital policy.
10 Any protective clothing required by hospital policy for specified drugs, such as antibiotics or cytotoxic drugs (see Chapter 12, Professional edition).

Procedure

Action	Rationale
1 Collect and check all equipment.	To prevent delays and enable full concentration on the procedure (E).
2 Check that the packaging of all equipment is intact.	To ensure sterility. If the seal is damaged, discard (NPSA 2007:C).
3 Wash hands with bactericidal soap and water or bactericidal alcohol handrub.	To prevent contamination of medication and equipment (DH 2007: C).
4 Prepare needle(s), syringe(s), etc., on a tray or receiver.	To contain all items in a clean area (E).
5 Inspect all equipment.	To check that none is damaged; if so, discard or report to Medicines and Health Care Products Regulatory Agency (MHRA) (C).
6 Consult the patient's prescription chart, and ascertain the following: (a) Drug. (b) Dose. (c) Date and time of administration. (d) Route and method of administration. (e) Diluent as appropriate. (f) Validity of prescription. (g) Signature of doctor.	To ensure that the patient is given the correct drug in the prescribed dose using the appropriate diluent and by the correct route (NMC 2008a: C; NPSA 2007: C).

Procedure guidelines (cont.)

7 Check all details with another nurse if required by hospital policy.	To minimize any risk of error (NMC 2008a: C).
8 Select the drug in the appropriate volume, dilution or dosage and check the expiry date.	To reduce wastage. Treatment with medication that is outside the expiry date is dangerous. Drugs deteriorate with storage. The expiry date indicates when a particular drug is no longer pharmacologically efficacious (NPSA 2007: C).
9 Proceed with the preparation of the drug, using protective clothing if advisable.	To protect practitioner during preparation (NPSA 2007: C).
10 Take the prepared dose to the patient, whose identity is checked.	To prevent error and confirm patient's identity (NPSA 2005: C).
11 Evaluate the patient's knowledge of the medication being offered. If this knowledge appears to be faulty or incorrect, offer an explanation of the use, action, dose and potential side-effects of the drug or drugs involved.	A patient has a right to information about treatment (NMC 2008a: C).
12 Close room door or curtains if appropriate.	To ensure patient privacy and dignity (E).
13 Administer the drug as prescribed.	To ensure patient receives treatment (E).
14 Record the administration on appropriate charts.	To maintain accurate records, provide a point of reference in the event of any queries and prevent any duplication of treatment (NMC 2005: C; NMC 2008a: C; NPSA 2007: C).

Single-dose ampoule: solution preparation

Action	Rationale
1 Inspect the solution for cloudiness or particulate matter. If this is present, discard and follow hospital guidelines on what action to take, e.g. return drug to pharmacy.	To prevent the patient from receiving an unstable or contaminated drug (NPSA 2007: C).

2 Tap the neck of the ampoule gently.	To ensure that all the solution is in the bottom of the ampoule (NPSA 2007: C).
3 Cover the neck of the ampoule with a sterile topical swab and snap it open. If there is any difficulty a file may be required.	To minimize the risk of contamination. To prevent aerosol formation or contact with the drug which could lead to a sensitivity reaction. To reduce the risk of injury to the nurse (NPSA 2007: C).
4 Inspect the solution for glass fragments; if present, discard.	To minimize the risk of injection of foreign matter into the patient (NPSA 2007: C).
5 Withdraw the required amount of solution, tilting the ampoule if necessary.	To avoid drawing in any air (NPSA 2007: C).
6 Replace the sheath on the needle and tap the syringe to dislodge any air bubbles. Expel air. *Note*: replacing the sheath should **not** be confused with resheathing used needles. An alternative to expelling the air with the needle sheath in place would be to use the ampoule or vial to receive any air and/or drug.	To prevent aerosol formation (NPSA 2007: C). To ensure that the correct amount of drug is in the syringe (NPSA 2007: C).
7 Attach a new needle if required (and discard used needle into appropriate sharps container) or attach a plastic end cap.	To reduce the risk of infection. To avoid tracking medications through superficial tissues. To ensure that the correct size of needle is used for the injection. To reduce the risk of injury to the nurse (NPSA 2007: C).

Single-dose ampoule: powder preparation

Action	Rationale
1 Tap the neck of the ampoule gently.	To ensure that any powder lodged here falls to the bottom of the ampoule (NPSA 2007: C).
2 Cover the neck of the ampoule with a sterile topical swab and snap it open. If there is any difficulty a file may be required.	To minimize the risk of contamination. To prevent contact with the drug which could cause a sensitivity reaction. To prevent injury to the nurse (NPSA 2007: C).

299

Procedure guidelines *(cont.)*

3 Inject the correct diluent slowly into the powder within the ampoule.	To ensure that the powder is thoroughly wet before agitation and is not released into the atmosphere (NPSA 2007: C).
4 Agitate the ampoule.	To dissolve the drug (NPSA 2007: C).
5 Inspect the contents.	To detect any glass fragments or any other particulate matter. If present, continue agitation or discard as appropriate (NPSA 2007: C).
6 When the solution is clear withdraw the prescribed amount, tilting the ampoule if necessary.	To ensure the powder is dissolved and has formed a solution with the diluent. To avoid drawing in air (NPSA 2007: C).
7 Replace the sheath on the needle and tap the syringe to dislodge any air bubbles. Expel air.	To prevent aerosol formation. To ensure that the correct amount of drug is in the syringe (NPSA 2007: C).
8 Attach a new needle if required (and discard used needle into appropriate sharps container) or attach a plastic end cap.	To reduce the risk of infection. To avoid tracking medications though superficial tissues. To ensure that the correct size of needle is used for the injection. To reduce the risk of injury to the nurse (NPSA 2007: C).

300

Multidose vial: powder preparation

Action	Rationale
1 Remove the tamper evident seal and clean the rubber septum with the chosen antiseptic and let it air dry for at least 30 seconds.	To prevent bacterial contamination of the drug, as the plastic lid prevents damage and does not ensure sterility (NPSA 2007: C).

Use either of these methods for reconstitution:

Reconstitution method (a): 2–6

2 Insert a 21 G needle into the cap to vent the bottle (see Action figure 2a).	To prevent pressure differentials, which can cause separation of needle and syringe (NPSA 2007: C).
3 Inject the correct diluent slowly into the powder within the ampoule.	To ensure that the powder is thoroughly wet before it is shaken and is not released into the atmosphere (NPSA 2007: C).

4 Remove the needle and the syringe.	To enable adequate mixing of the solution (E).
5 Place a sterile topical swab over the venting needle (see Action figure 2b) and shake to dissolve the powder. *Note*: the nurse may encounter other presentations of drugs for injection, e.g. vials with a transfer needle, and should follow the manufacturer's instructions in these instances.	To prevent contamination of the drug or the atmosphere. To mix the diluent with the powder and dissolve the drug (NPSA 2007: C).
6 Inspect the solution for cloudiness or particulate matter. If this is present, discard. Follow hospital guidelines on what action to take, e.g. return drug to pharmacy.	To prevent patient from receiving an unstable or contaminated drug (NPSA 2007: C).

301

Reconstitution method (b): 7–13

7 With the needle sheathed draw into the syringe a volume of air equivalent to the required volume of solution to be drawn up.	To prevent bacterial contamination of the drug (NPSA 2007: C).
8 Remove the needle cover and insert the needle into the vial through the rubber septum.	To gain access to the vial (E).
9 Invert the vial. Keep the needle in the solution and slowly depress the plunger to push the air into the vial.	To create an equilibrium in the vial (NPSA 2007: C).
10 Release the plunger so that the solution flows back into the syringe (if a large volume of solution is to be withdrawn use a push pull technique).	To create an equilibrium in the vial (NPSA 2007: C).
11 Inject the diluent into the vial. Keeping the tip of the needle above the level of the solution in the vial, release the plunger. The syringe will fill with the air which has been displaced by the solution.	This 'equilibrium method' helps to minimize the build up of pressure in the vial.

Procedure guidelines *(cont.)*

12 With the needle and syringe in place, gently swirl the vial to dissolve all the powder.	To mix the diluent with the powder and dissolve the drug (NPSA 2007: C).
13 Inspect the solution for cloudiness or particulate matter. If this is present, discard. Follow hospital guidelines on what action to take, e.g. return drug to pharmacy.	To prevent patient from receiving an unstable or contaminated drug (NPSA 2007: C).

Withdrawal of medication from vial

14 Withdraw the prescribed amount of solution, and inspect for pieces of rubber which may have 'cored out' of the cap (see Action figure 2c). *Note*: coring can be minimized by inserting the needle into the cap, bevel up, at an angle of 45° to 60°. Before complete insertion of the needle tip, lift the needle to 90° and proceed (see Action figure 14).	To ensure that the correct amount of drug is in the syringe (NPSA 2007: C). To prevent the injection of foreign matter into the patient (NPSA 2007: C).
15 Remove air from syringe without spraying into the atmosphere by injecting air back into the vial (see Action figure 2d) or replace the sheath on the needle and tap the syringe to dislodge any air bubbles. Expel air.	To reduce risk of contamination of practitioner. To prevent aerosol formation (NPSA 2007: C).
16 Attach a new needle if required (and discard used needle into appropriate sharps container) or attach a plastic end cap.	To reduce the risk of infection. To avoid possible trauma to the patient if the needle has barbed. To avoid tracking medications through superficial tissues. To ensure that the correct size of needle is used for the injection (NPSA 2007: C).

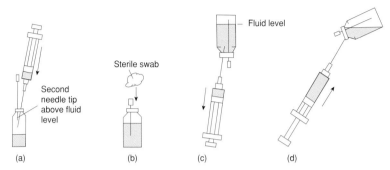

(a)   (b)   (c)   (d)

Action 2 Suggested method of vial reconstitution to avoid environmental exposure. (a) When reconstituting vial, insert a second needle to allow air to escape when adding diluent for injection. (b) When shaking the vial to dissolve the powder, push in second needle up to Luer connection and cover with a sterile swab. (c) To remove reconstituted solution, insert syringe needle and then invert vial. Ensuring that tip of second needle is above fluid, withdraw the solution. (d) Remove air from syringe without spraying into the atmosphere by injecting air back into vial.

303

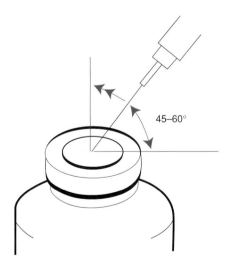

Action 14 Method to minimize coring.

Procedure guidelines *(cont.)*

Subcutaneous injection administration

Action	Rationale
1 Explain and discuss the procedure with the patient.	To ensure that the patient understands the procedure and gives his/her valid consent (Griffith & Jordan 2003: E; NMC 2006: C; NMC 2008b: C).
2 Consult the patient's prescription chart, and ascertain the following: (a) Drug. (b) Dose. (c) Date and time of administration. (d) Route and method of administration. (e) Diluent as appropriate. (f) Validity of prescription. (g) Signature of doctor.	To ensure that the patient is given the correct drug in the prescribed dose using the appropriate diluent and by the correct route (NMC 2008a: C; NPSA 2007: C).
3 Assist the patient into the required position.	To allow access to the appropriate injection site (Workman 1999: E).
4 Remove appropriate garments to expose the injection site.	To gain access for injection (Workman 1999: E).
5 Assess the injection site for signs of inflammation, oedema, infection and skin lesions.	To promote effectiveness of administration (Workman 1999: E). To reduce the risk of infection (Workman 1999: E). To avoid skin lesions and avoid possible trauma to the patient (Workman 1999: E).
6 Choose the correct needle size.	To minimize the risk of missing the subcutaneous tissue and any ensuing pain (Workman 1999: E).
7 Clean the injection site with a swab saturated with isopropyl alcohol 70%.	To reduce the number of pathogens introduced into the skin by the needle at the time of insertion. (For further information on this action see Skin preparation section, above.)

8 Gently pinch the skin up into a fold.	To elevate the subcutaneous tissue, and lift the adipose tissue away from the underlying muscle (Workman 1999: E).
9 Insert the needle into the skin at an angle of 45° and release the grasped skin (unless administering insulin when an angle of 90° should be used). Inject the drug slowly.	Injecting medication into compressed tissue irritates nerve fibres and causes the patient discomfort. The introduction of shorter insulin needles makes 90° the more appropriate angle (Trounce & Gould 2000: E).
10 Withdraw the needle rapidly. Apply pressure to any bleeding point.	To prevent haematoma formation (E).
11 Record the administration on appropriate sheets.	To maintain accurate records, provide a point of reference in the event of any queries and prevent any duplication of treatment (NMC 2005: C; NPSA 2007: C; NMC 2008a: C).
12 Ensure that all sharps and non-sharp waste are disposed of safely and in accordance with locally approved procedures. For example, sharps into sharps bin and syringes into yellow clinical waste bag.	To ensure safe disposal and to avoid laceration or other injury to staff (MHRA 2004: C; DH 2005b: C).

Intramuscular injection administration

Action	Rationale
1 Explain and discuss the procedure with the patient.	To ensure that the patient understands the procedure and gives his/her valid consent (Griffith & Jordan 2003: E; NMC 2006b: C; NMC 2008b: C).
2 Consult the patient's prescription sheet, and ascertain the following: (a) Drug. (b) Dose. (c) Date and time of administration. (d) Route and method of administration. (e) Diluent as appropriate. (f) Validity of prescription. (g) Signature of doctor.	To ensure that the patient is given the correct drug in the prescribed dose using the appropriate diluent and by the correct route (NMC 2008a: C; NPSA 2007: C).

Procedure guidelines *(cont.)*

3 Assist the patient into the required position.

To allow access to the injection site and to ensure the designated muscle group is flexed and therefore relaxed (Workman 1999: E).

4 Remove the appropriate garment to expose the injection site.

To gain access for injection (Workman 1999: E).

5 Assess the injection site for signs of inflammation, oedema, infection and skin lesions.

To promote effectiveness of administration (Workman 1999: E).
  To reduce the risk of infection (Workman 1999: E).
  To avoid skin lesions and avoid possible trauma to the patient (Workman 1999: E).

6 Clean the injection site with a swab saturated with isopropyl alcohol 70% for 30 seconds and allow to dry for 30 seconds (Workman 1999).

To reduce the number of pathogens introduced into the skin by the needle at the time of insertion, to prevent stinging sensation if alcohol is taken into the tissues upon needle entry (Workman 1999: E). (For further information on this action see Skin preparation section, above.)

7 Stretch the skin around the injection site.

To facilitate the insertion of the needle and to reduce the sensitivity of nerve endings (Workman 1999: E).

8 Holding the needle at an angle of 90°, quickly plunge it into the skin.

To ensure that the needle penetrates the muscle (Workman 1999: E).

9 Pull back the plunger. If no blood is aspirated, depress the plunger at approximately 1 ml every 10 seconds and inject the drug slowly. If blood appears, withdraw the needle completely, replace it and begin again. Explain to the patient what has occurred.

To confirm that the needle is in the correct position and not in a vein (Workman 1999: E). This allows time for the muscle fibres to expand and absorb the solution (Workman 1999: E).
  To prevent pain and ensure even distribution of the drug.

10 Wait 10 seconds before withdrawing the needle.	To allow the medication to diffuse into the tissue (Workman 1999: E).
11 Withdraw the needle rapidly. Apply pressure to any bleeding point.	To prevent haematoma formation (E).
12 Record the administration on appropriate charts.	To maintain accurate records, provide a point of reference in the event of any queries and prevent any duplication of treatment (NMC 2005: C; NMC 2008a: C; NPSA 2007: C).
13 Ensure that all sharps and non-sharp waste are disposed of safely and in accordance with locally approved procedures, e.g. put sharps into sharps bin and syringes into yellow clinical waste bag.	To ensure safe disposal and to avoid laceration or other injury to staff (MHRA 2004: C; DH 2005b: C).

307

Procedure guidelines   Rectal medication administration

Rectal preparations

For further information about the administration of rectal medication see the relevant sections in Chapter 11.

Procedure guidelines   Vaginal medication administration

Equipment

1 Disposable gloves.
2 Topical swabs.
3 Disposable sanitary pad.

4 Lubricating jelly.
5 Prescription chart.

Vaginal pessary insertion

Action

1 Explain and discuss the procedure with the patient.

Rationale

To ensure that the patient understands the procedure and gives her valid consent (Griffith & Jordan 2003: E; NMC 2006b: C; NMC 2008b: C).

Procedure guidelines (cont.)

2 Consult the patient's prescription sheet and ascertain the following:
  (a) Drug.
  (b) Dose.
  (c) Date and time of administration.
  (d) Route and method of administration.
  (e) Validity of prescription.
  (f) Signature of doctor.

To ensure that the patient is given the correct drug in the prescribed dose and by the correct route (NMC 2008a: C).

3 Select the appropriate pessary and check it with the prescription chart.

To ensure that the correct medication is given to the correct patient at the appropriate time (NMC 2008a: C; NPSA 2007: C).

4 Close room door or curtains keeping the patient covered as much as possible.

To ensure patient privacy and dignity (E).

5 Assist the patient into the appropriate position, either left lateral with buttocks to the edge of the bed or supine with the knees drawn up and legs parted.

To facilitate easy access to the vaginal canal and correct insertion of the pessary (Manufacturer's instruction: C).

6 Wash hands with bactericidal soap and water or bactericidal alcohol handrub, and put on gloves.

To minimize the risk of cross-infection (DH 2007: C).

7 Apply lubricating jelly to a topical swab and from the swab on to the pessary.

To facilitate insertion of the pessary and ensure the patient's comfort (Manufacturer's instruction: C).

8 Insert the pessary along the posterior vaginal wall and into the top of the vagina.
  Note: This procedure is best performed late in the evening when the patient is unlikely to get out of bed.

To ensure that the pessary is retained and that the medication can reach its maximum efficiency (Manufacturer's instruction: C).

9 Wipe away any excess lubricating jelly from the patient's vulval and/or perineal area with a topical swab.

To promote patient comfort (E).

10 Make the patient comfortable and apply a clean sanitary pad.	To absorb any excess discharge (E).
11 Remove and dispose of gloves safely and in accordance with locally approved procedures.	To ensure safe disposal (DH 2005b: C; MHRA: C).
12 Record the administration on appropriate charts.	To maintain accurate records, provide a point of reference in the event of any queries and prevent any duplication of treatment (NMC 2005: C; NMC 2008a: C; NPSA 2007: C).

Procedure guidelines   Topical applications of medication

Equipment

1 Clean non-sterile gloves.
2 Sterile topical swabs.

3 Applicators.

Procedure

Action	Rationale
1 Explain and discuss the procedure with the patient.	To ensure that the patient understands the procedure and gives his/her valid consent (Griffith & Jordan 2003: E; NMC 2006b: C; NMC 2008: C).
2 Check the patient's prescription chart.	To ensure that the patient is given the correct drug and dose (NMC 2008a: C).
3 Assist the patient into the required position.	To allow access to the affected area of skin (E).
4 Close room door or curtains if appropriate.	To ensure patient privacy and dignity (E).
5 Use aseptic technique if the skin is broken.	To prevent local or systemic infection (DH 2007: C).
6 If the medication is to be rubbed into the skin, the preparation should be placed on a sterile topical swab. The wearing of gloves may be necessary.	To minimize the risk of cross-infection. To protect the nurse (DH 2007: C).

Procedure guidelines *(cont.)*

7 If the preparation causes staining, advise the patient of this.	To ensure that adequate precautions are taken beforehand and to prevent unwanted stains (NMC 2008:C).
8 Record the administration on appropriate charts.	To maintain accurate records, provide a point of reference in the event of any queries and prevent any duplication of treatment (NMC 2005: C; NMC 2008a: C; NPSA 2007: C).

Procedure guidelines   Administration of medication in other forms

310

Procedure

Inhalation of medication

Action	Rationale
1 Explain and discuss the procedure with the patient.	To ensure that the patient understands the procedure and gives his/her valid consent (Griffith & Jordan 2003: E; NMC 2006b: C; NMC 2008b: C).
2 Seat the patient in an upright position if possible.	To permit full expansion of the diaphragm (E).

3 Consult the patient's prescription chart, and ascertain the following:
  (a) Drug.
  (b) Dose.
  (c) Date and time of administration.
  (d) Route and method of administration.
  (e) Diluent as appropriate.
  (f) Validity of prescription.
  (g) Signature of doctor.
	To ensure that the patient is given the correct drug in the prescribed dose using the appropriate diluent and by the correct route (NMC 2006b: C).

4 Administer only one drug at a time unless specifically instructed to the contrary.	Several drugs used together may cause undesirable reactions or they may inactivate each other (Jordan *et al.* 2003: E).
5 Measure any liquid medication with a syringe.	To ensure the correct dose (DH 2003d: C).

6 Clean any equipment used after use, and discard all disposable equipment in appropriate containers.

To minimize the risk of infection (DH 2007: C; MHRA: C).

7 Correct use of inhalers is essential (see manufacturer's information leaflet) and will be achieved only if this is carefully explained and demonstrated to the patient. If further advice is required, contact the hospital pharmacist.

Incorrect use may result in most of the dose remaining in the mouth and/or being expelled almost immediately. This renders treatment ineffective (Watt 2003: C; Manufacturer's instructions: C).

8 Record the administration on appropriate charts.

To maintain accurate records, provide a point of reference in the event of any queries and prevent any duplication of treatment (NMC 2005: C; NMC 2008a: C; NPSA 2007: C).

311

Gargling medication
Action

1 Throat irrigations should not be warmer than body temperature.

Rationale

Liquid warmer than body temperature may cause discomfort or damage tissue (E).

Nasal drop administration
Action

1 Explain and discuss the procedure with the patient.

Rationale

To ensure that the patient understands the procedure and gives his/her valid consent (Griffith & Jordan 2003: E; NMC 2006b: C; NMC 2008b: C).

2 Consult the patient's prescription sheet, and ascertain the following:
   (a) Drug.
   (b) Dose.
   (c) Date and time of administration.
   (d) Route and method of administration.
   (e) Validity of prescription.
   (f) Signature of doctor.

To ensure that the patient is given the correct drug in the prescribed dose and by the correct route (NMC 2006b: C).

3 Have paper tissues available.

To wipe away secretions and/or medication (E).

Procedure guidelines *(cont.)*

4 Ask the patient to blow their nose to clear the nasal passages if appropriate.	To ensure maximum penetration for the medication (E).
5 Hyperextend the patient's neck (unless clinically contraindicated, e.g. cervical spondylosis).	To obtain a safe optimum position for insertion of the medication (E).
6 Avoid touching the external nares with the dropper.	To prevent the patient from sneezing (E).
7 Request the patient to maintain his/her position for 1 or 2 minutes.	To ensure full absorption of the medication (E).
8 Each patient should have his/her own medication and dropper.	To minimize the risk of cross-infection (DH 2007: C).
9 Record the administration on appropriate charts.	To maintain accurate records, provide a point of reference in the event of any queries and prevent any duplication of treatment (NMC 2005: C; NMC 2008a: C; NPSA 2007: C).

Eye medications

For information on administering eye medications see Chapter 23.

Ear drop administration

Action	Rationale
1 Explain and discuss the procedure with the patient.	To ensure that the patient understands the procedure and gives his/her valid consent (Griffith & Jordan 2003: E; NMC 2006b: C; NMC 2008b: C).
2 Consult the patient's prescription chart and ascertain the following: (a) Drug. (b) Dose. (c) Date and time of administration. (d) Route and method of administration. (e) Validity of prescription. (f) Signature of doctor.	To ensure that the patient is given the correct drug in the prescribed dose using the appropriate diluent and by the correct route (NMC 2008a: C).
3 Ask the patient to lie on his/her side with the ear to be treated uppermost.	To ensure the best position for insertion of the drops (E).

4 Warm the drops to body temperature if allowed.	To prevent trauma to the patient (E).
5 Pull the cartilaginous part of the pinna backwards and upwards.	To prepare the auditory meatus for instillation of the drops (E).
6 Allow the drop(s) to fall in direction of the external canal.	To ensure that the medication reaches the area requiring therapy (E).
7 Request the patient to remain in this position for 1 or 2 minutes.	To allow the medication to reach the eardrum and be absorbed (E).
8 Record the administration on appropriate charts.	To maintain accurate records, provide a point of reference in the event of any queries and prevent any duplication of treatment (NMC 2005: C; NMC 2008a: C; NPSA 2007: C).

313

Procedure guidelines   Continuous infusion of intravenous drugs

This procedure may be carried out by the infusion of drugs from a bag, bottle or burette.

Equipment

1 Clinically clean receiver or tray containing the prepared drug to be administered.
2 Patient's prescription chart.
3 Recording chart or book as required by law or hospital policy.
4 Protective clothing as required by hospital policy for specific drugs.
5 Container of appropriate intravenous infusion fluid.
6 Swab saturated with isopropyl alcohol 70%.
7 Drug additive label.

Procedure

Action	Rationale
1 Explain and discuss the procedure with the patient.	To ensure that the patient understands the procedure and gives his/her valid consent (Griffith & Jordan 2003: E; NMC 2006b: C; NMC 2008b: C).

Procedure guidelines *(cont.)*

314

2 Inspect the infusion in progress.	To check it is the correct infusion being administered at the correct rate and that the contents are due to be delivered on time in order for the next prepared infusion bag to be connected. To check whether the patient is experiencing any discomfort at the site of insertion, which might indicate the peripheral device needs to be resited (NPSA 2007: C).
3 Before administering any prescribed drug check that it is due and has not already been given.	To protect the patient from harm (NPSA 2007: C).
4 Before administering any prescribed drug, consult the patient's prescription chart and ascertain the following: (a) Drug. (b) Dose. (c) Date and time of administration. (d) Route and method of administration. (e) Diluent as appropriate. (f) Validity of prescription. (g) Signature of doctor. (h) The prescription is legible.	To ensure that the patient is given the correct drug in the prescribed dose using the appropriate diluent and by the correct route. To protect the patient from harm (NMC 2008a: C; NPSA 2007: C). To comply with NMC (2007) *Standards for Medicines Management*.
5 Wash hands with bactericidal soap and water or bactericidal alcohol handrub, and assemble the necessary equipment.	To minimize the risk of infection (DH 2007: C).
6 Prepare the drug for injection described in the Procedure guidelines: Injections: administration.	To ensure the drug is prepared (NPSA 2007: C).
7 Check the name, strength and volume of intravenous fluid against the prescription chart.	To ensure that the correct type and quantity of fluid are administered (NMC 2008a: C; NPSA 2007: C).
8 Check the expiry date of the fluid.	To prevent an ineffective or toxic compound being administered to the patient (NPSA 2007: C).

9 Check that the packaging is intact and inspect the container and contents in a good light for cracks, punctures, air bubbles.

To check that no contamination of the infusion container has occurred (NPSA 2007: C).

10 Inspect the fluid for discoloration, haziness and crystalline or particulate matter.

To prevent any toxic or foreign matter being infused into the patient (NPSA 2007: C).

11 Check the identity and amount of drug to be added.
Consider:
(a) Compatibility of fluid and additive.
(b) Stability of mixture over the prescription time.
(c) Any special directions for dilution, e.g. pH, optimum concentration.
(d) Sensitivity to external factors such as light.
(e) Any anticipated allergic reaction.
If any doubts exist about the listed points, consult the pharmacist or appropriate reference works.

To minimize any risk of error. To ensure safe and effective administration of the drug. To enable anticipation of toxicities and the nursing implications of these (NPSA 2007: C).

315

12 Any additions must be made immediately before use.

To prevent any possible microbial growth or degradation (NPSA 2007: C).

13 Wash hands thoroughly using bactericidal soap and water or bactericidal alcohol handrub.

To minimize the risk of cross-infection (DH 2007: C).

14 Place infusion bag on flat surface.

To prevent puncturing the side of the infusion bag when making additions (NPSA 2007: C).

15 Remove any seal present.

To expose the injection site on the container (E).

16 Clean the site with the swab and allow it to dry.

To reduce the risk of contamination (NPSA 2007: C).

Procedure guidelines *(cont.)*

17 Inject the drug using a new sterile needle into the bag, bottle or burette. A 23 or 25 G needle should be used.	To minimize the risk of contamination. To enable resealing of the latex or rubber injection site (NPSA 2007: C).
18 If the addition is made into a burette at the bedside:	
(a) Avoid contamination of the needle and inlet port.	To minimize the risk of contamination (NPSA 2007: C).
(b) Check that the correct quantity of fluid is in the chamber.	To ensure the correct dilution (NPSA 2007: C).
(c) Switch the infusion off briefly.	To ensure a bolus injection is not given (NPSA 2007: C).
(d) Add the drug.	
19 Invert the container a number of times, especially if adding to a flexible infusion bag.	To ensure adequate mixing of the drug (NPSA 2007: C).
20 Check again for haziness, discoloration and particles. This can occur even if the mixture is theoretically compatible, thus making vigilance essential.	To detect any incompatibility or degradation (NPSA 2007: C).
21 Complete the drug additive label and fix it on the bag, bottle or burette.	To identify which drug has been added, when and by whom (NPSA 2007: C).
22 Place the container in a clean receptacle. Wash hands and proceed to the patient.	To minimize the risk of contamination (DH 2007: C).
23 Check the identity of the patient with the prescription chart and infusion bag.	To minimize the risk of error and ensure the correct infusion is administered to the correct patient (NPSA 2007: C).
24 Check that the contents of the previous container have been delivered.	To ensure that the preceding prescription has been administered (NPSA 2007: C).
25 Switch off the infusion. Place the new infusion bag on a flat surface and then disconnect empty infusion bag.	To ensure that the administration set spike will not puncture the side wall of the infusion bag (NPSA 2007: C; Finlay 2008: E).

26 Push the spike in fully without touching the spike and hang the new infusion bag on the infusion stand.	To reduce the risk of contamination (DH 2007: C).
27 Restart the infusion and adjust the rate of flow as prescribed.	To ensure that the infusion will be delivered at the correct rate over the correct period of time (NPSA 2007: C).
28 If the addition is made into a burette, the infusion can be restarted immediately following mixing and recording and the infusion rate adjusted accordingly.	To ensure that the infusion will be delivered correctly (NPSA 2007:C).
29 Ask the patient whether any abnormal sensations, etc., are experienced.	To ascertain whether there are any problems that may require nursing care and refer to medical staff where appropriate (E).
30 Discard waste, making sure that it is placed in the correct containers, e.g. sharps into a designated receptacle.	To ensure safe disposal and avoid injury to staff. To prevent reuse of equipment (MHRA 2004: C; DH 2005b: C).
31 Complete the patient's recording chart and other hospital and/or legally required documents.	To maintain accurate records. To provide a point of reference in the event of any queries. To prevent any duplication of treatment (NMC 2005: C).

Procedure guidelines   **Intermittent infusion of intravenous drugs**

Equipment

Equipment for this procedure is as described for the previous procedure (i.e. items 1–7), together with the following:

8 Intravenous administration set.

9 Intravenous infusion stand.

10 Clean dressing trolley.

11 Clinically clean receiver or tray.

12 Sterile needles and syringes.

13 20 ml for injection of a compatible flush solution, e.g. 0.9% sodium chloride or 5% dextrose.

14 Flushing solution to maintain patency plus sterile injection cap.

15 Alcohol-based lotion for cleaning injection site, e.g. chlorhexidine in 70% alcohol.

16 Alcohol-based hand wash solution or rub.

17 Sterile dressing pack.

18 Hypoallergenic tape.

Procedure guidelines *(cont.)*

Procedure

Action	Rationale
1 Explain and discuss the procedure with the patient.	To ensure that the patient understands the procedure and gives his/her valid consent (Griffith & Jordan 2003: E; NMC 2006c: C; NMC 2008b: C).
2 Before administering any prescribed drug, check that it is due and has not been given already. Check that the information contained in the prescription chart is complete, correct and legible.	To protect the patient from harm (NPSA 2007: C; NMC 2008a: C).
3 Before administering any prescribed drug, consult the patient's prescription chart and ascertain the following: (a) Drug. (b) Dose. (c) Date and time of administration. (d) Route and method of administration. (e) Diluent as appropriate. (f) Validity of prescription. (g) Signature of doctor. (h) The prescription is legible.	To ensure that the patient is given the correct drug in the prescribed dose using the appropriate diluent and by the correct route (NMC 2008a: C; NPSA 2007: C). To protect the patient from harm. To comply with NMC (2007) *Standards for Medicines Management*.
4 Prepare the intravenous infusion and additive as described for the previous procedure (i.e. items 2–13).	To ensure the drug is prepared correctly (NPSA 2007: C).
5 Prime the intravenous administration set with infusion fluid mixture and hang it on the infusion stand.	To ensure removal of air from set and check that tubing is patent. To prepare for administration (NPSA 2007: C).
6 Draw up 10 ml of compatible flush solution for injection in two separate syringes, using an aseptic technique.	To ensure sufficient flushing solution is available (E).
7 Draw up solution (as per hospital policy) to be used for maintaining patency, e.g. 0.9% sodium chloride.	To prepare for administration (E).

318

8 Place the syringes in a clinically clean receiver or tray on the bottom shelf of the dressing trolley.

To ensure top shelf is used for sterile dressing pack in order to minimize the risk of contamination (E).

9 Collect the other equipment and place it on the bottom shelf of the dressing trolley.

To ensure all equipment is available to commence procedure (E).

10 Place a sterile dressing pack on top of the trolley.

To minimize risk of contamination (E).

11 Check that all necessary equipment is present.

To prevent delays and interruption of the procedure (E).

12 Wash hands thoroughly using bactericidal soap and water or bactericidal alcohol handrub before leaving the clinical room.

To minimize the risk of cross-infection (DH 2007: C).

13 Proceed to the patient. Check patient's identity with prescription chart and prepared drugs.

To minimize the risk of error and ensure the correct drug is given to the correct patient (NMC 2008a; NPSA 2007: C).

14 Open the sterile dressing pack.

To minimize the risk of cross-infection (DH 2007: C).

15 Add lotion for cleaning the injection cap to the gallipot in order to wet the low-linting swabs.

To ensure the swabs can be used for cleaning when sufficient alcohol-based lotion is applied (E).

16 Wash hands with bactericidal soap and water or with a bactericidal alcohol handrub.

To minimize the risk of cross-infection. (DH 2007: C)

17 If peripheral device is in situ remove the patient's bandage and dressing.

To observe the insertion site (Dougherty 2008: E).

18 Inspect the insertion site of the device.

To detect any signs of inflammation, infiltration, etc. If present, take appropriate action (DH 2003c: C).

19 Wash hands as above (see item 16).

To minimize the risk of contamination (DH 2007: C).

Procedure guidelines *(cont.)*

20 Put on gloves, if appropriate.	To protect against contamination with hazardous substances, e.g. cytotoxic drugs (NPSA 2007: C).
21 Place a sterile towel under the patient's arm.	To create a sterile area on which to work (E).
22 (a) If using a needleless injection system, clean the cap with alcohol-soaked swabs.	To minimize the risk of contamination and maintain a closed system (Pratt *et al.* 2007: C).
(b) If using a non-injectable cap, clean the connection between the cap and the device/extension set then remove the cap while applying digital pressure at the point in the vein where the cannula tip rests.	To minimize the risk of contamination and to prevent blood spillage (E).
23 Inject gently 10 ml of 0.9% sodium chloride for injection.	To confirm the patency of the device (E).
24 Check that no resistance is met, no pain or discomfort is felt by the patient, no swelling is evident, no leakage occurs around the device and there is a good back-flow of blood on aspiration.	To ensure the device is patent (Dougherty 2008: E).
25 Connect the infusion to the device.	To commence treatment (E).
26 Open the roller clamp.	To check the infusion is flowing freely (E).
27 Check the insertion site and ask the patient if he/she is comfortable.	To confirm that the vein can accommodate the extra fluid flow and that the patient experiences no pain, etc. (E).
28 Adjust the flow rate as prescribed.	To ensure that the correct speed of administration is established (NPSA 2007: C).

320

29 Tape the administration set in a way that places no strain on the device, which could in turn damage the vein.	To reduce the risk of mechanical phlebitis or infiltration (Dougherty 2008: E).
30 If peripheral device is in situ cover it with a sterile topical swab and tape it in place.	To maintain asepsis (Dougherty 2008: E).
31 Remove gloves, if used.	To ensure disposal (E).
32 If the infusion is to be completed within 30 minutes, bandaging is unnecessary and the patient may be instructed to keep the arm resting on the sterile towel. Otherwise reapply bandage.	To reduce the risk of dislodging the device (E).
33 The equipment must be cleared away and new equipment only prepared when required at the end of the infusion.	To ensure that the equipment used is sterile prior to use (E).
34 Monitor flow rate and device site frequently.	To ensure the flow rate is correct and the patient is comfortable, and to check for signs of infiltration (NPSA 2007: C).
35 When the infusion is complete, wash hands using bactericidal soap and water or bactericidal alcohol handrub, and recheck that all the equipment required is present.	To maintain asepsis and ensure that the procedure runs smoothly (DH 2007: C; Finlay 2008: E).
36 Stop the infusion when all the fluid has been delivered.	To ensure that all of the prescribed mixture has been delivered and prevent air infusing into the patient (NPSA 2007: C).
37 Put on non-sterile gloves, if appropriate.	To protect against contamination with hazardous substances (E).

321

Procedure guidelines *(cont.)*

38 Disconnect the infusion set and flush the device with 10 ml of 0.9% sodium chloride or other compatible solution for injection. (A 'minibag' may be used to flush the drug through the tubing but the cost implications of this as well as the risk to patients on restricted intake should be considered before this is adopted routinely.)	To flush any remaining irritating solution away from the cannula (E).
39 Attach a new sterile injection cap if necessary.	To maintain a closed system (Hart 2008: E).
40 Flushing must follow.	To maintain the patency of the device (Dougherty 2008: E).
41 Clean the injection site of the cap with a swab saturated with chlorhexidine in 70% alcohol.	To minimize the risk of contamination (Hart 2008: E).
42 Administer flushing solution (using a 23 or 25 G needle if necessary) using the push pause technique and ending with positive pressure.	To maintain the patency of the device and if needle used enable reseal of the injection site (Dougherty 2008: E).
43 If a peripheral device is in situ cover the insertion site and cannula with a new sterile low-linting swab. Tape it in place. Apply a bandage.	To minimize the risk of contamination of the insertion site. To reduce the risk of dislodging the cannula (E).
44 Remove gloves, if used.	To ensure disposal (E).
45 Assist the patient into a comfortable position.	To ensure the patient is comfortable (E).
46 Record the administration on appropriate charts.	To maintain accurate records, provide a point of reference in the event of any queries and prevent any duplication of treatment (NMC 2005: C).
47 Discard waste, placing it in the correct containers, e.g. sharps into a designated container.	To ensure safe disposal and avoid injury to staff (MHRA 2004; DH 2005b; NHS Employers 2005).

Procedure guidelines   Injection (bolus or push) of intravenous drugs

This procedure may be carried out via any of the following:

1 The injection or Y site of an intravenous administration set.
2 An injection cap attached to any vascular access device.
3 An extension set, multiple adaptor or stopcock (one-, two- or three-way).

Equipment

1 Clinically clean receiver or tray containing the prepared drug(s) to be administered.
2 Patient's prescription chart.
3 Protective clothing as required by hospital policy or specific drugs.
4 Clean dressing trolley.
5 Clinically clean receiver or tray.
6 Sterile needles and syringes.
7 0.9% sodium chloride, 20 ml for injection or compatible solution.
8 Flushing solution, in accordance with hospital policy.
9 Alcohol-based solution for cleaning injection site, e.g. chlorhexidine in 70% alcohol.
10 Sterile dressing pack.
11 Hypoallergenic tape.
12 Sharps container.

Procedure

Action	Rationale
1 Explain and discuss the procedure with the patient.	To ensure that the patient understands the procedure and gives his/her valid consent (Griffith & Jordan 2003: E; NMC 2006c: C; NMC 2008b: C).
2 Before administering any prescribed drug, check that it is due and has not been given already. Check that the information contained in the prescription chart is complete, correct and legible.	To protect the patient from harm (NMC 2008: C).
3 Before administering any prescribed drug, consult the patient's prescription sheet and ascertain the following: (a) Drug. (b) Dose. (c) Date and time of administration. (d) Route and method of administration.	To ensure that the patient is given the correct drug in the prescribed dose using the appropriate diluent and by the correct route (NMC 2008a: C; NPSA 2007: C). To protect the patient from harm. To comply with NMC (2007) *Standards for Medicines Management*.

Procedure guidelines *(cont.)*

(e) Diluent as appropriate.
(f) Validity of prescription.
(g) Signature of doctor.
(h) The prescription is legible.

4 Select the required medication and check the expiry date.	Treatment with medication that is outside the expiry date is dangerous. Drugs deteriorate with storage. The expiry date indicates when a particular drug is no longer pharmacologically efficacious (NPSA 2007: C).
5 Wash hands with bactericidal soap and water or bactericidal alcohol handrub, and assemble necessary equipment.	To minimize the risk of infection (DH 2007: C).
6 Prepare the drug for injection as per procedure described earlier.	To prepare the drug correctly (E).
7 Prepare a 20 ml syringe of 0.9% sodium chloride (or compatible solution) for injection, as described, using aseptic technique.	To use for flushing between each drug (NPSA 2007: C).
8 Draw up flushing solution, as required by hospital policy.	To prepare for administration (E).
9 Place syringes in a clinically clean receptacle on the bottom shelf of the dressing trolley, along with the receptacle containing any drug(s) to be administered.	To ensure top shelf is used for sterile dressing pack in order to minimize the risk of contamination (E).
10 Collect the other equipment and place it on the bottom of the trolley.	To ensure all equipment is available to commence procedure (E).
11 Place a sterile dressing pack on top of the trolley.	To minimize the risk of contamination (E).
12 Check that all necessary equipment is present.	To prevent delays and interruption of the procedure (E).
13 Wash hands thoroughly.	To minimize the risk of infection (DH 2007: C).

14 Proceed to the patient and check identity with prescription chart and prepared drug.	To minimize the risk of error and ensure the correct patient (NPSA 2007: C).
15 Open the sterile dressing pack. Add lotion to wet the low-linting swab.	To gain access to equipment and to ensure the swab is soaked with cleaning solution (E).
16 Wash hands with bactericidal soap and water or with bactericidal alcohol handrub.	To reduce the risk of infection (DH 2007: C).
17 If a peripheral device is in situ, remove the bandage and dressing (if appropriate).	To observe the insertion site (E).
18 Inspect the insertion site of the device.	To detect any signs of inflammation, infiltration, etc. If present, take appropriate action (see Problem solving, below) (DH 2003c: C).
19 Observe the infusion, if in progress.	To confirm that it is infusing as desired (NPSA 2007: C) To prevent drug interaction. Some manufacturers may recommend that the drug is given into the injection site of a rapidly running infusion (NPSA 2007: C).
20 Check whether the infusion fluid and the drugs are compatible. If not, change the infusion fluid to 0.9% sodium chloride to flush between the drugs.	
21 Wash hands or clean them with an alcohol handrub.	To minimize the risk of infection (DH 2007: C).
22 Place a sterile towel under the patient's arm.	To create a sterile field (E).
23 Clean the injection site with a swab saturated with chlorhexidine in 70% alcohol and allow to dry.	To reduce the number of pathogens introduced by the needle at the time of the insertion. To ensure complete disinfection has occurred (Pratt *et al.* 2007: C).

Procedure guidelines *(cont.)*

24 Switch off the infusion or close the fluid path of a tap or stopcock.

To prevent excessive pressure within the vein. To prevent contact with an incompatible infusion fluid. To allow the nurse to concentrate on the site of insertion and injection (NPSA 2007: C).

25 If a peripheral device is in situ use a sterile 23 or 25 G needle if the injection is made through a resealable site and gently inject 0.9% sodium chloride. This may not be necessary if the patient has a 0.9% sodium chloride infusion in progress.

To enable resealing of the site at the end of the injection. To confirm patency of the vein. To prevent contact with an incompatible infusion solution (NPSA 2007: C).

26 Open the roller clamp of the administration set fully. Inject the drug at a speed sufficient to slow but not stop the infusion and inject the drug smoothly in the direction of flow at the specified rate.

To prevent a back-flow of drug up the tubing. To prevent excessive pressure within the vein. To prevent speed shock (NPSA 2007: C).

27 Ensure used needles and syringes are disposed of immediately into appropriate sharps container (or are returned to tray). Do not leave any sharps on opened sterile pack.

To reduce the risk of needlestick injury and to prevent contamination of pack (RCN 2005: C).

28 Observe the insertion site of the device throughout.

To detect any complications at an early stage, e.g. extravasation or local allergic reaction (Dougherty 2008: E).

29 Blood return and/or 'flashback' must be checked frequently throughout the injection (i.e. every 3–5 ml).

To confirm that the device is correctly placed and that the vein remains patent (Weinstein 2007: E).

30 Consult the patient during the injection about any discomfort, etc.

To detect any complications at an early stage, and ensure patient comfort (Dougherty 2008: E).

31 If more than one drug is to be administered, flush with 0.9% sodium chloride between administrations by restarting the infusion or changing syringes.

To prevent drug interactions (NPSA 2007: C).

32 At the end of the injection, flush with 0.9% sodium chloride by restarting the infusion or attaching a syringe containing 0.9% sodium chloride.	To flush any remaining irritant solution away from the device site (NPSA 2007: C).
33 Observe the insertion site of the cannula carefully.	To detect any complications at an early stage. Extra pressure within the vein caused by both fluid flow and injection of the drug may cause rupture of the vessel (Dougherty 2008: E).
34 After the final flush of 0.9% sodium chloride adjust the infusion rate as prescribed or open the fluid path of the tap/stopcock or use flushing solution.	To continue delivery of therapy. To maintain the patency of the cannula (Finlay 2008: E).
35 If a peripheral device is in situ cover the insertion site with new sterile low linting swab and tape it in place.	To minimize the risk of contamination of the insertion site (E).
36 Apply a bandage.	To reduce the risk of dislodging the cannula (E).
37 Assist the patient into a comfortable position.	To ensure the patient is comfortable (E).
38 Record the administration on appropriate charts.	To maintain accurate records, provide a point of reference in the event of any queries and prevent any duplication of treatment (NMC 2005: C).
39 Dispose of used syringes with needles, unsheathed, directly into a sharps container during procedure or place back on to plastic tray and then dispose of in a sharps container as soon as possible. *Do not* disconnect needle from syringe prior to disposal. Other waste should be placed into the appropriate plastic bags.	To avoid needlestick injury (MHRA 2004: C; NHS Employers 2005: C).

327

Problem solving: Injection and infusion of intravenous fluids and drugs

The problems associated with injection and infusion of intravenous fluids and drugs fall into two categories:

1 Local venous complications associated with the cannula insertion site.
2 Systemic problems which affect the whole patient, exerting effects on vital organs and their functions.

The nurse must regularly observe the insertion site, the infusion and the patient to detect any complications at the earliest possible moment and to prevent progression to more serious conditions. Early detection is aided by paying attention to the patient's comments of discomfort or pain. The patient's symptoms and physical signs both constitute reasons for resiting of the peripheral device or discontinuation of the infusion (Lamb & Dougherty 2008). Signs and symptoms are used as problem headings.

Problem	Possible causes	Preventive nursing measures	Suggested action
Infusion slows or stops.	Change in position of the following:		
	(a) Patient.	Check the height of the fluid container if the patient is active and receiving an infusion using gravity flow.	Adjust the height of the container accordingly. But the infusion should not hang higher than 1 m (above the patient) as the increased height will result in increased pressure and possible rupture of the vessel/device (Quinn 2008).
	(b) Limb.	Prevent by avoiding use of joints when inserting peripheral devices. Instruct the patient on the amount of movement permitted. Continued movement could result in mechanical phlebitis (Lamb & Dougherty 2008).	Move the arm or hand until infusion starts again. Secure the device, then bandage or splint the limb again carefully in the desired position. Take care not to cause damage to the limb.

Problem	Possible causes	Preventive nursing measures	Suggested action
	(c) Administration set.	Tape the administration set so that it cannot become kinked or occluded.	Check for kinks and/or compression if the patient is active or restless and correct accordingly.
	(d) Cannula.	Secure the cannula firmly to prevent movement. It may come into contact with the vein wall or a valve. Infusions sited in small veins are prone to this problem.	Remove the bandage and dressing and manoeuvre the peripheral device gently, without pulling it out of the vein, until the infusion starts again. Secure adequately.

Technical problems:

Problem	Possible causes	Preventive nursing measures	Suggested action
	(a) Negative pressure prevents flow of fluid.	Ensure that the container is vented using an air inlet.	Vent if necessary, using venting needle.
	(b) Empty container.	Check fluid levels regularly.	Replace the fluid container before it runs dry.
	(c) Venous spasm due to chemical irritation or cold fluids/drugs.	Dilute drugs as recommended. Remove solutions from the refrigerator a short time before use.	Apply a warm compress to soothe and dilate the vein, increase the blood flow and dilute the infusion mixture.
	(d) Injury to the vein.	Detect any injury early as it is likely to progress and cause more serious conditions (see below).	Stop the infusion and request resiting of the cannula.

Problem solving (cont.)

Problem	Possible causes	Preventive nursing measures	Suggested action
	(e) Occlusion of the device due to fibrin formation.	Maintain a continuous, regular fluid flow or ensure that patency is maintained by flushing. Instruct the patient to keep arm below the level of the heart if ambulant and attached to a gravity flow infusion.	**If peripheral device**: remove extension set/injection cap and attempt to flush the cannula gently using a 10 ml syringe of 0.9% sodium chloride. If resistance is met, stop and request a resiting of the peripheral device (see Chapter 45, Professional edition). **If central venous access device (CVAD)**: remove injection cap and attempt to flush the cannula gently using a 10 ml syringe of 0.9% sodium chloride. If resistance is met attempt to instil antifibrinolytic agent such as urokinase (see Chapter 45, Professional edition).
	(f) The cannula has become displaced either completely or partially, i.e. fluid or drug has leaked into the surrounding tissues (infiltration). If the drugs were vesicant in nature this would then be defined as extravasation.	Secure the cannula and tape the administration set so that no stress is placed on them. Instruct the patient on the amount of movement permitted (Fabian 2000).	Confirm that infiltration of drugs has/has not occurred by: (i) inspecting the site for leakage, swelling, etc.; (ii) testing the temperature of the skin: it will be cooler if infiltration has occurred; (iii) comparing the size of the limb with the opposite limb. (iv) Once infiltration has been confirmed, stop the infusion and request a resiting of the device. If the infusion is allowed to progress, discomfort and tissue damage will result. Apply cold or warm compresses to provide symptomatic relief, whichever provides the most comfort for the patient. Reassure the patient by explaining what is happening. Document in care plan and monitor site (Lamb & Dougherty 2008).

Problem	Possible causes	Preventive nursing measures	Suggested action
			(v) If extravasation, follow hospital policy and procedure (see Chapter 12, Main edition).
Erythema (inflammation) around the insertion site, and/or pain and swelling.	Phlebitis due to:	Observe the site regularly and use an assessment tool such as the VIP Scale to assess the site (Jackson 1998; DH 2003c). (See Figure 8.3)	Failure to detect and act when phlebitis is at an early stage, for whatever reason, will result in painful and incapacitating thrombophlebitis. Dislodgement of a thrombus could cause a pulmonary embolus (Lamb & Dougherty 2008; Weinstein 2008).
	(a) Sepsis.	Adhere to aseptic techniques when performing all intravenous procedures (RCN 2005)	Stop the infusion, remove the device and resite the device. Follow hospital policy about sending cannula tip for bacterial analysis. Clean the area and apply a sterile dressing. Check regularly. Document.
	(b) Chemical irritation.	Dilute drugs according to instructions. Check compatibilities carefully to reduce the risk of particulate formation. Administer the drugs as an infusion instead of a bolus injection. Be aware of the factors involved, e.g. pH (Lamb & Dougherty 2008). Apply local heat above the cannula site (Lamb & Dougherty 2008). Apply a glycerol trinitrate (GTN) patch to aid vasodilatation (Wright et al. 1985).	Stop the infusion and resite the device. If the infusion is allowed to progress, tissue damage and severe pain will result. Apply warm compresses to provide symptomatic relief. Encourage movement of the limb. Reassure the patient by explaining what has happened. Document.

331

Problem solving *(cont.)*

Problem	Possible causes	Preventive nursing measures	Suggested action
	(c) Mechanical irritation.	Secure the device and then bandage or splint the limb if the infusion is sited at a point of flexion. Use an extension set to minimize manipulation of the device. Instruct the patient on the amount of movement permitted (Campbell 1996; Jackson 1998; Taylor 2000).	Stop the infusion and remove the device. Resite the device. Although inflammation of this type progresses more slowly, it will cause discomfort. Provide symptomatic relief as above. Encourage movement and reassure the patient by explaining what has happened. Document.
	Infection with or without discharge.	Adhere to aseptic techniques when performing all intravenous procedures. Observe all recommendations for equipment changes, etc.	Stop the infusion, remove the peripheral device. Resite the peripheral device in opposite arm if possible. Follow hospital policy about sending device tip for bacterial analysis. If CVAD take a swab from exit site then clean the area and apply a sterile dressing. Check regularly. Observe the patient for signs of systemic infection.
	Cellulitis due to: (a) Sepsis. (b) Non-specific sterile inflammation.	As above.	As above. Due to the nature of the connective tissue any infection or inflammation spreads quickly, especially if the limb is oedematous.

Problem	Possible causes	Preventive nursing measures	Suggested action
	Local allergic reaction, e.g. flare reaction which occurs with anthracyclines such as doxorubicin.	Ask whether the patient has any allergies before administration of any drugs or fluids, including sensitivities to topical solutions, which may cause erythema at the site (NMC 2008a). Check whether the particular medication is commonly associated with local or venous flushing.	Observe the patient for systemic reaction. Treat the local area symptomatically. Reassure the patient. Inform medical staff. Document patient reaction.
Local oedema.	During infusion or injection: (a) Infiltration. (b) Phlebitis. (c) Extravasation of medication (see Chapter 12, Professional edition).	Secure the device and tape the administration set so that no stress is placed on the cannula. Use an extension set. Instruct the patient on the amount of movement permitted. Check regularly for swelling, e.g. tightness of bandages or around rings. Observe the patient carefully throughout drug administration.	Stop the infusion, remove the peripheral device then resite the device in opposite arm if possible. Apply warm compresses to provide symptomatic relief. Reassure the patient by explaining what is happening. Stop the injection immediately extravasation is suspected. Act in accordance with hospital policy. Some drugs may cause inflammation and supportive, symptomatic relief will be required. Others may have the potential to cause necrosis of tissue and further action may be necessary. Document.

333

Problem solving *(cont.)*

Problem	Possible causes	Preventive nursing measures	Suggested action
Oedema of the limb.	Infiltration.	Tape the device and administration set so that no stress is placed on the device, which in turn can lead to damage of the vein. Use an extension set. Instruct the patient on the amount of movement permitted. Check regularly for swelling, as above.	Stop the infusion, remove the peripheral device then resite the device in opposite arm if possible. Provide symptomatic relief and support. Reassure the patient.
	Circulatory overload.	Administer infusion fluids at the prescribed rate and do not make sudden alterations of flow. Use infusion equipment wherever possible and administration set with anti-free-flow systems. Be aware of the patient's renal and cardiac status. Monitor intake and output routinely (Lamb & Dougherty 2008; Weinstein 2007).	Slow the infusion. Monitor vital signs for increase in blood pressure and respirations. Place the patient in an upright position and keep him/her warm to promote peripheral circulation and relieve stress on the central veins. Reassure the patient. Notify a doctor immediately.
	Thrombosis.	Ensure the tip is located in correct position.	The patient may require ultrasound to diagnose a clot in the arm. If confirmed then the patient will require anticoagulation. The device may be removed.

Problem	Possible causes	Preventive nursing measures	Suggested action
Pain at the insertion site.	All of the previous listed conditions may be accompanied by soreness or pain.	As previously listed.	Provide local symptomatic relief, e.g. warmth, as required. Administer systemic analgesia, as prescribed, if necessary.
Pyrexia, rigors, tachycardia.	Septicaemia.	Adhere to aseptic techniques when performing all intravenous procedures. Inspect all equipment, infusion fluids, etc., before use. Observe recommendations for additives, equipment changes and general management. Avoid the use of equipment that can increase the risk of contamination, e.g. stopcocks (Finlay 2008; Lamb & Dougherty 2008).	Notify a doctor immediately. Follow hospital policy about sending equipment for bacterial analysis.
Decrease in blood pressure, tachycardia, cyanosis, unconsciousness.	Embolism: (a) Air.	Check the containers and change before they run through, especially bottles. Clear all air from tubing before commencing infusion. Check all connections regularly and make sure they are secure. Use infusion equipment with air in line detectors.	Turn the patient onto left side and lower the head of the bed to prevent air from entering the pulmonary artery. Notify a doctor immediately. Administer oxygen (RCN 2005; Lamb & Dougherty 2008; Weinstein 2007). Reassure the patient.

335

Problem solving *(cont.)*

Problem	Possible causes	Preventive nursing measures	Suggested action
	(b) Particle.	Check all infusion fluids before and after any additions have been made. Check drug compatibility and stability. Flush adequately between solutions. Observe the solution throughout the infusion for precipitate formation (Finlay 2008).	As above, but also change the container and administration set. Replace with new equipment and 0.9% sodium chloride infusion from a different batch. Follow hospital policy about sending contaminated fluid and equipment for bacterial analysis.
Itching, rash, shortness of breath.	Allergic reaction due to sensitivity to an intravenous fluid, additive or drug.	Ask the patient whether he/she has any allergies *before* administration of any drugs or fluids. Check whether the particular medication is commonly associated with any allergic reactions and observe the patient during treatment.	Stop drug infusion or injection and maintain the patency of the vascular access device using 0.9% sodium chloride. Notify a doctor immediately. Reassure the patient. Ensure that hydrocortisone and epinephrine are available. Document.
Flushed face, headache, congestion of the chest, possibly progressing to loss of consciousness.	Speed shock due to too rapid administration of drugs. May be a small volume (Lamb & Dougherty 2008; Weinstein 2007).	Administer drugs and infusion at the correct rate. Check the flow rate frequently. Use infusion equipment with anti-free-flow administration sets if the delivery rate is crucial.	As above.

337

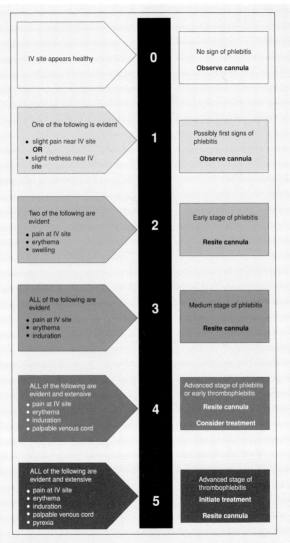

Figure 8.3 Vein infusion phlebitis scale (VIP Scale) (Jackson 1998).

References and further reading

Arduino, M.J. *et al.* (1997) Microbiological evaluation of needleless and needle access devices. *Am J Infect Control*, 25(5), 377–80.

Arndt, M. (1994) Research and practice: how drug mistakes affect self-esteem. *Nurs Times*, 90(15), 27–31.

Audit Commission (2001) *A Spoonful of Sugar: Medicines Management in NHS Hospitals.* Audit Commission, London.

Beyea, S.C. & Nicholl, L.S.H. (1995) Administration of medications via the intramuscular route: an integrative review of the literature and research based protocol for the procedure. *Appl Nurs Res*, 5(1), 23–33.

Bird, C. (1990) A prescription for self-care. *Nurs Times*, 86(43), 52–5.

BNF (2008) *British National Formulary*. BMJ Publishing Group Ltd, London.

Brenneis, C. *et al.* (1987) Local toxicity during subcutaneous infusion of narcotics. *Cancer Nurs*, 10(4), 172–6.

Bridge, J., Hemingway, S. & Murphy, K. (2005) Implications of non medical prescribing of controlled drugs. *Nurs Times*, 101(44), 32–3.

British Pharmacopoeia (2007) *British Pharmacopoeia*, The Stationary Office, London.

Brock, A.M. (1979) Self-administration of drugs in the elderly. *Nurs Forum*, 18(4), 340–57.

Brown, J., Moss, H. & Elliot, T. (1997) The potential for catheter microbial contamination from a needleless connector. *J Hosp Infect*, 36(3), 181–9.

Campbell, J. (1996) Intravenous drug therapy. *Prof Nurse*, 11(7), 437–42.

Central Health Services Council (1958) *Report of Joint Sub-Committee on the Control of Dangerous Drugs and Poisons in Hospitals* (Chairman J.K. Aitken). HMSO, London.

Cole, D. (1999) Selection and management of central venous access devices in the home setting. *J Intraven Nurs*, 22(6), 315–19.

Constans, T. *et al.* (1991) Hypodermoclysis in dehydrated elderly patients – local effects with and without hyaluronidase. *J Palliat Care*, 7(2), 10–12.

Cookson, S. *et al.* (1998) Increased blood stream infection rates in surgical patients associated with variation from recommended use and care following implementation of a needleless device. *Infect Control Hosp Epidemiol*, 19(1), 23–7.

Cresswell, J. (1999) *Nurse Prescribing Handbook*. Association of Nurse Prescribing and Community Nurse, UK.

Dann, T.C. (1969) Routine skin preparation before injection: an unnecessary procedure. *Lancet*, ii, 96–7.

Danzig, L.E. *et al.* (1995) Bloodstream infections associated with a needleless intravenous infusion system in patients receiving home infusion therapy. *JAMA*, 273(23), 1862–4.

Dawkins, L. *et al.* (2000) A randomised trial of winged Vialon cannulae and metal butterfly needles. *Int J Palliat Nurs*, 6(3), 110–16.

Deeks, P. & Byatt, K. (2000) Are patients who self-administer their medicines in hospital more satisfied with their care? *J Adv Nurs*, 31(2), 395–400.

DH (1988) *Guidelines for the Safe and Secure Handling of Medicines (The Duthie Report)*. HMSO, London.

DH (1989) *Report of the Advisory Group on Nurse Prescribing*. Crown One. HMSO, London.

DH (1998) *Review of Prescribing, Supply and Administration of Medicines. A Report on the Supply and Administration of Medicines under Group Protocols.* Crown Two. HMSO, London.

DH (1999) *Review of Prescribing, Supply and Administration of Medicines. Final Report.* Crown Three. HMSO, London.

DH (2000) Patient Group Directions (HSC 2000/026) Health and Safety Commission London.

DH (2001a) Guidelines for preventing infections associated with the insertion and maintenance of central venous catheters. *J Hosp Infect*, **47**(Suppl), S47–67.

DH (2001b) *National Service Framework for Older People.* HMSO, London.

DH (2003a) *Supplementary Prescribing.* National Health Service, London. (www.doh.gov.uk/supplementary prescribing).

DH (2003b) *Supplementary Prescribing by Nurses and Pharmacists within the NHS in England: a guide for implementation.* National Health Service, London.

DH (2003c) *Winning Ways: Working Together to Reduce Healthcare-Associated Infection in England.* Department of Health, London.

DH (2003d) *Building a Safer NHS for Patients: Improving Medication Safety.* Department of Health, London.

DH (2004) *Extending Independent Nurse Prescribing within the NHS in England: a Guide to Implantation.* Department of Health, London.

DH (2005a) *Saving Lives: A Delivery Programme to Reduce Healthcare-associated Infection including MRSA.* Department of Health, London.

DH (2005b) *Hazardous waste (England) regulations.* Department of Health, London.

DH (2006) *Improving Patients Access to Medicines – a Guide to Implementing Nurse and Pharmacist Independent Prescribing within the NHS in England.* Department of Health, London.

DHSS (1976) *Health Services Development, Addition of Drugs to Intravenous Fluids, HC(76)9 (Breckenridge Report).* HMSO, London.

Dickman, A., Schneider, J. & Varga, J. (2005) *The Syringe Driver: Continuous Infusions in Palliative Care*, 2nd edn. Oxford University Press, Oxford.

Dorr, T. & Von Hoff, D. (1993) *Cancer Chemotherapy Handbook*, 2nd edn. Appleton & Lange, Hemel Hempstead.

Dougherty, L. (2002) Delivery of intravenous therapy. *Nurs Stand*, **16**(16), 45–52.

Dougherty, L. (2008) Obtaining peripheral access. In: *Intravenous Therapy in Nursing Practice* (eds L. Dougherty & J. Lamb), 2nd edn. Blackwell Publishing, Oxford.

Downie, G., MacKenzie, J. & Williams, A. (Eds) (2000) Administration of medicines. In: *Pharmacology and Drugs Management for Nurses*, 2nd edn. Churchill Livingstone, London, pp. 495–557.

Epperson, E.L. (1984) Efficacy of 0.9% sodium chloride injection with and without heparin for maintaining indwelling intermittent injection sites. *Clin Pharm*, **3**, 626–9.

Fabian, B (2000) IV complications: Infiltration. *J Intraven Nurs*, **23** (4), 229–31.

Field, P.A. (1981) A phenomenological look at giving an injection. *J Adv Nurs*, **6**(4), 291–6.

Finlay, T. (2008) Safe administration of IV therapy. In: *Intravenous Therapy in Nursing Practice* (eds L. Dougherty & J. Lamb), 2nd edn. Blackwell Publishing, Oxford.

Gabriel, J. (2005) Vascular access: Indications and implications for patient care. *Nursing Standard*, **19** (26) 45–52.

339

Gatford, J. & Anderson, R. (1998) *Nursing Calculations*, 5th edn. Churchill Livingstone, Edinburgh.

Gladstone, J. (1995) Drug administration errors: a study into the factors underlying the occurrence and reporting of drug errors in a district general hospital. *J Adv Nurs*, **22**(4), 628–37.

Glynn, A. *et al.* (1997) *Hospital Acquired Infection – Surveillance Policies and Practice*. Central Public Health Laboratory, London.

Griffith, R. & Jordan, S. (2003) Administration of medicines part 1: the law and nursing. *Nurs Stand*, **18**(2), 47–53.

Hanchett, M. & Kung, L.Y. (1999) Do needleless intravenous systems increase the risk of infection? *J Intraven Nurs*, **22**(6), 117–21.

Hart, S. (2008) Infection control in IV therapy. In: *Intravenous Therapy in Nursing Practice* (eds L. Dougherty & J. Lamb), 2nd edn. Blackwell Publishing, Oxford.

Higgins, D. (2005) Drug Calculations. *Nurs Times*, **101**(46), 24–5.

HMSO (1968) *Medicines Act*. HMSO, London.

HMSO (1971) *Misuse of Drugs Act*. HMSO, London.

HMSO (2001) *Misuse of Drugs Regulations*. HMSO, London.

Hockley, J. *et al.* (1995) Audit to pinpoint IV drug administration pitfalls. *Nurs Times*, **91**(51), 33–4.

Hutton, M. (1998) Numeracy skills for IV calculations. *Nurs Stand*, **12**(43), 49–56.

Hyde, L. (2002) Legal and professional aspects of intravenous therapy. *Nurs Stand*, **16**(26), 39–42.

Hyde, L. (2008) Legal and professional aspects of IV therapy. In: *Intravenous Therapy in Nursing Practice* (eds L. Dougherty & J. Lamb), 2nd edn. Blackwell Publishing, Oxford.

Jackson, A. (1998) A battle in vein infusion phlebitis. *Nurs Times*, **94**(4), 68–71.

Jordan, S., Griffiths, H. & Griffith, R. (2003) Administration of medicines part 2: pharmacology. *Nurs Stand*, **18**(3), 45–54.

Kain, V. *et al.* (2006) Developing guidelines for syringe driver management. *Int J Palliat Nurs*, **12**(2), 60–8.

King, L. (2003) Subcutaneous insulin injection technique. *Nurs Stand*, **17**(34), 45–52.

Koivistov, V.A. & Felig, P. (1978) Is skin preparation necessary before insulin injection? *Lancet*, i, 1072–3.

Kuhn, M.M. (1989) *Pharmacotherapeutics. A Nursing Process Approach*, 2nd edn. F.A. Davis, Philadelphia.

Lamb, J. & Dougherty, L. (2008) Local and systemic complications of intravenous therapy. In: *Intravenous Therapy in Nursing Practice* (eds L. Dougherty & J. Lamb), 2nd edn. Blackwell Publishing, Oxford.

Latter, S. *et al.* (2005) *An Evaluation of Extended Formulary Independent Nurse Prescribing: Executive Summary of Final Report*. University of Southampton, Southampton.

Laverty, D., Mallett, J. & Mulholland, J. (1997) Protocols and guidelines for managing wounds. *Prof Nurse*, **13**(2), 79–80.

Lenz, C.L. (1983) Make your needle selection right to the point. *Nursing*, **13**(2), 50–1.

Luebke, M.A. *et al.* (1998) Comparison of the microbial barrier properties of a needleless and conventional needle based intravenous access system. *Am J Infect Control*, **26**, 437–41.

Luker, K. & Wolfson, D. (1999) Introduction. In: *Medicines Management for Clinical Nurses* (eds K. Luker & D. Wolfson). Blackwell Science, Oxford.

Luker, K.A. *et al.* (1998) Nurse–patient relationships: the context of nurse prescribing. *J Adv Nurs*, **28**, 235–42.

Mallett, J. *et al.* (1997) Nurse prescribing by protocol. *Nurs Times*, **93**(8), 50–2.

Martin, P.J. (1994) Professional updating through open learning as a method of reducing errors in the administration of medicines. *J Nurs Manage*, **2**(5), 209–12.

McClelland, B. (2007) *Handbook of Transfusion Medicine*, 3rd edn. HMSO, London.

McGraw, C. & Drennan, V. (2001) Self administration of medicine and older people. *Nurs Stand*, **15**(18), 33–6.

McHale, J. (2002) Extended prescribing: the legal implications. *Nurs Times*, **98**(32), 36–8.

Mendelson, M.H. *et al.* (1998) Study of a needleless intermittent intravenous access system for peripheral infusions: analysis of staff, patient and institutional outcomes. *Infect Control Hosp Epidemiol*, **19**(6), 401–6.

MHRA (2004) *Reducing Needlestick and Sharps Injuries*. Medicines and Healthcare Products Regulatory Agency, London.

MHRA (2005) *Consultation on Options for the Future of Independent Prescribing by Extended Formulary Nurse Prescribers*. Medicines and Healthcare Products Regulatory Agency, London.

Mitten, T. (2001) Subcutaneous drug infusions: a review of problems and solutions. *Int J Palliat Nurs*, **7**(2), 75–85.

Moriarty, D. & Hudson, E. (2001) Hypodermoclysis for rehydration in the community. *Br J Community Nurs*, **6**(9), 437–43.

NHS Employers (2005) *The Management of Health, Safety and Welfare Issues for NHS Staff*. NHS Confederation (Employers) Company, London.

NHS Executive (2000) *Health Service Circular HSC 2000/26. Patient Group Directions (England Only)*. SI 2000, No. 1919. NHS Executive, Leeds.

NHSE (1998a) *Nurse Prescribing. A Guide for Implementation*. HMSO, London.

NHSE (1998b) *Nurse Prescribing. Implementing the Scheme across England*. HSC 1998/232. HMSO, London.

NICE (2003) *Technology Appraisal Guidance No 57. Guidance on the Use of Continuous Subcutaneous Insulin Infusion for Diabetes*. National Institute for Health and Clinical Excellence, London.

Nicolson, H. (1986) The success of the syringe driver. *Nurs Times*, **82**, 49–51.

NMC (2001a) *Covert Administration of Medicines can be Justified*. Press statement, 5th September. Nursing and Midwifery Council, London.

NMC (2001b) *UKCC Position Statement on the Covert Administration of Medicines – Disguising Medicine in Food and Drink*. Nursing and Midwifery Council, London.

NMC (2001c) *Circular 25/2002*. Nursing and Midwifery Council, London.

NMC (2005) *Guidelines for Records and Record Keeping*. Nursing and Midwifery Council, London.

NMC (2006a) *Standards of Proficiency for Nurse and Midwife Prescribers*. Nursing and Midwifery Council, London.

NMC (2006b) *A–Z Advice Sheet Consent*. www.nmc.org.

NMC (2008a) *Standards for Medicines Management*. Nursing and Midwifery Council, London.

NMC (2008b) *The Code: Standards of Conduct, Performance and Ethics for Nurses and Midwives.* Nursing and Midwifery Council, London.

Noble-Adams, R. (1995) Dehydration: subcutaneous fluid administration. *Br J Nurs*, **4**(9), 488–94.

NPC (2001) *Maintaining Competency in Prescribing: an Outline Framework to Help Nurse Prescribers.* National Health Service, London.

NPC (2003a) *Supplementary Prescribing. A Resource to Help Healthcare Professionals to Understand the Framework and Opportunities.* National Health Service, London.

NPC (2003b) *Maintaining Competency in Prescribing: an Outline Framework to Help Nurse Supplementary Prescribers.* National Health Service, London.

NPSA (2005) *Wristbands for Hospital Inpatients Improves Safety (Safer Practice Notice 11).* NPSA, London.

NPSA (2006) *Ensuring Safer Practice with High Dose Ampoules of Morphine and Diamorphine, Alert No. 2006/12, 25th May.* NPSA, London.

NPSA (2007) *Promoting Safer Use of Injectable Medicines, Alert No. 2007/20, 28th March.* NPSA, London.

Osbourne, J., Blais, K. & Hayes, J.S. (1999) Nurses' perceptions: when is it a medication error? *J Nurs Admin*, **29**(4), 33–8.

Peragallo-Dittko, V. (1997) Rethinking subcutaneous injection technique. *Am J Nurs*, **97**(5), 71–2.

Perdue, L. (2001) Intravenous complications. In: *Intravenous Therapy: Clinical Principles and Practices* (eds J. Hankins *et al.*), 2nd edn. W.B. Saunders, Philadelphia, pp. 418–45.

Perucca, R. (2001) Obtaining vascular access. In: *Intravenous Therapy: Clinical Principles and Practices* (eds J. Hankins *et al.*), 2nd edn. W.B. Saunders, Philadelphia, pp. 375–88.

Pickstone, M. (1999) *A Pocketbook for Safer IV Therapy.* Medical Technology and Risk Series. Scitech Educational Ltd, Kent.

Pratt, R.J. *et al.* (2007) Epic 2: national evidence-based guidelines for preventing healthcare-associated infections in NHS hospitals in England. *J Hosp Infect*, **65**(1)(Suppl), S1–S12.

Quinn, C. (2008) Flow control. In: *Intravenous Therapy in Nursing Practice* (eds L. Dougherty & J. Lamb), 2nd edn. Blackwell Publishing, Oxford.

RCN (2005) *Standards for Infusion Therapy.* Royal College of Nursing, London.

Regnard, C.F. & Davies, A. (1986) *A Guide to Symptom Relief in Advanced Cancer.* Haigh and Hochland, Manchester.

Rochon, P. *et al.* (1997) A systematic review of the evidence for hypodermoclysis to treat dehydration in older people. *J Gerontol*, **52A**(3), M169–76.

Rodger, M.A. & King, L. (2000) Drawing up and administering intra-muscular injection: a review of the literature. *J Adv Nurs*, **31**(3), 574–82.

Royal Pharmaceutical Society of Great Britain (1997) *From Compliance to Concordance.* Royal Pharmaceutical Society of Great Britain, London.

Sasson, M. & Shvartzman, P. (2001) Hypodermoclysis: an alternative infusion technique. *Am Fam Physician*, **64**(9), 1575–8.

Sexton, J. (1999) The nurse's role in medicines administration – legal and procedural framework. In: *Medicines Management for Clinical Nurses* (eds K. Luker & D. Wolfson). Blackwell Science, Oxford.

Shepherd, M. (2002a) Medicines 2. Administration of medicines. *Nurs Times*, **98**(16), 45–8.

Shepherd, M. (2002b) Medicines 3. Managing medicines. *Nurs Times*, **98**(17), 43–6.

Shuttleworth, A. (2005) Are nurses ready to take on the BNF? *Nurs Times*, **101**(48), 29–30.

Simmonds, B.P. (1983) CDC guidelines for the prevention and control of nosocomial infections: guidelines for prevention of intravascular infections. *Am J Infect Control*, **11**(5), 183–9.

Taxis, K. & Barber, N. (2003) Ethnographic study on the incidence and severity of intravenous drug errors. *BMJ*, **326**, 684–7.

Taylor, N.J. (2000) Fascination with phlebitis. *Vasc Access Devices*, **5**(3), 24–8.

The Medicinal Products: Prescription by Nurse etc Act (1992).

Torre, M. (2002) Subcutaneous infusion: non-metal cannulae vs metal butterfly needles. *Br J Community Nurs*, **7**(7), 365–9.

Torrence, C. (1989) Intramuscular injection, part 1 and 2. *Surg Nurses*, **2**(5), 6–10; **2**(6), 24–7.

Treloar, A., Beats, B. & Philpot, M. (2000) A pill in the sandwich: covert medication in food and drink. *J R Soc Med*, **93**, 408–11.

Trissel, L.A. (2003) *Handbook on Injectable Drugs*, 12th edn. American Society of Health System Pharmacists, Bethesda, MD.

Trounce, J. & Gould, D. (2000) *Clinical Pharmacology for Nurses*, 16th edn. Churchill Livingstone, London.

Viola, R., Wells, G. & Peterson, J. (1997) The effects of fluid status and fluid therapy on the dying: a systematic review. *J Palliat Care*, **13**(4), 41–52.

Watt, S. (2003) Safe administration of medines to children: part 2. *Paediatr Nurs*, **15**(5), 40–4.

Weinstein, S.M. (2007) *Plumer's Principles and Practices of Intravenous Therapy*, 8th edn. Lippincott, Philadelphia.

Whittington, Z. (2008) Pharmacological aspects of IV therapy. In: *Intravenous Therapy in Nursing Practice* (eds L. Dougherty & J. Lamb), 2nd edn. Blackwell Publishing, Oxford.

Workman, B. (1999) Safe injection techniques. *Nurs Stand*, **13**(39), 47–52.

Wright, A. *et al.* (1985) Use of transdermal glyceryl trinitrate to reduce failure of intravenous infusion due to phlebitis and extravasation. *Lancet*, **ii**, 1148–50.

Multiple choice questions

1 **What does PGD stand for?**

 a Patient group drugs
 b Patient graded drugs
 c Patient group directive
 d Patient group direction

2 **What Act controls the import, export, production, supply, possession and manufacture of controlled drugs?**

 a Misuse of Drugs Act 2002
 b Medicines Act 1968
 c Misuse of Drugs Act 1971
 d Medicines Act 1986

3 **What injection should be available in all clinical areas where morphine or diamorphine is stored?**

 a Adrenaline
 b Maxalon
 c Saline
 d Naloxone

4 **In the majority of hospitals it is policy that medicine administration is carried out by:**

 a A registered nurse or student nurse
 b A registered nurse
 c A nurse, doctor or pharmacist
 d A registered nurse and healthcare assistant

5 Subcutaneous injections are given into:

   a   Gluteal muscle
   b   Deltoid muscle
   c   A vein
   d   Beneath the epidermis into fat and connective tissue

6 **Which of the following formulae can be used to work out how much drug volume is required from stock solution?**

   a   Prescribed dose multiplied by body weight
   b   Body weight divided by volume
   c   What you need, divided by what you have got, multiplied by volume of stock solution
   d   Volume required divided by duration

Answers to the multiple choice questions can be found in Appendix 3.

Chapter 9

Drug administration: delivery (infusion devices)

Definition

An infusion device is designed to accurately deliver measured amounts of fluid or drug via a number of routes (e.g. intravenous, subcutaneous or epidural) over a period of time. The infusion device is set at an appropriate rate to achieve the desired therapeutic response and prevent complications (Quinn 2000; Dougherty 2002; Medical Devices Agency 2003).

Indications

The nurse has a responsibility to determine when and how to use an infusion device to deliver hydration, drugs, transfusions and nutritional support, and how to select the appropriate device in order to manage the needs of the patient. Common types of infusion devices include: gravity infusion devices, gravity drip rate controllers, infusion pumps, syringe pumps, specialist pumps (e.g. patient controlled analgesia pumps, epidurals). The following factors should be considered when selecting an appropriate infusion delivery system (Quinn 2008):

1 Risk to the patient of:
   (a) Overinfusion.
   (b) Underinfusion.
   (c) Uneven flow.
   (d) Inadvertent bolus.
   (e) High pressure delivery.
   (f) Extravascular infusion.
2 Delivery parameters:
   (a) Infusion rate and volume required.
   (b) Accuracy required (over a long or short period of time).
   (c) Alarms required.

   (d) Ability to infuse into site chosen (venous, arterial, subcutaneous).

   (e) Suitability of device for infusing drug (e.g. ability to infuse viscous drugs).

3 Environmental features:

   (a) Ease of operation.

   (b) Frequency of observation and adjustment.

   (c) Type of patient (neonate, child, critically ill).

   (d) Mobility of patient.

Reference material

Infusion devices enable the delivery of a drug or fluid to a patient at a constant rate over a set period of time to achieve the desired therapeutic response. The process for infusional therapy includes:

- Prescription of the fluid or drug.
- Preparation of the infusion solution.
- Selection of the appropriate infusion device.
- Calculation and setting of the rate of infusion.
- Administration of the fluid to the patient.
- Monitoring and recording of the actual delivery.
- Disposal. (Medical Devices Agency 2003, p. 6.)

The nurse must have knowledge of the solutions, their effects, rate of administration, factors that affect flow of infusion, as well as the complications which could occur when flow is not controlled (Weinstein 2007). The nurse should have an understanding of which groups require accurate flow control in order to prevent complications (Box 9.1) and how to select the most appropriate device for

---

Box 9.1   Groups at risk of complications associated with flow control (adapted from Quinn 2008).

- Infants and young children.
- The elderly.
- Patients with compromised cardiovascular status.
- Patients with impairment or failure of organs, e.g. kidneys.
- Patients with major sepsis.
- Patients suffering from shock, whatever the cause.
- Postoperative or post-trauma patients.
- Stressed patients, whose endocrine homeostatic controls may be affected.
- Patients receiving multiple medications, whose clinical status may change rapidly.

Box 9.2   Complications of inadequate flow control (Quinn 2008).

Complications associated with overinfusion

- Fluid overload with accompanying electrolyte imbalance.
- Metabolic disturbances during parenteral nutrition, mainly related to serum glucose levels.
- Toxic concentrations of medications, which may result in a shock-like syndrome ('speed shock').
- Air embolism, due to containers running dry before expected.
- An increase in venous complications, e.g. chemical phlebitis, caused by reduced dilution of irritant substances (Weinstein 2007).

Complications associated with underinfusion

- Dehydration.
- Metabolic disturbances.
- A delayed response to medications or below therapeutic dose.
- Occlusion of a cannula/catheter due to slow flow or cessation of flow.

---

accuracy of delivery to best meet the patient's flow control needs (according to age, condition, setting and prescribed therapy) (Weinstein 2007).

The identification of risks is crucial, e.g. complex calculations, prescription errors (Dougherty 2002; Weinstein 2007) and the risks associated with the infusions, i.e. neo-natal risk infusions, high-risk infusion, low-risk infusions and ambulatory infusions (Quinn 2000; Medical Devices Agency 2003). The early detection of errors and infusion-related complications, e.g. over and underinfusion (Box 9.2) is imperative in order to instigate the appropriate interventions in response to an error or to manage any complications, as serious errors or complications can result in patient death (Quinn 2000; Dougherty 2002; NPSA 2003). Overinfusion accounts for about half of the reported errors involving infusion pumps with 80% due to user error rather than a fault with the device (Medical Devices Agency 2000). The use of infusion devices, both mechanical and electronic, has increased the level of safety in intravenous therapy. However, it is recommended that a clearly defined structure for management of infusion systems must exist within a hospital (Medical Devices Agency 2003; NPSA 2004; Department of Health, Social Services and Public Safety 2006; Health Care Standards Unit 2007a, b; NHS Litigation Authority 2007).

Criteria for selection of an infusion device:

- Rationalization of devices.
- Clinical requirement.

- Education.
- Compatibility with other equipment.
- Disposables.
- Product support.
- Costs.
- Service and maintenance.
- Regulatory issues, e.g. compliance with European Community Directives (Quinn 2000; Medical Devices Agency 2003; Department of Health, Social Services and Public Safety 2006; Health Care Standards Unit 2007a, b; NHS Litigation Authority 2007).

Strategies need to be developed for replacement of old, obsolete or inappropriate devices (Quinn 2000; Medical Devices Agency 2003; Department of Health, Social Services and Public Safety 2006; Health Care Standards Unit 2007a, b; NHS Litigation Authority 2007), planned service maintenance programmes and acceptance testing (Medical Devices Agency 2003).

'Fifteen million infusions are performed in the NHS every year and 700 unsafe incidents are reported each year with 19% attributed to user error' (NPSA 2004, p. 1). Between 1990 and 2000 there were 1485 incidents reported to the Medical Devices Agency which involved infusion pumps (Medical Devices Agency 2003). In 50% of incidents no cause was established. However, of the remaining incidents, 27% were attributed to user error (e.g. misloading of the administration set or syringe, setting the wrong rate, confusing pump type) and 20% to device-related issues (e.g. poor maintenance, cleaning) (Williams & Lefever 2000; Medical Devices Agency 2003). Syringe pumps have given rise to the most significant problems in terms of patient mortality and morbidity (Fox 2000; Medical Devices Agency 2003; NPSA 2003).

The high frequency of human error has highlighted the need for more formalized, validated, competency-based training and assessment (Pickstone 2000; Quinn 2000; Medical Devices Agency 2003; NPSA 2003, 2004). They must be familiar with the device they are using and not attempt to operate any device that they have not been fully trained to use (Murray & Glenister 2001; NPSA 2003). As a minimum, the training should cover the device, drugs and solutions, and the practical procedures related to setting up the device and problem solving (Medical Devices Agency 2000, 2003). Staff should also be made aware of the mechanisms for reporting faults with devices and procedures for adverse incident reporting within their trust and to the Medicines and Healthcare Products Regulatory Agency (MHRA) and the National Patient Safety Agency (NPSA) (MHRA 2006b).

A useful checklist (Table 9.1) has been produced by the Medical Devices Agency for staff to follow prior to using a medical device to ensure safe practice (Medical Devices Agency 2000, 2003).

349

Table 9.1 Checklist: How safe is your practice? Adapted from Medical Devices Agency (2000, p. 10; 2001, pp. 8 & 9).

- Have I been trained in the use of the infusion device?
- Was the training formalized and recorded or did I just pick it up as I went along?
- How was my competency in relation to the infusion device assessed?
- Have I read the user instructions on how to use the infusion device and am I familiar with any warning labels?
- When was the infusion device last serviced?
- Are there any signs of wear, damage or faults?
- Do I know how to set up and use the infusion device?
- Is the infusion device and any additional equipment in good working order?
- Do I know how the infusion device should perform and the monitoring that needs to be done to check its performance?
- Am I using the correct additional equipment, e.g. the appropriate disposable administration set for the infusion pump?
- Do I know how to recognize whether the infusion device has failed?
- Do I know what to do if the infusion device fails?
- Do I know how and to whom to report an infusion device-related adverse incident?
- Does checking the infusion device indicate it is functioning correctly and to the manufacturer's specification?
- What action should be taken if the infusion device is not functioning properly?
- Is there up-to-date documentation to record regular checking of the infusion device?
- What are the details (name and serial number) of the infusion device being used?
- What is the cleaning and/or decontamination procedure for the infusion device and what are my responsibilities in this process?
- Do I know how to report an adverse incident?
- Do I have access to MHRA Device Bulletins of relevance to my area of practice and do I read and take note of Hazard and Safety Notices?

Factors influencing flow rates

Once an infusion device is set up, the nurse should check the patient and the infusion rate regularly to ensure the prescribed flow rate is maintained (Medical Devices Agency 2003). The following factors may increase or decrease intravenous flow rates, particularly with mechanical devices using gravity flow, and should be taken into account when setting up an infusion device.

Type of fluid

The composition, viscosity and concentration of the fluid affects flow (Pickstone 1999; Quinn 2000; Springhouse 2005; Weinstein 2007). Irritating solutions may result in venospasm and impede the flow rate, this may be resolved by use of a warm pack over the cannula site and the limb (Springhouse 2005; Weinstein 2007).

Height of the infusion container

Intravenous fluids run by gravity and so any changes in the height of the container will alter the flow rate. The height of the container can be hung up to 1.5 m above the infusion site which will provide a hydrostatic pressure of 110 mmHg (Medical Devices Agency 2003; Springhouse 2005). One metre above the infusion site would create 70 mmHg of pressure, which is adequate to overcome venous pressure (normal range in an adult is 25–80 mmHg) (Pickstone 1999). Therefore any alterations in the patient's position may alter the flow rate and necessitate a change in the speed of the infusion to maintain the appropriate rate of flow (Perucca 2001; Weinstein 2007). Positioning of the patient will affect flow and patients should be instructed to keep the arm lower than the infusion, if the infusion is reliant on gravity (Quinn 2008).

Administration set

The flow rate of the infusion may be affected in several ways:

- Roller clamps or screw clamps, used to adjust and maintain rates of flow on gravity infusions, vary considerably in their efficiency and accuracy which is often dependent on a number of variables such as patient movement and height of infusion container (Perucca 2001). Roller clamps should be positioned on the upper third of the tubing near the fluid container, making access convenient for staff and out of the way of the patient to avoid accidental handling (Perucca 2001). The clamp should be repositioned periodically to prevent the tubing developing a memory (cold creep) where the tubing tries to retain its round shape and pushes the clamp open or where pinched tubing does not reopen (Perucca 2001; Medical Devices Agency 2003). The roller clamp should be used as the primary means of occluding the tubing even if there is an anti-free-flow device (Medical Devices Agency 2003).
- The inner diameter of the lumen and the length of tubing will also affect flow. Microbore sets have a narrow lumen, therefore flow is restricted to some degree. However, these sets may be used as a safeguard against 'runaway' or bolus infusions by either an integrated anti-siphon valve or anti-free-flow device (Quinn 2000; Perucca 2001; Weinstein 2007).
- Inclusion of other in-line devices, e.g. filters, may also affect the flow rate (Perucca 2001; Medical Devices Agency 2003).

Vascular access device

The flow rate may be affected by any of the following:

- The condition and size of the vein, e.g. phlebitis can reduce the lumen size and decrease flow (Weinstein 2007).
- The gauge of the cannula/catheter (Medical Devices Agency 2003; Springhouse 2005; Weinstein 2007).
- The position of the device within the vein, i.e. whether it is up against the vein wall.
- The site of the vascular access device, e.g. the flow may be affected by the change in position of a limb: such as a decrease in flow when a patient bends their arm if a cannula is sited over the elbow joint (Springhouse 2005).
- Kinking, pinching or compression of the cannula/catheter or tubing of the administration set may cause variation in the set rate (Medical Devices Agency 2003; Springhouse 2005).
- Restricted venous circulation, e.g. blood pressure cuff or the patient lying on the limb increases the risk of an occlusion of the device and may result in clot formation (Gabriel 1999; Quinn 2008).

The patient

Patients occasionally adjust the control clamp or other parts of the delivery system, for example, changing the height of the container, thereby making flow unreliable. Some pumps have tamper-proof features to minimize the risk of accidental manipulation of the infusion device (Perucca 2001) or unauthorized changing of infusion device controls (Amoore & Adamson 2003).

Infusion-related complications

Circulatory overload (isotonic fluid expansion)

A critical and common complication of intravenous therapy is circulatory overload, which is *isotonic fluid expansion*. It is caused by infusion of fluids of the same tonicity as plasma into the vascular circulation, for example sodium chloride 0.9%. As isotonic solutions do not affect osmolarity, water does not flow from the extracellular to the intracellular compartment. The result is that the extracellular compartment expands in proportion to the fluid infused (Weinstein 2007). Because of the electrolyte concentration, no extra water is available to enable the kidneys selectively to excrete and restore the balance.

If circulatory overload is detected early, treatment consists of withholding all fluids until excess water and electrolytes have been eliminated by the body and/or administration of diuretics to promote rapid diuresis (Weinstein 2007). However, careful monitoring should continue to prevent isotonic contraction occurring (where there is loss of fluid and electrolytes isotonic to the extracellular fluid such as blood and large volumes of fluid from diarrhoea and vomiting; Weinstein 2007). If fluid administration is allowed to continue unchecked, it can result in left-sided heart failure, circulatory collapse and cardiac arrest (Edwards 2001; Dougherty 2002).

Dehydration

Dehydration may be categorized either as hypertonic or hypotonic contraction and may be caused by underinfusion. Hypertonic contraction occurs when water is lost without corresponding loss of salts (Weinstein 2007) and occurs in patients unable to take sufficient fluids (elderly, unconscious or incontinent patients) or who have excess insensible water loss via skin and lungs or as a result of certain drugs in excess. Hypotonic contraction occurs when fluids containing more salt than water are lost and this results in a decrease in osmolarity of the extracellular compartment (Weinstein 2007).

It is important that the nurse recognizes the symptoms of overinfusion or underinfusion and certain factors should be considered when monitoring patients (Weinstein 2007) (Table 9.2).

353

Speed shock

Speed shock is a systemic reaction that occurs when a substance foreign to the body is rapidly introduced into the circulation (Weinstein 2007). This complication can manifest following administration of intravenous bolus injections or when large volumes of fluid are given too rapidly. This should not be confused with pulmonary oedema, which relates to the volume of fluid infused into the patient. Rapid, uncontrolled administration of drugs will result in toxic concentrations reaching vital organs. Toxicity may be manifested by an exaggeration of the usual pharmacological actions of the drug or by signs and symptoms specific for that drug or class of drugs. The most extreme toxic response which can occur if a drug is given at a dose or rate exceeding that recommended is termed the lethal response.

Signs of speed shock may include:

- Flushed face.
- Headache and dizziness.
- Congestion of the chest.
- Tachycardia and fall in blood pressure.
- Syncope.
- Shock.
- Cardiovascular collapse. (Perdue 2001; Weinstein 2007.)

Table 9.2 Monitoring overinfusion and underinfusion.

Type of fluid/ electrolyte imbalance	Patients at risk	Signs and symptoms	Treatment
Circulatory overload (isotonic fluid expansion)	Early postoperative or post-trauma patients, older people, those with impaired renal and cardiac function and children	■ Weight gain ■ A relative increase in fluid intake compared to output ■ A high bounding pulse pressure, indicating a high cardiac output ■ Raised central venous pressure measurements ■ Peripheral hand vein emptying time longer than normal. (Peripheral veins will usually empty in 3–5 seconds when the hand is elevated and will fill in the same length of time when the hand is lowered to a dependent position) ■ Peripheral oedema ■ Hoarseness ■ Dyspnoea, cyanosis and coughing due to pulmonary oedema and neck vein engorgement	If detected early: withholding all fluids until excess water and electrolytes have been eliminated by the body and/or administration of diuretics to promote rapid diuresis
Dehydration (hypertonic contraction or hypotonic contraction)	**Hypertonic** Elderly, unconscious or incontinent patients **Hypotonic** Infants are at greatest risk, especially if they have diarrhoea Loss of salt from various sources: excess diuresis, fistula drainage, burns, vomiting or sweating	**Hyper/Hypotonic contraction** ■ Weight loss **Hypercontraction** ■ Thirst (although this may be absent in the elderly) ■ Irritability and restlessness and possible confusion ■ Diminished skin turgor ■ Dry mouth and furred tongue **Hypocontraction** ■ Negative fluid balance ■ Weak, thready, rapid pulse rate ■ Increased 'hand filling time' ■ Increased skin turgor	Replacement of fluids and electrolytes

Prevention of speed shock involves the nurse having knowledge of the drug and the recommended rate of administration. When commencing an infusion using gravity flow, check that the solution is flowing freely before adjusting the rate. Movement of the patient or the device within the vessel can cause the infusion to flow more or less freely after a few minutes of setting the rate (Weinstein 2007). For high-risk medications an electronic flow control device is recommended (RCN 2005). Although most pumps have an anti-free-flow mechanism, always close the roller clamp prior to removing the set from the pump (Pickstone 1999; MHRA 2006a). If speed shock occurs, the infusion must be slowed down or discontinued. Medical staff should be notified immediately and the patient's condition treated as clinically indicated (Perdue 2001).

Siphonage

Uncontrolled flow from a syringe is called siphonage; this is a result of gravity or leakage of air into the syringe and administration set. Siphonage can occur whether or not the syringe is fixed into an infusion device (Pickstone 1999; Quinn 2000). It has been reported that, 'in practice, a 50 ml syringe attached to a length of administration set with an internal diameter of 3 mm has been shown to empty by siphonage in less than 1 minute' (Pickstone 1999, p. 57).

To minimize the risk of siphonage the following safe practice should be taken:

- The syringe (plunger and barrel) should be correctly located and secured.
- Intravenous administration extension sets should always be micro/narrow bore in diameter to increase the resistance to flow; wide-bore extension sets should be avoided.
- Position of the syringe pump should always be the same level as the infusion site (Medical Devices Agency 2003).
- The use of extension sets with an integral anti-siphonage valve (Quinn 2000; Medical Devices Agency 2003).

Paediatric considerations

The MHRA classify infusion devices into categories of infusion risk. Neonatal infusions are the highest risk category, high-risk infusions are typically the infusion of fluids in children where accuracy of the flow rate is essential (Medical Devices Agency 2003). Infusion therapy within the paediatric setting requires very specific skills (Sundquist 2001). Competency in calculation of paediatric dosages, maintaining a stringent fluid balance, use of paediatric-specific devices and management of complications are paramount.

Table 9.3   Therapy categories and performance parameters.

Therapy category	Therapy description	Patient group	Critical performance parameters
A	Drugs with narrow therapeutic margin	Any	Good long-term accuracy Good short-term accuracy
	Drugs with short half-life	Any	Rapid alarm after occlusion Small occlusion bolus
	Any infusion given to neonates	Neonates	Able to detect very small air embolus (volumetric pumps only) Small flow rate increments Good bolus accuracy Rapid start-up time (syringe pumps only)
B	Drugs, other than those with a short half-life	Any except neonates	Good long-term accuracy Alarm after occlusion
	Total parenteral nutrition Fluid maintenance Transfusions	Volume sensitive except neonates	Small occlusion bolus Able to detect small air embolus (volumetric pumps only) Small flow rate increments
	Diamorphine	Any except neonates	Bolus accuracy
C	Total parenteral nutrition Fluid maintenance Transfusions	Any except volume sensitive or neonates	Long-term accuracy Alarm after occlusion Small occlusion bolus Able to detect air embolus (volumetric pumps only) Incremental flow rates

Crown copyright material is reproduced with the permission of the Controller of HMSO and Queen's Printer for Scotland. Medical Devices Agency (2003).

Principles of equipment selection and application

The MHRA, formerly the Medical Devices Agency, has made recommendations on the safety and performance of infusion devices in order to enable users to make the appropriate choice of equipment to suit most applications (Medical Devices Agency 2003). The classification system is divided into three major categories according to the potential risks involved. These are shown in Table 9.3. A pump

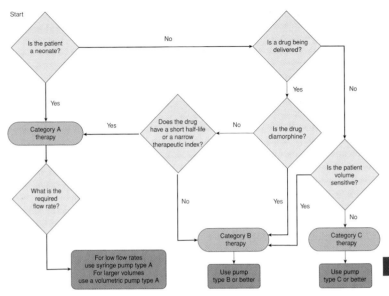

Figure 9.1   Decision tree for selection of infusion device. Crown copyright material is reproduced with the permission of the Controller of HMSO and Queen's Printer for Scotland. Medical Devices Agency (2003).

suited to the most risky category of therapy (A) can be safely used for the other categories (B and C). A pump suited to category B can be used for B and C, whereas a pump with the lowest specification (C) is suited only to category C therapies (Medical Devices Agency 2003) (Figure 9.1). Hospitals are required to label each infusion pump with its category and it is necessary to know the category of the proposed therapy and match it with a pump of the same or better category. A locally produced list of drugs/fluids by their categories will need to be provided to all device users (Medical Devices Agency 2003).

Requirements of devices

Accuracy of delivery

In order to meet requirements for high-risk and neonatal infusions, pumps must be accurate to within ±5% of the set rate when measured over a 60-minute period

(Perucca 2001; Medical Devices Agency 2003). They also have to satisfy short-term, minute-to-minute accuracy requirements, which determine smoothness and consistency of output (Medical Devices Agency 2003).

Occlusion response and pressure

Flow will occur if the pressure at the tip of an intravascular device is just fractionally above the pressure in the vein; the pressure does not need to be excessive. In an adult peripheral vein pressure is approximately 25 mmHg, while in a neonate it measures 5 mmHg (Quinn 2000). Most pumps have a variable pressure setting which allows the user to use their own judgement about the pressure needed to deliver therapy safely. It can be set as low as 100–250 mmHg (2–5 psi) for infusions of vesicants or routine infusions via healthy veins (Perucca 2001) or a maximum of 500 mmHg (10 psi) in positional central venous catheters. Flow is dependent upon pressure divided by resistance. If long extension sets of small internal bore are used, the resistance to flow will increase (Pickstone 1999; Quinn 2000). If an administration set occludes the resistance increases and the infusion will not flow into the vein. The longer the occlusion occurs, the greater the pressure and the pump will continue to pump until an occlusion alarm is activated. There are two types of occlusions defined: upstream, between the pump and the container, and downstream, which is between the pump and the patient. An upstream occlusion alarms when a vacuum is created in the upstream tubing or full reservoir, due to collapsed or empty plastic fluid container or clamped/kinking tubing. A downstream occlusion is when the pressure required by the pump exceeds a certain psi limit (Perucca 2001).

Pumps alarm at a pressure termed 'occlusion alarm pressure' and many pumps allow the user to set the pressure within a range (Medical Devices Agency 2003). Therefore the time it takes to alarm depends on the rate of flow: high rates alarm more quickly. When the alarm is activated, a certain amount of stored bolus will be present and it is important that what could be a potentially large bolus is not released into the vein. The release of the stored bolus could lead to rupture of the vein or constitute overinfusion, which may be detrimental to the patient particularly if it is a critical medication (Amoore & Adamson 2003; Medical Devices Agency 2003). For a syringe pump, to prevent a bolus being delivered to the patient, the clamp should not be opened as this will release the bolus: the first action is to remove the pressure by opening the syringe plunger clamp and then deal with the occlusion.

Air-in-line detectors are designed to detect only visible or microscopic 'champagne' bubbles. They should not create anxiety over small particles of air but alert the nurse to the integrity of the system. Most air bubbles detected are too small to have a harmful effect; however, the nurse should clarify the cause of any alarms (Perucca 2001; Medical Devices Agency 2003).

The Medical Devices Agency (2003) has set performance criteria for infusion pumps (see Table 9.3).

Infusion devices

Gravity infusion devices

Gravity flow

Gravity infusion devices depend entirely on gravity to deliver the infusion. The system consists of an administration set containing a drip chamber and a roller clamp to control the flow, which is usually measured by counting drops (Pickstone 1999). The indications for use are:

- Administration of drugs or fluids where adverse effects are not anticipated and which do not need to be infused with absolute precision.
- Where the patient's condition does not give cause for concern and no complication is predicted.

The flow rate is calculated using a formula that requires the following information: the volume to be infused; the number of hours the infusion is running over; and the drop rate of the administration set (which will differ depending on type of set). The number of drops per millilitre is dependent on the type of administration set used and the viscosity of the infusion fluid. Increased viscosity causes the size of the drop to increase. For example, crystalloid fluid administered via a solution set is delivered at the rate of 20 drops/ml; the rate of packed red cells given via a blood set will be calculated at 15 drops/ml.

The rate of administration of a continuous or intermittent infusion may be calculated from the following equation (Pickstone 1999):

$$\frac{\text{Volume to be infused}}{\text{Time in hours}} \times \frac{\text{Drop rate}}{60\,\text{minutes}} = \text{Drops per minute}$$

In this equation, 60 is a factor for the conversion of the number of hours to the number of minutes.

Advantages and disadvantages

The advantages of the gravity flow system are that it is simple to set up. It is low cost and the infusion of air is less likely than with electronic devices (Pickstone 1999). However, the system does require frequent observation and adjustment due to:

- The tubing changing shape over time.
- Creep or distortion of tubing made of polyvinyl chloride (PVC).

- Fluctuations of venous pressure which can affect the flow of the solution.
- The roller clamp can be unreliable, leading to inconsistent flow rates.

There can also be variability of drop size, and if the roller clamp is inadvertently left open free flow will occur. Infusion rates with viscous fluids can be reduced (particularly if administered via small cannulae) and there is a limitation on the type of infusion as it is not suitable for arterial infusions: this is because viscosity and arterial flow offer a high resistance to flow which cannot be overcome by gravity flow (Pickstone 1999; Quinn 2008).

Gravity drip rate controllers

A controller is a mechanical device that operates by gravity. These devices use standard solution sets and although they look much like a pump, they have no pumping mechanism. The desired flow rate is set in drops per minute and controlled by battery or mains powered occlusion valves (Medical Devices Agency 2003).

Advantages and disadvantages

Although they can maintain a drip rate within 1%, volumetric accuracy is not guaranteed and many of the disadvantages associated with gravity flow still remain. The main advantages are they are relatively inexpensive and can usually use standard gravity sets. They also incorporate some audible and visual alarm systems (Medical Devices Agency 2003).

Infusion pumps

These devices pump fluid from an infusion bag or bottle via an administration set (Quinn 2008).

Volumetric pumps

A volumetric pump works by calculating the volume delivered. This is achieved when the pump measures the volume displaced in a 'reservoir'. The reservoir is an integral component of the administration set. The pump calculates that every fill and empty cycle of the reservoir delivers a given amount of solution (Perucca 2001). The mechanism of action may be piston generated or linear peristaltic: where fingers in the pump move in a wave-like manner pushing the fluid out of the chamber (Pickstone 1999). The indications for use are all large volume infusions, both venous and arterial.

Most volumetric pumps have a linear peristaltic pumping mechanism, although some use cassettes. All are mains and battery powered, with the rate selected in millilitres per hour. The accuracy of flow is usually within 5% when measured over a period of time, which is more than adequate for most clinical applications (Pickstone 1999; Medical Devices Agency 2003).

Advantages and disadvantages

These pumps are able to overcome resistance to flow by increased delivery pressure and do not rely on gravity. This generally makes the performance of pumps predictable and capable of accurate delivery over a wider range of flow rates (Medical Devices Agency 2003).

The pumps also incorporate a wide range of features including air-in-line detectors, variable pressure settings and comprehensive alarms such as end of infusion, keep vein open (KVO, where the pump switches to a low flow rate, e.g. 5 ml/h, in order to continue flow to prevent occlusion of the device) and low battery. Many have a secondary infusion facility, which is to allow for intermittent therapy, e.g. antibiotics. The pump is programmed to switch to a secondary set and, when completed, it reverts back to the primary infusion at the previously set rate. The changing hospital environment has led to an increased demand on volumetric pumps, which in turn has resulted in the development of multichannel and dual-channel infusion pumps. These pumps may consist of two devices with an attached housing or of several infusion channels within a single device (Perucca 2001).

The disadvantages are that these are usually relatively expensive and often dedicated administration sets are required. The use of the wrong set could result in error even if the pump appears to work. Some are complicated to set up, which can also lead to errors (Medical Devices Agency 2003).

Syringe pumps

Syringe pumps are low-volume, high-accuracy devices designed to infuse at low flow rates. The plunger of a syringe containing the substance to be infused is driven forward by the syringe pump at a controlled rate to deliver it to the patient (Medical Devices Agency 2003).

Syringe pumps are useful where small volumes of highly concentrated drugs need to be infused (Pickstone 1999). The volume for infusion is limited to the size of the syringe used in the device, which is usually a 60-ml syringe, but most pumps will accept different sizes and brands of syringe. These devices are calibrated for delivery in millilitres per hour (Weinstein 2007).

Advantages and disadvantages

Syringe pumps are mains and/or battery powered, are usually easy to operate, and tend to cost less than volumetric pumps. The alarm systems are becoming more comprehensive but include low battery, end of infusion and syringe clamp open alarm. Most of the problems associated with the older models, for example free flow, mechanical backlash (slackness which delays the start-up time of the infusion) and incorrect fitting of the syringe, have been eliminated in the newer models (Pickstone 1999; Medical Devices Agency 2003). The risk of free flow is minimized by the use of an anti-siphonage valve which may be integral to the administration set (Pickstone 1999). Despite the use of an anti-siphonage valve, the clamp of the administration set must still be used (Medical Devices Agency 2003). Where mechanical backlash is an issue and there is a prime or purge option, this should be used at the start of the infusion to take up the mechanical slack (Amoore *et al.* 2001).

Specialist pumps

Patient-controlled analgesia pumps

Patient-controlled analgesia (PCA) devices are typically syringe pumps (although some are based on volumetric designs) (Medical Devices Agency 2003). The syringe pump forces down on the syringe piston, collapsing the syringe at a preset rate, but the distinguishing feature is the ability of the pump to deliver doses on demand, which occurs when the patient pushes a button (Perucca 2001). Whether or not the dose is delivered is determined by preset parameters in the pump. That is, if the maximum amount of drug over a given period of time has already been delivered, a further dose cannot be delivered.

362

PCA pumps are useful for patients who require analgesia. PCA pumps are used more in the acute setting, but are also useful in ambulatory situations.

Infusion options of a PCA pump are usually categorized into three types:

- Basal: a 'baseline' rate can be accompanied by intermittent doses requested by patients. This aims to achieve pain relief with minimal medication, but not necessarily to achieve a pain-free state (Perucca 2001).
- Continuous: designed for the patient who needs maximum pain relief without the option of demand dosing, e.g. epidural.
- Demand: drug delivered by intermittent infusion when button is pushed and can be used alone or supplemented by the basal rate. Doses can be limited by a designated maximum amount (Perucca 2001).

The PCA pump can dispense a bolus dose, with an initial bolus dose being called a loading dose. This may benefit patients as the one time dose is significantly higher than a demand dose in order to achieve immediate pain relief.

Advantages and disadvantages

These devices offer a 'lock-out' feature (when a key or a combination of numbers is necessary to gain access to pump controls), which is designed for patient safety. These pumps have an extensive memory capability which can be accessed through the display via a printer or computer (Medical Devices Agency 2003). This facility is critical for the pump's effective use in pain relief (Perucca 2001), as it enables the clinician to determine when and how often demand is made by a patient and what total volume has been infused (Perucca 2001). It has also been shown that they increase patient satisfaction, patients require less sedation, their anxiety is reduced and so are their nursing needs and time in hospital (Ripamonti & Bruera 1997).

Anaesthesia pumps

These are syringe pumps designed for delivery of anaesthesia or sedation and must only ever be used for that purpose. They should be restricted to operating theatres or critical care units and should be clearly labelled. They infuse at a very high flow rate and have a high-rate bolus facility in order to deliver the induction dose of anaesthesia quickly (Dolan 1999). There are new types of anaesthesia pumps that are available, total intravenous anaesthesia (TIVA) and target controlled infusion (TCI), which have been designed to control the induction, maintenance and reversal phases of anaesthesia (Absalom & Struys 2006).

Epidural pumps

363

These pumps are a method of providing analgesia (most commonly a combination of opioids and anaesthetic agents) via a fine catheter inserted directly into the epidural space. As a form of analgesia delivery, the efficacy of the epidural route has been well highlighted (Wheatley *et al.* 2001; Block *et al.* 2003; Werawatganon & Charuluxanun 2005).

Ambulatory infusion devices

Ambulatory devices are small devices which were developed to allow patients more freedom and to enable the patient to continue with normal activities or to move unencumbered by a large infusion device (Perucca 2001). Ambulatory devices range in size and weight and are used for small volumes of drugs and are mainly designed for patients to wear and use when ambulant. The solution containers are often more cumbersome than the actual pump itself. Due to their size, the number of alarms may be more limited. Considerations for selection of an ambulatory device include the following:

- Type of therapy.
- Patient's ability to understand how to manage the infusion device.
- Drug stability.
- Frequency of doses.
- Reservoir volumes required.
- Control of flow/flow rates.

- Type of access.
- Cost effectiveness.
- Portability.
- Convenience.

Ambulatory pumps fall into two categories: mechanical and battery-operated infusion devices.

Mechanical infusion devices

These are simple and compact but may not necessarily be cost effective as they are usually disposable. The mechanism for delivery is by balloon or simple spring, or they may be gas-powered.

Elastomeric balloons

These are made of a soft rubberized material capable of being inflated to a predetermined volume and the drug is then administered over a very specific infusion time. The balloon is encapsulated inside a rigid transparent container which may be round or cylindrical. The rate of infusion is not controlled by the balloon but by the diameter of the restricting outlet located in the preattached tubing. It is designed for single use that supplies the patient's need for a single dose infusion of drugs, e.g. intermittent small volume parenteral therapies such as delivery of antibiotics. Its small size causes little disruption to the patient's daily activities and it tends to be well tolerated (Perucca 2001).

Spring mechanism

Spring coil piston syringes have a spring which powers the plunger of a syringe in the absence of manual pressure. The volume is restricted by the size of the syringe, which is usually prefilled. The spring coil container tends to be a multidose, small-volume administration device and is a combination of a spring coil in a collapsible flattened disk. Its shape can accommodate many therapies and volumes (Perucca 2001).

Battery-operated infusion devices

Battery-operated pumps are small and light enough to be carried around by the patient without interfering with most everyday activities. They are operated using rechargeable or alkaline batteries but, owing to their size, the available battery capacity tends to be low. The length of time the battery lasts is often dependent on the rate the pump is set at. Most give an output in the form of a small bolus delivered every few minutes. Most devices have an integral case or pouch which allows the pump and the reservoir/syringe to be worn with discretion by the patient. There are two types: ambulatory volumetric infusion pumps and syringe drivers.

Ambulatory volumetric infusion/syringe pumps

An ambulatory volumetric infusion/syringe pump is an infusion device which pumps in the same way as a large volumetric pump, but by nature of its size it is portable and useful in the ambulatory setting (hospital or home care).

This pump is suitable for patients who have been prescribed continuous infusional treatment for a period of time, for example from 4 days to 6 months, and enables the patients, where appropriate, to receive treatment at home, because it is small and portable.

The advantages of the ambulatory pump are:

- Able to deliver drugs continuously or intermittently.
- Infusion routes: central, peripheral venous, epidural, intra-arterial, intrathecal and subcutaneous.
- Delivery of drugs accurately over a set period of time.
- Improving potential outcomes of treatment by delivering treatment continuously.
- Heightening the patient's independence and control by allowing them to be at home and participate in their own care.
- Is compact, light and easy to use.
- Has audible alarm systems.

The disadvantages are:

- It may require the insertion of a central venous access device, which has associated complications and problems.
- It could malfunction at home, which could be distressing and dangerous for the patient.
- In spite of its ease of use, some patients may not be able to cope with it at home.
- Patients may have to adapt their lifestyle to cope with living with a pump continuously.

Syringe drivers

A syringe driver is a portable battery-operated infusion device. It is used to deliver drugs at a predetermined rate via the appropriate parenteral route and is suited for symptom management, and palliative care (Dickman *et al*. 2005). The syringe driver should be used for patients who are unable to tolerate oral medication, for example, in nausea and vomiting, dysphagia, intestinal obstruction, local disease or sometimes in intractable pain which is unrelieved by oral medications and

365

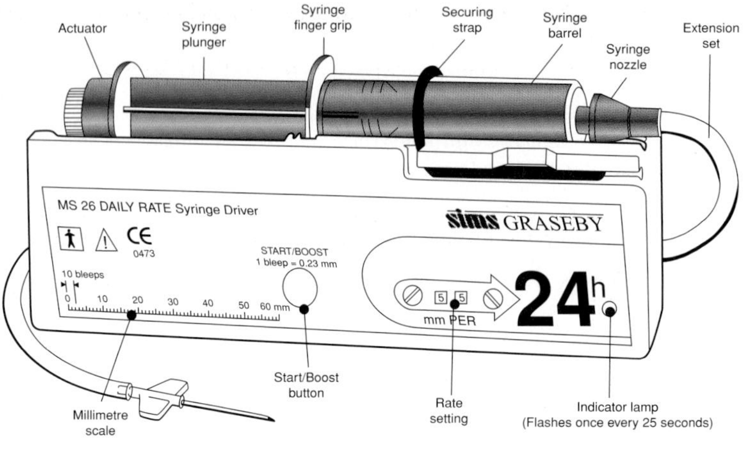

Figure 9.2   Sims (Graseby) Medical MS26 daily rate syringe driver.

where rapid dose titration is required. Drugs administered by subcutaneous infusion include opioid analgesics, antiemetics, anxiolytic sedatives, corticosteroids, non-steroidal anti-inflammatory drugs and anticholinergic drugs (Dickman *et al.* 2005).

The Sims (Graseby) Medical MS16A and MS26 syringe drivers are typical examples of the drivers in use; however, other types are available and nurses should follow the manufacturer's instruction manual for details of their use. The MS16A allows drug administration on an hourly rate. This driver is clearly marked with a pink '1 h' in the bottom right hand corner of the driver. The MS26 delivers drugs on a 24-hourly rate. This driver is clearly marked with a yellow '24 h' in the bottom right hand corner of the driver (Figure 9.2). It is important that users are aware that the MS16A syringe driver is calibrated in millimetres per hour, and the MS26 is calibrated in millimetres per day. Confusion between the two drivers in relation to rate settings has resulted in fatal errors (Dickman *et al.* 2005; MHRA 2006b). Most sizes and brands of plastic syringes can be used with these drivers; however, it is recommended to use Luer–Lok syringes to avoid leakage or accidental disconnection.

The advantages of the syringe driver are:

- It avoids the necessity of intermittent injections.
- Mixtures of drugs may be administered.
- Infusion timing is accurate, which is particularly advantageous in the community where the ability to constantly monitor the rate is not feasible.

- The device is lightweight and compact, allowing mobility and independence.
- Rate can be increased.
- Simple calculations of dosage are required over a 12- or 24-hour period.
- It allows patients to spend more time at home with their symptoms managed effectively.

The disadvantages are:

- The patient may become psychologically dependent on the device.
- Inflammation or infection may occur at the insertion site of the subcutaneous cannula.
- The rate calculation differs between the Sims (Graseby) Medical MS16A and MS26 syringe drivers and this can be confusing for the nurse.
- The alarm system of some syringe drivers, e.g. the Sims (Graseby), operates only if the plunger is obstructed. It does not alert the nurse if the flow is too rapid or is too slow.

Improving infusion device safety

A high frequency of human error is reported in the use of infusion device systems, so competence-based training in the use of devices is advocated for users of infusion device systems (Medical Devices Agency 2003; NPSA 2004). By rationalizing the range of infusion device types within organizations and the establishment of a centralized equipment library, the number of patient safety incidents will be reduced (Medical Devices Agency 2003; NPSA 2004). Smart infusion pumps reduce pump programming errors by the setting of pre-programmed upper and lower dose limits for specific drugs. The pump will alert the nurse when setting the infusion device if the pump has been set outside of the pre-set dose limits (Wilson & Sullivan 2004; Keohane *et al.* 2005; Weinstein 2007). Whatever infusion device is used, the need to monitor the patient and the device remain paramount for patient safety.

367

Summary

There are many infusion control devices available ranging from the simple to the complex and nurses should have a sound knowledge of how the device works or seek assistance from a colleague. Careful calculation and control of flow rates are essential as delivery of fluids and medications are critical for patient safety. Standardization of equipment reduces confusion and therefore reduces the risk of user error (Medical Devices Agency 2003; NPSA 2003, 2004; Department of Health, Social Services and Public Safety 2006; MHRA 2006b; Health Care Standards Unit 2007a, b; NHS Litigation Authority 2007).

Procedure guidelines **Syringe driver: monitoring and infusion**

Appropriate education/teaching material, e.g. syringe driver instruction manual and guidelines on problem solving, is required for both the patients and staff (Medical Devices Agency 2003: C).

Action

1 Monitor the following:
- At start of infusion – record date, time, start volume, infusion rate setting, name of person setting up infusion.
- Based upon the type of infusion and patient's condition; however at a minimum these should be carried out 15 minutes and 1 hour after the initial set up and thereafter a minimum of every 4 hours.
- Device must be checked at the start of each shift and/or when setting up an infusion.

Infusion device and infusion checks:

- Check and record the date, time, rate and volume remaining and that the battery/syringe driver is working.
- Record any reasons for changing of the drug, dose, rate setting of syringe driver or site.
- Check subcutaneous site for:
  (a) Pain/discomfort.
  (b) Swelling/induration.
  (c) Erythema.
  (d) Leakage of fluid.
  (e) Bleeding.

Rationale

To detect any errors and infusion related complications (Pickstone 1999: E; Quinn 2000: E; Dougherty 2002: E; Medical Devices Agency 2003: C; Dickman *et al.* 2005: E).

Accurate documentation of the site, rate, flow, start time and drugs used is imperative in order to avoid confusion and errors among staff (Quinn 2000: E; Dougherty 2002: E; Medical Devices Agency 2003: C; Dickman *et al.* 2005: E; NMC 2005: C; NMC 2006a: C; NMC 2008a: C).

2 Ask the patient to report any complaints of pain and tenderness at the infusion site and if they experience any change in their symptoms or have new symptoms.

To ascertain whether there are any problems that may require nursing care and refer to medical staff where appropriate (E).

Problem solving: Syringe drivers

Problem	Possible causes	Preventive nursing measures	Suggested action
Infusion pump alarming:			
(a) Air detected	Air bubbles in administration set.	Ensure all air is removed from all equipment prior to use.	Remove all air from the administration set and restart the infusion.
(b) Tube misload	Administration set has been improperly loaded.	Ensure set is loaded correctly.	Check that the set is loaded correctly and reload if necessary.
(c) Upstream occlusion	Closed clamp, obstruction or kink in the administration set is preventing fluid flow.	Ensure the container/fluid bag has been adequately pierced by the administration spike.	Inspect the administration set and restart the infusion.
		Ensure that the tubing is taped to prevent kinking.	If tubing is kinked, reposition, tape and restart infusion.
		Ensure the regulating (roller) clamp is open.	Check the administration set and open the clamp; restart the infusion.
(d) Downstream occlusion	Phlebitis/infiltration or extravasation.	Observe site regularly for signs of swelling, pain and erythema.	Remove peripheral device, provide symptomatic relief where appropriate. Initiate extravasation procedure. Resite as appropriate.
	Closed distal clamp.	Ensure clamps are open.	Locate distal occlusion, restart infusion.

Problem solving (cont.)

Problem	Possible causes	Preventive nursing measures	Suggested action
(e) KVO alert (keep vein open)	The volume infused is complete and the device is infusing at the KVO rate.	Programme in a new volume as appropriate.	Do not turn the device off. Allow KVO mode to run to maintain patency of device. Prepare new infusion or discontinue as appropriate.
Infusion devices malfunctioning (electrical/ mechanical)	Not charging at mains.	Ensure that the device is kept plugged in where appropriate.	Change device and remove device from use until fully charged. Send to works department to check plug.
	Low battery.	Check lead is pushed in adequately.	
	Batteries keep requiring replacement.	Do not use small rechargeable batteries in ambulatory devices.	
	Technical fault.	Ensure all infusion devices are serviced regularly.	Remove infusion device from use and contact biomedical engineering (BME) department or relevant personnel.
	Device soiled inside mechanism.	Maintain equipment and keep clean and free from contamination.	Remove administration set, wipe pump, reload. Do not use alcohol-based solutions on internal mechanisms.
Unstable infusion device	Mounted on old, poorly maintained stands.	Ensure that stands are maintained and kept clean. Replace old stands.	Remove device from stand. Remove stand and send to works department for repair.
	Mounted on incorrect stands.	Ensure the correct stands are used.	Check the stand and change to appropriate stand.
	Equipment not balanced on stand.	Ensure that all equipment is balanced around the stand.	Remove devices and attach to two stands if necessary. Balance equipment.

Problem	Possible causes	Preventive nursing measures	Suggested action
Under/ overinfusion	Technical fault with equipment.	Ensure regular servicing of devices.	Remove device from use immediately and label to prevent further use. Report incident to medical staff and nursing staff. Report to appropriate person, e.g. nurse specialist or an electro-biomedical engineer for checking. Complete an incident form. Inform head of risk management and MHRA as appropriate.
	Incorrect rate setting.	Ensure that the rate is calculated prior to commencing infusion. Check infusion rate regularly within the first hour and at start of each shift to ensure correct rate is set.	Check patient's condition. Inform medical staff and senior member of nursing staff.

References and further reading

Absalom, A. & Struys, M. (2006) *An Overview of TCI & TIVA*. Academia Press, Ghent, Belgium.

Amoore, J. *et al.* (2001) Syringe pumps and start up time: ensuring safe practice. *Nurs Stand*, **15**(17), 43–5.

Amoore, J. & Adamson, L. (2003) Infusion devices: characteristics, limitations and risk management. *Nurs Stand*, **17**(28), 45–52.

Block, B.M. *et al.* (2003) Efficacy of postoperative analgesia: a meta-analysis. *JAMA*, **290**, 2455–63.

Department of Health, Social Services and Public Safety (2006) *Controls Assurance Standards: Medical Devices and Equipment Management*. www.dhsspsni.gov.uk/medical_devices_06_pdf. Accessed 27/11/06.

DH (2003) *Building a Safer NHS for Patients: Improving Medication Safety*. Department of Health, London.

DH (2005) *Hazardous waste (England) regulations*. Department of Health London.

Dickman, A., Schneider, J. & Varga, J. (2005) *The Syringe Driver: Continuous Subcutaneous Infusions in Palliative Care*, 2nd edn. Oxford University Press, Oxford.

Dougherty, L. (2002) Delivery of intravenous therapy. *Nurs Stand*, **16**(16), 45–56.

Edwards, S. (2001) Regulation of water, sodium and potassium: implications for practice. *Nurs Stand*, **15**(22), 36–45.

Fox, N. (2000) Armed and dangerous. *Nurs Times*, **96**(44), 24–6.

Gabriel, J. (1999) Long term central venous access. In: *Intravenous Therapy in Nursing Practice* (eds L. Dougherty & J. Lamb). Churchill Livingstone, Edinburgh, pp. 301–31.

Griffith, R. & Jordan, S. (2003) Administration of medicines part 1: the law and nursing. *Nurs Stand*, **18**(2), 47–53.

Health Care Standards Unit (2007a) *First Domain – Safety (Info Bank) C4b*. www.hcsu.org.uk/index.php?option=com_content&task=view&id=197&Itemid=109. Accessed 28/08/07.

Health Care Standards Unit (2007b) *Updated signpost C4b*. www.hcsu.org.uk/index.php?option=com_content&task=view&id=309&Itemid=111. Accessed 28/03/07.

Keohane, C.A. *et al.* (2005) Intravenous medication safety and smart infusion systems. *J Infus Nurs*, **28**(5), 321–8.

Lamb, J. (1999) Local and systemic complications of intravenous therapy. In: *Intravenous Therapy in Nursing Practice* (eds L. Dougherty & J. Lamb). Churchill Livingstone, Edinburgh, pp. 163–93.

Medical Devices Agency (2000) *Equipped to Care*. Medical Devices Agency, London. www.mhra.gov.uk/home/idcplg?IdcService=SS_GET_PAGE&useSecondary=true&ssDocName=CON007425&ssTargetNodeId=575. Accessed 28/3/07.

MDA (2001) *Devices in Practice – guide for health and social care professionals*. www.mhra.gov.uk/home/idcplg?IdcService=SS_GET_PAGE&useSecondary=true&ssDocName=CON007423&ssTargetNodeId=575. Accessed 28/3/07.

Medical Devices Agency (2003) *Infusion Systems Device Bulletin*. DB 9503. Medical Devices Agency, London. www.mhra.gov.uk/home/idcplg?IdcService=SS_GET_PAGE&useSecondary=true&ssDocNameCON007321&ssTargetNodeId=572. Accessed 23/03/07.

MHRA (2004) *Reducing Needlestick and Sharps Injuries*. Medicines and Healthcare Products Regulatory Agency, London.

MHRA (2006a) *Free-flow situations*. www.mhra.gov.uk/home/idcplg?IdcService=GET_FILE&dID=20057&noSaveAs=0&Rendition=WEB. Accessed 03/06.

MHRA (2006b) *Reporting adverse incidents and disseminating medical device alerts*. DB2006 (01). www.mhra.gov.uk/home/idcplg?IdcService=SS_GET_PAGE&useSecondary=true&ssDocName=CON007304&ssTargetNodeId=572. Accessed 27/11/06.

Murray, W. & Glenister, H. (2001) How to use medical devices safely. *Nurs Times*, **97**(43), 36–8.

NHS Litigation Authority (2007) *NHSLA Risk Management Standards for Acute Trusts*. www.nhsla.com/NR/rdonlyres/F9DA791B-AF6D-4198-AC49-EE9B81A91B17/0/NHSLARiskManagementStandardsforAcuteTrusts200708website.doc. Accessed 28/08/07.

NMC (2005) *Guidelines for Records and Record Keeping*. Nursing and Midwifery Council, London.

NMC (2006a) *Medicines Management A–Z Advice Sheet*. Nursing and Midwifery Council. www.nmc-uk.org/aFrameDisplay.aspx? DocumentID=1801. Accessed 27/11/06.

NMC (2006b) *A–Z Advice Sheet Consent*. www.nmc.org.

NMC (2008a) *Standards for Medicines Management*. Nursing and Midwifery Council, London.

NMC (2008b) *The Code: Standards of Conduct, Performance and Ethics for Nurses and Midwives*. Nursing and Midwifery Council, London.

NPSA (2003) *Risk Analysis of Infusion Devices*. National Patient Safety Agency, London.

NPSA (2004) *Safer Practice Notice 01: Infusion Devices*. National Patient Safety Agency. www.npsa.nhs.uk/site/media/documents/526_npsa_saferpractice_01.pdf. Accessed 27/11/06.

NPSA (2007) *Promoting Safer Use of Injectable Medicines, Alert no.2007/20*. www.npsa.nhs.uk/site/media/documents/2602_0434_injectables_meds_alert_v20.pdf. Accessed 28/03/07.

Perdue, M.B. (2001) Intravenous complications. In: *Infusion Therapy in Clinical Practice* (eds J. Hankin *et al.*), 2nd edn. W.B. Saunders, Philadelphia, pp. 418–45.

Perucca, R. (2001) Types of infusion therapy equipment. In: *Infusion Therapy in Clinical Practice* (eds J. Hankin *et al.*), 2nd edn. W.B. Saunders, Philadelphia, pp. 300–33

Pickstone, M. (1999) *A Pocketbook for Safer IV Therapy*. Medical Technology and Risk Series. Scitech, Kent.

Pickstone, M. (2000) Using the technology triangle to assess the safety of technology-controlled clinical procedures in critical care. *Int J Intens Care*, 7(2), 90–6.

Pratt, R.J. *et al.* (2007) Epic 2: National evidence-based guidelines for preventing healthcare-associated infections in NHS hospitals in England. *J Hosp Infect*, **65**(Suppl), S2–12.

Quinn, C. (2000) Infusion devices: risks, functions and management. *Nurs Stand*, **14**(26), 35–41.

Quinn, C. (2008) Intravenous flow control and infusion devices. In: *Intravenous Therapy in Nursing Practice*, 2nd edn (eds L. Dougherty & J. Lamb). Blackwell Publishing, Oxford, pp. 197–224.

RCN (2005) *Standards for Infusion Therapy. RCN IV: Therapy Forum November 2005*. Royal College of Nursing, London.

Ripamonti, C. & Bruera, E. (1997) Current status of patient controlled analgesia in cancer patients. *Oncology*, **11**(3), 373–80.

Springhouse (2005) *Intravenous Therapy Made Incredibly Easy*, (ed. L. Bruck), 3rd edn. Lippincott, Williams & Wilkins, Philadelphia.

Sundquist, S.B. (2001) Didactic components of a comprehensive paediatric competency programme. *J Infus Nurs*, **24**(6), 367–74.

Weinstein, S. (2007) *Plumer's Principles and Practices of Intravenous Therapy*, 8th edn. Lippincott, Williams & Wilkins, Philadelphia.

Werawatganon, T. & Charuluxanun, S. (2005) Patient controlled intravenous opioid analgesia versus continuous epidural analgesia for pain after intra-abdominal surgery. *Cochrane Database of Systematic Reviews* 2005, Issue 1. CD004088.

Wheatley, R., Schug, S. & Watson, D. (2001) Safety and efficacy of postoperative epidural analgesia. *Br J Anaesth*, **87**(1), 47–61.

Williams, C. & Lefever, J. (2000) Reducing the risk of user error with infusion pumps. *Prof Nurse*, **15**(6), 382–4.

Wilson, K. & Sullivan, M. (2004) Preventing medication errors with smart infusion technology. *Am J Health Syst Pharm*, **61**(2), 177–83.

Multiple choice questions

1   The height of an intravenous infusion container when administering an intravenous infusion:

    a   Will alter the rate of flow of the infusion, decreasing in speed the further the distance from the infusion site

    b   Must be lower than the patient arm to prevent extravasation

    c   Will alter the rate of flow of the infusion, increasing in speed as it becomes higher above the infusion site

    d   Has no affect on the rate of the infusion

2   Which of the following statements is correct?

    a   A PCA pump can be used for administration of blood

    b   Syringe drivers can be used to give large volumes of intravenous fluids rapidly

    c   A gravity infusion device should be used for a critically ill patient

    d   Syringe drivers can be used to give small volumes of intravenous fluids slowly

3   Which of the following infusion devices would be used to deliver a low volume?

    a   Gravity drip rate controller

    b   Syringe driver

    c   Volumetric pump

    d   PCA pump

Answers to the multiple choice questions can be found in Appendix 3.

Chapter 10

Elimination: bladder lavage and irrigation

Definitions

Lavage

Bladder lavage is the manual washing out of the bladder with sterile fluid (Evans & Godfrey 2000).

Catheter maintenance solution

Catheter maintenance solution is a prepacked sterile reagent (usually 50 ml) that is allowed to drain into the bladder under gravity. The fluid is retained in the bladder (by clamping sterile reagent tube) for a specified time (usually 15 minutes) and then allowed to drain out under gravity (Evans & Godfrey 2000).

Irrigation

Bladder irrigation is the continuous washing out of the bladder with sterile fluid, usually 0.9% normal saline (Ng 2001).

Indications

Bladder lavage, catheter maintenance solutions and irrigation are indicated for the following reasons:

Lavage

- To clear an obstructed catheter.
- To remove the potential sources of obstruction, e.g. blood clots or sediment from infection (Evans & Godfrey 2000).

Catheter maintenance solutions

- To minimize recurrent catheter blockage due to encrustation.
- Reduce urethral trauma from encrustation on catheter removal (Getliffe 1996a).

Irrigation

- To prevent the formation and retention of blood clots, e.g. following prostatic surgery.
- On rare occasions to remove heavily contaminated material from a diseased urinary bladder (Scholtes 2002; Fillingham & Douglas 2004; Cutts 2005).

Reference material

Solutions used for lavage and irrigation

A number of prepacked sterile washout solutions or, as they are now commonly called, catheter maintenance solutions are available for cleaning the bladder; these include the following:

- 0.9% sodium chloride: used for mechanical flushing to remove tissue debris and small blood clots.
- Chlorhexidine 0.02%: used to prevent or reduce bacterial growth, in particular *Escherichia coli* and *Klebsiella*.
- Mandelic acid (1%): used to prevent the growth of urease-producing bacteria by acidifying the urine.
- 6% citric acid solution, 'solution R': used to dissolve persistent crystallization in the catheter or bladder.
- 3.23% citric acid and magnesium oxide solution, 'Suby G': used to prevent and/or dissolve crystallization in the catheter or bladder (Rew & Woodward 2001).

The selection of a particular solution will depend on its therapeutic properties in relation to the patient's needs.

The agent most commonly recommended for lavage and irrigation is 0.9% sodium chloride and should be used in every case unless an alternative solution is prescribed. 0.9% sodium chloride is isotonic; consequently it does not affect the body's fluid or electrolyte levels, enabling large volumes of the solution to be used as necessary (Cutts 2005). In particular, 3-litre bags of 0.9% sodium chloride are available for irrigation purposes.

Although not a common complication, absorption of irrigation fluid can occur during bladder irrigation. This can produce a potentially critical situation, as absorption leads to electrolyte imbalance and circulatory overload (Getliffe 1996a). Absorption is most likely to occur in theatre where glycine irrigation fluid, devoid of sodium or potassium, is forced under pressure into the prostatic veins (Forristal & Maxfield 2004). The 0.9% sodium chloride can not be used during surgery as it contains electrolytes which interfere with diathermy (Gilbert & Gobbi 1989). However, the risk of absorption still remains while irrigation continues postoperatively. For this reason it is important that fluid balance is monitored carefully during irrigation (Scholtes 2002).

Sterile water should never be used to irrigate the bladder as it will be readily absorbed by osmosis; however, it may be used as a purely mechanical means to flush out catheters for patients at home (Addison 2000).

Bladder lavage has been used in the management of catheter associated infections, catheter encrustation and blockage (Getliffe 1996a). However, potential risks to the bladder arise from the procedure itself and/or the solution used and there is considerable confusion and controversy surrounding its use in practice (Getliffe 1994b, 1996a; Rew 1999; Pomfret *et al.* 2004). Varying levels of knowledge have been found among nurses with regard to the type of washout fluid to use in specific circumstances and also the frequency of administration (Bailey 1991; Castledine 2001; Pomfret *et al.* 2004; Castledine 2006).

Catheter-associated infection

Catheter-associated urinary tract infections are a common complication occurring in over 90% of patients within 4 weeks of catheterization (Jewes *et al.* 1988). The risk of catheter-associated bacteriuria increases by 5–8% a day during catheterization (Mulhall *et al.* 1988) and is inevitable in long-term patients (Getliffe 1996b). Antibiotics will not prevent infection in long-term catheterized patients and their use is not recommended unless systemic symptoms are present (Simpson 2001). Bladder lavage using antibiotic or antiseptic solutions (chlorhexidine, noxythiolin, povidone iodine and acetic acid) have been commonly used to prevent, reduce or treat urinary tract infections (Getliffe, 2004). However, studies have shown that chlorhexidine may in fact remove sensitive bacteria in the normal urethral flora, allowing subsequent colonization by resistant organisms (Davies *et al.* 1987; Stickler *et al.* 1987; King & Stickler 1992). Furthermore, reviews of alternative solutions (noxythiolin, povidone iodine and acetic acid) and various antibiotics have been shown to be ineffective against a number of commonly occurring pathogens; therefore their use in long-term catheterized patients is not advocated (Stickler & Chawla 1987; Stickler 1990).

Catheter-associated urinary infections are difficult to treat as bacteria adhere to the surface of the catheter in the form of a biofilm (Costerton *et al.* 1999; Trautner & Darouiche 2004). Whilst antimicrobials may successfully kill bacteria in the urine, bacteria in the biofilm are generally less susceptible to these agents; consequently, they may still persist following treatment and potentially restart the cycle of infection (Gristina *et al.* 1987; Stickler *et al.* 1987).

377

Three theories have been suggested to explain why this may happen:

- Microbial secretions 'bind' the biofilm to the surface, making it difficult to remove and for antibiotic and antiseptic agents to penetrate (Getliffe 1996b; Liedl 2001).

- Cells in the biofilm exist in a slow-growing or starved state and are therefore not very susceptible to many antimicrobial agents (Getliffe 1996b; Liedl 2001).

- The micro-organisms in the biofilm undergo cellular changes so they develop into a different phenotype that has different sensibility to antibiotic agents from their free-living counterparts (Liedl 2001).

As yet there is no catheter material that resists biofilm formation in the clinical setting (Getliffe 1996b; Morris *et al.* 1997; Rew & Woodward 2001); however, all-silicone catheters have been found to take longer to become encrusted than the silicone-coated, Teflon and latex catheters (Kunin *et al.* 1987) (see Chapter 13).

Catheter encrustations and blockages

Recurrent catheter encrustation and blockage is a common problem with approximately 50% of catheterized patients being susceptible (Kohler-Ockmore 1992; Getliffe 1994a). Catheter blockage may occur as the result of detrusor spasm, twisted drainage tubing or constipation, but the most common reason is the formation of encrustation on the catheter surface and within its lumen with deposits of mineral salts from the urine (Getliffe 1996a; Godfrey & Evans 2000; Rew & Woodward 2001). Catheter encrustations form on any catheter surface in contact with urine, including the catheter tip and balloon, as well as the catheter lumen (Getliffe *et al.* 2000).

Several studies have shown that catheter encrustations are caused by the interaction of bacteria and urinary pH (Burr & Nusbeibeh 1995; Choong *et al.* 1999; Mathur *et al.* 2006). Catheter encrustations commonly consist of magnesium, ammonium phosphate (struvite) and calcium phosphate (apatite) deposits (Getliffe 1996b; McCarthy & Hunter 2001), which precipitate from urine when it becomes alkaline during infection from urease-secreting micro-organisms (Mobley & Warren 1987; Getliffe 1996a; Evans & Godfrey 2000). The urease producers implicated most commonly in catheter encrustations are of the *Proteus* species, in particular *Proteus mirabilis* (Getliffe 1996b; Stickler & Hughes 1999; Liedl 2001).

The development of catheter encrustations may lead to:

- Blockage of the catheter lumen.
- Bypassing of urine.
- Retention of urine.
- Pain and patient distress.
- Unnecessary catheter changes (Rew 1999; Getliffe 2004).

Getliffe's (1994a) study attempted to identify characteristics of patients who were at greater risk of obstructing their catheters. Patients who 'blocked' their catheters were found to have high urinary pH and ammonia concentrations. High ammonia concentration and alkaline urine are found when urine is infected with urease producing micro-organisms, such as *P. mirabilis*. Significantly more females were classed as 'blockers'; this may be due to the greater risks females have of developing catheter-associated urinary infections (Kennedy *et al.* 1983), as the shorter female urethra may allow more rapid colonization. 'Blockers' were also found to be significantly less mobile than 'non-blockers'. There was no significant relationship noted between non-blockers and high average daily fluid intake; this study therefore does not support the advice conventionally given to 'drink plenty' to reduce mineral precipitation.

There have been very few clinical studies about the use of bladder maintenance solutions to dissolve the minerals which cause encrustation and increase catheter life. The 0.9% sodium chloride has been shown to have no effect in dissolving encrustations, but it may, through the mechanical effect of flushing, dislodge debris (Flack 1993).

A study carried out by Kennedy *et al.* (1992) showed that citric acid solution with (Suby G) and without magnesium oxide (solution R) administered twice weekly for 3 weeks did not have a demonstrable effect in preventing crystal formation. However, 6% citric acid solution R has been shown to dissolve fragments of struvite renal calculi following lithotripsy (Holden & Rao 1991). Catheter encrustations may be dissolved using this solution but potential inflammatory tissue reactions of the urothelium limit its use (Getliffe 1996a). Getliffe (1996a) suggests it may be used prior to catheter removal to dissolve external encrustations, which cause pain and tissue trauma on withdrawal of the catheter. Getliffe's (1994b) in vitro study suggested that mandelic acid solution may be particularly effective in reducing encrustation.

Mandelic acid 1% has been shown to be effective in removing *Pseudomonas* species from the urine of catheterized patients, although it needs to be used twice a day for a long period (on average 19 days). It has also shown to be a biocidal agent against some biofilms of single or mixed bacterial species (Stickler & Hewitt 1991). This agent is thought to have a dual role, first in reducing urinary pH and second in dissolving struvite and calcium phosphate deposits. However, tissue reactions to mandelic acid 1% in clinical situations have yet to be demonstrated, as does its efficacy in the presence of urinary elements such as mucin and organic debris (Getliffe 1996a; Rew 1999).

Potential risks to the bladder urothelium associated with bladder maintenance solutions have raised concerns (Getliffe 1996a). Dilute acid solutions have been shown to remove the surface layer of mucus in the bladder (Parsons *et al.* 1970) and an increased shedding of urothelial cells has been observed following washouts with both acidic and neutral pH solutions (Elliot *et al.* 1989; Kennedy *et al.* 1992). This infers that both chemical irritation and physical force of instillation can be potential risk factors in disrupting bladder urothelium (Getliffe 2004). This highlights the importance of administering prepackaged maintenance solutions by gravity and not manually using a bladder syringe in order to minimize mechanical damage (Gates 2000).

There have been few clinically-based studies of the use of catheter maintenance solutions on which to base decisions on the optimum volume and frequency of bladder washouts. As the aim of a bladder washout is to remove encrustation from the catheter and not (as is commonly thought) the bladder, it has been suggested that 'mini' washouts regularly performed would be effective at reducing encrustations and minimizing irritant effects on the bladder (Getliffe 1994a; Getliffe & Dolman 2003; Yates 2004). A catheter lumen holds 4–5 ml of fluid; therefore, smaller volumes of 10–20 ml would still completely fill the catheter lumen and bathe the catheter tip. Therefore the bladder mucosa would not be exposed to large volumes of washout solution (Getliffe 2004). Getliffe (1994a) suggests that washouts could then be performed more frequently without increasing the risk of tissue damage. This suggestion has been supported by an in vitro study by Getliffe *et al.* (2000). Two sequential washouts with 50 ml of Suby G retained for 15 minutes were found to be significantly better at removing encrustations than a single washout of 100 ml; however, this theory is yet to be tested in a clinical setting. Despite the controversy surrounding the use of bladder maintenance solutions, an audit undertaken by several Primary Care Trusts and reported by Pomfret *et al.* (2004) showed that they are still widely used, although practice is varied and inconsistent. These findings highlight the need for researchers to undertake clinical-based studies in order that specific bladder lavage guidelines can be established to guide nursing practice (NICE 2003; Yates 2004; Pomfret & Mackenzie 2005; McNulty *et al.* 2006).

Patient assessment

There are a number of risks associated with bladder lavage (including introducing infection) and the procedure should not be undertaken lightly (McCarthy & Hunter 2001; NICE 2003). Prior to taking a decision to use bladder maintenance solutions, patients should be assessed and a catheter history should be noted (Rew 1999). The guiding principle for effective catheter management always involves addressing the individual needs of the patient (Godfrey & Evans 2000). Assessment of all aspects of catheter care should be taken, including:

- Patient activity and mobility (catheter positioning, catheter kinking).
- Diet and fluid intake.
- Standards of patient hygiene.
- Patients' and/or carers' ability to care for the catheter (Getliffe 1996a; Rew 1999; Ng 2001; Rew 2005).

Newly catheterized patients should be monitored to ascertain how long the catheter remains in situ before showing signs of blockage, without any interference with prophylactic washouts. A catheter history should be established, and documented, to enable future care to be planned (Rew 1999). In order to develop a distinct pattern of catheter history, Norberg *et al.* (1983) suggest that 3–5 consecutive catheters should be observed before treatment, if needed, is instigated. For patients with a history of encrustation, the use of pH indicator papers is also recommended to assist in the assessment of urine alkalinity. This can be used in conjunction with the collection of a urine specimen for microbiological analysis to identify any specific organisms, which may require systemic antibiotics (Rew 2005). To minimize the risk of introducing infection and to ensure the urine sample is fresh, the aforementioned investigations should be collected directly from the catheter at weekly catheter bag changes and where possible taken at the same time of day each week considering that urinary pH changes throughout the day (Rew 2005) (see Chapter 13).

An important aspect of management, for patients where a clear pattern of catheter history can be established, is the scheduling of catheter changes prior to likely blockages (Getliffe 1996b; Yates 2004). In patients where no clear pattern emerges, or for whom frequent catheter changes are traumatic, acidic bladder washouts can be beneficial in reducing catheter encrustations (Getliffe 1996a; Rew 1999; McCarthy & Hunter 2001; Yates 2004). The administration of catheter maintenance solutions to eliminate catheter encrustation can also be timed to coincide with catheter bag changes (every 5–7 days) so that the catheter system is not opened more than necessary (Yates 2004).

Catheters used for irrigation

A three-way urinary catheter must be used for irrigation in order that fluid may simultaneously be run into, and drained out from, the bladder (Getliffe 1996a; Ng 2001; Cutts 2005). A large-gauge catheter (16–24) is often used to accommodate any clot and debris which may be present. This catheter is commonly passed in theatre when irrigation is required, e.g. after prostatectomy (Forristal & Maxfield 2004). Occasionally if a patient is admitted with a heavily contaminated bladder, e.g. blood clots, bladder irrigation may be started on the ward. If the patient has a two-way catheter, this must be replaced with a three-way type (Scholtes 2002) (Fig. 10.1).

It is recommended that a three-way catheter is passed if frequent intravesical instillations of drugs or antiseptic solutions are prescribed and the risk of catheter obstruction is not considered to be very great. In such cases the most important factor is minimizing the risk of introducing infection and maintaining a closed urinary drainage system, for which the three-way catheter allows.

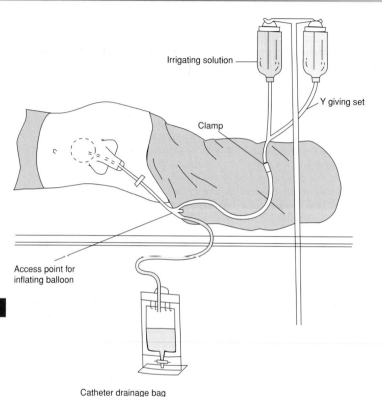

Catheter drainage bag

Figure 10.1 Closed urinary drainage system with provision for intermittent or continuous irrigation.

Procedure guidelines **Bladder lavage**

Equipment

1 Sterile dressing pack.
2 Sterile catheter tip syringe, 60 ml.
3 Sterile jug.
4 Antiseptic solution.
5 Bactericidal alcohol handrub.
6 Clamp.

7 New catheter bag (for balloon two-way catheter) or sterile spigot (for three-way catheter).
8 Sterile receiver.
9 Sterile solution for lavage.
10 Absorbent sheet.

Procedure

Action	Rationale
1 Explain and discuss the procedure with the patient.	To ensure that the patient understands the procedure and gives his/her valid consent (P; NMC 2006: C).
2 Screen the bed. Ensure that the patient is in a comfortable position allowing access to the catheter.	For the patient's privacy and to reduce the risk of cross-infection. Curtains are drawn at this stage so that dust and airborne organisms disturbed by the curtains do not settle on the sterile field (DH 2005a: C).
3 Perform the procedure using an aseptic technique.	To minimize the risk of infection (DH 2005a: C). (For further information on aseptic technique see Chapter 4.)
4 If necessary, draw up solutions using a 60-ml syringe, preferably with needle adapter. Cap the syringe and place it in a sterile receiver.	It is easier to draw up solutions from vials in the clinical area than at the bedside (E).
5 Take the trolley to the bedside, disturbing the screens as little as possible. Open the outer wrappings of packs and put them on the top shelf of the trolley.	To minimize airborne contamination. To begin to prepare equipment for procedure (E).
6 Prepare the sterile field. Pour the lavage solution into the sterile jug.	To prepare equipment for procedure (E).
7 Place absorbent sheet under the catheter junction and clamp the catheter. Wash hands with bactericidal alcohol handrub.	To prevent leakage when the catheter is disconnected. To reduce the risk of infection (DH 2005a: C).
8 Put on sterile gloves, place sterile towel under the junction of the catheter and the tubing of the drainage bag and disconnect them.	To create a sterile field and reduce the risk of cross-infection (DH 2005a: C). When the patient has a three-way catheter the drainage bag will not need disconnecting as the washout fluid is injected through the side-arm of the catheter. This should be spigotted off after use and the fluid remaining in the bladder will drain into the catheter bag (E).

383

Procedure guidelines *(cont.)*

9 Clean gloved hands with a bactericidal alcohol handrub. Clean around the end of the catheter with sterile low-linting gauze and an antiseptic solution.	To remove surface organisms from gloves and catheter and thus reduce the risk of introducing infection into the catheter (DH 2005a: C).
10 Draw up the irrigating fluid into the bladder syringe and insert the nozzle into the end of the catheter.	To prepare syringe for lavage (E).
11 Release the clamp on the catheter and gently inject the contents of the syringe into the bladder, trying not to inject air.	Rapid injection of fluid could be uncomfortable for the patient. Large volumes of air in the bladder cause distension and discomfort (Getliffe 1994a: R 5).
12 Remove the syringe and allow the bladder contents to drain by gravity into a receiver placed on a sterile towel.	To allow catheter to drain gently (E). To reduce risk of cross-infection (DH 2005a: C).
13 Repeat steps 11 and 12 of the procedure until the washout is complete or the returning fluid is clear.	To ensure the bladder is free of contaminants (Getliffe 1994a: R 5).
14 If the fluid does not return naturally, aspirate gently with the syringe.	Gentle suction is sometimes required to remove obstructive material from the catheter. If suction is applied too forcefully the urothelium may be sucked into the eyes of the catheter, preventing drainage and causing pain and trauma which may predispose to infection (Lowthian 1991: R 5; Macaulay 2004: R 5).
15 Connect a new catheter bag or sterile spigot if a three-way catheter is in place, and allow the remaining fluid to drain out.	A closed drainage system must be re-established as soon as possible to reduce the risk of bacterial invasion through the catheter (E).

16 If the solution is to remain in the bladder, the catheter should be clamped when all the fluid has been injected and the clamp released after the desired period.

To allow solution to act on bladder mucosa/catheter (E).

17 Measure the volume of washout fluid returned and compare it with the volume of fluid injected. Record any discrepancies of volume in the appropriate documents.

To keep an accurate record of urinary output and to observe for catheter obstruction (E).

18 Make the patient comfortable, remove equipment, clean the trolley, and wash hands.

To reduce the risk of cross-infection (DH 2005a: C).

Procedure guidelines **Urinary catheter: maintenance solution administration**

Equipment

1 Sterile dressing pack.
2 Antiseptic solution.
3 Bactericidal alcohol handrub.
4 Absorbent sheet.
5 New catheter bag.
6 Catheter maintenance solution.

Procedure

Action

1 Explain and discuss the procedure with the patient.

Rationale

To ensure that the patient understands the procedure and gives his/her valid consent (P; NMC 2006: C).

2 Screen the bed. Ensure that the patient is in a comfortable position, allowing the nurse access to the catheter.

For the patient's privacy and to reduce the risk of cross-infection (DH 2005a: C). Curtains are drawn at this stage so that dust and airborne organisms disturbed by the curtains do not settle on the sterile field (DH 2005a: C).

3 Perform the procedure using aseptic technique.

To minimize the risk of infection (DH 2005a: C). (For further information on aseptic technique see Chapter 4.)

Procedure guidelines *(cont.)*

4 Take the trolley to the bedside, disturbing the screens as little as possible. Open the outer wrappings of packs and put them on the top shelf of the trolley.

To minimize airborne contamination (DH 2005a: C). To begin to prepare the equipment for the procedure.

5 Remove outer packaging from catheter maintenance solution and place both 50 ml sterile solution containers on to the sterile field. Warm solution to body temperature by immersing package in water.

To prepare equipment for the procedure. Two 50 ml maintenance solution containers have been found to be the most effective way of treating encrustation (Getliffe *et al.* 2000: R 2b).
   Warm solutions to prevent bladder spasm (Rew 1999: R 5).

6 Expose the whole length of the catheter and observe for any signs of discharge, meatal problems and length of catheter in patient. (If patient is using a leg bag, remove straps and place bag on the bed before exposing the catheter.) Place the absorbent pad under catheter drainage bag junction.

To prepare patient for procedure (P). To detect for signs of infection, skin excoriation or displacement of catheter. If any signs noted report to medical staff as appropriate (C).

386

7 Wash hands with bactericidal rub and put on sterile gloves. Place sterile towel under catheter junction.

To reduce the risk of infection (DH 2005a: C).

8 Slide clamp on solution container tubing to closed, remove the security ring on the solution container connection port and loosen cover from the connection port.

To prevent fluid loss when connection port is opened (C). To prepare equipment (C).

9 Squeeze the end of the catheter together just above the connection to the drainage bag. Disconnect the drainage bag, keeping the catheter squeezed. Remove the cover from the connecting port on the solution container and insert it into the catheter. Release the catheter.

To prevent urine leaking from the catheter (E).

10 Slide the clamp open on the solution container, raise the bag slightly above the level of the bladder and allow the required amount of the solution to flow into the bladder. Gentle pressure may be needed initially to start the flow.

Rapid instillation of fluid could be uncomfortable for the patient (P). Administering maintenance solution via gravity and not physical force will reduce the risk of damage to the bladder mucosa (Getliffe *et al.* 2000: R 2b; Rew 2005: R 5).

Instil maximum of 50 ml solution or to bladder capacity.

To avoid by-passing (Getliffe & Dolman 2003: R 2b).

Where instillation is being used to dissolve encrustation, a second instillation may be performed.

This is more effective in dissolving encrustation (Getliffe *et al.* 2000: R 2b).

---

11 If the fluid is to be retained for a period of time close the clamp and place the bag on the bed. Reposition the covers and ensure the patient is comfortable for the required time (P).

To allow the solutions time to act on the catheter encrustations (Evans & Godfrey 2000: R 5). For the patient's privacy and comfort (P).

---

12 When the solution is to be removed, ensure the bag is below the level of the bladder, open the clip and allow the solution to drain back.

For gravity to help facilitate drainage (E).

---

13 When all the solution has drained back out of the bladder, close the clamp, disconnect the solution container and connect a new drainage bag. Note the amount of fluid returned.

To prevent spillage of solution. To re-establish closed drainage system (E).

---

14 Make the patient comfortable, remove and dispose of equipment, clean the trolley and wash hands.

To reduce risk of cross-infection (DH 2005a: C).

---

15 Sign prescription chart. Document that catheter maintenance solution has been administered and note any complication or problems encountered with the procedure.

To maintain accurate records. Provide a point of reference in the event of any queries and prevent duplication of treatment (E).

Procedure guidelines   **Continuous bladder irrigation**

Equipment

1 Sterile dressing pack.
2 Antiseptic solution.
3 Bactericidal alcohol handrub.
4 Clamp.
5 Sterile irrigation fluid.

6 Disposable irrigation set.
7 Infusion stand.
8 Sterile jug.
9 Absorbent sheet.

Procedure
Commencing bladder irrigation

Action	Rationale
1 Explain and discuss the procedure with the patient.	To ensure that the patient understands the procedure and gives his/her valid consent (NMC 2006: C; NMC 2008: C).
2 Screen the patient and ensure that he/she is in a comfortable position allowing access to the catheter.	For the patient's privacy and to reduce the risk of cross-infection. Curtains are drawn at this stage so that dust and airborne organisms disturbed by the curtains do not settle on the sterile trolley (DH 2005a: C).
3 Perform the procedure using an aseptic technique.	To minimize the risk of infection (DH 2005a: C). (For further information on aseptic technique see Chapter 13.)
4 Open the outer wrappings of the pack and put it on the top shelf of the trolley.	To prepare equipment (E).
5 Insert the end of the irrigation giving set into the fluid bag and hang the bag on the infusion stand. Allow fluid to run through the tubing so that air is expelled.	To prime the irrigation set so that it is ready for use. Air is expelled in order to prevent discomfort from air in the patient's bladder (E).
6 Clamp the catheter and place absorbent sheet under the catheter junction.	To prevent leakage of urine through the irrigation arm when the spigot is removed (E). To contain any spillages.

388

7	Clean hands with a bactericidal alcohol handrub. Put on gloves.	To minimize the risk of cross-infection (DH 2005a: C).
8	Place a sterile paper towel under the irrigation inlet of the catheter and remove the spigot.	To create a sterile field. To prepare catheter for connection to irrigation set (Scholtes 2002: R 5).
9	Discard the spigot and gloves.	To prevent reuse and reduce risk of cross-infection (DH 2005a: C).
10	Put on sterile gloves. Clean around the end of the irrigation arm with sterile low-linting gauze and an antiseptic solution.	To remove surface organisms from gloves and catheter and to reduce the risk of introducing infection into the catheter (DH 2005a: C).
11	Attach the irrigation giving set to the irrigation arm of the catheter. Keep the clamp of the irrigation giving set closed.	To prevent overdistension of the bladder, which can occur if fluid is run into the bladder before the drainage tube has been unclamped (Scholtes 2002: R 5).
12	Release the clamp on the catheter tube and allow any accumulated urine to drain into the catheter bag. Empty the urine from the catheter bag into a sterile jug.	Urine drainage should be measured before commencing irrigation so that the fluid balance may be monitored more accurately (Scholtes 2002: R 5).
13	Discard the gloves.	These will be contaminated, having handled the cathether bag (DH 2005a, b: C).
14	Set irrigation at the required rate and ensure that fluid is draining into the catheter bag.	To check that the drainage system is patent and to prevent fluid accumulating in the bladder (C).
15	Make the patient comfortable, remove unnecessary equipment and clean the trolley.	To reduce the risk of cross-infection (DH 2005a: C).
16	Wash hands.	To reduce the risk of cross-infection (DH 2005a: C).

Procedure guidelines *(cont.)*

Care of the patient during bladder irrigation

Action	Rationale
1 Adjust the rate of infusion according to the degree of haematuria. This will be greatest in the first 12 hours following surgery (average fluid input is 6–9 litres during the first 12 hours, falling to 3–6 litres during the next 12 hours). The aim is to obtain a drainage fluid which is rosé in colour.	To remove blood from the bladder before it clots and to minimize the risk of catheter obstruction and clot retention. (Scholtes 2002: R 5.)
2 Check the volume in the drainage bag frequently when infusion is in progress, e.g. half-hourly or hourly, or more frequently as required.	To ensure that fluid is draining from the bladder and to detect blockages as soon as possible, also to prevent overdistension of the bladder and patient discomfort (C, P). To empty catheter drainage bags before they reach capacity.
3 Using rubber-tipped 'milking' tongs, 'milk' the catheter and drainage tube, as required.	To remove clots from within the drainage system and to maintain an efficient outlet (Lowthian 1991: R 5).
4 Record the fluid balance chart accurately. The fluid balance of all patients having bladder irrigation must be monitored.	So that urine output is known and any related problems, e.g. renal dysfunction, may be detected quickly and easily (E).

390

Bladder irrigation recording chart

The bladder irrigation recording chart (Figure 10.2) is designed to provide an accurate record of the patient's urinary output during the period of irrigation.

Procedure for use of chart

Record the time (column A) and the fluid volume in each bag of irrigating solution (column B) as it is put up.

When the irrigating fluid has all run from the first bag into the bladder, record the original volume in the bag in column C. Record the corresponding time in

Patient name:			Hospital no:		
(A) Date and time	(B) Volume put up	(C) Volume run in	(D) Total volume out	(E) Urine	(F) Urine running total
10/7/06	2000				
10.00					
10.30			700		
11.10			850		
11.40		2000	600		
			2150	150	150
11.45	2000				
12.30			500		
13.15			700		
14.20		2000	800		
			2400	400	550
14.25	2000				
15.30			850		
17.00	Irrigation stopped	1200	800		
			1650	450	1000

Figure 10.2   Bladder irrigation recording chart.

column A. Do not attempt to estimate the fluid volume run-in while a bag is in progress as this will be inaccurate. If, however, a bag is discontinued, the volume run-in can be calculated by measuring the volume left in the bag and deducting this from the original volume. This should be recorded in column C (Scholtes 2002).

The catheter bag should be emptied as often as is necessary, the volume being recorded in column D and the corresponding time in column A. The catheter bag must also be emptied whenever the bag of irrigating fluid is empty, and the volume recorded in column D.

When each bag of fluid has run through, add up the total volume drained by the catheter in column D, and write this in red. Subtract from this the total volume run-in (column C) to find the urine output (D − C = E). Write this in column E. Draw a line across the page to indicate that this calculation is complete and continue underneath for the next bag.

Problem solving

Problem	Cause	Suggested action
Fluid retained in the bladder when the catheter is in position.	Fault in drainage apparatus, e.g.:	
	Blocked catheter	'Milk' the tubing. Wash out the bladder with 0.9% sodium chloride (E).
	Kinked tubing	Straighten the tubing (E).
	Overfull drainage bag	Empty the drainage bag (E).
	Catheter clamped off	Unclamp the catheter (E).
Distended abdomen related to an overfull bladder during the irrigation procedure.	Irrigation fluid is infused at too rapid a rate.	Slow down the infusion rate (E).
	Fault in drainage apparatus.	Check the patency of the drainage apparatus (E).
Leakage of fluid from around the catheter.	Catheter slipping out of the bladder.	Insert the catheter further in (E). Decompress balloon fully to assess the amount of water necessary. Refill balloon until it remains in situ, taking care not to overfill beyond safe level (see manufacturer's instructions) (E).
	Catheter too large or unsuitable for the patient's anatomy.	If leakage is profuse or catheter is uncomfortable for the patient, replace the catheter with one of smaller size (E).
Patient experiences pain during the lavage or irrigation procedure.	Volume of fluid in the bladder is too great for comfort.	Reduce the fluid volume within the bladder (E).

Problem	Cause	Suggested action
	Solution is painful to raw areas in the bladder.	Inform the doctor. Administer analgesia as prescribed (E).
Retention of fluid with or without distended abdomen, with or without pain.	Perforated bladder.	Stop irrigation. Maintain in recovery position. Call medical assistance (E). Monitor vital signs. Monitor patient for pain, tense abdomen (E).

For further details, see Chapter 13, Problem solving: Urinary catheter.

References and further reading

Addison, R. (2000) *Bladder Washout/Irrigation/Instillations. A Guide for Nurses.* Braun Medical, Sheffield.

Bailey, S. (1991) Using bladder washouts. *Nurs Times*, **87**(24), 75–6.

Burr, R.G. & Nusbeibeh, I. (1995) The blocking urinary catheter: the role of variation in urine flow. *Br J Urol*, **76**, 61–5.

Castledine, G. (2001) Case 42: Bladder washout – Staff nurse who carried out a bladder washout using Diet Coke. *Br J Nurs*, **10**(3), 144.

Castledine, G. (2006) Nurse whose inexperience and negligence in bladder washout put her patient at risk. *Br J Nurs*, **15**(3), 141.

Choong, S.K.S. *et al.* (1999) The physicochemical basis of urinary catheter encrustation. *Br J Urol*, **83**, 770–5.

Costerton, J.W. *et al.* (1999) Bacterial biofilms: a common cause of persistent infections. *Science*, **284**, 1318–22.

Cox, A.J. *et al.* (1987) Calcium phosphate in catheter encrustation. *Br J Urol*, **59**, 159–63.

Cutts, B. (2005) Developing and implementing a new bladder irrigation chart. *Nurs Stand*, **20**(8), 48–53.

Davies, A.J. *et al.* (1987) Does instillation of chlorhexidine into the bladder of catheterised geriatric patients help reduce bacteriuria? *J Hosp Infect*, **9**, 72–5.

DH (2005a) *Saving Lives: A Delivery Programme to Reduce Healthcare Infection including MRSA.* Department of Health, London.

DH (2005b) *Hazardous waste (England) regulations.* Department of Health, London.

Dudley, M.N. & Barriere, S.L. (1981) Antimicrobial irrigations in the prevention and treatment of catheter-related urinary tract infections. *Am J Hosp Pharm*, **38**, 59–65.

Elliot, T.S. (1990) Disadvantages of bladder irrigation in catheterized patients. (Brief research report.) *Nurs Times*, **86**, 52.

Elliot, T.S. *et al.* (1989) Bladder irrigation or irritation? *Br J Urol*, **64**, 391–4.

Evans, A. & Godfrey, H. (2000) Bladder washouts in the management of long-term catheters. *Br J Nurs*, **9**(14), 900–4.

Ferrie, B.G., Glen, E.S. & Hunter, B. (1979) Long-term urethral catheter drainage. *Br Med J*, **2**(6197), 1046–7.

Fillingham, S. & Douglas, J. (2004) *Urological Nursing*, 3rd edn. Bailliere Tindall, Edinburgh.

Flack, S. (1993) Finding the best solution. *Nurs Times*, **11**, 68–74.

Forristal, H. & Maxfield, J. (2004) Prostatic problems. In: *Urological Nursing* (eds S. Fillingham & J. Douglas), 3rd edn. Bailliere Tindall, London, pp. 161–84.

Gates, A. (2000) The benefits of irrigation in catheter care. *Prof Nurse*, **16**(1), 835–8.

Getliffe, K.A. (1994a) The characteristics and management of patients with recurrent blockage of long-term urinary catheters. *J Adv Nurs*, **20**, 140–9.

Getliffe, K.A. (1994b) The use of bladder wash-outs to reduce urinary catheter encrustation. *Br J Urol*, **73**, 696–700.

Getliffe, K.A. (1996a) Bladder instillations and bladder washouts in the management of catheterized patients. *J Adv Nurs*, **23**, 548–54.

Getliffe, K.A. (1996b) Care of urinary catheters. *Nurs Stand*, **11**(11), 47–54.

Getliffe, K.A. (2004) The effect of acidic maintenance solutions on catheter longevity. *Nurs Times*, **100**(16), 32–4.

Getliffe, K.A. & Dolman, M. (2003) *Promoting Continence: A Clinical and Research Resource*, 2nd edn. Bailliere Tindall, London.

Getliffe, K., Hughes, S.C. & Le Claire, M. (2000) The dissolution of urinary catheter encrustation. *Br J Urol*, **85**(1), 60–4.

Gilbert, V. & Gobbi, M. (1989) Bladder irrigation (principles and methods). *Nurs Times*, **85**, 40–2.

Godfrey, H. & Evans, H. (2000) Management of long-term urethral catheters: minimizing complications. *Br J Nurs*, **9**(2), 74–80.

Griffith, D.P. & Musher, O.N. (1976) Urease: the primary cause of infection induced urinary stones. *Invest Urol*, **13**(5), 346–82.

Gristina, A.G. *et al.* (1987) Adhesive colonisation of biomaterials and antibiotic resistance. *Biomaterials*, **8**, 423–6.

Hedelin, H. *et al.* (1984) The composition of catheter encrustations, including the effects of allopurinol treatment. *Br J Urol*, **56**, 250–4.

Holden, D. & Rao, P.N. (1991) Management of staghorn stones using a combination of lithotripsy, percutaneous nephrolithotomy and solution R irrigation. *Br J Urol*, **67**, 13–17.

Jewes, L.A. *et al.* (1988) Bacteriuria and bacteraemia in patients with long-term indwelling catheters: a domiciliary study. *J Med Microbiol*, **26**, 61–5.

Kennedy, A.P. *et al.* (1983) Factors relating to the problems of long-term catheterization. *J Adv Nurs*, **8**, 207–12.

Kennedy, A.P. *et al.* (1992) Assessment of the use of bladder washouts/instillations in patients with long term indwelling catheters. *Br J Urol*, **70**, 610–15.

King, J.B. & Stickler, D.J. (1992) The effects of repeated instillations of antiseptics on catheter-associated urinary tract infections. *Urol Res*, **20**, 403–7.

Kohler-Ockmore, J. (1992) Urinary catheter complications. *J District Nurs*, **10**(8), 18–20.

Kunin, C.M., Chin, Q.A. & Charnbers, S. (1987) Formation of encrustation on in-dwelling urinary catheters in the elderly. *J Urol*, **77**(3), 347–51.

Liedl, B. (2001) Catheter-associated urinary tract infections. *Curr Opin Urol*, **11**(1), 75–9.

Lowthian, P. (1991) Using bladder syringes sparingly. *Nurs Times*, **87**(10), 61–4.

Macaulay, D. (2004) Urinary drainage systems. In: *Urological Nursing* (eds. S. Fillingham & J. Douglas), 2nd edn. Bailliere Tindall, London, pp. 90–130.

Mathur, S. *et al.* (2006) Prospective study of individuals with long-term urinary catheters colonized with *Proteus* species. *Br J Urol*, **97**, 121–8.

McCarthy, K. & Hunter, I. (2001) Importance of pH monitoring in the care of long-term catheters. *Br J Nurs*, **10**(19), 1240–6.

McNulty, C.A.M. *et al.* (2006) Urinary catheterization in care homes for older people; self-reported questionnaire audit of catheter management by care home staff. *J Hosp Infect*, **26**, 29–36.

Mobley, H.L.T. & Warren, J.W. (1987) Urease positive bacteriuria and obstruction of long-term urinary catheters. *J Clin Microbiol*, **25**, 2216–17.

Morris, N.S., Stickler, D.J. & Winters, C. (1997) Which indwelling urethral catheters resist encrustations by *Proteus mirabilis* biofilms? *Br J Urol*, **80**, 58–63.

Mulhall, A.B., Chapman, R.G. & Crow, R.A. (1988) Bacteriuria during indwelling urethral catheterisation. *J Hosp Infect*, **11**(3), 253–62.

Ng, C. (2001) Assessment and intervention knowledge of nurses in managing catheter patency in continuous bladder irrigation following TURP. *Urol Nurs*, **21**(2), 97–108.

NICE (2003) *Infection Control. Prevention of Health Care-associated Infection in Primary and Community Care. Clinical Guidance 2.* National Institute for Health and Clinical Excellence, London.

NMC (2005) *Guidelines for Records and Record Keeping.* Nursing and Midwifery Council, London.

NMC (2006) *A–Z Advice Sheet Consent.* www.nmc.org.

NMC (2008) *The Code: Standards of Conduct, Performance and Ethics for Nurses and Midwives.* Nursing and Midwifery Council, London.

Norberg, B., Norberg, A. & Parkhede, U. (1983) The spontaneous variation in catheter life in long-stay geriatric patients with in-dwelling catheters. *Gerontology*, **29**, 332–5.

Parsons, C.L., Mulholland, S.G. & Anwar, H. (1970) Antibacterial activity of bladder surface mucin duplicated by exogenous glycosaminoglycan (heparin). *Infect Immun*, **25**, 552–4.

Pomfret, I. & Mackenzie, R. (2005) Questioning practice – the need for research in continence care. *J Comm Nurs*, **19**(11), 32–5.

Pomfret, I. *et al.* (2004) Using bladder instillations to manage indwelling catheters. *Br J Nurs*, **13**(5), 261–7.

Rao, G.G. & Elliott, T.S.J. (1988) Bladder irrigation. *Age Ageing*, **17**(6), 373–8.

Rew, M. (1999) Use of catheter maintenance solutions for long-term catheters. *Br J Nurs*, **8**(11), 708–15.

Rew, M. (2005) Caring for catheterized patients: urinary catheter maintenance. *Br J Nurs*, **14**(2), 87–92.

Rew, M. & Woodward, S. (2001) Troubleshooting common problems associated with long-term catheters. *Br J Nurs*, **10**(12), 764–74.

Roe, B.H. (1989) Use of bladder washouts: a study of nurses' recommendations. *J Adv Nurs*, **14**(6), 494–500.

Roe, B.H. (1990) The basis for sound practice. *Nurs Stand*, **4**, 25–7.

Scholtes, S. (2002) Management of clot retention following urological surgery. *Nurs Times*, **98**(28), 48–50.

Simpson, L. (2001) Indwelling urethral catheters. *Nurs Stand*, **15**(46), 47–54.

Stickler, D.J. (1990) The role of antiseptics in the management of patients undergoing short term indwelling bladder catheterisation. *J Hosp Infect*, **16**, 89–108.

Stickler, D.J. & Chawla, J.C. (1987) The role of antiseptics in the management of patients with long term indwelling bladder catheters. *J Hosp Infect*, **10**, 219–28.

Stickler, D.J. & Hewitt, P. (1991) Activity of antiseptic against biofilms of mixed bacterial species growing on silicone surfaces. *Eur J Microbiol Infect*, **10**, 416–21.

Stickler, D.J. & Hughes, G. (1999) Ability of *Proteus mirabilis* to swarm over urethral catheters. *Eur J Clin Microbiol Infect Dis*, **18**(3), 206–8.

Stickler, D.J. *et al*. (1981) Some observations on the activity of three antiseptics used as bladder irrigants in the treatment of UTI in patients with indwelling catheters. *Paraplegia*, **19**, 325–33.

Stickler, D.J., Clayton, C.L. & Chawla, J.C. (1987) The resistance of urinary tract pathogens to chlorhexidine bladder washouts. *J Hosp Infect*, **10**, 28–39.

Trautner, B.W. & Darouiche, R.O. (2004) Role of biofilm in catheter-associated urinary tract infection. *Am J Inf Con*, **32**(3), 177–83.

Yates, A. (2004) Crisis management in catheter care. *J Comm Nurs*, **18**(5), 28–30.

Multiple choice questions

1 Bladder lavage is carried out:

   a   To prevent infection
   b   To clear an obstructed catheter or remove potential sources of obstruction
   c   To make a catheter last longer
   d   For patient comfort

2 Bladder irrigation is carried out:

   a   After prostatic surgery
   b   To prevent infection
   c   After prostatic surgery and on rare occasions to remove material from a heavily diseased bladder
   d   Because the patient asks

3 Catheter related infection occurs in:

   a   Over 50% of patients within 2 weeks of catheterization
   b   Over 90% of patients within 4 weeks of catheterization
   c   9% of patients within 24 hours of catheterization
   d   All patients after 6 weeks of catheterization

4 Prior to bladder lavage you should clean around the end of the catheter with:

   a   Cotton wool and sterile water
   b   Sterile low-linting gauze and an antiseptic solution
   c   Gauze and saline
   d   Alcohol swab

Answers to the multiple choice questions can be found in Appendix 3.

Chapter 11

Elimination: bowel care

Definitions

Diarrhoea

Diarrhoea results when the balance between absorption, secretion and intestinal motility is disturbed (Hogan 1998). It has been defined as an abnormal increase in the quantity, frequency and fluid content of stool and associated with urgency, perianal discomfort and incontinence (Basch 1987), and is characterized by at least three loose, liquid stools per day (Bell 2004; NANDA-I 2007).

Constipation

Constipation results when there is a delayed movement of intestinal content through the bowel (Walsh 1997). It has been defined as persistent, difficult, infrequent or incomplete defecation, which may or may not be accompanied by hard, dry stools (Norton 2006; NANDA-I 2007).

Reference material

Bowel elimination is a sensitive issue and providing effective care and management for problems associated with it can be problematic. The difficulties associated with this can be minimized if the nurse seeks to respect the patient's dignity when carrying out procedures such as assisting them with using a bedpan or a commode.

Many patients are too embarrassed to discuss bowel function and will often delay reporting problems, despite the sometimes severe impact these symptoms have on their quality of life (Cadd *et al.* 2000). Generally complaints will be either that the patient has diarrhoea or is constipated. These should be seen as symptoms of some underlying disease or malfunction and managed accordingly.

Procedure guidelines   **Bedpan use: assisting a patient**

Equipment

1 Disposable apron and gloves.

2 Slipper bedpan and paper cover.

3 Toilet paper.

4 Manual handling equipment as appropriate.

5 Additional nurse if required.

6 Wash bowl, warm water, disposable wipes and a towel.

Procedure

Action	Rationale
1 Carry out appropriate manual handling assessment prior to commencing procedure and establish whether an additional nurse or equipment such as a hoist are necessary.	To maintain a safe environment.
2 Take the equipment to the bedside and explain the procedure to the patient.	To ensure that the patient understands the procedure and gives his/her valid consent (NMC 2006: C; NMC 2008b: C).
3 Close door/draw curtains around the patient's bed area.	To maintain privacy and dignity and avoid any unnecessary embarrassment for the patient (P).
4 Remove the bedclothes and, providing there are no contra-indications (e.g. if patient is on flat bed rest), assist the patient into an upright sitting position.	An upright, 'crouch like' posture is considered anatomically correct for defecation and poor posture adopted while using a bedpan has been shown to cause extreme straining during defecation. Patients should therefore be supported with pillows in order to achieve an upright position on the bedpan (Taylor 1997: E).
5 Ask the patient to raise their hips/buttocks and insert the bedpan beneath the patient's pelvis, ensuring that the wide end of the bedpan is between the legs, and the narrow is beneath the buttocks.	A slipper bedpan provides more comfort for a patient who is unable to sit upright on a conventional bedpan (Nicol *et al.* 2004: E).

399

Procedure guidelines *(cont.)*

6 Offer patients the use of pillows and encourage them to lean forward slightly.

To provide support and optimize positioning for defecation (Taylor 1997: E).

7 If the patient is unable to adopt a sitting/upright position, then roll them onto one side, using appropriate manual handling equipment, and insert a slipper bedpan with the narrow/flat end underneath their buttocks and wide end between their legs. Then roll the patient onto their back and so onto the bedpan.

8 Once the patient is on the bedpan, encourage them to move their legs slightly apart and check to ensure that their positioning is correct.

To avoid any spillage onto the bed clothes and reduce risk of contamination and cross-infection.

9 Cover the patient's legs with a sheet.

To maintain privacy and dignity (P).

10 Ensure that toilet paper and call bell are within patient's reach and leave the patient, but remain nearby.

To maintain privacy and dignity (P).

11 When the patient has finished using the bedpan, bring washing equipment to the bedside, remove the bedpan, and replace paper cover. Assist patient with cleaning perianal area using warm water and soap. Apply a small amount of barrier cream to the perineal/buttock area if appropriate.

Talcum powder should not be used and barrier creams should be applied sparingly, gently layered on in the direction of the hair growth rather than rubbed into the skin (Le Lievre 2002: E).

12 Offer a bowl of water for the patient to wash their hands.

For infection control and patient's comfort (P).

13 Ensure bedclothes are clean, straighten sheets and rearrange pillows, assisting patient to a comfortable position. Ensure call bell is within reach of the patient.

For patient comfort (P).

14 Take bedpan to the dirty utility (sluice) room and where necessary, measure urine output and note characteristics (see Bristol Stool Form Chart: Figure 11.1) and amount of faeces.	To monitor and evaluate patient's elimination patterns (E).
15 Dispose of contents safely and place bedpan in the washer/disposal unit.	To reduce any risk of contamination or cross-infection.
16 Remove disposable apron and gloves. Wash hands using soap and water/alcohol handrub.	For infection control.
17 Record any urine output/bowel action in patient's documentation.	To maintain accurate documentation.

Procedure guidelines **Commode use: assisting a patient**

Equipment

1 Disposable apron and gloves.
2 Commode with conventional bedpan inserted below seat.
3 Toilet paper.
4 Manual handling equipment as appropriate.
5 Additional nurse if required.
6 Wash bowl, warm water, disposable wipes and a towel.

Procedure

Action	Rationale
1 Carry out appropriate manual handling assessment prior to commencing procedure and ensure that patient's weight does not exceed the maximum recommended for commode (see manufacturer's guidelines).	To maintain a safe environment.
2 Take the equipment to the bedside and explain the procedure to the patient.	To ensure that the patient understands the procedure and gives his/her valid consent (NMC 2006: C; NMC 2008b: C).

Procedure guidelines *(cont.)*

3 Close door/draw curtains around the patient's bed area.	To maintain privacy and dignity and avoid any unnecessary embarrassment for the patient (P).
4 Remove the commode cover. Assist the patient out of the bed/chair and onto the commode.	
5 Ensure the patient's feet are positioned directly below their knees and flat on the floor. The use of a small footstool and/or pillows may help to achieve a comfortable position.	An upright, crouching posture is considered anatomically correct for defecation. Pillows and a footstool can provide support and optimize positioning for defecation (Taylor 1997: E).
6 Once the patient is on the commode, encourage them to move their legs slightly apart and check to ensure that their positioning is correct.	To avoid any spillage and reduce risk of contamination and cross-infection.
7 Cover the patient's knees with a towel or sheet.	To maintain privacy and dignity (P).
8 Ensure that toilet paper and call bell are within patient's reach and leave the patient, but remain nearby.	To maintain privacy and dignity (P).
9 When the patient has finished using the commode, bring washing equipment to the bedside. Assist patient with cleaning perianal area using toilet paper and, where necessary, warm water and soap. Apply a small amount of barrier cream to the perineal/buttock area if appropriate.	Talcum powder should not be used and barrier creams should be applied sparingly, gently layered on in the direction of the hair growth rather than rubbed into the skin (Le Lievre 2002: E).
10 Offer a bowl of water for the patient to wash their hands.	For infection control and patient's comfort (P).
11 Assist the patient to stand and walk to bed/chair, ensuring that they are comfortably positioned. Ensure call bell is within reach of the patient.	For patient comfort (P).

12 Replace cover on the commode and return to the dirty utility (sluice) room.	To reduce any risk of contamination or cross-infection and to avoid patient embarrassment.
13 Remove pan from underneath the commode and where necessary, measure urine output, and note characteristics (see Bristol Stool Form Chart: Figure 11.1) and amount of faeces.	To monitor and evaluate patient's elimination patterns (E).
14 Dispose of contents safely and place pan in the washer/disposal unit. Clean commode using warm, soapy water.	For infection control.
15 Remove disposable apron and gloves. Wash hands using soap and water/alcohol hand rub.	For infection control.
16 Record any urine output/bowel action in patient's documentation.	To maintain accurate documentation.

The nurse's priority is to effectively assess the nature and cause of the problem, to help find appropriate solutions and to inform and support the patient. This requires sensitive communication skills to dispel embarrassment and ensure a shared understanding of the meanings of the terms used by the patient (Smith 2001).

Anatomy and physiology

This section will consider the normal structure and function of the bowel, which includes the small and large intestine. The small intestine begins at the pyloric sphincter of the stomach, coils through the abdomen and opens into the large intestine at the ileocaecal junction. It is approximately 6 m in length and is divided into three segments: the duodenum (25 cm), jejunum (2.5 m) and ileum (3.5 m) (Thibodeau & Patton 2007). The mucosal surface of the small intestine is covered with finger-like processes called villi, which increase the surface area available for absorption and digestion. A number of digestive enzymes are also secreted by the small intestine (Tortora & Derrickson 2008).

Movement through the small bowel is divided into two types, namely segmentation and peristalsis, and is controlled by the autonomic nervous system.

Segmentation refers to the localized contraction of the intestine, which mixes the intestinal contents and brings particles of food into contact with the mucosa for absorption. Once the majority of a meal has been absorbed through this process, intestinal content is then pushed along the small intestine by repeated peristaltic wave-like actions. Intestinal content usually remains in the small bowel for 3–5 hours (Tortora & Derrickson 2008).

The total volume of fluid, including ingested liquids and gastrointestinal secretions, that enters the small intestine daily is about 9.3 litres. The small intestine is responsible for absorbing around 90% of the nutrients, electrolytes and water within this volume by diffusion, facilitated diffusion, osmosis and active transport (Tortora & Derrickson 2008). Water is able to move across the intestinal mucosa in both directions, but is influenced by the absorption of nutrients and electrolytes. As various electrolytes and nutrients are actively transported out of the lumen, they create a concentration gradient, promoting water absorption, via osmosis, in order to maintain an osmotic balance between intestinal fluid and blood. This ultimately leads to only about 1 litre of effluent passing through into the colon (Wood 1996; Thibodeau & Patton 2007; Tortora & Derrickson 2008).

From the ileocaecal sphincter to the anus the colon is approximately 1.5–1.8 m in length. Its main function is to eliminate the waste products of digestion by the propulsion of faeces towards the anus. In addition, it produces mucus to lubricate the faecal mass, thus aiding its expulsion. Other functions include the absorption of fluid and electrolytes, including sodium and potassium, the storage of faeces and the synthesis of vitamins B and K by bacterial flora (Thibodeau & Patton 2007; Tortora & Derrickson 2008).

Faeces consist of the unabsorbed end products of digestion, bile pigments, cellulose, bacteria, epithelial cells, mucus and some inorganic material. They are normally semi-solid in consistency and contain about 70% water (Tortora & Derrickson 2006). The colon absorbs about 2 litres of water in 24 hours, so if faeces are not expelled they will gradually become hard due to dehydration and more difficult to expel. If there is insufficient roughage (fibre) in the faeces, colonic stasis occurs, which leads to continued water absorption and further hardening of the faeces. The movement of faeces through the colon towards the anus is by mass peristalsis, a gastro colic reflex initiated by the presence of food in the stomach, which begins at the middle of the transverse colon and quickly drives the colonic contents into the rectum. This mass peristaltic movement generally occurs 3–5 times a day (Perdue 2005). In response to this stimulus, faeces move into the rectum (Norton 1996b; Taylor 1997; Tortora & Derrickson 2008). The rectum is very sensitive to rises in pressure, even of 2–3 mmHg, and distension will cause a perineal sensation with a subsequent desire to defecate. A co-ordinated reflex empties the bowel from mid-transverse colon to the anus. During this phase the diaphragm, abdominal and levator ani muscles contract and the glottis closes. Waves of peristalsis occur in the distal colon and the anal sphincter relaxes, allowing the evacuation of faeces (Tortora & Derrickson 2008). The stimulus to defecate varies in individuals according to habit, and if a decision is made to delay defecation, the stimulus disappears and a process of retroperistalsis occurs whereby the faeces moves back into the sigmoid colon (Perdue 2005). If these natural reflexes are inhibited on a regular basis they are eventually suppressed and reflex defecation is inhibited, resulting in such individuals becoming severely constipated.

Diarrhoea

The term diarrhoea originates from the Greek for 'to flow through' (Bell 2004) and can be characterized according to its onset and duration (acute or chronic) or by type (e.g. secretory, osmotic or malabsorptive). Sudden onset acute diarrhoea is very common, usually self-limiting, lasts less than 2 weeks and often requires no investigation or treatment (Shepherd 2000). The causes of acute diarrhoea include:

- Dietary indiscretion (eating too much fruit, alcohol misuse).
- Allergy to food constituents.
- Infective (King 2002):
  - (a) Travel-associated.
  - (b) Viral.
  - (c) Bacterial (usually associated with food).
  - (d) Antibiotic-related.
- Contrast media for screening purposes (Taylor 1997; Campbell & Lunn 1999).

Chronic diarrhoea generally lasts longer than 2 weeks and may have more complex origins (Hogan 1998). Chronic causes include (Taylor 1997; Fallon & O'Neill 1997):

- Inflammatory bowel disease, e.g. ulcerative colitis, Crohn's disease.
- Malabsorption, e.g. coeliac disease, tropical sprue.
- Organic disease, e.g. neoplasms, diverticulitis.
- Endocrine disorders, e.g. thyrotoxicosis, diabetes, carcinoid tumours.
- Intestinal obstruction including faecal obstruction.
- Miscellaneous colitis including pseudomembranous colitis, radiation enteritis, gut reaction and drug therapy, e.g. laxatives, antibiotics, chemotherapy.

Diarrhoea can have profound physiological and psychosocial consequences on a patient. Severe or extended episodes of diarrhoea may result in dehydration, electrolyte imbalance and malnutrition. Patients not only have to cope with increased frequency of bowel movement but may have abdominal pain, cramping, proctitis and anal or perianal skin breakdown. Food aversions may develop or patients may stop eating altogether as they anticipate subsequent diarrhoea following intake. Consequently this may lead to weight loss and malnutrition. Fatigue, sleep disturbances, feelings of isolation and depression are all common consequences for those experiencing diarrhoea (Hogan 1998). Patients with a stoma may also need to change their appliances more frequently and skin excoriation may occur which can exacerbate distress (Campbell & Lunn 1999). The impact of severe diarrhoea should not be underestimated; it is highly debilitating and may cause patients on long-term therapy to be noncompliant resulting in a potentially life-threatening problem (Kornblau *et al.* 2000).

Assessment

The cause of diarrhoea needs to be identified before effective treatment can be instigated. This may include clinical investigations such as stool cultures for bacterial, fungal and viral pathogens or a more formal medical evaluation of the gastrointestinal tract (Kornblau *et al.* 2000).

Ongoing nursing assessment is essential for ensuring individualized management and care. The lack of a systematic approach to assessment and poor documentation causes problems in effective management of diarrhoea (Cadd *et al.* 2000; Smith 2001). Nurses need to be aware of contributing factors and be sensitive to patients' beliefs and values in order to provide holistic care. A comprehensive assessment is therefore essential and should include:

1 History of onset, frequency and duration of diarrhoea.
2 Consistency, colour and form of stool including the presence of blood, fat, mucus. Stools can be graded using a scale such as the Bristol Stool Form Chart (Figure 11.1), where diarrhoea would be classified as types 6 or 7 (Longstreth *et al.* 2006).
3 Symptoms associated with diarrhoea, e.g. pain, nausea, vomiting, fatigue, weight loss, fever.
4 Recent lifestyle changes, emotional disturbances, or travel abroad.
5 Fluid intake and dietary history including any cause and effect relationships between food consumption and bowel action.
6 Normal medication, including recent antibiotics, laxatives or chemotherapy.
7 Effectiveness of antidiarrhoeal medication (dose and frequency).
8 Significant past medical history, e.g. bowel resection, pancreatitis, pelvic radiotherapy.

THE BRISTOL STOOL FORM SCALE

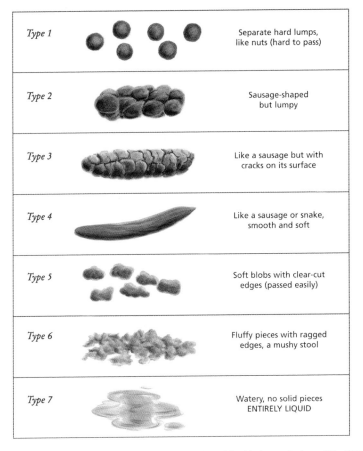

Type 1		Separate hard lumps, like nuts (hard to pass)
Type 2		Sausage-shaped but lumpy
Type 3		Like a sausage but with cracks on its surface
Type 4		Like a sausage or snake, smooth and soft
Type 5		Soft blobs with clear-cut edges (passed easily)
Type 6		Fluffy pieces with ragged edges, a mushy stool
Type 7		Watery, no solid pieces ENTIRELY LIQUID

Figure 11.1 Bristol Stool Form Chart. Reproduced by kind permission of Dr K.W. Heaton, Reader in Medicine at the University of Bristol. © 2000 Norgine Ltd.

9 Hydration status (e.g. evaluation of mucous membranes and skin turgor).
10 Perianal or peristomal skin integrity.
11 Stool cultures for bacterial, fungal and viral pathogens.
12 Patient's preferences and own coping strategies including non-pharmacological interventions and their effectiveness.
(Taylor 1997; Hogan 1998; Cadd *et al.* 2000; Kornblau *et al.* 2000; King 2002; Chelvanayagam & Norton 2004.)

Management

Once the cause of diarrhoea has been established, management should be focused on resolving the cause of the diarrhoea and providing physical and psychological support for the patient. Most cases of chronic diarrhoea will resolve once the underlying condition is treated, e.g. drug therapy for Crohn's disease, or with dietary management for coeliac disease. Episodes of acute diarrhoea, usually caused by bacteria or viruses, generally resolve spontaneously and are managed by symptom control and the prevention of complications (Shepherd 2000).

All episodes of acute diarrhoea must be considered potentially infectious until proved otherwise. The risk of spreading the infection to others can be reduced by adopting universal precautions such as wearing of gloves, aprons and gowns, disposing of all excreta immediately and, ideally, nursing the patient in a side room with access to their own toilet (King 2002). Advice should always be sought from infection control teams.

The prevention and/or correction of dehydration is the first step in managing an episode of diarrhoea. Simple steps to encourage patients to drink include:

- Providing drinks to suit individual taste preferences.
- Adding ice to drinks.
- Ice-lollies.
- Using china cups or glass instead of plastic or polystyrene cups.

Dehydration can be corrected by using oral rehydration solutions, or by intravenous fluids and electrolytes.

Antimotility drugs such as loperamide or codeine phosphate may be useful in some cases, for example in blind loop syndrome and radiation enteritis. These drugs reduce gastrointestinal motility to relieve the symptoms of abdominal cramps and reduce the frequency of diarrhoea (Shepherd 2000). It is important to rule out any infective agent as the cause of diarrhoea before using any of these drugs as they may make the situation worse by slowing the clearance of the infective agent (Taylor 1997). Occasionally intractable diarrhoea may be reduced by a subcutaneous infusion of octreotide, but this is more commonly indicated in patients with a high output of diarrhoea from a stoma (Fallon & O'Neill 1997).

Preserving the patient's privacy and dignity is essential during episodes of diarrhoea. The nurse has an important role in minimizing the patient's distress by adjusting language and using terms that are appropriate to the individual to reduce embarrassment (Smith 2001) and by listening to the patient's preference for care (Cadd *et al.* 2000).

It is important that the patient has easy access to clean toilet and washing facilities and that requests for assistance are answered promptly. Skin care is also essential to prevent bacteria present in faecal matter from destroying the skin's cellular defences and causing skin damage. This is particularly important with diarrhoea since it has high levels of faecal enzymes that come into contact with the perianal skin (Le Lievre 2002). The anal area should be gently cleaned with warm water immediately after every episode of diarrhoea (Taylor 1997). Soap should be avoided, unless it is an emollient, to avoid excessive drying of the skin and gentle patting of the skin is preferred for drying to avoid friction damage. Talcum powder should not be used and barrier creams should be applied sparingly, gently layered on in the direction of the hair growth rather than rubbed into the skin (Le Lievre 2002).

Constipation

Constipation occurs when there is either a failure of colonic propulsion (slow colonic transit), or a failure to evacuate the rectum (rectal outlet delay) or a combination of these problems (Norton 1996a; Teahon 1999; Norton 2006). The management of constipation depends on the cause and there are numerous possible causes, with many patients being affected by more than one causative factor (Figure 11.2). While constipation is not life-threatening it does cause a great deal of distress and discomfort. Particularly, constipation can be associated with abdominal pain or cramps, feelings of general malaise or fatigue and feelings of bloatedness. Nausea, anorexia, headaches, confusion, restlessness, retention of urine, faecal incontinence and halitosis may also be present in some cases (Norton 1996b; Maestri-Banks 1998).

It has been estimated that up to 27% of a given population experience constipation (Cook *et al.* 1999; Longstreth *et al.* 2006). There is a lack of consensus amongst both health care professionals and the general public as to what actually constitutes constipation (Perdue 2005; Norton 2006). Over recent years a set of international criteria (Rome Criteria) have been developed and recently revised (Longstreth *et al.* 2006) which can help to more accurately and consistently define constipation. According to the new Rome III Criteria an individual who is diagnosed with constipation should report having at least two of the following symptoms within the last 3 months where those symptoms began at least 6 months prior to diagnosis (Longstreth *et al.* 2006; Norton 2006.):

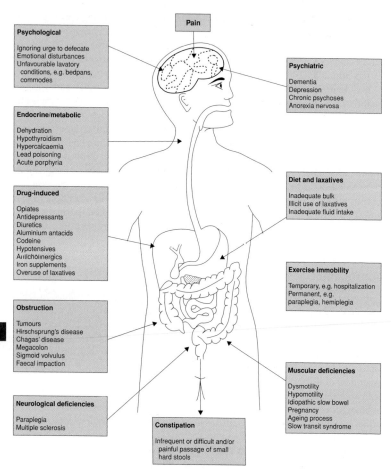

Figure 11.2   Classification of constipation: combined sources.

- Straining for at least 25% of the time.
- Lumpy or hard stool for at least 25% of the time.
- A sensation of incomplete evacuation for at least 25% of the time.
- A sensation of anorectal obstruction or blockage for at least 25% of the time.
- Manual manoeuvres used to facilitate defecation at least 25% of the time (e.g. manual evacuation).

- Less than three bowel movements a week.
- Also, in such patients loose stools are rarely present without the use of laxatives.

The myth of daily bowel evacuation being essential to healthy living has persisted through the centuries. It is thought that less than 10% of the population has a bowel evacuation daily (Edwards *et al.* 2003). This myth has resulted in laxative abuse becoming one of the commonest types of drug abuse in the Western world. The annual cost to the National Health Service (NHS) of prescribing medications to treat constipation is in the region of $45 million (DH 2005a). An individual's bowel habit is dictated by their diet, lifestyle and environment, and the notion of what is a 'normal' bowel habit varies considerably. Studies have revealed that in the USA and UK 95–99% of people pass at least three stools per week (Ehrenpreis, 1995) and normal bowel movement has been defined as ranging between three times a day and three times a week (Nazarko 1996). Given that there is such a wide normal range it is important to establish the patient's usual bowel habit and the changes that may have occurred.

Assessment

It is of vital importance that nurses adopt a proactive preventative approach to the assessment and management of constipation. Kyle *et al.* (2005a) have recently developed the Eton Scale, a constipation risk assessment tool. Whilst testing of the tool's sensitivity and reliability is still being carried out, it highlights the key risk factors that should be considered and provides advice and suggested actions according to the individual's level of risk. There are a variety of factors that may affect normal bowel functioning which should be considered within an assessment, including:

- Nutritional intake/recent changes in diet.
- Fluid intake.
- Mobility, e.g. lack of exercise.
- Medication, e.g. analgesics, antacids, iron supplements, tricyclic antidepressants.
- Lack of privacy, e.g. having to use shared toilet facilities, commodes or bedpans.
- Medical condition, including disease process or symptoms, e.g. cancer, vomiting.
- Radiological investigations of the bowel involving the use of barium.
- Change in patient's normal routine/lifestyle/home circumstances.
- Change in psychological status, e.g. depression.

(Fallon & O'Neill, 1997; Maestri-Banks 1998; Christer *et al.* 2003; Edwards *et al.* 2003; Thompson *et al.* 2003; Kyle *et al.* 2005a.)

In addition to the identification of these risk/contributing factors, it is important to take a careful history of a patient's bowel habits, taking particular note of the following:

1   Any changes in the patient's usual bowel activity. How long have these changes been present and have they occurred before?
2   Frequency of bowel action.
3   Volume, consistency and colour of the stool. Stools can be graded using a scale such as the Bristol Stool Form Chart (see Figure 11.1) where constipation would be classified as types 1 or 2 (Longstreth *et al.* 2006).
4   Presence of mucus, blood, undigested food or offensive odour.
5   Presence of pain or discomfort on defecation.
6   Use of oral or rectal medication to stimulate defecation and its effectiveness.

A digital rectal examination can also be performed, providing the nurse has received suitable training or instruction, to assess the contents of the rectum and to identify conditions which may cause discomfort such as haemorrhoids or anal fissures (Winney 1998; Hinrichs & Huseboe 2001; Peate 2003; RCN 2006).

Management

The effective treatment of constipation relies on the cause being identified by thorough assessment, as described above. Constipation can be categorized as primary, secondary or iatrogenic (Perdue 2005). Factors that lead to the development of primary constipation are extrinsic or lifestyle-related and include:

- An inadequate diet (low fibre).
- Poor fluid intake.
- A lifestyle change.
- Ignoring the urge to defecate.

Constipation that is attributed to an intrinsic, disease process or conditions such as anal fissures, colonic tumours or hypercalcaemia is classified as secondary constipation, whereas iatrogenic constipation generally results from treatment or medication (Perdue 2005). Constipation of unknown cause must be investigated in order to ensure that appropriate treatment is instigated (Taylor 1997; Teahon 1999).

Dietary manipulations may help to resolve mild constipation, although it is much more likely to help prevent constipation from recurring. Increasing dietary fibre increases stool bulk, which in turn improves peristalsis and stool transit time. This results in a softer stool being delivered to the rectum (Norton 1996b). The Government's strategy on food and health (DH 2005b) aims to increase the UK average daily fibre intake from the current 13.8 g to 18.0 g (this recommended amount is based on the Englyst method [DH 1998; British Nutrition Foundation 2004]). There are two types of fibre: insoluble is contained in foods such as wholegrain bread, brown rice, fruit and vegetables and soluble is contained in foods such as oats, pulses, beans and lentils. It is recommended that fibre should be taken from a variety of both soluble and insoluble foods and eaten at times spread throughout the day (Teahon 1999; Edwards *et al.* 2003; British Nutrition Foundation 2004; Food Standards Agency 2006). Care should be taken to increase dietary fibre intake gradually as bloating and abdominal discomfort can result from a sudden increase, particularly in the older person and those with slow-transit constipation (Cummings 1994; Norton 1996a; Bush 2000; Edwards *et al.* 2003). Other sources of dietary laxatives can be encouraged with care, for example prunes contain diphenylisatin and onions contain indigestible sugars (Norton 1996a).

Dietary changes need to be taken in combination with other lifestyle changes. Daily fluid intake should be between 2.0 and 2.5 litres (Taylor 1997; Teahon 1999; Day 2001). Fruit juices such as orange and prune juice can help stimulate bowel activity (Winney 1998) and coffee has been shown to stimulate colonic motor and bowel activity (Brown *et al.* 1990; Addison 1999a). The motor response takes place within minutes of drinking coffee and can last for up to 90 minutes (Addison 2000a). There is a need for further studies to examine the role of dietary manipulations in the management of constipation, particularly the function of dietary fibre and fluid intake (Addison 2000b).

Patients should be advised not to ignore the urge to defecate and to allow sufficient time for defecation (Norton 1996a). It is important that the correct posture for defecation is adopted; crouching or a 'crouch like' posture is considered anatomically correct (Taylor 1997) and the use of a foot stool by the toilet may enable patients to adopt a better defecation posture (Norton 1996a; Taylor 1997; Edwards *et al.* 2003). The use of the bedpan should always be avoided if possible as the poor posture adopted while using a bedpan has been shown to cause extreme straining during defecation (Taylor 1997). Patients should be supported with pillows to enable them to achieve an upright position if the use of a bedpan is unavoidable.

Where possible patients should be encouraged to increase their level of exercise; physical activity has been found to have a positive effect on peristalsis, particularly after eating (Thompson *et al.* 2003). Therapies such as homeopathy and reflexology can also be utilized (Emly *et al.* 1997; Rankin-Box 2000; Edwards *et al.* 2003). However, overall laxatives are the most commonly used treatment for constipation (Table 11.1). In general they should be used as a short-term measure to help relieve an episode of constipation as long-term use can perpetuate constipation and a dependence on laxatives can develop (Butler 1998).

Table 11.1 Types of laxative.

Type of laxative	Example	Brand names and sources
Bulk producers	Dietary fibre Mucilaginous polysaccharides Methylcellulose	Bran, wholemeal bread, Fybogel (ispaghula), Normacol (sterculia)
Stool softeners	Synthetic surface active agents, liquid paraffin	Agarol, Dioctyl, Petrolager, Milpar
Osmotic agents	Sodium, potassium and magnesium salts	Magnesium sulphate, milk of magnesia, lactulose
Stimulant laxatives	Sodium picosulphate, glycerin	Senna, Senokot, bisacodyl, Dulcolax, co-danthrusate, Picolax, glycerol

Laxatives

Laxatives can be defined simply as substances that cause evacuation of the bowel by a mild action (Mosby 2006). A laxative with a mild or gentle effect is also known as an aperient and one with a strong effect is referred to as a cathartic or a purgative. Purgatives should be used only in exceptional circumstances, i.e. where all other interventions have failed, or when they are prescribed for a specific purpose. The aim of laxative treatment is to achieve comfortable rather than frequent defecation and, wherever possible, the most natural means of bowel evacuation should be employed with preference given to use of oral laxatives where appropriate (Fallon & O'Neill 1997; Perdue 2005). The many different types of laxatives available may be grouped into four types according to the action they have (see Table 11.1).

Bulking agents

Bulking agents are usually the first line of laxative treatment and work by retaining water and promoting microbial growth in the colon, increasing faecal mass and stimulating peristalsis (Peate 2003). Ispaghula husk (Isogel, Regulan) and sterculia (Normacol) both trap water in the intestine by the formation of a highly viscous gel which softens faeces, increases weight and reduces transit time (Butler 1998). These agents need plenty of fluid in order to work (2–3 litres per day), so their appropriateness should be questioned for those with advanced cancer, or for the older patient (Maestri-Banks 1998; Hinrichs & Huseboe 2001; Perdue 2005). They also take a few days to exert their effect (Maestri-Banks 1998) and so are not suitable to relieve acute constipation. Also, they are contraindicated in some patients, including those who have bowel obstruction, faecal impaction, acute abdominal pain, reduced muscle tone, or those who have had recent bowel surgery. Increasing the bulk may worsen impaction, lead to increased colonic faecal loading or even intestinal obstruction (Norton 1996a), and in some cases may increase the risk of faecal incontinence. Other potentially harmful effects include malabsorption of minerals, calcium, iron and fat-soluble vitamins, and reduced bioavailability of some drugs (Taylor 1997). Another problem initially is that bulk laxatives tend to distend the abdomen, often making the individual feel full and uncomfortable. Sometimes this leads to temporary anorexia (Taylor 1997).

Stool softeners

Stool softening preparations, such as docusate sodium and glycerol (glycerin) suppositories act by lowering the surface tension of faeces which allows water to penetrate and soften the stool (Hinrichs & Huseboe 2001; Peate 2003). They may also have a weak stimulatory effect (Barrett 1992), but drugs of this type are often given in combination with a chemical stimulant (Shepherd 2000). Softening agents usually take 1–3 days to work (Day 2001).

Liquid paraffin acts as a lubricant as well as a stool softener by coating the faeces and allowing easier passage. However, its use should be avoided as there are a number of problems associated with this preparation. The use of liquid paraffin interferes with the absorption of fat-soluble vitamins and can also cause skin irritation, changes to the bowel mucosa and accidental inhalation of droplets of liquid paraffin may result in lipoid pneumonia (Maestri-Banks 1998; Peate 2003; BNF 2007).

415

Osmotic agents

These may be divided into two subgroups: lactulose and magnesium preparations. Lactulose is a synthetic disaccharide which exerts an osmotic effect in the small bowel. Distension of the small bowel induces propulsion which in turn reduces transit time. Colonic bacteria metabolize lactulose into a short chain organic salt which is then absorbed; therefore the osmotic effect does not continue throughout the colon (Barrett 1992). This process of metabolism also produces gas which in turn stimulates colonic movements and increases bacterial growth. This results in increased stool weight and thus colonic transit time is shortened (Spiller 1994). However, bowel action may still take up to 3 days to occur following administration (Shepherd 2000) and flatulence, cramps and abdominal discomfort are associated with high dosages. Magnesium preparations also exert an osmotic effect on the gut and additionally they stimulate the release of cholecystokinin. This encourages intestinal motility and fluid secretion (Nathan 1996). They have a rapid effect, working within 2–6 hours, so fluid intake is important with these preparations as patients may experience diarrhoea and dehydration (Hinrichs &

Huseboe 2001). These preparations should be avoided in patients with renal or hepatic impairment (Taylor 1997).

Stimulant laxatives

Laxatives including bisacodyl, danthron and senna stimulate the nerve plexi in the gut wall increasing peristalsis and promoting the secretion of water and electrolytes in the small and large bowel (Maestri-Banks 1998; Shepherd 2000; Peate 2003). Abdominal cramping may be increased if the stool is hard and a stool softener may be used in combination with this group of drugs (Taylor 1997; ABPI 1999). Long-term use of these laxatives should be avoided, except for patients on long-term opiates, as they may lead to impaired bowel function such as atonic non-functioning (cathartic) colon (Taylor 1997; ABPI 1999; Hinrichs & Huseboe 2001).

Preparations containing danthron are restricted to certain groups of patients, i.e. the elderly, the terminally ill and some cardiac patients, as some studies on rodents have indicated a potential carcinogenic risk (Taylor 1997; ABPI 1999; Shepherd 2000). Danthron preparations should not be used for incontinent patients, especially those with limited mobility, as prolonged skin contact will colour the skin pink or red and superficial sloughing of the discoloured skin will occur (Taylor 1997; ABPI 1999).

416 Enemas

Definition

An enema is the administration of a substance in liquid form into the rectum, either to aid bowel evacuation or to administer medication (Higgins 2006). Administration requires skill and knowledge from the practitioner and adherence to the Nursing and Midwifery Council (NMC) (2008a) *Standards for Medicines Management*.

Indications

Enemas may be prescribed for the following reasons:

- To clean the lower bowel before surgery; X-ray examination of the bowel using contrast medium or before endoscopy examination.
- To treat severe constipation when other methods have failed.
- To introduce medication into the system.
- To soothe and treat irritated bowel mucosa.
- To decrease body temperature (due to contact with the proximal vascular system).

- To stop local haemorrhage.
- To reduce hyperkalaemia (calcium resonium).
- To reduce portal systemic encephalopathy (phosphate enema).

Contraindications

Enemas are contraindicated under the following circumstances:

- In paralytic ileus.
- In colonic obstruction.
- Where the administration of tap water or soap and water enemas may cause circulatory overload, water intoxication, mucosal damage and necrosis, hyperkalaemia and cardiac arrhythmias.
- Where the administration of large amounts of fluid high into the colon may cause perforation and haemorrhage.
- Following gastrointestinal or gynaecological surgery, where suture lines may be ruptured (unless medical consent has been given).
- Frailty.
- Proctitis.
- The use of micro-enemas and hypertonic saline enemas in patients with inflammatory or ulcerative conditions of the large colon.
- Recent radiotherapy to the lower pelvis unless medical consent has been given (Davies 2004).

417

Reference material

Types of enemas

Evacuant enemas

An evacuant enema is a solution introduced into the rectum or lower colon with the intention of it being expelled, along with faecal matter and flatus, within a few minutes. The osmotic activity increases the water content of the stool so that rectal distension follows and induces defecation by stimulating rectal motility (Barrett 1992; Roe 1994).

The following solutions are often used:

- Phosphate enemas with standard or long rectal tubes in single-dose disposable packs. Although these are often used for bowel clearance before X-ray examination and surgery, there is little evidence to support their use due to the associated risks and contraindications. Davies (2004) and Bowers (2006) highlight the risk of phosphate absorption resulting from pooling of the enema due to lack of evacuation and also the risk of rectal injury caused by the enema tip. Studies have found that if evacuation does not occur, patients may suffer from hypovolaemic shock, renal failure and oliguria. When using this type of enema it is vital that good fluid intake is encouraged and maintained.

- Dioctyl sodium sulphosuccinate 0.1%, sorbitol 25% in single-dose disposable packs, are used to soften impacted faeces.
- Sodium citrate 450 mg, sodium alkylsulphoacetate 45 mg, sorbic acid 5 mg in single-dose disposable packs.

Retention enemas

A retention enema is a solution introduced into the rectum or lower colon with the intention of being retained for a specified period of time. Two types of retention enema are in common use:

- Arachis oil (may be obtained in a single-dose disposable pack). This needs to be used cautiously as it is contraindicated in patients with peanut allergies (Day 2001).
- Prednisolone.

Enemas containing arachis oil enhance the lubricating process, as well as softening impacted faeces (Butler 1998). These work by penetrating faeces, increasing the bulk and softness of stools. They work most effectively when warmed to body temperature and retained for as long as possible (Clarke 1988).

All types of enemas need to be prescribed and checked against the prescription before administration. It is essential that the implications and procedure are fully explained to the patient, so as to relieve anxiety and embarrassment.

418

Procedure guidelines   Enema administration

. . . .

Equipment

1 Disposable incontinence pad.
2 Disposable gloves.
3 Topical swabs.

4 Lubricating jelly.

5 Rectal tube and funnel (if not using a commercially prepared pack).
6 Solution required or commercially prepared enema.

. . . .

Procedure

Action	Rationale
1 Explain and discuss the procedure with the patient.	To ensure that the patient understands the procedure and gives his/her valid consent (NMC 2006: C; NMC 2008b: C).

. . . .

2 Ensure privacy.	To avoid unnecessary embarrassment to the patient (P).
3 Allow patient to empty bladder first if necessary.	A full bladder may cause discomfort during the procedure (Higgins 2006: E).
4 Ensure that a bedpan, commode or toilet is readily available.	In case the patient feels the need to expel the enema before the procedure is completed (P).
5 Warm the enema to room temperature by immersing in a jug of hot water.	Heat is an effective stimulant of the nerve plexi in the intestinal mucosa. An enema at room temperature or just above will not damage the intestinal mucosa. The temperature of the environment, the rate of fluid administration and the length of the tubing will all have an effect on the temperature of the fluid in the rectum (E).
6 Assist the patient to lie on the left side, with knees well flexed, the upper higher than the lower one, and with the buttocks near the edge of the bed.	This allows ease of passage into the rectum by following the natural anatomy of the colon. In this position gravity will aid the flow of the solution into the colon. Flexing the knees ensures a more comfortable passage of the enema nozzle or rectal tube (Higgins 2006: E).
7 Place a disposable incontinence pad beneath the patient's hips and buttocks.	To reduce potential infection caused by soiled linen. To avoid embarrassing the patient if the fluid is ejected prematurely following administration (P).
8 Wash hands with bactericidal soap and water or bactericidal alcohol handrub, and put on disposable gloves.	To minimize the risk of cross-infection (DH 2005c: C).
9 Place some lubricating jelly on a topical swab and lubricate the nozzle of the enema or the rectal tube.	This prevents trauma to the anal and rectal mucosa which reduces surface friction (Higgins 2006: E).

Procedure guidelines *(cont.)*

10 Expel excessive air from enema and introduce the nozzle or tube slowly into the anal canal while separating the buttocks. (A small amount of air may be introduced if bowel evacuation is desired.)	The introduction of air into the colon causes distension of its walls, resulting in unnecessary discomfort to the patient. The slow introduction of the lubricated tube will minimize spasm of the intestinal wall (evacuation will be more effectively induced due to the increased peristalsis) (C).
11 Slowly introduce the tube or nozzle to a depth of 10.0–12.5 cm.	This will bypass the anal canal (2.5–4.0 cm in length) and ensure that the tube or nozzle is in the rectum (C).
12 If a retention enema is used, introduce the fluid slowly and leave the patient in bed with the foot of the bed elevated by 45° for as long as prescribed.	To avoid increasing peristalsis. The slower the rate at which the fluid is introduced the less pressure is exerted on the intestinal wall. Elevating the foot of the bed aids in retention of the enema by the force of gravity (C).
13 If an evacuant enema is used, introduce the fluid slowly by rolling the pack from the bottom to the top to prevent backflow, until the pack is empty or the solution is completely finished.	The faster the rate of flow of the fluid the greater the pressure on the rectal walls. Distension and irritation of the bowel wall will produce strong peristalsis which is sufficient to empty the lower bowel (Higgins 2006: E).
14 If using a funnel and rectal tube, adjust the height of the funnel according to the rate of flow desired.	The forces of gravity will cause the solution to flow from the funnel into the rectum. The greater the elevation of the funnel, the faster the flow of fluid (E).
15 Clamp the tubing before all the fluid has run in.	To avoid air entering the rectum and causing further discomfort (E).
16 Slowly withdraw the tube or nozzle.	To avoid reflex emptying of the rectum (E).
17 Dry the patient's perineal area with a gauze swab.	To promote patient comfort and avoid excoriation (P).
18 Ask the patient to retain the enema for 10–15 minutes before evacuating the bowel.	To enhance the evacuant effect (C).

19 Ensure that the patient has access to the nurse call system, is near to the bedpan, commode or toilet, and has adequate toilet paper.

To enhance patient comfort and safety. To minimize the patient's embarrassment (P).

20 Remove and dispose of equipment.

To minimize risk of cross-infection (DH 2005c: C).

21 Wash hands.

To minimize risk of cross-infection (DH 2005c: C)

22 Record in the appropriate documents that the enema has been given, its effects on the patient and its results (colour, consistency, content and amount of faeces produced, using the Bristol Stool Form Chart [see Figure 11.1]).

To monitor the patient's bowel function (Gill 1999: C).

23 Observe patient for any adverse reactions (Peate 2003).

To monitor the patient for complications (Peate 2003: C).

Problem solving: Enema administration

Problem	Cause	Suggested action
Unable to insert the nozzle of enema pack or rectal tube into the anal canal.	Tube not adequately lubricated. Patient in an incorrect position. Patient apprehensive and embarrassed about the situation. Patient unable to relax anal sphincter.	Apply more lubricating jelly. Ask the patient to draw knees up further towards the chest. Ensure adequate privacy and give frequent explanations to the patient about the procedure. Ask the patient to take deep breaths and 'bear down' as if defecating (E).
Unable to advance the tube or nozzle into the anal canal.	Spasm of the canal walls.	Wait until spasm has passed before inserting the tube or nozzle more slowly, thus minimizing spasm. Ask patient to take slow deep breaths to help to relax (E).

Problem solving *(cont.)*

Problem	Cause	Suggested action
Unable to advance the tube or nozzle into the rectum.	Blockage by faeces.	Withdraw tubing slightly and allow a little solution to flow and then insert the tube further.
	Blockage by tumour.	If resistance is still met, stop the procedure and inform a doctor (E).
Patient complains of cramping or the desire to evacuate the enema before the end of the procedure.	Distension and irritation of the intestinal wall produce strong peristalsis sufficient to empty the lower bowel.	Stop instilling the enema fluid and wait with the patient until the discomfort has subsided (E).
Patient unable to open bowels after an evacuant enema.	Reduced neuromuscular response in the bowel wall.	Inform the doctor that the enema was unsuccessful and reassure the patient (E).

Suppositories

422

Definition

A suppository is a medicated solid formulation that melts at body temperature when inserted into the rectum (Moppett & Parker 1999).

Indications

The use of suppositories is indicated under the following circumstances:

- To empty the bowel prior to certain types of surgery and investigations.
- To empty the bowel to relieve acute constipation or when other treatments for constipation have failed.
- To empty the bowel before endoscopic examination.
- To introduce medication into the system.
- To soothe and treat haemorrhoids or anal pruritus.

Contraindications

The use of suppositories is contraindicated when one or more of the following pertain:

- Chronic constipation, which would require repetitive use.
- Paralytic ileus.
- Colonic obstruction.
- Malignancy of the perianal region.
- Low platelet count.
- Following gastrointestinal or gynaecological operations, unless on the specific instructions of the doctor.

Reference material

Administration of suppositories

The use of suppositories dates back to about 460 BC. Hippocrates recommended the use of cylindrical suppositories of honey smeared with ox gall (Hurst 1970). The torpedo-shaped suppositories commonly used today came into being in 1893, when it was recommended that they were inserted apex (pointed end) first (Moppett 2000).

This practice has been questioned by Abd-el-Maeboud *et al.* (1991) who suggest that suppositories should be inserted blunt end first. This advice is based on anorectal physiology; if a suppository is inserted apex first the circular base distends the anus and the lower edge of the anal sphincter fails to close tightly. The normal squeezing motion (reverse vermicular contraction) of the anal sphincter therefore fails to drive the suppository into the rectum. These factors can lead to anal irritation and expulsion of the suppository (Moppett 2000). The study by Abd-el-Maeboud *et al.* (1991) remains the only research evidence supporting this practice. Whilst their work demonstrated that patients found insertion and retention of suppositories much easier and more comfortable using the base-first method, the isolated nature of this research means that manufacturers' instructions continue to recommend apex end first. Therefore this area of practice remains somewhat unclear: the Abd-el-Maeboud *et al.* (1991) study, coupled with the anatomical and physiological rationale would imply that blunt end first is preferential.

There are several different types of suppository available. Retention suppositories are designed to deliver drug therapy, e.g. analgesia, antibiotic, non-steroidal anti-inflammatory drug (NSAID). Those designed to stimulate bowel evacuation include glycerine, bisacodyl and sodium bicarbonate. Lubricant suppositories, e.g. glycerine, should be inserted directly into the faeces and allowed to dissolve. They have a mild irritant action on the rectum and also act as faecal softeners (BNF 2007). However, stimulant types, such as bisacodyl, must come into contact with the mucous membrane of the rectum if they are to be effective as they release carbon dioxide causing rectal distension and thus evacuation.

423

Procedure guidelines Suppository administration

Equipment

1 Disposable incontinence pad.
2 Disposable gloves.
3 Topical swabs or tissues.
4 Lubricating jelly.

5 Suppository(ies) as required (check prescription before administering a medicinal suppository, e.g. aminophylline).

Procedure

Action

1 Explain and discuss the procedure with the patient. If you are administering a medicated suppository, it is best to do so after the patient has emptied his/her bowels.

Rationale

To ensure that the patient understands the procedure and gives his/her valid consent (NMC 2006: C; NMC 2008b: C). To ensure that the active ingredients are not impeded from being absorbed by the rectal mucosa or that the suppository is not expelled before its active ingredients have been released (Moppett 2000: E).

2 Ensure privacy.

To avoid unnecessary embarrassment to the patient (P).

3 Ensure that a bedpan, commode or toilet is readily available.

In case of premature ejection of the suppositories or rapid bowel evacuation following their administration (P).

4 Assist the patient to lie on the left side, with the knees flexed, the upper higher than the lower one, with the buttocks near the edge of the bed.

This allows ease of passage of the suppository into the rectum by following the natural anatomy of the colon. Flexing the knees will reduce discomfort as the suppository is passed through the anal sphincter (Moppett 2000: E).

5 Place a disposable incontinence pad beneath the patient's hips and buttocks.

To avoid unnecessary soiling of linen, leading to potential infection and embarrassment to the patient if the suppositories are ejected prematurely or there is rapid bowel evacuation following their administration (E).

6 Wash hands with bactericidal soap and water or bactericidal alcohol handrub, and put on gloves.	To reduce the risk of cross-infection (DH 2005c: C).
7 Place some lubricating jelly on the topical swab and lubricate the blunt end of the suppository if it is being used to obtain systemic action. Separate the patient's buttocks and insert the suppository blunt end first, advancing it for about 2–4 cm. Repeat this procedure if a second suppository is to be inserted.	Lubricating reduces surface friction and thus eases insertion of the suppository and avoids anal mucosal trauma. Research has shown that the suppository is more readily retained if inserted blunt end first (Abd-el-Maeboud et al. 1991). (For further information, see Suppositories section, above.) The anal canal is approximately 2–4 cm long. Inserting the suppository beyond this ensures that it will be retained (Abd-el-Maeboud et al. 1991: R 2b).
8 Once suppository(ies) has been inserted, clean any excess lubricating jelly from the patient's perineal area.	To ensure the patient's comfort and avoid anal excoriation (Moppett 2000: E).
9 Ask the patient to retain the suppository(ies) for 20 minutes, or until he/she is no longer able to do so. If a medicated suppository is given, remind the patient that its aim is not to stimulate evacuation and to retain the suppository for at least 20 minutes or as long as possible.	This will allow the suppository to melt and release the active ingredients. Inform patient that there may be some discharge as the medication melts in the rectum (Henry 1999: E).
10 Remove and dispose of equipment. Wash hands.	To reduce risk of infection (DH 2005c: C).
11 Record that the suppository(ies) have been given, the effect on the patient and the result (amount, colour, consistency and content, using the Bristol Stool Chart [see Figure 11.1]) in the appropriate documents.	To monitor the patient's bowel function (Gill 1999: C).
12 Observe patient for any adverse reactions.	To monitor for any complictions (Peate 2003: E).

425

References and further reading

Abd-el-Maeboud, K.H., El-Naggar, T. & El-Hawi, E.M.M. (1991) Rectal suppositories: commonsense mode of insertion. *Lancet*, **338**, 798–800.

ABPI (1999) *ABPI Compendium of Data Sheets and Summaries of Product Characteristics 1999–2000*. Datapharm Publications, Leatherhead, Surrey.

Addison, R. (1999a) Practical procedures for nurses No. 37.1. Fluid intake and continence care. *Nurs Times*, **95**(49).

Addison, R. (1999b) Practical procedures for nurses No. 33.1. Digital rectal examination 1. *Nurs Times*, **95**(40).

Addison, R. (2000a) Fluid intake: how coffee and caffeine affect continence. *Nurs Times*, **96**(40) (Suppl), 7–8.

Addison, R. (2000b) Fluids, fibre and constipation. *Nurs Times*, **96**(31) (Suppl), 11–12.

Addison, R. & White, M. (2002) Spinal injury and bowel management. *Nurs Times*, **98**(4), 61.

Amir, I. *et al.* (1998) Bowel care for the individual with spinal cord injury: comparison of four approaches. *Spinal Med*, **21**(1), 21–4.

Barrett, J.A. (1992) Faecal incontinence. In: *Clinial Nursing Practice. The Promotion and Management of Continence* (ed. B. Roe). Prentice Hall, New York, pp. 196–219.

Basch, A. (1987) Symptom distress changes in elimination. *Semin Oncol Nurs*, **3**(4), 287–92.

Bell, S. (2004) Investigations and management of chronic diarrhoea in adults. In: *Bowel Continence Nursing* (eds C. Norton & S. Chelvanayagam). Beaconsfield Publishers, Beaconsfield, Bucks, pp. 92–102.

BNF (2007) *British National Formulary Volume 54; 1.6.3: Faecal Softeners*. BMJ Publishing and the Royal Pharmaceutical Society of Great Britain, London.

Bowers, B. (2006) Evaluating the evidence for administering phosphate enemas. *Br J Nurs*, **15**(7), 378–81.

British Nutrition Foundation (2004) Dietary fibre. www.nutrition.org.uk. Accessed 9/8/06.

Brown, S.R., Cann, P.A. & Read, N. (1990) Effect of coffee on distal colon function. *Gut*, **31**, 450–53.

Bush, S. (2000) Fluids, fibre and constipation. *Nurs Times*, **96**(31) (Suppl), 11–12.

Butler, M. (1998) Laxatives and rectal preparations. *Nurs Times*, **94**(3), 56–8.

Cadd, A. *et al.* (2000) Assessment and documentation of bowel care management in palliative care: incorporating patient preferences into the care regimen. *J Clin Nurs*, **9**, 228–35.

Campbell, T. & Lunn, D. (1999) Colorectal cancer. Part 3 patient care. *Prof Nurse*, **15**(2), 117–21.

Chelvanayagam, S. & Norton, C. (2004) Nursing assessment of adults with faecal incontinence. In: *Bowel Continence Nursing* (eds C. Norton & S. Chelvanayagam). Beaconsfield Publishers, Beaconfield, Bucks, pp. 45–62.

Christer, R., Robinson, L. & Bird, C. (2003) Constipation: causes and cures. *Nurs Times*, **99**(25), 26–7.

Clarke, B. (1988) Making sense of enemas. *Nurs Times*, **84**(30), 40–4.

Cook, T. *et al.* (1999) The conservative management of constipation in adults. *J Assoc Chart Physiother Women's Health*, **85**, 24–8.

Crawshaw, A. (2004) How to establish a rectal irrigation service. *Gastrointest Nurs*, **2**(2), 29–31.

426

Cummings, J.H. (1994) Non-starch polysaccharides (dietary fibre) including bulk laxatives in constipation. In: *Constipation* (eds M.A. Kamm & J.E. Lennard-Jones). Wrightson Biomedical, Petersfield, Hampshire, pp. 307–314.

Davies, C. (2004) The use of phosphate enemas in the treatment of constipation: use of laxatives. *Br J Nurs*, **12**(19), 1130–6.

Day, A. (2001) The nurse's role in managing constipation. *Nurs Stand* **16**(8), 41–4.

DH (1998) *Nutritional Aspects of the Development of Cancer. Report on Health and Social Subjects 48*. HMSO, London.

DH (2005a) *Prescription Cost Analysis: England 2004*. HMSO, London.

DH (2005b) *Choosing a Better Diet: A Food and Health Action Plan*. HMSO, London.

DH (2005c) *Saving Lives: Delivery Programme to Reduce Healthcare Associated Infection including MRSA*. Department of Health, London.

DH (2005d) *Hazardous waste (England) regulations*. Department of Health, London.

Edwards, C., Dolman, M. & Horton, N. (2003) Down, down and away! An overview of adult constipation and faecal incontinence. In: *Promoting Continence. A Clinical and Research Resource* (eds K. Getliffe & E. Dolman), 2nd edn. Bailliere Tindall, London, pp. 185–226.

Ehrenpreis, E.D. (1995) Definitions and epidemiology of constipation. In: *Constipation. Etiology, Evaluation and Management* (eds S.D. Wexner & D.C.C. Bartolo). Butterworth Heinemann, Philadelphia, pp. 3–8.

Emly, M., Wilson, L. & Darby, J. (1997) Abdominal massage for adults with learning disabilities. *Nurs Times*, **97**(30) (Suppl), 61–2.

Fallon, M. & O'Neill, B. (1997) Clinical review. ABC of palliative care: constipation and diarrhoea. *BMJ*, **315**, 1293–6.

Food Standards Agency (2006) Starchy foods – fibre. www.eatwell.gov.uk/healthydiet/nutritionessentials/starchfoods/. Accessed 9/8/06.

Gardiner, A. (2004) Rectal irrigation for relief of functional bowel disorders. *Nurs Stand*, **19**(9), 39–42.

Gill, D. (1999) Practical procedures for nurses. Stool specimen assessment, Part 1: Assessment. *Nurs Times*, **96**, 26.

Harrison, P. (2000) *HDU/ICU Managing Spinal Injury: Critical Care*. Spinal Injuries Association, London.

Henry, C. (1999) The advantages of using suppositories. *Nurs Times*, **95**(17), 50–51.

Higgins, D. (2006) How to administer an enema. *Nurs Times*, **102**(20), 24–5.

Hinrichs, M. & Huseboe, J. (2001) Research-based protocol: management of constipation. *J Gerontol Nurs*, **27**(2), 17–28.

Hogan, C.M. (1998) The nurse's role in diarrhoea management. *Oncol Nurs Forum*, **25**(5), 879–86.

Hurst, A. (1970) *Selected Writings of Sir Arthur Hurst (1989–1944)*. Ballantyne, Spottiswode.

King, D. (2002) Determining the cause of diarrhoea. *Nurs Times*, **98**(23) (Suppl), 47–8.

Kornblau, A. *et al.* (2000) Management of cancer treatment-related diarrhea: issues and therapeutic strategies. *J Pain Symptom Manage*, **19**(2), 118–29.

Kyle, G. *et al.* (2005a) The Eton Scale: a tool for risk assessment for constipation. *Nurs Times*, **101**(18 Suppl), 50–1.

Kyle, G., Oliver, H. & Prynn, P. (2005b) *The Procedure for the Digital Removal of Faeces. Guidelines 2005.* Norgine, Uxbridge, UK.

Le Lievre, S. (2002) An overview of skin care and faecal incontinence. *Nurs Times,*, **98**(4) (Suppl), 58–9.

Longstreth, G.F. *et al.* (2006) Functional bowel disorders. *Gastroenterology*, **130**, 1480–91.

Maestri-Banks, A. (1998) An overview of constipation – causes and treatment. *Int J Palliat Nurs*, **4**(6), 271–5.

Moppett, S. (2000) Which way is up for a suppository? *Nurs Times*, **96**(19 Suppl), 12–13.

Moppett, S. & Parker, M. (1999) Insertion of a suppository. (Practical procedures for nurses, part 29). *Nurs Times*, **95**(23), supplement.

Mosby (2006) *Mosby's Dictionary of Medicine, Nursing and Health Professions.* Mosby Elsevier, St. Louis, MO.

NANDA-I (2007) *Nursing Diagnoses: Definitions and Classifications 2007–2008.* North American Nursing Diagnosis Association International, Philadelphia.

Nathan, A. (1996) Laxatives. *Pharm J*, **257**, 52–5.

Nazarko, L. (1996) Preventing constipation in older people. *Prof Nurse*, **11**(12), 816–18.

Nicol, M., Barin, C., Bedford-Turner, S. (2000) *Essential Nursing Skills.* Mosby International, Edinburgh.

NMC (2006) *A–Z Advice Sheet Consent.* www.nmc.org.

NMC (2008a) *Standards for Medicines Management.* Nursing and Midwifery Council, London.

NMC (2008b) *The Code: Standards of Conduct, Performance and Ethics for Nurses and Midwives.* Nursing and Midwifery Council, London.

Norton, C. (1996a) The causes and nursing management of constipation. *Br J Nurs*, **5**(20), 1252–8.

Norton, C. (1996b) *Nursing for Continence*, 2nd edn. Beaconsfield Publishers, Beaconsfield, Bucks.

Norton, C. (2006) Constipation in older patients: effects on quality of life. *Br J Nurs*, **15**(4), 188–92.

Peate, I. (2003) Nursing role in the management of constipation: use of laxatives. *Br J Nurs*, **12**(19), 1130–6.

Perdue, C. (2005) Managing constipation in advanced cancer care. *Nurs Times*, **101**(21), 36–40.

Petticrew, W. (1997) Treatment of constipation in older people. *Nurs Times*, **93**(48), 55–6.

Powell, M. & Rigby, D. (2000) Management of bowel dysfunction: evacuation difficulties. *Nurs Stand*, **14**(47), 47–54.

Rankin-Box, D. (2000) An alternative approach to bowel disorders. *Nurs Times*, **96**(19 Suppl), 24–5.

RCN (2006) *Digital Rectal Examination and Manual Removal of Faeces: Guidance for Nurses.* Royal College of Nursing, London.

Rigby, D. (2003) Manual evacuation of faeces. *Nurs Times*, **99**(1) (Suppl), 48.

Roe, B. (1994) *Clinical Nursing Practice: The Promotion and Management of Continence.* Prentice Hall, New York.

Shepherd, M. (2000) Treating diarrhoea and constipation. *Nurs Times*, **96**(6) (Suppl), 15–16.

Smith, S. (2001) Evidence-based management of constipation in the oncology patient. *Eur J Oncol Nurs*, **5**(1), 18–25.

Spiller, R.C. (1994) *Diarrhoea and Constipation*. Libra Pharmaceuticals, Petroc Press, Reading, Berks.

Taylor, C. (1997) Constipation and diarrhoea. In: *Nursing in Gastroenterology* (eds L. Bruce & T.M.D. Finlay). Churchill Livingstone, Oxford, pp. 27–54.

Teahon, E. (1999) Constipation. In: *Essential Coloproctology for Nurses* (eds T. Porret & N. Daniel). Whurr, London, pp. 206–221.

Thibodeau, G. & Patton, K.T. (2007) *Anatomy and Physiology*, 6th edn. Mosby Elsevier, St Louis, MO.

Thompson, M.J. *et al.* (2003) Management of constipation. *Nurs Stand*, **18**(14–16), 41–2.

Tortora, G.A. & Derrickson, B. (2008) *Principles of Anatomy and Physiology*, 12th edn. John Wiley & Sons, New York.

Walsh, M. (1997) *Watson's Clinical Nursing and Related Sciences*, 5th edn. Bailliere Tindall, London.

Weisner, P. & Bell, S. (2004) Bowel dysfunction: assessment and management in the neurological patient. In: *Bowel Continence Nursing* (eds C. Norton & S. Chelvanayagam). Beaconsfield Publishers, Beaconsfield, Bucks.

Weller, B. (1989) *Encyclopaedic Dictionary of Nursing and Health Care*. Bailliere Tindall, Eastbourne.

Winney, J. (1998) Constipation. *Nurs Stand*, **13**(11), 49–56.

Withell, B. (2000) A protocol for treating acute constipation in the community setting. *Br J Community Nurs*, **5**(3), 110–17.

Wood, S. (1996) Nutrition and the short bowel syndrome. In: *Stoma Care Nursing: A Patient-Centred Approach* (ed. C. Myres). Edward Arnold, London, pp. 79–89.

Multiple choice questions

1 Acute diarrhoea can be described as:

   a Sudden onset lasting up to 24 hours
   b Gradual onset and lasts up to 1 week
   c Sudden onset lasting up to a month
   d Sudden onset lasting less than 2 weeks

2 Chronic diarrhoea may have complex origins which may include:

   a Dietary, e.g. too much fruit or alcohol
   b Bowel disease, e.g. ulcerative colitis, Crohn's disease
   c Bacterial infection
   d Antibiotic related

3 If a patient is admitted with diarrhoea of unknown cause if possible they should be nursed in:

   a An open ward near the nurses' station
   b A side room with access to a toilet
   c A 4-bedded bay near the toilet
   d Any of the above

4 Constipation can be categorized as primary, secondary or iatrogenic. Primary causes are:

   a Inadequate diet and poor fluid intake
   b Ignoring the urge to defecate and lifestyle change
   c A lifestyle change and inadequate diet
   d Inadequate diet, poor fluid intake, lifestyle change, ignoring the urge to defecate

5 The daily recommended fluid intake to help maintain normal bowel habits is:

   a 3 litres
   b 3–3.5 litres
   c 1–1.5 litres
   d 2–2.5 litres

6 **Suppositories should be inserted:**

   a As quickly as possible
   b Pointed end first
   c Either way
   d Blunt end first

Answers to the multiple choice questions can be found in Appendix 3.

Chapter 12

Elimination: stoma care

Definition

'Stoma' is a word of Greek origin meaning 'mouth' or 'opening' (Taylor 2005). A bowel or urinary stoma is usually created by bringing a section of bowel out on to the abdominal wall as a diversionary procedure because the urinary or colonic tract beyond the position of the stoma is no longer viable.

Indications

Stoma care is required for the following purposes:

- To collect urine or faeces in an appropriate appliance.
- To achieve and maintain patient comfort and security.
- To maintain good skin and stoma hygiene (Black 1997).

Reference material

Types of stoma

Colostomy

A colostomy may be formed from any section of the large bowel (sigmoid, descending, transverse or ascending). Its position in the colon will dictate the output and consistency of faeces. Stomas formed in the sigmoid colon produce a semi-formed or formed stool; stoma formed higher in the colon will produce a more liquid stool. Colostomies may be permanent or temporary and either an 'end' or 'terminal' (Figure 12.1) or a defunctioning or loop colostomy (Figure 12.2). Temporary colostomies may be raised to divert the faecal output, either to allow healing of an anastomosis further along the colon, to relieve a distal obstruction or bowel injury, or to allow healing of colonic or rectoanal disease (Taylor 2005). With a defunctioning loop colostomy the colon

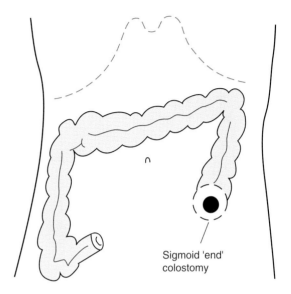

Figure 12.1   Sigmoid 'end' colostomy.

is exteriorized; a rod or bridge may be used to maintain a hold on the abdominal surface then the bowel is opened and mucocutaneous sutures are inserted to form the stoma (Black 2000b). Such a rod or bridge is usually removed
5–10 days after insertion (Figure 12.2). A further operation will be required to
close this stoma when it is no longer needed, i.e. when the anastomosed bowel
has healed. The term 'defunctioning' is used to indicate that the bowel distal
to the stoma is being rested (Borwell 1994; Myers 1996; Black 2000b; Taylor
2000).

Ileostomy

An ileostomy is formed when a section of ileum, usually the last 20 cm, is brought
out onto the abdominal wall, the ileum is everted to form a spout which allows the
effluent to drain into an appliance (Black 2000a) (Figure 12.2). Ileostomies may
be permanent (usually end) or temporary (usually loop). Temporary ileostomies
are often formed to allow healing of an anastomosis lower down in the bowel; to
allow healing of an ileo-anal pouch or to aid healing of diseased bowel (Taylor
2005). It is important that the proximal (active) side of a loop ileostomy has
a spout to enable the effluent to drain into an appliance. Rods or bridges may

433

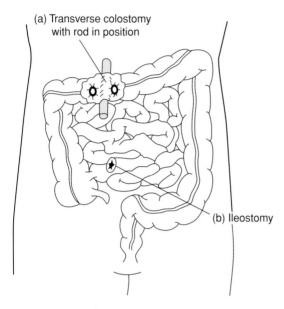

Figure 12.2   (a) Transverse colostomy and (b) ileostomy.

be used as with loop colostomies. In some cases of ulcerative colitis, the whole colon (total colectomy) may be removed; these patients may have an ileal–anal pouch constructed. To form these pouches the terminal ileum is fashioned into a reservoir and brought down and attached to the anus.

Urostomy (ileal loop, ileal conduit, colonic conduit)

A urostomy is formed when the bladder is removed or diseased. A section of ileum is isolated, along with its mesentery vessels, the remaining ends of the ileum are anastamosed to restore continuity. The isolated section is mobilized, the proximal end is closed and the ureters, once resected from the bladder, are implanted at this end. The distal end is brought out on to the surface of the abdominal wall and everted to form a spout (Figure 12.3) as in an ileostomy (Fillingham & Fell 2004; Black 2000b). Although urostomies are usually formed from ileum, the colon may also be utilized (Fillingham & Fell 2004). Urine from a urostomy will contain mucus from the bowel used in its construction (Taylor 2005).

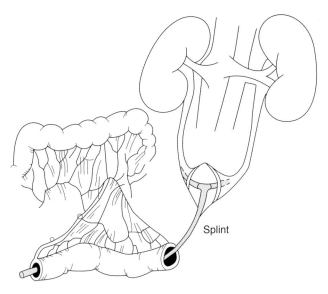

Figure 12.3 Urostomy.

Other types of urinary diversion

Other types of urinary diversion include ureterostomy, a procedure that brings the ureters out onto the abdominal wall together (one stoma) or separately (two stomas). This may be a permanent or temporary procedure, it may be used for ill patients with poor renal function and when less extensive abdominal surgery is indicated. Stomas formed in this way are often small and flush to the abdomen. They are prone to stenosis and it is often difficult to maintain a leak-proof appliance (Fillingham & Fell 2004). It may be possible for some patients with bladder disease to have a continent diversion. For further information on these continent urinary diversions, see Chapter 16, Professional edition.

Indications for bowel stoma

- Cancer of the bowel.
- Cancer of the pelvis.
- Trauma.
- Neurological damage.

435

- Congenital disorders.
- Ulcerative colitis.
- Crohn's disease.
- Diverticular disease.
- Familial polyposis coli.
- Intractable incontinence.
- Fistula.
- Radiation enteritis.

Indications for urinary stoma

- Cancer of the bladder.
- Cancer of the pelvis.
- Trauma.
- Congenital disorders.
- Neurological damage.
- Fistula.
- Intractable incontinence (Black 1994a; Taylor 2005).

Preoperative preparation, assessment and care

Physical preparation of the patient will vary according to the type of operation and the policies of individual surgeons and hospitals. This will involve the usual preparation for anaesthesia (see Chapter 22), preparation of the area of the body involved and of the bowel. Other specific procedures may also be included (Winkley 1998).

Psychological preparation of the individual facing stoma surgery should begin as soon as surgery has been considered, preferably by utilizing the skills of a trained stoma care nurse. Boore (1978), Hayward (1978), Ivimy (1997) and Beddows (1997) have illustrated the importance of preoperative information and explanation in reducing postoperative physical and psychological stress. It is important that the information and discussions are tailored to the individual's needs, taking into account their level of anxiety and distress (Borwell 1997c). Ongoing assessment of the patient's understanding of the information given should be carried out and documented.

Information-giving and discussion with patients about their stoma and lifestyle start preoperatively and continue throughout the patient's stoma experience. Preoperatively patients want information about the proposed surgical procedure and on a number of practical issues about living with a stoma including diet; lifestyle and work; appearance of stoma; stoma appliances and how to obtain them; relationships and sexual function (Kelly & Henry 1992). The aims of these interactions are as follows:

436

1 To help the individual with a stoma to return to his/her previous place in society whenever possible.

2 To help in the process of adapting to a changed body image. Patients' involvement with preoperative decision making positively influences their postoperative adjustment (Price 1990; Salter 1997; Black 2000a; Brown & Randle 2005).

3 To reduce anxiety. The patient's perception of life with a stoma may have a positive or detrimental influence on rehabilitation. Exploration of their understanding of stomas may reveal misunderstandings and commonly held myths which can be corrected. Patients may be aware of others in their social network who have a stoma: it is important to discuss their perceptions of these ostomates (Salter 1992; Bryant 1993; Brown & Randle 2005).

4 To explain that the presence of a stoma itself need not adversely affect any previous quality of life such as hobbies, work, social life or any other interests, although the underlying disease which has led to the stoma might (Salter 1992).

5 To prepare the patient for the appearance and likely behaviour pattern of the stoma (Pullen 1998; Cronin 2005).

6 To reassure patients that they will be able to manage an appliance whatever the environment (Salter 1995).

7 To assure patients that they will be supported fully while in hospital and that continuing support will be available in the community (Salter 1995; Pullen 1998).

Such preoperative education has been shown to increase co-operation and trust and reduce anxiety, the length of time the patient remains in hospital and the amount of postoperative analgesia required (Wade 1989). Family and/or close friends may also be involved, when appropriate, on agreement with the patient (Price 1996).

It is important to determine whether a patient will be able to manage a stoma by assessing the following:

- Visual capability.
- Manual dexterity.
- Physical limitations/disabilities, e.g. Parkinson's disease, arthritis, loss of an upper limb.
- Skin conditions.
- Abnormal contours, e.g. the changes that occur with spina bifida.
- Mental state, including previous psychiatric disorders, coping strategies, attitudes to body/stoma, memory.
- Sociocultural, e.g. occupation, social and sporting activities, family and social support, culture and religion.

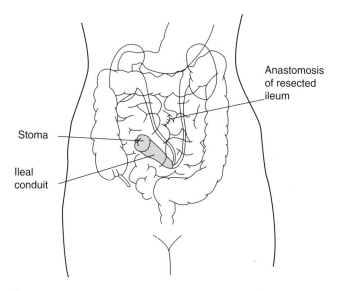

Figure 12.4   Position of stoma.

Siting of the stoma is one of the most important preoperative tasks to be carried out by the doctor, stoma care nurse or ward nurse with appropriate knowledge and skills (Figures 12.4 & 12.5). This minimizes future difficulties such as interference by the stoma with clothes, or skin problems caused by leakage of the appliance due to a badly sited stoma (e.g. on the waistline or in a body crease) (Bass *et al.* 1997; Erwin-Toth & Barrett 1997; Qin & Bao-Min 2001). When siting the stoma, consideration should be given to the following:

1   A flat area of the skin to facilitate safe adhesion of the appliance.
2   Avoidance of bony prominences such as hips and ribs which may interfere with the adhesion of the appliance, or pendulous breasts which may obscure the stoma from the patient's view, making self-care impossible.
3   Avoidance of skin creases, especially in the region of the groin or the umbilicus, to avoid urine or faecal matter tracking along the skin creases.
4   Avoidance of scars, which may cause skin creases that may lead to leakages.
5   Avoidance of waistline or belt areas, as patient's clothing may put pressure on the stoma which may lead to leaks or trauma.

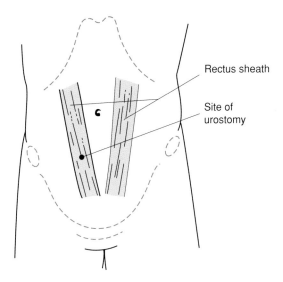

Figure 12.5   Site of urostomy.

6   Maintenance of the stoma within the rectus sheath, as this reduces the risk of herniation later (Myers 1996; Erwin-Toth & Barrett 1997; Sjodahl *et al.* 1998). The muscle may be identified by asking the patient to lie flat, then to raise the head. The muscle may also be palpated and easily felt when the patient coughs.

7   Ideally, the patient should be able to see the stoma site (Blackley 1998).

The patient must be observed while lying, sitting in a comfortable chair, with the abdominal muscles relaxed, and standing (Erwin-Toth & Barrett 1997). Consideration must be given to any bending or lifting involved with the patient's work and any other activities in which the patient partakes. Account must also be taken of any weight gain or loss in the postoperative period, as this may change the contours of the abdomen and hence the position of the stoma.

Personnel who may be expected to provide information

- Medical staff.
- Stoma care nurse.
- Nursing staff on ward.
- Primary health care team.

- Another suitable ostomate. 'Visitors' are trained by the voluntary associations and, ideally, should be of similar age, sex and background to the patient to enable the patient to discuss problems of adapting to life with a stoma (Rheaume & Gooding 1991; Mowdy 1998).

Useful aids

- Information booklets.
- Samples of the various appliances.
- Diagrams.
- Audio tapes.
- DVDs.

These aids are valuable to reinforce and clarify the verbal information.

Postoperative period

Stoma function

Colostomy function

In the first few days a sigmoid colon stoma will produce haemaserous fluid and wind. By day 5 there should be some faecal fluid and then by day 7–14 semi-formed stool (Cottam 1999). A closed appliance may be used. In the case of a stoma formed in the transverse colon, only a small amount of water will be reabsorbed from the faecal matter, so the faecal matter will be unformed. This means a drainable pouch will need to be used.

Patients with a sigmoid colostomy may find that wholemeal foods assist in producing a formed stool once or twice daily (Myers 1996; Black 1998). Medications that reduce peristaltic action, e.g. codeine phosphate, may also be used to control diarrhoea. The only means of controlling a sigmoid colostomy, however, is by regular irrigation or by use of a Conseal plug system. Stoma care nurses will need to assess patients before teaching them how to perform the irrigation procedure or to use Conseal plugs.

Ileostomy function

For the first few days the stoma will produce haemaserous fluid and wind. By days 5–10 there will be brown faecal matter (Cottam 1999). The fluid output after surgery can be as much as 1500 ml/24 hours but this will gradually reduce to 500–850 ml/24 hours as the bowel settles down (Black 2000a). Sometimes the output from a stoma remains high (>1000 ml/24 hours), which may be due to the amount of small bowel removed at surgery or an underlying bowel condition; these patients require careful management. It is important that fluid balance recordings are made and serum electrolyes are measured as they are at risk of sodium and/or magnesium depletion (Burch 2004). Patients with high output stoma may need to be managed by specialist teams which include gastroenterologists, dietitians and stoma care nurses. The effluent takes on a porridge-like consistency when a normal intake of food is established. A drainable appliance is therefore used. The effluent contains enzymes, which will excoriate the skin, therefore if the pouch leaks it must be changed promptly to prevent skin breakdown. The effluent cannot be controlled and is often more active after meals (Myers 1996; Black 1997). Sometimes medication, e.g. codeine or loperamide, which reduces peristaltic action, may be used to control excessive watery output.

Urostomy/ileal conduit function

Urine will dribble from the stoma every 20–30 seconds and it starts draining immediately. Normal output is 1500 ml/24 hours (Cottam 1999), but may be less after periods of reduced fluid intake, e.g. at night. Urinary stents (fine-bore catheters) may be in place from the ureters past the anastomosis and out of the stoma. They are placed to maintain patency and protect the suturing until primary healing is completed (Black 2000b). Stents are left in situ for 7–10 days.

Irrigation

Irrigation is a method of controlling the output of a colostomy by means of washing out the stoma with warm tap water (with the use of a coned irrigation set), every 24–48 hours.

The advantage of successful colostomy irrigation is that there is no stool leakage between irrigations (Davis 1996; Black 2000b). Patients who wish to use irrigation will be taught how to do it by their stoma care nurses.

Postoperative stages

441

Stage I

In theatre, an appropriately sized transparent drainable appliance should be applied, which should be left on for approximately 2 days. For the first 48 hours postoperatively, the stoma should be observed for signs of ischaemia or necrosis, the stoma colour (a pink and healthy appearance indicates a good blood supply), size and stoma output should be noted, as should the presence of any devices, i.e. ureteric stents, or bridge with a loop stoma (Kirkwood 2006). The drainable appliance should always be emptied frequently, gas should be allowed to escape and the appliance should not be allowed to get more than half full with effluent. If the appliance becomes too full, leaks may occur and the weight from the effluent or the pressure from gas may cause the appliance to fall off (Black 1997). A leak-proof, odour resistant well-fitted appliance at this time does much to promote patient confidence (Kirkwood 2006). The first time a bowel stoma acts the type, appearance, quantity and consistency of the matter passed should be recorded; this includes any flatus that may be passed (Kirkwood 2006).

Immediately postoperatively patients would not be expected to perform their own stoma care but would be encouraged to observe the nurse caring for them and discuss it with the nurse. During appliance changes observations should be made of:

- Stoma: colour, size and general appearance, i.e. oedematous, flush with abdomen, retracted.
- Peristomal skin: presence of any erythema, broken areas, rashes.
- Stoma/skin margin (mucocutaneous margin): sutures intact, tension on sutures, separation of stoma edge from skin (mucocutaneous separation).

Any abnormalities should be reported to the stoma care nurse and medical staff (Black 2000b; Burch 2004; Kirkwood 2006).

Viewing the stoma may be difficult for the patient, who may be very aware of other people's reaction to it (Price 1993). The patient's reaction to their stoma should be observed and recorded.

Stage II

As the patient's condition improves they should be encouraged to participate in the care of their stoma. A demonstration change of the appliance should be given with a full explanation of the principles of stoma care. This will be followed by further opportunities to discuss any problems or raise new queries. Care procedures should be divided into small successive stages and patients should be given support to work through these stages until they are able to take on the care of their stoma. Provided the patient agrees, it is useful to involve the patient's partner or close friends or relatives at this stage. Their acceptance of the stoma may encourage the patient and help to restore the patient's self-esteem (Salter 1995). They may now be ready to discuss appliances and choose the one that they wish to use at home. Preparation for discharge will be discussed (Black 1994b; Heywood Jones 1994).

Stage III

Ideally, the patient should now be independent, eating a normal diet, be ready for discharge and should be competent in stoma care.

If the family or close friends are closely involved during all stages and are supportive, patients are better able to adapt to the threat of mutilating surgery and altered pattern of elimination (Price 1993). The family or close friends are also likely to require support and information so that they are in a position to help the ostomate. Acceptance of the stoma is a gradual process and, on discharge from hospital, patients may only be beginning to adapt to life with a stoma (Salter 1997).

Specific discharge plans

Follow-up support

The patient is discharged with adequate supplies until a prescription is obtained from the general practitioner. Written reminders are provided of how to care for the stoma, how to obtain supplies of appliances, and any other information that may be required. The patient should have details of non-medical stoma clinics, details about the relevant agencies and information about voluntary associations. Arrangements should also have been made for a home visit from the stoma care nurse and/or the community nurse (Blackley 1998; Cronin 2005).

Obtaining supplies

All National Health Service (NHS) patients with a permanent stoma are entitled to free prescriptions for their stoma care products, and should complete the relevant forms for exemption from payment. Appliances can then be obtained from the local chemist, free home delivery services or directly from the appropriate manufacturers.

Diet

All patients should be encouraged to eat a wide variety of foods. Our digestive system reacts in an individual way to different foods and so it is important that patients try a wide range of foods on several occasions and that none should be specifically avoided (Bridgewater 1999). Patients can then make decisions about different foods based on their own experience of their own reaction. Explanations of how the gut functions, how it has been changed since surgery and the effects certain foodstuffs may cause should be given.

443

Colostomy and ileostomy formation means the loss of the anal sphincter so passage of wind cannot be controlled. High-fibre foods such as beans and pulses produce wind as they are broken down in the gut; hence individuals who eat large quantities of these foodstuffs may be troubled by wind. There are several non-food causes of wind, such as chewing gum, eating irregularly and drinking fizzy drinks, which should be considered before blaming a particular food (Bridgewater 1999). Eating yoghurt or drinking buttermilk may help reduce wind for these patients. Green vegetables, pulses and spicy food are examples of foods that may cause colostomy and ileostomy output to increase or become watery. Boiled rice, smooth peanut butter, apple sauce and bananas are some of the foods that may help thicken stoma output (Bridgewater 1999; Black 2000b).

Some foods, e.g. tomato skin and pips, may be seen unaltered in the output from an ileostomy (Hulten & Palselius 1996; Black 1997; Blackley 1998). Celery, dried fruit, nuts and potato skins are some of the foods which can temporarily block ileostomies (Bridgewater 1999; Black 2000b). The blockage is usually related to the amount eaten (Wood 1998). The offending food can be tried at another time in small quantities, ensuring it is chewed well and not eaten in a hurry (Bridgewater 1999).

There are no dietary restrictions with a urostomy. It must be stressed, however, that an adequate fluid intake must be maintained to minimize the risk of urinary tract infection. The recommended fluid intake for all individuals is 1.5–2.0 litres per day (Bridgewater 1999). Fluid intake should be increased in hot weather or at times when there is an increase in sweating, e.g. exercise, fever. Beetroot, radishes, spinach and some food dye may discolour urine; some drugs may also have this effect, e.g. metronidazole, nitrofurantoin. Urine may develop a strong odour following consumption of asparagus or fish (Bridgewater 1999).

Fear of malodour

This is a common fear for patients with bowel stomas, often based on hearsay or experience with other ostomists in hospital or the community. Appliances are odour free when fitted correctly. Flatus may be released via charcoal filters and deodorizers are available. The individual must be reassured, however, that any problems that occur postoperatively will be investigated, with a good possibility of their being solved by such means as the use of alternative appliances (Black 2000b; Burch 2004).

Sex and the ostomate

The possibility of sexual impairment for both men and women after stoma surgery depends on the nature of the operation, and the ensuing damage to the nerves and tissues involved. The psychological impact of the surgery and its effect on the individual's body image must also be taken into consideration. Surgery that results in physical sexual disability will have psychological repercussions, while some sexual difficulties may be of psychological origin (Salter 1996; Borwell 1997c; Black 2004). Impairment may be permanent or temporary. In the latter case, resolution of the difficulty may take anything up to 2 years. Pre- and postoperative counselling should be offered for both patient and partner.

All patients may experience loss of libido and sexual desire. Ejaculatory disturbances occur following cystectomy so men facing this surgery should be offered sperm banking prior to surgery. Erectile dysfunction is a common complication of pelvic surgery and there are a number of treatment options available. These include oral medications (sildenafil, tadalafil, vardenafil), sublingual apomorphine, intraurethral and intracavernosal aprosdadil, vacuum devices and penile implants (Ashford 1998; Newey 1998; Kirby *et al.* 1999).

Female patients may experience dyspareunia; this may be due to narrowing or shortening of the vagina, a reduction in the volume of vaginal secretions or changes in genital sensations (Schover 1986; Borwell 1999; Black 2004). The use of a lubricant, adopting different positions during lovemaking or encouraging greater relaxation by extending foreplay may help resolve painful intercourse (Bryant 1993; Borwell 1999; Black 2004).

Useful references on the psychological and sexual aspects of care may be found in Borwell (1997b, c), Huish *et al.* (1998), Wells (2000) and Heath and White (2001).

Stoma appliances and accessories

Many of the appliances now available are very similar in style, colour and efficiency and often there is very little to choose between them when the time comes for the ostomate to decide what to wear.

The aim of good stoma care is to return patients to their place in society (Black 1994b). One of the ways in which this can be facilitated is to provide them with a safe, reliable appliance. This means that there should be no fear of leakage or odour and the appliance should be comfortable, unobtrusive, easy to handle and disposable. The ostomate should be allowed a choice from the management systems available. It is also important to identify and manage problems with the stoma or peristomal skin early. When choosing the appropriate management system for the new ostomate, factors which need to be considered include:

- Type of stoma.
- Type of effluent.
- Patient's cognitive ability.
- Manual dexterity.
- Lifestyle.
- Condition of peristomal skin.
- Siting of stoma.
- Patient preference (Black 2000a; Kirkwood 2006).

445

Management systems available: pouches, plugs and irrigation

Pouches

Although some people whose stomas were created several years ago are wearing non-disposable rubber bags, most appliances used today are made from an odour-proof plastic film. These pouches usually adhere to the body by a hydrocolloid wafer or flange (Taylor 2000). Pouches may be opaque or clear and often have a soft backing to absorb perspiration. They usually have a built-in integral filter containing charcoal to neutralize any odour.

Choosing the right size

It is important that the flange of the appliance fits snugly around the stoma within 0.3 cm of the stoma edge (Kirkwood 2006). This narrow edge is left exposed so that the appliance does not rub on the stoma. Stoma appliances usually come with measuring guides to allow for choice of size. During the initial weeks following surgery the oedematous stoma will gradually reduce in size and the appliances will have to be changed accordingly.

Fear of malodour

Pouches usually have a built-in integral filter containing charcoal to neutralize any odour when flatus is released; therefore, smell is only noticeable when emptying or changing an appliance (Rudoni & Sica 1999). There are also various deodorizers available.These come in the form of drops or powders that may be put into the pouch or sprays, which can be sprayed into the air just before changing or emptying the pouch (Burch & Sica 2005). The individual should be reassured that any problems with odour or leakage will be investigated and that in most circumstances the problem will be solved with alternative appliances or accessories (Bryant 1993; Black 1997).

Types of pouch

The type of pouch used will depend on the type of stoma and effluent expected.

Closed pouches are mainly used when formed stool is expected, e.g. sigmoid colostomy (Figure 12.6c). These pouches have a flatus filter and need to be changed once or twice a day.

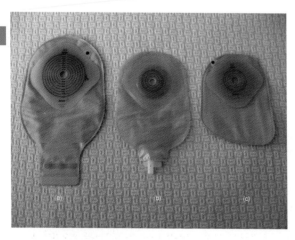

Figure 12.6 Stoma equipment. (a) Drainable bowel stoma pouch; (b) urostomy pouch; (c) closed bag.

Drainable pouches are used when the effluent is fluid or semi-formed, i.e. ileostomy or transverse colostomy (Figure 12.6a). These pouches have specially designed filters, which are less likely to become blocked or leak faecal fluid. These pouches need to be emptied regularly and the outlet rinsed carefully and then closed with a clip or 'roll-up' method. They may be left on for up to 3 days.

Urostomy pouches have a drainage tap for urine and should be emptied regularly (Figure 12.6b). They can be attached to a large bag and tubing for night drainage. These pouches can remain on for up to 3 days.

One- or two-piece systems

All types of pouch (closed, drainable or with a tap) as described above fall into one of two broad categories: one-piece or two-piece systems.

- **One-piece**. This comprises a pouch attached to an adhesive wafer that is removed completely when the pouch is changed. This is an easy system for an ostomate with dexterity problems, e.g. arthritis, peripheral neuropathy, to handle.
- **Two-piece**. This comprises a wafer onto which a pouch is clipped or stuck. It can be used with sore and sensitive skin because when the pouch is removed the flange is left intact and so the skin is left undisturbed.

Plug system

Patients with colostomies may be able to stop the effluent by inserting a plug into the stoma lumen. This plug swells in the moist environment and behaves as a seal. This system should only be introduced by a stoma nurse specialist (Taylor 2000).

447

Accessories

The specific products in this section have been mentioned as examples of what aids are available and reference to them is not necessarily intended as a recommendation.

Solutions for skin and stoma cleaning

Mild soap and water, or water only, is sufficient for skin and stoma cleaning. It is important that all soap residues are removed as they may interfere with pouch adhesion. Detergents, disinfectants and antiseptics cause dryness and irritation and should not be used. The stoma is not a wound or a lesion and should be regarded as a resited urethra or anus.

Skin barriers

1 **Creams:**

Unless made specifically for use on peristomal skin, creams should not be used, as the residual surface film of grease prevents adherence of the appliance. Creams usually have a soothing and moisturizing effect.

Use: For sensitive skin, as a protective measure.

Method: Use sparingly; massage gently into the skin until completely absorbed; excess grease may be wiped off with a soft tissue.

Example: Chiron barrier cream (aluminium chlorohydrate 2% in an emulsified base) (ABPI 1999).

Precaution: Not to be used on broken or sore skin.

2 **Protective films:**

Use: Act as a film on the skin, first to prevent irritation and, second, to give protection as it is removed with the adhesive of the bag, thus preventing removal of the stratum corneum of the skin. Most of the newer films do not contain alcohol so may be used on broken skin, although some of the older preparations do.

Method: Swab impregnated wipe or foam applicator on to skin; dries quickly. There is also a spray available.

Examples: Cavilon no sting barrier film, LBF, Skinsafe non-sting protective film.

Precaution: If preparation contains alcohol do not use on broken skin as it will cause stinging (ABPI 1999).

3 **Protective wafers:**

Use: These are hypoallergenic and are designed to cover and protect skin, and allow healing if the skin is sore or broken. They may be useful in cases of skin reaction or allergy to the adhesive or an appliance.

Method: The wafers may be cut with the aid of a template (pattern) to the required shape and fitted on to the skin. The appliances are then attached to the wafer. The rim of the wafer should not press against the stoma but should fit to 0.5 cm around it.

Examples: Stomahesive or Comfeel type of wafers. Stomahesive is composed of gelatin, pectin, sodium carboxymethylcellulose and polyisobutylene (Martindale 1993); it adheres painlessly to normal, erythematous, moist or broken skin; it is available in three sizes.

Precautions: Allergy may occur, but rarely.

4 **Seals/washers:**

Use: These are used to provide skin protection around the stoma; they will protect a smaller area than the wafers mentioned above. They are also useful to fill in 'dips' or 'gulleys' in the skin. They can be used to extend the wear time of an appliance when a stoma has a corrosive output which quickly breaks down the inner edge of a baseplate.

Method: Like the wafers, they have an adhesive side and may be applied directly to the skin. They form an integral part of some of the appliances.

Examples: Salts, cohesive seals, Dansac washers.

Precautions: As for protective wafers above.

5 **Pastes:**
Use: Useful to fill in crevices and 'gulleys' in the skin to provide a smooth surface for an appliance.

Method: Stomahesive: a syringe may be used to apply paste. Either leave for 60 seconds after applying to the skin, when the surface will be dry, making the paste easier to mould into the skin contour, or apply with a spatula, or wet the finger first to prevent the paste sticking and mould the paste immediately. It will sting on raw areas as it contains alcohol. Apply a little Orahesive powder to these areas first.

Examples: Stomahesive paste, soft paste.

6 **Protective paste:**
Use: To protect raw areas. Does not contain alcohol so will not cause irritation (useful for fistula problems). *Method*: Orabase, similar to Stomahesive paste in composition but with the addition of liquid paraffin. Liquid paraffin will inhibit adhesives sticking so care must be taken to ensure Orabase paste is not applied under appliances.

Example: Orabase paste.

449

7 **Powders:**
Use: For protection of sore or raw areas without impeding adhesion of the appliance.

Method: Sprinkle on affected areas.

Example: Orahesive powder.

8 **Adhesive preparations:**
Use: Only required when appliance does not adhere well to the skin, e.g. because of leakage, uneven site, or if abdominal fistulae present.

Method: The individual products differ considerably in their method of application and it is recommended that the user consults the manufacturer's instructions.

Example: Saltair solution.

9 **Adhesive removers:**

Use: If patient finds removing stoma appliance uncomfortable or residue from a hydrocolloid appliance is left on the peristoma skin.

Method: Swab skin with impregnate wipe at the edge of baseplate which should begin to lift; as baseplate lifts swab the skin under baseplate until baseplate has been removed or spray area.

Examples: Appeel wipes and spray, Lift wipes and bottle, Ostoclear sachets or spray.

Precaution: Some adhesive removers contain alcohol and therefore should not be used on broken skin. Those listed in the example do not contain alcohol (there are other non alcohol containing products available).

10 **Stoma baseplate securing tape:**

Uses: Used when baseplate is having difficulty in adhering fully such as with parastoma hernia, prolapsed stomas and badly sited stomas such as those near bony prominences.

Method: Apply to edge of baseplate that is having difficulty adhering.

Examples: Hydroframe, SecuPlast, Ostofix flange security tape.

11 **Thickening agents:**

Uses: To help solidify loose stoma output and so reduce pouch noise (Burch & Sica 2005).

Method: Place sachets, capsules or gel in pouch.

Examples: Morform sachet, Gel-X capsules, OstoSorb gel.

12 **Convex devices:**

Use: These devices are designed to be used with retracted stomas. The convex shape allows a greater seal round the stoma by filling in any crevices caused by retraction, scars or skin creases. The convexity pushes the peristomal skin down and causes the stoma to protrude a little. There is now a wide range of convex products available which all apply different levels of pressure to the peristoma skin. These include inserts, seals, soft convex flanges and rigid convex flanges.

Examples: Adapt ring Convex inserts, soft seal range of appliances, impression range of appliances.

Precautions: Changes to peristomal skin can result due to the result of convexity and patients should be taught to observe for this (Burch & Sica 2005). Bruising and ulceration are signs of skin damage (Wyss 2004); pyoderma gangrenosum is also associated with pressure on the peristomal skin due to convex appliances (Lyon & Beck 2001).

Deodorants

1 **Aerosols:**

Use: To absorb or mask odour.

Method: One or two puffs into the air before emptying or removing appliance.

Examples: Limone, Naturcare, FreshAire.

2 **Drops and powders:**

Use: For deodorizing bag contents.

Method: Before fitting pouch or after emptying and cleaning drainable pouch, squeeze tube two or three times.

Examples: Ostobon deodorant powder, Nodor S drops, Saltair No-roma.

Procedure guidelines Stoma care

These procedural guidelines contain the basic information needed for changing a stoma appliance. Modifications may be made according to the following factors:

1 The place of change, i.e. bathroom, bedside, availability of sink, etc.

2 The person changing the appliance, i.e. nurse, patient or carer.

3 Type of appliance used, e.g. one- or two-piece, closed or drainable.

4 Any accessories used, e.g. adhesive remover, barrier creams, seal/washer.

Equipment

1 Clean tray holding:
   (a) Tissues, wipes.
   (b) New appliance.
   (c) Measuring device/template.
   (d) Scissors.
   (e) Disposal bags for used appliances, tissues and wipes.
   (f) Relevant accessories, e.g. adhesive remover, protective film, seals/washers.
2 Bowl of warm water.
3 Soap (if desired).
4 Jug for contents of appliance.
5 Gloves. This practice should be explained to patients so that they do not feel it is just because they have a stoma that gloves are worn. (It is recognized that it could be difficult to attach an appliance with gloves in situ [due to adhesive], but once the stoma has been cleaned of excreta and blood, gloves may be removed to apply bag.)

Procedure

Action	Rationale
1 Explain and discuss the procedure with the patient.	To ensure that the patient understands the procedure and gives his/her valid consent (NMC 2006: C; NMC 2008: C). To familiarize the patient with the procedure.

Procedure guidelines (*cont.*)

2 Ensure that the patient is in a suitable and comfortable position where the patient will be able to watch the procedure, if well enough. A mirror may be used to aid visualization.

To allow good access to the stoma for cleaning and for secure application of the stoma bag. The patient will become familiar with the stoma and will also learn much about the care of the stoma by observation of the nurse (Bryant 1993: P).

3 Use a small protective pad to protect the patient's clothing from drips if the effluent is fluid and apply gloves for nurse's protection.

Avoids the necessity for renewing clothing or bedclothes and demoralization of the patient as a result of soiling (E).

4 If the bag is of the drainable type, empty the contents into a jug before removing the bag.

For ease of handling the appliance and prevention of spillage (E).

5 Remove the appliance. Peel the adhesive off the skin with one hand while exerting gentle pressure on the skin with the other.

To reduce trauma to the skin. Erythema as a result of removing the appliance is normal and quickly settles (Broadwell 1987: C).

6 Fold appliance in two to ensure no spillage and place in disposal bag.

To ensure safe disposal according to environmental policy (E; DH 2005b: C).

7 Remove excess faeces or mucus from the stoma with a damp tissue.

So that the stoma and surrounding skin are clearly visible (E).

8 Examine the skin and stoma for soreness, ulceration or other unusual phenomena. If the skin is unblemished and the stoma is a healthy red colour, proceed.

For the prevention of complications or the treatment of existing problems (E).

9 Wash the skin and stoma gently until they are clean.

To promote cleanliness and prevent skin excoriation (E).

10 Dry the skin and stoma gently but thoroughly.

The appliance will attach more securely to dry skin (E & C).

11	Measure the stoma, cut appliance leaving 3 mm clearance. Apply a clean appliance.	Appliance should provide skin protection. The aperture should be cut just a little larger than the stoma so that effluent can not cause skin damage This should be no more than 3 mm from the stoma (Kirkwood 2006: C).
12	Dispose of soiled tissues and the used appliance in a disposable bag and place it in an appropriate plastic bin. At home the bag should be placed in a plastic bag tied and disposed of in a rubbish bag.	To ensure safe disposal (E).
13	Wash hands thoroughly using bactericidal soap and water or bactericidal alcohol handrub.	To prevent spread of infection by contaminated hands.

Problem solving: Stoma care

Stoma

Problem	Cause	Suggested action
Leakage of urine or faeces	Ill-fitting appliance.	Remeasure stoma and ensure a snug-fitting appliance. Prepare template for future use.
	Skin creases or 'gulleys' preventing correct application of adhesive. Infrequent emptying of drainable bag leading to stress on adhesion.	Build up indented areas and fill in gulleys to create a smooth surface, e.g. using paste. Drainable bags should be emptied frequently, e.g. 2–3-hourly if necessary.
Sore skin	Leakage. Skin reaction to adhesive.	As above. Change to an appliance from another manufacturer or apply a protective square between skin and adhesive. Anti-inflammatory agents may be required for very severe reactions.
	Poor hygiene.	Improve the technique of nurses, patient or carers.

Problem solving *(cont.)*

Problem	Cause	Suggested action
Odour	Ill-fitting appliance; lack of seal between skin and adhesive. Poor hygiene. Poor technique, e.g. when emptying drainable bag.	Fit the appliance with care. Consider a change of the type of appliance. Improve the technique of nurses, patient or carers. Empty the bag, then rinse the end with water to ensure that it is clean before closing.

Urostomy specimen

Stoma specimen of urine contaminated. Ileum perforated during specimen collection.	Contaminants introduced during specimen collection. Catheter too hard or inserted too roughly.	Take a repeat specimen, observing aseptic procedure and cleaning the stoma well. Report to a doctor immediately.
Difficulty passing catheter into conduit.	Small degree of retraction of ileum.	Apply gentle pressure to the area around the stoma to make it protrude.
	Unpredictable direction of ileum.	Gently insert your little (gloved) finger into the stoma to determine the direction of the conduit. Insert the catheter tip along this line.

Useful addresses

Association for Spina Bifida and Hydrocephalus (ASBAH), 42 Park Road, Peterborough PE1 2UQ (Tel. 01733 555988), website: www.asbah.org.

Colostomy Association, 15 Station Road, Reading, Berkshire RG1 1LG (Tel. 0118 9391537 or 0800 5876744), website: www.colostomyassociation.org.uk.

IA (Ileostomy and Internal Pouch Support Group), Peremill House, 1–5 Mill Road, Ballyclare, Co. Antrim BT39 9DR (Tel. 028 9334 4043 or 0800 01847244).

Urostomy Association (The), Central Office, Foxglove Avenue, Uttoxeter, Staffs ST14 8UN (Tel. 08452412159), www.uagbi.org.

References and further reading

ABPI (1999) *Compendium of Data Sheets and Summaries of Product Characteristics 1999–2000*. Datapharm Publications, London.

Ashford, L. (1998) Erectile dysfunction. *Prof Nurse*, **13**(9), 603–8.

Bass, E.M. *et al.* (1997) Does preoperative stoma marking and education by the enterostomal therapist affect outcome? *Dis Colon Rectum*, **40**(4), 440–2.

Beddows, J. (1997) Alleviating pre-operative anxiety in patients: a study. *Nurs Stand*, **11**(37), 35–8.

Black, P. (2000a) Practical stoma care. *Nurs Stand*, **14**(41), 47–55.

Black, P. (2000b) *Holistic Stoma Care*. Bailliere Tindall, London.

Black, P.K. (1994a) Stoma care: a practical approach. *Nurs Stand*, **8**(34), RCN Nurs Update, Learning Unit 045.

Black, P.K. (1994b) Choosing the correct stoma appliance. *Br J Nurs*, **3**(11), 545–6, 548, 550.

Black, P.K. (1997) Practical stoma care. *Nurs Stand*, **11**(47), 49–55.

Black, P.K. (1998) Update. Colostomy. *Prof Nurse*, **13**(12), 851–7.

Black, P.K. (2004) Osychological, sexual and cultural issues for patients with a stoma. *Br J Nurs*, **13**(12), 692–7.

Blackley, P. (1998) *Practical Stoma, Wound and Continence Management*. Research Publications, Australia.

Boore, J.R.P. (1978) *A Prescription for Recovery: The Effect of Preoperative Preparation of Surgical Patients on Postoperative Stress, Recovery and Infection*. Royal College of Nursing, London.

Borwell, B. (1994) Colostomies and their management. *Nurs Stand*, **8**(45), CE article 332, 49–55.

Borwell, B. (1997a) Ileo-anal pouch surgery and its after-care. *Community Nurse*, **3**(7) 15–20.

Borwell, B. (1997b) The psychosexual needs of a stoma patient. *Prof Nurse*, **12**(4), 250–5.

Borwell, B. (1997c) Psychological considerations of stoma care nursing. *Nurs Stand*, **11**(48), 49–55.

Borwell, B. (1999) Sexuality and stoma care. In: *Stoma Care in the Community. A Clinical Resource for Practitioners* (ed. P. Taylor). Nursing Times Books, London, pp. 110–135.

Bridgewater, S.E. (1999) Dietary considerations. In: *Stoma Care in the Community. A Clinical Resource for Practitioners* (ed. P. Taylor). Nursing Times Books, London, pp. 187–202.

Broadwell, D.C. (1987) Peristomal skin integrity. *Nurs Clin North Am*, **22**(2), 321–32.

Brown, H. & Randle, J. (2005) Living with a stoma: a review of the literature. *J Clin Nurs*, **14**.

Bryant, R.A. (1993) Ostomy patient management: care that engenders adaptation. *Cancer Invest*, **11**(5), 565–77.

Burch, J. (2004) The management and care of people with stoma complications. *Br J Nurs*, **13**(6), 307–18.

Burch, J. & Sica, J. (2005) Stoma care accessories: an overview of a crowded market. *Br J Community Nurs*, **10**(1), 24–31.

Cottam, J. (1999) Recovering after stoma surgery (Know How series). *Community Nurse*, **5**(9), 24–5.

Cronin, E. (2005) Best practice in discharging patients with a stoma. *Nurs Times*, **101**(47), 67–8.

Davis, K. (1996) Irrigation technique. In: *Stoma Care Nursing – A Patient-Centred Approach* (ed. C. Myers). Arnold, London, pp. 136–145.

DH (2005a) *Saving Lives: A Delivery Programme to Reduce Healthcare Infection including MRSA*. Department of Health, London.

DH (2005b) *Hazardous waste (England) regulations*. Department of Health, London.

Erwin-Toth, P. & Barrett, P. (1997) Stoma site marking: a primer. *Ostomy Wound Manag*, **43**(4), 18–25.

Fillingham, S. & Fell, S. (2004) Urological stomas. In: *Urological Nursing*, (eds S. Fillingham & J. Douglas), 2nd edn. Bailliere Tindall, London, pp. 207–225.

Hayward, J. (1978) *Information – A Prescription Against Pain*. Royal College of Nursing, London.

Heath, H. & White, I. (2001) *The Challenge of Sexuality in Health Care*. Blackwell Science, London.

Heenan, A.L.J. (1996) Two piece stoma systems. *Prof Nurse*, **11**(5), 313–14.

Heywood Jones, I. (1994) Skills update. Stoma care. *Community Outlook*, **4**(12), 22–3.

Horn, S. (1991) Nursing patients with a continent urinary diversion. *Nurs Stand*, **4**(21), 24–6.

Huish, M., Kumar, D. & Stones, C. (1998) Stoma surgery and sex problems in ostomates. *Sex Marital Ther*, **13**(3), 311–28.

Hulten, L. & Palselius, I. (1996) Are dietary restrictions necessary for ileostomy surgery? *Eurostoma*, **13**, 20.

Ivimy, A. (1997) Postoperative recovery is influenced by preoperative care. *Eurostoma*, **17**, 8–9.

Kelly, L. (1995) Patients becoming people. *J Community Nurs*, **9**(8), 12–16.

Kelly, M.P. & Henry, T. (1992) A thirst for practical knowledge: stoma patients' opinions of the services they receive. *Prof Nurse*, **7**(6), 350–6.

Kirby, R., Carson, C. & Goldstein, I. (1999) *Erectile Dysfunction: A Clinical Guide*. Isis Medical Media, Oxford.

Kirkwood, L. (2006) Postoperative stoma care and the selection of appliances. *J Community Nurs*, **20**(3), 12–18.

Leaver, R. (1996) Continent urinary diversions: the Mitrafanoff principle. In: *Stoma Care Nursing – A Patient-Centred Approach* (ed. C. Myers). Arnold, London, pp. 166–79.

Lyon, C.C. & Beck, M.H. (2001) Dermatitis. In: *Abdominal Stomas and their Skin Disorders* (eds C.C. Lyon & A.J. Smith). Martin Duntitz, London, pp. 41–96.

Martindale (1993) *The Extra Pharmacopoeia* (ed. J.E.F. Reynolds), 13th edn. Pharmaceutical Press, London.

Mowdy, S. (1998) The role of the WOC nurse in an ostomy support group. *J Wound Ostomy Continence Nurs*, **25**, 51–4.

Myers, C. (1996) *Stoma Care Nursing – A Patient-Centred Approach*. Arnold, London.

Newey, J. (1998) Causes and treatment of erectile dysfunction. *Nurs Stand*, **12**(47), 39–40.

NMC (2006) *A–Z Advice Sheet Consent*. www.nmc.org.

NMC (2008) *The Code: Standards of Conduct, Performance and Ethics for Nurses and Midwives*. Nursing and Midwifery Council, London.

Ortiz, H. *et al.* (1993) Does the frequency of colostomy hernia depend on the colostomy location in the abdominal wall? *World Council Enterost Ther J*, **13**(2), 13–14.

Price, B. (1990) *Body Image Nursing: Concepts and Care*. Prentice Hall, New York.

Price, B. (1993) Profiling the high risk altered body image patient. *Senior Nurse*, **13**(4), 17–21.

Price, B. (1996) Practical support roles for relatives of stoma patients. *Eurostoma*, **16**, 10–11.

Pullen, M. (1998) Support role. *Nurs Times*, **94**(47).

Qin, W. & Bao-Min, Y. (2001) The relationship between site selection and complications in stomas. *World Council Enterost Ther*, **21**(2), 10–12.

Rheaume, A. & Gooding, B.A. (1991) Social support, coping strategies, and long term adaptation to ostomy among self-help group members. *J Enterost Ther*, **18**, 11–15.

Rudoni, C. & Sica, J. (1999) NaturCare from AlphaMed: the non-scented ostomy deodorant. *Br J Nurs*, **8**(17), 1168–70.

Salter, M. (1992) Body image: the person with a stoma, Part 1. *Wound Manage*, **2**(2), 8–9.

Salter, M. (1995) Guest editorial: some observations on body image. *World Council Enterost Ther*, **15**(3), 4–7.

Salter, M. (1996) Sexuality and the stoma patient. In: *Stoma Care Nursing – A Patient-Centred Approach* (ed. C. Myers). Arnold, London, pp. 203–219.

Salter, M. (1997) *Altered Body Image: The Nurse's Role*. Bailliere Tindall, London.

Schover, L.R. (1986) Sexual rehabilitation of the ostomy patient. In: *Ostomy Care and the Cancer Patient* (eds D.B. Smith & D.E. Johnson). Grune & Stratton, Orlando, pp. 103–19.

Sjodahl, R. *et al.* (1998) Parastoma hernias in relation to site of abdominal stoma. *Br J Surg*, **75**, 569–72.

Taylor, P. (2000) Choosing the right stoma appliance for a colostomy. *Nurse Prescrib Commun Nurse*, **6**(9), 35–8.

Taylor, P. (2005) An introduction to stomas: reasons for their formation. *Nurs Times*, **101**(29), 63–4.

Topping, A. (1990) Sexual activity and the stoma patient. *Nurs Stand*, **4**(41), 24–6.

Wade, B. (1989) Nursing care of the stoma patient. *Surg Nurse*, **2**(5), Suppl, ix–xii.

Wells, D. (2000) *Caring for Sexuality in Health and Illness*. Churchill Livingstone, London.

Willis, J. (1995) Stoma care principles and product type. *Nurs Times*, **91**(2), 43–5.

Winkley, M. (1998) Pre-operative fasting. *Nurs Times*, **94**(40), 56.

Wood, S. (1998) Nutrition and stoma patients. *Nurs Times*, **94**(48), 65–67.

Wyss, H. (2004) Retracted stoma and the optimisation of convex ostomy products. *World Council Enterost Ther J*, **24**(3), 26–8.

Multiple choice questions

1 **A colostomy may be formed from any section of:**

   a   Bowel
   b   Large bowel
   c   Ileum
   d   Ureters

2 **When siting a stoma the areas that should be avoided are:**

   a   Waistline or belt areas
   b   Bony prominences, skin crease or pendulous breasts
   c   Scars
   d   All of the above

3 **Following formation of a stoma these observations should be made:**

   a   Colour, size, general appearance.
   b   Colour, size, general appearance, state of peristomal skin
   c   Colour, size, general appearance, state of peristomal skin, stoma/skin margin
   d   Colour, size, drainage

4 **When deciding on a suitable management system for a new stoma the following need to be considered:**

   a   Type of stoma, type of effluent, manual dexterity
   b   Type of effluent, cognitive ability, manual dexterity, type of stoma, lifestyle
   c   Lifestyle, site of stoma, type of effluent, condition of peristomal skin, manual dexterity, cognitive ability, type of stoma, patient preference
   d   Patient preference, type of stoma, type of effluent, site of stoma, manual dexterity

5 The stoma and peristomal skin should be cleaned with:

   a   Sterile water
   b   0.9% sodium chloride
   c   Mild soap and water
   d   Antiseptic solution

6 Following discharge home patients with a stoma can obtain their supplies:

   a   From their local chemist
   b   Direct from the manufacturers
   c   Free from local chemist, free home delivery or direct from manufacturer
   d   From their local chemist and direct from manufacturer

Answers to the multiple choice questions can be found in Appendix 3.

Chapter 13

Elimination: urinary

Definition

'A catheter is a hollow tube that is used to remove fluid from, or instil fluid into, a body cavity or viscus' (Pomfret 1996, p. 245). Urinary catheterization is the insertion of a specially designed tube into the bladder using aseptic technique, for the purpose of draining urine, the removal of clots/debris, and the instillation of medication.

Indications

Male

In the male, urinary catheterization may be carried out for the following reasons:

- To empty the contents of the bladder, e.g. before or after abdominal, pelvic or rectal surgery and before certain investigations.
- To determine residual urine.
- To allow irrigation of the bladder.
- To bypass an obstruction.
- To relieve retention of urine.
- To introduce cytotoxic drugs in the treatment of papillary bladder carcinomas.
- To enable bladder function tests to be performed.
- To measure urinary output accurately, e.g. when a patient is in shock, undergoing bone marrow transplantation or receiving high-dose chemotherapy.
- To relieve incontinence when no other means is practicable.

Female

In the female, urinary catheterization may be carried out for the nine reasons listed above and for two further reasons:

- To empty the bladder before childbirth, if
- To avoid complications during the insertion
  sium) into the cervix/womb.

Reference material

Catheter selection

A wide range of urinary catheters are available, made
and with different design features. Careful assessmei _____ .ite
material, size and balloon capacity will ensure that _____ ._iected is as
effective as possible, that complications are minimized ._. that patient comfort
and quality of life are promoted (Pomfret 1996; Robinson 2001). Types of catheter
are listed in Table 13.1 and illustrated in Figure 13.1, together with their suggested
use. Catheters should be used in line with the manufacturer's recommendations,
in order to avoid product liability (RCN 1994).

Balloon size

In the 1920s, Fredrick Foley designed a catheter with an inflatable balloon to keep
it positioned inside the bladder. Balloon sizes vary from 2.5 ml for children to

Table 13.1   Types of catheter.

Catheter type	Material	Uses
Balloon (Foley) two-way catheter: two channels, one for urine drainage; second, smaller channel for balloon inflation	atex, PTFE coated latex, silicone elastomer coated, 100% silicone, hydrogel coated	Most commonly used for patients who require bladder drainage (short-, medium- or long-term)
Balloon (Foley) three-way irrigation catheter: three channels, one for urine; one for irrigation fluid; one for balloon inflation	atex, PTFE coated latex, silicone, plastic	To provide continuous irrigation (e.g. after prostatectomy). Potential for infection is reduced by minimizing need to break the closed drainage system (Gilbert & Gobbi 1989; Mulhall *et al.* 1993)
Non-balloon (Nelaton) or Scotts, or intermittent catheter (one channel only)	PVC and other plastics	To empty bladder or continent urinary reservoir intermittently; to instil solutions into bladder

PTFE, polytetrafluoroethylene; PVC, polyvinylchloride.

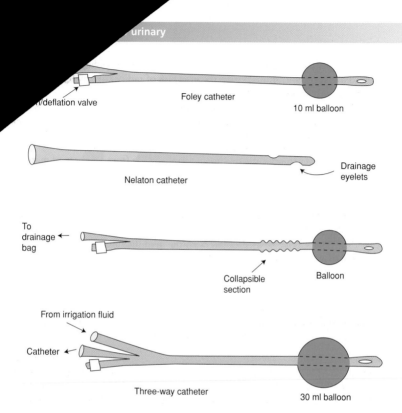

Foley catheter

10 ml balloon

Inflation/deflation valve

Nelaton catheter

Drainage
eyelets

To
drainage
bag

Collapsible
section

Balloon

From irrigation fluid

Catheter

Three-way catheter

30 ml balloon

Figure 13.1 Catheter types.

30 ml. The latter is used to aid haemostasis after prostatic surgery. Large balloon catheters (30 ml) weigh approximately 48 g, causing pressure on the bladder neck and pelvic floor and potential damage to these structures (Kristiansen *et al.* 1983; Pomfret 2000; Robinson 2001). These catheters are associated with leakage of urine, pain and bladder spasm as they can cause irritation to the bladder mucosa and trigone (Stewart 1998; Robinson 2001). Large balloons are inclined to sit higher in the bladder, allowing a residual pool of urine to collect below the balloon, providing a reservoir for infection (Getliffe 1996; Pomfret 2000).

Consequently, a 5–10 ml balloon is recommended for adults and a 3–5 ml balloon for children. Care should be taken to use the correct amount of water to fill the balloon because too much or too little may cause distortion of the catheter tip. This may result in irritation and trauma to the bladder wall consequently causing pain, spasm, bypassing and haematuria. If under inflated, one or more of the drainage eyes may become occluded or the catheter may become dislodged. Over inflation risks rupturing the balloon and leaving fragments of balloon inside the bladder (Pomfret 2000; Robinson 2001).

Catheter balloons ought to be filled only with sterile water. Tap water and 0.9% sodium chloride should not be used as salt crystals and debris may block the inflation channel, causing difficulties with deflation. Any micro-organisms which may be present in tap water can pass through the balloon into the bladder (Falkiner 1993; Stewart 1998).

Catheter size

Urethral catheters are measured in charrières (ch). The charrière is the outer circumference of the catheter in millimetres and is equivalent to three times the diameter. Thus a 12 ch catheter has a diameter of 4 mm.

Potential side-effects of large-gauge catheters include:

- Pain and discomfort.
- Pressure ulcers, which may lead to stricture formation.
- Blockage of paraurethral ducts.
- Abscess formation (Edwards *et al.* 1983; Crow *et al.* 1986; Roe & Brockle-hurst 1987; Blandy & Moors 1989; Winn 1998).

The most important guiding principle is to choose the smallest size of catheter necessary to maintain adequate drainage (McGill 1982). If the urine to be drained is likely to be clear, a 12 ch catheter should be considered. Larger gauge catheters may be necessary if debris or clots are present in the urine (Pomfret 1996; Winn 1998).

Length of catheter

463

There are three lengths of catheter currently available:

- Female length: 23–26 cm.
- Paediatric: 30 cm.
- Standard length: 40–44 cm.

The shorter female length catheter is often more discreet and less likely to cause trauma or infections because movement in and out of the urethra is reduced. Infection may also be caused by the longer catheter looping or kinking (Pomfret 2000; Robinson 2001). In obese women or those in wheelchairs, however, the inflation valve of the shorter catheter may cause soreness by rubbing against the inside of the thigh, and the catheter is more likely to pull on the bladder neck; therefore, the standard length catheter should be used (Pomfret 2000; Godfrey & Evans 2000; Evans *et al.* 2001).

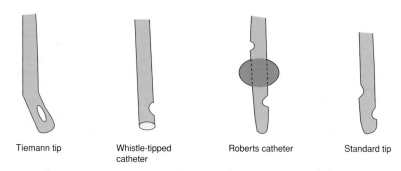

Tiemann tip   Whistle-tipped   Roberts catheter   Standard tip
                catheter

Figure 13.2   Catheter tips.

Tip design

Several different types of catheter tip are available in addition to the standard round tip (Figure 13.2). Each tip is designed to overcome a particular problem:

- The *Tieman-tipped catheter* has a curved tip with one to three drainage eyes to allow greater drainage. This catheter has been designed to negotiate the membranous and prostatic urethra in patients with prostatic hypertrophy.
- The *whistle-tipped catheter* has a lateral eye in the tip and eyes above the balloon to provide a large drainage area. This design is intended to facilitate drainage of debris, e.g. blood clots.
- The *Roberts catheter* has an eye above and below the balloon to facilitate the drainage of residual urine.

464

Catheter material

A wide variety of materials are used to make catheters. The key criterion in selecting the appropriate material is the length of time the catheter is expected to remain in place. Three broad timescales have been identified:

- Short-term (1–14 days).
- Short- to medium-term (2–6 weeks).
- Medium- to long-term (6 weeks–3 months).

Patients should be assessed individually as to the ideal time to change their catheters. The use of a catheter diary will help to ascertain a pattern of catheter blockages so changes can be planned accordingly.

The principal catheter materials are as follows.

1 *Polyvinylchloride (PVC)*. Catheters made from PVC or plastic are quite rigid. They have a wide lumen, which allows a rapid flow rate; however, their rigidity may cause some patients discomfort. They are mainly used for intermittent catheterization or postoperatively. They are recommended for short-term use only (Pomfret 1996).

2 *Latex*. Latex is a purified form of rubber and is the softest of the catheter materials. It has a smooth surface, with a tendency to allow crust formation. Latex absorbs water and consequently the catheter may swell, reducing the diameter of the internal lumen and increasing its external diameter (Pomfret 2000; Robinson 2001). It has been shown to cause urethral irritation (Wilksch *et al.* 1983) and therefore should only be considered when catheterization is likely to be short-term. Hypersensitivity to latex has been increasing in recent years (Woodward 1997) and latex catheters have been the cause of some cases of anaphylaxis (Young *et al.* 1994). Woodward (1997) suggests that patients should be asked whether they have ever had an adverse reaction to rubber products before catheters containing latex are utilized.

3 *Teflon (polytetrafluoroethylene [PTFE]) or silicone elastomer coatings*. A Teflon or silicone elastomer coating is applied to a latex catheter to render the latex inert and reduce urethral irritation (Slade & Gillespie 1985). Teflon or silicone elastomer coated catheters are recommended for short- or medium-term catheterization.

4 *All silicone*. Silicone is an inert material which is less likely to cause urethral irritation. Silicone catheters are not coated, and therefore have a wider lumen. The lumen of these catheters, in cross-section, is crescent or D-shaped, which may induce formation of encrustation (Pomfret 1996). Because silicone permits gas diffusion, balloons may deflate and allow the catheter to fall out prematurely (Studer 1983; Barnes & Malone-Lee 1986). These catheters may be more uncomfortable as they are more rigid than the latex-cored types (Pomfret 2000). All silicone catheters are suitable for patients with latex allergies. Silicone catheters are recommended for long-term use.

465

5 *Hydrogel coatings*. Catheters made of an inner core of latex encapsulated in a hydrophilic polymer coating have recently been developed. The polymer coating is well tolerated by the urethral mucosa, causing little irritation. Hydrogel coated catheters become smoother when rehydrated, reducing friction with the urethra. They are also inert (Nacey & Delahunt 1991), and are reported to be resistant to bacterial colonization and encrustation (Roberts *et al.* 1990; Woollons 1996). Hydrogel coated catheters are recommended for long-term use.

6 The *conformable catheter* is designed to conform to the shape of the female urethra, and allows partial filling of the bladder. The natural movement of the

urethra on the catheter, which is collapsible, is intended to prevent obstructions (Brocklehurst *et al.* 1988). They are made of latex and have a silicone elastomer coating. Conformable catheters are approximately 3 cm longer than conventional catheters for women.

Research into new types of catheter materials is ongoing, particularly examining materials that resist the formation of biofilms and reduce instances of urinary tract infections. Catheters coated with a silver alloy have been shown to prevent urinary tract infections (Saint *et al.* 1998). However, the studies that demonstrated this benefit were all small scale and a number of questions about the long-term effects of using such catheters, such as silver toxicity, need to be addressed. Argyria is a condition caused by the deposition of silver locally or systemically in the body, and can give rise to nausea, constipation and loss of night vision (Cymet 2001). As these catheters are much more expensive a cost-effectiveness analysis should also be carried out before they are used more widely (Best Practice 2000; Centre for Reviews and Dissemination Reviewers 2002). Further research in this area has implied that the use of these silver alloy catheters may be beneficial when catheterization is in high-risk patients, e.g. diabetic and intensive care patients (Saint *et al.* 2000), and used for short periods, 2–14 days, with particular regard to women (Saint *et al.* 2000; Lai & Fontecchio 2002). The Cochrane Collaboration analysed all the research trials on this issue and was fairly dismissive of the quality of the data achieved; however, the implication is that the financial cost may be worthwhile in specifically selected cases (Brosnahan *et al.* 2006). The Department of Health (DH), Rapid Review Panel has identified this product as being of potential value and it is under review.

Anaesthetic lubricating gel

466

The use of anaesthetic lubricating gels is well recognized for male catheterization, but there is some controversy in their use for female catheterization. In male patients the gel is instilled directly into the urethra and then external massage is used to move the gel down its length, unless a conforming gel such as instillagel is used and then this is not necessary. In female patients the anaesthetic lubricating gel or plain lubricating gel is applied to the tip of the catheter only, if it is used at all. It has been suggested that most of the lubricant is wiped off the catheter at the urethral introitus so therefore it fails to reach the urethral tissue (Muctar 1991).

These differences in practice imply that catheterization is a painful procedure for men but is not so for women. This assumption is not based on any empirical evidence or on any biological evidence. Other than the differences in length and route, the male and female urethra are very similar except for the presence of lubricating glands in the male urethra (Tortora & Derrickson 2008). The absence of these lubricating glands in the female urethra suggests that there is perhaps a greater need for the introduction of a lubricant. Women have complained of pain and discomfort during catheterization procedures (Mackenzie & Webb 1995), suggesting that the use of anaesthetic lubricating gels must be reconsidered (BAUN 2000; Woodward 2005). The literature does highlight a couple of issues on the use of lignocaine gel. Firstly where and how it is applied: if not instilled for long enough, i.e. more than 4 minutes, it will have only a lubricating affect (Association for Continence Advice 2003; Tanabe *et al.* 2004); and if the gel is not instilled up the urethra it will not dilate or anaesthetize it (NICE 2003; Bardsley 2005). There is a need for caution with the use of lignocaine in the elderly, those with cardiac dysrhythmias and those with sensitivity to the drug, as there is a danger of injury to the urothelial lining of the urethra during the procedure, allowing systemic absorption of the drug (BNF 2006).

Trauma can occur during catheterization, which in turn can increase the risk of infection. Using single use lubrication gels with antiseptic properties can reduce these risks (Pratt *et al.* 2001; BNF 2006). Since there is a lack of research to clarify the efficacy of lubricating gels, practice must be based on the research evidence that is available and the physiology and anatomy of the urethra.

Infections

Catheter-associated infections are the most common hospital-acquired infection, possibly accounting for up to 35–40% of all hospital infection (Roadhouse & Wellstead 2004). The maintenance of a closed drainage system is central in reducing the risk of catheter-associated infection. It is thought that micro-organisms reach the bladder by two possible routes: from the urine in the drainage bag or via the space between the catheter and the urethral mucosa (Gould 1994; Getliffe 1995). The most common sites where bacteria may enter the system are illustrated in Figure 13.2. To reduce the risk of infection it is important to keep manipulations of the closed system to a minimum; this includes unnecessary emptying, changing the drainage bags or taking samples. Before handling catheter drainage systems, hands must be decontaminated and a pair of clean non-sterile gloves should be worn (Pratt *et al.* 2001). All urine samples should only be obtained via the specially designed sampling ports using an aseptic technique.

Urine drainage bags should only be changed according to clinical need, i.e. when that catheter is changed or if the bag is leaking, or at times dictated by the manufacturer's instructions, for example every 5–7 days (Wilson 1998; Pratt *et al.* 2001). Urine drainage bags positioned above the level of the bladder and full bags cause urine to reflux which is associated with infection. Therefore bags should always be positioned below the level of the bladder to maintain an unobstructed flow and emptied appropriately. Urine drainage bags should be hung on suitable stands to avoid contact with the floor. In situations when dependent drainage is not possible, the system should be clamped until dependent drainage can be resumed (Kunin 1997). When emptying drainage bags, clean separate containers should be used for each patient and care should be taken to avoid contact between the drainage tap and the container (Pratt *et al.* 2001) (see Figure 13.3).

467

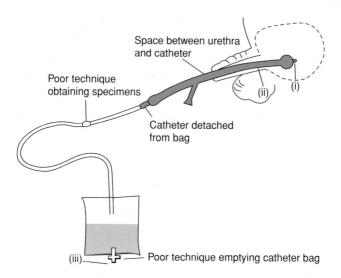

Space between urethra
and catheter

Poor technique
obtaining specimens

Catheter detached
from bag

(ii)

(i)

(iii)——— Poor technique emptying catheter bag

Figure 13.3 Common sites of cross-infection in a catheterized patient. (i) On catheter tip during insertion. (ii) Migration on the inside of the catheter via biofilm. (iii) Connection points of linked systems.

Meatal cleaning

Cleaning the urethral meatus, where the catheter enters the body, is a nursing procedure intended to minimize infection of the urinary tract. Studies examining the use of a variety of antiseptic, antimicrobial agents or soap and water found that there was no reduction in bacteriuria when using any of these preparations for meatal cleaning compared to routine bathing or showering (Pratt *et al.* 2001). Further studies support the view that vigorous meatal cleaning is unnecessary and may increase the risk of infection (Saint & Lipsky 1999). Therefore it is recommended that routine personal hygiene is all that is needed to maintain meatal hygiene (Pratt *et al.* 2001).

Drainage bags

A wide variety of drainage systems are available. Selecting a system involves consideration of the reasons for catheterization, the intended duration, the wishes of the patient, and infection control issues (Wilson & Coates 1996).

Urine drainage bags are available in a wide selection of sizes ranging from the large 2 litre capacity bag, which is used more commonly in non-ambulatory patients and overnight, to 350–750 ml leg bags. There are also large drainage bags that incorporate urine-measuring devices, which are used when very close monitoring of urine output is required.

There are a number of different styles of body-worn or leg bags. They allow patients greater mobility; they can be worn under the patient's own clothes and therefore are much more discreet, helping to preserve the patient's privacy and dignity. Shapes vary from oblong to oval and some have cloth backing for greater comfort in contact with the skin. Others are ridged to encourage an even distribution of urine through the bag, resulting in better conformity to the leg. The length of the inlet tube also varies (direct, short, long and adjustable length) and the intended position on the leg, i.e. thigh, knee or lower leg, determines which length is used. The patient should be asked to identify the most comfortable position. Several different tap designs exist and patients must have the manual dexterity to operate the mechanism. Most leg bags allow for larger 1–2 litre bags to be connected via the outlet tap, to increase capacity for night-time use.

Leg drainage bags

A variety of supports are available for use with these bags, including sporran waist belts, leg holsters, knickers/pants and leg straps (Roe 1992).

Leg straps

The use of thigh straps (e.g. Simpla G-Strap) helps to immobilize the catheter and thus reduce the trauma potential to the bladder neck and urethra. It is particularly appropriate for men, due to the longer length and weight of the tube being used; however, some women may also find the extra support more comfortable.

Catheter valves

469

Catheter valves, which eliminate the need for drainage bags, are also available. The valve allows the bladder to fill and empty intermittently, and is particularly appropriate for patients who require long-term catheterization, as they do not require a drainage bag.

Catheter valves are only suitable for patients who have good cognitive function, sufficient manual dexterity to manipulate the valve and an adequate bladder capacity. It is important that catheter valves are released at regular intervals to ensure that the bladder does not become over distended. (These valves must not be used on patients following certain operations to the prostate or bladder, as pressure caused by the distending bladder may cause perforation or rupture; in most of these instances the urethral catheter is only required for a short period of time and free drainage is the preferred method.) As catheter valves preclude free drainage they are unlikely to be appropriate for patients with uncontrolled detrusor over-activity, ureteric reflux or renal impairment (Fader *et al.* 1997). Catheter valves are designed to fit with linked systems so it is possible for patients to connect to a drainage bag. This may be necessary when access to toilets may be limited, for example overnight or on long journeys.

Catheter valves are licensed by the DH to remain in situ for 5–7 days, and this corresponds with most manufacturers' recommendations (Pomfret 1996). Little research into the advantages and disadvantages of catheter valves has been completed.

Suprapubic catheterization

Suprapubic catheterization is the insertion of a catheter through the anterior abdominal wall into the dome of the bladder. The procedure is performed under general or local anaesthesia, using a percutaneous system (Kirkwood 1999). A number of different suprapubic catheters are available. A trocar is used with all types of catheters in order to make the tract through which the catheter is threaded. Specifically designed catheters incorporate a fixing plate, which requires sutures to secure the catheter to the skin of the abdomen. For long-term use a Foley catheter is adequate. Large charrière size (18–22 ch) hydrogel coated or 100% silicone catheters are recommended (Winder 1994).

Suprapubic catheterization does offer some advantages over urethral catheterization. There is a reduction in the risk of patients developing urinary tract infection, as the bacterial count on the abdominal skin is less than around the perineal and perianal areas, although bacteriuria and encrustation still occur in susceptible patients (Winn 1998; Simpson 2001). Urethral integrity is retained and it allows for the resumption of normal voiding after surgery. Clamping the suprapubic catheter allows urethral voiding to occur, and the clamp can be released if voiding is incomplete. Pain and catheter-associated discomfort are reduced. Patient satisfaction is increased as, for some, their level of independence is increased and sexual intercourse can occur with fewer impediments (Hammarsten & Lindquist 1992; Barnes *et al.* 1993; Fillingham & Douglas 2004; Wilson 1998).

There are a number of risks and disadvantages associated with suprapubic catheterization:

- Bowel perforation and haemorrhage at the time of insertion.
- Infection, swelling, encrustation and granulation at insertion site.
- Pain, discomfort or irritation for some patients.
- Bladder stone formation and possible long-term risk of squamous cell carcinoma.
- Urethral leakage (Addison & Mould 2000).

Caring for a suprapubic catheter is the same as for a urethral catheter. Immediately following insertion of a suprapubic catheter, aseptic technique should be employed to clean the insertion site. Dressings may be required if secretions soil clothing, but they are not essential. Once the insertion site has healed (7–10 days), the site and catheter can be cleaned during bathing using soap, water and a clean cloth (Fillingham & Douglas 2004).

Intermittent self-catheterization

Intermittent self-catheterization (ISC) is not a new technique, although it has become noticeably more popular in recent years.

The procedure involves the episodic introduction of a catheter into the bladder to remove urine. After this the catheter is removed, leaving the patient catheter-free between catheterizations. In hospital this should be a sterile procedure because of the risks of hospital-acquired infection. However, in the patient's home a clean technique may be used (Wilson 1998; Lapides *et al.* 2002). Catheterization should be carried out as often as necessary to stop the bladder becoming over-distended and to prevent incontinence (Bennett 2002). How frequent this is depends on the individual but may vary from once a week, to once a day, to 4–6 times a day.

The advantages of intermittent catheterization over indwelling urethral catheterizations include improved quality of life, as patients are free from bulky pads or indwelling catheters and drainage bags, greater patient satisfaction and greater freedom to express sexuality. In addition, urinary tract complications are minimized and normal bladder function is maintained (Webb *et al.* 1990; Bakke & Malt 1993; Chai *et al.* 1995; Bakke *et al.* 1997).

Patients suitable for intermittent self-catheterization include:

- Those with a bladder capable of storing urine without leakage between catheterizations.
- Those who can comprehend the technique.
- Those with a reasonable degree of dexterity and mobility to position themselves for the procedure and manipulate the catheter.
- Those who are highly motivated and committed to carry out the procedure (Colley 1998).
- Those who have a willing partner to perform the technique (i.e. if agreeable to both).
- This procedure may be required by patients who have undergone continent reconstruction to manage initial postoperative incontinence. Patients with a Mitrofanoff reconstruction will need to perform this procedure for life (see Chapter 16, Professional edition).

Nelaton catheters are generally used to carry out intermittent self-catheterizations. These catheters are available in standard, female and paediatric lengths and in charrière sizes 6–24; as they are not left in the bladder they do not have a balloon (Winder 1995). They are normally manufactured from plastic but there is also a non-PVC, chlorine-free catheter obtainable. Some Nelaton catheters are coated with a lubricant which is activated by soaking the catheter in water for a short while; others are packaged with a lubricant gel which coats the catheter as it slides out of the packaging. These catheters are for single use only. Uncoated catheters, which require separate lubrication, may be reused by a single patient for up to a week, but the catheter must be rinsed in running water and properly dried after use; between uses it should be kept in a clean bag or container (Lapides *et al.* 1972; Barton 2000).

Procedure guidelines Urinary catheterization

Equipment

1 Sterile catheterization pack containing gallipots, receiver, low-linting swabs, disposable towels.
2 Disposable pad.

3 Sterile gloves.
4 Selection of appropriate catheters.
5 Sterile anaesthetic lubricating jelly.
6 Universal specimen container.

7 0.9% sodium chloride or antiseptic solution.
8 Bactericidal alcohol handrub.
9 Hypoallergenic tape or leg strap for tethering.
10 Sterile water.
11 Syringe and needle.
12 Disposable plastic apron.
13 Drainage bag and stand or holder.

Procedure
Urinary catheterization: male

Action	Rationale
1 Explain and discuss the procedure with the patient.	To ensure that the patient understands the procedure and gives his valid consent (NMC 2006: C; NMC 2008: C).
2 (a) Screen the bed.	To ensure patient's privacy. To allow dust and airborne organisms to settle before the field is exposed (DH 2005a: C).
(b) Assist the patient to get into the supine position with the legs extended.	To ensure the appropriate area is easily accessible (E).
(c) Do not expose the patient at this stage of the procedure.	To maintain patient's dignity and comfort (NMC 2008: C).
3 Wash hands using bactericidal soap and water or bactericidal alcohol handrub.	To reduce risk of infection (DH 2005a: C).

472

4	Put on a disposable plastic apron.	To reduce risk of cross-infection from micro-organisms on uniform (DH 2005a: C).
5	Prepare the trolley, placing all equipment required on the bottom shelf.	The top shelf acts as a clean working surface (E).
6	Take the trolley to the patient's bedside, disturbing screens as little as possible.	To minimize airborne contamination (DH 2005a: C).
7	Open the outer cover of the catheterization pack and slide the pack onto the top shelf of the trolley.	To prepare equipment (E).
8	Using an aseptic technique, open the supplementary packs.	To reduce the risk of introducing infection into the bladder (NICE 2003: C).
9	Remove cover that is maintaining the patient's privacy and position a disposable pad under the patient's buttocks and thighs.	To ensure urine does not leak onto bedclothes (E).
10	Clean hands with a bactericidal alcohol handrub.	Hands may have become contaminated by handling the outer packs (DH 2005a: C.
11	Put on sterile gloves.	To reduce risk of cross-infection (NICE 2003: C).
12	Place sterile towels across the patient's thighs and under buttocks.	To create a sterile field.
13	Wrap a sterile topical swab around the penis. Retract the foreskin, if necessary, and clean the glans penis with 0.9% sodium chloride or an antiseptic solution.	To reduce the risk of introducing infection to the urinary tract during catheterization (E).
14	Insert the nozzle of the lubricating jelly into the urethra. Squeeze the gel into the urethra, remove the nozzle and discard the tube. Massage the gel along the urethra.	Adequate lubrication helps to prevent urethral trauma. Use of a local anaesthetic minimizes the discomfort experienced by the patient (Bardsley 2005: P).

473

Procedure guidelines (cont.)

15 Squeeze the penis and wait approximately 5 minutes.

To prevent anaesthetic gel from escaping. To allow the anaesthetic gel to take effect (E).

16 Grasp the penis behind the glans, raising it until it is almost totally extended. Maintain grasp of penis until the procedure is finished.

This manoeuvre straightens the penile urethra and facilitates catheterization (Stoller 1995: P). Maintaining a grasp of the penis prevents contamination and retraction of the penis.

17 Place the receiver containing the catheter between the patient's legs. Insert the catheter for 15–25 cm until urine flows.

The male urethra is approximately 18 cm long (Bardsley 2005: P).

18 If resistance is felt at the external sphincter, increase the traction on the penis slightly and apply steady, gentle pressure on the catheter. Ask the patient to strain gently as if passing urine.

Some resistance may be due to spasm of the external sphincter. Straining gently helps to relax the external sphincter (E).

19 Either remove the catheter gently when urinary flow ceases, or:
   (a) When urine begins to flow, advance the catheter almost to its bifurcation.

Advancing the catheter ensures that it is correctly positioned in the bladder (E).

   (b) Gently inflate the balloon according to the manufacturer's direction, having ensured that the catheter is draining properly beforehand.

Inadvertent inflation of the balloon in the urethra causes pain and urethral trauma (Getliffe 2003: E).

   (c) Withdraw the catheter slightly and attach it to the drainage system.

   (d) Support the catheter, if the patient desires, either by using a specially designed support, e.g. Simpla G-Strap, or by taping the catheter to the patient's leg. Ensure that the catheter does not become taut when patient is mobilizing or when the penis becomes erect. Ensure that the catheter lumen is not occluded by the fixation device or tape.

To maintain patient comfort and to reduce the risk of urethral and bladder neck trauma. Care must be taken in using adhesive tapes as they may interact with the catheter material (Pomfret 1996: P; Fillingham & Douglas 2004: E).

474

Action	Rationale
20 Ensure that the glans penis is clean and then reduce or reposition the foreskin.	Retraction and constriction of the foreskin behind the glans penis (paraphimosis) may occur if this is not done (Pomfret 2003: E).
21 Make the patient comfortable. Ensure that the area is dry.	If the area is left wet or moist, secondary infection and skin irritation may occur (Pomfret 2003: E).
22 Measure the amount of urine.	To be aware of bladder capacity for patients who have presented with urinary retention. To monitor renal function and fluid balance. It is not necessary to measure the amount of urine if the patient is having the urinary catheter routinely changed (Pomfret 2003: E).
23 Take a urine specimen for laboratory examination, if required (see Chapter 28).	For further information, see the Procedure guidelines: Urine specimen collection: catheter (CSU), below.
24 Dispose of equipment in a yellow plastic clinical waste bag and seal the bag before moving the trolley.	To prevent environmental contamination. Yellow is the recognized colour for clinical waste (DH 2005b: C).
25 Draw back the curtains.	
26 Record information in relevant documents; this should include reasons for catheterization, date and time of catheterization, catheter type, length and size, amount of water instilled into the balloon, batch number, manufacturer, any problems negotiated during the procedure, and a review date to assess the need for continued catheterization or date of change of catheter.	To provide a point of reference or comparison in the event of later queries (NMC 2005: C; NMC 2008: C).

475

Urinary catheterization: female

Action	Rationale
1 Explain and discuss the procedure with the patient.	To ensure that the patient understands the procedure and gives her valid consent (NMC 2006: C; NMC 2008: C).

Procedure guidelines *(cont.)*

2 (a) Screen the bed.	To ensure patient's privacy. To allow dust and airborne organisms to settle before the sterile field is exposed (DH 2005a: C).
(b) Assist the patient to get into the supine position with knees bent, hips flexed and feet resting about 60 cm apart.	To enable genital area to be seen (E).
(c) Do not expose the patient at this stage of the procedure.	To maintain the patient's dignity and comfort (NMC 2008: C).
3 Ensure that a good light source is available.	To enable genital area to be seen clearly (E).
4 Wash hands using bactericidal soap and water or bactericidal alcohol handrub.	To reduce risk of cross-infection (DH 2005a: C).
5 Put on a disposable apron.	To reduce risk of cross-infection from micro-organisms on uniform (DH 2005a: C).
6 Prepare the trolley, placing all equipment required on the bottom shelf. (Also see Catheter selection section, above.)	To reserve top shelf for clean working surface (E).
7 Take the trolley to the patient's bedside, disturbing screens as little as possible.	To minimize airborne contamination (DH 2005a: C).
8 Open the outer cover of the catheterization pack and slide the pack on the top shelf of the trolley.	To prepare equipment (E).
9 Using an aseptic technique, open supplementary packs.	To reduce risk of introducing infection into the urinary tract (E).
10 Remove cover that is maintaining the patient's privacy and position a disposable pad under the patient's buttocks.	To ensure urine does not leak onto bedclothes (E).

11 Clean hands with a bactericidal alcohol handrub.	Hands may have become contaminated by handling of outer packs, etc (DH 2005a: C).
12 Put on sterile gloves.	To reduce risk of cross-infection (DH 2005a: C).
13 Place sterile towels across the patient's thighs.	To create a sterile field (E).
14 Using low-linting swabs, separate the labia minora so that the urethral meatus is seen. One hand should be used to maintain labial separation until catheterization is completed.	This manoeuvre provides better access to the urethral orifice and helps to prevent labial contamination of the catheter (E).
15 Clean around the urethral orifice with 0.9% sodium chloride or an antiseptic solution, using single downward strokes.	Inadequate preparation of the urethral orifice is a major cause of infection following catheterization. To reduce the risk of cross-infection (DH 2005a: C).
16 Insert the nozzle of the lubricating jelly into the urethra.Squeeze the gel into the urethra, remove the nozzle and discard the tube. Allow 5 minutes for the gel's antiseptic and anaesthetic effect to occur.	Adequate lubrication helps to prevent urethral trauma. Use of a local anaesthetic minimizes the patient's discomfort (Woodward 2005: P).
17 Place the catheter, in the receiver, between the patient's legs.	To provide a temporary container for urine as it drains (E).
18 Introduce the tip of the catheter into the urethral orifice in an upward and backward direction. If there is any difficulty in visualizing the urethral orifice due to vaginal atrophy and retraction of the urethral orifice, the index finger of the 'dirty' hand may be inserted in the vagina, and the urethral orifice can be palpated on the anterior wall of the vagina. The index finger is then positioned just behind the urethral orifice. This then acts as a guide, so the catheter can be correctly positioned (Jenkins 1998). Advance the catheter until 5–6 cm has been inserted.	The direction of insertion and the length of catheter inserted should bear relation to the anatomical structure of the area (E).

477

Procedure guidelines (cont.)

19 Either remove the catheter gently
   when urinary flow ceases, or:

   (a) Advance the catheter 6–8 cm.

   This prevents the balloon from becoming
   trapped in the urethra.

   (b) Inflate the balloon according to
   the manufacturer's directions,
   having ensured that the catheter
   is draining adequately.

   Inadvertent inflation of the balloon within
   the urethra is painful and causes urethral
   trauma (Getliffe 2003: P).

   (c) Withdraw the catheter slightly
   and connect it to the drainage
   system.

   (d) Support the catheter, if the
   patient desires, either by using a
   specially designed support, e.g.
   Simpla G-Strap, or by taping the
   catheter to the patient's leg.
   Ensure that the catheter does not
   become taut when patient is
   mobilizing. Ensure that the
   catheter lumen is not occluded
   by the fixation device or tape.

   To maintain patient comfort and to
   reduce the risk of urethral and bladder
   neck trauma. Care must be taken in using
   adhesive tapes as they may interact with
   the catheter material (Pomfret 1996: P).

20 Make the patient comfortable and
   ensure that the area is dry.

   If the area is left wet or moist, secondary
   infection and skin irritation may occur (E).

21 Measure the amount of urine.

   To be aware of bladder capacity for
   patients who have presented with urinary
   retention. To monitor renal function and
   fluid balance. It is not necessary to
   measure the amount of urine if the patient
   is having the urinary catheter routinely
   changed (Fillingham & Douglas 2004: E).

22 Take a urine specimen for laboratory
   examination if required.

   For further information, see the procedure
   on collection of a catheter specimen of
   urine, below.

23 Dispose of equipment in a yellow
   plastic clinical waste bag and seal
   the bag before moving the trolley.

   To prevent environmental contamination.
   Yellow is the recognized colour for
   clinical waste (DH 2005b: C).

24 Draw back the curtains.

25 Record information in relevant documents; this should include reasons for catheterization, date and time of catheterization, catheter type, length and size, amount of water instilled into the balloon, batch number, manufacturer, any problems negotiated during the procedure and a review date to assess the need for continued catheterization or date of change of catheter.

    Note: beware of patient having a vasovagal attack. This is caused by the vagal nerve being stimulated so that the heart slows down, leading to a syncope faint. If it happens, lie the patient down in the recovery position. Inform doctors.

To provide a point of reference or comparison in the event of later queries (NMC 2005: C.

Procedure guidelines   Urine specimen collection: catheter (CSU)

Equipment

1 Swab saturated with isopropyl alcohol 70%.
2 Gate clip.
3 Sterile syringe and needle.
4 Universal specimen container.

Procedure

Action	Rationale
1 Explain and discuss the procedure with the patient.	To ensure that the patient understands the procedure and gives his/her valid consent (NMC 2006: C; NMC 2008: C).
2 Screen the bed.	To ensure the patient's privacy (NMC 2008: C).
3 Only if there is no urine in the tubing, clamp the tubing below the rubber cuff until sufficient urine collects. (An access point is now available on catheter bags.)	To obtain an adequate urine sample (E).

Procedure guidelines *(cont.)*

4 Wash hands using bactericidal soap and water or bactericidal alcohol handrub.	To reduce risk of infection (DH 2005a: C).
5 Clean the access point with a swab saturated with 70% isopropyl alchohol.	To reduce risk of cross-infection (DH 2005a: C).
6 Using a sterile syringe and needle (if necessary), aspirate the required amount of urine from the access point (see Action figure 6).	If the catheter bag or tubing is punctured it causes leakage carrying organisms with it. Specimens collected from the catheter bag may give false results due to organisms proliferating there (E).
Needle sampling port: insert the needle into the port at an angle of 45° and aspirate the required amount of urine, withdraw the needle.	To reduce the risk of the needle going straight through the tubing (E).
Needleless sampling port: insert the syringe firmly into the centre of the sampling port (following manufacturer's instructions). Aspirate the required amount of urine and disconnect the syringe.	To reduce the risk of needlestick injury (NMC 2008: C).
7 Reclean access point with a swab saturated with 70% isopropyl alchohol.	To reduce contamination of access point and to reduce risk of cross-infection (DH 2005a: C).
8 Place the specimen in a sterile container.	To ensure that only organisms for investigation are preserved (Fillingham & Douglas 2004: E).
9 Wash and dry hands with bactericidal soap and water.	To reduce risk of cross-infection (DH 2005a: C).
10 Unclamp if necessary.	To allow drainage to continue (E).
11 Make the patient comfortable.	
12 Label the container and dispatch it (with the completed request form) to the laboratory as soon as possible after sample is taken to allow more accurate results from culture.	To ensure the best possible conditions for laboratory tests (Fillingham & Douglas 2004: E).

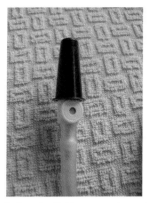

Action 6   Taking a specimen. Needle sampling port.

Procedure guidelines   Urinary catheter bag: emptying

Equipment

1 Swabs saturated with 70% isopropyl alcohol.
2 Sterile jug.

3 Disposable gloves.

Procedure

Action	Rationale
1 Explain and discuss the procedure with the patient.	To ensure that the patient understands the procedure and gives his/her valid consent (NMC 2006: C; NMC 2008: C).
2 Wash hands using bactericidal soap and water or bactericidal alcohol handrub, and put on disposable gloves.	To reduce risk of cross-infection (DH 2005a: C).
3 Clean the outlet valve with a swab saturated with 70% isopropyl alcohol.	To reduce risk of infection (DH 2005a: C).
4 Allow the urine to drain into the jug.	To empty drainage bag and accurately measure volume of contents (E).

Procedure guidelines *(cont.)*

5 Close the outlet valve and clean it again with a new alcohol-saturated swab.	To reduce risk of cross-infection (DH 2005a: C).
6 Cover the jug and dispose of contents in the sluice, having noted the amount of urine if this is requested for fluid balance records.	To reduce risk of environmental contamination (DH 2005a: C).
7 Wash hands with bactericidal soap and water.	To reduce risk of infection (DH 2005a: C).

Procedure guidelines   Urinary catheter removal

Equipment

1 Dressing pack containing sterile towel, gallipot, foam swab or non-linting gauze.

2 Disposable gloves.

3 Needle and syringe for urine specimen, specimen container.

4 Syringe for deflating balloon.

Procedure

Action	Rationale
1 Catheters are usually removed early in the morning.	So that any retention problems can be dealt with during the day (E).
2 Explain procedure to patient and inform him or her of potential post-catheter symptoms, i.e. urgency, frequency and discomfort, which are often caused by irritation of the urethra by the catheter.	So that patient knows what to expect, and can plan daily activity. For adequate flushing of bladder, especially to dilute and expel debris and infected urine, if present (Fillingham & Douglas 2004: C).
3 Clamp below the sampling port until sufficient urine collects. Take a catheter specimen of urine using the sampling port.	To obtain an adequate urine sample and to assess whether post-catheter antibiotic therapy is needed (DH 2005a: C).

482

4 Wearing gloves, use saline to clean the meatus and catheter, always swabbing away from the urethral opening.	To reduce risk of infection (DH 2005a: C).
In women, never clear from the perineum/vagina towards the urethra.	To help reduce the risk of bacteria from the vagina and perineum contaminating the urethra (E).
5 Release leg support.	For easier removal of catheter (E).
6 Having checked volume of water in balloon (see patient documentation), use syringe to deflate balloon.	To confirm how much water is in the balloon. To ensure balloon is completely deflated before removing catheter (E).
7 Ask patient to breathe in and then out; as patient exhales, gently (but firmly with continuous traction) remove catheter.	To relax pelvic floor muscles (E).
Male patients should be warned of discomfort as the deflated balloon passes through the prostate gland.	It is advisable to extend the penis as per the process for insertion to aid removal (E).
8 Clean meatus, tidy away equipment, and make the patient comfortable. Symptoms should resolve over the following 24–48 hours. If not, further investigation may be needed. Encourage patient to exercise and to drink 2–3 litres of fluid per day.	

Problem solving: Urinary catheter

With catheter in place

Problem	Cause	Suggested action
Urinary tract infection introduced during catheterization.	Faulty aseptic technique. Inadequate urethral cleaning. Contamination of catheter tip.	Inform a doctor. Obtain a catheter specimen of urine.
Urinary tract infection introduced via the drainage system.	Faulty handling of equipment. Breaking the closed system. Raising the drainage bag above bladder level.	Inform a doctor. Obtain a catheter specimen of urine.

Problem solving *(cont.)*

Problem	Cause	Suggested action
No drainage of urine.	Incorrect identification of external urinary meatus (female patients). Blockage of catheter.	Check that catheter has been sited correctly. In the female if catheter has been wrongly inserted in the vagina, leave the catheter in position to act as a guide, re-identify the urethra and catheterize the patient. Remove the inappropriately sited catheter.
Empty bladder.		Check patient's volaemic status. Increase fluid intake, whether oral or by other means to discount dehydration as the cause. On insertion of the new catheter, urine will drain.
Urethral mucosal trauma.	Incorrect size of catheter. Procedure not carried out correctly or skilfully. Movement of the catheter in the urethra. Creation of false passage as a result of too rapid insertion of catheter.	Recatheterize the patient using the correct size of catheter. Check the catheter support and apply or reapply as necessary. Nurse may need to remove the catheter and wait for the urethral mucosa to heal.
Inability to tolerate indwelling catheter.	Urethral mucosal irritation.	Nurse may need to remove the catheter and seek an alternative means of urine drainage.
	Psychological trauma.	Explain the need for and the functioning of the catheter.
	Unstable bladder. Radiation cystitis.	

Problem	Cause	Suggested action
Inadequate drainage of urine.	Incorrect placement of a catheter. Kinked drainage tubing. Blocked tubing, e.g. pus, urates, phosphates, blood clots.	Resite the catheter. Inspect the system and straighten any kinks. If a three-way catheter, such as a Foley, is in place, irrigate it. If an ordinary catheter is in use, milk the tubing in an attempt to dislodge the debris, then attempt a gentle bladder washout. Failing this, the catheter will need to be replaced; a three-way one should be used if the obstruction is being caused by clots and associated haematuria.
Fistula formation.	Pressure on the penoscrotal angle.	Ensure that correct strapping is used.
Penile pain on erection.	Not allowing enough length of catheter to accommodate penile erection.	Ensure that an adequate length is available to accommodate penile erection.
Paraphimosis.	Failure to retract foreskin after catheterization or catheter toilet.	Always retract the foreskin.
Formation of crusts around the urethral meatus.	Increased urethral secretions collect at the meatus and form crusts, due to irritation of urothelium by the catheter (Fillingham & Douglas 2004).	Correct catheter toilet.

485

Problem solving (cont.)

Problem	Cause	Suggested action
Leakage of urine around catheter.	Incorrect size of catheter.	Replace with the correct size, usually 2 ch smaller.
	Incorrect balloon size.	Select catheter with 10 ml balloon. Use Roberts tipped catheter.
	Bladder hyperirritability.	As a last resort, bladder hyperirritability can be reduced by giving diazepam or anticholinergic drugs.
Unable to deflate balloon.	Valve expansion. Valve displacement.	1 Check the non-return valve on the inflation/deflation channel. If jammed, use a syringe and needle to aspirate by means of the inflation arm above the valve.
	Channel obstruction.	2 Obstruction by a foreign body can sometimes be relieved by the introduction of a guidewire through the inflation channel.
		3 Inject 3.5 ml of dilute ether solution (diluted 50/50 with sterile water or 0.9% sodium chloride) into the inflation arm.
		4 Alternatively, the balloon can be punctured suprapubically using a needle under ultrasound visualization.
		5 Following catheter removal the balloon should be inspected to ensure it has not disintegrated, leaving fragments in the bladder. *Note*: steps 2–4 should be attempted by or under the directions of a urologist. The patient may require cystoscopy following balloon deflation to remove any balloon fragments and to wash the bladder out.
Dysuria.	Inflammation of the urethral mucosa.	Ensure a fluid intake of 2–3 litres per day. Advise the patient that dysuria is common but will usually be resolved once micturition has occurred at least three times. Inform medical staff if the problem persists.

Problem	Cause	Suggested action
Retention of urine.	May be psychological.	Encourage the patient to increase fluid intake. Offer the patient a warm bath. Inform medical staff if the problem persists.
	Urinary tract infection.	Encourage a fluid intake of 2–3 litres a day. Collect a specimen of urine. Inform medical staff if the problem persists. Administer prescribed antibiotics.

Penile sheaths

Definition

Penile sheaths are external devices applied over the penis that direct urine into a urinary drainage bag from where it can be conveniently emptied. They are used by men to manage urinary incontinence.

Indications

Penile sheaths may be used to relieve incontinence when no other means is practicable or when all other methods have failed.

Reference material

Penile sheaths (otherwise known as conveens) are only to be considered once other methods of promoting continence have failed, as the promotion and treatment of incontinence should be the primary concern of the nurse (Pomfret 2003). They should be considered as a preferable alternative to other methods of continence control, such as pads which quickly can become sodden (Pomfret 2003) and cause skin problems, and catheters, which have several potential complications (Fader *et al.* 2001).

The factors that are important in the selection of the sheath is that the sheath is comfortable to wear, adheres well to the skin, does not leak, and is easy to put on and take off (Continence Foundation 2005).

Size selection

Modern sheaths come in a variety of sizes and the correct size required can be determined by measuring the girth of the penile shaft. Some devices come with

487

a handy guide with different diameters cut into it so that the correct size can be easily determined. They are available from the manufacturers in a variety of different sizes, which generally increase in increments of 5–10 mm (Continence Foundation 2005).

Fixation

Over the years there have been a number of ways that sheaths have been attached to the penis. However, the main methods in current use follow two different approachs. First, the sheaths can be self-adhesive, in which the sheath itself has a section along its length with adhesive on the internal aspect of it that sticks to the penile shaft as it is applied. The second method is a double-sided strip of hypoallergenic or foam material applied in a spiral around the penis (which increases the surface area of the conveen adhered to the penis) and then the sheath is applied over the top.

Procedure guidelines   Penile sheath application

Equipment

1 Bowl of warm water and soap.
2 Non sterile gloves.
3 Selection of appropriate penile sheaths.
4 Bactericidal alcohol handrub.

5 Disposable plastic apron.
6 Drainage bag and stand or holder.
7 Hypoallergenic tape for tethering or leg strap.
8 Catheter leg bag.

Procedure

Action	Rationale
1 Explain and discuss the procedure with the patient.	To ensure that the patient understands the procedure and gives his valid consent (NMC 2006: C).
2 (a) Screen the bed.	To ensure patient's privacy. To allow dust and airborne organisms to settle before the field is exposed (NMC 2008: C).
(b) Assist the patient to get into the supine position with the legs extended.	To ensure the appropriate area is easily accessible (E).
(c) Do not expose the patient at this stage of the procedure.	To maintain patient's dignity and comfort (NMC 2008: C).

3	Wash hands using bactericidal soap and water or bactericidal alcohol handrub.	To reduce risk of infection (DH 2005a: C).
4	Put on a disposable plastic apron.	To reduce risk of cross-infection from micro-organisms on uniform (DH 2005a: C).
5	Prepare the trolley, placing all equipment required on the bottom	The top shelf acts as a clean working surface (E).
6	Take the trolley to the patient's bedside, disturbing screens as little as possible.	To minimize airborne contamination (DH 2005a: C).
7	Remove cover that is maintaining the patient's privacy and position a disposable pad under the patient's buttocks and thighs.	To ensure urine does not leak onto bedclothes (E).
8	Clean hands with a bactericidal alcohol handrub.	Hands may have become contaminated by handling the outer packs (DH 2005a: C).
9	Put on non-sterile gloves.	To reduce risk of cross-infection (DH 2005a: R).
10	Retract the foreskin, if necessary, and clean the penis with soap and water. Dry completely and reduce or reposition the foreskin.	To remove old adhesive and ensure sheath sticks to the skin and to prevent retraction and constriction of the foreskin behind the glans penis (paraphimosis) which may occur if this is not performed (Continence Foundation 2005: C).
11	Trim any excess pubic hair from around the base of the penis.	To prevent sheath from painfully pulling pubic hair when applied (Continence Foundation 2005: C).
12	Apply sheath following manufacturer's guidelines ensuring that there is a space between the glans penis and the sheath. Squeeze the sheath gently around the penile shaft.	To prevent the sheath from rubbing the glans penis and causing discomfort and potential skin irritation and to ensure sheath has adhered to penis (Pomfret 2003: C).
13	Connect catheter bag and ensure tubing is not kinked.	To facilitate drainage of urine into catheter bag (E).

489

Procedure guidelines *(cont.)*

14 Dispose of equipment in a yellow plastic clinical waste bag and seal the bag before moving the trolley.	To prevent environmental contamination. Yellow is the recognized colour for clinical waste (DH 2005b: C).
15 Draw back the curtains once the patient has been covered.	To maintain the patient's dignity (NMC 2008: C).
16 Record information in relevant documents; this should include reasons for applying penile sheath, date and time of application, sheath type, length and size, manufacturer, any problems negotiated during the procedure, and a review date to assess the need for reapplication.	To provide a point of reference or comparison in the event of later queries (NMC 2005b: C).

References and further reading

Addison, R. (2001) Intermittent self-catheterisation. *Nurs Times*, **97**(20), 67–9.

Addison, R. & Mould, C. (2000) Risk assessment in suprapubic catheterization. *Nurs Stand*, **14**(36), 43–6.

Association for Continence Advice (2003) *Notes on Good Practice*. Association for Continence Advice, London.

Bakke, A. & Malt, U.F. (1993) Social functioning and general well being in patients treated with clean intermittent catheterisation. *J Psychosom Res*, **37**(4), 371–80.

Bakke, A., Digranes, A. & Hoisaeter, P.A. (1997) Physical predictors of infection in patients treated with clean intermittent catheterisation: a prospective 7-year study. *Br J Urol*, **79**(1), 85–90.

Bardsley, A. (2005) Use of lubricant gels in urinary catheterisation. *Nurs Stand*, **20**(8), 41–6.

Barnes, D.G. *et al.* (1993) Management of the neuropathic bladder by supra-pubic catheterisation. *Br J Urol*, **72**, 169–72.

Barnes, K.E. & Malone-Lee, J. (1986) Long-term catheter management: minimising the problem of premature replacement due to balloon deflation. *J Adv Nurs*, **11**, 303–7.

Barton, R. (2000) Intermittent self-catheterisation. *Nurs Stand*, **15**(9), 1–9.

BAUN (2000) *Guidelines for Female Urethral Catheterisation using 2% Lignocaine Gel (Instillagel)*. British Association of Urological Nurses Fitwise, Bathgate, Scotland.

Bennett, E. (2002) Intermittent self-catheterisation and the female patient. *Nurs Stand*, **30**(17), 37–42.

Best Practice (2000) Management of short term indwelling urethral catheters to prevent urinary tract infections. *Best Practice*, **4**(1), 1–6.

Blandy, J.P. & Moors, J. (1989) *Urology for Nurses*. Blackwell Science, Oxford.

BNF (2006) *British National Formulary No 51*. British Medical Association and Royal Pharmaceutical Society of Great Britain, London.

Brocklehurst, J.C. *et al.* (1988) A new urethral catheter. *Br Med J*, **296**, 1691–3.

Brosnahan, J., Jull, A. & Tracy, C. (2006) Types of urethral catheters for management of short-term voiding problems in hospitalised adults (review). The Cochrane Collaboration. *The Cochrane Library*, Issue **2**. John Wiley & Sons, New York.

Centre for Reviews and Dissemination Reviewers (2002) *Management of Short Term Indwelling Urethral Catheters to Prevent Urinary Tract Infections: a Systematic Review. Database of Abstracts of Reviews of Effectiveness*. Centre for Reviews and Dissemination Reviewers, York.

Chai, T. *et al.* (1995) Compliance and complications of clean intermittent catheterisation in the spinal-cord injured patient. *Paraplegia*, **33**(3), 161–3.

Colley, W. (1998) Catheter care 1. *Nurs Times*, **94**(23), insert.

Continence Foundation (2005) Factsheet 2: penile sheaths. www.continence.foundation.org.uk. Accessed on 25/4/07.

Crow, R.A. *et al.* (1986) *A Study of Patients with an Indwelling Catheter and Related Nursing Practice*. Nursing Practice Unit, University of Surrey.

Cruickshank, J.P. & Woodward, S. (2001) *Management of Continence and Urinary Catheter Care*. Mark Allen, London.

Cymet, T. (2001) Do silver alloy catheters increase the risk of systemic argyria? *Arch Intern Med*, **161**(7), 1014–15.

DH (2005a) *Saving Lives: A Delivery Programme to Reduce Healthcare infection including MRSA*. Department of Health, London.

DH (2005b) *Hazardous waste (England) regulations*. Department of Health, London.

Doherty, W. (2000) Intermittent self-catheterisation: draining the bladder. *Nurs Times*, **96**(31), 13.

Edwards, L.E. *et al.* (1983) Post-catheterisation urethral strictures: a clinical and experimental study. *Br J Urol*, **55**, 53–6.

Evans, A., Painter, D. & Feneley, R. (2001) Blocked urinary catheters: nurses' preventive role. *Nurs Times*, **97**(1), 37–8.

Fader, M. *et al.* (1997) A multi-centre comparative evaluation of catheter valves. *Br J Nurs*, **6**(7), 359–67.

Fader, M. *et al.* (2001) Sheaths for urinary incontinence: a randomized trial. *Br J Urol*, **87**, 367–72.

Falkiner, F.R. (1993) The insertion and management of indwelling urethral catheters – minimising the risk of infection. *J Hosp Infect*, **25**, 79–90.

Fillingham, S. & Douglas, J. (2004) *Urological Nursing*, 3rd edn. Bailliere Tindall, London.

German, K. *et al.* (1997) A randomized cross-over study comparing the use of a catheter valve and a leg-bag in urethrally catheterised male patients. *Br J Urol*, **79**(1), 96–8.

Getliffe, K. (1995) Care of urinary catheters. *Nurs Stand*, **10**(1), 25–31.

Getliffe, K. (1996) Care of urinary catheters. *Nurs Stand*, **11**(11), 47–54.

Getliffe, K. (2003) Catheters and catheterisation. In: *Promoting Continence: a Clinical and Research Resource* (eds K. Getliffe & M. Dolman). Bailliere Tindall, London, pp. 259–301.

Gilbert, A. & Gobbi, M. (1989) Making sense of bladder irrigation. *Nurs Times*, **85**(16), 40–2.

Godfrey, H. & Evans, A. (2000) Management of long-term catheters: minimising complications. *Br J Nurs*, **9**(2), 74–81.

Gould, D. (1994) Keeping on tract. *Nurs Times* **90**(40), 58–64.

Hammarsten, J. & Lindquist, K. (1992) Supra-pubic catheter following transurethral resection of the prostate: a way to decrease the number of urethral strictures and improve the outcome of operation. *J Urol*, **147**, 648–52.

Jenkins, S.C. (1998) Digital guidance of female urethral catheterization. *Br J Urol*, **82**, 589–90.

Kirkwood, L. (1999) Taking charge. *Nurs Times*, **95**(6), 63–4.

Kristiansen, P. *et al.* (1983) Long-term urethral catheter drainage and bladder capacity. *Neurol Urodyn*, **2**, 135–43.

Kunin, C.M. (1997) *Urinary Tract Infections: Detection, Prevention and Management*, 5th edn. Williams and Wilkins, Baltimore.

Lai, K.K. & Fontecchio, S. (2002) Use of silver-hydrogel urinary catheters on the incidence of catheter-associated urinary tract infections in hospitalized patients. *Am J Infect Control*, **30**, 221–5.

Lapides, J. *et al.* (1972) Clean, intermittent self-catheterisation in the treatment of urinary tract disease. *J Urol*, **107**, 458–61.

Lapides, J. *et al.* (2002) Clean, intermittent self-catheterization in the treatment of urinary tract disease. *J Urol*, **167**(4), 1584–6.

Leaver, R. & Pressland, D. (2001) Intermittent self-catheterisation in urinary tract reconstruction. *Br J Community Nursing Nurs*, **6**(5), 253–8.

Mackenzie, J. & Webb, C. (1995) Gynopia in nursing practice: the case of urethral catheterization. *J Clin Nurs*, **4**, 221–6.

McGill, S. (1982) Catheter management: it's size that's important. *Nurs Mirror*, **154**, 48–9.

Milligan, F. (1999) Male sexuality and urethral catheterisations: a review of the literature. *Nurs Stand*, **13**(38), 43–7.

Moore, K. (1995) Intermittent self-catheterisation: research based practice. *Br J Nurs*, **4**(18), 1057–63.

Muctar, S. (1991) The importance of a lubricant in transurethral interventions. *Urologue (B)*, **31**, 153–5 [translation].

Mulhall, A.B. *et al.* (1993) Maintenance of closed urinary drainage systems: are practitioners aware of the dangers? *J Clin Nurs*, **2**, 135–40.

Nacey, J.N. & Delahunt, B. (1991) Toxicity study of first and second generation hydrogel-coated latex catheters. *Br J Urol*, **67**, 314–16.

NICE (2003) *Full Guidelines. Prevention of Healthcare Associated Infection in Primary and Community Care. Section 3. Urinary Catheterisation*. National Institute for Health and Clinical Excellence, London.

NMC (2005) *Guidelines for Records and Record Keeping*. Nursing and Midwifery Council, London.

NMC (2006) *A–Z Advice Sheet Consent*. www.nmc.org.

NMC (2008) *The Code: Standards of Conduct, Performance and Ethics for Nurses and Midwives*. Nursing and Midwifery Council, London.

Pomfret, I.J. (1996) Catheters: design, selection and management. *Br J Nurs*, **5**(4), 245–51.

Pomfret, I.J. (2000) Catheter care in the community. *Nurs Stand*, **22**(14), 46–51.

Pomfret, I.J. (2003) Back to basics: an introduction to continence issues. *J Community Nurs*, **16**(7), 36–41.

Pratt, R.J. *et al.* (2001) Guidelines for preventing infections associated with the insertion and maintenance of short-term indwelling urethral catheters in acute care. *J Hosp Infect*, **47**(Suppl), S39–46.

RCN (1994) *Guidelines on Male Catheterisation: the Role of the Nurse*. Royal College of Nursing, London.

Roadhouse, A.J. & Wellstead, A. (2004) The prevention of indwelling catheter related urinary tract infections – the outcome of a performance improvement project. *Br J Infection Control*, **5**(5), 22–23.

Roberts, J.A. *et al.* (1990) Bacterial adherence to urethral catheters. *J Urol*, **144**, 264–9.

Robinson, J. (2001) Urethral catheter selection. *Nurs Stand*, **25**(15), 39–42.

Roe, B.H. (1992) Use of indwelling catheters. In: *Clinical Nursing Practice: The Promotion and Management of Continence* (ed. B.H. Roe). Prentice Hall, Hemel Hempstead, pp. 177–191.

Roe, B.H. & Brocklehurst, J.C. (1987) Study of patients with indwelling catheters. *J Adv Nurs*, **12**, 713–18.

Ryan-Woolley, B. (1987) *Urinary Catheters: Aids for the Management of Incontinence*. King's Fund Project Paper No. 65. King's Fund, London.

Saint, S. (2002) How to prevent urinary catheter-related infections in the critically ill. *J Crit Illn*, **15**(8), 419–23.

Saint, S. & Lipsky, B.A. (1999) Preventing catheter-associated bacteriuria. Should we? Can we? How? *Arch Intern Med*, **159**, 800–8.

Saint, S. *et al.* (1998) The efficacy of silver alloy-coated urinary catheters in preventing urinary tract infection: a meta-analysis. *Am J Med*, **105**(3), 236–41.

Saint, S. *et al.* (2000) The potential clinical and economical benefits of silver alloy urinary catheters in preventing urinary tract infections. *Arch Intern Med*, **160**, 2670–5.

Simcare (1989) *Intermittent Self-Catheterization – A Guide for Patients' Families*. Simcare, Lancing.

Simpson, L. (2001) Indwelling urethral catheters. *Nurs Stand*, **15**(46), 47–54, 56.

Slade, N. & Gillespie, W.A. (1985) *The Urinary Tract and the Catheter: Infection and Other Problems*. John Wiley & Sons, Ltd, Chichester.

Stewart, E. (1998) Urinary catheters: selection, maintenance and nursing care. *Br J Nurs*, **7**(19), 1152–61.

Stoller, M. (1995) Retrograde instrumentation of the urinary tract. In: *Smith's General Urology* (eds E.A. Tanagho & J.W. McAninch). Prentice-Hall, London, pp. 160–171.

Studer, U.E. (1983) How to fill silicone catheter balloons. *Urology*, **22**, 300–2.

Tanabe, P. *et al.* (2004) Factors affecting pain scores during female urethral catheterization. *Acad Emerg Med*, **11**(6), 699–702.

Thakar, R. & Stanton, S. (2000) Management of urinary incontinence in women. *BMJ*, **323**(7272), 1326–31.

Tortora, G.A. & Derrickson, B. (2008) *Principles of Anatomy and Physiology*, 12th edn. John Wiley & Sons, Inc., New York.

Webb, R.J., Lawson, A.L. & Neal, D.E. (1990) Clean intermittent self-catheterisation in 172 adults. *Br J Urol*, **65**(1), 20–3.

Wilksch, J. *et al.* (1983) The role of catheter surface morphology and extractable cytotoxic material in tissue reactions to urethral catheters. *Br J Urol*, **55**, 48–52.

Wilson, M. (1998) Infection control. *Prof Nurse Study Suppl*, **13**(5), S10–13.

Wilson, M. & Coates, D. (1996) Infection control and urine drainage bag design. *Prof Nurse*, **11**(4), 245–52.

Winder, A. (1994) Suprapubic catheterisation. *Community Outlook*, **4**(12), 25–6.

Winder, A. (1995) Intermittent self catheterisation. *Community Nurs*, **9**(2), 24–8.

Winn, C. (1996) Catheterisation: extending the scope of practice. *Nurs Stand*, **10**(52), 49–56.

Winn, C. (1998) Complications with urinary catheters. *Prof Nurse Study Suppl*, **13**(5), S7–10.

Woodward, S. (1997) Complications of allergies to latex urinary catheters. *Br J Nurs*, **6**(4), 786–93.

Woodward, S. (2005) Use of lubricant in female urethral catheterization. *Br J Nurs*, **14**(19), 1022–3.

Woollons, S. (1996) Urinary catheters for long-term use. *Prof Nurse*, **11**(12), 825–32.

Young, A.E. *et al.* (1994) A case of latex anaphylaxis. *Br J Hosp Med*, **52**(11), 599–600.

Multiple choice questions

1 What catheter balloon size is recommended for adults?

   a   30 ml
   b   3–5 ml
   c   5–10 ml
   d   10–30 ml

2 What solution should be used to inflate the catheter balloon?

   a   0.9% sodium chloride
   b   Sterile water
   c   Tap water
   d   Any of the above

3 Catheter associated infections account for 35–40% of hospital infections. What is the most common way for infection to enter the closed system?

   a   Poor technique in emptying the catheter bag
   b   Poor technique in obtaining specimens
   c   Catheter detached from the bag
   d   All of the above

4 Prior to catheterization the urethral meatus should be cleaned with:

   a   Soap and water
   b   0.9% sodium chloride
   c   Antiseptic solution
   d   0.9% sodium chloride or antiseptic solution

5 **When removing a urethral catheter you should:**

    a   Take a catheter specimen of urine and clean the area

    b   Take a catheter specimen, clean the area and deflate the balloon

    c   Clean the area, deflate the balloon

    d   Take a catheter specimen of urine, clean the area, check the volume of water in the catheter and deflate

6 **Urine drainage catheter bags should be changed:**

    a   As per manufacturer's instructions

    b   Every day

    c   If leaking, when catheter is changed or at times recommended by manufacturer's directions

    d   When the patient asks

Answers to the multiple choice questions can be found in Appendix 3.

Chapter 14

Intrapleural drainage

Definitions

Any abnormal collection of fluid or air in the pleural space can compress the lung, causing it to collapse either partially or fully, which can seriously compromise ventilation and the mechanics of breathing (Allibone 2003). Intrapleural drainage is a method used to remove the collection of air, fluid, pus or blood from the pleural space in order to restore normal lung expansion and function (Hyde *et al.* 1997; McMahon-Parkes 1997).

An intrapleural drain is a length of tubing, made of clear, rigid yet pliable plastic, which may have a radiopaque strip incorporated into it that enables X-ray detection. It has a proximal and distal end. The proximal end is inserted into the pleura and has a number of holes at the insertion end which facilitate drainage. The distal end is connected to the drainage system (Marieb 2001) (Figure 14.1).

Indications

Indications for chest drain insertion

- Pneumothorax:
  - (a) in any ventilated patient;
  - (b) tension pneumothorax after initial needle relief;
  - (c) persistent or recurrent pneumothorax after simple aspiration;
  - (d) large secondary spontaneous pneumothorax in patients over 50 years.
- Malignant pleural effusion.
- Empyema and complicated parapneumonic pleural effusion.
- Traumatic haemopneumothorax.
- Postoperative, e.g. thoracotomy, oesophagectomy, cardiac surgery (Laws *et al.* 2003).
- Drainage of pleural effusions.
- Drainage of chyle (digested fat drained by the lymphatic system) (Adam & Osborne 2005).

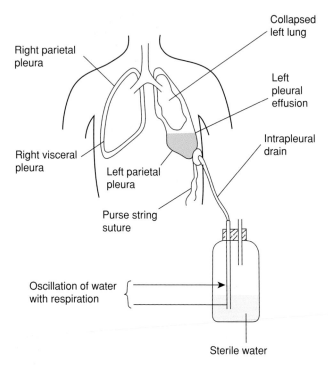

Figure 14.1   An intrapleural drain and underwater seal bottle are used to drain a left pleural effusion.

498   *Objectives in caring for the patient with intrapleural drains*

- To keep the system patent.
- To maintain sterility of the intrapleural drainage system and avoid introduction of bacteria into the intrapleural space.
- To keep the system upright and airtight (Kirkwood 2002).

Reference material

Anatomy and physiology of the pleura

Each lung is surrounded by a double membrane called the pleura. The outer membrane is the parietal pleura; this is attached to the thoracic (chest) wall and

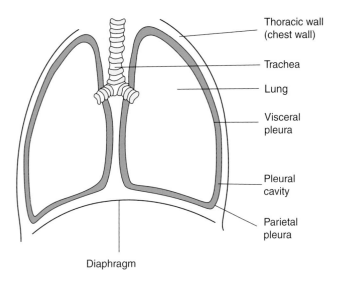

Thoracic wall
(chest wall)

Trachea

Lung

Visceral
pleura

Pleural
cavity

Parietal
pleura

Diaphragm

Figure 14.2   Relationship between pleural membranes, chest wall and lungs.

contains nerve receptors which detect pain. The inner membrane is the visceral pleura and this adheres to the lung covering the lung fissures, hilar bronchi and vessels (Figure 14.2). The pleurae are thin, serous and porous, which allows for movement of interstitial fluid across these membranes (Marieb 2001; Berne & Levy 2004; Hall &Guyton 2005; Tortora & Derrickson 2008).

Pleural space

A space exists between the parietal and visceral pleura commonly known as the pleural space, cavity or potential space. Approximately 3–5 ml of serous fluid produced by the pleurae fills this space, enabling the pleurae to move in unison with the chest wall on inspiration. In addition, the serous fluid enables the membranes to be held closely together by surface tension forces. A careful balance is required to control the amount of fluid present in the pleural space. This balance is maintained by the oncotic pressure across the pleurae and lymphatic drainage. Approximately 1–2 litres of fluid moves across the pleural space each day (Thelan *et al.* 1995).

The natural recoil tendency of the lungs during breathing causes them to try and collapse, but a negative pressure is required on the outside of the lungs to keep them expanded. This is provided by the pleurae. During respiration the intrapleural pressure will vary. Before inspiration the pressure within the pleural space is equal to -5 cmH$_2$O. During inspiration there is a decrease in the intrapleural pressure due to the diaphragm being drawn down and outward with expansion of the chest. The pressure falls to -7.5 cmH$_2$O, and this results in air being drawn in for gaseous exchange (Marieb 2001). During expiration the lung returns to its preinspiratory state by elastic recoil, with collapse of the chest wall and diaphragm and the exhalation of gas, resulting in a subsequent rise in the intrapleural pressure to -4 cmH$_2$O. If there is loss of the normal negative pressure, partial or total lung collapse can occur, which can then lead to a reduction in the capacity of the lung available for effective gaseous exchange (Marieb 2001; Berne & Levy 2004; Hall & Guyton 2005; Tortora & Derrickson 2008).

Conditions that require intrapleural drainage

Pneumothorax

This can be defined as air in the pleural cavity (Kumar & Clarke 2002). When the integrity of either pleural layer is breached, air can enter the pleural cavity, causing the lung to collapse down towards the hilum (Gallon 1998).

Spontaneous pneumothorax

Spontaneous pneumothorax is a collection of air or gas in the chest that causes the lung to collapse (MedlinePlus 2006). Spontaneous pneumothorax can occur as a result of trauma, surgery, central venous catheter insertion, during positive pressure ventilation, and in those individuals with lung conditions, e.g. asthma, chronic bronchitis, tuberculosis, pneumonia or carcinoma of the lung due to the mechanical and physiological processes of these conditions (MedlinePlus 2006). If left untreated a spontaneous pneumothorax can become a tension pneumothorax.

Tension pneumothorax

A tension pneumothorax is a complete collapse of the lung. It occurs when air enters but does not leave the space around the lung (pleural space). It is a life-threatening emergency that requires immediate treatment (MedlinePlus 2006).

Pleural effusion

This is defined as an excessive amount of fluid in the pleural space (Kumar & Clarke 2002). The fluid can be composed of malignant cells, or result from an accumulation of lymph in the pleural space (chylothorax) (Kozar & Adams 2005). An effusion occurs as a result of trauma, carcinoma, heart failure, hypoproteinaemia or pneumonia. Pleural effusions occur when an imbalance in pressure allows the flow of fluid into the pleural space to exceed its absorption (Chernecky & Shelton 2001).

Care should be taken when draining pleural effusions as complications can occur, such as re-expansion of pulmonary oedema (Tang *et al.* 2002). No more than 1500 ml should be drained at a time, clamping the tube to interrupt drainage for 1–2 hours before recommencing or slowed to about 500 ml/h depending on haemodynamic status (Laws *et al.* 2003). A chest X-ray should also be performed to ascertain correct position of the drain and to detect any complications (Tang *et al.* 2002).

If the patient's respiratory status worsens after chest drain insertion, and proper placement of tube has been confirmed, the possibility of re-expansion pulmonary oedema should be considered; if this is present, the pleural drainage should be limited to less than 1000 ml/day and the negative pleural pressure to 5 kPa (Deshpande *et al.* 2003).

Haemothorax

Haemothorax is a collection of blood in the space between the chest wall and the lung (the pleural cavity), usually the result of chest injury, trauma to the heart, lungs or major vessels or in a patient who has bled on anticoagulant therapy (MedlinePlus 2006).

Haemopneumothorax

Haemothorax may also be associated with pneumothorax. Depending on the amount of blood or air in the pleural cavity, a collapsed lung can lead to respiratory and haemodynamic failure (MedlinePlus 2006).

Empyema

This is defined as pus in the pleural space. Its main causes include rupture of an abscess of the lung, following pneumonia, pulmonary tuberculosis, or an infection following thoracic surgery (Kumar & Clarke 2002).

Collective signs and symptoms

The following signs and symptoms can occur in the conditions previously mentioned, individually or together depending on the patient's condition:

- Pallor.
- Cyanosis.

501

- Dyspnoea.
- Increasing respiratory rate.
- Reduced breath sounds on affected side.
- Dullness of air entry, on listening to the chest with stethoscope.
- Reduced chest movement on affected side.
- Decrease in peripheral tissue oxygen saturations.
- Pleuritic chest pain.
- Cardiovascular change, i.e. increasing heart rate, decreasing blood pressure due to compression of the mediastinum and in turn the heart and surrounding vessels (Kumar & Clarke 2002).

Drain insertion site

Before insertion of an intrapleural drain the patient should have a chest X-ray reviewed by the doctor. The chest X-ray will confirm the site of the pneumothorax or effusion to be drained. Patients who are receiving anticoagulation therapy or who have platelet abnormalities should have appropriate haematological investigations (international normalized ratio [INR] or activated partial thromboplastin ratio [APTR]) to ascertain whether correction is required prior to insertion of the drain (Tang *et al.* 2002). If the INR or APTR is too high, bleeding could occur if left untreated.

Intrapleural drains are usually inserted in the chest, in an area which is known as the 'triangle of safety'. The mid-axillary line borders this area posteriorly, the level of the nipple inferiorly and the lateral border of the pectoralis major interiorly (Hyde *et al.* 1997; Peek *et al.* 2000; Tang *et al.* 2002). Once the drain has been placed in any position within the 'triangle of safety', re-expansion of the lung occurs. However, in cases of intrapleural adhesions or localized collection of pus or fluids, the doctor will need to position the tip of the drain to assist drainage (Hyde *et al.* 1997; Tang *et al.* 2002).

502

Drain size

The size of tube used is dependent on the reason for drainage. Whilst no large randomized trials comparing small and large bore tubes have been performed, the optimum size of drainage catheter remains controversial (Laws *et al.* 2003).

In the past the use of a large bore drain was recommended to prevent the blockage of chest drains, particularly by thick malignant or infected fluid (Hyde *et al.* 1997). However, currently the majority of physicians prefer to use smaller catheters (10–14 French [F]) and some smaller studies have shown that these are often as effective as larger bore tubes (Clementsen *et al.* 1998; Patz 1998). Small bore drains are more comfortable and better tolerated by the patient (Laws *et al.* 2003).

Securing the drain

The British Thoracic Society (Laws *et al.* 2003) advises that purse string stitches should not be used as they cause pain by changing a linear wound into a circular one and leave an unsightly scar. Only large and medium bore drains require suturing; small gauge chest tubes do not usually require suturing. The suture material should be strong and non-absorbable to prevent breaking, such as silk, and a mattress suture should be employed rather than a purse string suture (Laws *et al.* 2003).

Stripping/milking of intrapleural drains

Milking and stripping of chest tubes to keep them patent has been studied, and has shown that this increases the negative pressure in the intrathoracic cavity to −100 to −400 cmH$_2$O and subsequently it seems that milking or stripping of chest tubes on a routine basis should be avoided (Kirkwood 2002). If a chest drain becomes occluded or blocked the tubing needs to be replaced rather than milking or stripping (Avery 2000).

Clamping of intrapleural drains

The British Thoracic Society Guidelines (Miller & Harvey 1993) discourage clamping of intrapleural drains as this can prevent air leaving the pleural space. This in turn can cause a pneumothorax which could progress to a life-threatening tension pneumothorax. There is also no need to clamp tubing when mobilizing or transporting patients to other departments as this may also cause a tension pneumothorax (Hyde *et al.* 1997; Henry *et al.* 2003). When changing the bottle system, it is necessary to clamp the drain for the shortest period of time possible and during this process the patient should be under close observation for any signs of deterioration in breathing (Brandt *et al.* 1994).

In cases of pneumothorax the chest drain should not be clamped at the time of its removal (Laws *et al.* 2003). The only time a non-bubbling chest drain should be momentarily clamped is in the event of disconnection, if there is damage to the drainage bottle, or to locate a leak in the drainage system (Avery 2000; Henry *et al.* 2003; Laws *et al.* 2003; Allibone 2005).

Drainage systems

Prepacked drainage systems are now available for drainage of pneumothoraces, haemothoraces or pleural effusions. The bottle has a screw top with two ports. One port has the underwater length of tubing attached. The second port has a shorter length of tubing attached which acts as the venting end and is exposed

503

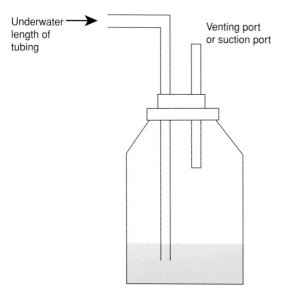

Underwater length of tubing →

Venting port or suction port

Figure 14.3　One-bottle system.

to air or could be attached to a suction unit. Venting prevents the build-up of pressure in the chest drainage system which could prevent evacuation of air or fluid (McMahon-Parkes 1997) (Figure 14.3).

The underwater seal occurs when there is adequate water in the bottle, usually 500 ml of water. The distal end of the intrapleural drain is then attached to the underwater seal port of the chest drain bottle and immersed 2.5 cm below the level of the water. Incoming air, bubbles through the water, which acts as a one-way valve and prevents the backflow of air into the intrapleural space (McMahon-Parkes 1997).

For more complicated pneumothoraces or haemothoraces a plastic multi-chamber system incorporates the above one-bottle system into one unit. There are three chambers: the first is for drainage, the second chamber is the underwater seal and the third chamber is the vacuum or suction control. When this system is set up, water is placed in the water seal chamber to the indicated mark, and also placed in the suction control chamber to the required level. This system is a great improvement on the previous systems and enables patient mobility (Pierce 1995) (Figure 14.4).

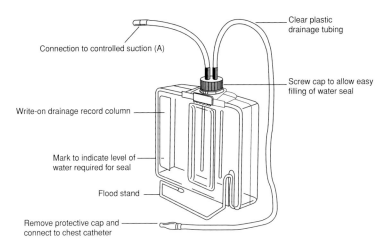

Connection to controlled suction (A)

Clear plastic
drainage tubing

Screw cap to allow easy
filling of water seal

Write-on drainage record column

Mark to indicate level of
water required for seal

Flood stand

Remove protective cap and
connect to chest catheter

Figure 14.4   Underwater chest drainage system.

Maintenance of drainage systems during and after insertion

When the drain is attached to the drainage bottle bubbling or swinging should be observed; this indicates that air is being evacuated from the pleural space. As the lung re-inflates, the bubbling should decrease. If bubbling continues, a leak may be present in the patient's lung. Causes of air leaks include:

■ Air in chest from a pneumothorax.
■ An eyelit from chest tube outside the chest wall.
■ Blocked drain may cause an air leak at puncture site.
■ Inadequate drain size.
■ Poor tube connections.
■ Poor seal around the entry site to the lung (Kirkwood 2002).

The presence of an air leak should be assessed. Bubbling can occur in the underwater seal compartment. If bubbling occurs when the patient coughs, this would usually indicate the leak is only minor. However, continuous bubbling would indicate a serious air leak in the system. The drain and tube should be inspected thoroughly down to the level of the underwater seal to eliminate any external problems such as loose tubing connections or poor seal around the drain at the insertion site. A chest X-ray should also be ordered to establish the position of the drain. Air leaks should be treated with caution and prompt action is required (such as referral to a specialist respiratory physician).

Tubing should be tailored to suit the patient's needs, allowing room to manoeuvre but preventing coiling and looping (Hyde *et al.* 1997; Avery 2000; Kirkwood 2002). Pleural effusion, impaired gas exchange and infection can also be caused by loops, coiling and kinks in the tubing as well as impeding drainage (Gorden *et al.* 1997; Kirkwood 2002) so regular inspection of tubing should be carried out.

There is debate about the most recent recommendations on taping the connection between the chest drainage bottle and drainage tubes (Godden 1998; Avery 2000), as the nurse may not be able to see if the connections have parted beneath the tape (Adam & Osborne 2005); however, without any additional method of security, such as tape, there is a risk of the drainage tubing becoming disconnected (Allibone 2005).

Dressings for insertion site

A simple dry dressing (low-linting gauze) should be applied around the drain and secured with adhesive tape during drainage and after removal of drain (Tang *et al.* 2002). Heavy strapping should be avoided as it can restrict chest movement. Dressings during the drainage procedure should be kept clean and dry and not removed until the drain is ready for removal (Tang *et al.* 1999; Avery 2000).

Pain control

On insertion of a chest drain, tissue damage occurs and this activates nerve fibres surrounding the insertion site (Gray 2000; Hilton 2004). While the drain is in place, the nerve fibres or tissue cannot heal. Therefore, the patient will experience pain throughout the insertion procedure and after the drain has been inserted (Tomlinson & Treasure 1997). Inadequate pain control can cause the patient to breathe incorrectly and the patient may try to avoid coughing, resulting in complications such as chest infections (Gray 2000). Risk can be reduced by chest physiotherapy from a physiotherapist (Gray 2000). In a study by Luketich (Luketich *et al.* 1998), 50% of patients experience pain levels of 9–10 on a scale of 0–10, with 10 being most pain imaginable. Therefore, prior to inserting an intrapleural drain unless contraindicated, premedication such as benzodiazepine or an opioid should be administered as prescribed (Laws *et al.* 2003). A comprehensive plan for pain control involving the patient and the health care professionals should be produced. Pain management should cover all stages of the intrapleural drainage process (Gray 2000):

- Insertion.
- Management of the intrapleural drain during the drainage process.
- Removal of the intrapleural drain.

Current protocols for the management of pain include patient-controlled analgesia, paravertebral blocks, non-steroidal anti-inflammatory drugs or transcutaneous electrical nerve stimulation (Allibone 2005).

Suction and its use

The addition of suction to the drainage system increases the negative pressure, enhancing lung re-expansion. A high-volume and low-pressure suction unit should be applied (Hyde *et al.* 1997; Tang *et al.* 2002) using pressure in the range of 5–15 kPa. The suction pressure should only be increased if the patient's pain is controlled and if the patient tolerates the increase. Once suction has been discontinued, the tubing to the underwater seal should be disconnected, otherwise this could cause positive pressure and may precipitate a tension pneumothorax (Tang *et al.* 2002) (see (A) in Figure 14.4). The suction unit should be cleaned by wiping it with a damp cloth and a mild disinfectant solution. Most suction units are fitted with a disposable air filter capsule, between the vacuum connector and the filter capsule mount. The filter prevents cross-infection and should be changed after each patient.

Chest drain removal

If a patient has had a pneumothorax, the chest drain should not be clamped at the time of its removal (Laws *et al.* 2003). The chest drain should be removed either while the patient is asked to perform a Valsalva manoeuvre or during expiration with a brisk firm movement while an assistant ties the mattress suture to close the wound (Laws *et al.* 2003). The Valsalva manoeuvre (asking the patient to hold their breath while trying to exhale out against a closed glottis, or bear down) increases the intrathoracic pressure which prevents air from entering the thoracic cavity on removal of the drain (McMahon-Parkes 1997; Avery 2000).

507

The decision to remove a drain is usually made by a medical practitioner based on the following criteria:

- Absence of an air leak into the chest drain bottle, usually noted when the patient exhales forcibly or coughs. When a patient is ventilated with positive pressure this will coincide with the expiration.
- Re-expansion of lung following previous discontinuation of any suction when there should be no air leak or drainage.

- The volume of fluid draining into the chest drain is minimal. Guidelines on what is minimal vary but less than 10 ml/h per drain has been suggested (Higgins 2006).
- There is no evidence of respiratory compromise or failure.
- There is no coagulation deficit or increased risk of bleeding (check latest coagulation results prior to removal).
- In many cases radiological evidence of the absence of air or fluid accumulation will be required before removal.

Advice should be sought from a medical practitioner if there is any doubt as to whether to remove a chest drain (Higgins 2006).

Procedure guidelines   Intrapleural drain insertion

Equipment

1 Sterile chest drain pack containing, gallipot, disposable towel, forceps, disposable scalpel and sterile low-linting gauze.
2 Suture material: silk.
3 Cleaning solution, chlorhexidine gluconate 0.5% in 70% alcohol.
4 Sterile gloves and gown.
5 Local anaesthetic, lidocaine 1%.
6 Syringes 2 × 10 ml.
7 Needles 1 × 21 gauge, 1 × 23 gauge.
8 Chest drain. Check appropriate size to be used for insertion.
9 Sterile dressing.
10 Tape.
11 Chest drain tubing.
12 Chest drain bottle.
13 Sterile water 1 litre bottle.
14 Chest drain clamps × 2.
15 Low vacuum suction pump if required.

Intrapleural drain insertion

Action	Rationale
1 Cleanse hands with alcoholic handrub. Hands to be cleansed before and after each patient contact.	To minimize the risk of infection (DH 2005a: C).
2 Explain and discuss the procedure with the patient.	To ensure the patient understands why and how the procedure is to be performed and gives his/her valid consent (Laws *et al.* 2003: C; NMC 2006: C).
Note: the procedure might have to be performed under emergency conditions.	A patient may have become acutely unwell, and so the procedure would prevent respiratory and cardiovascular collapse (Adam & Osborne 2005: E).

3 Administer analgesia prior to procedure after discussion with the doctor, about the type and route of administration. The analgesia should be given at least half an hour before the procedure.	To minimize any pain during the procedure and to ensure the patient is pain free and able to co-operate (Laws *et al.* 2003: C).
4 Administer sedation on doctor's instruction, if considered appropriate, e.g. for an anxious patient.	To relieve anxiety and allow the patient to relax and co-operate, and to enable the procedure to proceed (E).
5 Cleanse hands with alcoholic handrub.	To minimize the risk of infection (DH 2005a: C).
6 Prepare trolley, placing equipment on bottom shelf. Take to patient's bedside.	
7 Prime the underwater seal system with sufficient sterile water to cover the drainage tube. Cleanse hands with alcoholic handrub.	This prevents back flow of air or fluid into the pleural space, and marks the initial water level to allow measurement of subsequent drainage (Adam & Osborne 2005: E).
8 Assist doctor in setting up sterile procedure pack.	To minimize risk of infection and to have equipment ready (E).
9 Check the correct side of chest for drain insertion to optimize access to the triangle of safety.	To ensure drainage of correct side by checking the chest X-ray (O'Connor & Morgan 2005: E).
10 Position patient in preparation for the procedure. The patient may be positioned flat on the bed with the arm on the affected side placed behind his/her head away from the chest wall or abducted to 90°. If patient is able to sit upright, he/she can be positioned resting over a table supported by a pillow.	To facilitate insertion of the intrapleural drain. To aid patient comfort (Hyde *et al.* 1997: E).
11 Observe the patient throughout procedure, with attention to respiratory status including colour, respiratory rate, respiratory pattern, equal movement of chest and peripheral tissue oxygen saturations.	To look for any change in the patient's condition and report to the doctor, to ensure appropriate intervention, e.g. oxygen therapy (Laws *et al.* 2003: C).

509

Procedure guidelines (cont.)

Observe patient for any change to the cardiovascular system by alterations in heart rate or blood pressure.	To look for any change in the patient's condition and report to the doctor, to ensure appropriate intervention (Allibone 2003: E).
12 Communicate with the patient during the procedure and explain what is happening at each stage.	By communicating throughout the patient feels involved and informed (Laws *et al.* 2003: C).
13 Assist doctor in procedure as below:	
(a) The doctor will wash his hands with an antiseptic detergent and apply sterile gloves and a gown.	To minimize risk of infection (DH 2005a: C).
(b) The area for planned insertion of the drain will be cleaned with chlorhexidine gluconate 0.5% in alcohol and allowed to air dry.	To minimize risk of infection (DH 2005a: C).
(c) Local anaesthetic will be injected into the skin and deeper tissue (intercostal muscle and parietal pleura) along proposed insertion site.	To minimize the feeling of pain on drain insertion (Gray 2000: P).
(d) Wait 2–3 min for local anaesthetic to take.	To ensure local anaesthetic has been effective (E).
(e) An incision is then made with a scalpel to enable the intrapleural drain to be inserted.	To aid and ease the movement of the drain into the correct position (E).
(f) A finger may then be manoeuvred through to the parietal pleura to guide the drain into place, between the parietal and visceral pleurae in the pleural space for large bore chest tubes (Miller & Harvey 1993).	To aid the drain into the correct position (E). Exploration with a finger is felt to be unnecessary for the elective medical insertion of medium or small sized chest tubes (Laws *et al.* 2003: C).
(g) The drain is then clamped using two clamps until connected to the drainage system.	To prevent further lung collapse and entry of air (Laws *et al.* 2003: C).
(h) Connect the distal end of the drain to the drainage system and ensure that it is well supported and secured.	To allow for inflation of the lung or drainage of fluid, to ensure there is no movement of drain and that it remains in the correct position (Allibone 2003: E).
(i) The proximal end of the drain is secured and sutured in place with a mattress stitch. Unclamp chest drains.	To secure drain in position (Laws *et al.* 2003: C). Purse string stitches should no longer be used as they cause pain and unsightly scarring (Laws *et al.* 2003: C).

14 Clean the site and apply a dressing of gauze, then an occlusive dressing over the gauze.	To ensure site is well covered and sealed (Laws *et al*. 2003: C). To reduce risk of infection (DH 2005a: C).
15 Send patient for chest X-ray.	To ensure the correct position of the drain and to ensure that the lung has re-inflated (Laws *et al*. 2003: C).
16 Check the drain is well secured.	To prevent movement of drain or accidental disconnection of drain (Laws *et al*. 2003: C).
17 Monitor if there is bubbling/swinging of water in the bottle/tubing or drainage fluid and check there are no leaks around the site or that any loose connections exist within the drainage system.	To ensure there is no occlusion or leak which will prevent re-expansion of the lung or drainage of the fluid (Laws *et al*. 2003: C).
18 Record any bubbling, swinging and drainage on observation and fluid balance charts.	To keep acurate record of type of drainage on fluid balance chart (Laws *et al*. 2003: C; NMC 2005: C).
19 Ensure patient comfort following the procedure. Return the patient to an elevated position sitting in bed, well supported by pillows, and give further analgesia if required.	To ensure patient comfort in order to aid recovery and breathing (Allibone 2003: E).
20 Dispose of waste appropriately.	To reduce risk of cross-infection and sharps injury (DH 2005a: R Ia; DH 2005b: C).
21 Cleanse hands with alcoholic handrub.	Hands to be cleansed before and after each patient contact (DH 2005a: C).

Suction for intrapleural drainage

Action	Rationale
1 Cleanse hands with alcoholic handrub.	To minimize the risk of infection (DH 2005a: C).
2 Communicate with the patient during the application of suction and explain what is happening at each stage.	To keep the patient fully informed. To enable the patient to feel reassured (Laws *et al*. 2003: C).

Procedure guidelines *(cont.)*

3 Discuss analgesia management with the patient. Give analgesia to the patient as prescribed.	To ensure patient comfort (Gray 2000: P).
4 Prepare the suction unit, which should be low vacuum suction (bedside suction units are high volume and therefore not suitable).	To maintain safety, ensuring the suction is set at low pressure (Laws *et al.* 2003: C).
5 Connect tube A (see Figure 14.4) to the suction unit, as directed by the medical team. Adjust the suction to required level prescribed, usually −5 cmH$_2$O (Adam & Osborne 2005), or to a level that is tolerable for the patient.	To ensure patient comfort and to ensure suction is applied (E). Higher volumes of suction may injure lung tissue (Kirkwood 2002: E).
6 Position patient to aid comfort, ensuring the patient is pain free and relaxed.	To aid breathing for lung expansion. To aid patient comfort (Gray 2000: E).
7 Monitor intrapleural drainage and record amount.	To maintain patient safety by observing level of suction and amount of fluid drained (Allibone 2003: E).
8 Check suction unit is working and suction pressure is maintained according to doctor's orders.	To maintain patient safety (Laws *et al.* 2003: C).

Post-intrapleural-drain procedure

Action	Rationale
1 Observe patient for any change in respiratory status: (a) Colour. (b) Respiratory rate and pattern. (c) Unequal chest movement. (d) Peripheral tissue oxygen saturations. (e) Blood gases.	These symptoms may indicate a change of chest drain position, occlusion of the drain or recurrence of pneumothorax or collection of fluid (Laws *et al.* 2003: C).
Observe patient for any change in cardiovascular status: (a) Heart rate. (b) Blood pressure.	May indicate pressure on the cardiovascular system (Allibone 2003: E).

512

Observe patient for signs of infection:
(a) Temperature.
(b) Exit site.

Obtain appropriate specimens (see Chapter 28) and inform medical staff (Wilson 2006: E).

2 Ensure the drain remains well secured with suture and dressing.

To prevent movement of drain and ensure safety of patient (Laws *et al*. 2003: C).

3 Ensure the drain is well positioned with no loops or kinks.

To prevent occlusion of drain (Kirkwood 2002: E).

4 Ensure drain tubing is well supported at the side of the bed using tape and clamps.

To prevent drain pulling and dragging, causing trauma to the patient or movement of or the risk of the drain falling out.

5 Ensure drain tubing and connections are secure and attached to the drainage unit.

To ensure a sealed unit exists to prevent air entry into the pleura which could lead to further lung collapse (Kirkwood 2002: E).

6 Ensure a pair of clamps is available beside the patient in case of accidental disconnection.

To clamp drain and prevent further lung collapse (Laws *et al*. 2003: C).

7 Do not clamp drains other than in the case of accidental disconnection.

To prevent a high positive pressure that can be created when the drain is clamped and which can result in a tension pneumothorax (Laws *et al*. 2003: C).

8 Ensure chest drain remains at a level below the chest at all times.

This prevents backflow of fluid into the pleural space (Laws *et al*. 2003: C).

9 Do not milk or strip tubing, rather change tubing if there is an occlusion.

Milking or stripping can cause an increase in negative pressure which could result in damage to lung tissue (Laws *et al*. 2003: C).

10 Observe volume and type of drainage; is it clear/bloodstained, etc.? Record on a fluid chart and in the nursing notes. Continue to record whether the drain is bubbling or swinging. If volumes exceed 1500 ml within the first 2 hours, clamp the tubing for 1 hour and inform doctors.

To ensure monitoring of type and volume of fluid loss. To prevent re-expansion oedema and large volume loss causing relative hypovolaemia (Laws *et al*. 2003 C).

513

Procedure guidelines *(cont.)*

11 Ensure that when the patient is sitting in the chair that the tubing, if coiled, is lifted periodically.	To aid drainage without letting the bottle be lifted higher than the thoracic cavity (Allibone 2003: E).
12 Position patient comfortably in bed, sitting upright, well supported by pillows.	To aid patient comfort. To aid breathing and allow for full expansion of the lungs (Laws *et al.* 2003: C).
13 Change the position of the patient while in bed.	To reduce risk of breakdown in skin integrity (E).
14 Encourage mobilization of the patient, e.g. to sit in chair and also to walk aided by physiotherapist or nurse.	To encourage patient independence and prevent complications, e.g. pulmonary embolus, deep vein thrombosis, breakdown in skin integrity (Allibone 2003: C).
15 Ensure patient maintains mobility of arm on side of drain.	To prevent complications and reduce risk of immobility of arm.
16 Ensure patient remains pain free.	To relieve pain and aid recovery (Gray 2000: P).
17 Maintain patient hygiene and mouth care. Assist patient in washing/mouth care because of restriction of movement due to drain.	To aid patient comfort and reduce the risk of infection (DH 2005a: C).
18 Maintain normal oral and dietary intake.	To aid healing process. To reduce risk of dehydration and malnutrition. To reduce risk of infection (DH 2005a: C).
19 Maintain a normal sleep pattern.	To allow patient to rest and aid recovery (E).
20 Ensure patient is kept occupied, e.g. reading, watching television, listening to the radio.	To relieve boredom and aid recovery (E).

514

Procedure guidelines   Intrapleural drain: changing the bottle

Equipment

1 Cleaning solution, e.g. chlorhexidine in 70% alcohol.
2 Non-sterile gloves.
3 Tape.
4 Sterile chest drain bottle.
5 1 litre sterile water bottle.
6 Chest drain clamps × 2.
7 Procedure pack.

Changing intrapleural drain bottle

Action	Rationale
1 Cleanse hands with alcoholic handrub.	Hands to be cleansed before and after each patient contact (DH 2005a: C).
2 Explain and discuss the procedure with the patient.	To ensure the patient is well prepared, and to ensure their co-operation and consent (Laws *et al.* 2003: C; NMC 2006: C).
3 Cleanse hands with alcoholic rub and fill chest drain bottle to water fill line or until drainage tube is submerged in water.	To prevent infection and to prevent reflux of air or fluid into the lungs, and to create a water seal (Kirkwood 2002: E).
4 Undo the taping around the tubing.	
5 Clamp the tubing close to the chest wall with two clamps for the shortest time needed to change the bottles.	To prevent air entering the chest cavity causing a pneumothorax (Laws *et al.* 2003: C). Clamping the drain for long periods of time may increase the risk of pneumothorax (Laws *et al.* 2003: C).
6 Observe patient's breathing and respiratory status during the procedure.	To identify any respiratory deterioration early and report any abnormalities timely to medical team (Allibone 2005: E).

515

Procedure guidelines (cont.)

7 Clean tubing at the connection and remove full bottle and tubing and connect new bottle and tubing to clamped chest tube.	To prevent infection entering system during disconnection and connection of tubing (DH 2005a: C).
8 Ensure a secure connection, unclamp and tape.	To prevent bottle from falling over or disconnection causing air to re-enter the pleural cavity (Allibone 2005).
9 Ensure chest drain bottle is secure in metal stand on the floor.	
10 Cleanse hands with alcoholic rub.	
11 Document new bottle on fluid balance chart and in nursing documentation.	To keep accurate record of amounts drained (Allibone 2005: E; NMC 2005: C).
12 Observe patient for any changes in respiratory status as per previous instructions.	To identify any respiratory deterioration early and report any abnormalities to the medical team (Allibone 2005: E).

Procedure guidelines   Intrapleural drain removal

Equipment

1 Sterile dressing pack containing gallipot, gauze, sterile towel.
2 Cleaning solution, e.g. 0.9% sodium chloride.
3 Non-sterile gloves.
4 Stitch cutter.
5 Sterile dressing.
6 Tape.

Two nurses/assistants are required to facilitate safe removal of a chest drain. One is required to tie the suture and seal the site, and the other to remove the drain.

Intrapleural drain removal

Action	Rationale
1 Cleanse hands with alcoholic handrub.	Hands to be cleansed before and after each patient contact (DH 2005a: C).

2 Prepare patient for removal of the drain. Explain and discuss each step of the procedure with the patient.	To ensure the patient is well prepared, and to ensure their co-operation and consent (Laws *et al*. 2003: C; NMC 2006: C).
3 Encourage patient to practise breathing exercises, as these are required to help with the procedure. The patient should be instructed to take three deep breaths in and out and on the fourth breath to hold the breath in. It is on this breath that the drain will be removed, i.e. end of inspiration (Adam & Osborne 2005).	To prepare the patient and encourage co-operation (E). To allow the patient to practise the breathing exercises (E). To prevent the entry of air that can occur due to a negative intrathoracic pressure (Tomlinson & Treasure 1997; Allibone 2005: E).
4 In order to reduce the complication of recurrent pneumothorax, the Valsalva manoeuvre can be used. This requires patients to hold their breath and to bear down or try to breathe out against a closed glottis (Allibone 2005).	This increases the intrathoracic pressure, which reduces the possibility of air re-entering the pleural space through the drain site (Laws *et al*. 2003: C; Allibone 2005: E).
5 Clamping of chest drain prior to removal is not necessary.	Unnecessary clamping increases risk of pneumothorax (Laws *et al*. 2003: C; Adam & Osborne 2005).
6 Administer analgesia prior to procedure after discussion with doctor about the type and route of administration. The analgesia should be given at least half an hour before the procedure.	To minimize any pain during the procedure and to ensure the patient is pain free and able to co-operate (Gray 2000: P).
7 Administer sedation on doctor's instruction, if considered appropriate, e.g. for an anxious patient.	To relieve anxiety and allow the patient to relax and co-operate and to enable the procedure to go ahead (E).
8 Discontinue suction if in use and disconnect from venting/suction port.	To prevent a tension pneumothorax (Laws *et al*. 2003: C).

517

Procedure guidelines *(cont.)*

9 Cleanse hands with alcoholic handrub.	Hands need to be cleansed before and after each patient contact (DH 2005a: C).
10 Prepare trolley for procedure.	To aid the procedure (E).
11 Assist or set up the sterile procedure pack.	To minimize risk of infection and to have equipment ready (DH 2005a: C).
12 Position patient comfortably.	To aid patient comfort (E).
13 Place protective pad underneath the patient and drain.	To absorb any ooze from the drain. To reduce risk of contamination of the patient and bed clothing (E).
14 Cleanse hands with alcoholic handrub before touching the drain or dressing.	To reduce risk of infection (DH 2005a: C).
15 Remove dressing from around drain site, examine sutures present. (a) tube retaining suture (anchor suture) and (b) mattress suture; expose the ends of these sutures.	To prepare for drain removal and check what type of suture is present so that the suture can be used to form an airtight seal when the drain is removed (Adam & Osborne 2005: E).
16 Both assistants for the procedure must wash their hands with an antiseptic solution undertaking a full surgical scrub and apply gloves.	To reduce risk of infection (DH 2005a: C).
17 First nurse/assistant prepares mattress string suture and loosens ends ready to tie the suture when the drain is removed.	To prepare for drain removal (E).
18 Second nurse/assistant prepares and cuts the anchor suture and ensures the drain is mobile and ready to remove.	To prepare for drain removal (E).

19	Second nurse/assistant asks the patient to start deep breathing exercises: to take three deep breaths then hold his/her breath on the fourth one while the drain is pulled out steadily and smoothly. And ask the patient to perform the Valsalva manoeuvre.	To aid in drain removal. Deep breathing exercises can help to prevent a tension pneumothorax. If a drain is removed too quickly or without due care a pneumothorax can occur due to rupture of the pleura (Laws *et al*. 2003: C).
20	First nurse/assistant will then tie the mattress string suture securely to the skin.	To form an airtight seal and prevent air entry and formation of a pneumothorax (Laws *et al*. 2003: C).
21	Ask the patient to breath normally after tube is removed.	To assess if there is any air escaping from suture site (E).
22	Clean around site with 0.9% sodium chloride and apply an occlusive dressing, such as gauze soaked in flexible collodion or petroleum gauze under waterproof strapping.	To clean site, form an airtight seal and prevent air entry (E). To prevent an air leak if drain puncture site is not closed properly (Adam & Osborne 2005: E).
23	Ensure that the patient is sitting upright, and support with pillows.	To ensure patient comfort and aid respiration (Allibone 2005: E).
24	Dispose of waste appropriately.	To ensure safety and reduce risk of infection (DH 2005a: C; DH 2005b: C).
25	Document removal on fluid chart and in nursing notes.	To provide a point of reference for any queries (E).
26	A chest X-ray should be performed approximately 1 hour post-removal.	To check that a pneumothorax has not recurred (O'Connor & Morgan 2005: R 5).
27	Both the patient and the drain site should be monitored closely (Allibone 2005).	To observe for signs of respiratory distress secondary to reaccumulation of fluid/air in pleural cavity (Allibone 2005: E).
28	Cleanse hands with alcoholic handrub.	Hands need to be cleansed before and after each patient contact (DH 2005a: C).

519

Problem solving: Intrapleural drainage

Problem	Cause	Suggested action
Patient shows signs of respiratory distress, increased respiratory rate, uneven chest movement, decreasing peripheral tissue oxygen saturations.	Pneumothorax or tension pneumothorax.	Observe patient continually for change in vital signs. Inform doctor and administer oxygen. Prepare for reinsertion of chest drain.
Lack of drainage.	Kinking, looping or pressure on the tubing may cause reflux of fluid into the intrapleural space or may impede drainage, causing blocking of the intrapleural drain.	Check the system and straighten tubing as required. Secure the tubing to prevent a recurrence of the problem.
Fluid in drain not swinging.	Drain occluded due to position or occlusion.	Check no loops or kinks present in tubing. Lift drain, not higher than the patient's chest, to see if the obstruction will clear. Seek medical advice as the drain may need replacing.
Fluid in drain not bubbling.	Drain occluded or not correctly positioned.	Check no loops or kinks in the tubing. Lift tubing to see if it will clear.
Continual bubbling in chest drain bottle.	Air leak in system.	Check system for loose connections in tubing or around drainage unit. If no leak present in the drainage tubing the leak may be present in the lung. Inform doctor. Prepare chest drain insertion pack.
Leakage from drain site.	Bleeding or infection.	Remove the dressing and observe the site. Inform doctor, take swab. Clean and redress site. Discuss with medical team regarding prescription of antibiotic therapy.

520

Problem	Cause	Suggested action
Drainage from around drain site.	As a result of the insertion procedure. Incomplete closure with sutures. Infected insertion site.	Observe drain site, amount and type of drainage. Inform doctor. Take swab from site. Prepare suture pack to be available if required. Discuss with medical team regarding prescription of antibiotic therapy.
Accidental disconnection of the drainage tubing from the intrapleural drain.	Connections not secure.	Apply a clamp to the drain immediately in order to avoid air entering the pleural space. Re-establish the connection as soon as possible in order to re-establish drainage. If necessary, use a clean, sterile drainage tube; tubing may have been contaminated when it became disconnected. Report to the doctor, who may wish to X-ray.
		Record the incident in the relevant records. The patient may have been upset by the incident and will need reassurance.
Intrapleural drain falls out.	Drain not secure.	Pull the purse-string suture immediately to close the wound. Cover the wound with an occlusive sterile dressing. Check the patient's vital signs. Inform a doctor. The objective is to minimize the amount of air entering the pleural space. The drain will probably need reinserting. Prepare chest drain insertion pack. Reassure the patient with appropriate explanations.
Poor arm movement.	Restriction of arm movement due to position of drain.	Encourage movement of limb to keep mobile. Adjust analgesia as required.
Pain.	Drain pulling at site.	Try repositioning tubing, so that it is not dragging or irritating skin. Give analgesia as prescribed.

521

Problem solving *(cont.)*

Problem	Cause	Suggested action
Restricted mobility of patient.	Due to position of drain and attachment to the drainage unit.	Explore with the patient the movement that is possible and aid them where help is required. Encourage mobility, aid patient to sit in chair. Work in liaison with physiotherapist. Encourage patient to move in bed and change position.

References and further reading

Adam, S.K. & Osborne, S. (2005) Respiratory problems. In: *Critical Care Nursing*. 2nd edn. Oxford Medical Publications, Oxford, pp. 69–119

Allibone, L. (2003) Nursing management of chest drains. *Nurs Stand*, **17**(22), 45 54.

Allibone, L. (2005) Respiratory care. Principles for inserting and managing chest drains. *Nurs Times* **101** (42), 45–9.

Avery, S. (2000) Insertion and management of chest drains. *Nurs Times*, **96**, 3–6.

Berne, R.M. & Levy, M.N. (2004) Structure and function of the respiratory system. In: *Physiology*, 5th edn. Mosby, London, pp. 445–463

Brandt, M.L. *et al.* (1994) The paediatric chest tube. *Clin Intensive Care*, **5**(3), 123–9.

Chernecky, C. & Shelton, B. (2001) Pulmonary complications in patients with cancer: diagnostic and treatment information for the noncritical care nurse. *Am J Nurs*, **101**(5), 24A–24H.

Clementsen, P. *et al.* (1998) Treatment of malignant pleural effusion: pleurodesis using a small bore catheter. A prospective randomized study. *Respir Med*, **92**, 593–6.

Deshpande, K.S., Tortolani, A.J. & Kvetan, V. (2003) Troubleshooting chest tube complications: how to prevent, or quickly correct the major problems. *J Crit Illn*, **18**(6), 275–80.

DH (2005a) *Saving Lives: A Delivery Programme to Reduce Healthcare Associated Infection including MRSA*. Department of Health, London.

DH (2005b) *Hazardous waste (England) regulations*. Department of Health, London.

Gallon, A. (1998) Pneumothorax. *Nurs Stand*, **39**(10), 35–9.

Godden, J. (1998) Managing the patient with a chest drain: a review. *Nurs Stand*, **12**(32), 35–9.

Gorden, P.A., Norton, J.M. & Guerra, J.M. (1997) Positioning of chest drain tubes: effects on pressure and drainage. *Am J Crit Care*, **6**, 33–8.

Gray, E. (2000) Pain management for patients with chest drains. *Nurs Stand*, **14**(23), 40–4.

Grodzin, C.J. & Baik, R.A. (1997) Indwelling small pleural catheter needle thoracentesis in the management of large pleural effusions. *Chest*, **111**(4), 981–8.

Hall, J.E. and Guyton, A.C (2005) Pulmonary ventilation. In: *A Textbook of Medical Physiology*, 11th edn. W.B. Saunders, Philadelphia, pp. 471–482.

Henry, M., Arnold, T. & Harvey, J. (2003) British Thoracic Society guidelines for the management of spontaneous pneumothorax. *Thorax*, **58**, 39–52.

Higgins, D. (2006) Removal of chest drains. *Nurs Times*, **102**(13), 26–7.

Hilton, P. (2004) Evaluating the treatment options for spontaneous pneumothorax. *Nurs Times*, **100**(28), 32–3.

Hyde, J., Skyes, T. & Graham, T. (1997) Reducing morbidity from chest drains. *BMJ*, **314**(7085), 914–15.

Kirkwood, P. (2002) Ask the experts. *Crit Care Nurse*, **22**(4), 70–3.

Kozar, R. & Adams, S.D. (2005) Chylothorax. Emedicine from www.emedicine.com/med/topic381.htm. Accessed 28/08/07.

Kumar, P. & Clarke, C. (2002) *Clinical Medicine*. Mosby, St. Louis, MO.

Laws, D., Neville, E. & Duffy, J. (2003) British Thoracic Society guidelines for the insertion of a chest drain. *Thorax*, **58**, 53–9.

Luketich, J.D. *et al.* (1998) Chest tube insertion: a prospective evaluation of pain management. *Clin J Pain,* **14**, 152–4.

Marieb, E.N. (2001) The respiratory system. In: *Human Anatomy and Physiology*, 5th edn. John Wiley & Sons, Inc., New York. Pearson Education, San Francisco, CA. pp. 834–86.

McMahon-Parkes, K. (1997) Management of pleural drains. *Nurs Times*, **93**(52), 48–52.

MedlinePlus (2006) Medical encyclopedia. www.nlm.nih.gov/medlineplus/ency/article/000100.htm. Accessed 7/08/06.

Miller, A.C. & Harvey, J.E. (1993) Guidelines for the management of spontaneous pneumothorax. *BMJ*, **307**, 114–16.

NMC (2005) *Guidelines for Records and Record Keeping*. Nursing and Midwifery Council, London.

NMC (2006) *A–Z Advice Sheet Consent*. www.nmc.org.

O'Connor, A.R. & Morgan, W.E. (2005) Radiological review of pneumothorax. *BMJ*, **330**, 1493–7.

Parkin, C. (2002) A retrospective audit of chest drain practice in a specialist cardiothoracic centre and concurrent review of chest drain literature. *Nurs Crit Care*, **7**(1), 30–6.

Patz, E.F. (1998) Malignant pleural effusions: recent advances and ambulatory sclerotherapy. *Chest*, **113**(1, Suppl 1), 74–5.

Peek, G., Morcos, S. & Cooper, G. (2000) The pleural cavity. *BMJ*, **320**, 1318–21.

Pierce, L.N.B. (1995) *Guide to Mechanical Ventilation and Intensive Respiratory Care*. W.B. Saunders, London, Appendix 111, pp. 356–63.

Tang, A., Hooper, T. & Hassan, R. (1999) A regional survey of chest drains: evidence based practice? *Postgrad Med J*, **75**(886), 471–4

Tang, A., Vellissaris, T. & Weeden, D. (2002) An evidence based approach to drainage of pleural cavity: evaluation of best practice. *J Eval Clin Pract*, **8**(3), 333–40.

Thelan, L.A. *et al.* (1995) *Critical Care Nursing–Diagnosis and Management*, 2nd edn. Mosby, St. Louis, MO.

Tomlinson, M.A. & Treasure, T. (1997) Insertion of a chest drain: how to do it. *Br J Hosp Med*, **58**(6), 248–52.

Tooley, C. (2002) The management and care of chest drains. *Nurs Times*, **98**(26), 48–50.

Tortora, G.J. & Derrickson, B. (2008) The respiratory system. In: *Principles of Anatomy and Physiology*, 12th edn. John Wiley & Sons, Inc., New York, Hoboken NJ, pp. 846–94.

Van Le, L. *et al.* (1994) Pleural effusions: outpatient management of pigtail catheter chest tubes. *Gynecol Oncol*, **54**, 215–7.

Wilson, J. (2006) *Infection Control in Clinical Practice*. Bailliere Tindall, London.

Yeam, I. & Sassoon, C. (1997) Haemothorax and chylothorax. *Curr Opin Pulmon Med*, **3**(4), 310–14.

Multiple choice questions

1 Patients will require insertion of an intrapleural drain for:

   a   Pneumothorax
   b   Drainage of pleural effusion
   c   Post thoracotomy
   d   All of the above

2 A pneumothorax can be defined as:

   a   Pain in the chest cavity
   b   Air in the pleural cavity
   c   Fluid in the pleural cavity
   d   Pus in the pleural cavity

3 Before insertion of an intrapleural drain *all* patients need what investigation?

   a   Blood test
   b   MRI scan
   c   Chest X-ray
   d   CT scan

4 When an intrapleural drain is attached to the drainage bottle, which of the following would you expect to see?

   a   Bubbling or swinging of the water required for the seal
   b   Bubbling or swinging of the water that reduces over time
   c   Bubbling or swinging of the water that increases over time
   d   No movement of the water required for the seal

Answers to the multiple choice questions can be found in Appendix 3.

Chapter 15

Last offices

Definition

Nursing care should not stop when the patient dies. Last offices, sometimes referred to as 'laying out', is the term for the nursing care given to a deceased patient which demonstrates continued respect for the patient as an individual (NMC 2008) and in contemporary society it is focused on attending to health, safety and legal requirements, making the body safe to handle and pleasant for others to see, whilst also respecting religious beliefs and cultural norms.

Reference material

In many societies, the care and preparation of the deceased is carried out only by close family members. In others it is undertaken by certain specialized individuals within the community (Clark 2000). For example, amongst orthodox Jews, the *chevra kadisha* or Burial Society of each community, made up of volunteers, cares for the deceased and prepares them for burial (Helman 2007). However in the UK, where of all recorded deaths, 66% of patients die in hospital (ONS 2000), it is common practice for nurses who have cared for the individual before death to care for the body after death, prior to it leaving the hospital ward or department (Berry & Griffie 2004).

There is documented evidence of nurses caring for the bodies of their deceased patients dating back to the nineteenth century (Wolf 1988). However, contemporary nursing practice is somewhat different to that of our predecessors who were required to cleanse the body of the deceased, plugging, packing and tying the patient's orifices to prevent the leakage of body fluids (Pearce 1963). Today emphasis is given to the legal issues surrounding death, the removal of invasive, defunct equipment, washing and grooming, and ensuring the correct identification of the body (Costello 2004). Such practices are being asserted by end-of-life care tools such as the Liverpool Care Pathway for the Dying (Ellershaw & Wilkinson 2003), which is fast gaining national momentum and demonstrating improvements to the care of the dying and care after death.

Whilst the procedure of last offices has its foundation in traditional cultures and has become a nursing ritual that does not have a heavy weight of research-based evidence (Cooke 2000), the administration of last offices can have symbolic meaning for nurses and can be a fulfilling experience as it is the final demonstration of respectful, sensitive care given to a patient (Nearney 1998) and also the family (Speck 1992). Last offices can mark the social transition of the person, the biological death of the patient, and begins the process of handing over care to the family and funeral director. Therefore, last offices can be considered as an important act in the rite of passage or *rite de passage* in moving the deceased into the world of the dead (Van Gennep 1972) that people in all cultures recognize. Whilst we may not be able to locate a scientific evidence base for this clinical nursing procedure, there is a strong cultural requirement to continue with it as, 'Rituals serve to express symbolic meanings important to groups of people functioning within a subculture' (Wolf 1988, p. 59). And whilst in contemporary nursing practice and education there is a move away from ritualistic practice as it is considered as irrational and unscientific (Philpin 2002), the procedure of last offices remains a notable exception. However, this is not to say that nurses carrying out last offices do it, 'without thinking about it in a problem solving way' (Walsh & Ford 1989, p. 9) or in a way that does not recognize the individual needs of the deceased and their carers. Instead these are carried out with insight into the meanings attached to the accomplishment of this aspect of nursing care (Philpin 2002).

In administering last offices, nurses need to know the legal requirements for care of the dead and it is essential that the correct procedures are followed. Every effort should be made to accommodate the wishes of the patient's relatives (Neuberger 2004).

It is impossible to understand the laws and prohibitions about handling human bodies after death without having some idea of what that particular person's religion or philosophy has to say about the nature of human life and its value (Neuberger 1999). As the UK today is a multicultural and multifaith society, this offers a great challenge to nurses who need to be aware of the different religious and cultural rituals that may accompany the death of a patient. There are considerable cultural variations within and between people of different faiths, ethnic backgrounds and national origins and their approach to death and dying (Neuberger 1999). Whilst those who have settled in a society where there is a dominant faith or culture other than their own appear to increasingly adopt that dominant culture, in many ways they retain, almost deliberately to emphasize differences, their different practices at times of birth, marriage or death (Neuberger 1999). Approaches to death and dying also reveal as much of the attitude of society as a whole as they do about individuals within that society (Field *et al.* 1997).

Practices relating to last offices will vary depending on the patient's cultural background and religious practices (Nearney 1998). The following sections provide a guide to cultural and religious variations in attitudes to death and how individuals may wish to be treated. The information that follows is not designed to be a chapter of comparative theology. Nor is it a 'factfile' (Gunaratnam 1997; Smaje & Field 1997; Gilliat-Ray 2001) of information on culture and religion that seeks to give concrete information. Such a 'factfile' would not be appropriate as we need to be aware that whilst death and death-related beliefs, rituals and traditions can vary widely from each specific cultural group, within any given religious or cultural group there may be varying degrees of observance of these issues (Green & Green 2006) from orthodox to the agnostic and atheist. Our motivation to categorize individuals into groups with clearly defined norms can lead to a lack of understanding of the complexities of religious and cultural practice and can depersonalize individuals and their families (Smaje & Field 1997; Neuberger 1999).

Last offices for an expected death may be very different to those given to a patient who has died suddenly or unexpectedly (Docherty 2000) or in a critical care setting; therefore, these issues will be dealt with later in this chapter. In certain cases the patient's death may need to be referred to the coroner for further investigation and possible post-mortem (DH 2003). If those caring for the deceased are unsure about this, then the person in charge of the patient's care should be consulted before last offices are commenced. However, further advice on this is given in the Issues specific to critical care section, below.

Prior to the patient's death, whenever possible it is good practice to ascertain if the patient wishes to donate organs or tissue following their death. For further information on this visit: www.uktransplant.org.uk/urt.

Procedure guidelines   Last offices

Equipment

1 Disposable plastic aprons.
2 Disposable plastic gloves.
3 Bowl of warm water, soap, the deceased's own toiletries and face cloths or disposable wash cloths and two towels.
4 Disposable razor or the patient's own electric razor, comb and equipment for nail care.
5 Equipment for mouth care including equipment for cleaning dentures.

6 Identification labels ×2.
7 Documents required by law and organization policy, e.g. notification of death cards.
8 Shroud or patient's personal clothing: night-dress, pyjamas, clothes previously requested by patient, or clothes that comply with family/cultural wishes.

527

Procedure guidelines *(cont.)*

9 Body bag if required (i.e. in event of actual or potential leakage of bodily fluids and/or infectious disease) and labels for the body defining the nature of the infection/disease (HSE 2003: C).

10 Gauze, waterproof tape, dressings and bandages if wounds or intravenous/arterial lines and cannulae are present.

11 Disposable or washable receptacle for collecting urine if appropriate.

12 Plastic bags for clinical and household waste.

13 Sharps bin if appropriate.

14 Laundry skip and appropriate bags for soiled linen.

15 Clean bed linen.

16 Record books for property and valuables.

17 Bags for the patient's personal possessions.

Procedure

Action	Rationale
1 Inform the nurse in charge of the ward or unit and inform medical staff of the patient's death. Confirmation of death must be given. This is usually done by medical staff. If an expected death occurs in the event of medical staff not being available, it may be possible for the senior nurse on duty to confirm the death if an agreed local policy has been implemented (RCN 1996: C). An unexpected death must be confirmed by an attending medical officer. Confirmation of death must be recorded in a patient's medical, nursing notes and care pathway documentation if necessary.	A registered medical practitioner who has attended the deceased person during their last illness is required to give a medical certificate of the cause of death (Home Office 1971: C). The certificate requires the doctor to state on which date he/she last saw the deceased alive and whether or not he/she has seen the body after death.
2 Inform and offer support to relatives and/or next of kin. Offer support of Hospital Chaplain or other religious leader or other appropriate person, e.g. bereavement support officer. If relative(s) or next of kin are not contactable by telephone or by the GP, it may be necessary to inform the police of the death. Also inform other patients in the area of the patient's death.	To ensure relevant individuals are aware of patient's death. To provide sensitive care (Wilkinson & Mula 2003: E).

3 Ascertain if the patient had an infectious disease and whether this is notifiable or not. There are additional requirements for patients with blood-borne infections; therefore, the senior nurse on duty should be consulted and local infection control policy adhered to. Placing the deceased in a body bag is advised for all notifiable diseases and a number of non-notifiable infectious diseases (i.e. human immunodeficiency virus [HIV] and transmissible spongiform encephalopathies, e.g. Creutzfeldt–Jakob disease).

Certain extra precautions are required when handling a patient who has died from an infectious disease. However, the deceased will pose no greater threat of an infectious risk than when they were alive. It is assumed that staff will have practised universal precautions when caring for all patients, and this practice must be continued when caring for the deceased patient (HSE 2003: C).

4 Last offices should be carried out within 2–4 hours of death.

Rigor mortis can occur relatively soon after death, and this time is shortened in warmer environments (Berry & Griffie 2006: E).

5 If possible determine from the family or carers, the patient's previous wishes for care after death.

Some families and carers may wish to assist with last offices, and within certain cultures it may be unacceptable for anyone but a family member or religious leader to wash the patient (Green & Green 2006: P & C). Families and carers should be supported and encouraged to participate if possible as this may help to facilitate the grieving process (Berry & Griffie 2006: E).

6 Wash hands and put on disposable gloves and disposable plastic apron.

Personal protective equipment (PPE) must be worn when performing last offices, and is used to both protect yourself and all of your patients from the risks of cross-infection (RCN 2005: C).

529

7 If the patient is on a pressure-relieving mattress or device, consult the manufacturer's instructions before switching off or changing settings.

Nurses must act at all times to maintain the patient's safety when using a pressure-relieving mattress or device (RCN 2003: C & E).

Procedure guidelines *(cont.)*

8 Lay the patient on his/her back with the assistance of two nurses (adhering to your own organization's Manual Handling policy). Remove all but one pillow. Support the jaw by placing a pillow or rolled-up towel on the chest or underneath the patient's jaw. Do not bind the patient's jaw with bandages as this can leave pressure marks on the face which can be difficult to remove. Remove any mechanical aids such as syringe drivers, heel pads, etc. Apply guaze and tape to syringe driver sites and document disposal of medication (adhering to your own organization's Disposal of Medication policy). Straighten the patient's limbs.

To maintain the patient's privacy and dignity (NMC 2008: C) and for future nursing care of the body. A body with flexed limbs can be difficult to fit easily into a mortuary trolley, mortuary fridge or coffin and can cause additional distress to any carers who wish to view the body. However, if the body cannot be straightened, force should not be used as this can be corrected by the funeral director (Green & Green 2006: E).

9 Close the patient's eyes by applying light pressure to the eyelids for 30 seconds. If this is unsuccessful then a little sticky tape such as micropore can be used, and leaves no mark. Alternatively, moistened cotton wool may be used to hold the eyelids in place.

To maintain the patient's dignity (NMC 2008: C) and for aesthetic reasons. Closure of the eyelids will also provide tissue protection in case of corneal donation (Green & Green 2006: E).

10 Drain the bladder by applying firm pressure over the lower abdomen. Have a disposable or washable receptacle at the ready to collect urine. Therefore the practice of tying a bandage round a penis is not necessary and many families may find this practice unacceptable.

Because the body can continue to excrete fluids after death (Green & Green 2006: E).

11 Leakages from the oral cavity, vagina and bowel can be contained by the use of suctioning, drainage and incontinence pads respectively. Patients who do continue to have leakages from their orifices after death should be placed in a body bag following last offices. The packing of orifices can cause damage to the body and should only be done by professionals, e.g. mortuary technicians who have received specialist training.	Leaking orifices pose a health hazard to staff coming into contact with the body (HSE 2003: C; Green & Green 2006: E). Ensuring that the body is clean will demonstrate a continued respect for the patient's dignity (NMC 2008: C). The packing of orifices is considered unnecessary as it increases the rate of bacterial growth and therefore increases odour when these areas of the body are not allowed to drain naturally (Berry & Griffie 2006: E).
12 Exuding wounds or unhealed surgical scars should be covered with a clean absorbant dressing and secured with an occlusive dressing. Stitches and clips should be left intact. Stomas should be covered with a clean bag.	The dressing will absorb any leakage from the wound site (Naylor et al. 2001: R 2b). Open wounds and stomas pose a health hazard to staff coming into contact with the body (RCN 2005: C).
13 Remove drainage tubes, etc. unless otherwise stated, and document actions and any tubes remaining, e.g. central venous access device which should not be removed by nursing staff. Open drainage sites need to be sealed with an occlusive dressing (e.g. Tegaderm).	Open drainage sites pose a health hazard to staff coming into contact with the body (RCN 2005: C). When a death is being referred to the coroner or for post-mortem, all lines, devices and tubes should be left in place (Green & Green 2006: C).
14 Wash the patient, unless requested not to do so for religious/cultural reasons or carer's preference. Male patients should be shaved unless they chose to wear a beard in life. If shaving a man apply water-based emollient cream to the face.	For hygenic and aesthetic reasons. As a mark of respect and point of closure in the relationship between nurse and patient (Cooke 2000: C). To prevent brown streaks on the skin (Ashford and St. Peter's Hospitals NHS Trust 2005: E).
15 It may be important to family and carers to assist with washing, thereby continuing to provide the care given in the period before death.	It is an expression of respect and affection, and part of the process of adjusting to loss and expressing grief (Berry & Griffie 2006: E).
16 Clean the patient's mouth using a foam stick to remove debris and secretions. Clean dentures and replace them in the mouth if possible.	For hygenic and aesthetic reasons (Cooke 2000: C).

Procedure guidelines *(cont.)*

17 Remove all jewellery (in the presence of another nurse) unless requested by the patient's family to do otherwise. Jewellery remaining on the patient should be documented on the 'notification of death' form. Record the jewellery and other valuables in the patient's property book and store the items according to local policy. Avoid the use of the names of precious metals or gems when describing jewellery to prevent later confusion. Instead use terms such as 'yellow metal' or 'red stone'. Rings left on the body should be secured with tape, if loose.

To meet with legal requirements, cultural practices and relatives' wishes (Green & Green 2006: C).

18 Dress the patient in personal clothing or white garment, traditionally called a shroud, depending on organizational policy or relatives' wishes.

For aesthetics for family and carers viewing the body or religious or cultural reasons and to meet family's or carer's wishes (Green & Green 2006: C).

19 Ensure a correct hospital or organizational irremovable patient identification label is attached to the patient's wrist and attach a further identification label to one ankle. Complete any documents such as notification of death cards. Copies of such cards are usually required (refer to hospital policy for details). Tape one securely to clothing or shroud.

To ensure correct and easy identification of the body in the mortuary (Green & Green 2006: C).

20 Wrap the body in a sheet, ensuring that the face and feet are covered and that all limbs are held securely in position.

To avoid possible damage to the body during transfer and to prevent distress to colleagues, e.g. portering staff (Green & Green 2006: E).

21 Secure the sheet with tape.

Pins must not be used as they are a health and safety hazard to staff (Nearney 1998: E; Travis 2002: E).

22 Place the body in a sheet and then a body bag if leakage of body fluids is a problem or is anticipated, or if the patient has certain infectious diseases (see Chapter 5).	Actual or potential leakage of fluid, whether infection is present or not, poses a health hazard to all those who come into contact with the deceased patient. The sheet will absorb excess fluid (HSE 2003: C).
23 Tape the second notification of death card to the outside of the sheet (or body bag).	For ease of identification of the body in the mortuary (Green & Green 2006: E).
24 Request the portering staff to remove the body from the ward and transport to the mortuary.	Decomposition occurs rapidly, particularly in hot weather and in overheated rooms. Many pathogenic organisms survive for some time after death and so decomposition of the body may pose a health and safety hazard for those handling the body (Cooke 2000: E). Autolysis and growth of bacteria are delayed if the body is cooled.
25 Screen off area where removal of the body will occur.	To avoid causing unnecessary distress to other patients, relatives and staff (Nearney 1998: E; Travis 2002: E).
26 Remove gloves and apron. Dispose of equipment according to local policy and wash hands.	To minimize risk of cross-infection and contamination (DH 2001: R 1a).
27 Record all details and actions within the nursing documentation.	To record the time of death, names of those present, and names of those informed (NMC 2008: C).
28 Transfer property, patient records, etc. to the appropriate administrative department.	The administrative department cannot begin to process the formalities such as the death certificate or the collection of property by the next-of-kin until the required documents are in its possession (Green & Green 2006: C; NMC 2005: C).

533

Issues specific to critical care

Critical care, accident and emergency and other such acute settings present further issues related to last offices. These are in addition to those listed above.

Issues starting with verification of death may differ; therefore, senior nursing and medical staff should be consulted before commencing last offices.

Additional practices may need to be carried out if the patient is a donor patient, particularly in the case of brain stem death (DH 1998). It is important to liaise with the transplant co-ordinator to ascertain before last offices if there are specific preparations required. In the case of a coroner-led post-mortem there may also be specific preparations required (DH 2003). Senior nursing staff or the coroner's office should be consulted to establish if this is necessary before undertaking last offices.

Procedure guidelines   Last offices: additional considerations in critical care

The following should be considered in addition to the same numbered action in the procedures listed above in Procedure guidelines: Last offices.

Procedure

Action	Rationale
3 High-risk infectious patients should be marked as such, e.g. patient with HIV, hepatitis B, on the accompanying forms, and should have hazard labels on the body bag and on the patient. Linen and waste should be treated as infected. In the case of tuberculosis, there is still a risk of expirational transmission after death. This phenomenon should be considered and communicated, especially to mortuary staff or nurses who may re-prepare the patient for a viewing at a later point in time. In certain cases (i.e. typhus, SARS [Severe Acute Respiratory Syndrome], yellow fever, anthrax, plague, rabies and smallpox) viewing should not be permitted given the high risk of transmission. In the case of highly infectious patients (e.g. notifiable) packing should be considered.	Rolling the patient in last offices may force expiration and facilitate transmission of tuberculosis. The risk of transmission remains after death in certain notifiable diseases (typhus, SARS, yellow fever, anthrax, plague, rabies and smallpox) (HSAC 2003: C). Packing may reduce the risk of transmission.

4 If the patient is not to be referred to the coroner then remove all invasive and non-invasive attachments to the patient, such as: central venous access lines, peripheral venous access lines, Swan–Ganz catheters, tracheal tubes (tracheostomy/ endotracheal [ET]), drains. If a coroner's case, cap off lines and ensure no possibility of leakage. Do not remove any invasive lines.

The coroner may need to see exactly what state the patient was in at the time death and what could have contributed to cause of death (DH 2003: C). Documentation ensures that there is a record of invasive equipment in situ for the patient notes and the coroner.

11 All deceased critical care patients should be placed in a zipped plastic (body) bag. Absorbent sheets (incontinence pads) may be placed either side of the head.

There is an increased likelihood of critical care patients leaking (Travis 2002: E).

12 Consider leaving intact recent surgical dressings for wounds that could potentially leak, e.g. large amputation wounds. Reinforcement of the dressing should be sufficient.

Certain surgical wounds may have been carefully dressed in theatre and disturbing them in order to redress may precipitate leakage (Travis 2002: E).

13 Document tubes/equipment remaining, e.g. tunneled skin catheters, pacemaker, implantable cardioverter defibrillators (ICDs).

Documentation ensures that there is a record of equipment still *in situ* (Travis 2002: E).

16 Apply petroleum jelly to lips and perioral area. Suction oropharynx if patient previously intubated/had a tracheostomy.

Even if the patient is not obviously leaking from the oral cavity, secretions may accumulate in the oropharynx in previously intubated and tracheostomy patients. Petroleum jelly may prevent skin excoriation/corrosion if stomach contents aspirate (Travis 2002: E).

535

Problem solving: Last offices

Problem	Suggested action
Relatives not present at the time of the patient's death.	Inform the relatives as soon as possible of the death. Consider also that they may want to view the body before last offices are completed.
Relatives or next-of-kin not contactable by telephone or by the general practitioner.	If within the UK, local police will go to next-of-kin's house. If abroad, the British Embassy will assist.
Death occurring within 24 hours of an operation.	All tubes and/or drains must be left in position. Spigot any cannulae or catheters. Treat stomas as open wounds. Leave any endotracheal or tracheostomy tubes in place. Post-mortem examination will be required to establish the cause of death. Any tubes, drains etc., may have been a major contributing factor to the death.
Unexpected death.	As above. Post-mortem examination of the body will be required to establish the cause of death.
Unknown cause of death.	As above.
Patient brought into hospital who is already deceased.	As above, unless patient seen by a medical practitioner within 14 days before death. In this instance the attending medical officer may complete the death certificate if he/she is clear as to the cause of death.
Patient with leaking wounds/orifices with or without infection present. Patient with hepatitis B or who is HIV positive.	For further information see Chapter 5.
Patient who dies after receiving systemic radioactive iodine.	For further information see Chapter 36, Professional edition.

536

Problem	Suggested action
Patient who dies after insertion of gold grains, colloidal radioactive solution, caesium needles, caesium applicators, iridium wires or iridium hair pins.	Inform the physics department as well as appropriate medical staff. Once a doctor has verified death, the sources are removed and placed in a lead container. A Geiger counter is used to check that all sources have been removed. This reduces the radiation risk when completing the last offices procedures. Record the time and date of removal of the sources.
Patient and/or relative wishes to donate organs/tissues for transplantation.	Patients with malignancies can only donate corneas (with certain exceptions) and in some cases, heart valves and tracheas. Ultimately, this is a clinician-led decision. Contact local transplant co-ordinator as soon as decision is made to donate organs/tissue and before last offices is attempted. Obtain verbal and written consent from the next-of-kin, as per local policy. Prepare body as per transplant co-ordinator's instructions (UK Transplant, 2007).
Patient to be moved straight from ward to undertakers.	Contact senior nurse for hospital. Contact local Registry Office as release of Certificate for Burial or Cremation ('green' document) needs to be obtained. Liaise with chosen funeral directors and the deceased's family. Perform last offices as per religious/cultural/family wishes. Obtain written authority for removal of body by the funeral directors, from the next-of-kin. Document all actions and proceedings (Travis 2002: C).
Relatives want to see the body after removal from the ward.	Inform the mortuary staff in order to allow time for them to prepare the body. The body will normally be placed in the hospital viewing room. Ask relatives if they wish for a chaplain or other religious leader or appropriate person to accompany them. As required, religious artefacts should be removed from or added to the viewing room. The nurse should check that the body and environment are presentable before accompanying the relatives into the viewing room. The relatives may want to be alone with the deceased but the nurse should wait outside the viewing room in order that support may be provided should the relatives become distressed. After the relatives have left, the nurse should contact the portering service who will return the body to the mortuary.

Procedure guidelines Last offices: requirements for people of different religious faiths

The following are only guidelines: individual requirements may vary even among members of the same faith. Varying degrees of adherence and orthodoxy exist within all the world's faiths. The given religion of a patient may occasionally be offered to indicate an association with particular cultural and national roots, rather than to indicate a significant degree of adherence to the tenets of a particular faith. If in doubt, consult the family members concerned.

Bahai

1 The body of the deceased should be treated with respect. Bahai relatives may wish to say prayers for the deceased person, but normal last offices performed by nursing staff are quite acceptable.

2 Bahai adherents may not be cremated or embalmed, nor may they be buried more than an hour's journey from the place of death. A special ring will be placed on the finger of the patient and should not be removed.

3 Bahais have no objection to post-mortem examination and may leave their bodies to scientific research or donate organs if they wish.

4 Further information can be obtained from the nearest Assembly of the Bahais (see telephone directory). Alternatively, contact:
  National Spiritual Assembly of the Bahais of the United Kingdom
  27 Rutland Gate, London SW7 1PD
  Tel: 020 7590 8792
  Email: nsa@bahai.org.uk
  Website: www.bahai.org.uk

Buddhism

1 There is no prescribed ritual for the handling of the corpse of a Buddhist person, so customary laying out is appropriate. However, a request may be made for a Buddhist monk or nun to be present.

2 As there are a number of different schools of Buddhism, relatives should be contacted for advice as some sects have strong views on how the body should be treated.

3 When the patient dies, inform the monk or nun if required (the patient's relatives often take this step). The body should not be moved for at least 1 hour if prayers are to be said.

4 There are unlikely to be objections to post-mortem examination and organ donation, although some Far Eastern Buddhists may object to this.

5 The patient's body should be wrapped in an unmarked sheet.

6 Cremation is preferred.

7 For further information contact:
  Dennis Sibley
  The Buddhist Hospice Trust
  1 Laurel House, Trafalger Road
  Newport, Isle of Wight, PO30 1QN
  Tel: 01983 526945
  Email:
  dsibley@buddhisthospice.org.uk

Christianity

1 There are many denominations and degrees of adherence within the Christian faith. In most cases customary last offices are acceptable.

2 Relatives may wish staff to call the hospital chaplain, or minister or priest from their own church to either perform last rites or say prayers.

3 Some Roman Catholic families may wish to place a rosary in the deceased patient's hands and/or a crucifix at the patient's head.

4 Some orthodox families may wish to place an icon (holy picture) at either side of the patient's head.

5 For further information consult the hospital chaplain or consult the telephone directory for the local denominational minister or priest.
Alternatively, contact:
Hospital Chaplaincies Council
Church House, Great Smith Street, London SW1 3NZ
Tel: 020 7898 1894
Useful website:
www.nhs-chaplaincy-spiritualcare. org.uk

Humanism

1 Humanism is an approach to life based on reason and a sense of a common humanity with a recognition that moral values are founded within human nature and experience alone (BBC 2006). Therefore Humanism is not a religion but a rationalist non-religious approach to life. Humanism affirms that human beings have the right and responsibility to give meaning and shape to their own lives (BBC 2006).

2 Therefore, individuals who define themselves as Humanists should as far as possible, like all other patients, be involved in decisions relating to their care before and after death.

3 For further information contact:
British Humanist Association
1 Gower Street, London WC1E 6HD
Tel: 020 70793582
Email: info@humanism.org.uk
Website: www.humanism.org.uk

539

Procedure guidelines *(cont.)*

Hinduism

1 If required by relatives, inform the family priest or one from the local temple. If unavailable, relatives may wish to read from the *Bhagavad Gita* or make a request that staff read extracts during the last offices.

2 The family may wish to carry out or assist in last offices and may request that the patient is dressed in his or her own clothes. If possible, the eldest son should be present. A Hindu may like to have leaves of the sacred Tulsi plant and Ganges water placed in his/her mouth by relatives before death. It is therefore imperative that relatives are warned that the patient's death is imminent. Relatives of the same sex as the patient may wish to wash his/her body, preferably in water mixed with water from the River Ganges. If no relatives are present, nursing staff of the same sex as the patient should wear gloves and apron and then straighten the body, close the eyes and support the jaw before wrapping in a sheet. The body should not be washed. Do not remove sacred threads or jewellery.

3 The patient's family may request that the patient be placed on the floor and they may wish to burn incense.

4 The patient is usually cremated as soon as possible after death. Post-mortems are viewed as disrespectful to the deceased person, and so are only carried out when strictly necessary. Consult the wishes of the family before touching the body.

5 For further information contact the nearest Hindu temple (see telephone directory) or:

> National Council of Hindu Temples (UK)
> 40 Stoke Row, Coventry CV2 4JP
> Email: info@hinducouncil.org
> Useful website:
> www.hinducouncil.org

Jainism

1 The relatives of a Jainist patient may wish to contact their priest to recite prayers with the patient and family.

2 The family may wish to be present during the last offices and also to assist with washing. However, not all families will want to perform this task.

3 The family may ask for the patient to be clothed in a plain white gown or shroud with no pattern or ornament and then wrapped in a plain white sheet. They may provide the gown themselves.

4 Post-mortems may be seen as disrespectful, depending on the degree of orthodoxy of the patient. Organ donation is acceptable.

5 Cremation is arranged whenever possible within 24 hours of death.

6 Orthodox Jains may have chosen the path of *Sallekhana*, that is, death by ritual fasting. Sallekhana is rarely practised today although it may still have an influence on the Jain attitude to death.

7 For further information contact:
The Institute of Jainology
Unit 18, Silicon Business Centre,
26 Wandsworth
    Road, Greenford, Middlesex
UB6 7JZ
Tel: 020 8997 2300
The Jain Centre
32 Oxford Street, Leicester LE1 5XU
Tel: 0116 254 3091
Useful website: www.jainism.org

Jehovah's Witness

1 Routine last offices are appropriate. Relatives may wish to be present during last offices, either to pray or to read from the Bible. The family will inform staff should there be any special requirements, which may vary according to the patient's country of origin.
2 Jehovah's Witnesses usually refuse post-mortems unless absolutely necessary. Organ donation may be acceptable.

3 Further information can be obtained from the nearest Kingdom Hall (see telephone directory) or:
The Medical Desk
The Watch Tower Bible and Tract Society
Watch Tower House, The Ridgeway, London
    NW7 1RN
Tel: 020 8906 2211
Email: his@wtbts.org.uk

Judaism

1 The family will contact their own Rabbi if they have one. If not, the hospital chaplaincy will advise. Prayers are recited by those present.
2 Traditionally the body is left for about 8 minutes before being moved while a feather is placed across the lips and nose to detect any signs of breath.
3 Usually close relatives will straighten the body, but nursing staff are permitted to perform any procedure for preserving dignity and honour.
Wearing gloves, the body should be handled as little as possible but nurses may:

(a) Close the eyes.
(b) Tie up the jaw.
(c) Put the arms parallel and close to the sides of the body leaving the hands open. Straighten the patient's legs.
(d) Remove tubes unless contraindicated.
Patients must not be washed and should remain in the clothes in which they died. The body will be washed by a nominated group, the Holy Assembly, which performs a ritual purification.

541

Procedure guidelines *(cont.)*

4 Watchers stay with the body until burial (normally completed within 24 hours of death). In the period before burial a separate non-denominational room is appreciated, where the body can be placed with its feet towards the door.

5 It is not possible for funerals to take place on the Sabbath (between sunset on Friday and sunset on Saturday). If death occurs during the Sabbath, the body will remain with the watchers until the end of the Sabbath. Advice should be sought from the relatives. In some areas, the Registrar's office will arrange to open on Sundays and Bank Holidays to allow for the registration of death where speedy burial is required for religious reasons. The Jewish Burial Society will know whether this service is offered in the local area.

6 Post-mortems are permitted only if required by law. Organ donation is sometimes permitted.

7 Cremation is unlikely but some non-orthodox Jews are now accepting this in preference to burial.

8 For further information, contact:
The Burial Society of the United Synagogue
Tel: 020 8343 3456
The Office of the Chief Rabbi (Orthodox)
735 High Road, North Finchley, London WC1N 9HN
Tel: 020 8343 6301

Reform Synagogues of Great Britain
The Sternberg Centre for Judaism
80 East End Road, Finchley, London N3 2SY
Tel: 020 8349 4731

Union of Liberal and Progressive Synagogues
Montagu Centre, 21 Maple Street, London
W1T 4BE

Mormon (Church of Jesus Christ of the Latter Day Saints)

1 There are no special requirements, but relatives may wish to be present during the last offices. Relatives will advise staff if the patient wears a one or two piece sacred undergarment. If this is the case, relatives will dress the patient in these items.

2 For further information contact the nearest Church of Jesus Christ of Latter Day Saints (see telephone directory) or:
The Church of Jesus Christ of Latter Day Saints
751 Warwick Road, Solihull, West Midlands B91 3DQ
Tel: 0121 712 1200
Useful website: www.ldschurch.org

Muslim (Islam)

1 Where possible, the patient's bed should be turned so that their body (head first) is facing Mecca. If the patient's bed cannot be moved, then the patient can be turned on to their right side so that the deceased's face is facing towards Mecca.

2 Many Muslims object to the body being touched by someone of a different faith or opposite sex. If no family members are present, wear gloves and close the patient's eyes, support the jaw and straighten the body. The head should be turned to the right shoulder and the body covered with a plain white sheet. The body should not be washed nor the nails cut.

3 The patient's body is normally either taken home or taken to a mosque as soon as possible to be washed by another Muslim of the same sex. Burial takes place preferably within 24 hours of death. Cremation is forbidden. Post-mortems are permitted only if required by law. Organ donation is not always encouraged, although in the UK a Fatwa (religious verdict) was given by the UK Muslim Law Council which now encourages Muslims to donate organs.

4 For further information contact:
   IQRA Trust
   3rd Floor, 16 Grosvenor Crescent,
   London SW1X 7EP
   Tel: 020 7838 7987
   Email: info@iqratrust.org
   Website: www.iqratrust.org.uk

Rastafarian

1 Customary last offices are appropriate, although the patient's family may wish to be present during the preparation of the body to say prayers.

2 Permission for organ donation is unlikely and post-mortems will be refused unless absolutely necessary.

3 Useful website: www.rastafarian.net

Sikhism

1 Family members (especially the eldest son) and friends will be present if they are able.

2 Usually the family takes responsibility for the last offices, but nursing staff may be asked to close the patient's eyes, support the jaw, straighten the body and wrap it in a plain white sheet.

3 Do not remove the '5 *ks*', which are personal objects sacred to the Sikhs:
   Kesh: do not cut hair or beard or remove turban.

   Kanga: do not remove the semi-circular comb, which fixes the uncut hair.
   Kara: do not remove bracelet worn on the wrist.
   Kaccha: do not remove the special shorts worn as underwear.
   Kirpan: do not remove the sword: usually a miniature sword is worn.

4 The family will wash and dress the deceased person's body.

5 Post-mortems are only permitted if required by law. Sikhs are always cremated.

543

Procedure guidelines *(cont.)*

6 Organ donation is permitted but some Sikhs refuse this as they do not wish the body to be mutilated.

7 For further information contact the nearest Sikh temple or Gurdwara (see telephone directory). Alternatively, contact:

    Sikh Missionary Society UK
    10 Featherstone Road, Southall, Middlesex UB2 5AA

Tel: 020 8574 1902
Sikh Educational and Cultural Association (UK)
Sat Nam Kutia, 18 Farncroft, Gravesend, Kent
    DA11 7LT
Tel: 01474 332356
Useful website:
www.bbc.co.uk/religion/religions/sikhism

Zoroastrian (Parsee)

1 Customary last offices are often acceptable to Zoroastrian patients.

2 The family may wish to be present during, or participate in, the preparation of the body.

3 Orthodox Parsees require a priest to be present, if possible.

4 After washing, the body is dressed in the *Sadra* (white cotton or muslin shirt symbolizing purity) and *Kusti* (girdle woven of 72 strands of lambs' wool symbolizing the 72 chapters of the *Yasna* [Liturgy]).

5 Relatives may cover the patient's head with a white cap or scarf.

6 It is important that the funeral takes place as soon as possible after death.

7 Burial and cremation are acceptable. Post-mortems are forbidden unless required by law.

8 Organ donation is forbidden by religious law.

9 For further information contact:
    The Zoroastrian Trust Funds of Europe
    440 Alexandra Avenue, Harrow, Middlesex HA2 9TL
    Tel: 020 8866 0765
    Fax: 020 8868 4572
    Email: secretary@ztfe.com
    Useful website:
    www.bbc.co.uk/religion/religions/zoroastrian

544 References

Ashford and St. Peter's Hospitals NHS Trust (2005) *Last Offices Nursing Procedure*. Ashford and St Peter's Hospitals NHS Trust, Kent.

Berry, P. & Griffie, J. (2006) Planning for the actual death. In: *Textbook of Palliative Nursing* (eds B. R. Ferrell & N. Coyle), 2nd edn. Oxford University Press, Oxford, pp. 561–77.

Clark, D. (2000) Death in Staithes. In: *Death, Dying and Bereavement* (eds D. Dickenson, M. Johnson & J.S. Katz). Sage Publications, London, pp. 4–9.

Cooke, H. (2000) *A Practical Guide to Holistic Care at the End of Life*. Butterworth Heinemann, Oxford.

Costello, J. (2004) *Nursing the Dying Patient: Caring in Different Contexts*. Palgrave Macmillan, Basingstoke, Hants.

DH (1998) *A Code of Practice for the Diagnosis of Brain Stem Death*. Department of Health, London. Available at: www.dh.gov. uk/assetRoot/04/03/54/62/04035462.pdf. Accessed 14/07/06

DH (2001) Standard principles for preventing hospital acquired infections. *J Hosp Infect*, **47**(Suppl), S21–7.

DH (2003) *A Guide to the Post-mortem Examination Procedure*. Department of Health, London.

Docherty, B. (2000) Care of the dying patient. *Prof Nurse*, **15**(12), 752.

Ellershaw, J. & Wilkinson, S. (2003) *Care of the Dying. A Pathway to Excellence*. Oxford University Press, Oxford.

Field, D., Hockley, J. & Small, N. (1997) *Death, Gender and Ethnicity*. Routledge, London.

Gilliat-Ray, S. (2001) Sociological perspectives on the pastoral care of minority faiths in hospital. In: *Spirituality in Health Care Contexts* (ed. H. Orchard). Jessica Kingsley Publishers, London, pp. 135–46.

Green, J. & Green, M. (2006) *Dealing with Death: A Handbook of Practices, Procedures and Law*, 2nd edn. Jessica Kingsley Publishers, London.

Gunaratnam, Y. (1997) Culture is not enough: a critique of multiculturalism in palliative care. In: *Death, Gender and Ethnicity* (eds D. Field, J. Hockley & N. Small). Routledge, London, pp. 166–86.

HSAC (2003) *Safe Working and the Prevention of Infection in the Mortuary and Post-mortem Room*. Health and Safety Executive Books, London.

HSE (2003) *Safe Working and the Prevention of Infection in the Mortuary and Post-mortem Room*. Health and Safety Executive Books, London.

Helman, C.J. (2007) *Culture, Health and Illness*, 5th edn. Arnold, London.

Home Office (1971) *Report of the Committee on Death Certification and Coroners*. CMND 4810. HMSO, London.

Howarth, G. & Jupp. P.C. (eds) (1996) *Contemporary Issues in the Sociology of Death, Dying and Disposal*. Macmillan, Basingstoke.

Naylor, W., Laverty, D. & Mallett, J. (2001) *The Royal Marsden Hospital Handbook of Wound Management in Cancer Care*. Blackwell Science, Oxford.

Nearney, L. (1998) Last offices, part 1. *Nurs Times*, **94**(26), Insert.

Neuberger, J. (1999) Cultural issues in palliative care. In: *Oxford Textbook of Palliative Medicine* (eds D. Doyle, G. Hanks & N. MacDonald). Oxford University Press, Oxford, pp. 777–80.

Neuberger, J. (2004) *Caring for People of Different Faiths*. Radcliffe Medical Press, Abingdon, Oxon.

NMC (2005) *Guidelines for Records and Record Keeping*. Nursing and Midwifery Council, London.

NMC (2008) *The Code: Standards of Conduct, Performance and Ethics for Nurses and Midwives*. Nursing and Midwifery Council, London.

ONS (2000) NHS hospital activity by NHS Regional Office area, 2000–01. www.statistics.gov.uk. Accessed 3/5/06.

Pearce, E. (1963) *A General Textbook of Nursing*. (First published 1937.) Faber & Faber, London.

Philpin, S. (2002) Rituals and nursing: a critical commentary. *J Adv Nurs*, **38**(2), 144–51.

RCN (1996) *Verification of Death by Registered Nurses.* Issues in Nursing and Health, 38. Royal College of Nursing, London.

RCN (2003) *The Use of Pressure Relieving Devices (Beds, Mattresses and Overlays) for the Prevention of Pressure Ulcers in Primary and Secondary Care.* Royal College of Nursing, London.

RCN (2005) *Good Practice in Infection Prevention and Control. Guidance for Nursing Staff.* Royal College of Nursing, London.

Seale, C. (1998) *Constructing Death. The Sociology of Dying and Bereavement.* Cambridge University Press, Cambridge.

Smaje, C. & Field, D. (1997) Absent minorities? Ethnicity and the use of palliative care services. In: *Death, Gender and Ethnicity* (eds D. Field, J. Hockley & N. Small). Routledge, London, pp. 142–65.

Speck, P. (1992) Care after death. *Nurs Times,* **88**(6), 20.

Travis, S. (2002) *Procedure for the Care of Patients Who Die in Hospital.* Royal Marsden NHS Trust, London.

UK Transplant (2007) Direct communication with UK transplant (February 2007 and August 31st 2007). See www.uktransplant. org.uk for information.

Van Gennep, A. (1972) *The Rites of Passage.* Chicago University Press, Chicago.

Walsh, M. & Ford, P. (1989) *Nursing Rituals, Research and Rational Action.* Butterworth Heinemann, Oxford.

Wilkinson, S. & Mula, C. (2003) Communication in care of the dying. In: *Care of the Dying: A Pathway to Excellence* (eds J. Ellershaw & S. Wilkinson). Oxford University Press, Oxford, pp. 74–89.

Wolf, Z. (1988) *Nurses' Work: The Sacred and the Profane.* University of Pennsylvania Press, Philadelphia.

Further reading on religious faiths

Commission for Racial Equality (1999) *CRE Factsheet: Ethnic Minorities in Britain.* CRE, London.

Eliade, M. & Couliano, I.P. (2000) *The Harper Collins Concise Guide to World Religions.* Harper, San Francisco.

Karmi, G. (1996) *The Ethnic Health Handbook. A Factfile for Health Care Professionals.* Blackwell Science, Oxford.

Keene, M. (2002) *World Religions.* Lion Publishing, Oxford.

North Kent Council for Interfaith Relations (2002) *The Spiritual and Pastoral Care of Patients in Hospital and Their Relatives.* North Kent Council for Interfaith Relations, Kent.

Rankin, J., Brown, A. & Gateshill, P. (1992) *Ethics and Religions.* Longman, London.

Sampson, C. (1982) *The Neglected Ethic: Religious and Cultural Factors in the Care of Patients.* McGraw-Hill, Maidenhead.

Bahai faith

Smith, P. (1998) *The Bahai Religion: a Short Introduction to its History and Teachings.* George Ronald, Oxford.

Smith, P. (2000) *A Concise Encyclopaedia of the Bahai Faith*. Oneworld Publications, Oxford.

Buddhism

Gyatso, G.K. (2001) *Introduction to Buddhism: An Explanation of the Buddhist Way of Life*. Tharpa Publications, Ulverston, Cumbria.
Hagan, S. (1997) *Buddhism: Plain and Simple*. Penguin, London.
Maguire, J. (2001) *Essential Buddhism: A Guide to Beliefs and Practices*. Pocket Books, New York.
Northcott, N. (2002) Nursing with dignity, part 2. Buddhism. *Nurs Times*, **98**(10), 36–8.
Sibley, D. (1997) Caring for dying Buddhists. *Int J Palliat Nurs*, **3**(1), 26–30.
Snelling, J. (1998) *The Buddhist Handbook: A Complete Guide to Buddhist Teaching and Practice*. Rider, London.
Stokes, G. (2000) *Buddha: A Beginner's Guide*. Hodder & Stoughton, London.
Williams, P. (1989) *Mahayana Buddhism*. Routledge, London.

Christianity

Anon (1992) *The Holy Bible*. Hodder & Stoughton, London.
Christmas, M. (2002) Nursing with dignity, part 3. Christianity I. *Nurs Times*, **98**(11), 37–9.
Cross, F.L. & Livingstone, E.L. (1997) *The Oxford Dictionary of the Christian Church*. Oxford University Press, Oxford.
Edwards, D.L. (1999) *What Anglicans Believe*. Mowbray, London.
Grenz, S.J. (1998) *What Christians Believe and Why*. Paternoster Press, Carlisle.
Littleton, M. (2001) *Jesus*. John Knox Press, Westminster.
McManners, J. (ed.) (2002) *The Oxford History of Christianity*. Oxford Paperbacks, Oxford.
Papadopoulos, I. (2002) Nursing with dignity, part 4. Christianity II. *Nurs Times*, **98**(12), 36–7.
Stott, J. (2002) *Basic Christianity*. Intervarsity Press, London.
Ware, T. (1997) *The Orthodox Church*. Penguin, London.

Hinduism

Cross, S. (2002) *Way of Hinduism*. Thorsons, London.
Flood, G. (2001) *An Introduction to Hinduism*. Cambridge University Press, Cambridge.
Henley, A. (1983) *Caring for Hindus and Their Families: Religious Aspects of Care*. National Extension College, Cambridge.
Jootun, D. (2002) Nursing with dignity, part 7. Hinduism. *Nurs Times*, **98**(15), 38–40.
Klostermaier, K.K. (2000) *Hinduism: A Short History*. Oneworld Publications, Oxford.
Laungani, P. (1997) Death in a Hindu family. In: *Death and Bereavement Across Cultures* (eds C. Parkes, P. Laungani & B. Young). Routledge, London, pp. 52–72.
Wordsworth Classics (1997) *The Bhagavad Gita*. Wordsworth, Herts.

Humanism

BBC (2006) Religion & ethics – Humanism. www.bbc.co.uk/religion/ religions/atheism/types/humanism.shtml. Accessed 16/8/06.

Jainism

Dundas, P. (2002) *The Jains*. Routledge, London.

Jehovah's Witnesses

Cumberland, W.H. (1986) The Jehovah's Witness tradition. In: *Caring and Curing: Health and Medicine in the Western Religious Traditions* (eds R. Numbers & D. Amundsen). Macmillan, New York, pp. 468–85.

Simpson, J. (2002) Nursing with dignity, part 9. Jehovah's Witnesses. *Nurs Times*, 98(17), 36–7.

The Watch Tower (2007) Medical care and blood [online] Available: www.watchtower.org/e/medical_care_and_blood.htm. Accessed 5/09/07.

Judaism

Collins, A. (2002) Nursing with dignity, part 1. Judaism. *Nurs Times*, 98(9), 33–5.

Katz, J.S. (1996) Caring for dying Jewish people in a multicultural/religious society. *Int J Palliat Nurs*, 2(1), 43–7.

Lancaster, B. (1997) *The Elements of Judaism*. Element, London.

Neuberger, J. (1999) Spiritual issues. Judaism and palliative care. *Eur J Palliat Care*, 6(5), 166–8.

Neusner, J. (2002) *Judaism*. Penguin, London.

Wigoder, N., Skolnick, F. & Himelstein, S. (2002) *The New Encyclopaedia of Judaism*. New York University Press, New York.

Wood, C. (2002) *Living Judaism*. Heinemann Library, New York.

Mormonism

Bush, L.E. (1986) The Mormon tradition. In: *Caring and Curing: Health and Medicine in the Western Religious Traditions* (eds R. Numbers & D. Amundsen). Macmillan, New York, pp. 397–420.

Eliason, E.A. (ed.) (2001) *Mormons and Mormonism*. University of Illinois Press, Illinois.

Muslim faith

Akhtar, S. (2002) Nursing with dignity, part 8. Islam. *Nurs Times*, 98(16), 40–2.

Gordon, M.S. (2002) *Islam*. Duncain Baird, London.

Henley, A. (1982) *Caring for Muslims and Their Families: Religious Aspects of Care*. National Extension College, Cambridge.

Horrie, C. & Chippindale, P. (2001) *What is Islam? A Comprehensive Introduction*. Virgin, London.

Lewis, P. (1994) *Islamic Britain*. I.B. Tauris, London.

Penguin Classics (1999) *The Koran*. Penguin, London.
Ruthven, M. (2000) *Islam: A Very Short Introduction*. Oxford University Press, Oxford.
Sarwas, G. (1998) *Islam: Beliefs and Teachings*. Muslim Educational Trust, London.
Sheikh, A. & Gatrad, A.R. (2000) *Caring for Muslim Patients*. Radcliffe Medical Press, Oxford.

Paganism

Prout, C. (1992) Paganism. *Nurs Times*, **88**(33), 42–3.

Rastafarianism

Barrett, L.E. (1997) *The Rastafarians*. Beacons Press, Boston.
Baxter, C. (2002) Nursing with dignity, part 5. Rastafarianism. *Nurs Times*, **98**(13), 42–3.

Sikhism

Cole, W.O. & Sambhi, P. (1995) *The Sikhs. Their Religious Beliefs and Practices*. Sussex Academic Press, London.
Gill, B.K. (2002) Nursing with dignity, part 6. Sikhism. *Nurs Times*, **98**(14), 39–41.
Henley, A. (1983) *Caring for Sikhs and Their Families: Religious Aspects of Care*. National Extension College, Cambridge.
Kalsi, S.S. (1999) *The Simple Guide to Sikhism*. Global Books, New Jersey.
Mayled, J. (2002) *Living Religions. Living Sikhism*. Heinemann Library, New York.
Sambi, S.P. & Cole, W.O. (1990) Caring for Sikh patients. *Palliat Med*, 4, 229–33.
Shackle, C., Mandair, A. & Singh, G. (eds) (2000) *Sikh Religion: Culture and Ethnicity*. Routledge Curzon, New York.
Singh, D. & Smith, A. (2001) *Religions of the World*. Hodder Wayland, Hove.

Zoroastrianism

Boyce, M. (2001) *Zoroastrianism*. Routledge Curzon, New York.
Clark, P. (1998) *Zoroastranism*. Sussex Academic Press, London.
Hinnells, J.R. (1996) *Zoroastrians in Britain*. Clarendon Press, Oxford.
Kreyenbroek, P.G. (2001) *Living Zoroastrianism*. Routledge Curzon, New York.

Multiple choice questions

1 **Last offices refers to:**

   a Washing the deceased
   b Washing the deceased and removing unnecessary equipment
   c Washing and grooming the deceased, understanding of the legal issues around death, removing unnecessary equipment, correctly labelling the body
   d Washing and grooming the deceased, correctly labelling the body

2 **In what situation would all lines, endotracheal tubes and other equipment be left *in situ* ?**

   a If the relatives are not with the patient
   b If the death is referred to the coroner
   c If you are short of staff
   d If the death occurs at night

3 **Who is able to confirm death?**

   a Any nurse
   b A senior nurse if there is an agreed local policy, a registered medical practitioner
   c A registered medical practitioner
   d A senior nurse

4 **Jewellery should be removed from the deceased:**

   a By a nurse unless otherwise requested by relatives
   b Only if requested
   c By a nurse in the presence of another nurse
   d By the funeral director

Answers to the multiple choice questions can be found in Appendix 3.

Chapter 16

Lumbar puncture

Definition

Lumbar puncture is a medical procedure which involves withdrawing cerebrospinal fluid (CSF) by the insertion of a hollow spinal needle with a stylet into the lumbar subarachnoid space (Hickey 2003). It may be used for either therapeutic or diagnostic purposes (Barker & Chao 2002).

Indications

A lumbar puncture and withdrawal of CSF, with or without the introduction of therapeutic agents, is performed for the following purposes.

- *Diagnosis*: CSF is normally a crystal clear, colourless and sterile liquid which resembles water. Analysis of the CSF for cells not normally present may be made to determine the presence of a pathological process (Price & Madhusudan 2002). In addition, CSF pressure can be measured (Barker & Chao 2002).
- *Introduction of therapeutic agents*: for example, antibiotics or cytotoxic intrathecal chemotherapy in the presence of malignant cytology (Hickey 2003; Tervit & Phillips 2006). Since 2001 all UK trusts that undertake to administer intrathecal cytotoxic chemotherapy must ensure safe practice guidelines have been introduced and that they are fully compliant with National Guidelines on the Safe Administration of Intrathecal Chemotherapy (DH 2001).
- *Introduction of spinal anaesthesia for surgery* (Hickey 2003).
- *Introduction of radiopaque contrast medium*: used to provide radiopaque pictures (myelograms) of the spinal cord (Blows 2002). Myelograms are useful in diagnosing spinal lesions and in helping to plan surgery by isolating the level of the lesion.

Contraindications

The procedure should not be undertaken in the following circumstances.

- In patients where raised intracranial pressure (ICP) is suspected or present due to the risk of 'brain herniation' (Lindsay & Bone 2004; Belford 2005).
- In patients with papilloedema, bacterial meningitis or deteriorating neurological symptoms, where raised ICP or an intracranial mass is suspected. In this situation, neuroimaging (computed tomography [CT] or magnetic resonance imaging [MRI] scan) should be undertaken prior to lumbar puncture in order to avoid resultant potentially fatal brainstem compression, herniation or coning (Belford 2005). However, a normal CT scan does not always ensure that it is safe to perform a lumbar puncture, until better non-invasive procedures to monitor ICP become available and are routinely used, the decision to proceed must be left to clinical expertise and judgement (Hickey 2003).
- Local skin infection may result in meningitis by passage of the bacteria from the skin to the CSF during the procedure (Hickey 2003). Cutaneous or osseous infection at the site of the lumbar puncture may be considered an absolute contraindication (Hickey 2003).
- In patients who are unable to co-operate or who are too drowsy to give a history. Patient co-operation is essential to carry out a baseline neurological examination and to minimize the potential risk of trauma associated with this procedure (Barker & Chao 2002).
- In patients who have severe degenerative spinal joint disease. In such cases difficulty will be experienced both in positioning the patient and in accessing between the vertebrae (Hickey 2003).
- In those patients undergoing anticoagulant therapy or who have coagulopathies or thrombocytopenia (less than 50×10^9/litre). These patients are at increased risk of bleeding and therefore coagulopathies and thrombocytopenia must be corrected prior to undertaking lumbar puncture (Lindsay & Bone 2004).

Reference material

Anatomy and physiology

The spinal cord lies within the spinal column, beginning at the foramen magnum and terminating about the level of the first lumbar vertebra (Marieb 2004) (Figure 16.1). Like the brain, the spinal cord is enclosed and protected by the meninges, that is, the dura mater, arachnoid mater and pia mater (Barker 2002). The dura and arachnoid mater are separated by a potential space known as the subdural space. The arachnoid and pia mater are separated by the subarachnoid

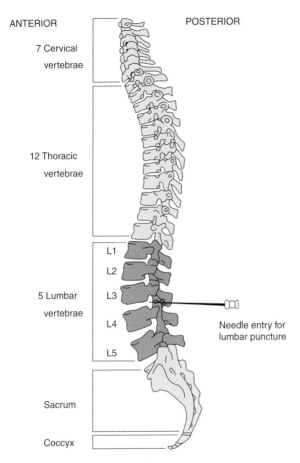

ANTERIOR

POSTERIOR

7 Cervical
vertebrae

12 Thoracic
vertebrae

L1
L2
5 Lumbar
vertebrae
L3
L4

Needle entry for
lumbar puncture

L5

Sacrum

Coccyx

Figure 16.1 Lateral view of spinal column and vertebrae, showing needle entry site for lumbar puncture.

space which contains the CSF (Allan 2002). Below the first lumbar vertebra the subarachnoid space contains CSF, the filum terminale and the cauda equina (the anterior and posterior roots of the lumbar and sacral nerves) (Weldon 1998). So as to avoid damage to the spinal cord, it is imperative that lumbar puncture is performed below the first lumbar vertebra where the cord terminates (Figure 16.2).

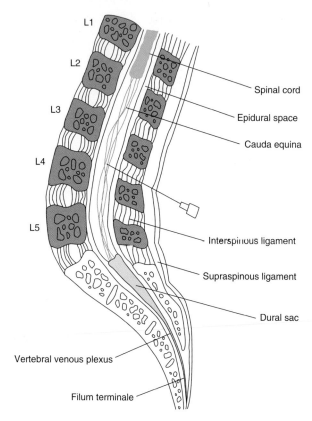

Figure 16.2 Lumbar puncture. Sagittal section through lumbosacral spine. The most common site for lumbar puncture is between L3 and L4 and between L4 and L5 as the spinal cord terminates at L1.

The cord serves as the main pathway for the ascending and descending fibre tracts that connect the peripheral and spinal nerves with the brain (Barker 2002; Marieb 2004). The peripheral nerves are attached to the spinal cord by 31 pairs of spinal nerves.

Cerebrospinal fluid

CSF is formed primarily by filtration and secretion from networks of capillaries, called choroid plexuses, located in the ventricles of the brain. Eventually,

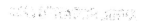

absorption takes place through the arachnoid villi, which are finger-like projections of the arachnoid mater that push into the dural venous sinuses. CSF is clear, colourless and slightly alkaline, with a specific gravity of 1007 (Hickey 2003). In an adult, approximately 500 ml of CSF are produced and reabsorbed each day (Weldon 1998), with 120–150 ml present at one time. CSF constituents include:

- Water.
- Mineral salts.
- Glucose.
- Protein (16–45 mg/dl).
- Urea and creatinine (Hickey 2003).

The functions of CSF include:

- To act as a shock absorber.
- To carry nutrients to the brain.
- To remove metabolites from the brain.
- To support and protect the brain and spinal cord.
- To keep the brain and spinal cord moist (Hickey 2003).

Sampling and CSF pressure

The amount of CSF withdrawn for sampling depends on the investigation required. In practice, approximately 5–10 ml of CSF is usually withdrawn, although investigations for cell count and Gram stain can be performed using 1 ml (Barker & Chao 2002). The pressure of CSF can be measured at the time of lumbar puncture using a manometer. Normal CSF pressure falls within a range of 100–150 mm (Lindsay & Bone 2004). Spinal pressure may be raised in the presence of cerbrovascular accident, a space-occupying lesion or bacterial meningitis (Barker & Chao 2002).

Abnormalities of CSF

- A red discoloration of the CSF is indicative of the presence of blood, which is an abnormal finding. If the presence of blood is caused by a traumatic spinal tap, the blood will usually clot and the fluid clear as the procedure continues. If the presence of blood is due to subarachnoid haemorrhage, no clotting will occur (Lindsay & Bone 2004).
- Turbid or cloudy CSF is indicative of the presence of a large number of white cells or protein and is an abnormal finding. The causes of such turbidity include infection or the secondary infiltration of the meninges with malignant disease, e.g. leukaemia or lymphoma (Hoffbrand *et al.* 2001).

555

- The presence of different types of blood cells in the CSF can be diagnostic of a variety of neurological disorders, e.g.:

  (a) Erythrocytes are indicative of haemorrhage.
  (b) Polymorphonuclear leucocytes are indicative of meningitis or cerebral abcess.
  (c) Monocytes are indicative of a viral or tubercular meningitis or encephalitis.
  (d) Lymphocytes present in larger numbers are indicative of viral meningitis or infiltration of the meninges by malignant disease.
  (e) The presence of leukaemic blast cells is indicative of infiltration of the meninges by leukaemia.
  (f) Viral, bacterial or fungal cultures from the CSF sample are indicative of infection.

  (Allan 2002; Barker & Chao 2002; Hickey 2003).

Investigations

A number of tests can be performed on CSF to aid diagnosis (Lindsay & Bone 2004).

- *Culture and sensitivity*. Identifying the presence of micro-organisms would confirm the diagnosis of bacterial/fungal meningitis or a cerebral abscess. The isolation of the causative organism would enable the initiation of appropriate antibiotic or antifungal therapy.
- *Virology screening*. Isolation of a causative virus would enable appropriate therapy to be initiated promptly.
- *Serology for syphilis*. Tests include: Wasserman test (WR), venereal disease research laboratory (VDRL) and *Treponema pallidum* immobilization (TPI) test.
- *Protein*. The total amount of protein in CSF should be 15.45 mg/dl (154.5 μg/ml). Proteins are large molecules which do not readily cross the blood–brain barrier. There is normally more albumin (80%) than globulin in CSF as albumins are smaller molecules (Fischbach 2003). Raised globulin levels are indicative of multiple sclerosis, neurosyphilis, degenerative cord or brain disease. However, raised levels of total protein can be indicative of meningitis, encephalitis, myelitis or the presence of a tumour (Hickey 2003).
- *Cytology*. Central nervous system tumours or secondary meningeal disease tend to shed cells into the CSF, where they float freely. Examination of these cells morphologically after lumbar puncture will determine whether the tumour is malignant or benign (Fischbach 2003).

Complications associated with lumbar puncture

- Infection (inadvertently introduced during procedure: there is a greater risk in the presence of neutropenia) (Hart 2006).
- Haemorrhage/localized bruising (may be caused by a traumatic procedure or in the presence of thrombocytopenia or a coagulopathy) (Barker & Chao 2002; Lindsay & Bone 2004).
- Transtentorial or tonsillar herniation (if Queckenstedt's test is carried out in the presence of raised ICP) (Belford 2005).
- Headache. Frequency of post-lumbar puncture headache varies among studies and between diagnostic and therapeutic procedures. The following risk factors have been identified: young age; female gender; and the presence of headache before or at the time of the lumbar puncture (Evans *et al.* 2000). Less certain risk factors include low body mass index and previous experience of post-lumbar puncture headache (Evans *et al.* 2000). Research also suggests that the size of the needle used for the lumbar puncture may contribute to headache as a large gauge needle, such as an 18 gauge, may create a larger dural opening and the tip may tear dural fibres, delaying puncture closure. To minimize the risk of headache, a 25-gauge blunt-ended needle is recommended (Connolly 1999).
- Backache.
- Leakage from puncture site (Hickey 2003).
- The combination of intrathecal methotrexate with radiotherapy may cause arachnoiditis (irritation of the meninges), cerebral atrophy and necrosing encephalopathy (Vasey & Evans 2002). Arachnoiditis has also been reported when administering intrathecal methylprednisolone (Latham *et al.* 1997).

The role of the nurse

The role of the nurse in caring for a patient undergoing a lumbar puncture procedure may include helping to explain the procedure to the patient, preparing the patient, supporting both patient and physician during the procedure and close follow-up monitoring. Education and support are essential as the patient may have concerns about this invasive procedure (Barker & Chao 2002). Preparation may include advising the patient to empty their bowels and bladder to ensure comfort, and correct and comfortable positioning during the procedure. Follow-up care will include: neurological observations; monitoring for issues such as difficulties with voiding, raised temperatures, headaches and discomfort. Analgesia and reassurance may be required (Allan 2002).

Procedure guidelines **Lumbar puncture**

Equipment

1 Antiseptic skin-cleaning agents, e.g. chlorhexidine in 70% alcohol or isopropyl alcohol.
2 Selection of needles and syringes.
3 Local anaesthetic, e.g. lidocaine 1%.
4 Sterile gloves.
5 Sterile dressing pack.
6 Lumbar puncture needles of assorted sizes.
7 Disposable manometer.

8 Three sterile specimen bottles. (These should be labelled 1, 2 and 3. The first specimen, which may be bloodstained due to needle trauma, should go into bottle 1. This will assist the laboratory to differentiate between blood due to procedure trauma and that due to subarachnoid haemorrhage.)
9 Plaster dressing.

Procedure

Action	Rationale
1 Explain and discuss the procedure with the patient.	To ensure that the patient understands the procedure and gives his/her valid consent (Barker & Chao 2002: E; NMC 2006: C).
2 Patient should empty his/her bladder and bowels before procedure.	To ensure comfort (Barker & Chao 2002; Hickey 2003: E).
3 Assist patient into required position on a firm surface:	To ensure maximum widening of the intervertebral spaces and thus easier access to the subarachnoid space (Lindsay & Bone 2004: E).
(a) Lying (see Action figure 3): ■ One pillow under the patient's head. ■ On side with knees drawn up to the abdomen and clasped by the hands. ■ Support patient to maintain this position.	To avoid sudden movement by the patient which would produce trauma (Barker & Chao 2002: E).
(b) Sitting: ■ Patient straddles a straight back chair so that his/her back is facing the doctor. ■ Patient folds arms on the back of the chair and rests head on them.	This position may be used for those patients unable to maintain the lying position. It allows more accurate identification of the spinous processes and thus the intervertebral spaces (Barker & Chao 2002; Hickey 2003: E).

4 Continue to support, explain care and observe the patient throughout the procedure.

To facilitate psychological and physical well being (Barker & Chao 2002: E).

5 Assist doctor as required; doctor will proceed to:

To monitor any physical or psychological changes.

(a) Clean the skin with the antiseptic cleaning agent.

To ensure the removal of skin flora to minimize the risk of infection (Lindsay & Bone 2004: E).

(b) Identify the area to be punctured and infiltrate the skin and subcutaneous layers with local anaesthetic.

To minimize discomfort from the procedure (Barker & Chao 2002: E).

(c) Introduce a spinal puncture needle between the second and third lumbar vertebrae and into the subarachnoid space.

This is below the level of the spinal cord but still within the subarachoid space (Lindsay & Bone 2004: E).

(d) Ensure that the subarachnoid space has been entered and attach the manometer to the spinal needle, if required.

To obtain a CSF pressure reading (normal pressure is 100–150 mmH$_2$O) (Hickey 2003; Lindsay & Bone 2004: E).

(e) Obtain the appropriate specimens of CSF (approx. 10 ml) for analysis. Cell count and Gram stain can be perfomed using 1 ml of fluid.

To establish diagnosis (Hickey 2003: E).

(f) If intrathecal medication is to be instilled, drug and dose must be checked and administered safely acording to National Guidelines (DH 2003).

To ensure the correct drug and dosage of drug is safely administered (DH 2003: C; Coward & Cooley 2006).

(g) Withdraw the spinal needle once specimens have been obtained, appropriate pressure measurements taken and intrathecal medication administered.

To minimize the risks of the procedure (Barker & Chao 2002: E).

(h) Careful precaution should be taken when administering cytotoxic drugs and disposing of cytotoxic waste.

To protect patient and clinicians (Coward & Colley: E; DH 2005: C).

Procedure guidelines *(cont.)*

6 When the needle is withdrawn, apply pressure over the lumbar puncture site using a sterile topical swab.

To maintain asepsis and to stop blood and CSF flow (Hickey 2003: E).

7 When all leakage from the puncture site has ceased, apply a plaster dressing.

To prevent secondary infection (Allan 2002; Barker & Chao 2002: E).

8 Make the patient comfortable. He/she should lie flat or the head should be tilted slightly downwards. Time to lie flat varies from hospital to hospital, but it is usually around 4 hours if there is no headache. If the procedure has been done in an outpatient setting the patient may be discharged home after 1–2 hours but with clear instructions to lie flat in transport and at home, and to report any of the following: leakage from the site, headaches or backaches.

To avoid headache and decrease the possibility of brainstem herniation (coning) due to a reduction in CSF pressure (Barker & Chao 2002; Hickey 2003: E).

9 Remove equipment and dispose of as appropriate.

To prevent the spread of infection and reduce risk of needle stick injury (Allan 2002: E).

10 Record the procedure in the appropriate documents.

To promote continuity of care and provide an accurate record for future reference (Allan 2002: E; NMC 2005: C).

11 Ensure the specimens are labelled appropriately and sent with the correct forms to the laboratory.

To ensure that the correct results are returned to the appropriate patient's notes (Barker & Chao 2002: E).

12 Patient should be monitored for the next 24 hours with careful observation of the following:

   (a) Leakage from the puncture site.

There may be a small amount of bloodstained oozing. The presence of clear fluid should be reported immediately to the doctor, especailly if accompanied by fluctuation of other symptoms (level of consciousness, motor changes, problems voiding), as it may be a cerebrospinal leak (Barker & Chao 2002: E).

   (b) Headache.

Not unusual following lumbar puncture and may be due to loss of CSF or irritation of the spinal roots. Usually relieved by lying flat and, if ordered by the doctor, a mild analgesic (Hickey 2003: E).

   (c) Backache.

As above.

   (d) Neurological observations/vital signs.

These may indicate signs of change in ICP (Hickey 2003: E). (For further information on neurolgical observations and vital signs, see Chapter 19.)

13 Encourage a fluid intake of 2–3 litres in 24 hours.

To replace lost fluid. Patient may have difficulty micturating due to procedure and supine position (Allan 2002; Hickey 2003: E).

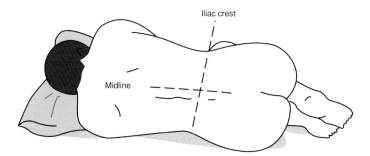

Iliac crest

Midline

Action 3 Position for lumbar puncture. Head is flexed onto chest and knees are drawn up.

Problem solving: Lumbar puncture

Problem	Cause	Suggested action
Pain down one leg during the procedure.	A dorsal nerve root may have been touched by the spinal needle.	Inform doctor, who will probably move the needle. Reassure patient.
Headache following procedure (may persist for up to a week).	Removal of the sample of CSF.	Reassure patient that it is a transient symptom. Ensure that he/she lies flat for specified period of time. Encourage a high fluid intake to replace fluid lost during procedure. Administer analgesics as ordered. If headache is severe and increasing, inform a a doctor: there is a possibility of persistent CSF leak or rising ICP (Barker & Chao 2002).
Backache following procedure.	(a) Removal of the sample of CSF. (b) Position required for puncture.	Reassure patient that it is usually a transient symptom. Ensure that he/she lies flat for appropriate period of time. Administer analgesic as ordered (Hickey 2003).
Fluctuation of neurological observations, i.e. level of consciousness, pulse, respirations, blood pressure or pupillary reaction.	Herniation (coning) of the brainstem due to the decrease of ICP. (Raised ICP is a contraindication to lumbar puncture.)	Observe patient constantly for signs of alteration in ICP. The frequency may be decreased as patient's condition allows. Report any fluctuations in these observations to a doctor immediately (Barker & Chao 2002).
Leakage from the puncture site.	(a) Resolution of bleeding. (b) Leakage of CSF.	(a) No further action required (b) Report immediately to a doctor, especially if accompanied by fluctuation in neurological observations (see Chapter 19) (Barker & Chao 2002).

References and further reading

Allan, D. (2002) Caring for the patient with a disorder of the nervous system. In: *Watson's Clinical Nursing and Related Sciences* (ed. M. Walsh), 6th edn. Balliere Tindall, Edinburgh, pp. 665–746.

Barker, E. (2002) Neuroanatomy and physiology of the nervous system. In: *Neuroscience Nursing: A Spectrum of Care* (ed. E. Barker), 2nd edn. Mosby, Phildaelphia, pp. 3–50.

Barker, E. & Chao, W.P. (2002) Neurodiagnostic and laboratory studies. In: *Neuroscience Nursing: A Spectrum of Care* (ed. E. Barker), 2nd edn. Mosby, Phildaelphia, pp. 99–130.

Belford, K. (2005) Central nervous cancers. In: *Cancer Nursing: Principles and Practice* (eds C.H. Yarbro, M.H, Frogge & M. Goodman), 6th edn. Jones & Bartlett, Boston, pp. 1089–136.

Blows, W. (2002) Diagnostic investigations, part 1: lumbar puncture. *Nurs Times*, **98**(36), 25–6.

Connolly, M.A. (1999) Clinical snapshot. Postdural puncture headache. *Am J Nurs*, **99**(11), 48–9.

Coward, M. & Cooley, H.M. (2006) Chemotherapy. In: *Nursing Patients with Cancer: Principles and Practice* (eds N. Kearney & A. Richardson). Elsevier, Edinburgh, pp. 283–302.

DH (2001) *National Guidance on the Safe Administration of Intrathecal Chemotherapy.* HSC 2001/022. Department of Health, London.

DH (2003) *Updated National Guidance on the Safe Administration of Intrathecal Chemotherapy.* HSC 2003/10. Department of Health, London.

DH (2005) *Hazardous waste (England) regulations.* Department of Health, London.

Evans, R.W. *et al.* (2000) Assessment: prevention of post-lumbar puncture headaches: report of the Therapeutics and Technology Assessment Subcommittee of the American Academy of Neurology. *Neurology*, **55**(7), 909–14.

Fischbach, F.T. (2003) *A Manual of Laboratory Diagnostic Tests*, 7th edn. Lippincott, Philadelphia.

Hart, S. (2006) Prevention of infection. In: *Nursing in Haematological Oncology* (ed. M. Grundy), 2nd edn. Balliere Tindall, Edinburgh, pp. 321–38.

Hickey, J. (ed) (2003) Cerebrospinal fluids and spinal procedures. In: *The Clinical Practice of Neurological and Neuroscience Nursing*, 5th edn. Lippincott, Philadelphia, pp. 89–91.

Hoffbrand, A.V., Moss, P.A.H. & Petit, J.E. (2006) *Haematology*, 5th edn. Blackwell Publishing, Oxford.

Latham, J.M. *et al.* (1997) The pathological effects of intrathecal betamethasone. *Spine*, **22**(14), 1558–62.

Lindsay, K.W. & Bone, I. (2004) *Neurology and Neurosurgery Illustrated*, 4th edn. Churchill Livingstone, Edinburgh.

Marieb, E.N. (2004) *Human Anatomy & Physiology*, 6th edn. Pearson, San Francisco.

NMC (2005) *Guidelines for Records and Record Keeping.* Nursing and Midwifery Council, London.

NMC (2006) *Z–Z Advice Sheet Consent.* www.nmc.org.

Price, C.G.A. & Madhusudan, S. (2002) Non Hodgkin's lymphoma. In: *Treatment of Cancer* (eds P. Price & K. Sikora), 4th edn. Arnold, London, pp. 977–95.

Richards, P. (1992) Monitoring of cerebral function. *Br J Hosp Med*, **48**(7), 390–2.

563

Scurr, M., Judson, I. & Root, T. (2005) Combination chemotherapy and chemotherapy principles. In: *The Royal Marsden Hospital Handbook of Cancer Chemotherapy* (eds D. Brighton & M. Wood). Elsevier, Edinburgh, pp. 17–30.

Tervit, S. & Phillips, K. (2006) Chemotherapy. In: *Nursing in Haematological Oncology* (ed. M. Grundy), 2nd edn. Balliere Tindall, Edinburgh, pp. 173–200.

Vasey, P. A. & Evans, J. (2002) Principles of Chemotherapy and Drug Development. In: *Treatment of Cancer* (eds P. Price & K. Sikora) 4th edn. Arnold, London, pp. 103–29.

Weldon, K. (1998) Anatomy and physiology of the nervous system. In: *Neuro-Oncology for Nurses* (ed. D. Guerrero). Whurr, London, pp. 1–28.

Multiple choice questions

1 Lumbar puncture and withdrawal of cerebrospinal fluid are performed for which of the following reasons?

    a   Diagnosis
    b   Introduction of therapeutic or anaesthetic agents
    c   Introduction of radiopaque contrast medium
    d   All of the above

2 The pressure of cerebrospinal fluid can be measured at the time of the lumbar puncture using a:

    a   Sphygmomanometer
    b   Manometer
    c   Thermometer
    d   CSF measurement meter

3 How many specimen bottles are required when performing a lumbar puncture?

    a   1
    b   4
    c   3
    d   2

4 In what position should the patient be placed for a lumbar puncture?

    a   Prone
    b   On side with knees drawn up to abdomen and clasped hands
    c   Supine
    d   Semi-prone

5 Patients should remain lying flat following a lumbar puncture for:

    a   24 hours
    b   12 hours
    c   4 hours
    d   As long as they want

6 Following a lumbar puncture the patient should be observed for:

    a   Headache
    b   Change in level of consciousness
    c   Leakage from puncture site
    d   All of the above

Answers to the multiple choice questions can be found in Appendix 3.

Chapter 17

Nutritional support

Definition

Nutritional support refers to any method of giving nutrients which encourages an optimal nutritional status. It includes modifying the types of foods eaten, dietary supplementation, enteral tube feeding and parenteral nutrition (National Collaborating Centre for Acute Care 2006).

Indications

Nutritional support should be considered for anybody unable to maintain their nutritional status by taking their usual diet.

- Patients unable to eat their usual diet (e.g. because of anorexia, mucositis, taste changes or dysphagia, see Problem solving, below) should be given advice on modifying their diet.
- Patients unable to meet their nutritional requirements, despite dietary modifications, should be offered oral nutritional supplements.
- Patients unable to take sufficient food and dietary supplements to meet their nutritional requirements should be considered for an enteral tube feed.
- Patients unable to eat at all should have an enteral tube feed. Reasons for complete inability to eat include carcinoma of the head and neck area or oesophagus, surgery to the head or oesophagus, radiotherapy treatment to the head or neck, and fistulae of the oral cavity or oesophagus.
- Parenteral nutrition (PN) may be indicated in patients with a non-functioning or inaccessible gastrointestinal (GI) tract who are likely to be 'nil by mouth' for 5 days or longer. Reasons for a non-functioning or inaccessible GI tract include bowel obstruction, short bowel syndrome, gut toxicity following bone marrow transplantation or chemotherapy, major abdominal surgery, uncontrolled vomiting and enterocutaneous fistulae. Enteral nutrition should always be considered as the first option when considering nutritional support.

Patients in any group may have an increased requirement for nutrients due to an increased metabolic rate, as found in patients with burns, major sepsis, trauma or cancer cachexia (Bozzetti 2001; Thomas 2001). Patients should have nutritional requirements estimated prior to the start of nutritional support and should be monitored regularly.

Reference material

Nutrition screening

Identification of patients who are malnourished or who are at risk of malnutrition is an important first step in the patient's nutritional care. There are a number of screening tools available which consider different aspects of nutritional status. Subjective global assessment (SGA) is a comprehensive assessment but necessitates more time and expertise to carry out than most screening. Some more simple screening tools, including the malnutrition universal screening tool (MUST) (BAPEN 2003b), based on the patient's body mass index, weight loss and illness score are less time consuming. Other tools may be specific to the patient's age or diagnosis (Kondrup *et al.* 2003). The most important feature of using any screening tool is that patients identified as requiring nutritional assessment or intervention have a nutritional care plan initiated and are referred to the dietitian for further advice if appropriate.

Assessment of nutritional status

Before the initiation of nutritional support the patient must be assessed. The purpose of assessment is to identify whether a patient is undernourished, the reasons why this may have occurred and to provide baseline data for planning and evaluating nutritional support (National Collaborating Centre for Acute Care 2006). It is useful to use more than one method of assessing nutritional status. For example, a dietary history may be used to assess the adequacy of a person's diet but does not reflect actual nutritional status, whereas percentage weight loss does give an indication of nutritional status. However, percentage weight loss taken in isolation gives no idea of dietary intake and likelihood of improvement or deterioration in nutritional status (National Collaborating Centre for Acute Care 2006).

568 ### Nutrient intake

Nutrient intake can be assessed by a diet history (Thomas & Bishop 2007). A 24-hour recall may be used to assess recent nutrient intake and a food chart may be used to monitor current dietary intake. A diet history may also be used to provide information on food frequency, food habits, preferences, meal pattern, portion sizes, the presence of any eating difficulty and changes in food intake (Reilly 1996). A food chart where all current food and fluid taken is recorded is a useful method for monitoring nutritional intake, especially in the hospital setting or when dietary recall is not reliable (Thomas & Bishop 2007).

Body weight and weight loss

Body mass index (BMI) or comparison of a patient's weight with a chart of ideal body weight gives a measure of whether the patient has a normal weight, is overweight or underweight, and may be calculated from weight and height using the following equation:

$$\text{BMI} = \frac{\text{Weight (kg)}}{\text{Height (m)}^2}$$

Tables are available to allow the rapid and easy calculation of BMI (BAPEN 2003b). These comparisons, however, are not a good indicator of whether the patient is at risk nutritionally, as an apparently normal weight can mask severe muscle wasting.

Of greater use is the comparison of current weight with the patient's usual weight. Percentage weight loss is a useful measure of the risk of malnutrition:

$$\% \text{ Weight loss} = \frac{\text{Usual Weight} - \text{Actual Weight}}{\text{Usual Weight}} \times 100$$

A patient would be identified as malnourished if they had any of the following:

- BMI less than 18.5 kg/m^2.
- Unintentional weight loss greater than 10% within the last 3–6 months.
- BMI less than 20 kg/m^2 and unintentional weight loss greater than 5% within the last 3–6 months.

(National Collaborating Centre for Acute Care 2006.)

Sick children should have their weight and height measured frequently. It may be useful to measure on a daily basis (Shaw & Lawson 2007). These measurements must be plotted onto centile charts. A single weight or height cannot be interpreted as there is much variation of growth within each age group. It is a matter of concern if a child's weight begins to fall across the centiles or if the weight plateaus.

Obesity and oedema may make interpretation of body weight difficult; both may mask loss of lean body mass and potential malnutrition (Pennington 1997). Accurate weighing scales are necessary for measurement of body weight. Patients who are unable to stand may require sitting scales for weight to be measured.

It is often not appropriate to weigh palliative care patients who may experience inevitable weight loss as disease progresses. Psychologically it may be difficult for patients to see that they are continuing to lose weight. Measures of nutritional status such as clinical examination and current food intake may still be used in addition to measures of body weight.

Skinfold thickness

Skinfold thickness measurements can be used to assess stores of body fat. They are rarely used in routine nutritional assessment due to the insensitivity of the technique and the variation between measurements made by different observers. They are more appropriate for long-term assessments or research purposes and the technique should only be used by practitioners who are practiced in using skinfold thickness calipers because of the potential for intra-investigator variation in results (Durnin & Wolmersley 1974). Calipers are used to measure the thickness of subcutaneous fat at four sites: the triceps, biceps, subscapular and supra-iliac. The measurements can be used to determine the percentage of body fat of a person (Durnin & Wolmersley 1974). Percentage charts for skinfold thickness measurements may be used to assess nutritional status (Thomas & Bishop 2007, Appendix 6.4).

Bioelectrical impedance

Bioelectrical impedance analysis (BIA) is a simple, non-invasive and relatively inexpensive technique for measuring body composition (Janssen *et al.* 2000). The procedure involves the patient lying down for a period of 5–10 minutes while electrodes are connected to the hand and foot and a small undetectable electrical current is passed through the body. The speed at which this current travels through the body is influenced by the amount of water contained within the different body compartments. Tissues with a high water content (e.g. skeletal muscle) have a high electrical conductivity, whilst those with low water content (i.e. fat) act as poor conductors. BIA machines thus measure the impedance of the current as it passes through the subject. This information is then used in combination with prediction equations to calculate the volume or mass of different body compartments, which is then displayed electronically (Kyle *et al.* 2004a).

BIA is a technique which works well in healthy subjects but is of limited use in individuals with abnormal hydration status (e.g. severe dehydration or ascites) and is also less reliable at the extremes of BMI ranges (Kyle *et al.* 2004b). It is most suitable for research studies where body composition of groups of subjects is measured or for monitoring changes in nutritional status over a period of time (Buchholz *et al.* 2004). Importantly it is contraindicated in patients fitted with a pacemaker where the alternative skinfold thickness measurements should be used. The more expensive BIA machines also provide a measurement called 'phase angle' which has been shown to be of prognostic value in human immunodeficiency virus (HIV) (Schwenk *et al.* 2000) and advanced pancreatic and colorectal cancer patients (Gupta *et al.* 2004a, b).

Clinical examination

Observation of the patient may reveal signs and symptoms indicative of nutritional depletion.

- *Physical appearance*: emaciated, wasted appearance, loose clothing/jewellery.
- *Oedema*: will affect weight and may mask the appearance of muscle wastage. May indicate plasma protein deficiency and is often a reflection of the patient's overall condition rather than a measure of nutritional status.
- *Mobility*: weakness and impaired movement may result from loss of muscle mass.
- *Mood*: apathy, lethargy and poor concentration can be features of undernutrition.
- *Pressure sores and poor wound healing*: may reflect impaired immune function as a consequence of undernutrition and vitamin deficiencies (Thomas & Bishop 2007).

Specific nutritional deficiencies may be identifiable in some patients. For example, thiamine deficiency characterized by dementia is associated with high alcohol consumption. Rickets is seen in children with vitamin D deficiency.

Subjective global assessment

Subjective global assessment (SGA) is a clinical score, which can be obtained by a trained observer using a standardized questionnaire along with a physical examination, focused on nutritional status (Detsky *et al*. 1987). The questionnaire includes questions about food intake, physical symptoms and weight loss and therefore encompasses a number of methods of assessing nutritional status. Adaptations of the original tool have been produced including the Patient-Generated Subjective Global Assessment aimed specifically at patients with cancer (Huhmann & Cunningham 2005).

Biochemical investigations

Biochemical tests carried out on blood may give information on the patient's nutritional status. The most commonly used are:

- *Plasma proteins*. Changes in plasma albumin may arise due to physical stress, changes in circulating volume, hepatic and renal function, shock conditions and septicaemia. Plasma albumin and changes in plasma albumin are not a direct reflection of nutritional intake and nutritional status as it has been shown that these may remain unchanged despite changes in body composition (National Collaborating Centre for Acute Care 2006). In addition, albumin has a long half-life of 21 days, so it cannot reflect recent changes in nutritional

571

intake. It may be useful to review serum albumin concentrations in conjunction with C-reactive protein (CRP), which is an acute phase protein produced by the body in response to injury or trauma. CRP greater than 10 mg/l and serum albumin less than 30 g/l suggests 'illness'. CRP less than 10 mg/l and serum albumin less than 30 g/l suggests protein depletion (Elia 2001). Pre-albumin and retinol binding protein levels are more sensitive measures of nutrition support, reflecting recent changes in dietary intake rather than nutritional status. However, they may be expensive to measure (Nataloni *et al.* 1999).

- *Haemoglobin.* This is often below haematological reference values in malnourished patients (men: 13.5–17.5 g/dl; women: 11.5–15.5 g/dl). This can be due to a number of reasons, such as loss of blood from circulation, increased destruction of red blood cells or reduced production of erythrocytes and haemoglobin, e.g. due to dietary deficiency of iron or folate.

- *Serum vitamin and mineral levels.* Clinical examination of the patient may suggest a vitamin or mineral deficiency. For example, gingivitis may be due to a deficiency of vitamin C, vitamin A, niacin or riboflavin. Goitre is associated with iodine deficiency, and tremors, convulsions and behavioural disturbances may be caused by magnesium deficiency (Shenkin 2001). Serum vitamin and mineral levels are rarely measured routinely, as they are expensive and often cannot be performed by hospital laboratories.

- *Immunological competence.* Total lymphocyte count may reflect nutritional status although levels may also be depleted with malignancy, chemotherapy, zinc deficiency, age and non-specific stress (Bodger & Heatley 2001).

If a patient is considered to be malnourished by one or more of the above methods of assessment then a referral to a dietitian should be made immediately (Burnham & Barton 2001).

Calculation of nutritional requirements

Energy requirements may be calculated using equations such as those derived by Schofield (1985), which take into account weight, age, sex, activity level and clinical injury, e.g. post-surgery, sepsis or ventilator dependency. An easier and more appropriate method is to use body weight and allowances based on the patient's clinical condition (Table 17.1). Careful adjustments may be necessary in cases of oedema or obesity, in order to avoid overfeeding (Horgan & Stubbs 2003).

Fluid and nitrogen (or protein) requirements can be calculated in a similar way. If additional nitrogen is being given in situations where losses are increased, for example due to trauma, GI losses or major sepsis, then additional energy intake is required to assist in promoting a nitrogen balance. Improvement in nitrogen balance is the single nutritional parameter most consistently associated

Table 17.1 Guidelines for estimation of patient's daily energy and protein requirements (per kilogram body weight).

	Normal	**Pyrexia or extreme sepsis**
Energy (kcal)	25	25–35
(kJ)	105	105–146
Nitrogen (g)	0.17 (0.14–0.2)	0.2–0.3
Protein (g)	1 (0.87–1.25)	1.25–1.87
Fluid (ml)	30–35	30–35 plus 2–2.5 ml per 1°C in temperature above 37°C

with improved outcome, and the primary goal of nutrition support should be the attainment of nitrogen balance (Gidden & Shenkin 2000). Additional fluid of 500–750 ml is necessary for every 1°C rise in temperature in pyrexial patients (Thomas 2001).

Vitamin and mineral requirements calculated as detailed in the Committee on Medical Aspects of Food Policy (COMA) Report 41 on dietary reference values (DH 1991) apply to groups of healthy people and are not necessarily appropriate for those who are ill. A patient deficient in a vitamin or mineral may benefit from additional supplements to improve a condition. For example, a malnourished patient with poor wound healing may benefit from an increase in vitamin C and zinc, although the evidence is controversial (ter Riet *et al.* 1995; Thomas 1997; Desneves *et al.* 2005). Macronutrient and micronutrient requirements for children are also listed in the Committee on Medical Aspects of Food Policy (COMA) Report 41 on dietary reference values (DH 1991). Calculations are usually done with the reference nutrient intake (RNI). The child's actual body weight, not the expected body weight, is used when calculating requirements. This is to avoid excessive feeding. For a very small child, the height age instead of the chronological age is the basis of calculation (Shaw & Lawson 2007).

Planning nutritional support

Many factors, including being in hospital, need to be taken into consideration when planning nutritional support. Within the *Essence of Care* framework (DH 2001a), food and nutrition were identified by patients as a fundamental area of care that is frequently unsatisfactory within the National Health Service (NHS).

Clinical benchmarking (DH 2001a) and the *Better Hospital Food* programme (NHS 2001) aim to address common problems that patients experience whilst in hospital. Box 17.1 outlines the benchmark for food and nutrition, identifying specific factors that need to be considered when reviewing service provision, in order to promote better practice.

Box 17.1 Food and nutrition benchmark (*food* includes drinks) (DH 2001).

Agreed patient/client-focused outcome: patients/clients are enabled to consume food (orally) which meets their individual needs

Indicators/information that highlight concerns which may trigger the need for benchmarking activity:

- Patient satisfaction surveys
- Complaints figures and analysis
- Audit results: including catering audit, nutritional risk assessments, documentation audit, environmental audit (including dining facilities)
- Contract monitoring, e.g. wastage of food, food handling and/or food hygiene training records

- Ordering of dietary supplements/special diets
- Audit of available equipment and utensils
- Educational audits/student placement feedback
- Litigation/Clinical Negligence Scheme for Trusts
- Professional concern
- Media reports
- Sustainable Food and the NHS (Kings Fund Research Summary 2005), Food and Nutritional Care in Hospitals (Council of Europe 2003)

Factor	Benchmark of best practice
1 Screening/assessment to identify patients'/clients' nutritional needs	Nutritional screening progresses to **further assessment for all** Patients/clients identified as **'at risk' using a screening** tool that assesses body mass index and weight changes, **e.g. MUST** (National Collaborating Centre for Acute Care 2006)
2 Planning, implementation and evaluation	Plans of care based on **ongoing nutritional assessments** are of care for those patients who required advised,implemented and evaluated nutritional assessment
3 A conducive environment (acceptable sights, smells and sounds)	The environment is **conducive to** enabling the **individual** patients/clients to eat. Implementation of Protected Mealtimes
4 Assistance to eat and drink	Patients/clients **receive the care and assistance** they require with eating and drinking. Provision of eating aids where appropriate

5 Obtaining food	Patients/clients/carers, **whatever their communication needs**, have sufficient information to enable them to obtain their food. Examples include the NHS menu provision and utilizing menu translation services
6 Food provided	Food that is provided by the service **meets the needs and preferences** of individual patients/clients through audit of patient feedback and equality and diversity co-operatives
7 Food availability	Patients/clients have set meal times. Flexibility is also important, ensuring **a replacement meal is offered** if a meal is missed and patients **can access a lighter meal or snacks** at any time
8 Food presentation	Food is presented to patients/clients in a way that takes in to account portion capacity and what **appeals to them as individuals**
9 Monitoring	The amount of food patients actually eat is **monitored, recorded** and leads to **action** when cause for concern
10 Eating to promote health	**All opportunities** are used to encourage the patients/clients to eat to **promote their own health**

Other factors which may influence future food intake (e.g. surgery, chemotherapy or radiotherapy) also need to be taken into consideration when planning nutritional support, as clinical experience shows these may exert a deleterious effect on appetite and the ability to maintain an adequate nutritional intake (Newman *et al.* 1998)

Dietary supplements

These may be used to improve an inadequate diet or may be used as a sole source of nutrition if taken in sufficient quantity.

Sip feeds

These come in a range of flavours, both sweet and savoury, and are presented as a powder in a packet or ready prepared in a can, bottle or carton. Sip feeds contain whole protein, hydrolysed fat and carbohydrates. Most are called 'complete feeds' since they provide all protein, vitamins, minerals and trace elements to meet requirements if a prescribed volume is taken (Thomas & Bishop 2007). Others may be aimed at specific needs, for example high protein.

Energy supplements

Carbohydrates

Glucose polymers in powder or liquid form contain approximately 350 kcal (1442 kJ) per 100 g and 187–299 kcal (770-1232 kJ) per 100 ml respectively. Powdered glucose polymer is virtually tasteless and may be added to anything in which it will dissolve, e.g. milk and other drinks, soup, cereals and milk pudding; liquid glucose polymers may be fruit flavoured or neutral (Thomas & Bishop 2007). Such supplements would be used to increase the energy content of the diet.

Fat

Fat may be in the form of long-chain triglycerides (LCT) or medium-chain triglycerides (MCT) and comes as a liquid which can be added to food and drinks. These oils provide 416–772 kcal (1714-3181 kJ) per 100 ml: the oils with a lower energy value are presented in the form of an emulsion and those with a higher energy value are presented as pure oil (Thomas & Bishop 2007).

Mixed fat and glucose polymer solutions and powders are available and provide 150 kcal per 100 ml or 486 kcal per 100 g, depending on the relative proportion of fat and carbohydrates in the product.

Products containing MCT are used in preference to those containing LCT where a patient suffers from GI impairment causing malabsorption. Patients require specific advice about their use to ensure that they are introduced into the diet slowly and GI tolerance is assessed (Thomas & Bishop 2007).

Always check with the manufacturer for the exact energy content of products.

Note: products containing a glucose polymer are unsuitable for patients with diabetes mellitus.

Protein supplements

These come in the form of a powder and provide 55–90 g protein per 100 g. Protein supplement powders may be added to any food or drink in which they will dissolve, e.g. milk, fruit juice, soup, milk pudding.

Energy and protein supplements are not used in isolation as these would not provide an adequate nutritional intake. They are used in conjunction with sip feeds and a modified diet. The detailed nutritional compositions of dietary supplements are available from the manufacturers.

Vitamin and mineral supplements

When dietary intake is poor a vitamin and mineral supplement may be required. This can often be given as a one-a-day tablet supplement that provides 100% of the dietary reference values. Care should be taken to avoid unbalanced supplements or those containing amounts larger than the dietary reference value (FSA 2003).

Modification of diet

Practical information on modification of diet can be found in the Royal Marsden Hospital Patient Information Series *Eating Well When You Have Cancer – A Guide for Cancer Patients* (Royal Marsden NHS Trust 2002). See also Table 17.2.

Enteral tube feeding

While the majority of patients will be able to meet their nutritional requirements orally, there is a group of individuals who will require enteral tube feeding either in the short term or on a more permanent basis. Several different feeding tubes are available.

Types of enteral feed tubes

Nasogastric/nasoduodenal/nasojejunal

Nasogastric feeding is the most commonly used enteral tube feed and is suitable for short-term feeding, i.e. 2–4 weeks (National Collaborating Centre for Acute Care 2006). Fine-bore feeding tubes should be used whenever possible as these are more comfortable for the patient than wide-bore tubes. They are less likely to cause complications such as rhinitis, oesophageal irritation and gastritis (Payne-James *et al.* 2001). Polyurethane or silicone tubes are preferable to polyvinylchloride (PVC) as they withstand gastric acid and can stay in position longer than the 10–14 day lifespan of the PVC tube (Payne-James *et al.* 2001).

A wire introducer is provided with many of the tubes to aid intubation. The position of the nasogastric tube can be checked using two methods:

- Chest X-ray.
- Testing of aspirate with pH indicator paper.

A chest X-ray must be used to confirm the position of the tube in high risk groups such as patients with oesophageal or head and neck tumours, who have impaired swallowing or who are unconscious because they are at higher risk of misplacement of the nasogastric tube. All other patients should have the position of the tube checked with syringed aspirate of gastric content. This should have a pH less than 5.5 (NPSA 2005). In accordance with National Patient Safety

Table 17.2 Suggestions for modification of diet.

Eating difficulty	Dietary modification
Anorexia	Serve small meals and snacks, e.g. twice daily snack options Make food look attractive with garnish Fortify foods with butter, cream or cheese to increase energy content of meals Use alcohol, steroids, megestrol acetate or medroxyprogesterone as an appetite stimulant Encourage food that patient prefers Offer nourishing drinks between meals. In hospital consider a 'cocktail' drinks round.
Sore mouth	Offer foods that are soft and easy to eat Avoid dry foods that require chewing Avoid citrus fruits and drinks Avoid salt and spicy foods Allow hot food to cool before eating
Dysphagia	Offer foods that are soft and serve with additional sauce or gravy Some foods may need to be blended: make sure food is served attractively Supplement the diet with nourishing drinks between meals
Nausea and vomiting	Have cold foods in preference to hot as these emit less odour Keep away from cooking smells Sip fizzy, glucose-containing drinks Eat small frequent meals and snacks that are high in carbohydrate (e.g. biscuits and toast) Try ginger drinks and ginger biscuits
Early satiety	Eat small, frequent meals. In hospital access an 'out of hours' meal service Avoid high-fat foods which delay gastric emptying Avoid drinking large quantities when eating Use prokinetics, e.g. metoclopramide, to encourage gastric emptying

578

Agency (NPSA) guidance the following methods should **not** be used to confirm the position of a feeding tube:

- Auscultation of air insufflated through the feeding tube ('whoosh test').
- Testing the pH of the aspirate using blue litmus paper.

- Interpreting the absence of respiratory distress as an indicator of the correct positioning.
- Monitoring bubbling at the end of the tube.
- Observing the appearance of feeding tube aspirate.

In addition to the initial confirmation, the tube should be checked on a daily basis in the following situations:

- Before administering each feed.
- Before giving medication.
- Following episodes of vomiting, retching or coughing as it is likely the tube may be displaced.
- Following evidence of tube displacement (e.g. the tube appears visibly longer).

If a pH of below 5.5 is not obtained then it is highly likely that the tube has become displaced. The medical team should be contacted as the tube may need to be replaced. For further details on checking nasogastric tubes please refer to the full NPSA guidance or to local policy.

Gastrostomy

A gastrostomy may be more appropriate than a nasogastric tube where feeding is for medium- or long-term feeding. It avoids delays in feeding and discomfort associated with tube displacement (National Collaborating Centre for Acute Care 2006). Suitable patients are those undergoing radical or hyperfractionated radiotherapy to the neck or children with solid tumours. They will require long-term enteral feeding because the treatment is intensive and prolonged. A gastrostomy tube may be placed endoscopically (percutaneous endoscopically placed gastrostomy [PEG]) or radiologically (radiologically inserted gastrostomy [RIG]). They are made from polyurethane or silicone and are therefore suitable for short- or long-term feeding. A flange, flexible dome, inflated balloon or pigtail sits within the stomach and holds the tube in position. The use of conventional balloon urinary catheters is now outdated, particularly as these are at risk of allowing gastric acid to leak at the tube entry site. However, gastrostomy tubes held in place with an inflatable balloon have the benefit over urinary catheters of being less likely to leak and are also made from polyurethane or silicone rather than from PVC. Clinical trials have shown that complications with PEG tubes, such as leakage, are rare (Riera *et al*. 2002).

For long-term feeding (i.e. longer than 1 month), a gastrostomy tube may be replaced with a button which is made from silicone. The entry site for feeding is flush with the skin, making it neat and less obvious than a gastrostomy tube. This is more cosmetically acceptable, especially for teenagers, but does require a certain amount of manual dexterity from the patient (Thomas & Bishop 2007).

The button is held in place by a balloon or dome inside the stomach (Griffiths 1996).

PEG tubes may be placed while the patient is sedated; thereby avoiding the risks associated with general anaesthesia.

Certain groups of patients are not suitable for endoscopy; in these cases a RIG can be used. They are indicated for oesophageal patients with bulky tumours where it would be difficult to pass an endoscope and also for head and neck patients whose airway would be obstructed by an endoscope. There is also documented risk of the endoscope seeding the tumour to the gastrostomy site when it pulls the tube past a bulky tumour although this is a rare complication (Pickhardt *et al.* 2002).

Jejunostomy

A jejunostomy is preferable to a gastrostomy if a patient has undergone upper GI surgery or has severe delayed gastric emptying; in some cases it can be used to feed a patient with pyloric obstruction (Thomas & Bishop 2007). Fine-bore feeding jejunostomy tubes may be inserted with the use of a jejunostomy kit, which consists of a needle-fine catheter. The use of needles and an introducer wire allows a fine-bore polyurethane catheter to be inserted into a loop of jejunum. Alternatively, some gastrostomy tubes allow the passage of a fine-bore tube into the jejunum.

Enteral feeding equipment

The administration of enteral feeds may be as a bolus, intermittent or continuous infusion, via gravity drip or pump-assisted (Table 17.3). There are many enteral feeding pumps available which vary in their range of flow rate from 1 ml to 300 ml per hour. The following systems may be used for feeding via a pump or gravity-drip:

- Feed is decanted into plastic bottles or PVC bags. The administration set may be an integral part of the bag. The feed is sterile until opened and decanting feed into reservoirs will increase the risk of contamination of the feed from handling (Payne-James *et al.* 2001). Malnourished and immunocompromised patients are particularly at risk from contamination and infection so this method of administration should be avoided where possible.
- The 'ready to hang system' has a glass bottle, plastic bottle or pack attached directly to the administration set. The bottles and packs are available in different types of feeds and sizes for flexibility. This is a closed sterile system. It has been shown to be successful in preventing exogenous bacterial contamination (Payne-James *et al.* 2001).

Table 17.3 Methods of administering enteral feeds.

Feeding regimen	Advantages	Disadvantages
Continuous feeding via a pump	Easily controlled rate Reduction of GI complications	Patient connected to the feed for majority of the day May limit patient's mobility
Intermittent feeding via gravity or a pump	Periods of time free of feeding Flexible feeding routine May be easier than managing a pump for some patients	May have an increased risk of GI symptoms, e.g. early satiety Difficult if outside carers are involved with the feed
Bolus feeding	May reduce time connected to feed Very easy Minimum equipment required	May have an increased risk of GI symptoms May be time consuming

GI, gastrointestinal.

Enteral feeds

Commercially prepared feeds should be used for nasogastric, gastrostomy or jejunostomy feeding. Available in liquid or powder form, they have the advantage of being of known composition and are sterile when packaged.

1 Whole protein/polymeric feeds contain protein, hydrolysed fat and carbohydrate and so require digestion. These may provide 1.0–1.5 kcal/ml (see manufacturer's specifications). As the energy density of the feed increases so does the osmolarity. Hyperosmolar feeds tend to draw water into the lumen of the gut and can contribute to diarrhoea if given too rapidly. Fibre may be beneficial for maintaining gut ecology and function, rather than promoting bowel transit time (Thomas & Bishop 2007).

2 Feeds containing MCT. In some whole protein feeds a proportion of the fat or LCT may be replaced with MCT. The feed often has a lower osmolarity, and is therefore less likely to draw fluid from the plasma into the gut lumen. MCT is transported via the portal vein rather than the lymphatic system. These feeds are suitable for patients with fat malabsorption and maybe steatorrhoea (Cummings 2000).

3 Chemically defined/elemental feeds. These contain free amino acids, short-chain peptides or a combination of both as the nitrogen source. They are often low in fat or may contain some fat as MCT. Glucose polymers provide the main energy source. These feeds require little or no digestion and are suitable

for those patients with impaired GI function (Thomas & Bishop 2007). They are hyperosmolar and low in residue.

4   Special application feeds. Low protein and mineral feeds may be used for patients with liver or renal failure. High-fat, low-carbohydrate feeds may be used for ventilated patients because less carbon dioxide is produced per calorie intake compared with a low-fat, high-carbohydrate feed.

   Very high energy and protein feeds may be used where nutritional requirements are exceptionally high, e.g. burns, severe sepsis. These feeds contain approximately double the amount of energy and protein compared to standard whole protein feeds.

5   Paediatric feeds are designed for children 1–12 years old and/or 8–45 kg in weight. The protein, vitamin and mineral profile is suitable for children. Generally they are lower in osmolarity than adult feeds. The whole protein/polymeric feeds are based on cow's milk but are lactose free. Some of these feeds may contain dietary fibre. These feeds provide 1.0–1.5 kcal/ml for children who require additional energy and protein in a smaller volume. Protein hydrolysate feeds and elemental feeds are used in conditions such as food allergies or malabsorption. Some specialist centres use these feeds for enteral feeding during bone marrow transplants as children may have malabsorption caused by gut mucositis. The osmolarity of these feeds is higher than whole protein feeds. They need to be introduced carefully (Thomas & Bishop 2007).

6   Immune modulating feeds. There is evidence to show that the addition of glutamine, arginine or omega-3 fatty acids, if given preoperatively, may benefit post-surgical GI patients (Braga *et al.* 2002).

Up-to-date information on the exact composition of dietary supplements and enteral feeds can be obtained from the manufacturers.

Monitoring enteral tube feeding

In order to avoid complications and ensure optimal nutritional status, it is important to monitor the following in patients on enteral tube feeds:

- Oral intake.
- Body weight.
- Urea and electrolytes.
- Blood glucose.
- Full blood count.
- Fluid balance.
- Tolerance to feed, e.g. nausea, fullness and bowel activity.
- Quantity of feed taken.
- Care of tube.
- Care of stoma site.

Complications of enteral tube feeding

The type and frequency of complications related to tube feeding depend on the access route, underlying disease state, the feeding regimen and the patient's metabolic state (Payne-James *et al.* 2001) (Table 17.4).

Home enteral feeding

Some patients who are established on tube feeding in hospital also require enteral tube feeding at home. A multidisciplinary approach is needed for a successful discharge usually involving a dietitian, doctor, ward nurse, community nurse and general practitioner. The patient's circumstances and the ability of the patient or carers to manage the feed must be considered when the patient's discharge is being planned. Adequate time should be allowed in the hospital setting for patients to become fully accustomed to the techniques of feed administration and care of the feeding tube, prior to discharge home. Patients should also be given written information to reinforce the education they receive prior to discharge (BAPEN 1994a).

Support in the form of the general practitioner, community nurse and community dietetic services should be established before discharge. A multidisciplinary discharge meeting may be of benefit to both the patient and the professionals involved. Many of the commercial feed companies organize for the patient's feed and equipment to be delivered to the patient's home, after consultation with the local community services (BAPEN 1994a). The hospital or community dietitian can arrange this. Early notification of discharge is essential as it usually takes a minimum of 7 days to set this up.

Termination of enteral tube feeding

It is important to ensure that an individual is able to meet their nutritional requirements orally prior to termination of the feed. Ideally, the feeds should be reduced gradually, according to the dietary intake (BAPEN 1999). It may be useful to maintain an overnight feed while the patient is establishing oral intake.

Parenteral nutrition

Parenteral nutrition (PN) is the direct infusion into a vein, of solutions containing the essential nutrients in quantities to meet all the daily needs of the patient (Furst *et al.* 2001). While enteral feeding is the preferred route of nutritional support in terms of cost and mechanical, septic and metabolic complications (National Collaborating Centre for Acute Care 2006), PN may be indicated for patients with a prolonged ileus, uncontrolled vomiting or diarrhoea, severe radiation enteritis, short bowel syndrome or GI obstruction.

583

Table 17.4 Complications that may occur during enteral feeding.

Complication	Cause	Solution
Aspiration	Regurgitation of feed due to poor gastric emptying Incorrect placement of tube	Medication to improve gastric emptying, e.g. metoclopramide Check tube placement Ensure patient has head at 45° during feeding
Nausea and vomiting	Related to disease/treatment Medication such as antibiotics, analgesia, etc. Poor gastric emptying Rapid infusion of feed	Antiemetics Reduce infusion rate Change from bolus to intermittent feeding
Diarrhoea	Medication such as antibiotics, chemotherapy, laxatives Radiotherapy to pelvis Disease-related, e.g. pancreatic insufficiency Gut infection	Antidiarrhoeal agent If possible discontinue antibiotics, avoid microbiological contamination of feed or equipment. Treat disease or manage symptoms Send stool sample to check for gut infection
Constipation	Inadequate fluid intake Immobility Use of opiates or other medication causing gut stasis Bowel obstruction	Check fluid balance and correct if necessary Administer laxatives/bulking agents If possible encourage mobility If in bowel obstruction, discontinue feed
Abdominal distension	Poor gastric emptying Rapid infusion of feed Constipation or diarrhoea	Gastric motility agents Reduce rate of infusion If possible encourage mobility Treat constipation or diarrhoea
Blocked tube	Inadequate flushing or failure to flush feeding tube Administration of medication via the tube	Prevent blockages by flushing with 30–50 ml water before and after feeds or medication Use liquid or finely crushed medications If blocked, try warm water, soda water, sodium bicarbonate, fizzy soft drink, enzyme preparations

Route of administration

The traditional method of access is a central venous catheter. Central venous access is required because PN solutions are hyperosmolar and there is a risk of thrombophlebitis associated with feeding into peripheral veins (Wilson & Jordan 2001; Springhouse Corporation 2002). However, it has been shown that with care and attention, peripheral veins can be used to provide short-term peripheral PN (National Collaborating Centre for Acute Care 2006). This would be via a midline or a peripheral cannula. For the administration of PN the device should be placed in the largest vein possible, usually in the forearm away from a joint with rotation of the site every 48–72 hours (Shaw 2008) (see Chapter 45, Professional edition).

The major hazard associated with the delivery of PN via a central venous catheter is infection. Therefore, catheter insertion should take place using strict aseptic technique either within theatre or at the bedside (Hamilton *et al.* 1995; Fitzsimmons 1997; Benton & Marsden 2002; Weinstein 2007). A skin-tunnelled catheter is the catheter of choice for long-term nutrition but peripherally inserted central canulas (PICCs) or non-tunnelled central venous catheters can also be used in the short term. The number of lumens will depend on the patient's peripheral venous access and the number of additional therapies required. It is recommended that the minimum number of lumens is used but if additional intravenous access is required then a double or triple lumen catheter should be inserted and then one lumen should be dedicated for use with PN. If using a single lumen device, routine blood sampling and additional infusions should be carried out independently, using a separate cannula if necessary (Davidson 2005).

PN solution

The basic components of a PN regimen are provided by solutions of:

- *Amino acids* (nitrogen source). Commercially available solutions provide both essential amino acids, usually in proportions to meet requirements, and non-essential amino acids, such as alanine and glycine.
- *Glucose* (carbohydrate energy source). Glucose is the carbohydrate source of choice. It provides 3.75 kcal/g (1545 kJ/g).
- *Fat emulsion* (fat energy source). Fat generates 9 kcal/g (37 kJ/g) and its inclusion in PN is necessary to provide essential fatty acids. Fat usually provides 30–50% of non-nitrogen energy. Nitrogen: non-nitrogen energy is usually provided in the ratio of 1 : 150–200. An insufficient energy supply from carbohydrate and fat will encourage the use of nitrogen for energy.

- *Electrolytes*, e.g. sodium, potassium, calcium.
- *Vitamins*. Both water-soluble and fat-soluble vitamins are required.
- *Trace elements*, e.g. zinc, copper, chromium, selenium (Thomas & Bishop 2007).

Choice of a PN regimen

PN is usually administered from a single infusion container in which all the requirements for a 24-hour feed are premixed. Such infusions are available as standard ready prepared bags that require the addition of vitamins, minerals and trace elements or individual bags may be made to a particular prescription and purchased from a compounding unit.

The regimen for a particular patient should be formulated according to the patient's needs for energy and nitrogen (see calculation of nutritional requirements, Table 17.1). The majority of commercial vitamin and mineral preparations aim to meet both short- and long-term requirements although appropriate monitoring is required to ensure that nutritional requirements are met.

Standard PN regimens may be suitable for some patients who require short-term nutritional support or do not appear to have excessively altered nutritional requirements.

The choice of such regimens depends on the patient's body weight and nutritional requirements. To allow for the possible need to vary the constituents of the infusion in response to changes in the patient's electrolyte or nutritional requirements, PN solutions should be ordered daily. Once compounded, most PN preparations last up to 7 days (Weinstein 2007) and need to be stored in a refrigerator. However, some triple chamber PN bags can be stored at ambient temperatures and require mixing prior to administration. These bags generally require the addition of vitamins, minerals and trace elements under aseptic conditions.

PN should be introduced slowly in the seriously ill or injured with no more than 50% of requirements given in the first 24–48 hours (National Collaborating Centre for Acute Care 2006).

Delivery of PN and recommendations for intravenous management

Administration sets should always be changed every 24 hours (Wilson & Jordan 2001; Springhouse Corporation 2002; Pratt *et al.* 2007), using an aseptic technique. Existing injection sites on the administration set should never be used for the giving of additional medications as PN is incompatible with numerous medications. Drugs may bind to the nutrients or the PN bag reducing their availability.

Table 17.5 Monitoring of patients receiving parenteral nutrition. National Collaborating Centre for Acute Care (2006).

- Daily initially, reducing to twice weekly when stable
- Inspect catheter entry site daily for signs of infection or inflammation
- Inspect site of peripheral cannulae for signs of phlebitis (peripherally fed patients)
- Assess general condition daily
- Record temperature and blood pressure daily initially then as needed

If any additional medications, blood products or central venous pressure (CVP) readings are required then they should be given via a separate lumen or via a peripheral device.

A volumetric infusion pump must be used to ensure accurate delivery of PN. No bag should be used for longer than 24 hours (Wilson & Jordan 2001; Springhouse Corporation 2002) and rates should never be adjusted more than ±10% (Weinstein 2007).

If the infusion must be discontinued the catheter should be flushed and patency maintained. The risk of infection increases if the infusion is disconnected from the central venous device; therefore, it is not advisable to disconnect PN until the whole daily requirement has been administered (Pratt *et al.* 2007).

Monitoring of PN

During intravenous feeding monitoring is necessary to detect and minimize complications (Tables 17.5 & 17.6). Once feeding is established and the patient is biochemically stable then the frequency of monitoring may be reduced if the clinical condition of the patient permits. Additional patient monitoring such as 24-hour urine collection for urinary urea, nitrogen and serum zinc, copper or selenium may be carried out where indicated, e.g. in severe malnutrition or when PN is used for prolonged periods of time (Weinstein 2007).

Metabolic complications of PN

Metabolic complications should be detected by appropriate monitoring. Some more common complications are:

- *Fluid overload.* This may occur when other blood products and fluids are given concurrently. It may be possible to reduce the volume of a 24-hour bag of PN while maintaining the nutritional content. Pharmacy can advise on the feasibility of making such regimens.

Table 17.6 Biochemical monitoring of parenteral nutrition. National Collaborating Centre for Acute Care (2006).

Parameter	Frequency	Rationale	Interpretation
Sodium, potassium, urea, creatinine	Baseline Daily until stable then 1 or 2 times a week	Assessment of renal function, fluid status and Na and K status	Interpret with knowledge of fluid balance and medication
Glucose	Baseline 1 or 2 times a day (or more if needed) until stable then weekly	Glucose intolerance is common	Good glycaemic control is necessary
Magnesium, phosphate	Baseline Daily if risk of refeeding syndrome Three times a week until stable Then weekly	Depletion is common and under recognized	Low concentrations indicate poor status
Liver function tests including International Normalized Ratio	Baseline Twice weekly until stable Then weekly	Abnormalities common during parenteral nutrition	Complex, may be due to sepsis, other disease or nutritional intake
Calcium, albumin	Baseline then weekly	Hypocalcaemia or hypercalcaemia may occur	Correct measured serum calcium concentration for albumin Hypocalcaemia may be secondary to Mg deficiency Low albumin reflects disease not protein status

C-reactive protein	Baseline Then 2 or 3 times a week until stable	To assess the presence of an acute phase reaction The trend of results is important
Full blood count and mean cell volume	Baseline 1 or 2 times a week until stable then weekly	Anaemia due to iron or folate deficiency is common Effects of sepsis may be important
Iron, ferritin	Baseline Then every 3–6 months	Iron deficiency common in long-term parenteral nutrition Iron status difficult if acute phase reaction (Fe decreases and ferritin increases)
Folate, B_{12}	Baseline Then every 2–4 weeks	Iron deficiency is common Serum folate/B_{12} sufficient, with full blood count

Monitoring of trace elements such as selenium, zinc, copper and manganese should be carried out if patients are on long-term parenteral nutrition, for example for periods longer than 1 month.

Table 17.7 Criteria for determining patients at risk of refeeding problems (National Collaborating Centre for Acute Care 2006).

Patient has one or more of the following	Patient has two or more of the following
BMI < 16 kg/m²	BMI < 18.5 kg/m²
Unintentional weight loss > 15%	Weight loss > 10%
Very little nutritional intake for > 10 days	Very little nutritional intake for > 5 days
Low levels of postassium, phosphate or magnesium prior to feeding	A history of alcohol abuse or drugs including insulin, chemotherapy, antacids or diuretics

BMI, body mass index.

- *Hyperglycaemia.* This may occur due to stress-induced insulin resistance or carbohydrate overload. A simultaneous sliding scale insulin infusion may be required. Failure to recognize hyperglycaemia may result in osmotic diuresis.
- *Hypoglycaemia.* Abrupt cessation of PN may result in a rebound hypoglycaemia. A reduction in infusion rate to half the rate prior to stopping the infusion may help prevent this occurring.
- *Azotaemia.* Raised plasma urea may indicate renal dysfunction or dehydration. Alterations in the nitrogen and non-protein energy content of the PN may be required, or an increase in fluid input (Payne-James *et al.* 2001).
- *Hypophosphataemia.* This is associated with excessive glucose infusion and the refeeding syndrome in malnourished patients (Thorell & Nordenström 2001). It is necessary to correct phosphate levels by providing additional phosphate prior to feeding. Phosphate levels should be monitored daily at the start of feeding.

Other complications such as metabolic acidosis, electrolyte disturbances, hyperammonaemia, hypernatraemia and hypokalaemia may require a review of the PN solution, rate of administration, additional fluids, blood products and drugs.

Termination of PN

590

PN should not be terminated until oral or enteral tube feeding is well established (Weinstein 2007). The patient needs to be established on an adequate oral or enteral tube feed before the PN is discontinued (National Collaborating Centre for Acute Care 2006). It is important that all members of the multidisciplinary team are involved in the decision to terminate PN and that enteral intake is monitored sufficiently.

Elective removal of central venous catheter

See Chapter 45, Professional edition.

Home PN

There are few indications for home PN. It may be necessary in patients who have complete intestinal failure or insufficient functioning bowel to maintain an adequate nutritional status via the enteral route, e.g. short bowel syndrome due to Crohn's disease or radiation enteritis. The cost of home parenteral feeding is high and requires intensive training with an efficient and comprehensive back-up service. It is recommended that only hospitals which have the appropriate facilities to train patients and provide the necessary care in case of an emergency should be involved in home PN. There is national guidance as to the training, provision and appropriate support for such patients which should be consulted prior to any discharge of patients receiving PN (BAPEN 1994a; DH 2002).

Multidisciplinary team

It is important that all members of the multidisciplinary team, including dietitian, nurse, doctor, pharmacist, catering department and community services, are involved in the patient's nutritional care to ensure a thorough and co-ordinated approach to nutritional management (BAPEN 1994b; National Collaborating Centre for Acute Care 2006).

Procedure guidelines **Weighing the patient**

Accurate weighing and correct documentation of the patient's weight may be necessary, for example for nutrition screening or planning of drug dosage.

Equipment

1 Scales (either sitting or standing) that are calibrated and positioned on a level surface. If electronic or battery scales are used then they must be connected to the mains or have appropriate working batteries prior to the patient getting on the scales.

591

Procedure

Action	Rationale
1 Position the scales for easy access and apply the brakes (if appropriate).	To ensure that the patient can get on and off the scales easily and to avoid accidents should the scales move (E).

Procedure guidelines *(cont.)*

2 Ask the patient to remove shoes and outdoor garments. The patient should be wearing light indoor clothes only.	Outdoor clothes and shoes will add additional weight and make it difficult to obtain an accurate body weight (E).
3 Ensure that the scales record zero then ask the patient to stand on scales (or sit if using sitting scales). Ask the patient to remain still and check that the patient is not supporting any weight on any object, e.g. wall, stick or feet on the floor.	To record an accurate weight (E).
4 Note the reading on the scale and record immediately taking care that it is legible. Check with the patient that the weight reflects their expected weight and that the weight is similar to previous weights recorded.	To check that the weight is correct. If the weight is not as expected then the patient should be re-weighed (E).

Procedure guidelines   **Feeding an adult**

An essential part of providing diet for a patient is to ensure that the patient is able to consume the food and fluid in a safe and pleasant environment. Some patients may require assistance with feeding or drinking and a system should be in place to ensure that these patients receive the required attention at each meal time and beverage that is provided (Nicol *et al.* 2000).

Equipment

1 Appropriate environment for eating, preferably at a dining table with chair or the patient should be positioned where the patient can sit up as much as possible in a supported midline position.
2 Clean table or tray.
3 Chair for the nurse or carer to sit with the patient.
4 Appetising meal that complies with any dietary restriction that is relevant to the patient. For example, these may include allergies, texture modifications, religious or cultural dietary requirements.

Procedure

Action	Rationale
1 Ensure the patient is comfortable, i.e. has an empty bladder, clean hands, clean mouth and if applicable clean dentures.	To make the mealtime a pleasant experience (E).
2 Wash hands thoroughly with soap and water.	Hands must be cleansed before and after patient contact to minimize cross-infection (DH 2005: C).
3 Obtain the correct food, drink, cutlery and napkin.	To prevent errors with the wrong food being served to the patient (E).
4 Protect the patient's clothing with a napkin.	To maintain dignity and cleanliness (E).
5 Assist the patient to take appropriate portions of food at the correct temperature. Tailor the size of each mouthful to the individual patient. Allow the patient to chew and swallow food before giving the next mouthful.	To make the mealtime a pleasant experience. To ensure that swallowing is not compromised if the patient feels that they must hurry with the meal (E).
6 Avoid asking questions when the patient is eating but check between mouthfuls that the food is suitable and patient is able to continue with the meal.	To reduce the risk of aspirating, which may be increased if speaking whilst eating (E).
7 Use the napkin to remove particles of food or drink from the patient's face.	To maintain dignity and cleanliness (E).
8 Ask the patient when they wish to have a drink. Tip the glass or cup gently so that the flow of liquid is controlled or use a straw if this is helpful. Take care with hot drinks to avoid offering these when too hot to drink.	To give the opportunity for the patient to swallow (E). Hot liquids may scald the patient.
9 Encourage the patient to take as much food as they feel able to eat but do not press if they have indicated that they have eaten sufficient.	To improve nutritional intake but also maintain patient dignity and choice (E).

Procedure guidelines *(cont.)*

10 After the meal assist the patient to meet hygiene needs; for example, wash hands and face and clean teeth.	To maintain patient dignity (E).

Procedure guidelines **Nasogastric intubation with tubes without using an introducer, e.g. a Ryle's tube**

It is recommended that a nasogastric tube designed for feeding purposes be used wherever possible, e.g. fine-bore feeding tube, rather than a Ryle's tube which is used for drainage of gastric contents.

Equipment

1 Clinically clean tray.
2 Nasogastric tube that has been stored in a deep freeze for at least half an hour before the procedure is to begin, to ensure a rigid tube that will allow for easy passage.
3 Topical gauze.
4 Lubricating jelly.

5 Hypoallergenic tape.
6 20 ml syringe.
7 Indicator strips, e.g. pH Fix, 0–6, Fisher Scientific.
8 Receiver.
9 Spigot.
10 Glass of water.

Procedure

Action

Rationale

1 Explain and discuss the procedure with the patient.

To ensure that the patient understands the procedure and gives his/her valid consent (E; NMC 2006: C).

2 Arrange a signal by which the patient can communicate if he/she wants the nurse to stop, e.g. by raising his/her hand.

The patient is often less frightened if he/she feels able to have some control over the procedure (E).

3 Assist the patient to sit in a semi-upright position in the bed or chair. Support the patient's head with pillows.
Note: The head should not be tilted backwards or forwards (Rollins 1997).

To allow for easy passage of the tube. This position enables easy swallowing and ensures that the epiglottis is not obstructing the oesophagus (E).

4 Mark the distance which the tube is to be passed by measuring the distance on the tube from the patient's ear lobe to the bridge of the nose plus the distance from the ear lobe to the bottom of the xiphisternum.	To indicate the length of tube required for entry into the stomach (E).
5 Wash hands with bactericidal soap and water or bactericidal alcohol handrub, and assemble the equipment required.	Hands must be cleansed before and after patient contact to minimize cross-infection (DH 2005: R 1a).
6 Check the patient's nostrils are patent by asking him/her to sniff with one nostril closed. Repeat with the other nostril.	To identify any obstructions liable to prevent intubation (E).
7 Lubricate about 15–20 cm of the tube with a thin coat of lubricating jelly that has been placed on a topical swab.	To reduce the friction between the mucous membranes and the tube (E).
8 Insert the proximal end of the tube into the clearer nostril and slide it backwards and inwards along the floor of the nose to the nasopharynx. If an obstruction is felt, withdraw the tube and try again in a slightly different direction or use the other nostril.	To facilitate the passage of the tube by following the natural anatomy of the nose (E).
9 As the tube passes down into the nasopharynx, ask the patient to start swallowing and sipping water, enabling the tube to pass into the oesophagus (R).	To focus the patient's attention on something other than the tube. The swallowing action closes the glottis and crico-pharyngeal sphincter opens enabling the tube to pass into the oesophagus (Groher 1997: R 5).
10 Advance the tube through the pharynx as the patient swallows until the tape-marked tube reaches the point of entry into the external nares. If the patient shows signs of distress, e.g. gasping or cyanosis, remove tube immediately.	Distress may indicate that the tube is in the bronchus. However, absence of distress is ineffective for detecting a misplaced tube (NPSA 2005: C).

Procedure guidelines *(cont.)*

11 Secure the tube to the nostril with adherent dressing tape, e.g. Elastoplast (Burns *et al.* 1995). If this is contraindicated, a hypoallergenic tape should be used. An adhesive patch (if available) will secure the tube to the cheek.	To hold the tube in place. To ensure patient comfort (E).
12 Check the position of the tube to confirm that it is in the stomach by using the following methods:	
(a) Taking an X-ray of chest and upper abdomen.	To confirm placement of radiopaque nasogastric tube. X-ray of radiopaque tubes is the most accurate confirmation of position and is the method of choice in patients with altered anatomy, those who are aspirating or are unconscious with no gag reflex (NPSA 2005: C).
(b) Aspirating 2 ml of stomach contents and testing with pH indicator strips (Rollins 1997). When aspirating fluid for pH testing, wait at least 1 hour after a feed or medication has been administered (either orally or via a tube). Before aspirating, flush the tube with 20 ml of air to clear other substances (Metheny *et al.* 1993). A pH level of 5.5 is unlikely to be pulmonary aspirate and is considered appropriate to proceed to feed through the tube (Metheny 2004; NPSA 2005).	Indicator strips to be used should have gradations of 0.5 or paper with a range of 0–6 or 1–11 to distinguish between gastric acid and bronchial secretions (NPSA 2005: C). To prove an accurate test result because the feed or medication may raise the pH of the stomach. Wait at least 1 hour before aspirating to enable the feed or medication to be absorbed, otherwise an inaccurate test will be obtained (NPSA 2005: C).
(c) If a pH of 6.0 or above is obtained or there is doubt over the result in the range of pH 5–6 then feeding must **not** commence. The nasogastric tube may need to be repositioned or checked with an X-ray.	There is an increased risk of the nasogastric tube being incorrectly placed (NPSA 2005: C).

13 The following methods **must not** be used to test the position of a nasogastric feeding tube: auscultation (introducing air into the nasogastric tube and checking for a bubbling sound via a stethoscope, also known as the 'whoosh test'), use of litmus paper or absence of respiratory distress.

These tests are not accurate or reliable as a method of checking the position of a nasogastric tube as they have been shown to give false positive results (Metheny 2004; NPSA 2005: C).

Procedure guidelines Jejunostomy feeding tube care

This procedure should be performed daily to maintain skin integrity and detect any problems early, e.g. infection, skin breakdown.

Equipment

1 Sterile procedure pack containing gallipot, low-linting gauze.

2 Sterile 0.9% sodium chloride.

Procedure

Action	Rationale
1 Explain and discuss the procedure with the patient.	To ensure that the patient understands the procedure and gives his/her valid consent (E; NMC 2006: C).
2 Perform procedure using aseptic technique.	To minimize the risk of cross-infection (DH 2005: C) (for further information see Procedure guidelines: Aseptic technique, Chapter 4).
3 Remove post-procedural dressing if in place. Observe peristomal skin and stoma site for signs of infection, irritation or excoriation.	To gain access to stoma site. To detect complications early and instigate appropriate treatment (Lynch & Fang 2004: R 5).
4 Clean the stoma site with a sterile solution such as 0.9% sodium chloride. Using low-linting gauze dry the area thoroughly.	To remove any exudate, to prevent infection and skin excoriation (E).

597

Procedure guidelines *(cont.)*

5 Check that the sutures on the retention device are intact. If not, advise medical staff and arrange for the retention device to be resutured.

To prevent accidental removal of the jejunostomy tube (E).

6 Secure the jejunostomy tube to the skin with hypoallergenic tape. The site may be covered with a dry dressing or left uncovered.

To prevent the weight of the tube pulling on the exit site (E).

7 Advise the patient not to use moisturizing creams or talcum powder.

To prevent infection and/or irritation to the skin (E).

Procedure guidelines **Enteral feeding tubes: administration of medication**

Equipment

1 50 ml enteral or catheter-tipped syringe.
2 Tap water or sterile water (for jejunostomy tubes or for patients who are immunosuppressed) (NICE 2003). Water should be fresh and kept covered.

3 Mortar and pestle or tablet crusher if tablets are being administered (BAPEN 2003a: C).

Procedure

Action

1 Check whether patient can take medication orally, whether medication is necessary or if it can be temporarily suspended.

Rationale

If patient can take medication orally this reduces the risk of tube blockage (BAPEN 2003a: C).

2 Consider whether an alternative route can be used, e.g. buccal, transdermal, topical, rectal or subcutaneous.

If patient can take medication via an alternative route this reduces the risk of tube blockage (BAPEN 2003a: C).

3 Check drug is absorbed from the site of delivery.	Some drugs may not be absorbed directly from the jejunum (BAPEN 2003a: C).
4 Clean hands with bactericidal soap and water or alcoholic handgel. Put on non-sterile gloves.	To minimize cross-infection and protect the practitioner from gastric/intestinal contents (DH 2005: C).
5 Stop the enteral feed and flush the tube with at least 30 ml of water (sterile water for jejunostomy administration), using an enteral or catheter-tipped syringe.	To clear the tube of enteral feed as this may cause a blockage or interact with medications. Sterile water should be used for jejunostomy tubes as water is bypassing the protective acidic environment of the stomach (E).
6 Where there is an absolute contraindication for medicine to be taken with feed: (a) Stop the feed 1–2 hours before and 2 hours after administration (this will depend on the drug), e.g. for phenytoin administration, stop feed 2 hours before and 2 hours after.	To avoid interaction with enteral feed.
(b) Consult with the dietitian to prescribe a suitable feeding regimen.	To ensure that the patient's nutritional requirements are met in the time available around medicine administration (BAPEN 2003a: C).
7 Prior to preparation, check with the pharmacist which medicines should never be crushed.	Some medications are not designed to be crushed. These include: (a) Modified-release tablets: absorption will be altered by crushing, possibly causing toxic side-effects. (b) Enteric-coated tablets: the coating is designed to protect the drug against gastric acid. (c) Cytotoxic medicines: this will risk exposing the practitioner to the drug.
8 Prepare each medication to be given separately. Volumes greater than 10 ml may be drawn up in a 50 ml syringe and administered via the tube. For small volumes (less than 10 ml) follow step 11.	To avoid interaction between different medications and to ensure solubility (BAPEN 2003a: C).

599

Procedure guidelines *(cont.)*

(a) Soluble tablets: dissolve in
10–15 ml water.

(b) Liquids: shake well. For thick
liquids mix with an equal volume
of water.

(c) Tablets: crush using a mortar and
pestle or tablet crusher and mix
with 10–15 ml water.

9 Never add medication directly to the enteral feed.	To avoid interaction between medicines and feed (BAPEN 2003a: C).
10 Administer the medication through the tube via a 50 ml syringe. Rinse the tablet crusher or mortar with 10 ml water, draw up in a 50 ml syringe and flush this through the tube.	To ensure the whole dose is administered (BAPEN 2003a: C).
11 If volumes of less than 10 ml are required the dose should be measured in a 10 ml oral syringe. The plunger of a 50 ml syringe should be removed and the 50 ml syringe connected with the enteral tube. The dose should then be administered into the barrel of the 50 ml syringe and the 10 ml syringe rinsed with water, which should also be administered via the barrel of the 50 ml syringe.	To ensure the whole dose is administered (BAPEN 2003a: C).
12 If more than one medicine is to be administered, flush between drugs with at least 10 ml of water to ensure that the drug is cleared from the tube.	To avoid interactions between medicines (BAPEN 2003a: C).
13 Flush the tube with at least 30 ml water following the administration of the last drug.	To avoid medicines blocking the enteral tube (BAPEN 2003a: C).
14 If the patient is on a fluid restriction or for a paediatric patient, consult the dietitian and pharmacist about the quantity of water to be given before and after medication.	To ensure that the patient does not exceed their fluid restriction or requirements (BAPEN 2003a: C).

Problem solving: Swallowing difficulties

Supervision of patients with swallowing difficulties is important, and in some cases patients may require support at meal times, or when drinking, to carry out the recommended strategies. It is important for nurses to participate in educational programmes for patients and carers in order to encourage awareness of the implications of dysphagia. Anxieties associated with dysphagia should be allayed and confidence to undertake safe eating and drinking techniques built up. Patients may experience one or a number of the following problems.

Problem	Cause	Prevention	Suggested action
Patient experiencing difficulties with drinking and/or eating (which may lead to dehydration, insufficient nutritional intake and compromised airway).	(a) *Mechanical*. Patients who have undergone surgery and/or radiotherapy to the oral cavity, pharynx, larynx, or trachea (including temporary or permanent tracheostomy) are likely to experience swallowing difficulties of a temporary or more persistent nature (Figure 17.1) (Royal College of Speech and Language Therapists 2006: C).		Refer to specialist speech and language therapist (SLT) for full assessment and management plan. Refer to dietitian for nutritional assessment and management plan.
	(b) *Neurological*. Patients who have tumours which affect the subcortical, cerebral and brainstem area (and thus the cranial nerves) may present with symptoms of dysphagia. These symptoms will continue as long as the disease and/or treatment effects are evident (Royal College of Speech and Language Therapists 2006: C).		

Problem solving *(cont.)*

Problem	Cause	Prevention	Suggested action
	(c) *Oesophageal obstruction or dysfunction*. Patients who have tumours of the upper GI tract may well experience discomfort and difficulty with the oesophageal phase of the swallow. The only way to alleviate oesophageal difficulties is through medical or surgical management. Swallowing therapy is not indicated in these circumstances, although the specialist speech and language therapist may be able to offer advice to minimize the patient's difficulties or their risk of aspiration, reflux or backflow by altering food consistencies or advising on alternative swallow strategies (E).		
Dehydration and/or difficulty in maintaining adequate hydration.	Thin liquids (e.g. water) are difficult for the patient with dysphagia to manage. Watery liquids do not retain their cohesion in the mouth and therefore pass swiftly into the pharynx. Patients may avoid liquids of this consistency and become dehydrated.	Identify patients who are at risk.	Seek medical advice on the appropriateness of intravenous hydration. A referral to a specialist SLT: to advise on other liquid consistencies; safe swallow techniques and exercises. These may help the patient to increase oral intake.

Problem	Cause	Prevention	Suggested action
Difficulty in maintaining a clear airway (may be severe enough to block airway in tracheostomy patients).	Inability to manage secretions, indicated by drooling and/or gurgly voice. Tracheostomy patients may feel breathing is laboured (Royal College of Speech and Language Therapists 2006).	Monitor patient's progress carefully and regularly and liaise with the speech and language therapist about any changes noted.	Following assessment by specialist speech and language therapist, adjusting the patient's position may help (e.g. sitting posture and head position before and after swallowing). Oral suction may be required (see Chapter 29).
Patient requires nutritional support and/or alternative feeding method.	Dysphagia and/or disease process leading to inadequate nutrition.	All patients with dysphagia should be fully assessed by a dietitian to ensure current nutritional requirements are met by nutritional support, alternative feeding method, normal diet, or a combination of these.	Nutritional support and/or alternative feeding method may be indicated following discussion with members of the multidisciplinary team. Following assessment by a specialist speech and language therapist, recommendations may be made about sitting posture, head position, and consistency of food and drink. These will be individually tailored to the patient's needs. Nursing staff should monitor progress carefully, noting changes and reporting them to the appropriate professional.
Dysphagia in oral and/or pharyngeal stages of swallowing, related to head position and/or structural or neurological deficits.	Patients with tumours of the upper GI tract may experience difficulty with the oesophageal phase of the swallow; patients with tumours affecting the brainstem/cranial nerves will experience dysphagia (Royal College of Speech and Language Therapists 2006).		Proceed as advised by the specialist speech and language therapist. Their advice may include modifications in posture. Safe swallow manoeuvres, modifying consistencies and exercises to optimize function.

603

Problem solving *(cont.)*

Problem	Cause	Prevention	Suggested action
Selecting suitable food and/or drink.	Not all members of the multidisciplinary team and/or catering and other staff may be aware of the extent of the patient's swallowing difficulties (E).	Liaise with specialist speech and language therapist, dietitian and catering.	Provide food and drink of a consistency which will not exacerbate the patient's problems. This might include soft foods, thickened liquids, or purées. Food and drink must be individually tailored to suit the patient.

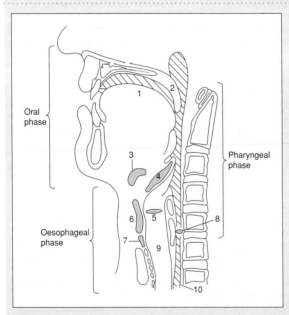

Figure 17.1   The normal swallow. (1, tongue; 2, soft palate; 3, hyoid bone; 4, epiglottis; 5, vocal cords; 6, thyroid cartilage; 7, cricoid cartilage; 8, pharyngoesophageal sphincter; 9, trachea; 10, oesophagus.) The oral, pharyngeal and oesophageal phases are separate but highly co-ordinated (Groher 1997; Logemann 1998).

References and further reading

BAPEN (1994a) *Enteral and Parenteral Nutrition in the Community* (ed. M. Elia). British Association for Parenteral and Enteral Nutrition, Maidenhead.

BAPEN (1994b) *Organisation of Nutritional Support in Hospitals* (ed. D.B.A. Silk). British Association for Parenteral and Enteral Nutrition, Maidenhead.

BAPEN (1996) *Current Perspectives on Parenteral Nutrition in Adults* (ed. C.R. Pennington). British Association for Parenteral and Enteral Nutrition, Maidenhead.

BAPEN (1999) *Current Perspectives on Enteral Nutrition in Adults* (ed. C.A. McAtear). British Association for Parenteral and Enteral Nutrition, Maidenhead.

BAPEN (2003a) Tube feeding and your medicines: a guide for patients and carers. www.bapen.org.uk. Accessed 24/9/07

BAPEN (2003b) *Malnutrition Universal Screening Tool 'MUST' Report*. British Association for Parenteral and Enteral Nutrition, Maidenhead.

Benton, S. & Marsden, C. (2002) Training nurses to place tunnelled central venous catheters. *Prof Nurse*, **17**(9), 531–5.

Bodger, K. & Heatley, R.V. (2001) The immune system and nutrition support. In: *Artificial Nutritional Support in Clinical Practice* (eds J. Payne-James, G. Grimble & D. Silk), 2nd edn. Greenwich Medical Media, London, pp. 137–48.

Bond, S. (1997) *Eating Matters*. Centre for Health Services Research, University of Newcastle, Newcastle upon Tyne.

Bozzetti, F. (2001) Nutrition support in patients with cancer. *Artificial Nutritional Support in Clinical Practice* (eds J. Payne-James, G. Grimble & D. Silk), 2nd edn. Greenwich Medical Media, London, pp. 639–80.

Braga, M. *et al.* (2002) Preoperative oral arginine and n-3 fatty acid supplementation improves the immunometabolic host response and outcome after colorectal resection for cancer. *Surgery*, **132**, 805–14.

Buchholz, A.C., Bartok, C. & Schoeller, D.A. (2004) The validity of bioelectrical impedance models in clinical populations. *Nutr Clin Prac*, **19**, 433–46.

Bumpers, H.L. *et al.* (2003) Unusual complications of long-term percutaneous gastrostomy tubes. *J Gastrointest Surg*, **7**, 917–20.

Burke, A. (1997) *Hungry in Hospital*? Association of Community Health Councils for England and Wales, London.

Burnham, R. & Barton, S. (2001) The role of the nutrition support team. In: *Artificial Nutritional Support in Clinical Practice* (eds J. Payne-James, G. Grimble & D. Silk), 2nd edn. Greenwich Medical Media, London, pp. 241–53.

Burns, S.M. *et al.* (1995) Comparison of nasogastric tube securing methods and tube types in medical intensive care patients. *Am J Crit Care*, **4**(3), 198–203.

Cook (UK) Limited (2007) Radiologically inserted gastrostomy and gastrojejunostomy. www.cookmedical.com/esc/educationResource. do?id=Video_Tape. Accessed 24/9/07.

Council of Europe (2003) Food and nutritional care in hospitals: how to prevent undernutrition. Council of Europe www.coe.int. Accessed 24/9/07

Cummings, J.H. (2000) Nutritional management of diseases of the gut. In: *Human Nutrition and Dietetics* (eds J.S. Garrow, W.P.T. James & A. Ralph), 10th edn. Churchill Livingstone, Edinburgh, pp. 547–73.

Davidson, A. (2005) Management and effects of parenteral nutrition. *Nurs Times*, **101**(42), 28–31.

Desneves, K.J. *et al.* (2005) Treatment with supplementary arginine, vitamin C and zinc in patients with pressure ulcers: a randomized controlled trial. *Clin Nutr*, **24**(6), 979–87.

Detsky, A.S. *et al.* (1987) What is subjective global assessment of nutritional status? *J Parent Enteral Nutr*, **11**, 8–13.

DH (1991) *Dietary Reference Values for Food Energy and Nutrients for the United Kingdom.* COMA Report 41. HMSO, London.

DH (2001a) *Essence of Care – Patient Focused Benchmarking for Health Care Professionals.* Department of Health, London.

DH (2001b) Guidelines for preventing infections associated with the insertion and maintenance of central venous catheters. *J Hosp Infect*, **47**(S), S47–67.

DH (2002) *Specialised Services National Definitions Set (2nd edition) Home Parenteral Nutrition (HPN) (adult) – Definition No 12.* Department of Health, London.

DH (2005) *Saving Lives: A Delivery Programme to Reduce Healthcare Associated Infection including MRSA.* Department of Health, London.

Dorries, C.P. (2004) *Coroner's Report.* H.M. Coroner, South Yorkshire (West), 27 April 2004.

Durnin, J.B. & Wolmersley, J. (1974) Body fat assessed from total body density and its estimation from skinfold thickness: measurements on 481 men and women aged from 16 to 72 years. *Br J Nutr*, **32**, 77–9.

Elia, M. (2001) Metabolic response to starvation, injury and sepsis. In: *Artificial Nutritional Support in Clinical Practice* (eds J. Payne-James, G. Grimble & D. Silk), 2nd edn. Greenwich Medical Media, London, pp. 1–24.

Fitzsimmons, C.L. (1997) Central venous catheter placement – extending the role of the nurse. *J R Coll Phys*, **31**(5), 533–5.

FSA (2003) Safe upper levels for vitamins and minerals. Expert Group on vitamins and minerals. FSA, London.

Furst, P., Kuhn, K.S. & Stehle, P. (2001) Parenteral nutrition substrates. In: *Artificial Nutritional Support in Clinical Practice* (eds J. Payne-James, G. Grimble & D. Silk), 2nd edn. Greenwich Medical Media, London, pp. 401–34.

Gidden, F. & Shenkin, A. (2000) Laboratory support of the clinical nutrition service. *Clin Chem Lab Med*, **38**(8), 693–714.

Griffiths, M. (1996) Single-stage percutaneous gastrostomy button insertion: a leap forward. *J Parent Enteral Nutr*, **20**(3), 237–9.

Groher, M. (1997) *Dysphagia: Diagnosis and Management*, 2nd edn. Butterworth Heinemann, Boston.

Gupta, D. *et al.* (2004a) Bioelectrical impedance phase angle as a prognostic indicator in advanced pancreatic cancer. *Br J Nutr*, **92**(6), 957–62.

Gupta, D. *et al.* (2004b) Bioelectrical impedance phase angle in clinical practice: implications for prognosis in advanced colorectal cancer. *Am J Clin Nutr*, **80**(6), 1634–8.

Hamilton, H., O'Byrne, M. & Nicholai, L. (1995) Central lines inserted by clinical nurse specialists. *Nurs Times*, **91**(17), 38–9.

Heymsfield, S.B. & Matthews, D. (1994) Body composition: research and clinical advances – 1993 A.S.P.E.N. research workshop. *J Parent Enteral Nutr*, **18**(2), 91–103.

Horgan, G.W. & Stubbs, J. (2003) Predicting basal metabolic rate in the obese is difficult. *Eur J Clin Nutr*, **57**, 335–40.

Huhmann, M.B. & Cunningham, R.S. (2005) The importance of nutritional screening in cancer related weight loss. *Lancet Oncol*, **6**, 334–3.

Janssen, I. *et al.* (2000) Estimation of skeletal muscle mass by bioelectrical impedance analysis. *J Appl Physiol*, **89**, 456–71.

Kings Fund Research Summary (2005) Sustainable food and the NHS. www.kingsfund.org.uk/publications/kings_fund_publications/sustainable_food.html. Accessed 24/9/07

Kondrup, J. *et al.* (2003) ESPEN Guidelines for nutrition screening 2002. *Clin Nutr*, **22**(4), 415–21.

Kyle, U.G. *et al.* (2004a) Bioelectrical impedance analysis – part I: review of principles and methods. *Clin Nutr*, **23**, 1226–43.

Kyle, U.G. *et al.* (2004b) Bioelectrical impedance analysis – part II: utilization in clinical parctice. *Clin Nutr*, **23**, 1430–53.

Logemann, J. (1998) *The Evaluation and Treatment of Swallowing Disorders*, 2nd edn. College Hill Press, San Diego.

Loser, C.H.R. *et al.* (2005) ESPEN guidelines on artificial enteral nutrition – Percutaneous endoscopic gastrostomy (PEG). *Clin Nutr*, **24**, 848–61.

Lynch, C.R. & Fang, J.C. (2004) Prevention and management of complications of percutaneous endoscopic gastrostomy (PEG) tubes. *Practical Gastroenterology Series*, **22**, 66–76.

Metheny, N.A. (2004) Monitoring feeding tube placement – a literature review. *Nutr Clin Pract*, **19**, 487–95.

Metheny, N.A. & Titler, M.G. (2001) Assessing placement of feeding tubes. *Am J Nurs*, **101**(5), 36–45.

Metheny, N. *et al.* (1993) Effectiveness of pH measurements in predicting tube placement: an update. *Nurs Res*, **42**(6), 324–31.

Nataloni S. *et al.* (1999) Nutritional assessment in head injured patients through the study of rapid turnover visceral proteins *Clin Nutr*, **18**, 247–51.

National Collaborating Centre for Acute Care (2006) Nutrition support in adults: oral nutrition support, enteral tube feeding and parenteral nutrition. National Collaborating Centre for Acute Care, London. www.rcseng.ac.uk/publications/docs/nutrition_support_guidelines.html. Accessed 24/9/07.

Newman, L.A. *et al.* (1998) Eating and weight changes following chemoradiation therapy for advanced head and neck cancer. *Arch Otolaryngol Head Neck Surg*, **124**, 589–92.

NHS (2001) *Better Hospital Food. The NHS Recipe Book Implementation Support Pack*. HMSO, London.

NICE (2003) *Care during Enteral Feeding. Infection Control – Prevention of Health Care Associated Infection in Primary and Community Care. Clinical Guideline 2*. National Institute for Health and Clinical Excellence, London.

Nicol, M. *et al.* (2000) *Essential Nursing Skills*. Moseby, Elsevier Ltd, London.

NMC (2006) *A–Z Advice Sheet Consent*. www.nmc.org.

NPSA (2005) Reducing the harm caused by misplaced nasogastric feeding tubes. www.npsa.nhs.uk/health/display?contentId=4216. Accessed 24/9/07.

Nutricia Clinical Care (1996) *The Flocare Gastrostomy Range: a Guide to Professional Care*. Nutricia Clinical Care, Cow & Gate Nutricia, Trowbridge.

Payne-James, J., Grimble, G. & Silk, D. (2001) Enteral nutrition: tubes and techniques of delivery. In: *Artificial Nutritional Support in Clinical Practice* (eds J. Payne-James, G. Grimble & D. Silk), 2nd edn. Greenwich Medical Media, London, pp. 281–302.

Pennington, C.R. (1997) Disease and malnutrition in British hospitals. *Proc Nutr Soc*, **56**, 393–407.

Pickhardt, P.J., Rohrmann, C.A. Jr & Cossentino, M.J. (2002) Stomal metastases complicating percutaneous endoscopic gastrostomy: CT findings and the argument for radiologic tube placement. *Am J Roentgenol*, **179**(3), 735–9.

Pratt, R.J. *et al.* (2007) Epic 2: National evidence-based guidelines for preventing healthcare-associated infections in NHS hospitals in England. *J Hosp Infect*, **65**(1) (Suppl), S2–S12.

Reilly, H. (1996) Nutrition in clinical management: malnutrition in our midst. *Proc Nutr Soc*, **55**, 841–53.

Riera, L. *et al.* (2002) Percutaneous endoscopic gastrostomy in head and neck cancer patients. *J Otorhinolaryngol Relat Spec*, **64**(1), 32–4.

Rollins, H. (1997) A nose for trouble. *Nurs Times*, **93**(49), 66–7.

Royal College of Speech & Language Therapists (2006) Communicating quality 3: guidance on best practice in service organisation and provision. www.rcslt.org. Accessed 24/9/07.

Royal Marsden NHS Trust (2002) *Eating Well When You Have Cancer – A Guide for Cancer Patients*. Royal Marsden NHS Trust, London.

Schofield, W.N. (1985) Predicting basal metabolic rate. New standards and review of previous work. *Hum Nutr Clin Nutr*, **39C**(Suppl 15), 5–41.

Schwenk A. *et al.* (2000) Phase angle from bioelectrical impedance analysis remains an independent predictive marker in HIV-infected patients in the era of highly active antiretroviral treatment. *Am J Clin Nut*, **72**(2), 496–501.

Shaw, C. (2008) Parenteral nutrition. In: *Intravenous Therapy in Nursing Practice* (eds L. Dougherty & J. Lamb), 2nd edn. Blackwell Publishing, Oxford.

Shaw, V. & Lawson, M. (2007) Nutritional assessment, dietary requirements and feed supplementation. In: *Clinical Paediatric Dietetics* (eds V. Shaw & M. Lawson), 3rd edn. Blackwell Publishing, Oxford, pp. 3–20.

Shenkin, A. (2001) Adult micronutrient requirements. In: *Artificial Nutritional Support in Clinical Practice* (eds J. Payne-James, G. Grimble & D. Silk), 2nd edn. Greenwich Medical Media, London, pp. 193–212.

Springhouse (2002) Parenteral nutrition. In: *IV Therapy Made Incredibly Easy*. Springhouse Corporation, Philadelphia, pp. 269–302.

ter Reit, G., Kessels, A.G. & Knipschild, P.G. (1995) Randomised clinical trial of ascorbic acid in the treatment of pressure ulcers. *J Clin Epidemiol*, **48**(12), 1453–60.

Thomas, B. & Bishop, J. (2007) *Manual of Dietetic Practice*, 4th edn. Blackwell Publishing, Oxford.

Thomas, D.R. (1997) Specific nutritional factors in wound healing. *Adv Wound Care*, **10**(4), 40–3.

Thorell, A. & Nordenström, J. (2001) Metabolic complications of parenteral nutrition. In: *Artificial Nutritional Support in Clinical Practice* (eds J. Payne-James, G. Grimble & D. Silk), 2nd edn. Greenwich Medical Media, London, pp. 445–59.

Weinstein, S.M. (2007) Parenteral nutrition. In: *Principles and Practice of Intravenous Therapy* (ed. S.M. Weinstein), 8th edn. Lippincott, Philadelphia.

Wilson, J.M. & Jordan, N.L. (2001) Parenteral nutrition. In: *Infusion Therapy in Clinical Practice* (eds J. Hankin *et al.*). W.B. Saunders, Philadelphia, pp. 209–247.

Multiple choice questions

1 Which of the following is the most appropriate strategy to encourage a patient with a sore mouth to eat?

   a   Offer fizzy drinks
   b   Allow hot food to cool before eating
   c   Eat frozen food
   d   Offer citrus based foods and drinks

2 'Direct infusion into a vein, of solutions containing the essential nutrients in quantities to meet all the daily needs of the patient.' This is a definition of which type of feeding?

   a   Parenteral nutrition
   b   Infusional feeding
   c   Enteral feeding
   d   Jejunal feeding

3 What does BMI stand for?

   a   Body measurement index
   b   Body mass indictors
   c   British measurement index
   d   Body mass index

4 Which of the following is NOT a sign of malnourishment?

   a   BMI less than 18.5 kg/m^2
   b   BMI less than 22 kg/m^2
   c   Unintentional weight loss greater than 10% within the last 3–6 months
   d   BMI less than 20 kg/m^2 and unintentional weight loss greater than 5% within the last 3–6 months

5 A major hazard associated with parenteral feeding is which of the following?

   a   Embolism
   b   Blockage
   c   Infection
   d   Dislodgement

6 When inserting a nasogastric tube how should the patient be positioned?

   a   Semi-upright
   b   Lying on left hand side
   c   Sitting with head tilted forward
   d   Sitting with head tilted backwards

Answers to the multiple choice questions can be found in Appendix 3.

Chapter 18

Observations

Pulse

Definition

The pulse is a pressure wave that is transmitted through the arterial tree with each heart beat following the expansion and recoil of arteries during each cardiac cycle (Marieb & Hoehn 2007). A pulse can be palpated in any artery that lies close to the surface of the body (Figure 18.1). The radial artery at the wrist is easily accessible and therefore frequently used; there are several other clinically important areas for monitoring the pulse such as the carotid, femoral and brachial plexus (Marieb & Hoehn 2007).

Indications

The pulse is taken for the following reasons:

- To gather information on the heart rate, pattern of beats (rhythm) and amplitude (strength) of pulse.
- To determine the individual's pulse on admission as a base for comparing future measurements.
- To monitor changes in pulse.

(Marieb & Hoehn 2007).

Reference material

In health the arterial pulse is one of the measurements used to assess the effects of activity, postural changes and emotions on the heart rate. In ill health the pulse can be used to assess the effects of disease, treatments and response to therapy. Each time the heart beats it pushes blood through the arteries. The pumping action of the heart causes the walls of the arteries to expand and distend, causing

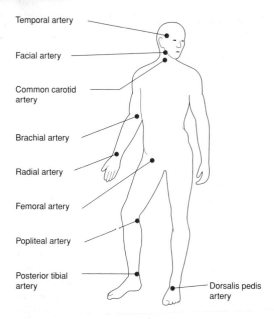

Temporal artery

Facial artery

Common carotid
artery

Brachial artery

Radial artery

Femoral artery

Popliteal artery

Posterior tibial
artery

Dorsalis pedis
artery

Figure 18.1 Body sites where pulse is most easily palpated. The pulse can be felt in arteries lying close to the body surface.

a wave-like sensation which can then be felt as the pulse (Marieb & Hoehn 2007). The pulse is measured by lightly compressing the artery against firm tissue and by counting the number of beats in a minute.

The pulse is palpated to note the following:

- Rate.
- Rhythm.
- Amplitude.

Rate

The normal pulse rate varies in different client groups as age-related changes affect the pulse rate. The approximate range is illustrated in Table 18.1 (Weber & Kelley 2003).

The pulse may vary depending on the posture of an individual. For example, the pulse of a healthy man may be around 66 beats per minute when he is lying

Table 18.1 Normal pulse rates per minute at various ages. From Weber & Kelley (2003).

Age	Approximate range
1 week–3 months	100–160
3 months–2 years	80–150
2–10 years	70–110
10 years–adult	55–90

down; this increases to 70 beats per minute when sitting up, and 80 beats per minute when he stands suddenly (Marieb & Hoehn 2007).

The rate of the pulse of an individual with a healthy heart tends to be relatively constant. However, when blood volume drops suddenly or when the heart has been weakened by disease, the stroke volume declines and cardiac output is maintained only by increasing the rate of heart beat.

Cardiac output (CO) is the amount of blood pumped out by each heart ventricle in 1 minute, while the stroke volume is the amount of blood pumped out by a ventricle with each contraction. The relationship between these and the heart rate is expressed in an equation (see below). Using normal resting values for heart rate (75 beats per minute) and stroke volume (70 ml per beat) the average adult cardiac output can be calculated (Marieb & Hoehn 2007):

$$\text{Cardiac output} = \text{Heart rate} \times \text{Stroke volume}$$

The heart rate and hence pulse rate are influenced by various factors acting through neural, chemical and physically induced homeostatic mechanisms (Figure 18.2):

- Neural changes in heart rate are caused by the activation of the sympathetic nervous system which increases heart rate, while parasympathetic activation decreases heart rate (Thibodeau & Patton 2007).
- Chemical regulation of the heart is affected by hormones (adrenaline and thyroxine) and electrolytes (sodium, potassium and calcium) (Thibodeau & Patton 2007). High or low levels of electrolytes, particularly potassium, magnesium and calcium, can cause an alteration in the heart's rhythm and rate.
- Other factors that influence heart rate are age, sex, exercise and body temperature (Marieb & Hoehn 2007).

613

Tachycardia   Is defined as an abnormally fast heart rate, over 100 beats per minute in adults. This may result from a raised body temperature, increased sympathetic response due to physical/emotional stress, certain drugs or heart

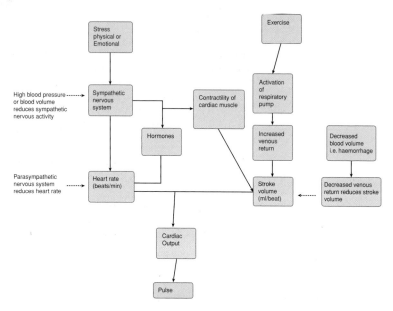

Figure 18.2 Influence of neural, chemical and physical factors on cardiac output and hence pulse.

disease (Marieb & Hoehn 2007). Because tachycardia occasionally promotes fibrillation, persistent tachycardia is considered pathological (Marieb & Hoehn 2007).

Bradycardia (slow)   Is a heart rate slower than 60 beats per minute (Marieb & Hoehn 2007). It may be the result of a low body temperature, certain drugs or parasympathetic nervous system activation. It is also found in fit athletes when physical and cardiovascular conditioning occurs (Marieb & Hoehn 2007). This results in hypertrophy of the heart with an increase in its stroke volume. These heart changes result in a lower resting heart rate but with the same cardiac output (Marieb & Hoehn 2007). If persistent bradycardia occurs in an individual as a result of ill health, this may result in inadequate blood circulation to body tissues. A slowing of the heart rate accompanied by a rise in blood pressure is one of the indications of raised intracranial pressure (Marieb & Hoehn 2007).

Rhythm   The pulse rhythm is the sequence of beats. In health, these are regular. The co-ordinated action of the muscles of the heart in producing a regular heart rhythm is due to the ability of cardiac muscle to contract inherently without nervous control (Marieb & Hoehn 2007). The co-ordinated action of the muscles in the heart results from two physiological factors:

- Gap junctions in the cardiac muscles which form interconnections between adjacent cardiac muscles and allow transmission of nervous impulses from cell to cell (Marieb & Hoehn 2007).
- Specialized nerve-like cardiac cells that form the nodal system. These initiate and distribute impulses throughout the heart, so that the heart beats as one unit (Marieb & Hoehn 2007). The nodal system is comprised of the sinoatrial node, atrioventricular node, atrioventricular bundle and the Purkinje fibres.

The sinoatrial node is the pacemaker, initiating each wave of contraction. This sets the rhythm for the heart as a whole (Figure 18.3). Its characteristic rhythm is called *sinus rhythm*.

Defects in the conduction system of the heart can cause irregular heart rhythms, or arrhythmias, resulting in uncoordinated contraction of the heart.

Fibrillation is a condition of rapid and irregular contractions. A fibrillating heart is ineffective as a pump (Marieb & Hoehn 2007).

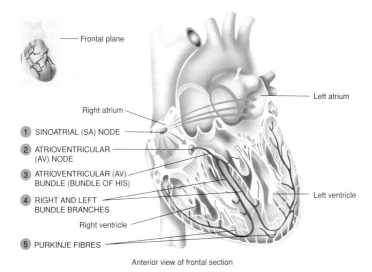

Figure 18.3 The conduction system of the heart. Autorhythmic fibres in the sinoatrial (SA) node, located in the right atrial wall, act as the heart's pacemaker, initiating cardiac action potentials that cause contraction of the heart's chambers. The conduction system ensures that the chambers of the heart contract in a co-ordinated manner. (Redrawn from Tortora & Derrickson (2007) with permission).

- *Atrial fibrillation* is a disruption of rhythm in the atrial areas of the heart occurring at extremely rapid and uncoordinated intervals. The rapid impulses result in the ventricles not being able to respond to every atrial beat and, therefore, the ventricles contract irregularly (Adam & Osborne 2005). There are many causes of this condition, but the following are the most common: (i) ischaemic heart disease; (ii) acute illness; (iii) electrolyte abnormality; and (iv) thyrotoxicosis.

- *Ventricular fibrillation* is an irregular heart rhythm characterized by chaotic contraction of the ventricles at very rapid rates (Adam & Osborne 2005). Ventricular fibrillation results in cardiac arrest and death if not reversed with defibrillation and the injection of adrenaline (epinephrine). The cause of this condition is often myocardial infarction (MI), electrical shock, acidosis, electrolyte disturbances and hypovolaemia (Resuscitation Council UK 2005).

Body fluids are good conductors of electricity so it is possible through electrocardiography to observe how the currents generated are transmitted through the heart. The electrocardiograph provides a graphic representation and record (electrocardiogram [ECG]) of electrical activity as the heart beats. The ECG makes it possible to identify abnormalities in electrical conduction within the heart. Changes in the pattern or timing of the deflection in the ECG may indicate problems with the heart's conduction system, such as those caused by MI (Marieb & Hoehn 2007). Examples of conduction abnormalities are shown in Figure 18.4a–d.

Amplitude

Amplitude is a reflection of pulse strength and the elasticity of the arterial wall. This varies because of the alternating strong and weak ventricular contractions (Bickley & Szilagyi 2007). The flexibility of the artery of the young adult feels different from the hard artery of the patient suffering from arteriosclerosis. It takes some clinical experience to appreciate the differences in amplitude. However, it is important to be able to recognize major changes such as the faint flickering pulse of the severely hypovolaemic patient or the irregular pulse in cardiac arrhythmias.

Assessing gross pulse irregularity

Paradoxical pulse is a pulse that markedly decreases in amplitude during inspiration. On inspiration, more blood is pooled in the lungs and so decreases the return to the left side of the heart; this affects the consequent stroke volume. A paradoxical pulse is usually regarded as normal, although in conjunction with such features as hypotension and dyspnoea, it may indicate cardiac tamponade (Bickley & Szilagyi 2007).

When there is a gross pulse irregularity, it may be useful to use a stethoscope to assess the apical heart beat. This is done by placing the diaphragm of the

(a)

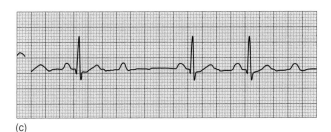

(b)

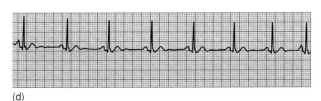

(c)

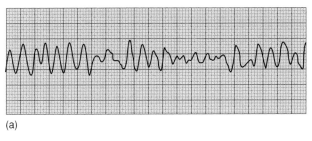

(d)

Figure 18.4 Normal and abnormal ECG tracings. **(a)** Coarse ventricular fibrillation. **(b)** Junctional tachycardia. **(c)** ECG complexes too small; cardiac monitor did not recognize QRS complexes resulting in continuous false asystole alarms. Also difficulties may be encountered interpreting cardiac arrhythmias when the gain is set too low. **(d)** Second degree AV block Mobitz type 2.

617

stethoscope over the apex of the heart and counting the beats for 60 seconds. A second nurse should record the radial pulse at the same time. The deficit between the two should be noted using, for example, different colours on the patient's chart to indicate the apex and radial rates (Docherty 2002).

Conditions where a patient's pulse may need careful monitoring are described below:

- Postoperative and critically ill patients require monitoring of the pulse to assess for cardiovascular stability. The patient's pulse should be recorded preoperatively in order to establish a baseline and to make comparisons. Hypovolaemic shock post-surgery from the loss of plasma or whole blood results in a decrease in circulatory blood volume. The resulting acceleration in heart rate causes a tachycardia that can be felt in the pulse. The greater the loss in volume the more thready the pulse is likely to feel.
- Blood transfusions require the careful monitoring of the pulse as an incompatible blood transfusion may lead to a rise in pulse rate (BCSH 1999) (see Chapter 30).
- Patients with local or systemic infections or inflammatory reactions require monitoring of their pulse to detect sepsis/severe sepsis. This is characterized by a decrease in the mean arterial pressure (MAP) and a rise in pulse rate (Marieb & Hoehn 2007).
- Patients with cardiovascular conditions require regular assessment of the pulse to monitor their condition and the efficacy of medications.

Note: even where the patient has continuous ECG monitoring, such as in coronary care, Accident and Emergency (A&E) and intensive care unit (ITU), it is still essential to manually feel a pulse to determine amplitude and volume and whether the pulse is irregular.

Procedure guidelines   **Pulse measurement**

Equipment

1 A watch that has a second hand.

Procedure

Action	Rationale
1 Wash hands and dry hands.	To prevent cross-infection (DH 2005: C).
2 Explain and discuss the procedure with the patient.	To ensure that the patient understands the procedure and gives his/her valid consent (NMC 2006: C; NMC 2008: C).
3 Where possible, measure the pulse under the sameconditions each time.	To ensure continuity and consistency in recording (E).

4 Ensure that the patient is comfortable and relaxed. *Note*: If the patient has taken any medication, this may alter the pulse rate.	To ensure that the patient is comfortable (E).
5 Place the first, second or third finger along the appropriate artery and apply light pressure until the pulse is felt (see Action figure 5).	The fingertips are sensitive to touch. Practitioners should be aware that the thumb and forefinger have pulses of their own and therefore these may be mistaken for the patient's pulse (Docherty & Coote 2006: E).
6 Press gently against the peripheral artery being used to record the pulse.	The radial artery is usually used as it is often the most readily accessible (Bickley & Szilagyi 2007: E).
7 The pulse should be counted for 60 seconds.	Sufficient time is required to detect irregularities or other defects (Bickley & Szilagyi 2007: E).
8 Record the pulse rate on appropriate documentation.	To monitor differences and detect trends; any irregularities should be brought to the attention of the appropriate senior nursing and medical teams (NMC 2008: C).

Note: In children under 2 years of age, the pulse should not be taken in this way; the rapid pulse rate and small area for palpation can lead to inaccurate data. The heart rate should be assessed by utilizing a stethoscope and listening to the apical heart beat.

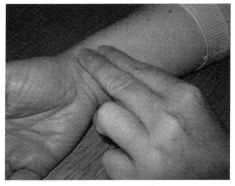

Action 5 Taking a pulse.

Blood pressure

Definition

Blood pressure may be defined as the force exerted by blood against the walls of the vessels in which it is contained (Marieb & Hoehn 2007). Variations in blood pressure gradient provide the circulation with the force that keeps the blood moving through the body (Marieb & Hoehn 2007). Blood pressure is usually expressed in terms of millimetres of mercury (mmHg).

Indications

Blood pressure is measured for one of two reasons:

- To determine the patient's blood pressure on admission as a baseline for comparison with future measurements.
- To monitor fluctuations in blood pressure.

(Marieb & Hoehn 2007).

Reference material

Blood flow is the volume of blood flowing through a vessel at a given time from the heart. Blood flow is equivalent to cardiac output (Marieb & Hoehn 2007). **Resistance** is the friction that occurs as the blood passes through the differently sized vessels, and impacts on the blood flow and cardiac output (Marieb & Hoehn 2007). There are three important sources of resistance: blood viscosity, vessel length and vessel diameter (Figure 18.5a, b).

Viscosity is the internal resistance to flow and may be thought of as the 'stickiness' of a fluid (Thibodeau & Patton 2007). Blood is more viscous than water due to the elements of plasma proteins and cells that form its constituent parts, and consequently blood moves more slowly. The longer the **vessel length,** the greater the resistance encountered. The relationship between vessel length and viscosity is often constant; however, **vessel diameter** changes frequently and is an important factor in altering peripheral resistance (Thibodeau & Patton 2007). In a small blood vessel more of the fluid is in contact with the vessel walls which results in increased friction. Arterioles are the major determinants of peripheral resistance because they are small-diameter blood vessels which can expand in response to neural and chemical controls (Thibodeau & Patton 2007).

Normal blood pressure is maintained by neural, chemical and renal controls, providing the constant blood flow around the body crucial for organ function. The neural controls operate via reflex arcs (Marieb & Hoehn 2007) derived from stretch receptors found in the wall of the proximal arterial tree, especially in the region of the aortic arch and carotid sinuses. When arterial pressure rises, there is increased stimulation of these nerve endings. The increased number of impulses

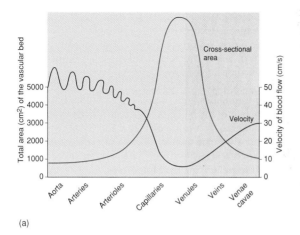

(a)

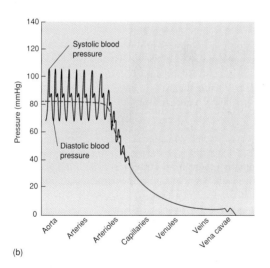

(b)

Figure 18.5 **(a)** Relationship between velocity (speed) of blood flow and total cross-sectional area in different types of blood vessels. Velocity of blood flow is slowest in the capillaries because they have the largest total cross-sectional area. **(b)** Blood pressures in various parts of the cardiovascular system. The dashed line is the mean (average) blood pressure in the aorta, arteries and arterioles. Blood pressure rises and falls with each heartbeat in blood vessels leading to capillaries. (Redrawn from Tortora & Derrickson (2007) with permission.)

along the vagus and glossopharyngeal nerves leads to reflex vagal slowing of the heart and reflex release of vasoconstrictor tone in the peripheral blood vessels. The resulting fall in cardiac output and the reduction of peripheral resistance tend to restore the blood pressure to the normal value. A fall in the arterial pressure decreases the stimulation of the arterial stretch receptors. The reflex tachycardia and vasoconstriction that ensue tend to raise the blood pressure to its normal value, forming a continuous homeostatic process (Marieb & Hoehn 2007). When the oxygen content of the blood drops sharply, chemoreceptors in the aortic arch transmit impulses to the vasomotor centre and reflex constriction occurs. The rise in blood pressure that follows helps to increase blood return to the heart and lungs (Marieb & Hoehn 2007). Renal regulation provides a major long-term mechanism of influencing blood pressure. When there is a fall in arterial pressure this results in chemical changes which lead to the release of the enzyme renin. Renin triggers a series of enzymic reactions that result in the formation of angiotensin, a powerful vasoconstrictor chemical. Angiotensin also stimulates the adrenal cortex to release aldosterone, a hormone that increases renal reabsorption of sodium. The sodium, in turn, increases the volume of water reabsorbed by the kidneys; such retention of fluid and vasoconstriction of blood vessels raises arterial pressure (Marieb & Hoehn 2007).

Blood pressure varies not only from moment to moment but also in the distribution between various organs and areas of the body. It is lowest in neonates and increases with age, weight gain, stress and anxiety (Marieb & Hoehn 2007). Shock, MI and haemorrhage are factors that cause a fall in blood pressure as they reduce cardiac output and peripheral vessel resistance or they diminish venous return after fluid loss (Figure 18.6).

Normal blood pressure

Normal blood pressure generally ranges from 100/60 to 140/90 mmHg. Blood pressure can fluctuate within a wide range and still be considered normal (Marieb & Hoehn 2007).

Systolic pressure

The systolic blood pressure is the peak pressure of blood in the arteries and is caused by the contraction of the ventricle. The systolic blood pressure averages around 120 mmHg in adults (Marieb & Hoehn 2007).

Diastolic pressure

The diastolic pressure is the minimum pressure of the blood against the wall of the vessel following closure of the aortic valve and is taken as a direct indication of blood vessel resistance (Marieb & Hoehn 2007).

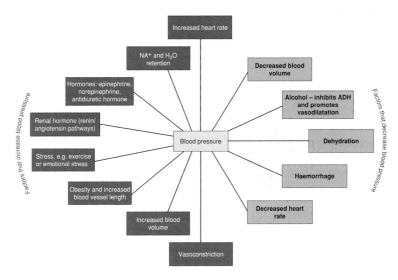

Figure 18.6   Factors that lead to a change in blood pressure. (Redrawn from Tortora & Derrickson (2007) with permission.)

Hypotension

Hypotension or low blood pressure is generally defined in adults as a systolic blood pressure below 100 mmHg (Marieb & Hoehn 2007). Hypotension often reflects individual variations; however, it may indicate orthostatic hypotension, i.e. postural changes that result in a lack of normal reflex response leading to a low blood pressure, or it may be the first indicator of a shock condition, e.g. septic shock, cardiogenic, hypovolaemic or toxic shock syndrome (Marieb & Hoehn 2007).

Hypertension

Hypertension is an elevation in the blood pressure and may be an acute or chronic physiological response (Marieb & Hoehn 2007). Hypertension may be a temporary response to fever, physical exertion or stress. NICE (2006) describes hypertension as persistently raised blood pressure over 140/90 mmHg. The British Hypertension Society recommends that patients who have:

- sustained blood systolic blood pressure of greater than or equal to 160 mmHg or;
- sustained diastolic blood pressure of greater than or equal to 100 mmHg,

should be commenced on antihypertensive drug treatment. Williams *et al.* (2004) further states that patients with blood pressures between 140 and 159 mmHg systolic should be offered hypertensive drug treatment if other risk factors are present, i.e. evidence of cardiovascular disease or diabetes.

Persistent hypertension is a common disease and approximately 30% of people over the age of 50 years are hypertensive (Marieb & Hoehn 2007).

Mean arterial pressure

The mean arterial pressure is the average pressure required to push blood through the circulatory system. This can be determined electronically or mathematically as well as by using an intra-arterial catheter and mercury mano-meter.

Mathematically, for example:

Mean arterial pressure (MAP) = (Systolic blood pressure [SBP]
— Diastolic blood pressure [DBP]/3) + DBP

(Adam & Osborne 2005).

A blood pressure of 130/85 mmHg gives a MAP of 100 mmHg.

Methods of recording and equipment

There are two main methods for recording the blood pressure: direct and indirect. **Direct** methods are more accurate than indirect methods. The most accurate method of measuring blood pressure involves the insertion of a minute pressure transducer unit into an artery for transmission of a waveform or digital display on a monitor. The most commonly used techniques involve placing a cannula in an artery and attaching a pressure-sensitive device to the external end (Adam & Osborne 2005).

Patients who need to be constantly monitored, e.g. in theatres, high-dependency and intensive care units, may require such devices to be used. In such patients it is essential to have an early knowledge of any change in the blood pressure, as this may indicate deterioration in the patient's condition and requires prompt treatment.

The **indirect** method is the auscultatory method. This procedure is used to measure blood pressure in the brachial artery of the arm (Evans *et al.* 2004) (Figure 18.7).

624 The sphygmomanometer

The sphygmomanometer consists of a compression bag enclosed in an unyielding cuff, and inflating bulb, pump or other device by which the pressure is increased,

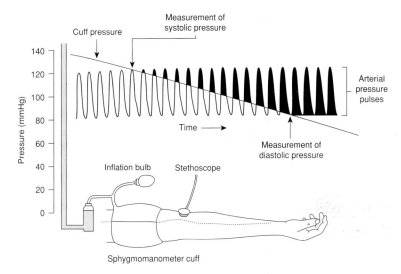

Figure 18.7 Using a sphygmomanometer, and the appearance and disappearance of Korotkoff's sounds.

a manometer from which the applied pressure is read, and a control valve to deflate the system (Valler-Jones & Wedgbury 2005).

Manual sphygmomanometers

While mercury sphygmomanometers have been the standard method for recording blood pressure, there are concerns regarding the safety and impact on the environment of medical devices containing mercury. Following a report by the European Commission on the decommissioning of mercury (Maxon 2004), there has been no ban on the use of medical devices containing mercury in the UK. However, the Medicines and Healthcare Regulatory Agency recommends, 'the selection of mercury-free products when the opportunity arises' (MHRA 2005, p. 4). If mercury sphygmomanometers are used they should be in good repair, staff should be properly trained in their use and in the event of mercury spillage or disposal, proprietary kits should be available to help contain the spillage and minimize the risk of mercury vapour forming. While in use, the measuring tube of the manometer should be kept in a vertical position, otherwise substantial errors can occur (Campbell *et al.* 1990; Beevers *et al.* 2001b). Local policies and the manufacturer's recommendations should be followed.

The most common types of error for mercury sphygmomanometers are:

- Rapid deflation of the cuff during measurement.
- Improper placement (e.g. mercury column not vertical).
- Perished rubber tubing (McAlister & Straus 2001).
- Defective valves (Beevers *et al*. 2001b).

The other widely used type of manual sphygmomanometer is the aneroid sphygmomanometer. This is a mechanical device that measures the cuff pressure using a bellows connected to the cuff via rubber tubing. The pressure inside the bellows is transferred to a dial via a system of gears and levers (Beevers *et al*. 2001a). This type of sphygmomanometer can be calibrated properly, but is susceptible to inaccuracies or damage that would not be apparent to the user (O'Brien *et al*. 2001). The most common types of error for aneroid sphygmomanometers are:

- Non-zeroed or bent indicators.
- Cracked face plates.
- Perished rubber tubing (McAlister & Straus 2001).

In addition, there are sources of error common to all methods of manual blood pressure measuring:

- Systematic error (e.g. lack of concentration, poor hearing, inattention to audible or visual cues).
- Failure to interpret the Korotkoff sounds correctly (discussed later in this section).
- Terminal digit preference (tendency to record blood pressures ending in '5' or '0').
- Bias (e.g. recording a blood pressure corresponding to what would be expected for the patient, not the actual reading) (Beevers *et al*. 2001b).

Non-invasive automated sphygmomanometers

Automated devices to measure blood pressure have been available for some time now. Devices are manufactured for a variety of different purposes, including home use. Generally, devices intended for home use are not found to be accurate or reliable enough for clinical use (O'Brien *et al*. 2001). The British Hypertension Society and the US Association for the Advancement of Medical Instrumentation (AAMI) regularly check blood pressure measuring devices and publish recommendations for their use.

Automatic blood pressure monitors are often oscillometric devices, where the measurement of blood pressure is based on the variations of pressure in the cuff caused by the pulsing of the artery directly underneath it (Berger 2001). For this reason, placement of the cuff over the artery is essential for accurate blood pressure reading.

As with all medical devices, use should be in accordance with the procedures recommended by the manufacturer. The principles of measuring an accurate blood pressure using an electronic device will be similar to manual recording of blood pressure with regard to patient factors such as positioning, choice and placement of the cuff. All medical devices should be properly serviced and maintained and may need calibration at intervals. Guidance should be sought from the manufacturer.

Users of electronic sphygmomanometers should also be aware that errors in measurement (for example, if there is a weak, thready or irregular pulse) may not be readily obvious to the operator and that manual blood pressure measurement may be indicated. Those patients with muscular tremors may also experience inaccurate blood pressure readings (Beevers *et al.* 2001a).

Parts of a sphygmomanometer

Cuff
The cuff is made of washable material that encircles the arm and encloses the inflatable rubber bladder. It is secured around the arm or leg by wrapping its tapering end to the encircling material, usually by Velcro.

Inflatable bladder
A bladder that is too short and/or too narrow will give falsely high pressures. The European Society of Hypertension recommends that the centre of the bladder should cover the brachial artery and that the bladder length should be 80% of the arm circumference and the width at least 40% (O'Brien *et al.* 2003).

Control valve, pump and rubber tubing
The control valve is a common source of error. It should allow the passage of air without excessive pressure needing to be applied on the pump. When the valve is closed it should hold the mercury at a constant level and, when released, it should allow a controlled fall in the level of mercury. The rubber tubing should be long (approximately 80 cm) and with airtight connections that can easily be separated to allow rapid deflation if required.

In reviewing the methods for sphygmomanometer inaccuracies, both Campbell *et al.* (1990) and Markandu *et al.* (2000) found that errors in technique and equipment malfunction accounted for differences in readings of more than 15 mmHg. Carney *et al.* (1995) also found when evaluating 463 sphygmomanometers that only 58% were in working order.

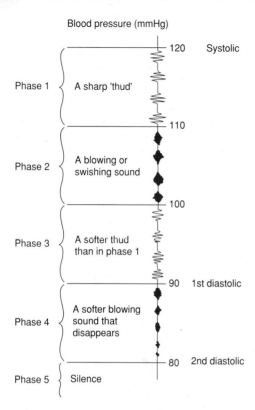

Figure 18.8   Korotkoff's sounds.

The stethoscope

Using the stethoscope it is possible to identify a series of five phases as blood pressure falls from the systolic to the diastolic. These phases are known as Korotkoff's sounds (Figure 18.8) (Thibodeau & Patton 2007).

Korotkoff's sounds form five phases:

1   The appearance of faint, clear tapping sounds which gradually increase in intensity.
2   The softening of sounds, which may become swishing.
3   The return of sharper sounds which become crisper but never fully regain the intensity of the phase 1 sounds.

4   The distinct muffling sound which becomes soft and blowing.
5   The point at which all sound ceases.

(Evans *et al.* 2004).

When the cuff pressure has fallen to just below the systolic pressure, a clear but often faint tapping sound suddenly appears in sequence with each cardiac contraction. The sound is produced by the transient and turbulent blood flowing through the brachial artery during the peak of each systole.

As the pressure in the cuff is reduced further, the sound becomes louder, but when the artery is no longer constricted and the blood flows freely, the sounds become muffled and then can no longer be heard. The diastolic pressure is usually defined as the cuff pressure at which the sounds disappear (Marieb & Hoehn 2007).

The stethoscope's diaphragm should be placed lightly over the point of maximal pulsation of the brachial artery (Petrie *et al.* 1997; Beevers, *et al.* 2001b; Valler-Jones & Wedgbury 2005). The diaphragm is designed to amplify low-frequency sounds such as Korotkoff's sounds (Valler-Jones & Wedgbury 2005). Excessive pressure on the stethoscope's diaphragm may partially occlude the brachial artery and delay the occurrence of Korotkoff's sounds. For this reason the diaphragm should not be tucked under the edge of the cuff (Valler-Jones & Wedgbury 2005).

Practical considerations

Much recent research has focused on the faulty techniques employed when blood pressures are taken (Campbell *et al.* 1990; Bogan *et al.* 1993; Kemp *et al.* 1994; Torrance & Serginson 1996; Gillespie & Curzio 1998; Beevers *et al.* 2001b). Blood pressure readings are altered by various factors that influence the patient, the techniques used and the accuracy of the sphygmomanometer. The variability of any readings can be reduced by an improved technique and by taking several readings (Campbell *et al.* 1990; Markandu *et al.* 2000). In 1981 Thompson discussed the methodology of blood pressure recording and identified poor technique and observer bias as possible sources of error. He concluded that many nurses were inadequately trained in blood pressure measurement and that more attention needed to be paid to this area. In 1996, Beevers & Beevers (1996) found that observer error could be reduced if techniques for measuring blood pressure were taught repeatedly during medical and nursing training. Furthermore, the techniques should be reinforced regularly.

Similar conclusions were found in studies by Mancia *et al.* (1987), Feher & Harris St. John (1992) and Torrance & Serginson (1996). Poor technique due to inadequate education can cause marked variation in the accuracy of measurements and can lead to inappropriate treatment decisions (Kemp *et al.* 1994; Markandu *et al.* 2000).

Regular servicing of equipment is crucial for reducing errors. Valler-Jones & Wedgbury (2005) recommend that mercury sphygmomanometers are serviced every 6–12 months, while aneroid sphygmomanometers should be serviced every 3–6 months.

Ambulatory blood pressure monitoring allows the measurement of trends in the patient's blood pressure over a longer period. For the assessment of hypertensive patients it is increasingly regarded as an important tool to assess blood pressure during normal daily activity (McAlister & Straus 2001; Williams *et al.* 2004). Ambulatory blood pressure is increasingly regarded as superior to individual blood pressure readings.

Clinical considerations

Variations in the procedure and frequency of taking blood pressure may be required in different patient groups with differing conditions. With a child it is important that the correctly sized cuff is used and that the average of repeated measurements is recorded. Low diastolic pressures are common in children and thus the pressure at muffling (Korotkoff phase 4) may be difficult to determine.

Low diastolic pressures are common in elderly patients who may have atherosclerosis, and in patients with an increased cardiac output, i.e. as a result of pregnancy, exercise or hypothyroidism.

Patients with venous access devices or shunts for dialysis in their arms or superior vena cava obstruction may be unsuitable for upper arm measurements of blood pressure; however, the blood pressure may be measured in the leg or forearm. For this procedure the patient lies prone and a thigh or large cuff is used, its bladder centered over the posterior popliteal artery. The stethoscope diaphragm should be applied on the artery below the cuff. Systolic blood pressure is normally 20–30 mmHg higher in the leg than in the arm. The right sized cuff should be used for obtaining the blood pressure using the forearm, and the bladder should be centered over the radial artery below the elbow, and the cuff wrapped in a similar manner to the normal procedure. The stethoscope diaphragm should be positioned over the radial artery about 2.5 cm above the wrist. Forearm blood pressure measurements may vary significantly from an upper arm measurement, and therefore it is important to document cuff size and location (Hill & Grim 1991).

Patients who have had breast surgery with lymph node dissections and/or radiotherapy, or have lymphoedema should not have their blood pressure recorded on the affected side. This is due to the increased frailty of tissue in the area and the risk of developing lymphoedema. Patients should be told to only have their blood pressure taken on the unaffected arm or legs (Yarbro *et al.* 2005).

Conditions where a patient's blood pressure may need careful monitoring are described below:

- Patients with consistent hypotension as this could lead to renal failure.
- Hypertension is never diagnosed on a single blood pressure reading. Blood pressures are monitored to evaluate the condition of the patient and the effectiveness of medication (Williams *et al.* 2004; Marieb & Hoehn 2007).
- Postoperative and critically ill patients require monitoring of blood pressure to assess for cardiovascular stability. The patient's blood pressure should be recorded preoperatively in order to establish a baseline for comparison.
- Patients receiving intravenous infusions may require blood pressure monitoring to observe for circulatory overload. Certain chemotherapy protocols use protracted amounts of intravenous fluids. In this group of patients diuretics are frequently used to reduce the increase in blood volume which results in a rise in blood pressure. Careful monitoring of blood pressure, weight, kidney function and electrolytes is imperative to prevent fluid overload and electrolyte imbalance (Marini & Wheeler 2006).
- Patients with local or systemic infections or neutropenia require monitoring of their blood pressure in order to detect septicaemic shock. This is characterized by a change in the capillary epithelium and vasodilatation due to circulating cell mediation (Bone 1996), which permits loss of blood and plasma through capillary walls into surrounding tissues. The decrease in the circulating volume of blood results in impaired tissue perfusion, culminating in cellular hypoxia (Thibodeau & Patton 2007).

Box 18.1   Measuring blood pressure – ten top tips (MHRA 2006)

---

1   Ensure that only clinically validated equipment is purchased and all sphygmomanometers are checked regularly: mercury devices at least 12 monthly and aneroid devices at least twice a year
2   Availability of different cuff sizes encourages cuffs being used appropriately
3   High blood pressure on the basis of anxiety should not be ruled out
4   BP should initially be measured in both arms and the arm with higher reading should be used in subsequent measurements
5   Ensure the arm is supported
6   Try to measure at the same time of day where possible
7   Be alert to 'white coat effect'
8   Remember ambulatory blood pressure measurement average day time values will be lower than hospital/surgery readings
9   Remember variability is high and blood pressure readings in patients may differ depending on time of day
10 Measurement of blood pressure by any other method is less reliable in the presence of arrhythmias

Procedure guidelines **Blood pressure (manual)**

Blood pressure should be measured in both arms initially (BHS 2006; NICE 2006). A considerable number of people (particularly the elderly) can have large variations between arms. The arm with the highest reading should be the one used (Williams *et al.* 2004). Refer to Box 18.1 for recommendations from the Medicines and Healthcare Products Regulatory Agency (MHRA) 2006 for guidelines of best practice when taking patients' blood pressure.

Equipment

1 Sphygmomanometer.

2 Stethoscope.

Action	Rationale
1 Explain to the patient that blood pressure is to be taken and discuss the procedure.	To ensure that the patient understands the procedure and gives his/her consent (NMC 2006: C; NMC 2008: C).
2 Wash hands using bactericidal soap and water or bactericidal alcohol handrub, and dry.	To minimize the risk of infection (DH 2005: C).
3 Allow the patient to rest for 5 minutes either supine or seated in quiet room with comfortable temperature.	To ensure an accurate reading is obtained. Normally blood pressure readings are measured with the patient in a sitting position (BHS 2006: C).
4 Ensure that tight or restrictive clothing is removed from the arm.	To obtain a correct reading (BHS 2006: C).
5 Ensure that the upper arm is supported and positioned at heart level, with the palm of the hand facing upwards (BHS 2006).	To obtain an accurate reading. Measurements made with the arm dangling by the hip can be 11–12 mmHg higher than those made with the arm supported and the cuff at heart level. Measurements made with the arm raised can be falsely high (Beevers *et al.* 2001b: C).
6 Use a cuff that covers 80% of the circumference of the upper arm (BHS 2006).	To obtain a correct reading (BHS 2006: C).

7 Apply the cuff of the sphygmomanometer snugly around the arm, ensuring that the centre of the bladder covers the brachial artery. The lower edge of the cuff should be 2–3 cm above the arterial pulse in the antecubital fossa (Valler-Jones & Wedgbury 2005).	To obtain a correct reading (BHS 2006: C). To prevent inaccurate result due to the pressure being exerted by the cuff on the brachial artery (Valler-Jones & Wedgbury 2005: E).
8 Position the manometer within 1 m of the patient, and where it can be seen at eye level (BHS 2006).	To prevent the cuff tubing hanging down and causing a risk of being caught by objects or by the operator. The manometer should be at eye level to obtain an accurate recording (BHS 2006: C).
9 Instruct the patient to stop eating, talking, etc., during blood pressure measurement.	Activity, including eating or talking, will cause an inaccurate high blood pressure to be recorded (BHS 2006: C).
10 Inflate the cuff until the radial pulse can no longer be felt. This provides an estimation of the systolic pressure. Deflate the cuff completely and wait 15–30 seconds before continuing to measure (Hill & Grim 1991).	A low systolic pressure may be reported in patients who have an auscultatory gap. This is when Korotkoff's sounds disappear shortly after the systolic pressure is heard, and resume well above what corresponds to the diastolic pressure. About 5% of the population have an auscultatory gap and it is most common in those with hypertension (Hill & Grim 1991: E). This error can be avoided if the systolic pressure is first estimated by palpation (Hill & Grim 1991: E).
11 The cuff is then inflated to a pressure 30 mmHg higher than the estimated systolic pressure.	Pressure exerted by the inflated cuff prevents the blood from flowing through the artery (BHS 2006: C).
12 The diaphragm of the stethoscope should be placed over the pulse point of the brachial artery (see Action figure 12).	Apply just enough pressure on the stethoscope to keep it in its place over the brachial artery. Excessive pressure can distort sounds or make them persist for longer than normal (BHS 2006: C).

633

Procedure guidelines *(cont.)*

13 Deflate the cuff at 2 mmHg per second or per heart beat (Perloff *et al.* 1993).

At a slower rate of deflation venous congestion and arm pain can develop, resulting in a falsely low reading. At faster rates of deflation the mercury may fall too quickly, resulting in an imprecise reading (BHS 2006: C).

14 The measurement of systolic blood pressure is when a minimum of two clear repetitive tapping sounds can be heard. Diastolic pressure is measured at the point when the sound can no longer be heard.

To ensure that an accurate reading is obtained (BHS 2006: C).

15 A record should be made of the systolic and diastolic pressures and comparisons made with previous readings. It should be recorded which arm was used to take the blood pressure. Any irregularities should be brought to the attention of the medical team.

The average of two or more blood pressure readings is often taken to represent a patient's normal blood pressure.

Taking more than one measurement reduces the influence of anxiety and may provide a more accurate record (Williams *et al.* 2004: C).

Documentation should be done immediately to reduce the risk of error (Williams *et al.* 2004: C).

16 Remove the equipment and clean after use.

To reduce the risk of cross-infection (DH 2005: C).

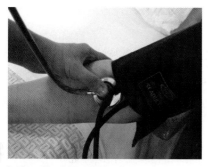

Action 12   Manual blood pressure reading technique.

Respiration

Definition

The respiration system is a tube with many branches that end in millions of tiny hair-filled sacs called alveoli (Richardson 2006b; Tortora & Derrickson 2008). The respiratory system includes the nose, and nasal cavity, pharynx, larynx, trachea, bronchi and their smaller branches, and the lungs, which contain the terminal air sacs, or alveoli (Marieb & Hoehn 2007). The airways have three main functions (Richardson 2006b):

- To facilitate gaseous exchanges to and from the lungs.
- To protect the lungs from the entry of any foreign matter.
- To control the heat and humidity of gases.

The function of the respiratory system is to supply the body with oxygen and remove carbon dioxide. This is achieved by the diffusion of gases between the air in the alveoli of the lungs and the blood in the alveolar capillaries (Marieb & Hoehn 2007).

Indications

The respiration rate is evaluated:

- To determine a baseline respiratory rate for comparisons.
- To monitor changes in oxygenation or in respiration.
- To evaluate the patient's response to medications or treatments that affect the respiratory system.

(Tortora & Derrickson 2008).

Reference material

The body cells require a continuous supply of oxygen to carry out their vital functions and this is provided by respiration (Marieb & Hoehn 2007). To accomplish respiration, four distinct events must occur:

1 Ventilation is where air is moved into and out of the lungs so that gas in the air sacs is replenished.
2 Gaseous exchange between the blood and the alveoli.
3 Oxygen and carbon dioxide are transported to and from the lungs by the cardiovascular system. This is called respiratory transportation.
4 Internal respiration is the cellular respiration that occurs in the cell where oxygen is utilized and carbon dioxide produced.

Control of respiration

Respiratory centre

The respiratory centre generates the basic pattern of breathing. Located in the brain, it is made up of groups of nerve cells in the reticular endothelial system of the medulla oblongata. Regular impulses are sent by these cells to the motor neurones via the anterior horn of the spinal cord, which supplies the intercostal muscles and the diaphragm (Thibodeau & Patton 2007). When the motor neurones are stimulated, the muscles contract and inspiration occurs. When the neurones are inhibited, the muscles relax and expiration follows.

Although the respiratory centre generates the basic rhythm, the depth and rate of breathing can be altered in response to the body's changing needs. The most important factors are those of nervous and chemical control (Figure 18.9).

Nervous control

Lung tissue is stretched on inspiration and this stimulates afferent fibres in the vagus nerve. These impulses cause inspiration to cease and expiration occurs. Emotion, pain and anxiety also cause an increased respiratory rate (Marieb & Hoehn 2007).

Chemical control

An increase in the amount of carbon dioxide in the blood supplying the respiratory centre stimulates the respiratory centre and breathing becomes faster and deeper (Tortora & Derrickson 2008).

During exercise, carbon dioxide is produced in the muscles by the oxidation of carbohydrate. The amount of carbon dioxide in the blood increases and this stimulates the respiratory centre, producing an increase in depth and rate of respiration. More oxygen is made available in the alveoli for the blood to transport to the muscles, at the same time eliminating more carbon dioxide.

Any substance that, like carbon dioxide, lowers the pH of the blood will stimulate the respiratory centre. Figure 18.9 illustrates the factors influencing the rate and depth of breathing.

Patients with respiratory disease, e.g. emphysema and chronic bronchitis, who maintain high levels of carbon dioxide, will have arterial oxygen levels below 9 kPa (see Chapter 27). This is termed the 'hypoxic drive'. This chronic elevation of the partial pressure of carbon dioxide results in the chemoreceptors becoming unresponsive to this chemical stimulus. The change in respiratory drive results in respiration being stimulated by decreases in oxygen levels rather than levels of carbon dioxide (Marieb & Hoehn 2007). This may be detrimental to the patient's respiration if oxygen is administered therapeutically at high levels.

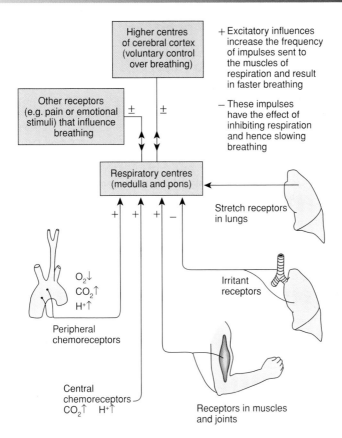

Figure 18.9 Factors influencing rate and depth of breathing.

Ventilation

Ventilation results from pressure changes transmitted from the thoracic cavity to the lungs (Figure 18.10). Inspiration is initiated by contraction of the diaphragm and external intercostal muscles, resulting in the rib cage rising up, and the thrusting forward of the sternum. The ribs also swing outwards, expanding the volume of the thorax (Marieb & Hoehn 2007). Because the lungs adhere tightly to the thoracic wall, attached by the layers of parietal and visceral pleura, this increases

637

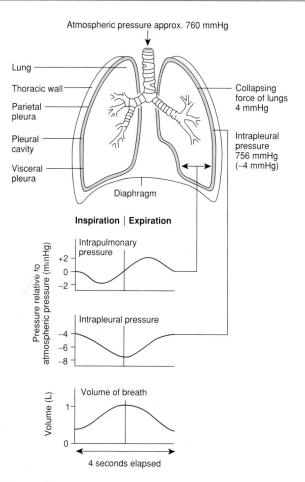

Figure 18.10   Intrapulmonary and intrapleural pressure relationships. Ventilation occurs due to pressure changes transmitted from the thoracic cavity to the lungs.

the intrapulmonary volume (Marieb & Hoehn 2007). Gases travel from an area of high pressure to areas of low pressure. The increased intrapulmonary volume results in a negative pressure of 1–3 mmHg less than the atmospheric pressure (Marieb & Hoehn 2007). The resulting pressure gradient causes air to rush into the lungs (Figure 18.11).

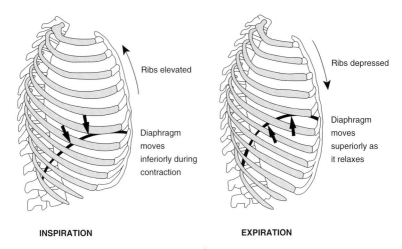

Ribs elevated

Diaphragm
moves
inferiorly during
contraction

INSPIRATION

Ribs depressed

Diaphragm
moves
superiorly as
it relaxes

EXPIRATION

Figure 18.11 Changes in thoracic volume during breathing.

Expiration is largely passive, occurring as the inspiratory muscles relax and the lungs recoil as a result of their elastic properties (Marieb & Hoehn 2007). When intrapulmonary pressure exceeds atmospheric pressure this compresses the microscopic air sacs (alveoli) and an expiration of gases occurs.

A method commonly used to measure the volume of air exchanged during breathing is a **spirometer** (spiro = breathe; meter = measuring device). The record of these results is called a **spirogram** (Figure 18.12).

At rest, a healthy adult averages 12 breaths a minute, with each inhalation and exhalation moving about 500 ml of air into and out of the lungs. The volume of one breath is called the **tidal volume**. Therefore, the **minute ventilation** (**MV**) is the total volume of air inhaled and exhaled each minute which is the respiratory rate multiplied by the tidal volume which equates to 6 litres per minute (Tortora & Derrickson 2008).

Disease that affects the pleura of the individual may influence ventilation. A chest wound or rupture of the visceral pleura may allow air to enter the pleural space from the respiratory tract. The presence of air in the intrapleural space is referred to as a pneumothorax. Pleurisy, inflammation of the pleura where secretion of pleural fluid declines, causes a stabbing pain with each inspiration. Alternatively, an excessive increase in pleural secretions may hinder breathing (Marieb & Hoehn 2007). Air in the pleural space results in lung collapse (atelectasis). This affects the intrapulmonary pressure and hence ventilation.

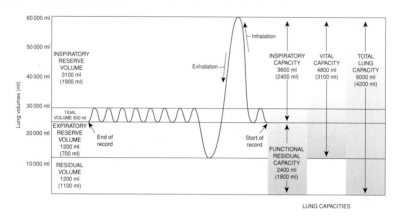

Figure 18.12 Spirogram of lung volumes and capacities. The average values for a healthy adult male and female are indicated, with values for a female in parentheses. Note that the spirogram is read from right (start of record) to left (end of record). Lung capacities are combinations of various lung volumes.

The degree to which the lungs stretch and fill during inspiration and return to normal during expiration is due to the compliance and elasticity of lung tissue. Lung compliance depends on the elasticity of lung tissue and the flexibility of the thorax (Marieb & Hoehn 2007). When this is impaired, expiration becomes an active process, requiring the use of energy. The diseases that lower lung compliance are characterized by changes in the lung parenchyma. Examples include emphysema and fibrosing alveolitis, as a result of intrinsic or extrinsic means:

- **Intrinsic:**
    - severe infection;
    - rheumatoid arthritis;
    - systemic lupus erythematosus (SLE).
- **Extrinsic:**
    - pneumoconiosis;
    - psitticosis;
    - asbestosis;
    - oxygen fibrosis.

(Marieb & Hoehn 2007.)

In emphysema the lungs become progressively less elastic and more fibrous, which hinders both inspiration and expiration. The increased muscular activity results in greater energy required to breathe.

Compliance is diminished by any factor that:

■ Reduces the natural resilience of the lungs.
■ Blocks the bronchi or respiratory passageways.
■ Impairs the flexibility of the thoracic cage.

Friction in the air passageways causes resistance and affects ventilation (Thibodeau & Patton 2007). Normally, airway resistance is reduced so that minimal opposition to airflow occurs. However, any factor that amplifies airway resistance such as the presence of mucus, tumour or infected material in the airways demands that breathing movements become more strenuous (Marieb & Hoehn 2007).

Respiratory volumes

The amount of air that is breathed varies depending on the condition of inspiration and expiration. Information about a patient's respiratory status can be gained by measuring various lung capacities, which consist of the sum of different respiratory volumes.

Tidal volume

The tidal volume (TV) is the amount of air inhaled or exhaled with each breath under resting conditions (about 500 ml) (Marieb & Hoehn 2007).

Inspiratory reserve volume

The inspiratory reserve volume (IRV) is the amount of air that can be inhaled forcibly after a normal tidal volume inhalation (about 3100 ml) (Marieb & Hoehn 2007).

Expiratory reserve volume

The expiratory reserve volume (ERV) is the maximum amount that can be exhaled forcibly after a normal tidal volume exhalation (about 1200 ml) (Marieb & Hoehn 2007).

Residual volume

641

The residual volume (RV) is the amount of air remaining in the lungs after a forced expiration (about 1200 ml).

Respiratory capacities

Respiratory capacities are measured for diagnostic purposes. They consist of two or more respiratory lung volumes (Marieb & Hoehn 2007).

Total lung capacity

The total lung capacity (TLC) is the amount of air in the lungs at the end of a maximum inspiration (Marieb & Hoehn 2007):

$$TLC = TV + IRV + ERV + RV \text{ (6000 ml)}.$$

Vital capacity

The vital capacity (VC) is the maximum amount of air that can be expired after a maximum inspiration (Marieb & Hoehn 2007):

$$VC = TV + IRV + ERV \text{ (4800 ml)}.$$

Inspiratory capacity

The inspiratory capacity (IC) is the maximum amount of air that can be inspired after a normal expiration (Marieb & Hoehn 2007):

$$IC = TV + IRV \text{ (3600 ml)}.$$

Functional residual capacity

The functional residual capacity (FRC) is the amount of air remaining in the lungs after a normal tidal volume expiration (Marieb & Hoehn 2007):

$$FRC = ERC + RV \text{ (2400 ml)}.$$

Dead space

A percentage of the inspired air (about 120 ml) fills the respiratory passageways and does not contribute to gaseous exchange. This is termed the anatomical dead space (Marieb & Hoehn 2007).

Gaseous exchange

Oxygen in the inspired air enters while carbon dioxide leaves the blood in the lungs in the process of ventilation. These gases move in opposite directions in the alveoli by the mechanism of diffusion (Marieb & Hoehn 2007). Adjacent to the alveoli is a dense vascular network. Oxygen moves into the alveolar capillaries and carbon dioxide moves out (Figure 18.13). This process is called gaseous

Gas exchanges occurring at the tissues

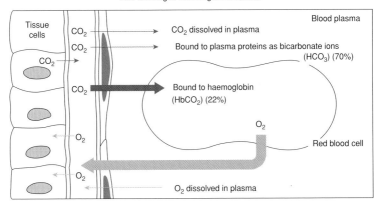

Gas exchanges occurring at the lungs

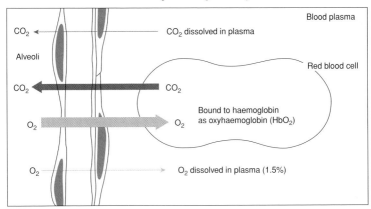

Figure 18.13 Transport and exchange of carbon dioxide and oxygen.

exchange. Factors influencing this process include the partial pressure gradients, the width of the respiratory membrane and the surface area available (Marieb & Hoehn 2007).

The gaseous composition of the atmosphere and alveoli is demonstrated in Table 18.2. The atmosphere consists almost entirely of oxygen and nitrogen; the alveoli contain more carbon dioxide and water vapour and considerably less

643

Table 18.2   Composition of gas in the atmosphere and alveoli.

	Atmosphere inspired (%)	Alveoli (%)
Oxygen	20.9	13.7
Carbon dioxide	0.04	5.2
Nitrogen	78.6	74.9
Water	0.46	6.2

oxygen. These different figures reflect the following processes (Marieb & Hoehn 2007):

- Gaseous exchange in the lungs.
- Humidification of air by the respiratory passageways.
- The mixing of alveolar gas that occurs with each breath.

Respiratory transportation

Oxygen is carried in the blood in two ways, bound to the haemoglobin within the red blood cells and dissolved in plasma. Haemoglobin carries 98.5% of the oxygen from the lungs and the tissues. The amount of oxygen bound to haemoglobin depends on several factors (Marieb & Hoehn 2007):

- The partial pressure of oxygen (PaO_2) and the partial pressure of carbon dioxide ($PaCO_2$) in the blood. The gradient of partial pressure influences the rates of diffusion, the oxygen gradient being steeper than that of carbon dioxide. Carbon dioxide is transported from the tissue primarily as bicarbonate ions in the plasma (70%), whereas only small amounts are transported by haemoglobin in the red blood cells (22%) (Marieb & Hoehn 2007).
- The blood pH influences the affinity of haemoglobin for oxygen: as the pH decreases, as in acidosis, the amount of oxygen unloaded in the tissues increases (Marieb & Hoehn 2007).
- As body temperature rises above normal levels, the affinity of haemoglobin for oxygen declines, and therefore oxygen unloading is enhanced. This effect is seen in localized temperature changes such as inflammation (Marieb & Hoehn 2007).

Diseases that reduce the oxygen-carrying ability of the blood, whatever the cause, are termed anaemia. This is characterized by oxygen blood levels that are inadequate to support normal metabolism (Marieb & Hoehn 2007). Common causes of anaemia include:

- Insufficient number of red cells, including destruction of red cells, haemorrhage and bone marrow failure.
- Decreases in haemoglobin content, including iron deficiency anaemia and pernicious anaemia.
- Abnormal haemoglobin, including thalassaemia and sickle cell anaemia (Marieb & Hoehn 2007).

Internal respiration

Internal respiration is the exchange of gases that occurs within the tissues between the capillaries and the cells. Carbon dioxide enters the blood and oxygen moves into the cells (see Figure 18.13).

Hypoxia is the result of an inadequate amount of oxygen delivered to body tissues. The blue coloration of tissues and mucosal membranes is termed cyanosis (Marieb & Hoehn 2007).

Lung defence mechanisms

The upper airway is designed to warm, humidify and filter inspired air. The nasal passages absorb noxious gases and trap inhaled particles. Smaller particles are removed by the cough reflex.

Observation of respiration

Respirations in an individual should be observed for rate, depth and pattern of breathing (Marieb & Hoehn 2007) (Table 18.4).

Rate

Rate and depth determine the type of respiration. The normal rate at rest is approximately 14–18 breaths per minute in adults and is faster in infants and children (Table 18.3). The ratio of pulse rate to respiration rate is approximately 5 : 1 (Marieb & Hoehn 2007).

Table 18.3 Respiratory rates. From Weber & Kelley (2003).

Age	Average rate/minute
Birth–6 months	30–50
6 months–2 years	20–30
3–10 years	20–28
10–18 years	12–20
Adult	15–20

Table 18.4 Respiratory assessment procedure.

Observation	Rationale
Rate and regularity of respiration	Very slow or rapid breathing may be a sign of oxygenation or underlying change, for example due to sepsis
Observe for signs of respiratory effort: ■ Nasal flaring ■ Pursed lips ■ Use of accessory muscles such as the shoulder or neck muscles (sternomastoid or scalene)	These signs may show that the patient is making extra effort in breathing and may indicate changes in the respiratory status before other observations (e.g. oxygen saturation or rate)
Listen for cough or wheezing	Dry cough may be caused by viral infection, bronchial carcinoma or congestive cardiac failure Moist cough may be due to chronic bronchitis or asthma or bacterial infection Wheezing is caused by bronchospasm or bronchial obstruction
Assess respiratory history including smoking history, history of asthma, exertional shortness of breath or other respiratory symptoms	These factors will alert the nurse to potential patient problems or concurrent conditions
Assess sputum	White or opalescent sputum may be produced by asthmatics or patients with chronic bronchitis, but does not necessarily indicate infection Thick viscous sputum that is coloured indicates infection and should be sent for microbiology culture and sensitivity Frothy sputum indicates pulmonary oedema Haemoptysis can occur with infection, pulmonary embolism, malignant disease or trauma

Changes in the rate of ventilation may be defined as follows. *Tachypnoea* is an increased respiratory rate, seen in fever, for example, as the body tries to rid itself of excess heat. Respirations increase by about 7 breaths per minute for every 1°C rise in temperature above normal. They also increase with pneumonia, other obstructive airway diseases, respiratory insufficiency and lesions in the pons of the brainstem (Marieb & Hoehn 2007).

Bradypnoea is a decreased but regular respiratory rate, such as that caused by the depression of the respiratory centre in the medulla by opiate narcotics, or by a brain tumour.

Depth

The depth of respiration is the volume of air moving in and out with each respiration. This tidal volume is normally about 500 ml in an adult and should be constant with each breath. A spirometer is used to measure the precise amount (see Respiratory capacities section, above). Normal, relaxed breathing is effortless, automatic, regular and almost silent (Marieb & Hoehn 2007).

Dyspnoea is undue breathlessness and an awareness of discomfort with breathing. There are several types of dyspnoea (Tortora & Derrickson 2008).

- Exertional dyspnoea is shortness of breath on exercise and is seen with heart failure.
- Orthopnoea is a shortness of breath on lying down which is relieved by the patient sitting upright. This is often caused by left ventricular failure of the heart.
- Paroxysmal nocturnal dyspnoea is a sudden breathlessness that occurs at night when the patient is lying down and is often caused by pulmonary oedema and left ventricular failure (Bickley & Szilagyi 2007).

Pattern

Changes in the pattern of respiration are often found in disorders of the respiratory control centre. Examples of changes in respiratory pattern follow.

Hyperventilation is an increase in both the rate and depth of respiration. This follows extreme exertion, fear and anxiety, fever, hepatic coma, midbrain lesions of the brainstem, and acid–base imbalance such as diabetic ketoacidosis (Kussmaul's respiration) or salicylate overdose (in both of these situations the body compensates for the metabolic acidosis by increased respiration), as well as an alteration in blood gas concentration (either increased carbon dioxide or decreased oxygen) (Tortora & Derrickson 2008). The breathing pattern is normally regular and consists of inspiration, pause, longer expiration and another pause; this, however, may be altered by some defects and diseases. In adults, more than 20 breaths per minute is considered moderate, more than 30 is severe (Marieb & Hoehn 2007).

Apnoeustic respiration is a pattern of prolonged, gasping inspiration, followed by extremely short, inefficient expiration, seen in lesions of the pons in the midbrain.

Cheyne–Stokes respiration is periodic breathing, characterized by a gradual increase in depth of respiration followed by a decrease in respiration, resulting in apnoea.

Biot's respiration is an interrupted breathing pattern, like Cheyne–Stokes respiration, except that each breath is of the same depth. It may be seen with spinal meningitis or other central nervous system conditions.

Conditions where a patient's respirations may need careful monitoring are described below:

- Patients with conditions that affect respiration, such as those described in the text, require monitoring of respiration to evaluate their condition and the effectiveness of medication.

- Postoperative and critically ill patients require monitoring of respiration. The patient's respiration should be recorded preoperatively in order to make significant comparisons. The breathing is observed to assess for the return to normal respiratory function.

- Patients receiving oxygen inhalation therapy or receiving artificial respiration require monitoring of breathing to assess respiratory function.

Oxygen saturation

Oxygen is transported to the body's tissues in the blood. The red blood cells contain haemoglobin molecules that bind with oxygen in the lungs and transport it to the tissues where it is released. When oxygen combines with haemoglobin it forms oxyhaemoglobin. Each haemoglobin molecule has the potential to bind with four oxygen molecules. When all the binding sites for oxygen are used then the haemoglobin is saturated with oxygen.

The oxygen saturation reading is a measure of the percentage of haemoglobin molecules saturated with oxygen. The normal arterial oxygen saturation is approximately 95–98% (Woodrow 1999).

Pulse oximetry

Pulse oximetry works on the principle that blood saturated with oxygen is a different colour from blood depleted of oxygen. The probe for a pulse oximeter contains a red light source and a detector. These shine through the tissues of the body and work together to measure the colour difference between oxygenated and unoxygenated blood. The machine detects the pulse from an arterial blood source and is able to calculate the percentage of oxygen saturation by combining the detected colour changes of the blood combined with the detected pulse of the artery (Harper 2004). Because of the way the pulse oximeter works, it is susceptible to error if it is not able to accurately measure the transmission of light through the tissues or detect the pulse of the artery (Harper 2004).

Indications for pulse oximetry

- Monitoring effectiveness of oxygen therapy.
- During sedation or anaesthesia.
- During transportation of patients who are unwell and require oxygenation assessment.
- Haemodynamic instability (e.g. cardiac failure or MI) (Howell 2002).
- Respiratory illness (e.g. asthma, chronic obstructive pulmonary disease [COPD]) (Place 2000).
- Monitoring during administration of respiratory depressant drugs, e.g. opiate epidural or patient-controlled analgesia.

Possible sources of error

Light transmission:

- Barriers or obstruction, e.g. nail varnish, dirt, foreign objects, bright or fluorescent room lighting, intravenous dyes used in imaging (Harper 2004; Keenan 1995).

Pulse detection:

- Movement, rigors or shivering, poor circulation, atrial fibrillation (Woodrow 1999), vasoconstriction, arterial constriction, shock, cardiac arrest hypothermia (Howell 2002).

Limitations of pulse oximetry and oxygen saturation

Oxygen saturation is only one factor in oxygenation of the tissues. In anaemia it is possible to have high oxygen saturation readings, but inadequate amounts of oxygen reaching the tissues. Carbon monoxide (CO) exposure will lead to uptake of CO molecules in preference to oxygen (O_2). As carboxyhaemoglobin is also bright red it can lead to significant overestimation of oxygen saturation when using pulse oximeters (Howell 2002).

Procedure guidelines **Pulse oximetry**

Equipment

1 Pulse oximeter. 2 Alcohol swab.

Intermittent readings

Assess the patient observing correct placement of probe and for underlying problems identified above that may be influencing the reading.

Continuous readings

If the oxygen saturation monitoring is to be continuous, leaving the probe on one digit for protracted periods of time may cause pressure damage to either the skin or nail bed. There is also possibility of developing burns from the probe.

The MHRA (2001) advises to reposition the probe at least 4-hourly, or more frequently if specified by manufacturer's instructions.

Procedure

Action	Rationale
1 Explain to the patient that an oxygen saturation reading is needed and obtain consent to continue.	To ensure the patient understands the procedure and is able to provide valid consent (NMC 2006: C; NMC 2008: C).
2 Ensure that the patient is comfortable and warm enough, especially if continuous monitoring is needed.	To maintain patient comfort. Shivering will interfere with the pulse oximeter reading (Jevon 2000: E).
3 Wash and dry hands.	To minimize the risk of cross-infection (DH 2005: C).
4 Make sure the probe and equipment are clean and in good working order.	To minimize the risk of cross-infection and ensure accuracy of recording (DH 2005: C; Jevon 2000: E).
5 Select a suitable area for the probe (usually finger) and place the probe as directed by the manufacturer's instructions (see Action figure 5).	Proper function of the pulse oximeter will only be possible if the probe is placed as intended by the manufacturer (Grap 2002: E).
6 Switch the pulse oximeter machine on.	

7 Make sure that the probe sensor is detecting the pulse and that it corresponds to the patient's pulse. This will usually be indicated by a beep in time with each detected pulse or a graphical indication of the pulse on a display panel.

To ensure that the probe is detecting the pulse (Grap 2002: C).

8 Take the reading of the oxygenation saturation and document this in the patient's notes. Make a note of any oxygen administration.

To provide a written record of the patient's condition and therapy (NMC 2008: C).

9 Ensure that any abnormal reading or observation is reported to the medical team.

To ensure that any patient problems are communicated (NMC 2008: C).

10 Once oxygen saturation monitoring is completed, clean equipment and return to storage as appropriate.

Cleaning of the equipment, including the probe, will minimize the risk of cross-infection. Proper storage, including initiating battery recharging, will ensure that the equipment is ready for use when next required (DH 2005: C).

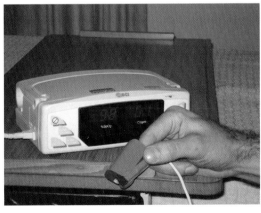

Action 5   Positioning of probe.

Peak flow

Definition

Peak expiratory flow rate (PEFR or peak flow) is a measurement of the highest rate at which air can be expelled from the lungs through an open mouth (Booker 2004).

Reference material

Peak flow can be used as an indication of any restriction in the airway. It is a useful aid in diagnosing and monitioring asthma and respiratory conditions (GINA 2006). PEFR is one aspect of lung function assessment and is usually used in conjunction with assessment of the lung volume and other factors to give a more complete indication of lung function (Booker 2004).

Timing of peak flow readings

For patients with asthma, the Global Initiative for Asthma (GINA) (GINA 2006) recommends measuring peak flows morning and evening before treatment is taken. In addition, a peak flow measurement should be taken 30 minutes after morning medications or nebulizers. Constriction of the airways will decrease the amount of air that can pass through and this will result in a lowered peak flow. Bronchodilators act to open the airways and allow a faster flow of air, resulting in an increase in peak flow (GINA 2006).

Factors affecting peak flow

A patient's peak flow will vary due to age, sex and ethnic origin. Respiratory problems such as asthma, COPD or emphysema will also result in a reduction in peak flow. Assessment of any impairment should be against a recognized chart of normal values (Figure 18.14) or against the patient's best recorded measurements (GINA 2006). In general, the result for a normal adult would be 400–600 litres per minute (Edmond 2002).

In patients with asthma the peak flow reading will usually vary over time and in response to medication. Any significant deterioration in peak flow may signal the onset of acute severe asthma (Box 18.2).

In the event of any life-threatening feature or pulse oximetry of less than 92%, arterial blood gases should be measured.

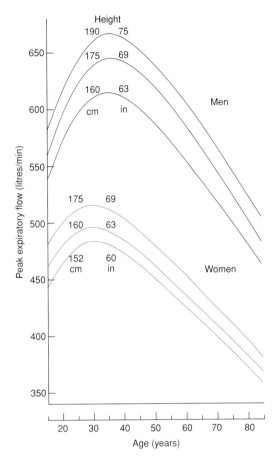

Figure 18.14   Chart of normal adult PF values. From Gregg & Nunn (1989) with permission from *BMJ*.

Blood gas markers for a severe life-threatening asthma attack are:

- Normal or high $PaCO_2$ (5–6 kPa/36–45 mmHg).
- Severe hypoxia, PaO_2 less than 8 kPa/60 mmHg regardless of oxygen therapy.
- Low pH or high H^+.

Box 18.2   Recognition and assessment of asthma (Edmond 2002)

Features of acute severe asthma:

- Peak flow < (less than or equal to) 50% of the predicted value (see Figure 18.14) or best readings.
- Unable to finish sentence in one breath.
- Respirations > (greater than or equal to) 25 breaths per minute.
- Pulse over 110 beats/min.

Life-threatening features:

- Peak flow < (less than) 33% of predicted or best readings.
- Cyanosis, silent chest or feeble respiratory effort.
- Bradycardia or hypotension.
- Confusion, exhaustion or coma.

Severe and life-threatening asthma attacks can occur without patient distress. Not all features above may be evident, but if one or more symptoms are noted and there is a deterioration, the medical team should be contacted urgently (GINA 2006).

Procedure guidelines   **Peak flow reading using manual peak flow meter**

Equipment

1 Peak flow meter.

2 Observation chart.

Procedure

Action	Rationale
1 Explain the procedure to the patient and obtain consent.	To ensure the patient understands the procedure and gives valid consent (NMC 2006: C; NMC 2008: C).
2 Establish patient's current and best peak flow readings or predicted peak flow.	To allow for comparison and assessment of the patient's reading (Baillie 2001: E).
3 Wash and dry hands.	To minimize cross-infection (DH 2005: C).
4 Collect and assemble equipment. Attach mouthpiece to meter if required (see specific documentation).	

5 Move the indicator to the zero mark prior to reading.	To ensure the reading is accurate (Baillie 2001: E).
6 Sit patient in upright/usual position for readings.	To ensure consistency of readings (Baillie 2001: E).
7 Ask the patient to take a deep breath in and place their lips around the mouthpiece (see Action figure 7).	To ensure accuracy of reading (Dickinson & Martindale 2002: E).
8 Ask the patient to breathe out through the peak flow meter as hard as possible.	To ensure accuracy of reading (Baillie 2001: E).
9 Take a note of the reading. Readings may vary, so repeat process three times in total and use the best of the three readings.	To ensure accuracy of readings (Baillie 2001: C; Dickinson & Martindale 2002).
10 Return the patient to a comfortable position.	
11 Discard the used mouthpiece (if appropriate), wash your hands and store the peak flow meter ready for next use.	To minimize cross-infection (DH 2005: C).
12 Record the highest peak flow reading in the patient record, noting time of reading and any nebulized therapy. Inform medical staff of any abnormality in the reading.	To provide an accurate record of assessment (Baillie 2001: E).

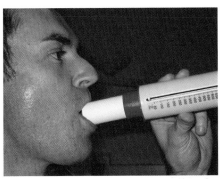

Action 7   Manual peak flow meter technique.

Temperature

Definition

Body temperature represents the balance between heat production and heat loss (Marieb & Hoehn 2007). All body tissues produce heat depending on how metabolically active they are. When the body is resting, most heat is generated by the heart, liver, brain and endocrine organs (Marieb & Hoehn 2007).

Indications

Monitoring the patient's temperature is an important aspect of nursing assessment. Temperature needs to be measured accurately and monitored effectively to enable temperature changes to be detected quickly and any necessary intervention commenced (Watson 1998). Measurement of body temperature is carried out for two reasons:

- To determine the patient's temperature on admission as a baseline for comparison with future measurements.
- To monitor fluctuations in temperature.

Reference material

All tissues produce heat as a result of cell metabolism, and this is increased by exercise and activity (Marieb & Hoehn 2007). Body temperature is usually maintained between 36.0 and 37.5°C regardless of changes in the environment (Tortora & Derrickson 2008). Humans have the ability through homeostasis to ensure the core temperature that remains constant in spite of environmental changes. The body core generally has the highest temperature while the skin is the coolest (Figure 18.15). Core temperature reflects the heat of arterial blood and represents the balance between the heat generated by body tissues in metabolic activity and that lost through various mechanisms (Marieb & Hoehn 2007).

The core body temperature is set and closely regulated by the thermoregulatory centre of the hypothalamus. This comprises a group of neurones in the anterior and posterior portions, referred to as the preoptic area (Tortora & Derrickson 2008), which works as a thermostat (Figure 18.16). A relatively constant temperature is maintained by homeostasis, which is a constant process of heat gain and heat loss. The body requires stability of its temperature to produce an optimum environment for biochemical and enzymic reactions to maintain cellular function. Body temperature above or below this normal range affects total body function (Marieb & Hoehn 2007). A temperature above 41°C can cause convulsions and a temperature of 43°C renders life unsustainable.

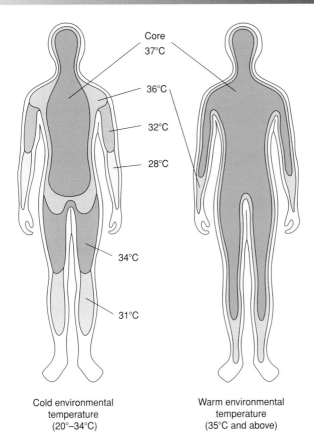

Core
37°C

36°C

32°C

28°C

34°C

31°C

Cold environmental
temperature
(20°–34°C)

Warm environmental
temperature
(35°C and above)

Figure 18.15 Body core and skin temperatures.

Heat is gained through metabolic activity of the body, especially of the muscles and liver. Heat loss is achieved through the skin by the processes of radiation, convection, conduction and evaporation (Marieb & Hoehn 2007).

Various factors cause fluctuations of temperature:

- The body's circadian rhythms cause daily fluctuations. The body temperature is higher in the evening than in the morning (Marieb & Hoehn 2007). Minor & Waterhouse (1981) recorded a difference of 0.5–1.5°C between morning and evening measurements.

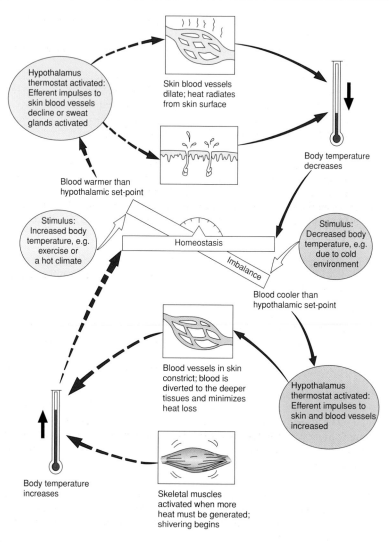

Figure 18.16 Mechanisms of body temperature regulation.

- Ovulation can elevate the body's temperature as it influences the basal metabolic rate (Tortora & Derrickson 2008).
- Exercise and eating cause an elevation in temperature (Marieb & Hoehn 2007).
- Extremes of age affect a person's response to environmental change. The young or elderly are unable to maintain an efficient equilibrium. Thermoregulation is inadequate in the newborn and especially in low-birth-weight babies. In older people there is an increased sensitivity to cold and the body temperature is generally lower (Nakamura *et al.* 1997).

Hypothermia   Hypothermia is defined as a core temperature of 35°C that causes the metabolic rate to decrease (Trim 2005). Hypothermia may be classified as mild (32–35°C), moderate (28–32°C) and severe (less than 28°C) (Cuddy 2004). This occurs when the body loses more heat and is subsequently unable to maintain homeostasis (Neno 2005). If the temperature does fall below 35°C, the patient will start to shiver severely (Edwards 1997). However, hypothermia frequently escapes detection due to symptoms being non-specific and an oral thermometer's failure to record in the appropriate range (Marini & Wheeler 2006). It can occur in all ages, but the elderly are at particular risk, and is often multifactorial in origin. It can arise as a result of:

- Environmental exposure.
- Medications that can either alter the perception of cold, increase heat loss through vasodilatation or inhibit heat generation, e.g. alcohol, paracetamol.
- Metabolic conditions, e.g. hypoglycaemia and adrenal insufficiency.
- The exposure of the body and internal organs during surgery and the use of drugs which dampen the vasoconstrictor response (Marini & Wheeler 2006).

Surgical patients having procedures greater than 1 hour have increased disruptions to normal homeostatic mechanisms resulting in a drop of temperature. Complications can include cardiovascular ischaemia, delayed wound healing and increase risk for wound infections and increase in postoperative recovery time (Wagner 2006).

Hyperthermia   Pyrexia is defined as a significant rise in body temperature (Marieb & Hoehn 2007). Sudden temperature elevations usually indicate infection. However, other life-threatening non-infectious causes of fever are often overlooked (Table 18.5).

Fever caused by pyrexia is the result of the internal thermostat resetting to higher levels. This resetting of the thermostat is the result of the action of pyrogens, which are chemical substances now known to be cytokines. Cytokines are chemical mediators, which are involved in cellular immunity (Marieb & Hoehn

Table 18.5 Non-infectious causes of hyperthermia.

Agonist drugs	Malignancy
Alcohol withdrawal	Malignant hyperthermla
Anticholinergic drugs	Neuroleptic malignant syndrome
Allergic drug or transfusion reaction	Pheochromocytoma
Autonomic insufficiency	Salicylate intoxication
Crystalline arthritis (gout)	Status epilepticus
Drug allergy	Stroke or central nervous system damage
Heat stroke	Vasculitis
Hyperthyroidism	

2007). They enhance the immune response and are released from white blood cells, injured tissues and macrophages. This causes the hypothalamus to release prostaglandins, which in turn reset the hypothalamic thermostat. The body then promotes heat-producing mechanisms such as vasoconstriction. Heat loss is reduced, the skin becomes cool and the person 'shivers'. This is often called a rigor (Marieb & Hoehn 2007). A rigor is marked by shivering and the patient complains of feeling cold. The temperature quickly rises as a result of the normal physiological response to cold. This results in the following physiological changes:

- Thermoreceptors in the skin are stimulated, resulting in vasoconstriction. This decreases heat loss through conduction and convection.
- Sweat gland activity is reduced to minimize evaporation.
- Shivering occurs, muscles contract and relax out of sequence with each other, thus generating heat.
- The body increases catecholamine and thyroxine levels, elevating the metabolic rate in an attempt to increase temperature.

(Marieb & Hoehn 2007.)

All of these changes contribute to a rise in metabolism with an increase in carbon dioxide excretion and the need for oxygen. This leads to an increased respiratory rate. When the body temperature reaches its new 'setpoint' the patient no longer complains of feeling cold, shivering ceases and sweating commences.

There are several grades of pyrexia, and these are described in Table 18.6.

There are different methods for lowering body temperature. Antipyretics, including paracetamol, can mask the function of the hypothalamus, by reducing the temperature while masking the underlying signs of disease (Cuddy 2004). It is thought that these drugs inhibit the inflammatory action of prostaglandins, affecting the hypothalamus by temporarily resetting the thermostat to normal levels. However, these drugs must be used with caution in patients with established liver

Table 18.6 Grades of pyrexia.

Low-grade pyrexia	Normal to 38°C	Indicative of an inflammatory response due to a mild infection, allergy, disturbance of body tissue by trauma, surgery, malignancy or thrombosis
Moderate to high-grade pyrexia	38–40°C	May be caused by wound, respiratory or urinary tract infections
Hyperpyrexia	40°C and above	May arise because of bacteraemia, damage to the hypothalamus or high environmental temperatures

disease or a history of gastric bleeding as they can cause gastric irritation and put an increased strain on a diseased liver to break down the drug.

Fanning is of benefit for moderate to high pyrexias. Fanning and tepid sponging are not recommended while the patient's temperature is still rising as this will only make the patient feel colder, cause distress (Sharber 1997) and cause the peripheral thermoreceptors to detect a decrease in temperature that leads the hypothalamus to initiate heat-gaining activities such as shivering and peripheral vasoconstriction (Krikler 1990).

Recordings of body temperature are an index of biological function and are a valuable indicator of a patient's health.

Temperature recording sites

Traditionally, the mouth, axilla or rectum have been the preferred sites for obtaining temperature readings. This is due to their accessibility. With the development of new technology the use of the tympanic membrane is increasingly popular, as it is less invasive and provides rapid results (Burke 1996). It has been suggested that tympanic membrane thermometers give a more accurate representation of actual body temperature, as the tympanic membrane lies close to the temperature regulation centre in the hypothalamus and shares the same artery (Van Staaij *et al.* 2003).

Oral

To most accurately measure the temperature orally, the thermometer is placed in the posterior sublingual pocket of tissue at the base of the tongue (Torrance & Semple 1998). It is important that the thermometer is placed in this region and not in the area under the front of the tongue, as there may be a temperature difference of up to 1.7°C between these areas. This temperature difference is due to the sublingual pockets being protected from the air currents, which cool the frontal areas (Neff *et al.* 1989).

This area is in close proximity to the thermoreceptors which respond rapidly to changes in the core temperature, hence changes in core temperatures are reflected quickly here (Carroll 2000; Stevenson 2004).

Oral temperatures are affected by the temperatures of ingested foods and fluids, smoking and by the muscular activity of chewing. It has been shown that oxygen therapy does not affect the oral temperature reading (Hasler & Cohen 1982; Lim-Levy 1982). A respiratory rate that exceeds 18 breaths per minute, together with a patient who smokes, will also reduce the core temperature values (Knies 2003). Oral thermometers should not be used with confused patients because of the risk of injury (Watson 1998).

Rectal

The rectal temperature is often higher than the oral temperature because this site is more sheltered from the external environment. Rectal thermometry has been demonstrated in clinical trials to be more accurate than oral or axillary thermometry; however, it is not advocated due to its invasive nature (Trim 2005). While other more precise methods can still detect fever, the rectal method offers greater precision. However, the presence of soft stool may separate the thermometer from the bowel wall and give a false reading, especially if the central temperature is changing rapidly. In infants this method is not recommended as it carries a risk of rectal ulceration or perforation (Jensen *et al.* 1994).

A rectal thermometer should be inserted at least 4 cm in an adult to obtain the most accurate reading.

Axillary

The axilla is considered less desirable than the other sites because of the difficulty in achieving accurate and reliable readings (Evans *et al.* 2004) as it is not close to major vessels, and skin surface temperatures vary more with changes in temperature of the environment (Woollens 1996). It is usually only used for patients who are unsuitable for, or who cannot tolerate, oral thermometers, e.g. after general anaesthetic, or patients with mouth injuries (Edwards 1997).

To take an axillary temperature reading, the thermometer should be placed in the centre of the armpit, with the patient's arm firmly against the side of the chest. It is important that the same arm is used for each measurement as there is often a variation in temperature between left and right (Heindenreich & Giuffe 1990).

Whichever route is used for temperature measurement, it is important that this is then used consistently, as switching between sites can produce a record that is misleading or difficult to interpret.

Time for recording temperatures

The average person experiences circadian rhythms which make their highest body temperature occur in the late afternoon or early evening, i.e. between 4 PM and 8 PM. The most sensitive time for detecting pyrexias appears to be between 7 PM and 8 PM (Angerami 1980). Samples *et al.* (1985) found the highest temperature between 5 PM and 7 PM. These studies suggest the most useful time to measure and detect an abnormal temperature would be approximately 6 PM. This should be considered when interpreting variations in 4- or 6-hourly observations, and when taking once-daily temperatures.

Types of thermometer

A variety of thermometers are now available, from clinical glass thermometers with oral or rectal bulbs to the electronic sensor thermometer to the tympanic thermometer. Until recently, mercury in glass thermometers continued to be used, even though it has been shown they are unable to detect temperatures lower than 34.5°C (94°F) or higher than 40.5°C (105°F) (Khorshid *et al.* 2005). The MHRA (2005) advises that, for safety, equipment with mercury should be replaced where possible. They are also slow to respond to temperature changes (Marini & Wheeler 2006). O'Toole (1997) also highlights that mercury thermometers present a risk to patients of developing an infection. Therefore by using ones with disposable covers the risk of cross-infection is reduced. The use of electronic devices is therefore preferable where there are extremes of temperature or where there are temperature fluctuations. Other types of thermometer include those listed by Docherty (2000):

- Single-use plastic-coated strips with heat-sensitive recorders (dots) which change colour to indicate the temperature (record from 35.5°C to 40.4°C).
- Digital analogue probe thermometers with plastic disposable sheets (record from 32°C to 42°C).
- Invasive thermometers attached to a pulmonary artery catheter (record from 0°C to 50°C) (O'Toole 1997; Braun *et al.* 1998).

Tympanic membrane thermometer

Tympanic thermometers are small hand-held devices that have a disposable probe that is inserted into the patient's ear canal. The sensor at the end of the probe records the infrared radiation (IRR) that is emitted by the membrane, as a result of its warmth, and converts this into a temperature reading presented on a digital screen (Jevon & Jevon 2001). The probe is protected by a disposable cover, which is changed between patients to prevent cross-infection (Gallimore 2004). Van Staaij *et al* (2003) suggest that tympanic thermometers give a more accurate representation of actual body temperature because the tympanic membrane lies close to the temperature regulation centre in the hypothalamus and shares the same artery.

A common problem with using tympanic thermometers is poor technique (Gilbert *et al.* 2002), leading to inaccurate temperature measurements. The placement of the probe to fit snugly within the ear canal (see Figure 18.17) is crucial as differences between the opening of the ear canal and the tympanic membrane can be as much as 2.8°C (Hudek *et al.* 1998). Jevon and Jevon (2001) highlight other causes of false readings, which include dirty or cracked probe lens, incorrect installation of the probe cover and short time intervals between measurements (less than 2–3 minutes).

Conditions where a patient's temperature requires careful monitoring

1 Patients with conditions that affect basal metabolic rate, such as disorders of the thyroid gland, require monitoring of body temperature. Hypothyroidism is a condition where an inadequate secretion of hormones from the thyroid gland results in a slowing of physical and metabolic activity; thus the individual has a decrease in body temperature. Hyperthyroidism is excessive activity of the thyroid gland; a hypermetabolic condition results, with an increase in all metabolic processes. The patient complains of a low heat tolerance. Thyrotoxic crisis is a sudden increase in thyroid hormones and can cause a hyperpyrexia (Walsh 2002).

2 Postoperative and critically ill patients require monitoring of temperature. The patient's temperature should be observed preoperatively in order to make any significant comparisons. In the postoperative period the nurse should observe the patient for hyperthermia or hypothermia as a reaction to the surgical procedures (Wagner 2006).

3 Patients with a susceptibility to infection, for example those with a low white blood cell count (less than 1000 cells/mm^3), or those undergoing radiotherapy, chemotherapy or steroid treatment, will require a more frequent observation of temperature. The fluctuation in temperature is influenced by the body's response to pyrogens. Immunocompromised patients are less able to respond to infection. Bacteraemia means a bacterial invasion of the bloodstream. Septic shock is a circulatory collapse as a result of severe infection. Pyrexia may be absent in those who are immunosuppressed or in the elderly (Neno 2005).

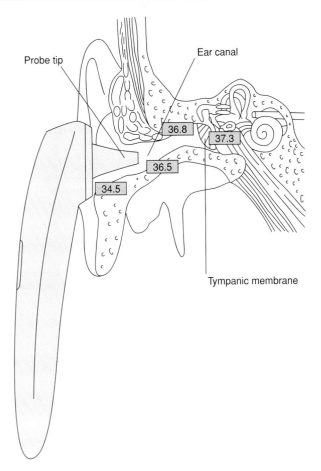

Probe tip

Ear canal

36.8

37.3

36.5

34.5

Tympanic membrane

Figure 18.17 Tympanic membrane thermometer.

4   Patients with a systemic or local infection require monitoring of temperature to assess development or regression of infection.
5   Pyrexia can occur when patients are receiving a blood transfusion but severe transfusion reactions usually occur within the first 15 minutes of starting (BCSH 1999).

Procedure guidelines   **Temperature measurement**

Equipment

1 Tympanic membrane thermometer.

2 Disposable probe covers.

Procedure

Action	Rationale
1 Explain and discuss procedure with the patient.	To ensure that the patient understands the procedure and gives his/her valid consent (NMC 2006: C; NMC 2008: C).
2 Wash and dry hands.	To minimize the risks of cross-infection and contamination (DH 2005: C).
3 Document to ensure the same ear is used for consecutive readings.	Anatomical differences between the two ears can result in a difference of up to 1°C (Jevon & Jevon 2001: C).
4 Remove thermometer from the base unit and ensure the lens is clean and not cracked. Use a dry wipe to clean if required.	Alcohol-based wipes should not be used as this can lead to a false low temperature measurement (Jevon & Jevon 2001: E).
5 Place disposable probe cover on the probe tip, ensuring the manufacturer's instructions are followed.	The probe cover protects the tip of the probe and is necessary for the functioning of the instrument (Jevon & Jevon 2001: E).
6 Gently place the probe tip in the ear canal to seal the opening, ensuring a snug fit.	To prevent air at the opening of the ear from entering it, causing a false low temperature measurement (Bayham *et al.* 1996: C; Jevon & Jevon 2001: E).
7 Press and release SCAN button.	To commence the instrument scanning (Bayham *et al.* 1996: C).
8 Remove probe tip from the ear as soon as the thermometer display reads DONE, usually indicated by beeps.	Measurement usually complete within 2 seconds (Bayham *et al.* 1996: C).
9 Read the temperature display.	Document in the patient's records (Jevon & Jevon 2001: C; NMC 2008: C).
10 Press RELEASE/EJECT button to discard probe cover.	Probe covers are for single use only (Jevon & Jevon 2001: E).
11 Wipe thermometer clean and replace in base unit.	To reduce the risk of cross-infection (DH 2005: C).

Urinalysis

Definition

Urinalysis is the analysis of the volume and physical, chemical and microscopic properties of urine which informs the practitioner about the state of the body (Tortora & Derrickson 2008).

Indications

The composition of urine can change dramatically as a result of disease processes. It may contain red blood cells, glucose, proteins, white blood cells or bile (Marieb & Hoehn 2007). The presence of such abnormalities in urine is an important warning sign of illness and may be helpful in clinical assessment in the following ways:

- Screening: for systemic disease, for example, diabetes mellitus or renal conditions.
- Diagnosis: to confirm or exclude suspected conditions, for example urinary tract infection.
- Management and planning: to ascertain as a baseline, monitor progress of an existing condition and/or plan programme of care and medication (Wilson 2005).

Reference material

Urine is formed in the kidneys, which process approximately 180 litres of blood-derived fluid a day. Approximately 1% of this total actually leaves the body as urine, the rest returns to the circulation (Marieb & Hoehn 2007). Urine formation, and the simultaneous adjustment of blood composition, involves three processes (Marieb & Hoehn 2007) (Figure 18.18):

- Glomerular filtration.
- Tubular reabsorption.
- Tubular secretion.

Glomerular filtration occurs in the glomeruli of the kidney, which act as non-selective filters. Filtration occurs as a result of increased glomerular blood pressure caused by the difference in diameter between afferent and efferent arterioles. The effect is a simple mechanical filter that permits substances smaller than plasma proteins to pass from the glomeruli to the glomerular capsule (Marieb & Hoehn 2007).

667

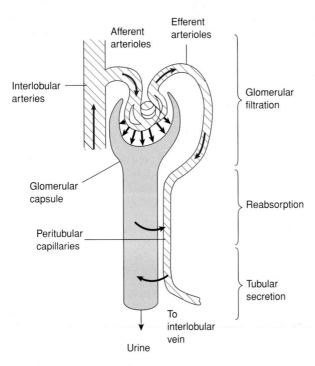

Figure 18.18   A nephron depicted diagrammatically to show the three major mechanisms by which urine is produced.

Tubular reabsorption then occurs, removing necessary substances from the filtrate and returning them to the peritubular capillaries. Tubular reabsorption is an active process that requires protein carriers and energy. Substances reabsorbed include nutrients and most ions. It is also a passive process, however, driven by electrochemical gradients. Substances reabsorbed in this way include sodium ions and water. Creatinine and the metabolites of drugs are not reabsorbed either because of their size, insolubility or a lack of carriers. Most of the nutrients, 80% of the water and sodium ions, and the majority of actively transported ions are reabsorbed in the proximal convoluted tubules (Marieb & Hoehn 2007).

Reabsorption is controlled by hormones. Aldosterone increases reabsorption of sodium (and hence also water), and antidiuretic hormone (ADH) enhances reabsorption of water in the collecting tubules (Marieb & Hoehn 2007).

Tubular secretion is both an active and a passive process in which the tubules excrete drugs, urea, excess ions and other substances into the filtrate. It plays an important part in maintaining the acid–base balance of blood (Marieb & Hoehn 2007).

Regulation of urine concentration and volume occurs in the loop of Henle, where the osmolarity of the filtrate is controlled. As the filtrate flows through the tubules the permeability of the walls controls how dilute or concentrated the resulting urine will be. In the absence of ADH, dilute urine is formed because the filtrate is not reabsorbed as it passes through the kidneys. As levels of ADH increase, the collecting tubules become more permeable and water moves out of the filtrate back into the blood. Consequently, smaller amounts of more concentrated urine are produced (Marieb & Hoehn 2007).

Characteristics of urine

Urine is typically clear, pale to deep yellow in colour and slightly acidic (pH 6) (Rigby & Gray 2005), though pH can change as a result of metabolic processes or diet. Vomiting and bacterial infection of the urinary tract can cause urine to become alkaline. Urinary specific gravity ranges from 1.001 to 1.035, according to how concentrated the urine is (Fillingham & Douglas 2003; Marieb & Hoehn 2007).

The colour of urine is due to a pigment called urochrome which is derived from the body's destruction of haemoglobin. The more concentrated urine is the deeper yellow it becomes. Changes in colour may reflect diet (e.g. beetroot or rhubarb), or may be due to blood or bile in the urine (Marieb & Hoehn 2007). Often fresh urine appears turbid (cloudy), indicating there may be an infection of the urinary tract. The urinary tract is the most common site of bacterial infection. There are many predisposing factors (Figure 18.19), the most common of which is instrumentation, that is, cystoscopy and urinary catheterization (Bayer Diagnostics 1997).

Bacteriuria is defined as the presence of bacteria in the urine (Rigby & Gray 2005). Urine specimens are rarely sterile, as a result of contamination with periurethral flora during collection. Infection is distinguished by counting the number of bacteria. Significant bacteriuria is defined as a presence of more than 10^5 organisms per ml of urine in the presence of clinical symptoms. Covert bacteriuria is the presence of more than 10^5 organisms per ml of urine without clinical symptoms (Marini & Wheeler 2006) (Figure 18.20).

Fresh urine smells slightly aromatic. This can change as a result of disease processes such as diabetes mellitus, when acetone is present in the urine, giving it a fruity smell. The composition of urine can change dramatically as a result of disease, and abnormal substances may be present. Urinalysis can identify many

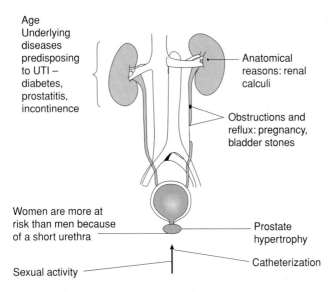

Figure 18.19 Diagramatic representation of predisposition to UTIs.

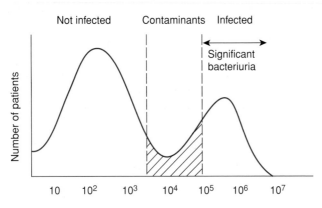

Figure 18.20 Significant bacteriuria. Specimens of urine are rarely sterile. A cut-off point is identified to distinguish true infection (significant bacteriuria) from effects of contamination from surrounding tissues.

of these substances, and should be part of every physical assessment (Cook 1996; Torrance & Elley 1998).

Renal clearance is the rate at which the kidneys clear a particular chemical from the plasma in a given time. Renal clearance tests are done to determine the glomerular filtration rate (GFR), which provides information about the amount of functioning renal tissue. Renal clearance tests are also done to detect glomerular damage and to follow the progress of renal disease (Marieb & Hoehn 2007).

Dipstick (reagent) tests

Strips that have been impregnated with chemicals are dipped quickly in urine and read as a means of testing urine. When dipped in urine, the chemicals react with abnormal substances and change colour. Although dipstick reagents have been primarily used as screening tools for protein or glucose in the urine, more sophisticated reagents are now available. These reagents test for nitrites and leucocyte esterase as indicators of bacterial infection. Leucocyte esterase is an enzyme from neutrophils not normally found in urine and is a marker of infection. Nitrites are produced by the bacterial breakdown of dietary nitrate, which is a waste product of protein metabolism (Rigby & Gray 2005). It is essential to use the strips according to the manufacturer's instructions and be aware of factors that may affect the results. These factors include specific drugs (Table 18.7), the quality of the urine specimen itself and the possibility that false negative results are possible.

In the microbiology laboratory, urine samples constitute about 40% of the total workload; of these, 70–80% of samples are not infected. This means that much time, energy and finances are wasted on unnecessary sample processing and investigation (Bayer Diagnostics 1997).

Further testing may be necessary, such as culture and sensitivity testing under laboratory conditions, to identify organisms responsible for infection and to determine the most effective treatment (Wilson 2005) (Table 18.8). Twenty-four hour collection is also used to measure substances such as steroids, white cells, electrolytes or to determine urine osmolarity (Tortora & Derrickson 2008).

Procedure guidelines   **Urinalysis**

. . . .

Procedure

Action	Rationale
1 Store reagent sticks in accordance with manufacturer's instructions. This is usually a dark dry place.	Tests may depend on enzymic reaction. To ensure reliable results (Bayer Diagnostics 2006: C).

. . . .

Procedure guidelines *(cont.)*

2 Explain and discuss the procedure with the patient.	To ensure that the patient understands the procedure and gives his/her valid consent (NMC 2006: C; NMC 2008: C).
3 Wash and dry hands.	To maintain infection control and prevent cross-infection (DH 2005: C).
4 Obtain clean specimen of fresh urine from patient.	Urine that has been stored deteriorates rapidly and can give false results (Bayer Diagnostics 2006: C).
5 Dip the reagent strip into the urine. The strip should be completely immersed in the urine and then removed immediately. Run edge of strip along the container. This will remove excess urine and prevent mixing of chemicals from adjacent reagent areas (Bayer Diagnostics 2006: C).	To remove any excess urine (Bayer Diagnostics 2006: C).
6 Hold the stick at an angle.	Urine reagent strips should not be held upright when reading them because urine may run from square to square, mixing various reagents (Bayer Diagnostics 2006: C).
7 Wait the required time interval before reading the strip against the colour chart (see Action figure 7).	The strips must be read at exactly the time interval specified, or the reagents will not have time to react, or may be inaccurate (Bayer Diagnostics 2006: C).

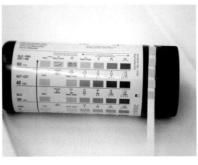

Action 7   Comparing urinalysis results.

Table 18.7 Routine observations of urine: possible indications and plan of action. Modified from Rigby and Gray (2005).

Observation	Possible indications	Plan of action
Colour		
Green	Pseudomonas infection, presence of bilirubin	Culture and microscopy
	Excretion of cytotoxic agents, e.g. Mitomycin or substances, e.g. Methylene Blue	Discard with care
Pink/Red	Blood	Culture and microscopy. If currently receiving chemotherapy, e.g. Ifosfamide, further mesna may need to be given. Discard with care
	Excretion of cytotoxic agents, e.g. Doxorubicin	
Orange	Excess urobiliogen, Rifampicin	Discard
Yellow	Bilirubin	Discard
Brown	Bilirubin	Discard
Odour		
Fishy	Infection	Culture and microscopy
Sweet smelling	Ketones	Culture and microscopy
Debris		
Cloudy	Infection, stale urine	Culture and microscopy
Sediment	Infection, contamination	Culture and microscopy

Blood glucose

Definition

The body regulates the blood glucose levels by producing insulin. Insulin's main effect is to lower the blood glucose level, but it also influences protein and fat metabolism. If the pancreas fails to produce sufficient insulin, the level of glucose in the blood will remain high. Conversely, if too much insulin is made, or given,

Table 18.8   How drugs may influence the results of reagent sticks.

Drug	Reagent test	Effect on the results
Ascorbic acid	Glucose, blood, nitrite	High concentrations may diminish colour
L-Dopa	Glucose	High concentrations may give a false negative reaction
	Ketones	Atypical colour
Nalidixic acid	Urobilinogen	Atypical colour
Probenacid		
Phenazopyridine (pyridium)	Protein	May give atypical colour
	Ketones	Coloured metabolites may mask a small reaction
	Urobilinogen, bilirubin	May mimic a positive reaction
	Nitrite	
Rifampicin	Bilirubin	Coloured metabolites may mask a small reaction
Salicylates (aspirin)	Glucose	High doses may give a false negative reaction

then the level of glucose in the blood remains low. For optimum cell function, blood glucose levels should be maintained normally at a level of 4–7 mmol/l (Ferguson 2005).

Indications

Blood glucose monitoring is used to indicate when blood glucose is not within the normal range. Conditions where a patient's blood glucose may need careful monitoring are:

- To make a diagnosis of diabetes mellitus, which is only confirmed following a glucose tolerance test (Burden 2001).
- In the acute management of unstable diabetic states: diabetic ketoacidosis, hyperosmolar non-ketotic coma and hypoglycaemia.
- To make a diagnosis of hypoglycaemia.
- To monitor and manage the treatment of both insulin-dependent diabetes mellitus (IDDM or type one) and non-insulin-dependent diabetes mellitus (NIDDM or type two).

Reference material

To maintain normal blood glucose levels, insulin and the counter-regulatory hormones, or stress hormones, must be in balance. These hormones, which include adrenaline, noradrenaline, cortisol, growth hormone and glucagon, are released in the event of stress (Sharp 1993).

During infection, major surgery or critical illness, people's regulatory hormone levels of cortisol, noradrenaline and glucagon will rise in response to the stressful event. This stimulates glycogen and fat breakdown, which causes the blood glucose levels to rise. In a healthy individual, insulin production would increase. In a person who is unable to raise his/her insulin levels, e.g. a diabetic, the result is hyperglycaemia (Curry & Weedon 1993). The majority of people who have diabetes will be known to be diabetic prior to this event, but as many as one million people in the UK have the condition and do not know it (Diabetes UK 2000). However, there may be a proportion who have had no history of such a disorder, only becoming diabetic in response to their primary illness and treatment. An example of this is steroid-induced diabetes. This diagnosis does not mean that they will remain a diabetic, but that they may need careful monitoring after their recovery.

Hypoglycaemia

Hypoglycaemia is described as a blood glucose level that is unable to meet the metabolic demands of the body (Marini & Wheeler 2006). Often young and healthy individuals can be asymptomatic during this inadequate level of glucose in the blood. Early symptoms are sweating, tremor, weakness, nervousness, tachycardia and hypertension. These symptoms depend upon not only the absolute blood glucose value but, also the rate of its decline. Severe hypoglycaemia causes mental disorientation, convulsions, unconsciousness and shock (Tortora & Derrickson 2008). The most common factors associated with hypoglycaemia include missed or delayed meals, eating less food at a meal than planned, vigorous exercise without carbohydrate compensation, taking too much diabetes medication (e.g. insulin) and drinking alcohol (Briscoe & Davis 2006).

Other causes of hypoglycaemia are:

- Infection, which can result in hepatic failure, renal insufficiency, depletion of muscle glycogen and starvation.
- Alcohol, which suppresses glyconeogenesis and nutritional intake. This induces a low insulin state, ketone production and fatty acid release.
- Hepatic failure, which can be due to tumour infiltration, cirrhosis or hepatic necrosis.
- Renal failure.

675

- Salicylate poisoning.
- Insulin-secreting tumours.
- Surgery.

(Marini & Wheeler 2006.)

Treatment should be by the administration of glucose. The route will depend on the conscious level of the individual and the treatment the patient has undergone. In all cases of hypoglycaemia it is vital to closely monitor the patient and recheck the serum glucose 1–2 hourly (Marini & Wheeler 2006).

Hyperglycaemia

When insulin is deficient or absent, blood glucose levels remain high after a meal. This is because insulin acts like a key, unlocking a door to allow glucose to enter the cell. If insulin is absent, the glucose is unable to enter most cells. When blood glucose levels rise, hyperglycaemic hormones are not released, but when glucose levels become excessive (hyperglycaemia) the person will feel nauseated, which precipitates the flight or fight response (Marieb & Hoehn 2007). The cells are starved of glucose and the body reacts inappropriately by producing reactions usually seen in states of fasting (hypoglycaemia). Processes such as glycogenolysis (the breakdown of glycogen to release glucose), lipolysis (the breakdown of stored fats into glycerol and fatty acids) and gluconeogenesis (the conversion of glycerol and amino acids into glucose) are instigated (Marieb & Hoehn 2007).

The blood glucose continues to rise and some of the glucose is excreted in the urine. As the level of glucose in the kidney increases, water reabsorption by the tubules becomes inhibited. This causes the body to excrete large amounts of urine (polyuria). The person will feel excessively thirsty (polydipsia) and will pass urine often and in large quantities. The person may also feel extremely hungry (polyphagia). The combination of polydipsia and polyuria will lead to dehydration, a fall in blood pressure and electrolyte imbalance. The acid–base imbalance caused by the loss of sodium (hyponatremia) and potassium (hypokalaemia) leads to the person complaining of symptoms spanning from muscle cramps, nausea, vomiting and diarrhoea to confusion, lethargy, cardiac events and coma (Marini & Wheeler 2006).

Even though there is excessive glucose in the body, the body cannot utilize it, so an alternative source of energy has to be found. To compensate, the body starts to break down its fats and protein stores for energy metabolism (Marieb & Hoehn 2007). Figure 18.21 summarizes the consequences of insulin deficiency. Fats are mobilized, which leads to high levels of fatty acids in the blood (lipidaemia). This can also cause sudden and dramatic weight loss. The fatty acid metabolites, known as ketones, accumulate in the blood more rapidly than they can be excreted or used. The blood pH will fall, resulting in ketoacidosis and ketones being excreted into the urine. If ketoacidosis is allowed to continue it

Organs/tissue involved	Organ/tissue responses to insulin deficiency	Resulting conditions:		Signs and symptoms
		In blood	In urine	
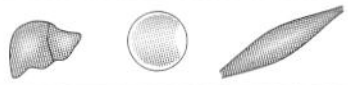	Decreased glucose uptake and utilization	Hyperglycaemia	Glycosuria	
	Glycogenolysis		Osmotic diuresis	Polydipsia (and fatigue, weight loss)
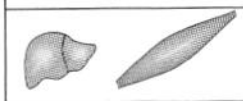	Protein catabolism and gluconeogenesis			Polyphagia
	Lipolysis and ketogenesis	Lipidaemia and ketoacidosis	Ketonuria	Acetone breath
				Hyperpnoea
			Loss of Na+, K+; electrolyte and acid–base imbalances	Nausea/vomiting/ abdominal pain
				Cardiac irregularities
				Central nervous system depression; coma

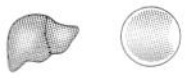

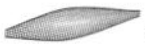

= Muscle   = Adipose tissue   = Liver

Figure 18.21 Consequences of insulin deficiency.

can become life-threatening as it disrupts all physiological processes, including oxygen transportation and heart activity. Depression of the nervous system leads to coma and death (Marieb & Hoehn 2007).

Diabetic ketoacidosis is a common but serious condition, the mortality of which remains significant, despite aggressive treatment (Marini & Wheeler 2006). It is a result of a deficiency of insulin and a high level of stress hormones. In the diabetic patient it is usually precipitated by a poor diet and inadequate medication and can be brought on by infection. Stroke, MI, trauma, pregnancy, pancreatitis and hypothyroidism are also potential precipitants (Marini & Wheeler 2006). The most prominent metabolic changes caused by ketoacidosis are metabolic acidosis and volume depletion.

Treatment involves fluid replacement, restoration of the acid–base imbalance and careful monitoring. If patients in a ketoacidotic state do not respond to fluid replacement and correction of the pH, then other conditions such as septic shock, bleeding, adrenal insufficiency, MI and pancreatitis should be considered, and treated accordingly (Marini & Wheeler 2006).

The administration of intravenous insulin should be titrated by an infusion device, and measurements of blood glucose should be taken 1–2 hourly in order to guide the rate of insulin and fluid delivery. If the blood glucose level does not fall within the first few hours it may indicate insulin resistance and the amount of insulin may need to be increased (Marini & Wheeler 2006).

Note: care needs to be taken in the rapid reversal of fluid loss and electrolyte imbalance. Excessive fluids can cause sudden acid–base shifts and exacerbate hypokalaemia. Central nervous system acidosis and arrhythmias are preventable with constant monitoring. Once urine flow is re-established, potassium should be given. Magnesium and phosphate levels in the blood should also be monitored. A common complication after aggressive treatment is hypoglycaemia.

Blood glucose monitoring

Monitoring a patient's blood glucose provides an accurate indication of how the body is controlling glucose metabolism. In the short term, monitoring can prevent hypoglycaemia and ketoacidosis, and in the long term it can significantly reduce the risk of complications which affect the vascular and neural pathways by helping to maintain near-normal glucose levels (UKPDS 1998).

An advantage of blood glucose testing is that the use of blood can inform people with diabetes that their blood sugar is low or high, whereas a urine test can only indicate instances of high blood sugar (Burden 2001). The immediacy of results allows patients to receive appropriate care and advice. Blood samples can be taken from capillary, venous or arterial routes. The vessel used will depend on the accessibility of obtaining the blood sample, the frequency of testing and the condition of the patient. However, a meta-analysis questions the clinical efficiency and effectiveness of blood glucose self-monitoring (Coster et al. 2000).

It is essential that both the correct equipment is used and the operator is trained and proficient in its operation. Many different monitoring devices are currently available. Nursing and medical research has now been undertaken to identify the most accurate and practicable equipment (Trajanoski et al. 1996; Chan et al. 1997; Cowan 1997; Rumley 1997; Kirk & Rheney 1998; Batki et al. 1999).

Current methods for testing blood glucose rely on finger pricking but non-invasive blood glucose monitoring devices are being developed which would enable automatic detection of hypoglycaemia or hyperglycaemia (American Diabetes Association 2001). Non-invasive monitoring means checking blood glucose levels without puncturing the skin for a blood sample. One device approved is worn like a wristwatch and measures blood glucose via interstitial fluid (Pickup 2000).

Point-of-care testing (POCT), sometimes referred to as near-patient testing, is any test performed for a patient by a health care professional outside the laboratory setting (MDA 2002a). There is a significant risk for errors to occur when using POCT. The Department of Health (DH) issued a hazard warning in 1987 and again in a 1996 safety notice. These warnings highlighted the need for formal training and strict quality control (DH 1996). Quality assurance in relation to POCT is defined as the measures taken to ensure the test results are reliable (MDA 2002a); this also aims to maintain the competency of all users. These hazard notices drew attention to the fact that a management or therapeutic decision based on an unreliable blood glucose result can prove fatal. Inaccurate results are often due to incorrect timing of the test, insufficient amount of blood taken and smearing of the sample (Heenan 1990). Staff undertaking POCT should be aware that certain patient conditions may lead to false and misleading results. The testing of blood glucose in the blood may be affected by the following:

- Hyperlipaemia (containing abnormal fat concentrations, for example cholesterol above 56.5 mmol/l). May elevate readings.
- Haematocrit values. If extremely high, i.e. above 55%, and blood glucose values are above 11 mmol/l, the value may be up to 15% too low. If the haematocrit level is low, i.e. less than 35%, the value may be up to 10% too high.
- Dialysis treatment. May elevate readings.
- Bilirubin values above 0.43 mmol/l, e.g. in jaundice. May elevate readings.
- Intravenous infusion of ascorbic acid (vitamin C). May depress readings.
- When there has been peripheral circulatory failure, e.g. following severe dehydration caused by hyperglycaemic–hyperosmolar state with or without ketoacidosis, hypotension, shock or peripheral vascular disease. In these cases the results of the blood sample taken from the peripheral blood, e.g. from a finger prick, may be much lower than laboratory measurements taken from venous or arterial sources. In these cases treatment should be based on laboratory measurements only (Sandler *et al.* 1990).

The DH report (1996) highlights that there must be standardization in training, reliability and quality control. In order to achieve this, the following aspects need to be considered when selecting POCT blood glucose monitoring equipment:

1 Equipment is designed for use by non-laboratory staff and is suitable for use in the clinical environment.
2 All the equipment used is compatible and will give reliable results.
3 The biochemistry laboratory is involved in the purchase and maintenance of the equipment. This may involve the purchase of one type of device from one company for the whole hospital, to reduce costs and provide standardization (Lowes 1995).
4 The product should be easy to use and the staff should be involved in the choice of the device (Kirk & Rheney 1998).
5 The ongoing cost and maintenance of the device need to be considered; this should include buying strips, control solutions and the replacement of devices (Kirk & Rheney 1998).
6 There are written standard operating procedures available and kept with the device.
7 Training is given to the operators and records are kept of this. After training the following learning outcomes should be demonstrated by the operator (MDA 2002a):

679

(a) Knowledge of the basic principle of measurement and normal ranges.
(b) The proper use of the equipment as laid down by the operating instructions and specifications (Bayne 1997).
(c) The consequences of improper use.
(d) Health and safety procedures for the collection of blood samples, i.e. to prevent spillage and needlestick injuries.
(e) The importance of complete documentation.
(f) Use of appropriate calibration and quality control techniques.
(g) An understanding that blood sugar analysis should only be used as a guide and a tool, with diagnosis and treatment decisions being based on confirmed laboratory results (DH 1996).

There is a requirement to monitor the quality of the results of the device and the person operating it. This is both a hospital and a government directive (MDA 2002a). Independent quality control should be carried out with the collaboration of the biochemistry laboratory. External auditing of quality control should be undertaken and this may be provided in the package offered by the company.

Procedure guidelines   Blood glucose monitoring

Only nursing staff who have obtained a certificate of training for the equipment should undertake this task.

Equipment

1 Blood glucose monitor.
2 Test strips.
3 Control solution.

4 Single-use safety lancets.
5 Gloves.

Procedure

Action	Rationale
1 Before taking the device to the patient the monitor needs to be checked for the following: (a) That one pack of test strips is open and has not been left exposed to the air and that they are in date. (b) That the monitor and the test strips have been calibrated together. (c) That if a new pack of strips is required, the monitor is recalibrated.	To ensure accuracy of the result. The quality control and checks have been carried out in order to ensure the safety of the patient (Roche Diagnostics 2004: C).

(d) That a high and low internal quality control test is carried out prior to any patient sample being measured.

(e) That the result of the internal quality control is recorded in the equipment log book and signed.

2 Explain the procedure to the patient. Some patients may want to look away at the sight of a needle.	The patient should be aware of the procedure in order to allay some of his/her anxieties, and to be able to co-operate in the procedure (NMC 2008: C).
3 Patients should be advised to wash their hands prior to blood sampling. The use of alcohol rub should be avoided. Encourage patients to keep their hands warm until sampling has been performed.	To ensure a non-contaminated result. To encourage good blood flow (Cowan 1997: E).
4 Ask the patient to sit or lie down.	To ensure the patient's safety as some patients may feel faint when blood is taken (Roche Diagnostics 2004: C).
5 Wash your hands, and put on gloves.	To minimize the risk of cross-infection. To minimize the risk of contamination (DH 2005: C).
6 Use a single-use lancet (DH 1996) and if the lancet has depth settings ensure correct setting (most commonly the middle setting (Roche Diagnostics 2004).	To minimize the risk of cross-infection and accidental needlestick injury. Disposable lancets are advised following an outbreak of hepatitis B in French and US hospitals (DH 1996; Roche Diagnositcs 2004: C).
7 Take a blood sample from the side of the finger using the lancet, ensuring that the site of piercing is rotated. Avoid frequent use of the index finger and thumb. The finger may bleed without assistance, or may need assistance by 'milking' to form a droplet of blood which is large enough to cover the test pad.	The side of the finger is used as it is less painful and easier to obtain a hanging droplet of blood. The site is rotated to reduce the risk of infection from multiple stabbing, the areas becoming toughened and to reduce pain (Roche Diagnostics 2004: C).

Procedure guidelines *(cont.)*

8 Apply the blood to the testing strip. Some test strips are hydrophilic and are dosed/filled from the side and are not dropped directly onto the strip.	The window on the test strip allows verification of a correctly dosed strip (Roche Diagnostics 2004: C).
9 Dispose of lancet in a container designed for sharps.	To reduce the risk of needlestick injury (Roche Diagnostics 2004: C).
10 Depending on the type of monitor, the procedure will differ. See individual manuals and hospital policies.	To ensure the accuracy of the result (Roche Diagnostics 2004: C).
11 Once the result is obtained, record immediately.	To ensure the accuracy of the result (Roche Diagnostics 2004: C).
12 Dispose of waste appropriately. Remove gloves and dispose.	To reduce the risk of cross-infection (DH 2005: C).
13 Make the patient comfortable and observe site of test for bleeding.	To ensure the patient's comfort (E).
14 Wash and dry hands.	To prevent cross-infection (DH 2005: C).

References and further reading

Adam, S. & Osborne, S. (2005) *Critical Care Nursing: Science and Practice*. Oxford University Press, Oxford.

American Diabetes Association (2001) Clinical practice recommendations. *Diabetes Care*, **24**, 580–2.

Angerami, E.L.S. (1980) Epidemiological study of body temperature in patients in a teaching hospital. *Int J Nurs Stud*, **17**, 91–9.

Armstrong, R.S. (2002) Nurse's knowledge of error in blood pressure measurement technique. *Int J Nurs Prac*, **8**(3), 118–26.

Baillie, L. (2001) *Developing Practical Nursing Skills*. Arnold, London.

Batki, A. *et al.* (1999) Selecting blood glucose monitoring systems. *Prof Nurse*, **14**(10), 715–23.

Bayer Diagnostics (1997) *Urinary Tract Infection*. Technical Information Bulletin No. 8. Bayer Diagnostics, Newbury.

Bayer Diagnostics (2006) *Your Practical Guide to Urine Analysis*. Bayer Diagnostics, Newbury.

Bayham, E. *et al.* (1996) *First Temp Genius. Clinical Considerations for Use of First Temp & First Temp Genius Infrared Tympanic Thermometers*. Sherwood Medical Company, USA.

Bayne, C. (1997) How sweet it is: glucose monitoring equipment and interpretation. *Nurs Manage*, **28**(9), 52–4.

BCSH (1999) The administration of blood and blood components and the management of transfused patients. *Transfus Med*, **9**, 227–38.

Beevers, M. & Beevers, G.B. (1996) Blood pressure measurement in the next century, a plea for stability. *Blood Press Monit*, **1**(2), 117–20.

Beevers, G., Lip, G.Y.H. & O'Brien, E. (2001a) Blood pressure measurement, part 1. Sphygmomanometry: factors common to all techniques. *BMJ*, **322**(7292), 981–5.

Beevers, G., Lip, G.Y.H. & O'Brien, E. (2001b) Blood pressure measurement, part 2. Conventional spyygmomanometry: technique of auscultatory blood pressure measurement. *BMJ*, **322**(7292), 1043–7.

Berger, A. (2001) How does it work? Oscillatory blood pressure monitoring devices. *BMJ*, **323**(7318), 9–19.

Bickley, L. & Szilagyi, P. (2007) *Bates' Guide to Physical Examination and History Taking*, 9th edn. Lippincott Williams & Wilkins, Philadelphia.

Bogan, B., Kritzer, S. & Deane, D. (1993) Nursing student compliance to standards for blood pressure measurement. *J Nurse Educ*, **32**(2), 90–2.

Bone, R.C. (1996) The pathogenesis of sepsis and rationale for new treatments. Proceedings of the International Intensive Care Conference, Barcelona.

Booker, R. (2004) Best practice in the use of spirometry. *Nurs Stand*, **19**(48), 149–54.

Braun, S.K., Preston, P. & Smith, R.N. (1998) Getting a better read on thermometry. *Reg Nur*, **61**(3), 57–60.

Briscoe, V.J & Davis, S.N. (2006) Hypoglycemia in type 1 and 2 diabetes: physiology, pathophysiology and management. *Clinical Diabetes*, **24**(3), 115–21.

British Hypertension Society (BHS) (2006) FACT FILE 01/2006. www.bhsoc.org/bhf-factfiles/bhf-factfile-Jan2006.doc. Accessed 21/11/07.

British Thoracic Society (2004) British guidelines on the management of asthma, revised edition. www.brit-thoracic.org.uk/guidelines%201997_asthma_html. Accessed 01/07.

British Thoracic Society Standards of Care Committee (1997) Current best practice for nebuliser treatment. *Thorax*, **52**(Suppl 2), S1-S3.

Burden, M. (2001) Diabetes blood glucose monitoring. *Nurs Times*, **97**(8), 36–9.

Burke, K. (1996) The tympanic membrane thermometer in paediatrics: a review of the literature. *Accid Emerg Nurs*, **4**(4), 190–3.

Campbell, N.R. *et al.* (1990) Accurate, reproducible measurement of blood pressure. *Can Med Assoc J*, **143**(1), 19–24.

Carney, S.L. *et al.* (1995) Hospital sphygmomanometer use; an audit. *J Qual Clin Pract*, **15**(1), 17–22.

Carroll, M. (2000) An evaluation of temperature measurement. *Nurs Stand*, **14**(44), 39–43.

Chan, J. *et al.* (1997) Accuracy, precision and user-acceptability of self blood glucose monitoring machines. *Diabetes Res Clin Pract*, **36**(2), 91–104.

Cook, R. (1996) Urinalysis: ensuring accurate urine testing. *Nurs Stand*, **10**(46), 49–55.

Coster, S. *et al.* (2000) Self monitoring in type 2 diabetes mellitus: a meta-analysis. *Diabet Med*, **17**(11), 755–61.

Cowan, T. (1997) Blood glucose monitoring devices. *Prof Nurse*, **12**(8), 593–7.

Cuddy, M. (2004) The effects of drugs on thermoregulation. *Advanced Practice in Acute Critical Care*, **15**(2), 238–53.

Curry, M. & Weedon, L. (1993) Balancing act. *Nurs Times*, **89**(23), 50–2.

DH (1996) *Extra-Laboratory Use of Blood Glucose Meters and Test Strips: Contraindications, Training and Advice to Users.* Medical Devices Agency Adverse Incident Centre Safety Notice 9616, June. Department of Health, London.

DH (2005) *Saving Lives: a Delivery Programme to Reduce Healthcare Associated Infection Including MRSA: Skills for Implementation.* Department of Health, London. See www.dh.gov.uk/publications. Accessed 01/07.

Diabetes UK (2000) *Diabetes in the UK – The Missing Millions.* Diabetes UK, London.

Dickinson, A. & Martindale, G. (2002) Caring for the patient with a respiratory disorder. In: *Watson's Clinical Nursing and Related Sciences* (ed. M. Walsh), 6th edn. Bailliere Tindal, Edinburgh, pp. 333–370.

Dobbin, K. (2002) Noninvasive blood pressure monitoring protocols for practice: applying research at the bedside. *Crit Care Nurse*, **22**(2), 123–4.

Docherty, B. (2000) Temperature recording. *Prof Nurse*, **16**(3), 943.

Docherty, B. (2002) Cardiorespiratory physical assessment for the acutely ill. *Br J Nurs*, **11**(11), 750–8.

Docherty, B. (2005) The arteriovenous system: part one, the anatomy. *Nurs Times*, **101**(34), 28–9.

Docherty, B. & Coote, S. (2006) Monitoring the pulse as part of the track and trigger. *Nurs Times*, **102**(43), 28–9. See www.nursingtimes.net/nursingtimes/pages/monitoringthepulse-aspartoftrackandtrigger. Accessed 18/12/06.

Edmonds, C. *et al.* (2006) Disorders of the respiratory system. In: *Nursing Practice, Hospital & Home, the Adult* (eds M. Alexander, J. Fawcett & P. Runciman). Churchill Livingstone, London, pp. 73–103.

Edwards, S. (1997) Measuring temperature. *Prof Nurse*, **13**(2), 55–7.

Edwards, S.L. (2000) Maintaining an adequate circulation. In: *Surgical Nursing Advanced Practice* (eds K. Manley & L. Bellman). Churchill Livingstone, London, pp. 507–37.

Edwards, L. & Manley, K.L. (1998) *Care of Adults in Hospital.* Edward Arnold, London.

Evans, D. *et al.* (2004) *Vital Signs.* The Joanna Briggs Institute, Australia.

Feher, M. & Harris St. John, K. (1992) Blood pressure measurement by junior hospital doctors: a gap in medical education? *Health Trends*, **24**(2), 59–61.

Ferguson, A. (2005) Blood glucose monitoring. *Nurs Times*, **101**(38), 28–9.

Fillingham, S. & Douglas, J. (2003) *Urological Nursing*, 3rd edn. Bailliere Tindal, London.

Gallimore, D. (2004) Reviewing the effectiveness of tympanic thermometers. *Nurs Times*, **100**(32), 32–5.

Gilbert, M., Barton, A.J. & Counsell, C.M. (2002) Comparison of oral and tympanic temperatures in adult surgical patients. *Appl Nurs Res*, **15**(1), 42–7.

Gillespie, A. & Curzio, J. (1998) Blood pressure measurement: assessing staff knowledge. *Nurs Stand*, **12**(23), 35–7.

GINA (2006) Global strategy for asthma management and prevention. www.ginasthma.org. Accessed 4/12/06.

Grap, M. (2002) Protocols for practice, applying research at the bedside. *Crit Care Nurse*, **22**(3), 69–74.

Gregg, I. & Nunn, A.J. (1989) New regression equations for predicting peak flow expiratory flow in adults. *BMJ*, **298**, 1068–70.

Harper, J. (2004) Post-anaesthesia care unit nurses' knowledge of pulse oximetry. *J Nurs Staff Dev*, **20**(4), 177–80.

Hasler, M. & Cohen, J. (1982) The effect of oxygen administration on oral temperature assessment. *Nurs Res*, **31**, 265–8.

Hatchett, R. (2000) Central venous pressure measurement. *Nurs Times*, **96**(15), 49–50.

Heenan, A. (1990) Blood glucose measurement. *Nurs Times*, **86**(4), 65–8.

Heindenreich, T. & Giuffe, M. (1990) Postoperative temperature measurement. *Nurs Res*, **39**(3), 153–5.

Henderson, N. (1997) Central venous lines. *Nurs Stand*, **11**(42), 49–56.

Hill, M.N. & Grim, C.M. (1991) How to take a precise blood pressure. *Am J Nurs*, **91**(2), 38–42.

Howell, M. (2002) The correct use of pulse oximetry in measuring oxygen status. *Prof Nurse*, **17**(7), 416–18.

Hudek, C.M., Gallo, B.M. & Morton, P.G. (1998). *Critical Care Nursing: a Holistic Approach*, 7th edn. Lippincott, New York.

Jensen, B.N. *et al.* (1994) The superiority of rectal thermometry to oral thermometry with regard to accuracy. *J Adv Nurs*, **20**, 660–5.

Jevon, P. (2000) Pulse oximetry – 2. *Nurs Times*, **96**(27), 43–4.

Jevon, P. & Jevon, M. (2001) Using a tympanic thermometer. *Nurs Times*, **97**(9), 43–4.

Keenan, J. (1995) Pulse oximetry (cardiology update). *Nurs Stand*, **9**, 35–55.

Kemp, F., Foster, C. & McKinlay, S. (1994) How effective is training for blood pressure measurement? *Prof Nurs*, **9**(8), 521–4.

Khorshid, L. *et al.* (2005) Comparing mercury-in-glass, tympanic and disposable thermometers in measuring body temperature in healthy young people. *J Clin Nurs*, **14**(4), 496–500.

Kirk, J. & Rheney, C. (1998) Important factors of blood glucose meters. *J Am Pharm Assoc*, **8**(2), 210–19.

Knies, R. (2003) Temperature measurement in acute care: the who, what, where, when, why, and how? www.enw.org/Research-Thermometry.htm. Accessed 30/1/07.

Krikler, S. (1990) Pyrexia: what to do about temperatures. *Nurs Stand*, **4**(25), 37–8.

Kumar, P. & Clark, M. (2005) *Clinical Medicine*, 6th edn. Elsevier Saunders, Edinburgh.

Lemery, R. *et al.* (2003) Anatomic description of Bachmann's bundle and its relation to the atria septum. *Am J Cardiol*, **91**(12), 1482–5.

Lim-Levy, F. (1982) The effect of oxygen inhalation on oral temperature. *Nurs Res*, **31**, 150–2.

Lowes, L. (1995) Accuracy in ward-based blood glucose monitoring. *Nurs Times*, **91**(13), 44–5.

Mancia, G. *et al.* (1987) Alerting reaction and rise in blood pressure during measurement by physician and nurse. *Hypertension*, **9**, 209–15.

Marieb, E.M. & Hoehn, K. (2007) *Human Anatomy and Physiology*. Pearson Benjamin Cummings, San Francisco.

Marini, J.J. & Wheeler, A.P. (2006) *Critical Care Medicine: the Essentials*. Lippincott Williams & Wilkins, Philadelphia.

Markandu, N.D. *et al.* (2000) The mercury sphygmomanometer should be abandoned before it is prescribed. *J Hum Hypertens*, **14**(3136), 31–6.

Maxon, P. (2004) Mercury flows in Europe and the World: the impact of decommissioned Chlor-Alkali plants. European Commission, Brussels.

McAlister, F.A. & Straus, S. (2001) Evidence based treatment for hypertension – measurement of blood pressure an evidence based review. *BMJ*, **322**, 908–11.

MDA (2002a) Self monitoring in type 2 diabetes mellitus: a meta-analysis. *Diabet Med*, **17**(11), 755–61.

MDA (2002b) *Management and Use of IVD Point-of-Care Test Devices*. Medical Devices Agency, London.

Metcalfe, H. (2000) Recording a 12-lead electrocardiogram – 1. *Nurs Times*, **96**(19), 43–4.

MHRA (2001) Tissue necrosis caused by pulse oximeter probes. SN2001(08). www.mhra.gov.uk/home. Go to publications and safety notices. Accessed 7/12/2006.

MHRA (2005) Report of the independent advisory group on blood pressure monitoring in clinical practice. www.mhra.gov.uk/home. Go to medical advice alerts. Accessed 7/12/06.

MHRA (2006) Medical device alert ref. MDA/2006/037. Blood pressure monitors and sphygmomanometers.www.mhra.gov. uk/home. Accessed 7/12/2006.

Minor, D.G. & Waterhouse, J.M. (1981) *Circadian Rhythms and the Human*. Wright, Bristol.

Mooney, G. (2003) What you need to know about central venous lines. *Nurs Times*, **99**(10), 28–29.

Morton, P.G., Tucker, T. & Van Rueden, R. (2005) *Critical Care Nursing: a Holistic Approach*, 8th edn. Lippincott Williams & Wilkins, Philadelphia.

Nakamura, K. *et al.* (1997) Oral temperatures in the elderly in nursing homes in summer and winter in relation to activities of daily living. *Int J Biometerol*, **40**(2), 103–6.

Neff, J. *et al.* (1989) Effect of respiratory rate, respiratory depth, and open versus closed mouth breathing on sublingual temperature. *Res Nurse Health*, **12**, 195–202.

Neno, R. (2005) Hypothermia: assessment, treatment and prevention. *Nurs Stand*, **19**(20), 47–52.

NICE (2006) *CG 34. Hypertension: Management of Hypertension in Adults in Primary Care*. National Institute of Health and Clinical Excellence, London.

NMC (2005) *Guidelines for Records and Record Keeping*. Nursing and Midwifery Council, London.

NMC (2006) *A–Z Advice Sheet Consent*. www.nmc.org.

NMC (2008) *The Code: Standards of Conduct, Performance and Ethics for Nurses and Midwives*. Nursing and Midwifery Council, London.

O'Brien, E. *et al.* (2001) Blood pressure measuring devices: recommendations of the European Society of Hypertension. *BMJ*, **322**(7285), 531–6.

O'Brien, E. *et al.* (2003) European Society of Hypertension recommendations for conventional, ambulatory and home blood pressure measurement. *J Hypertens*, **21**, 821–48.

O'Neill, D. & Le Grove, A. (2003) Monitoring critically ill patients in accident and emergency. *Nurs Times*, **99**(45), 32–5.

O'Toole, S. (1997) Alternatives to mercury thermometers. *Prof Nurse*, **12**(11), 783–6.

Perloff, D. *et al.* (1993) Human blood pressure determined by sphygmomanometry. *Circulation*, **88**(5), 2460–70.

Petrie, J.C. *et al.* (1997) *British Hypertension Society: Recommendations on Blood Pressure Measurement*, 2nd edn. British Hypertension Society, London.

Philip, J.P. & Kowery, P.R. (2001) *Cardiac Arrhythmia: Mechanisms, Diagnosis and Management*, 2nd edn. Lippincott Williams & Wilkins, Philadelphia.

Pickup, J. (2000) Sensitive glucose sensing in diabetes. *Lancet*, **355**(9202), 426–7.

Place, B. (2000) Pulse oximetry: benefits and limitations. *Nurs Times*, **96**(26), 42.

Resuscitation Council UK (2005) *Resuscitation Guidelines*. RCUK Publications, London.

Richardson, M. (2006a) The respiratory system. Part 1: nose, pharynx and larynx. *Nurs Times*, **102** (21), 24–5.

Richardson, M. (2006b) The respiratory system. Part 2: trachea to alveoli. *Nurs Times*, **102** (22), 24–5.

Rigby, D. & Gray, K. (2005) Understanding urine testing. *Nurs Times*, **101**(12), 60–1.

Roberts, A. (2002) The role of anatomy and physiology in interpreting ECGs. *Nurs Times*, **98**(20), 34–36.

Roche Diagnostics (2004) Accu-Chem Safe T-Pro Plus: Information Leaflet. Roche, East Sussex.

Rumley, A. (1997) Improving the quality of new patient blood glucose measurement. *Ann Clin Biochem*, **34**(Part 2), 281–6.

Samples, F. *et al.* (1985) Circaadian rhythms: basis for screening for fever. *Nurs Res*, **34**(6), 377–9.

Sandler, M. *et al.* (1990) Misleading capillary glucose measurements. *Pract Diab Int*, **7**, 210.

Sharber, J. (1997) The efficacy of tepid sponge bathing to reduce fever in young children. *Am J Emerg Med*, **15**(2), 188–92.

Sharp, S. (1993) Blood glucose monitoring in the intensive care unit. *Br J Nurs*, **2**(4), 209–14.

Sims, J. (1996) Making sense of pulse oximetry and oxygen dissociation curve. *Nurs Times*, **92**(1), 34–5.

Stevenson, T. (2004) Achieving best practice in routine observation of hospital patients. *Nurs Times*, **100**(30), 34–5.

Thibodeau, G. & Patton, K.T. (2007) *Anatomy and Physiology*, 6th edn. Mosby Elsevier, St. Louis MO.

Thompson, D.R. (1981) Recording patients' blood pressure: a review. *J Adv Nurs*, **6**(4), 283–90.

Torrance, C. & Elley, K. (1998) Urine testing 2 – urinalysis. *Nurs Times*, **94**(5), Supp 1–2.

Torrance, C. & Semple, M. (1998) Recording temperature. *Nurs Times*, **94**(2), Supp 1–2.

Torrance, C. & Serginson, E. (1996) Student nurses' knowledge in relation to blood pressure measurement by sphygmomanometry and auscultation. *Nurse Educ Today*, **16**(6), 397–402.

Tortora, G.J. & Derrickson, B. (2008) *Principles of Anatomy and Physiology*, 12th edn. John Wiley & Sons, Inc., New York.

Trajanoski, Z. *et al.* (1996) Accuracy of home blood glucose meters during hypoglycaemia. *Diabetes Care*, **19**(12), 1412–15.

Trim, J. (2005) Monitoring temperature. *Nurs Times*, **101**(20), 30–31.

Udwadia, F.E. (2005) *Principles of Critical Care*, 2nd edn. Oxford University Press, Oxford.

UKPDS (1998) Tight blood pressure control and risk of macrovascular and microvascular complications in type 2 diabetes. *BMJ*, **317**(7160), 703–13.

Valler-Jones, T. & Wedgbury, K. (2005) Measuring blood pressure using the mercury sphygmomanometer. *Br J Nurs*, **14**(3), 145–50.

Van Staaij, B.K. *et al.* (2003) Accuracy and feasibility of daily infrared tympanic membrane temperature measurements in identification of fever in children. *Int J Pediatr Otorhinolaryngol*, **67**, 1091–7.

Wagner, D. (2006) Unplanned perioperative hypothermia. *AORN J*, **83**(2), 470–6.

Walsh, M. (2002) *Watson's Clinical Nursing and Related Sciences*, 6th edn. Bailliere Tindall, London.

Watson, R. (1998) Controlling body temperature in adults. *Nurs Stand*, **12**(20), 49–55.

Weber, J. & Kelley, J. (2003) *Health Assessment in Nursing*, 2nd edn. Lippincott Williams & Wilkins, Philadelphia.

Williams, B. *et al.* (2004) Guidelines for management of hypertension: report of the fourth working party of the British Hypertension Society, BHS IV. *J Hum Hypertens*, **18**, 139–85.

Wilson, L.A. (2005) Urinalysis. *Nurs Stand*, **19**(35), 51–4.

Woodrow, P. (1999) Pulse oximetry. *Nurs Stand*, **13**(42), 42–6.

Woodrow, P. (2002) Central venous catheters and central venous pressure. *Nurs Stand*, **16**(26), 45–51.

Woollens, S. (1996) Temperature measurement devices. *Prof Nurse*, **11**(8), 541–7.

Yarbro, C.H., Frogge, M.H.M. & Goodman, M. (2005) *Cancer Nursing: Principles and Practice*, 6th edn. Jones and Barlett, Sudbury.

Multiple choice questions

1 A pulse can be palpated in any artery that lies close to a surface of the body. Which artery is the most frequently used to take a pulse?

   a Temporal
   b Radial
   c Brachial
   d Femoral

2 Which node in the heart acts as a natural pacemaker?

   a Sinoatrial
   b Atrioventricular
   c His bundle node
   d Lymph node

3 Hypertension (raised blood pressure) is a common problem. What percentage of people over 50 suffer from this condition?

   a 20%
   b 30%
   c 50%
   d 60%

4 Which gland regulates core temperature?

   a Adrenal gland
   b Pituitary gland
   c Hypothalamus gland
   d Endocrine gland

5   Urine is typically clear, pale to deep yellow in colour. What is its pH value?

    a   Slightly acidic
    b   Slightly alkali
    c   Neutral
    d   Very acidic

6   Finger pricking is the usual way to perform blood glucose monitoring. What should a patient be advised to do before pricking their finger for this observation?

    a   Clean finger with alcohol swab
    b   Wash hands
    c   Elevate hand
    d   Keep hand cold

7   When performing a manual blood pressure check what is the first thing that should be done?

    a   Ensure tight and restrictive clothes have been removed
    b   Ensure upper arm is supported and positioned at heart level
    c   Ensure the patient is lying flat
    d   Allow the patient to rest for 5 minutes

8   How do you monitor respiratory rate?

    a   Using a peak flow monitor
    b   Using a spirometer
    c   Observing the number of breaths taken over a minute
    d   Measuring the pulse and respiratory rate manually

9 Due to its accuracy and ease of gaining a reading, what is the preferred site for obtaining a temperature reading?

    a   Rectum
    b   Tympanic membrane
    c   Axilla
    d   Oral

10 Bradycardia (in an adult) is most accurately defined as which of the following?

    a   Abnormally fast heart rate over 100 beats per minutes
    b   Body temperature below 35 °C
    c   Irregular contractions of the heart
    d   Heart rate slower than 60 beats per minute

Answers to the multiple choice questions can be found in Appendix 3.

Chapter 19

Observations: neurological

Definition

Neurological observation relates to the assessment and evaluation of the integrity and function of an individual's nervous system (Rowley & Fielding 1991).

Indications

An accurate neurological assessment is essential in planning patient care. Neurological observations are required to monitor and evaluate changes in the nervous system by indicating trends, thus aiding diagnosis and treatment, which in turn may affect prognosis and rehabilitation (Carlson 2002a; Kaye 2005).

Reference material

Changes in neurological status can be rapid and dramatic or subtle, developing over minutes, hours, days, weeks or even months depending on the insult (Aucken & Crawford 1998). Therefore the frequency of neurological observations will depend upon the patient's condition and the rapidity with which changes are occurring or expected to occur.

Neurological function is assessed by observing five critical areas:

- Level of consciousness.
- Pupillary activity.
- Motor function.
- Sensory function.
- Vital signs.

Consciousness

Consciousness is a state of awareness of self and the environment and is dependent upon two components:

- Arousability.
- Awareness.

(Carlson 2002a.)

Arousability

This depends on the integrity of the reticular activating system (RAS). The core of nuclei which make up the RAS extends from the brainstem to the thalamic nuclei in the cerebral hemispheres (Figure 19.1). Thus cognitive ability depends on the ability of the cerebral cortex to permit reciprocal stimulation and conscious behaviour. Consciousness therefore depends on the intactness of the cerebral cortex and the RAS and their ability to communicate effectively (Carlson 2002b; Fairley & McLernon 2005).

Awareness

This requires an intact cerebral cortex to interpret sensory input and respond accordingly. This is the content of the consciousness (Scherer 1986; Bateman 2001).

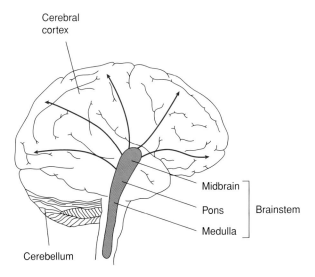

Cerebral cortex

Midbrain
Pons — Brainstem
Medulla

Cerebellum

Figure 19.1 Reticular activating system.

Levels of consciousness may vary and are dependent on the location and extent of any neurological damage (Aucken & Crawford 1998). Previous and/or co-existing problems should be heeded when noting levels of consciousness, for example deafness, hemiparesis/hemiplegia.

Level of consciousness

Alterations in level of consciousness can vary from slight to severe changes, indicating the degree of brain dysfunction (Aucken & Crawford 1998). Consciousness ranges on a continuum from alert wakefulness to deep coma with no apparent responsiveness. Therefore, nurses must ensure that families and friends are involved at initial history taking and throughout care so as to chronicle accurately any change in neurological symptoms.

Terms such as 'fully conscious', 'semiconscious', 'lethargic' or 'stuporous' to describe levels of consciousness are subjective and open to misinterpretation. Thus, level of consciousness is often measured using the Glasgow Coma Scale (GCS), which was developed in 1974 at the University of Glasgow by Teasdale and Jennett (1974) (Table 19.1; Figure 19.2). The GCS was designed to grade the severity of impaired consciousness in patients with traumatic head injuries or intracranial surgery (Aucken & Crawford 1998). The GCS is now used worldwide; it is objective and provides a reliable and easy-to-use measure of conscious level. For example, a GCS score less than 8 is equated with a state of coma (NICE 2003). When used consistently, the GCS provides a graphical representation that shows improvement or deterioration of the patient's conscious level at a glance (see Figure 19.2). The National Institute for Health and Clinical Excellence (NICE) (2003) advocates the use of the GCS for assessment and classification of all head injury patients.

Assessment of level of consciousness

Assessment using the GCS involves three phases (Teasdale & Jennett 1974):

1 Eye opening.
2 Evaluation of verbal response.
3 Evaluation of motor response.

Evaluation of eye opening

Eye opening indicates that the arousal mechanism in the brain is active. Eye opening may be: spontaneous; to speech, e.g. spoken name; to painful stimulus; or not at all. Arousal (eye opening) is always the first measurement undertaken when performing the GCS, as without arousal, cognition cannot occur (Aucken & Crawford 1998). It must, however, be remembered that swollen or permanently closed eyes (e.g. after tarsorrhaphy surgery in which the upper and lower eyelids

Table 19.1 Scoring activities of the Glasgow Coma Scale. Scores are added, with the highest score 15 indicating full consciousness. From Aucken and Crawford (1998) and Carlson (2002a).

Category	Score	Response
Eye opening:		
Spontaneous	4	Eyes open spontaneously without stimulation
To speech	3	Eyes open to verbal stimulation (normal, raised or repeated)
To pain	2	Eyes open with painful/noxious stimuli
None	1	No eye opening regardless of level of stimulation
Verbal response:		
Orientated	5	Able to give accurate information regarding time, person and place
Confused	4	Able to answer in sentences using correct language but cannot answer orientation questions appropriately
Inappropriate words	3	Uses incomprehensible words in a random or disorganized fashion
Incomprehensible sounds	2	Makes unintelligible sounds, e.g. moans and groans
None	1	No verbal response despite verbal or other stimuli
Best motor response:		
Obeys commands	6	Obeys and can repeat simple commands, e.g. arm raise
Localizes to pain	5	Purposeful movement to remove painful stimuli
Normal flexion	4	Withdraws extremity from source of pain, e.g. flexes arm at elbow without wrist rotation in response to painful stimuli
Abnormal flexion	3	Decorticate posturing (flexion of arms, hyperextension of legs) spontaneously or in response to noxious stimuli
Extension	2	Decerebrate posturing (limbs extended and internally rotated) spontaneously or in response to noxious stimuli
None	1	No response to noxious stimuli. Flaccid limbs

are partially or wholly joined to protect the cornea; Martin 2003) will not open and do not necessarily indicate a falling conscious level.

Evaluation of verbal response
Verbal response may be:

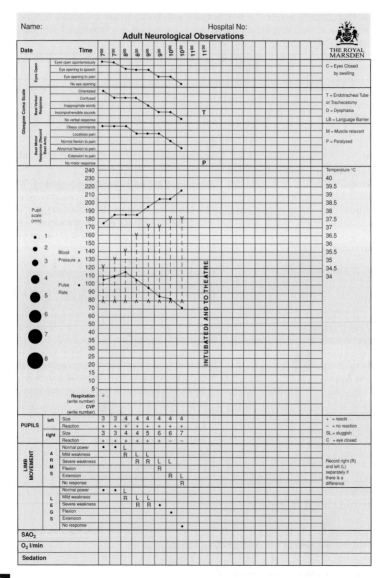

Figure 19.2 The Glasgow Coma Scale.

- *Orientated*: the patient is aware of self and environment.
- *Confused*: the patient's responses to questions are incorrect and patient is unaware of self or environment.
- *Inappropriate words:* the patient responds using intelligible words which are unsuitable as responses.
- *Incomprehensible*: the patient may moan and groan without recognizable words.
- *Absent*: the patient does not speak or make sounds at all.

The absence of speech may not always indicate a falling level of consciousness. The patient may not speak English (though he/she can still speak), may have a tracheostomy or may be dysphasic. The patient may have a motor (expressive) dysphasia, and therefore be able to understand but unable to find the right word, or a sensory (receptive) dysphasia, being unable to comprehend what is being told to them (Aucken & Crawford 1998; Shah 1999). At times patients with expressive dysphasia may also have receptive problems; therefore it is important to make an early referral to a speech and language therapist. The nurse should also bear in mind that some patients may need a lot of stimulation to maintain their concentration to answer questions, even though they can answer them correctly. It is, therefore, important to note the amount of stimulation that the patient required as part of the baseline assessment (Aucken & Crawford 1998).

Evaluation of motor response

To obtain an accurate picture of brain function, motor response is tested by using the upper limbs because responses in the lower limbs reflect spinal function (Aucken & Crawford 1998). The patient should be asked to obey commands; for example, the patient should be asked to squeeze the examiner's hands (both sides) with the best motor response recorded. The nurse should note power in the hands and the patient's ability to release the grip. This is because some patients with cerebral dysfunction, for example those with diffuse brain disease, may show an involuntary grasp reflex where stimulation of the palm of their hand causes them to grip (Aucken & Crawford 1998). If movement is spontaneous, the nurse should note which limbs move, and how, for example whether the movement is purposeful.

Response to painful stimulus may be:

- *Localized*: the patient moves the other hand to the site of the stimulus.
- *Flexor*: the patient's limb flexes away from pain.
- *Extensor*: the patient's limb extends from pain.
- *Flaccid*: no motor response at all.

(Aucken & Crawford 1998; Shah 1999.)

Application of painful stimuli

Painful stimuli should be employed only if the patient does not respond to firm and clear commands. It is always important that the least amount of pressure to elicit a response is applied so as to avoid bruising or paining the patient. As such, it should only be undertaken by experienced professionals (for suggested methods, see below).

As the ability to localize pain is lost, various responses may be observed when painful stimuli are applied (Carlson 2002a). It is important to note, when applying a painful stimulus, that the brain responds to central stimulation and the spine responds first to peripheral stimulation (Aucken & Crawford 1998).

Central stimulation can be applied in the following ways (Aucken & Crawford 1998; Carlson 2002a; Price 2002):

- *Trapezium squeeze*: using the thumb and two fingers, hold 5 cm of the trapezius muscle where the neck meets the shoulder and twist the muscle.
- *Supraorbital pressure*: running a finger along the supraorbital margin, a notch is felt. Applying pressure to the notch causes an ipsilateral (on that side) sinus headache. This method is not to be used if the facial or cranial bones are unstable, facial fractures are suspected, after facial surgery or if the assessor has sharp fingernails.
- *Sternal rub*: using the knuckles of a clenched fist to grind on the centre of the sternum. When applied adequately, marks are left on the skin as sternal tissue is tender and bruises easily. Please note that because of the danger of bruising, this method should not be used for repeated assessment but may be indicated if a decision as to whether to re-scan or alter management, e.g. proceed to surgery, is necessary.

Peripheral stimulation can be applied in the following way:

Place the patient's finger between assessor's thumb and a pencil or pen. Pressure is gradually increased over a few seconds until the slightest response is seen. Any finger can be used, although the third and fourth fingers are often most sensitive (Frawley 1990). Please note that because of the risk of bruising, pressure should not be applied to the nail bed. It must be remembered that nail bed pressure is a peripheral stimulus and should only be used to assess limbs that have not moved in response to a central stimulus (Aucken & Crawford 1998).

It cannot be overemphasized that the above methods of patient assessment should only be undertaken by appropriately qualified and trained nurses.

Evaluation of pupillary activity

Careful examination of the reactions of the pupils to light is an important part of neurological assessment (Table 19.2). The size, shape, equality, reaction to light (both direct and consensual responses, that is, the response from the eye

Table 19.2 Examination of pupils. From Fuller (2004).

Observation	Pupil size	Pupil reactiveness	Possible indication
Pupils equal	Pinpoint	——	Opiates or pontine lesion
	Small	Reactive	Metabolic encephalopathy
	Mid-sized	Fixed	Midbrain lesion
		Reactive	Metabolic lesion
Pupils unequal	Dilated	Unreactive	IIIrd nerve palsy
	Small	Reactive	Horner's syndrome

that is not directly exposed to light) and position of the eyes should be noted. Are the eyes deviated upwards or downwards? Are both eyes conjugate (moving together) or dysconjugate (not moving together)? Impaired pupillary accommodation (adjustment of the eye resulting in pupil constriction or dilation) signifies that the midbrain itself may be suffering from pressure exerted by a swelling mass in the brain. Pupillary constriction and dilation are controlled by cranial nerve III (oculomotor) and any changes may indicate pressure on this nerve or brainstem damage (Figure 19.3) (Fuller 2004).

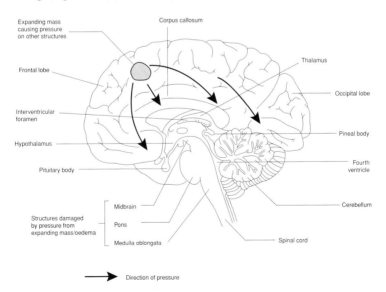

Figure 19.3 Diagrammatic representation of pressure from expanding mass and/or cerebral oedema.

It should be noted that 'normal' visual function depends on a full and conjugate range of eye movements (involving cranial nerves III, IV, VI) in addition to normally functioning optic and oculomotor nerves and an intact visual centre in the occipital cortex (Aucken & Crawford 1998).

Evaluation of motor function

Damage to any part of the motor nervous system can affect the ability to move. After assessing motor function on one side of the body the contralateral muscle group should also be evaluated to detect asymmetry. Motor function assessment involves an evaluation of the following:

- Muscle strength.
- Muscle tone.
- Muscle co-ordination.
- Reflexes.
- Abnormal movements.

(Aucken & Crawford 1998; Fuller 2004.)

Muscle strength

This involves testing the patient's muscle strength against the pull of gravity and then against one's own resistance. Changes in motor strength especially between right and left sides may indicate imminent neurological failure (Carlson 2002a).

Muscle tone

This involves flexing and extending the patient's limbs on both sides and noting how well such movements are resisted. Increased resistance would denote increased muscle tone and vice versa.

Muscle co-ordination

Any disease or injury that involves the cerebellum or basal ganglia will affect co-ordination. Assessment of hand and leg co-ordination can be achieved by testing the rapidity and rhythm of alternating movements and of point-to-point movements.

Reflexes

Among the most important reflexes are: blink, gag and swallow, oculocephalic and plantar:

- *Blink*: this is a protective reflex and can be affected by damage to the Vth cranial nerve (trigeminal) and the VIIth cranial nerve (facial). Absence of the corneal reflex (Vth and VIIth cranial nerves) may result in corneal damage. Facial weakness (VIIth cranial nerve) will affect eye closure.

- *Gag and swallow*: damage to the IXth cranial nerve (glossopharyngeal) and Xth cranial nerve (vagus) may impair protective reflexes. These two cranial nerves are always assessed together as their functions overlap. Muscle innervation of the palate is from the vagus, while sensation is supplied by the glossopharyngeal nerves (Aucken & Crawford 1998; Fuller 2004).

- *Oculocephalic*: this reflex is an eye movement that occurs only in patients with a severely decreased level of consciousness. In conscious patients this reflex is not present. When the reflex is present, the patient's eyes will move in the opposite direction from the side to which the head is turned. However, in patients with absent brainstem reflexes, the eyes will appear to remain stationary in the centre. Assessing this reflex should not be carried out if there is suspected instability of the cervical spine as this reflex can involve head movement which could exacerbate any spinal injury (Aucken & Crawford 1998).

- *Plantar*: Abnormalities of plantar reflex will help to locate the anatomical site of the lesion. Upgoing plantar (extension) reflex is termed 'positive Babinski' and indicates an upper motor neurone lesion. It should be noted that in babies under 1 year of age upgoing plantar is normal (Aucken & Crawford 1998).

Abnormal movements

When carrying out neurological observations, any abnormal movements such as seizures, tics and tremors must be noted.

Sensory functions

Constant sensory input enables an individual to alter responses and behaviour to suit the environment. When disease or injury damages the sensory pathways, the sensory responses are always affected. Any assessment of sensory function should include an evaluation of the following:

- Central and peripheral vision.
- Hearing and ability to understand verbal communication.
- Superficial sensations (light touch, pain) and deep sensations (muscle and joint pain, muscle and joint position).

(Carlson 2002a; Fuller 2004.)

Vital signs

It is recommended that assessments of vital signs should be made in the following order:

1 Respirations.
2 Temperature.
3 Blood pressure.
4 Pulse.

(See also Chapter 18.)

Respirations

Of these four vital signs, respiratory patterns give the clearest indication of how the brain is functioning because the complex process of respiration is controlled by more than one area of the brain. Any disease or injury that affects these areas may produce respiratory changes. The rate, character and pattern of a patient's respiration must be noted. Abnormal respiratory patterns are listed in Table 19.3.

Table 19.3 Abnormal respiratory patterns.

Type	Pattern	Significance
Cheyne–Stokes	Rhythmic waxing and waning of both rate and depth of respirations, alternating regularly with briefer periods of apnoea. Greater than normal respiration, i.e. 16–24 breaths per minute	May indicate deep cerebral or cerebellar lesions, usually bilateral; may occur with upper brainstem involvement
Central neurogenic hyperventilation	Sustained, regular, rapid respirations, with forced inspiration and expiration	May indicate a lesion of the low midbrain or upper pons areas of the brainstem
Apnoeustic	Prolonged inspiration with a pause at full inspiration; there may also be expiratory pauses	May indicate a lesion of the lower pons or upper medulla, hypoglycaemia or drug-induced respiratory depression
Cluster breathing	Clusters of irregular respirations alternating with longer periods of apnoea	May indicate a lesion of lower pons or upper medulla
Ataxic breathing	A completely irregular pattern with random deep and shallow respirations; irregular pauses may also appear	May indicate a lesion of the medulla

Constant re-evaluation of the patient's ability to maintain and protect their airway is a concern when there is evidence of reduced consciousness or coma (GCS score is less than 8). At this stage, muscles often become flaccid and the use of the recovery position may need to be considered. Patients who have deteriorated may require adjuncts to protect the airway and possibly artificial ventilation (Resuscitation Council (UK) 2006). Close working liaison with physiotherapists and speech and language therapists is important to minimize the danger of chest infections.

Temperature
Damage to the hypothalamus, the temperature-regulating centre, may result in grossly fluctuating temperatures (Fairley & McLernon 2005).

Blood pressure, pulse and respirations
Observations of blood pressure, pulse and respirations will provide evidence of increased intracranial pressure. When intracranial pressure is greater than 33 mmHg for even a short time, cerebral blood flow is significantly reduced. The resulting ischaemia stimulates the vasomotor centre, causing systemic blood pressure to rise. The patient becomes bradycardic and the respiratory rate falls. Abnormalities of blood pressure and pulse usually occur late, after the patient's level of consciousness has begun to deteriorate. This change in the blood pressure was first described by Cushing and is known as the Cushing reflex (Carlson 2002b).

Frequency of observations
The frequency and type of neurological observation are matters of much debate (Price 2002). It is therefore not possible to be prescriptive, as the frequency will depend on the underlying pathology and possible consequences. For example, in a patient with a head injury and a skull fracture there may be bruising to the brain (contusion), cerebral oedema and an extradural haemorrhage which may increase in size. The bruising and oedema may develop over a couple of days and gradually give rise to subtle neurological changes, whilst the extradural haemorrhage can develop very quickly and cause profound neurological changes over a matter of a few hours. Therefore such a patient may require frequent 30-minute GCS observations for the first 6 hours followed by 1–2-hourly observations for a further 48 hours. The nurse must be competent and take appropriate action if changes in the patient's neurological status occur, as well as reporting any subtle signs that may indicate deterioration, e.g. if the patient is incontinent, reluctant to eat, drink or initiate interaction. It should never be assumed that difficulty to rouse a patient is due to night-time sleep as even a deeply asleep patient with no focal deficit should respond to pain. Therefore if the patient requires an increased

Table 19.4 Frequency of observations.

Category	Frequency	Rationale
All patients diagnosed as suffering from neurological or neurosurgical conditions. Unconscious patients (including ventilated and anaesthetized)	At least 4-hourly, affected by the patient's condition. Frequency indicated by patient's condition	To monitor the condition of the patient so that any necessary action can be instigated. To monitor the condition closely and to detect trends so that appropriate action may be taken

amount of stimulus to achieve the same GCS score, this may also be a pointer to subtle deterioration (Table 19.4) (Aucken & Crawford 1998; Waterhouse 2005).

General points

The initial assessment of a patient should include a history (taken from relatives or friends if appropriate), including noting changes in mood, intellect, memory and personality, since these may be indicators of a long-standing problem, e.g. brain tumour (Belford 2005).

Visual acuity

The clarity or clearness of vision may be tested using Snellen's chart, which uses decreasing letter size, or newspaper prints, with and without glasses if worn.

Visual fields

Lesions at different points in the visual pathways affect vision (Table 19.5). It should be noted that loss of vision is always described with reference to the visual fields rather than the retinal fields (Weldon 1998).

Table 19.5 Visual pathways. From Fuller (2004).

Defect	Implication
Monocular field defects	Lesion anterior to optic chiasm
Bitemporal field defects	Lesion at the optic chiasm
Homonymous field defects	Lesion behind the optic chiasm
Congruous homonymous field defects	Lesion behind lateral geniculate bodies

Procedure guidelines **Neurological observations and assessment**

Note: the following describes a full neurological assessment. It may be inappropriate, unnecessary or impossible for the nurse to carry out all of the procedures every time the patient is observed.

Equipment

1 Pen torch.
2 Thermometer.
3 Sphygmomanometer.
4 Tongue depressor.

5 Low-linting swabs.
6 Patella hammer.
7 Neurotips™ (refer to action 27).
8 Two test tubes (refer to action 28).

Procedure

Action	Rationale
1 Inform the patient of the procedure, whether conscious or not, and explain and discuss the observations.	Sense of hearing is frequently unimpaired even in unconscious patients. It is important, as far as is possible, that the patient understands the procedure and gives his/her valid consent (DH 2001: C; NMC 2006: C).
2 Talk to the patient. Note whether he/she is alert and is giving full attention or whether he/she is restless or lethargic and drowsy. Ask the patient who he/she is, the correct day, month and year, where he/she is, and to give details about family.	To establish whether the patient's level of consciousness is deteriorating. If the patient is becoming disorientated, changes will occur in this order: (a) Disorientation as to time. (b) Disorientation as to place. (c) Disorientation as to person (Aucken & Crawford 1998: R 5).
3 Ask the patient to squeeze and release your fingers (include both sides of the body) and then to stick out their tongue.	To evaluate motor responses and to ensure that the responses are equal and are not reflexive (Carlson 2002a: R 5).
4 If the patient does not respond, apply painful stimuli. Suggested methods have been discussed earlier.	Responses grow less purposeful as the patient's level of consciousness deteriorates. As the condition worsens, the patient may no longer localize pain and respond to it in a purposeful way (Aucken & Crawford 1998: R 5).

Procedure guidelines *(cont.)*

5 Record, precisely, the findings, recording the patient's best response. Write exactly what stimulus was used, where it was applied, how much pressure was needed to elicit the response, and how the patient responded.

Vague terms can be easily misinterpreted. Accurate recording will enable continuity of assessment and comply with NMC guidelines (NMC 2005: C).

6 Extend both hands and ask the patient to squeeze your fingers as hard as possible. Compare grip and strength.

To test grip and ascertain strength. Record best arm in GCS chart to reflect best outcome (Carlson 2002a: R 5).

7 Darken the room, if necessary, or shield the patient's eyes with your hands.

To enable a better view of the eye (E).

8 Ask the patient to open their eyes. If the patient cannot do so, hold the eyelids open and note the size, shape and equality of the pupils.

To assess the size, shape and equality of the pupils as an indication of brain damage. Normal pupils are spherical, usually at mid-position and have a diameter ranging from 2 to 5 mm (Shah 1999: R 5).

9 Hold each eyelid open in turn. Move torch towards the patient from the side. Shine it directly into the eye. This should cause the pupil to constrict promptly.

To assess the reaction of the pupils to light. A normal reaction indicates no lesions in the area of the brainstem regulating pupil constriction (Aucken & Crawford 1998: R 5).

10 Hold both eyelids open but shine the light into one eye only. The pupil into which the light is not shone should also constrict.

To assess consensual light reflex. Prompt constriction indicates intact connections between the brainstem areas regulating pupil constriction (Scherer 1986: R 5).

11 Record unusual eye movements.

To assess cranial nerve damage (Aucken & Crawford 1998: R 5).

12 Note the rate, character and pattern of the patient's respirations.

Respirations are controlled by different areas of the brain. When disease or injury affects these areas, respiratory changes may occur (Carlson 2002a: R 5).

13 Take and record the patient's temperature at specified intervals.

Damage to the hypothalamus, the temperature-regulating centre in the brain, will be reflected in grossly abnormal temperatures (Fairley & McLernon 2005: R 5).

14 Take and record the patient's blood pressure and pulse at specified intervals.

To monitor signs of increased intracranial pressure. Hypertension and bradycardia usually occur late, after the patient's level of consciousness has begun to deteriorate. Call for medical assistance as soon as it is evident that there is a deterioration in the patient's level of consciousness (Scherer 1986: R 5; Tortora & Derrickson 2008: R 5).

15 Ask the patient to close the eyes and hold the arms straight out in front, with palms upwards, for 20–30 seconds. The weaker limb will 'fall away'.

To show weakness and difference in limbs (Carlson 2002a: R 5).

16 Stand in front of the patient and extend your hands. Ask the patient to push and pull against your hands. Ask the patient to lie on his/her back in bed. Place the patient's leg with knee flexed and foot resting on the bed. Instruct the patient to keep the foot down as you attempt to extend the leg. Then instruct the patient to straighten the leg while you offer resistance.

Note: if a patient cannot follow the instruction due to a language barrier or unconsciousness, observe spontaneous movements and note how strong they appear. Then, if necessary, apply painful stimuli.

To test arm strength. If one arm drifts downwards or turns inwards, it may indicate hemiparesis. To test flexion and extension strength in the patient's extremities by having patient push and pull against your resistance (Carlson 2002a: R 5).

17 Flex and extend all the patient's limbs. Note how well the movements are resisted.

To test muscle tone (Carlson 2002a: R 5).

Procedure guidelines *(cont.)*

18 Ask the patient to pat the thigh as fast as possible. Note whether the movements seem slow or clumsy. Ask the patient to turn the hand over and back several times in succession. Evaluate co-ordination. Ask the patient to touch the back of the fingers with the thumb in sequence rapidly.

To assess hand and arm co-ordination. The dominant hand should perform better (Carlson 2002a: R 5).

19 Extend one of your hands towards the patient. Ask the patient to touch your index finger, then his/her nose, several times in succession. Repeat the test with the patient's eyes closed.

To assess hand and arm co-ordination/cerebellar function (Carlson 2002a: R 5).

20 Ask the patient to place a heel on the opposite knee and slide it down the shin to the foot. Check each leg separately.

To assess leg co-ordination (Fuller 2004: R 5).

21 Ask the patient to look up or hold the eyelid open. With your hand, approach the eye unexpectedly or touch the eyelashes.

To test the corneal (blink) reflex (Fuller 2004: R 5).

22 Ask the patient to open the mouth, and hold down the tongue with a tongue depressor. Touch the back of the pharynx, on each side, with a low-linting swab.

To test the gag reflex (Fuller 2004: R 5).

23 Ask the patient to lie on his/her back in bed. Place your hand under the knee, raise and flex it. Tap the patellar tendon. Note whether the leg responds.

To assess the deep tendon knee-jerk reflex (Fuller 2004: R 5).

24 Stroke the lateral aspect of the sole of the patient's foot. If the response is abnormal (Babinski's response), the big toe will dorsiflex and the remaining toes will fan out.

To assess for upper motor neurone lesion (Fuller 2004: R 5).

25 Ask the patient to read something aloud. Check each eye separately. If vision is so poor that the patient is unable to read, ask the patient to count your upraised fingers or distinguish light from dark.	To test for visual acuity (Fuller 2004: R 5).
26 Occlude the ear with a low-linting swab. Stand a short way from the patient. Whisper numbers into the open ear. Ask for feedback. Repeat for both ears.	To test hearing and comprehension (Fuller 2004: R 5).
27 Ask the patient to close the eyes. Using the point of a Neurotip™ (sharp instrument for applying pressure) stroke the skin. Use the blunt end occasionally. Ask patient to tell you what is felt. See if the patient can distinguish between sharp and dull sensations.	To test superficial sensations to pain (Fuller 2004: R 5).
28 Ask the patient to close the eyes. Fill two test tubes with water: one warm, one cold. Touch the patient's skin with each test tube and ask patient to distinguish between them.	To test superficial sensations to temperature (Fuller 2004: R 5).
29 Stroke a low-linting swab lightly over the patient's skin. Ask the patient to say what he/she feels.	To test superficial sensations to touch (Fuller 2004: R 5).
30 Ask the patient to close the eyes. Hold the tip of one of the patient's fingers between your thumb and index finger. Move it up and down and ask the patient to say in which direction it is moving. Repeat with the other hand. For the legs, hold the big toe.	To test proprioception. *Definition of proprioception*: the receipt of information from muscles and tendons to the labyrinth that enables the brain to determine movements and the position of the body (Tortora & Derrickson 2008).

Procedure guidelines *(cont.)*

31 Should seizures (epilepsy/fits) occur, maintain airway if possible by placing the patient in the recovery position. Do not insert artificial airway into patient's mouth during the tonic/clonic phase. Record type of seizure, duration, any warning (aura) or incontinence the patient may have, as well as any postictal (after the fit) weakness (Todd's paralysis) or increase in drowsiness. Ensure the patient is closely observed until back to previous conscious level prior to ictus (fit). Anticonvulsants may be required as prescribed.	To maintain patient's safety and to assist in the diagnosis of any underlying pathology (E).

References and further reading

Aucken, S. & Crawford, B. (1998) Neurological observations. In: *Neuro-Oncology for Nurses* (ed. D. Guerrero). Whurr, London, pp. 29–65.

Bateman, D. (2001) Neurological assessment of coma. *J Neurol Neurosurg Psychiatry*, 71(Suppl 1), i13–17.

Belford, K. (2005) Central nervous system cancers. In: *Cancer Nursing: Principles and Practice* (eds C. Henke- Yarbro, M. Frogge & M. Goodman), 6th edn. Jones and Bartlett, Sudbury MA, pp. 1089–136.

Carlson, B.A. (2002a) Neurologic clinical assessment. In: *Critical Care Nursing: Diagnosis and Management* (eds L. Urden, K. Stacy & M. Lough), 4th edn. Mosby, St. Louis, pp. 645–57.

Carlson, B.A. (2002b) Neurologic anatomy and physiology. In: *Critical Care Nursing: Diagnosis and Management* (eds L. Urden, K. Stacy & M. Lough), 4th edn. Mosby, St. Louis, pp. 617–44.

DH (2001) Good practice in consent implemation guide: consent to examination or treatment. www.dh.gov.uk. Accessed 24/9/07.

Fairley, S. & McLernon S. (2005) Neurological problems. In: *Critical Care Nursing: Science and Practice* (eds Adam S. Osborne S.), 2nd edn. Oxford University Press, Oxford, pp. 285–327.

Frawley, P. (1990) Neurological observations. *Nurs Times*, 86(35), 29–34.

Fuller, G. (2004) *Neurological Examinations Made Easy*, 3rd edn. Churchill Livingstone, Edinburgh.

Jennett, B. & Teasdale G. (1984) *An Introduction to Neurosurgery*, 4th edn. William Heinemann Medical Books, London, pp. 23–9.

Kaye, A.H. (2005) Neurological assessment and examination. *Essential Neurosurgery*, 3rd edn. Blackwell Publishing, Oxford, pp. 1–14.

Lower, J. (2003) Using pain to assess neurological response. *Nursing*, **33**(6), 56–7.

Martin, E.A. (2003) *Oxford Concise Colour Medical Dictionary*, 3rd edn. Oxford University Press, Oxford.

NICE (2003) *Head Injury: Triage, Assessment, Investigation and Early Management of Head Injury in Infants, Children and Adults*. National Institute for Clinical Excellence, London.

NMC (2005) *Guidelines for Records and Record Keeping*. Nursing and Midwifery Council, London.

NMC (2006) *A–Z Advice Sheet Consent*. www.nmc.org.

Price, T. (2002) Painful stimuli and the Glasgow Coma Scale. *Nurs Crit Care*, **7**(1), 17–23.

Resuscitation Council (UK) (2006) Airway management and ventilation. In: *Advanced Life Support*, 5th edn. Resuscitation Council (UK), London, pp. 41–57.

Rowley, G. & Fielding, K. (1991) Reliability and accuracy of the Glasgow Coma Scale with experienced and inexperienced users. *Lancet*, **337**(8740), 535–8.

Scherer, P. (1986) The logic of coma. *Am J Nurs*, **86**, 542–9.

Shah, S. (1999) Neurological assessment. *Nurs Times*, **13**, 49–56.

Teasdale, G. & Jennett, B. (1974) Assessment of coma and impaired consciousness: a practical scale. *Lancet*, **2**, 81–4.

Tortora, G.J. & Derrickson B. (2008) *Principles of Anatomy and Physiology*, 12th edn. John Wiley & Sons Ltd, Chichester.

Waterhouse, C. (2005) The Glasgow Coma Scale and other neurological observations. *Nurs Stand* **19**(33), 56–64.

Weldon, K. (1998) Neurological observations. In: *Neuro-Oncology for Nurses* (ed. D. Guerrero). Whurr, London, pp. 1–28.

Multiple choice questions

1 The following is a definition of an abnormal respiratory pattern:

   Rhythmic waxing and waning of both rate and depth of respirations, alternating regularly with brief periods of apnoea.

   Which type of respiration is it?

   a Apnoeustic breathing
   b Ataxia breathing
   c Cheyne–Stokes breathing
   d Cluster breathing

2 The Glasgow Coma Scale is the worldwide recognized measure of consciousness and should be used for the assessment and classification of all patients with head injuries. A score of what is equated with coma?

   a Less than 20
   b Less than 12
   c Less than 8
   d Less than 2

3 What three aspects does the Glasgow Coma Scale assess?

   a Eye opening, verbal response, motor response
   b Eye opening, gag reflex, motor response
   c Verbal response, motor response, respiratory rate
   d Respiratory rate, eye opening and motor response

4 Careful examination of pupil reaction is a significant part of any neurological assessment. Which cranial nerve controls papillary constriction and dilation?

   a VIII
   b IX
   c I
   d III

5 **In order to complete a neurological assessment, which of the following equipment would be necessary?**

    a   Pen torch, thermometer, sphygmomanometer

    b   Patella hammer, thermometer, sharp object (Neuroitip)

    c   Tongue depressor, pen torch, thermometer

    d   All of the above

Answers to the multiple choice questions can be found in Appendix 3.

Chapter 20

Pain management and assessment

Definition

Pain is not a simple sensation but a complex phenomenon having both a physical and an affective (emotional) component. To reflect this, the International Association for the Study of Pain (IASP) (1994) published the following definition of pain: 'An unpleasant sensory and emotional experience associated with actual or potential tissue damage, or described in terms of such damage'. Pain is subjective and another favoured definition for use in clinical practice, proposed originally by McCaffery (1968) and cited in McCaffery (2000, p. 2), is: 'Pain is whatever the experiencing person says it is, existing whenever the experiencing person says it does'.

Many factors influence the expression of pain and may be associated with the patient, the nurse or the clinical environment (organizational aspects) (Carr & Mann 2000a).

Reference material

There are several ways to categorize the types of pain that occur; for example, acute or chronic, nociceptive (somatic or visceral) or neuropathic. It is increasingly recognized that acute and chronic pain may represent a continuum rather than distinct separate entities, combine different pain mechanisms and vary in duration (ANZCA and Faculty of Pain Medicine 2005).

Acute pain

The IASP has defined acute pain as: 'Pain of recent onset and probable limited duration. It usually has an identifiable temporal and causal relationship to injury or disease' (Ready & Edwards 1992, p. 1). Acute pain is produced by a wide range of physiological processes, and includes inflammatory, neuropathic, sympathetically maintained, visceral and cancer pain (Walker *et al.* 2006).

Chronic pain

Chronic pain is usually prolonged and defined as pain that exists for more than 3 months (IASP 1996). It is often associated with major changes in personality, lifestyle and functional ability (Foley 2004). Chronic pain occurs as a result of both cancer and non-malignant chronic conditions such as neuropathic, musculoskeletal, and chronic postoperative pain syndromes.

The term breakthrough pain is widely used. Within the medical literature other terms are referred to in the description of breakthrough pain including episodic pain, exacerbation of pain, pain flare, transient pain and transitory pain (Colleau 1999). This is further discussed below.

Assessment of pain

Assessment is a key step in the process of managing pain. The aim of assessment is to identify all the factors, physical and non-physical, that affect the patient's perception of pain. A comprehensive clinical assessment is essential to gain a thorough understanding of the patient's pain, select an appropriate analgesic therapy, evaluate the effectiveness of interventions and modify therapy according to the patient's response.

Acute pain assessment for surgical patients

For surgical pain to be controlled effectively, pain must be assessed regularly and systematically. The process of pain assessment begins before surgery and continues through to discharge.

Assessment of the psychosocial aspects of acute pain

A number of psychosocial factors can influence pain. Pain is an individual, multifactorial experience influenced by previous pain events, beliefs about pain and pain management, anxiety, mood and culture (ANZCA and Faculty of Pain Medicine 2005). Patients may be anxious about the outcome of the surgery or how pain will be controlled, particularly if they have bad memories of previous pain experiences (Audit Commission 1997; Carr & Mann 2000b). Anxiety in turn exacerbates pain by increasing muscle tension. Providing patients with appropriate support and information to address these concerns can reduce both anxiety and postoperative pain (Audit Commission 1997; Kalkman *et al.* 2003).

Assessment of pre-existing pain

Patients who have been taking regular opioid analgesics for a pre-existing chronic pain problem may require higher doses of analgesia to manage an acute pain episode (Macintyre 2001; Lewis & Williams 2005; Mehta & Langford 2006). It is therefore important to take a history of pre-existing pain and analgesic use so that appropriate analgesic measures can be planned in advance of surgery.

Assessment of location and intensity of pain

Location

Many complex surgical procedures involve more than one incision site and the nature and extent of pain at each site may vary. A careful assessment of the location and type of pain is required, because each pain problem may respond to different pain management techniques. Pain location may also help to determine why pain is exacerbated by certain movements or positions (Anderson & Cleeland 2003).

Intensity

As part of the assessment process it is important to assess the intensity of pain. Only then can the effects of any intervention be evaluated and care modified as appropriate. The simplest techniques for pain measurement involve the use of a verbal rating scale, numerical rating scale or visual analogue scale. Using one of these scales, patients are asked to match pain intensity to the scale.

Three principles apply to the use of these scales:

- The patient must be involved in scoring his/her own pain intensity. It provides the patient with an opportunity to express their pain intensity and also what it means to them and the effect it has on their lives. This is important because health care professionals frequently underestimate the intensity of a patient's pain and effectiveness of pain relief (Drayer *et al.* 1999; Loveman & Gale 2000; Idvall *et al.* 2002).
- Pain intensity assessment should incorporate different components of pain. This should include assessment of static (rest) pain and dynamic pain (on sitting, coughing or moving the affected part). For example, in a postoperative patient this is important to prevent complications of delayed recovery such as chest infections and emboli (deep vein thrombosis, pulmonary embolism) and to determine if analgesia is adequate for return of normal function (Macintyre & Ready 2001; Hobbs & Hodgkinson 2003).
- It is important to remember that a complete picture of a patient's pain cannot be derived solely from the use of a pain scale (Lawler 1997). Ongoing

communication with the patient is required to uncover and manage any psychosocial factors that may be affecting the patient's pain experience.

Chronic pain assessment

The prevalence of chronic pain is approximated at being between 30–50% among patients with cancer who are undergoing active treatment for a solid tumour and between 70 and 90% among those patients with advanced disease (Portenoy & Lessage 1999). For example, approximately two-thirds of advanced cancer patients will also complain of anorexia, one-half will have a symptomatic dry mouth and constipation, and one-third will suffer nausea, vomiting, insomnia, dyspnoea, cough or oedema (Donnelly & Walsh 1995). It is clear from these figures that chronic pain assessment cannot be seen in isolation; identification of all related symptoms is of equal importance as they will contribute to a lowered pain threshold (the lowest stimulus intensity at which a person perceives pain) and impaired pain tolerance (the greatest stimulus intensity causing pain that a person is prepared to tolerate) (Grond *et al.* 1996). Furthermore, chronic cancer pain is often multifactorial. Adequate pain assessment requires a comprehensive evaluation of all factors that play a significant role in the cancer pain experience (Zaza 2002).

A diagnosis of cancer does not necessarily mean that the malignant process is the cause of the pain. Pain in chronic cancer may be:

- Caused by the cancer itself.
- Caused by treatment.
- Associated with debilitating disease, such as a pressure ulcer.
- Unrelated to either the disease or the treatment, such as headache.

(Twycross & Wilcock 2001.)

It is imperative to ascertain the patients' current level of anxiety and depression and to understand each patient's own understanding of the meaning of pain (Foley 2004). The cause of *each* pain should therefore be identified carefully; many pains unrelated to the cancer will respond to specific treatment. If the pain is due to the cancer, then it is important to determine the precise mechanism of pain because treatment will vary accordingly. Patients with cancer may experience a range of psychological and spiritual problems that extend far beyond the experience of physical pain (Paz & Seymour 2004). The concept of total pain reminds practitioners that pain is a deeply personal experience and that one of the greatest challenges is for nurses to be able to facilitate the expression for each individual of that particular pain (Krishnasamy 2001). Pain assessment needs to acknowledge these facts and particular attention must be paid to factors that will modulate pain sensitivity (Table 20.1).

Table 20.1 Factors affecting pain sensitivity.

Sensitivity increased	Sensitivity lowered
Discomfort	Relief of symptoms
Insomnia	Sleep
Fatigue	Rest
Anxiety	Sympathy
Fear	Understanding
Anger	Companionship
Sadness	Diversional activity
Depression	Reduction in anxiety
Boredom	Elevation of mood

Assessment tools for acute and chronic pain

Accurate pain assessment is a prerequisite of effective control and is an essential component of nursing care. In the assessment process, the nurse gathers information from the patient that allows an understanding of the patient's experience and its effect on the patient's life. The information obtained guides the nurse in planning and evaluating strategies for care. Pain is rarely static; therefore, its assessment is not a one-time process but is ongoing.

Pain assessment is difficult to achieve. For example, the tendency suggested by both research and clinical practice is for the patient not to report any pain or to do so inadequately or inaccurately, minimizing the pain experience (McCaffery & Beebe 1989). Nurses are influenced by a number of variables when assessing the amount of pain a patient is suffering (Kitson 1994). Pargeon and Hailey (1999) demonstrated that health care providers usually over- or underestimate a patient's pain. It has also been suggested that nurses do not possess sufficient knowledge to care for patients in pain (McCaffery & Ferrell 1997; Drayer *et al.* 1999). A survey of over 3000 nurses (McCaffery & Robinson 2002) demonstrated that nurse education has improved confidence in the pain assessment process but that further education continues to be required in the pharmacology of pain medications and addressing nurses' fears of opioid addiction and respiratory depression, which continue to contribute to the under-treatment of pain.

A variety of pain assessment tools exist which can be used to assist nurses to assess pain and plan nursing care. They enable pain to be successfully assessed and monitored (Walker *et al.* 1987; McCaffery & Beebe 1989; Twycross *et al.* 1996) and improve communication between staff and patients (Raiman 1986). Higginson (1998, p. 150) notes that: 'Taking assessments directly from the patient is the most valid way of collecting information on their quality of life'. Encouraging patients to take an active role in their pain assessment by using pain tools helps to increase their confidence and makes them feel part of the pain management process.

Some degree of caution, however, must be exercised with the use of pain assessment tools. The nurse must be careful to select the tool that is most appropriate for a particular type of pain experience. For example, it would not be appropriate to use a pain assessment tool that had been designed for use with patients with chronic pain, to assess postoperative pain. Furthermore, pain tools should not be used totally indiscriminately. Walker *et al.* (1987) found that pain tools appeared to have little value in cases of unresolved or intractable pain.

The most commonly used pain assessment tools meet the following criteria (Fitzpatrick *et al.* 1998):

■ Simplicity: ease of understanding for all the patient groups.
■ Reliability: reliability of the tool when used in similar patient groups; results are reproducible and consistent.
■ Valid: the tool measures the patient's perception of pain.
■ Sensitivity: sensitivity of the tool to the patient's pain.
■ Accuracy: accurate and precise recording of data.
■ Interpretable: meaningful pain scores or data are produced.
■ Feasiblity/practicality: the degree of effort involved in using the tool is acceptable; a practical tool is more likely to be used by patients and nursing staff.

The use of pain assessment tools for acute pain has been shown both to increase the effectiveness of nursing interventions and to improve the management of pain (Scott 1994; Harmer & Davies 1998). Several pain assessment tools are available. Verbal Descriptor Scales (VDS) are based on numerically ranked words such as 'none', 'mild', 'moderate', 'severe' and 'very severe' for assessing both pain intensity and response to analgesia. Numerical Rating Scales (NRS) have both written and verbal forms. The written forms are described as either a vertical or a horizontal line with '0' indicating no pain located on one extremity of the line and '10' indicating severe pain at the other extremity. This type of scale is easily used as a verbal scale of 0–10 if patients are unable to see or focus on a written scale. Although originally published as a line with a scale of 0–10 there are many versions of it (Flaherty 1996). Since many of these scales focus on assessing the intensity of pain, it is important that nurses do not neglect to combine their use of these tools with an assessment of the patient's psychosocial needs.

For practical purposes, a combined pain assessment and observation chart is frequently used in the postoperative period. The Royal Marsden Hospital Postoperative Observation and Pain Assessment Chart is an example of one of these (Figure 20.1). The patient's assessment of their pain is recorded on the numerical

Patient Name: _____ Hosp. No.: _____ C.U./Consultant: _____

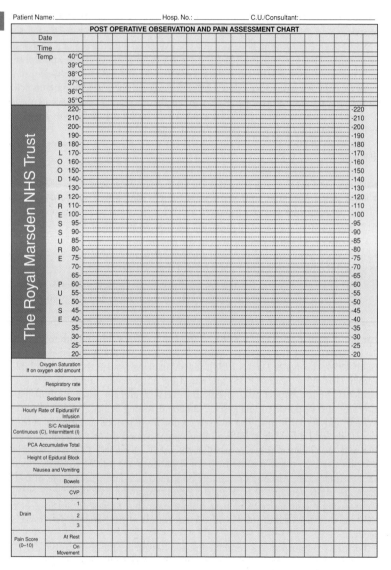

Figure 20.1 The Royal Marsden Hospital Postoperative Observation And Pain Assessment Chart.

rating pain scale at the bottom of the chart at the same time that other observations are carried out (usually 2–4 hourly but more frequently if pain is not controlled).

Other pain assessment tools have been developed to capture the multidimensional nature of pain. These specifically measure several features of the pain experience. This includes the location and intensity of pain, pattern of pain over time, the effect of pain on the patient's daily function and activities, the effect on the patient's mood and the ability to interact and socialize with others. Examples of these include the McGill Pain Questionnaire (MPQ) (Melzack 1975) and the Brief Pain Inventory (BPI) (Cleeland 1991). These are more commonly used in chronic pain assessment.

Neuropathic pain is defined as pain due to a disturbance of function or pathological change in a nerve (Merskey & Bogduk 1994). Patients may describe spontaneous pain (those that arise without detectable stimulation) and evoked pain (abnormal responses to stimuli) (Bennett 2001). The Leeds Assessment of Neuropathic Symptoms and Signs (LANSS) pain scale (Bennett 2001) was developed to more accurately assess this type of pain.

The Royal Marsden NHS Foundation Trust currently uses a patient held pain tool for patients with chronic cancer pain (Figure 20.2).

The need for effective acute pain control

There are several reasons why pain needs to be well-controlled following surgery, not least that patients have a right to expect adequate treatment of pain and that all members of the health care team have an ethical obligation to provide it (Audit Commission 1997). It is now known that under-treatment of acute pain coupled with the physiological response to surgery, known as the stress response, can have a number of adverse consequences (Macintyre & Ready 2001). Uncontrolled pain can lead to increased anxiety, fear, sleeplessness and muscle tension which further exacerbate pain. It can delay the recovery process by hindering mobilization and deep breathing, which increases the risk of a patient developing a deep vein thrombosis, chest infection or pressure ulcer. Pain can also lead to significant delays in gastric emptying and a reduction in intestinal motility (Macintyre & Ready 2001). With severe pain, activity of the sympathetic nervous system and the neuroendocrine 'stress response' cause platelet activation, changes in regional blood flow and stress on the heart. These can lead to impaired wound healing and myocardial ischaemia (Macintyre & Ready 2001). There is evidence to suggest that in the long term, poorly controlled acute pain may lead to the development of chronic pain. Perkins and Kehlet (2000) established that moderate to severe acute postoperative pain was a predictor for developing chronic pain after breast surgery, thoracic surgery and hernia repair.

The Royal Marsden NHS Trust
Patient Held Pain Chart

Surname:

First name:

Who completed the assessment:
(specify if nurse or family member helped)

Date of this assessment:

Instructions for use:

1. This chart is for you to complete (you may want your family or a nurse to help you)

2. Work through the questions in section 1 and 2 of the chart. Do ask for help if you are not clear about any of the questions.

3. When you get to section 3 use the instructions at the top of the sheet to help you keep an ongoing record of your pain and the effect of any pain treatments.

Please keep this chart with you because the nurses and doctors who are looking after you will use it to help manage your pain(s)

Section 1: Where is your pain?

Please draw on the body outlines below to show where you feel pain. Label each site A, B, C, etc. or use a different colour

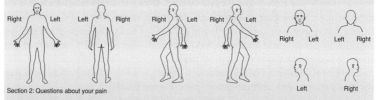

Section 2: Questions about your pain

How would you describe your pain(s) at the site(s) you drew on the body diagram? (e.g. aching, tender, sharp, shooting, burning).

What helps reduce your pain(s) at each site? (e.g. specific drugs, activities or treatments such as massage).

What makes your pain worse at each site? (e.g. specific activity or heat/cold).

How often do you get pain at each site? (e.g. all the time or at different times during the day).

How do you feel when you are in pain and how has it changed your daily activities? (e.g. moving, sleeping).

Section 3: Scoring and recording your pain scores

Pain Scores	Instructions for scoring and recording pain scores
0 = No pain 1–4 = Mild pain 5–6 = Moderate pain 7–9 = Severe pain 10 = Worst pain imaginable	1) In the column marked Pain scores use the scoring system shown here to record your pain score(s) at each site (see columns A, B, C, etc.) where you feel pain. 2) Score your pain at regular intervals. Do this before your pain treatments (e.g. analgesics/pain medicines, massage) and 30–45 minutes afterwards so that you can see if they have helped.

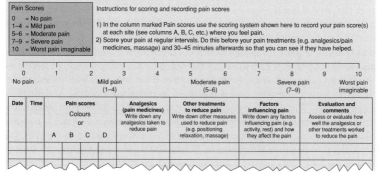

Figure 20.2   The Royal Marsden Hospital Patient Held Pain Chart.

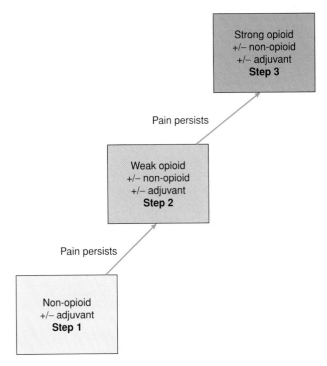

Figure 20.3   The Analgesic Ladder. Modified from WHO (1996).

Management of chronic pain

The control of pain is directed by the 'Analgesic Ladder', which was presented by the World Health Organization (WHO) in 1996 (Figure 20.3). The simple principles are such that pharmacological intervention begins on the first step of the ladder and proceeds upwards as and when the pain reaches a higher level and the current analgesia is no longer effective. Analgesia should be administered 'around the clock' (ATC) to enable chronic persistent pain to be controlled. It is important to remember that the patient will experience different types of pain due to different aetiological and physiological changes, manifested through the cancer trajectory (e.g. bone pain, neuropathic pain). It is important to make an assessment of each pain separately, since the pain may need to be managed in a different manner and one analgesic intervention will rarely be sufficient. Often the best practice is to combine the baseline analgesia with an appropriate adjuvant treatment in order to achieve maximum pain control (Table 20.2).

Table 20.2   The use of adjuvant drugs (co-analgesics).

Type	Use	Examples
Non-steroidal anti-inflammatory drugs (NSAIDs)	Bone pain Muscular pain Inflammation Visceral pain	Diclofenac Naproxen Ibuprofen
Steroids	Pressure Bone pain Inflammation Raised intracranial pressure	Dexamethasone Prednisolone
Tricyclic antidepressants	Neuropathic pain	Amitriptyline
Anticonvulsants		Sodium valproate Carbamazepine Gabapentin Pre Gabalin
Antibiotics	Infection	Flucloxacillin Trimethoprim
Benzodiazepines	Anxiety	Diazepam Clonazepam
Antispasmodics	Spasms	Baclofen
Bisphosphonates	Bone pain	Sodium clodronate Disodium pamidronate Zoledronic acid

Oral administration of therapeutic interventions may not always be appropriate. In chronic pain the European Association of Palliative Care (EAPC) recommends that if patients can no longer manage the oral route, the preferred alternative route is subcutaneous, which is simple and less painful than the intramuscular route (Hanks *et al.* 2001). In rare circumstances when rapid titration of analgesia is required the intravenous route may also be used if patients have established intravenous access.

Accurate ongoing assessment is imperative for efficient and effective pain control.

The management of pain following surgery

Since nurses, surgeons, anaesthetists, pain specialists, pharmacists and physiotherapists are all involved in the management of surgical pain, teamwork is essential.

Professionals must reach clear agreement as to their individual roles so that patients receive the best possible care from preadmission through to discharge (Audit Commission 1997).

A wide variety of pharmacological and non-pharmacological techniques are available for the management of surgical pain. The following basic principles apply to their use:

1 Tailor the treatments to:
   (a) Meet individual needs.
   (b) Prevent pain, rather than allowing it to become established.
2 Whenever possible, choose the simplest and safest techniques to achieve the desired level of pain relief (McQuay *et al.* 1997).
3 Use the WHO Analgesic Ladder (see Figure 20.3) to select the most appropriate analgesics for mild, moderate and severe acute pain.
4 Choose the most appropriate route for giving analgesia.
5 Combine techniques to provide balanced analgesia and enhance overall pain control (Kehlet 1997).
6 Ensure patients receive regular antiemetics to control postoperative nausea and vomiting. Vomiting increases muscle tension and exacerbates pain.

Acute pain

Pharmacological techniques

Opioid analgesics

Opioids are the first-line treatment for pain that follows major surgery. Inter-patient opioid requirements vary greatly (Macintyre & Jarvis 1996) and opioid doses need to be titrated carefully to achieve pain relief to suit each individual patient while minimizing any unwanted side-effects (McQuay *et al.* 1997; see Chronic pain section for further details on side-effects).

A number of opioids are used for controlling pain following surgery. These include morphine, diamorphine, fentanyl and oxycodone. The most common routes of opioid administration are intravenous, epidural, subcutaneous, intramuscular or oral.

Evidence for the concept of opioid rotation when patients have intolerable opioid related side-effects originates from cancer pain studies (Quigley 2004) but it may be a useful strategy to consider in the management of acute pain as well.

Intravenous analgesia

Continuous intravenous infusions of opioids such as morphine, diamorphine and fentanyl are effective for controlling pain in the immediate postoperative period. Their use is often restricted to critical care units where patients can be closely monitored because of the potential risk of respiratory depression (Macintyre &

Ready 2001). Compared with patient-controlled analgesia (PCA; see next paragraph) continuous infusions of opoids for acute pain management in a general ward setting resulted in a fivefold increase in the incidence of respiratory depression (Schug & Torrie 1993).

Patient-controlled analgesia (PCA) is an alternative and safer technique for giving intravenous opioids (usually morphine, diamorphine or fentanyl) in the ward environment (Sidebotham *et al*. 1997). With PCA, patients self-administer intermittent doses of opioids, by using an infusion pump and timing device. When in pain, the patient presses a button connected to the pump and a set dose of opioid is delivered (usually intravenously but it may also be given subcutaneously) to the patient (Macintyre & Ready 2001).

There are a number of advantages of using PCA:

- PCA is more likely to maintain reasonably constant blood concentrations of the opioid within the analgesic corridor. This is the blood level where analgesia is achieved without significant side-effects. The flexibility of PCA helps to overcome the wide interpatient variation in opioid requirements (Macintyre & Ready 2001).
- PCA allows patients to titrate analgesia against daily variations in the pain stimulus (Tye & Gell-Walker 2000). By using a PCA pump, patients can administer analgesia as soon as pain occurs and titrate the dose of analgesia according to increases and decreases in the pain stimulus. This is particularly helpful for controlling more intense pain during movement.
- PCA prevents delays in patients receiving analgesics (Chumbley *et al*. 2002).

Whilst PCA may be very effective for controlling pain for a number of patients undergoing surgery (Macintyre 2001), it is not suitable for the following groups (Tye & Gell-Walker 2000):

- Patients who are unable to activate the PCA device due to problems with dexterity or visual impairment.
- Patients who are unable to understand the concept of PCA, particularly the very young or patients who are confused.
- Patients who do not wish to take responsibility for their pain control.

(For further details about the use of PCA pumps see Chapter 9.)

Epidural analgesia

Epidural analgesia refers to the provision of pain relief by continuous administration of analgesic pharmacological agents (usually low concentrations of local anaesthetics and opioids) into the epidural space via an indwelling catheter (ANZCA and Faculty of Pain Medicine 2005). Giving analgesia epidurally is a particularly valuable technique for the prevention of postoperative pain in patients undergoing major thoracic, abdominal and lower limb surgery, and can sometimes be used to manage the pain associated with trauma. Commonly used opioids for epidural analgesia include fentanyl and diamorphine (Wheatley *et al.* 2001). Combinations of low concentrations of local anaesthetic agents and opioids have been shown to provide consistently superior pain relief compared with either drug alone (Macintyre & Ready 2001). Further details of this technique are given in Chapter 21.

Subcutaneous analgesia

Opioids are often given subcutaneously to manage chronic cancer pain. More recently, there has been an increase in the use of subcutaneous opioids for postoperative pain control. Both PCA- and nurse-administered opioid injections of morphine, diamorphine or oxycodone via an indwelling subcutaneous cannula have been used successfully to manage postoperative pain (Vijayan 1997). An advantage of giving analgesia subcutaneously is that it avoids the problems associated with maintaining intravenous access.

Intramuscular analgesia

Until the early 1990s regular 3–4-hourly intramuscular injections of opioids such as pethidine, morphine or preparations containing morphine (Omnopon) were routinely used for the management of postoperative pain. Because alternative techniques such as PCA and epidural analgesia are available, intramuscular analgesia is now used less frequently. Some useful algorithms have been developed to give guidance on titrating intramuscular analgesia (Harmer & Davies 1998; Macintyre & Ready 2001). Absorption via this route may be impaired in conditions of poor perfusion (e.g. in hypovolaemia, shock, hypothermia or immobility). This may lead to inadequate early analgesia (the drug cannot be absorbed properly and reach systemic circulation and forms a drug depot) and late absorption of the drug depot (where the drug has remained in the muscular tissue and is absorbed only once perfusion is restored) (ANZCA and Faculty of Pain Medicine 2005).

Oral analgesia

Oral opioids are used less frequently in the immediate postoperative period because many patients may be nil by mouth or on restricted oral intake for a period of time. Often this route is used if patients require strong analgesics following discontinuation of epidural or intravenous analgesia. Morphine is an ideal oral preparation because it is available as a tablet (Sevredol) or an elixir (Oramorph). Oxycodone can be given as second line opioid treatment if patients are allergic/sensitive to or fail to respond to morphine.

Opioids for mild to moderate pain and non-opioid analgesics

Paracetamol and paracetamol combinations

The use of non-opioid analgesics such as paracetamol or paracetamol combined with a weak opioid such as codeine is recommended for managing pain following minor surgical procedures or when the pain following major surgery begins to subside (McQuay *et al.* 1997). Paracetamol can also be given rectally if the oral route is contraindicated. An intravenous preparation of paracetamol is now available and can provide effective analgesia after surgical procedures (Romsing *et al.* 2002). It is more effective and of faster onset than the same dose given enterally. The use of the intravenous form should be limited to patients where the enteral route cannot be used.

Paracetamol taken in the correct dose of not more than 4 g per day is relatively free of side-effects. When used in combination with codeine preparations, the most frequent side-effect is constipation.

Tramadol

Another opioid for mild to moderate pain, which has been shown to be an effective analgesic for postoperative pain, is tramadol (McQuay & Moore 1998; Reicin *et al.* 2001). Although tramadol does have some side-effects, which include nausea and dizziness, it is free of non-steroidal anti-inflammatory drug (NSAID) side-effects and causes less constipation than codeine preparations and opioids (Bamigbade & Langford 1998). The combination of tramadol with paracetamol is more effective than either of the two components administered alone (McQuay & Edwards 2003).

Non-steroidal anti-inflammatory drugs

Non-steroidal anti-inflammatory drugs (NSAIDs) have been shown to provide better pain relief than paracetamol combinations for acute pain (McQuay *et al.* 1997). These drugs can be used alone or in combination with both opioid and non-opioid analgesics. Two commonly used NSAIDs are diclofenac, which can be administered orally, enterally or rectally, and ibuprofen, which is available only as an oral or enteral preparation. The disadvantage of both of these is that often side-effects such as coagulation problems, renal impairment and gastrointestinal disturbances limit their use. Newer COX 2-specific NSAIDs have the advantage that they are associated with similar analgesia and anti-inflammatory effects (Reicin *et al.* 2001) but have no effect on platelets or the gastric mucosa (Rowbotham 2000). As a result coagulation problems and gastrointestinal irritation are likely to be significantly reduced. However, recently several of these drugs have been withdrawn from the market due to long-term cardiovascular side-effects and it will take time for newer products with an improved safety profile to re-establish themselves in practice (ANZCA and Faculty of Pain Medicine 2005).

Nitrous oxide (Entonox)

Inhaled nitrous oxide provides analgesia that is short acting and works quickly. It has a special role in managing pain associated with wound dressings and drain removal (see Chapter 28, Professional edition on the use of Entonox).

Local anaesthetics

In addition to epidural analgesia, local anaesthetics may be used to block individual or groups of peripheral nerves during surgical procedures and to infiltrate surgical wounds at the end of an operation (Carroll & Bowsher 1993). Occasionally these techniques may be used to extend the duration of postoperative analgesia beyond the finite period that a single injection technique provides (ANZCA and Faculty of Pain Medicine 2005). Techniques include regular intermittent bolus doses or continuous infusions of local anaesthetic.

Non-pharmacological techniques for acute and chronic pain

Optimal pain control is more likely to be achieved by combining non-pharmacological techniques with pharmacological techniques. Despite the lack of research evidence to support the effectiveness of many non-pharmacological techniques, their benefits to patients and families should not be underestimated.

Psychological interventions

A number of simple psychological interventions can improve a patient's pain control by:

■ Reducing anxiety, stress and muscle tension.
■ Distraction (distraction plays a role in pain management by pushing awareness of pain out of central cognition).
■ Increasing control and pain-coping mechanisms.
■ Improving general well-being (Zarnegar & Daniel 2005).

Some simple interventions include the following.

Creating trusting therapeutic relationships

By creating trusting relationships with patients, nurses are instrumental in reducing anxiety and helping patients to cope with pain (Carr & Mann 2000b). Nurses can help to create a trusting relationship by:

■ Listening to the patient.
■ Believing the patient's pain experience (Seers 1996).
■ Acting as a patient advocate.
■ Providing patients with appropriate physical and emotional support.

The use of gentle humour

Pasero (1998) suggests that many patients find gentle humour an effective way of coping with pain. Humour may be particularly helpful prior to a painful procedure as it can have a lasting effect. In the clinical setting, humorous tapes, books and videos can be made available for patient use.

Information/education

Patient information/education can make all the difference between effective and ineffective pain relief. Information/education helps to reduce anxiety (Hayward 1975; Taylor 2001) and enables patients to make informed decisions about their care. Patients should be given specific information about why pain control is important, what to expect in terms of pain relief, how they can participate in their management and what to do if pain is not controlled. Some caution is required, however, because not all patients respond positively to the same level of information. Patients with high levels of anxiety may find that detailed information can increase their anxiety and influence their pain control. To avoid this, patients can be given a choice of whether or not they receive simple or detailed information (Mitchell 1997).

Relaxation

Whilst scientific evidence for the effectiveness of relaxation techniques is limited (Carroll & Seers 1998; Seers & Carroll 1998), a number of studies have shown benefits for patients experiencing pain (Sloman *et al.* 1994; Good *et al.* 1999; Lang *et al.* 2000). Payne (1995) describes several relaxation techniques ranging from simple breathing techniques to progressive muscle relaxation and more complex techniques. One simple relaxation technique script that has been adapted for use at The Royal Marsden Hospital is outlined in Box 20.1. This technique can be taught to patients and used during painful procedures or at times when the patient feels anxious or stressed. Patients should be encouraged to practise the technique to gain mastery.

Music

The use of taped music in the health care setting can also provide relaxation and distraction from pain (Beck 1991; Good 1996; Heiser *et al.* 1997; Good *et al.* 1999). Setting up a library of taped music (e.g. easy listening, classical) and having personal stereos available for patient use is a simple way to provide patients with relaxing music.

Art

Art therapies have also been used to assist the patient in moving the focus of attention away from the physical sensation of pain to other aspects of the person

---

Box 20.1 Simple relaxation technique script

Please note that breathing during this technique should be normal for the patient in their present condition.

1 Loosen any tight clothing and position yourself comfortably, either lying or sitting. Have your arms and legs uncrossed. Ensure your back and head are well supported.
2 Allow both your hands to rest on your abdomen, one on top of the other. It may be helpful to place a pillow on your lap for your hands to rest on.
3 Gently allow your eyes to close. Breathe normally in and out through your nose if you find this comfortable.
4 As you breathe in, be aware of your abdomen rising gently under your hands (do not force this movement).
5 As you breathe out, be aware of your abdomen relaxing under your hands.
6 Let your shoulders relax and drop down.
7 Let your jaw relax.
8 Now keep your attention softly focused on the rise and fall of your abdomen as this movement follows each breath.
9 Repeat steps 4–8 for between 3 and 5 minutes or longer if appropriate.

During the exercise
As you become aware of any thoughts that arise, let them go and just bring your attention back to the rise and fall of the abdomen. If you are still having difficulty focusing on the technique try saying the following phrases: 'I am relaxed' or 'I feel calm'.

To finish the exercise
Now slowly become aware of your surroundings, stretch out your fingers and toes, gently open your eyes and come back to the room.

(Trauger-Querry & Haghighi 1999). The skills of an art therapist are required to ensure the successful use of this intervention.

Physical interventions

In addition to psychological interventions, a number of physical interventions can be helpful in reducing pain.

Comfort measures

Simple comfort measures such as careful body positioning (for example, supporting a painful arm on a pillow) and the use of soft and therapeutic mattresses (Ballard 1997) can help to improve patient comfort and pain control.

Exercise

Both passive and active physical exercises may benefit patients by increasing range of motion (Feine & Lund 1997), preventing joint stiffness and muscle wasting which may further compound pain problems. Exercise should always be tailored to the patient's tolerance and stamina. A simple exercise regimen which is practised regularly and supervised by a therapist can help patients feel better and more in control as well as having benefits in terms of pain relief.

Rest

In addition to exercise, teaching patients to rest comfortably in any position when in pain is a meaningful action and the base from which a person can learn to move more easily (O'Connor & Webb 2002). A person with a terminal illness may experience restriction of movement and neuromuscular pain with increased tension. For these patients, learning to rest and letting go of any tension can be helpful. O'Connor and Webb (2002) describe a specific method for resting known as the Feldenkrais method. Using this, a person can be taught how to rest comfortably in any position: this may be lying down, sitting or standing.

Transcutaneous electrical nerve stimulation

Transcutaneous electrical nerve stimulation (TENS) is thought to work by sending a weak electrical current through the skin to stimulate the sensory nerve endings. Depending on the stimulation parameters used, TENS is thought to modulate pain impulses by closing the gate to pain transmission within the spinal cord by stimulating the release of natural pain-relieving chemicals in the brain and spinal cord (King 1999).

To date there is limited scientific evidence for the effectiveness of TENS. Despite this, many health care professionals use TENS for a variety of chronic pain conditions and support the view that this is a useful form of analgesia (Walsh 1997). In contrast, TENS has not been found to improve the control of acute pain following surgery (McQuay *et al.* 1997).

Acupuncture

This involves placing fine solid needles into the skin at acupoints or trigger points. Although the exact mechanism of action is unknown, acupuncture is believed to work in part by stimulating release of the body's own natural opioids. Although there is also limited scientific evidence for the pain-relieving effects of acupuncture, largely due to the poorly controlled studies (Ezzo *et al.* 2000), it is used widely and has an important role in pain management.

Heat therapies

For decades superficial heat therapy has been used to relieve a variety of muscular and joint pains, including arthritis, back pain and period pain. There is much anecdotal and some scientific evidence to support the usefulness of heat as an adjunct to other pain treatments (Akin *et al.* 2001; Nadler *et al.* 2002; Robinson *et al.* 2002).

Heat works by:

- Stimulating thermoreceptors in the skin and deeper tissues, thereby reducing the sensitivity to pain by closing the gating system in the spinal cord.
- Reducing muscle spasm.
- Reducing the viscosity of synovial fluid which alleviates painful stiffness during movement and increases joint range (Carr & Mann 2000b).

In the home environment people use a variety of different methods for applying heat therapies, such as warm baths, hot water bottles, wheat-based heat packs and electrical heating pads. In the hospital setting caution is required with this equipment as it does not reach health and safety standards (no even and regular temperature distribution) and there have been incidences of serious burns (Barillo *et al.* 2000). Carr and Mann (2000b) note that heat therapy should not be used immediately following tissue damage as it will increase swelling. The Medicines and Healthcare Products Regulatory Agency (MHRA 2005) has documented evidence of burns caused by using heat patches or packs and therefore urge caution in their use and also recommend regular checking of skin throughout therapy.

Cold therapies
Cold therapies can also be used to stimulate nerves and modulate pain (Carr & Mann 2000b). Cold may be particularly valuable following an acute bruising injury where it can help to reduce inflammation and limit further damage. Cold can be applied in the form of crushed ice or gel-filled cold packs which should be wrapped in a towel to protect the skin from an ice burn.

Chronic pain

Pharmacological techniques

Using the WHO Analgesic Ladder (1996)

The Analgesic Ladder was designed as a framework for the management of chronic pain (see Figure 20.3). There are several drugs available to manage chronic pain and the Analgesic Ladder allows the flexibility to choose from the range according to the patient's requirements and tolerance (Hanks *et al.* 2001).

Step 1: non-opioid drugs
Examples of non-opioid drugs include paracetamol, aspirin and NSAIDs that are effective for mild to moderate pain. These drugs are especially effective for musculoskeletal and visceral pain (Twycross & Wilcock 2001).

Step 2: opioids for mild to moderate pain

Examples of opioids for mild to moderate pain include codeine, dihydrocodeine, tramadol and oxycodone (steps 2 and 3). These drugs are used when adequate pain management is not achieved with the use of non-opioids and are usually used in combination formulations. It is not recommended to administer another analgesic from the same group if the drug being used is not controlling the pain. Uncontrolled pain needs to be assessed and managed with the titration of an opioid by moving up the Analgesic Ladder. The exception to this would be if the patient was experiencing intolerable side-effects on the weak opioid and an alternative drug may be beneficial.

In recent studies tramadol has been recognized as being efficacious in the management of chronic cancer pain of moderate severity (Davis *et al.* 2005). It is uncertain whether tramadol is more effective in neuropathic pain than other opioids for mild to moderate pain; one report suggests a reduction in allodynia (pain from stimuli which is not normally painful) (Sindrup & Jensen 1999; Twycross & Wilcock 2001). Nurses should be aware that there are circumstantial reports that suggest tramadol lowers seizure threshold, and therefore care needs to be taken in those patients who have a history of epilepsy, as well as any other medications that may contribute to the lowering of the seizure threshold for example tricyclic antidepressants and selective serotonin reuptake inhibitors (SSRIs) (Twycross & Wilcock 2001). Few patients with severe pain will achieve a satisfactory level of pain control with tramadol. It is available in immediate and modified release preparations.

Step 3: opioids for moderate to severe pain

Morphine A large amount of information and research is available concerning morphine and therefore it tends to be the drug of choice within this category (Hanks *et al.* 2001, 2004). It is available in oral, rectal, parenteral and intraspinal preparations. A recent study of 43 European Palliative Care Units showed that morphine was the most frequently used opioid for moderate to severe pain, with over 50% of patients taking oral or parenteral preparations (Klepstad *et al.* 2005). All strong opioids require careful titration from an expert practitioner. It is better to begin with a small dose, usually one that is equivalent to the previous medication, and increase gradually in conjunction with careful assessment of its effectiveness (Hanks *et al.* 2001). Titration begins with the immediate-release form which is available in tablet (Sevredol) or elixir (Oramorph) preparations, and once pain control is achieved the patient can be converted to a modified release preparation that acts over a 12- or 24-hour period (Zomorph or MXL respectively).

Breakthrough analgesia is administered using the equivalent 4-hourly dose of the immediate-release form. This dose can be given as required (hourly) and subsequent adjustments can be made to the modified form if the patient is requiring more than three breakthrough doses in a 24-hour period (Hanks *et al.* 2001).

Patients should be informed of potential side-effects such as constipation, nausea and increased sleepiness, in order to allay any fear. The patient should also be told that nausea and drowsiness are transitory and normally improve within 48 hours, but that constipation can be an ongoing problem and it is recommended that a laxative should be prescribed at the same time as the opioid is started. It is recommended that the most effective laxative for this group of patients is a combination of both a softening and a stimulating laxative (Davis *et al.* 2005).

Patients often have many concerns about commencing strong drugs such as morphine. Frequent fears centre around addiction and believing that its use signifies the terminal phase of the illness (McQuay 1999). Time should be taken to reassure patients and their families and provide verbal and written information. Although morphine is still considered to be the opioid drug of choice for moderate to severe pain (Hanks *et al.* 2001), alternative opioids allows the practitioner to carefully assess the patient on an individual basis and select the most appropriate opioid to use.

Durogesic (fentanyl)   Fentanyl is a strong opioid, available in a patch, which is recommended in patients who have stable pain requirements. Transdermal patches are available in 12 (new size), 25, 50, 75 or 100 μg. It is reported to have an improved side-effect profile in comparison to morphine (Ahmedzai & Brooks 1997), although some patients experience nausea and mild drowsiness (BMA/Royal Pharmaceutical Society of Great Britain 2008) and occasionally patients may develop a reaction to the adhesive in the patch (Ling 1997). Use of the patch has increased because it allows the patient freedom from taking tablets.

Changing of the patch is recommended every 3 days, and steady plasma levels are reported to be reached after 8–16 hours (Zech *et al.* 1994), although in some patients it may be necessary to change it more frequently. The patch should be applied to skin that is free from excess hair and any form of irritation and should not be applied to irradiated areas. It is advisable to change the location on the body to avoid an adverse skin reaction. Occasionally difficulties arise relating to the titration of the patch as each patch is equivalent to a range of morphine (Table 20.3). For breakthrough pain, if patients are able to take oral medications then an immediate release preparation, for example immediate release morphine sulphate (oramorph/sevredol), at the appropriate dose can be used. An immediate-release fentanyl lozenge is available for use in breakthrough or incident pain. The advantage of oral transmucosal fentanyl citrate (OTFC) is its fast onset via the buccal mucosa (5–15 minutes) and its short duration (up to 2 hours). It is available in a range of doses (200–1600 μg) but there is no direct relation between the baseline analgesia and the breakthrough dose. Titration can be difficult and lengthy

Table 20.3   Oral morphine conversion to Durogesic (fentanyl) patch.

4-hourly oral morphine dose (mg)	Durogesic patch strength (μg/hour)	24-hour morphine dose (mg)
20	25	135
25–35	50	135–224
40–50	75	225–314
55–65	100	315–404
70–80	125	405–494
85–95	150	495–584
100–110	175	585–674
115–125	200	675–764

A 12 μg/hour Durogesic DTrans (fentanyl transdermal system with matrix technology) patch has been introduced to aid dose titration between 25 and 75 μg/hour.

as the recommended starting dose is 200 μg with titration upwards (Portenoy *et al.* 1999).

Fentanyl is also available in parenteral preparations. There are potential problems with fentanyl due to dose limitations. The ampoules are available in 50 μg/1 ml. If the dose required is too large a volume to use in the syringe driver, then alfentanil may be a useful alternative (Dickman *et al.* 2002).

Palladone (hydromorphone)   Palladone (hydromorphone) is mostly used when patients experience unacceptable drowsiness with morphine. It is similar to morphine in its pharmacokinetic profile and it is approximately 5.0–7.5 times more potent than morphine. It is available in immediate-release and sustained-release preparations and titration occurs in the same manner as morphine (Hays *et al.* 1994).

The side-effects are similar to those of morphine (Ellershaw 1998).

Methadone   Methadone is a synthetic opioid developed more than 40 years ago (Riley *et al.* 2006). It is available in oral, rectal and parenteral preparations. There has been some reluctance amongst professionals to use methadone, which arose from the difficulties experienced in titrating the drug due to its long half-life (15 hours) that caused accumulation to occur, especially in the elderly (Gannon 1997). There are different methods of achieving effective titration (Gannon 1997); for example, one regimen is to calculate one-tenth of the total daily dose of morphine (maximum starting dose must not exceed 30 mg). Administer the methadone to the patient on an as-required basis but not within 3 hours of the last fixed dose. The total dose required over a 24-hour period is calculated after 5–6 days, divided and given as a two or three times daily regimen and this avoids the build-up of methadone within the body (Morley & Makin 1998). Titration is recommended within a hospital setting to ensure accurate administration. This can be difficult for patients because they have to experience pain before they are administered a dose of methadone in the titration period.

Methadone can be a cheap, effective alternative to morphine if titration is supervised by the specialist pain or palliative care team (Gardner-Nix 1996).

Methadone is particularly useful in patients with renal failure. Morphine is excreted via the kidneys and if renal failure occurs this may lead to the patient experiencing severe drowsiness as a result of culmination of morphine metabolites (Gannon 1997). Methadone is lipid soluble and is metabolized mainly in the liver. About half of the drug and its metabolites are excreted by the intestines and half by the kidneys.

Oxycodone   Oxycodone is available as an immediate or modified release tablet and titration should occur in the same way as morphine. Oxycodone is a useful opioid as an alternative to morphine (Riley *et al.* 2006). It has similar properties to morphine and can be administered orally, rectally, intraspinally and parenterally. Oxycodone has similar side-effects and it is usually given 4–6 hourly. Oxycodone has an analgesic potency of 1.5–2.0 times higher than morphine. It has similar side-effects to morphine, although oxycodone has been found to cause less nausea (Heiskanen and Kalso 1997) and significantly less itchiness (Mucci-LoRusso *et al.* 1998).

Diamorphine   Diamorphine is used parenterally in a syringe driver for the control of moderate to severe pain when patients are unable to take the oral form of morphine. It is calculated by dividing the total daily dose of oral morphine by three. Breakthrough doses are calculated by dividing the 24-hour dose of diamorphine by six and administering on an as-required basis (Hanks *et al.* 2004). A recent problem with the supply of Diamorphine nationally has resulted in centres using morphine sulphate or an alternative opioid as a substitute.

Nasal analgesia   It is suggested that the nasal route may be effective for a number of opioids (Hanks *et al.* 2004). Nasal diamorphine spray has been shown to provide effective pain relief in Accident and Emergency Departments in children and teenagers who are experiencing acute pain. This approach is being investigated in adult cancer patients with acute, episodic pain (Hanks *et al.* 2004).

Alfentanil   Alfentanil is also a useful alternative to diamorphine and is used as an alternative opioid for those patients who have renal impairment. The onset of action is rapid owing to a more rapid blood–brain equilibration. It is 10 times more potent than diamorphine (i.e. diamorphine 10 mg = alfentanil 1 mg). The breakthrough dose can be calculated as one-tenth of the 24-hour dose as opposed to the usual one-sixth. For example 1 mg of alfentanil over 24 hours will require a breakthrough dose of alfentanil 0.1 mg. It is beneficial when high doses are required as it comes in ampoules of 1 mg/2 ml and 5 mg/1 ml and smaller volumes can be used (Hill 1992).

Buprenorphine Buprenorphine is an alternative strong opioid available in a patch form. The patch has similar advantages to fentanyl but does not contain a reservoir of the drug. Instead it is contained in a matrix form with effective levels of the drug being reached within 24 hours. Titration is recommended with an alternative opioid initially and then transfer to the patch when stable requirements have been reached. The patches are available in strengths of 5, 10 and 20 μg/hour at a lower dose patch (Butrans) that should be worn continuously by the patient for 7 days. The higher dose patch (Transtec) of 35, 52.5 and 70 μg/hour is now licensed to be used up to 96 hours or twice weekly for patient convenience. Conversion is based on the chart supplied by the pharmaceutical company which demonstrates equivalent doses. Buprenorphine is also available as a sublingual tablet, which is titrated from 200 to 800 μg 6-hourly. Conversion is based on multiplying the total daily dose of buprenorphine by 100 to give the total daily dose of morphine (i.e. 200 μg buprenorphine/8-hourly = 600 μg buprenorphine/24 hours = 60 mg morphine/24 hours) (Budd 2002).

Cannabis Studies are currently taking place to examine the potential benefits of using cannabis for the management of chronic conditions, e.g. multiple sclerosis and cancer. Good-quality research is sparse (Wall *et al.* 2001) but there are a number of studies that allude to its benefits in managing chronic pain, spasticity and muscle spasms (Martyn 1995; Consroe 1997).

Breakthrough analgesia

Breakthrough pain refers to a transitory exacerbation of pain experienced by the patient who has relatively stable and adequately controlled background pain (Portenoy *et al.* 2004). There should not be a time limit on this type of prescription because it would need to be given when and if the patient demonstrated any signs of discomfort or pain (with the exception of renal failure where dosages would need to be limited).

Breakthrough doses are calculated on a 4-hour equivalence; for example, if a patient was prescribed 60 mg MXL (a modified form of morphine given once a day), the equivalent breakthrough dose would be 10 mg of the immediate-release formulation. If several breakthrough doses are required within a 24-hour period, then the background analgesia (long-acting form) would have to be increased (McMillan 2001). However, it is important to recognize the classifications of breakthrough pain, as increasing the background dose will not always be indicated.

Breakthrough pain can be classified as follows:

(a) Spontaneous pain: this type of pain occurs unexpectedly.
(b) Incident pain: this pain is related to specific events and can be classified into four categories (Davies 2006):

1 Volitional pain is precipitated by a voluntary act, for example walking.
2 Non-volitional pain is precipitated by an involuntary act, for example coughing.
3 Procedural is a type of pain related to a therapeutic intervention, for example wound dressing.
4 End-of-dose failure is related to analgesic dosing (declining analgesic levels).

The use of opioids in renal failure

Renal failure can cause significant and dangerous side-effects due to the accumulation of the drug. Basic guidelines for pain management in renal failure include:

- Reduce analgesia dose and/or dose frequency (6-hourly instead of 4-hourly).
- Select a more appropriate drug (non-renally excreted).
- Avoid modified release preparations.
- Seek advice from a specialist pain/palliative care team and/or pharmacist (Farrell & Rich 2000).

Adjuvant drugs (co-analgesics)

Adjuvant drugs are a miscellaneous group of drugs whose primary indication is for conditions other than pain which may however relieve pain in specific circumstances (Twycross & Wilcock 2001). Examples of this category of drugs include NSAIDs, steroids, antibiotics, antidepressants, anti-epileptics, N-methyl-D-aspartate (NMDA) receptor channel blockers, antispasmodics and muscle relaxants (Twycross & Wilcock 2001).

The WHO Analgesic Ladder recommends the use of these drugs in combination with non-opioids, opioids for mild to moderate pain and opioids for moderate to severe pain (see Table 20.2).

Cancer treatment interventions

In addition to pharmacological and non-pharmacological strategies, treatment of cancer pain may be managed most effectively with radiotherapy, surgery, chemotherapy, hormonal manipulation and bisphosphonates. Many palliative care units/hospices may not have access to these interventions and, indeed, careful consideration must be given to ensure that the advantages achieved from any proposed treatment are not outweighed by the potential side-effects and consequent poor quality of life. The aim of these treatments would be to reduce the overall size of the tumour(s), and therefore to improve symptom control; and this must be clearly indicated to the patient (Twycross & Wilcock 2001).

Opioids and driving

In 2004 a publication in *Palliative Medicine* offered guidance for professionals on the advice they should offer to patients who were taking opioids and driving. One of the contributors to the guidance was the medical advisor to the Driver and Vehicle Licensing Agency (DVLA) (Pease *et al.* 2004). Advice to patients should include:

(a)   A patient should not drive:
- For 5 days after starting or changing the dose of the recommended opioid.
- If they feel sleepy
- After drinking alcohol or taking strong opioids which have not been recommended by the doctor or non-medical prescriber, e.g. cannabis.
- On days when additional breakthrough medication of an opioid has been taken.

(b)   Patients can restart driving:
- After 5 days starting or changing the dose of the recommended opioid and if the patient does not feel sleepy. But the patient:
  - should make the first trip short;
  - on roads that the patient is familiar with;
  - at a time when the traffic is not too busy, and
  - have an experienced driver accompany the patient as this may be helpful.

(c)   Patients do not need to inform the DVLA about starting an opioid but may need to inform them of other aspects relating to their illness. The patient should be encouraged to inform their insurance company about their current state of health and current medications.

Anaesthetic interventions

Sometimes it is difficult to attain and maintain adequate pain control without significant side-effects and it is in situations such as this that anaesthetic interventions may be of benefit.

Effective control can be achieved by epidural or intrathecal (spinal) infusions:

- as single injections for simple nerve blocks or;
- regional nerve blocks which target individual nerves, plexuses or ganglia (Hicks & Simpson 2004).

Examples include managing pelvic pain and post-radiation brachial plexopathy. These interventions can be useful, but careful consideration and assessment must take place to ensure that any potential side-effects are discussed with the patient (anaesthetic interventions may severely limit the patient's activities) and that future planning is addressed with the patient and family as an epidural/intrathecal infusion may limit discharge options for the patient who is dying.

Conclusion

The management of acute and chronic pain is a constant challenge to the health care professional. Accurate assessment of the type and site of each pain, accompanied by careful monitoring and reviewing of any intervention, are essential in order to provide care that benefits the patient and does not impinge on his or her quality of life.

Nurses are in an ideal situation to promote a trusting relationship with the patient by encouraging the patient to express any concerns, thus allowing the patient adequate opportunities to work in partnership and be an active participant in his or her pain management programme.

Procedure guidelines **Pain control: assessment and education of patient prior to surgery**

Procedure

Action	Rationale
1 If patient has had previous surgery, ask for details of: (a) Previous and current pain control methods (pharmacological and non-pharmacological). (b) Effectiveness of these methods. (c) Experience of side-effects, such as nausea and vomiting.	To ensure previous experiences are taken into consideration when planning pain control. To allay any fears based on previous experience. To ensure care is planned to minimize side-effects such as nausea and vomiting (Audit Commission 1997: C).
2 Assess patient for pre-existing long-term pain problems. Obtain information on: (a) Pain type, location and intensity. (b) Use of analgesics.	To plan in advance of surgery the pain control methods that will be used to manage both the patient's long-term and anticipated postoperative pain (Lewis & Williams 2005: R 5).

3 Check patient suitability for various pain control methods, e.g. renal function, clotting abnormalities, dexterity, visual impairment.

To avoid the use of inappropriate pain control methods, e.g.:
(a) Diclofenac in renal impairment.
(b) Epidural analgesia with clotting abnormalities.
(c) PCAs, if lack of dexterity or visual impairment makes the patient incapable of pressing the demand button which is connected to the pump (Mehta & Langford: R 4).

4 Liaise with multidisciplinary team and patient to select most appropriate pain control method(s).

To ensure effective collaboration between the patient and team in order to optimize postoperative pain control (Halaszynski *et al.* 2004: R 4).

5 Explain and discuss with patient:
(a) How pain will be assessed and the use of a pain Scale.
(b) How pain will be controlled.

To allay anxiety and promote patient well-being and control.
To encourage active involvement in pain control. To give the patient a chance to ask questions (E).

(c) Goals for pain control at rest and on movement.

To ensure the patient understands the rationale for pain control during deep breathing and movement. This will help prevent postoperative complications, e.g. chest infections (Knoerl *et al.* 1999: R 3).

6 Provide patient with written information about pain control.

To support verbal information (Chumbley *et al.* 2002: R 4).

7 Where appropriate, demonstrate the use of pain control methods before surgery.

To ensure the patient has the skill and knowledge to effectively use the pain control methods chosen, e.g. PCAs (Chumbley *et al.* 2002: R 4).

Procedure

Action	Rationale
1 Explain the purpose of using the chart to the patient.	To ensure that the patient understands the procedure and gives his/her valid consent and co-operation (Witt-Sherman *et al.* 2004: R 4; NMC 2006: C).
2 Encourage the patient, where appropriate, to identify pain him/herself.	The body outline (see Figure 20.2) is a vehicle for the patient to describe his/her own pain experience (Witt-Sherman *et al.* 2004: R 4).
3 When it is necessary for the nurse to complete the chart, ensure that the patient's own description of his/her pain is recorded.	To reduce the risk of misinterpretation (E).
4 (a) Record any factors that influence the intensity of the pain, e.g. activities or interventions that reduce or increase the pain such as distractions or a heat pad.	Ascertaining how and when the patient experiences pain enables the nurse to plan realistic goals. For example, relieving the patient's pain during the night and while he/she is at rest is usually easier to achieve before relief from pain on movement (Davis & McVicker 2000: E).
(b) Record whether or not the patient is pain free at night, at rest or on movement.	To ascertain an understanding of the experience of pain for the patient (Twycross & Wilcock 2001: R 5).
(c) Record frequency of pain, what helps to relieve the pain, what makes the pain worse and how the patient feels when they are in pain.	
5 Index each site (A–D; see Figure 20.2) in whatever way seems most appropriate, e.g. shading or colouring of areas or arrows to indicate shooting pains.	This enables individual pain sites to be located (Witt-Sherman *et al.* 2004: R 4).

Procedure guidelines *(cont.)*

6 Give each pain site a numerical value according to the key to pain intensity or the pain scale and note time recorded.	To indicate the intensity of the pain at each site (Turk & Okifuji 1999: E).
7 Record any analgesia given and note route and dose.	To monitor efficacy of prescribed analgesia. (Twycross & Wilcock 2001: R 5)
8 Record any significant activities that are likely to influence the patient's pain.	Extra pharmacological or non-pharmacological interventions might be indicated (Turk & Okifuji 1999: E; RCN 2005: C).

Note: fixed times for reviewing the pain have been omitted intentionally to allow for flexibility. It is suggested that, initially, the patient's pain is reviewed by the patient and nurse every 4 hours. When a patient's level of pain has stabilized, recordings may be made less frequently, e.g. 12-hourly or daily. The chart should be discontinued if a patient's pain becomes totally controlled.

References and further reading

Ahmedzai, F. & Brooks, D. (1997) Transdermal Fentanyl versus Oral Morphine in Cancer Pain: Preference, Efficacy and Quality of Life. *J Pain Symptom Management* **13**, 254–61.

Akin, M. *et al.* (2001) Continuous low-level topical heat in the treatment of dysmenorrhea. *Obstet Gynecol*, **97**(3), 343–9.

Anderson, K.O. & Cleeland, C.S. (2003) The assessment of cancer pain. In: *Cancer Pain: Assessment and Management* (eds E.D. Bruera & R.K. Portenoy). Cambridge University Press, Cambridge, pp. 51–66.

ANZCA and Faculty of Pain Medicine (2005) *Acute Pain Management: Scientific Evidence*, 2nd edn. Australian and New Zealand College of Anaesthetists, Melbourne, Victoria, Australia.

Audit Commission (1997) *Anaesthesia under Examination*. Audit Commission, Oxford.

Ballard, K. (1997) Pressure-relief mattresses and patient comfort. *Prof Nurse*, **13**(1), 27–32.

Bamigbade, T. & Langford, R. (1998) Tramadol hydrochloride: an overview of current use. *Hosp Med*, **59**(5), 373–6.

Barillo, D. *et al.* (2000) Burns caused by medical therapy. *J Burn Care Rehabil*, **21**(3), 269–73.

Beck, S. (1991) The therapeutic use of music for cancer-related pain. *Oncol Nurse Forum*, **18**(8), 1327–37.

Bennett, M. (2001) The LANSS pain scale: the Leeds assessment of neuropathic symptoms and signs. *Pain*, **92**, 147–57.

BMA/Royal Pharmaceutical Society of Great Britain (2008) *British National Formulary*. Pharmaceutical Press, Oxford.

Budd, K. (2002) *Evidence-based Medicine in Practice. Buprenorphine: a Review*. Haywood Medical, London.

Carr, E. (1990) Post-operative pain: patient expectations and experiences. *J Adv Nurs*, **15**(1), 89–100.

Carr, E. & Mann, E. (2000a) Recognising the barriers to effective pain relief. In: *Pain: Creative Approaches to Effective Management*. Macmillan Press/Bournemouth University, London, pp. 109–29.

Carr, E. & Mann, E. (2000b) Managing chronic pain. In: *Pain: Creative Approaches to Effective Management*. Macmillan Press/Bournemouth University, London, pp. 81–108.

Carroll, D. & Bowsher, D. (1993) *Pain Management and Nursing Care*. Butterworth Heinemann, Oxford.

Carroll, D. & Seers, K. (1998) Relaxation for the relief of chronic pain: a systematic review. *J Adv Nurs*, **27**(3), 476–87.

Caunt, H. (1992) Reducing the psychological impact of postoperative pain. *J Nurs*, **1**(1), 13–19.

Chumbley, G.M., Hall, G.M. & Salmon, P. (2002) Patient-controlled analgesia: what information does the patient want? *J Adv Nurs*, **39**(5), 459–71.

Cleeland, C.S. (1991) The brief pain inventory. www.mdanderson. org/pdf/bpilong. Accessed 24/9/07.

Coda, B. *et al.* (1997) Comparative efficacy of patient-controlled administration of morphine, hydromorphone, or sufentil for the treatment of oral mucositis following bone marrow transplantation. *Pain*, **72**(3), 333–46.

Colleau, S.M. (1999) The significance of breakthrough pain in cancer. *Cancer Pain Release*, **12**, 1–4.

Consroe, P. (1997) The perceived effects of smoked cannabis on patients with multiple sclerosis. *Eur Neurol*, **38**(1), 44–8.

Davies, A. (2006) *Cancer-related Breakthrough Pain*. Oxford Pain Mnagement Library, Oxford.

Davis, B.D. & McVicker, A. (2000) Issues in effective pain control: from assessment to management. *Int J Palliat Nurs*, **6**(4), 162–9.

Davis, M., Glare, P. & Hardy, J. (2005) *Opioids in Cancer Pain*. Oxford University Press, Oxford.

Dickman, A., Littlewood, C. & Varga, J. (eds) (2002) Drug information. In: *The Syringe Driver. Continuous Subcutaneous Infusions in Palliative Care*. Oxford University Press, Oxford, pp. 11–58.

Donaldson, G. *et al.* (1997) Comparative efficacy of patient controlled administration of morphine, hydromorphone or sufentil for the treatment of oral mucositis following bone marrow transplantation. *Pain*, **72**(3), 333–46.

Donnelly, S. & Walsh, D. (1995) The symptoms of advanced cancer. *Semin Oncol*, **22**(2 Suppl 3), 67–72.

Drayer, R.A., Henderson, B.S. & Reidenberg, M. (1999) Barriers to better pain control in hospitalised patients. *J Pain Symptom Control*, **17**(6), 434–40.

Ellershaw, J. (1998) Hydromorphone: a new alternative to morphine. *Prescriber*, **9**(4), 21–7.

Ezzo, J. *et al.* (2000) Is acupuncture effective for the treatment of chronic pain? A systematic review. *Pain*, **86**(3), 217–25.

Farrell, A. & Rich, A. (2000) Analgesic use in patients with renal failure. *Eur J Palliat Care*, **7**(6), 201–5.

Field, L. (1996) Are nurses still underestimating patients' pain post-operatively? *Br J Nurs*, **15**(13), 778–84.

Feine, J. & Lund, J. (1997) An assessment of the efficacy of physical therapy and physical modalities for the control of chronic musculoskeletal pain. *Pain*, **71**(1), 5–23.

Fine, P.G. *et al.* (1991) An open label study of oral transdermal fentanyl citrate (OTFC) for the treatment of breakthrough cancer pain. *Pain*, **45**, 149–53.

Fitzpatrick R. *et al.* (1998) Evaluating a patient based outcome measure for use in clinical trials. *Health Technol Assess*, **21**, 95–102.

Flaherty, S.A. (1996) Pain measurement tools for clinical practice and research. *J Am Assoc Nurse Anesth*, **64**, 133–40.

Foley, K. (2004) Pain assessment and cancer pain syndromes. In: *Oxford Textbook of Palliative Medicine* (eds D. Doyle *et al.*), 3rd edn. Oxford Medical Publications, Oxford, pp. 298–316.

Gannon, C. (1997) The use of methadone in the care of the dying. *Eur J Palliat Care*, **4**(5), 152–8.

Gardner-Nix, J. (1996) Oral methadone for managing chronic non malignant pain. *J Pain Symptom Control*, **11**(5), 321–2.

Good, M. (1996) Effects of relaxation and music on postoperative pain: a review. *J Adv Nurs*, **24**, 905–14.

Good, M. *et al.* (1999) Relief of postoperative pain with jaw relaxation, music and their combination. *Pain*, **81**(1–2), 163–72.

Good, M. *et al.* (2005) Relaxation and music reduce pain following intestinal surgery. *Res Nurs Health*, **28**, 240–51.

Gould, T. *et al.* (1992) Policy for controlling pain after surgery: effect of sequential changes in management. *Br Med J*, **305**(6863), 1187–93.

Grond, S. *et al.* (1996) Assessment of cancer pain: a prospective evaluation. *Pain*, **64**(1), 107–14.

Halaszynski, T.M., Juda, R. & Silverman, D.G. (2004) Optimizing postoperative outcomes with efficient preoperative assessment and management. *Crit Care Med*, **32**(4), S76–86.

Hamrin, E., Sjostrom, B. & Unosson, M. (2002) Patient and nurse assessment of quality of care in postoperative pain management. *Qual Saf Health Care*, **11**, 327–34.

Hanks, G., Cherny, N. & Fallon, M. (2004) Opioid analgesic therapy. In: *Oxford Textbook of Palliative Medicine* (eds D. Doyle *et al.*), 3rd edn. Oxford Medical Publications, Oxford, pp. 316–342.

Hanks, G. & Expert Working Group of the European Association for Palliative Care (1996) Morphine in cancer pain: modes of administration. *Br Med J*, **3**(12), 823–6.

Hanks, G.W. (1991) Opioid-responsive and opioid non-responsive pain in cancer. *Br Med Bull*, **47**, 718–31.

Hanks, G.W. *et al.* (2001) Morphine and alternative opioids in cancer pain: the EAPC recommendations. *Br J Cancer*, **84**(5), 587–93.

Harmer, M. & Davies, K. (1998) The effect of education, assessment and a standardised prescription on postoperative pain management. *Anaesthesia*, **53**(5), 424–30.

Hays, H. *et al.* (1994) Comparative clinical efficacy and safety of immediate release and controlled release hydromorphone for chronic severe pain. *Cancer*, **74**(6), 1808–16.

Hayward, J. (1975) *Information, a Prescription against Pain, the Study of Nursing Care.* Research Project, Series 2(5). Royal College of Nursing, London.

Heiser, R. *et al.* (1997) The use of music during the immediate postoperative recovery period. *AORN J*, **65**(4), 777.

Heiskanen, T. & Kalso, E. (1997) Controlled-release oxycodone and morphine in cancer related pain. *Science Direct* **73**(1), 37–45.

Hicks, F. & Simpson, K.H. (eds) (2004) Regional nerve blocks. In: *Nerve Blocks in Palliative Care.* Oxford University Press, Oxford, pp. 53–55.

Higginson, I. (1998) Can professionals improve their assessments? *J Pain Symp Manage*, **15**(3), 149–50.

Hill, H.F. (1992) Patient controlled analgesic infusions: alfentanil versus morphine. *Pain*, **49**(3), 301–10.

Hobbs, G.J. & Hodgkinson, V. (2003) Assessment, measurement, history and examination. In: *Clinical Pain Management: Acute Pain* (eds D.J. Rowbotham & P.E. Macintyre). Arnold Publishers, London pp. 93–112.

IASP (1994) IASP pain terminology. www.iasp-pain.org/terms. Accessed 17/7/06.

IASP (1996) Classification of chronic pain. *Pain*, **3**(Suppl), 51–226.

Idvall, E. *et al.* (2002) Patient and nurse assessment of quality of care in postoperative pain management. *Qual Saf Health Care*, **11**, pp. 327–34.

Kalkman, C.J. *et al.* (2003) Preoperative prediction of severe postoperative pain. *Pain*, **105**, 415–23.

Kehlet, H. (1997) Multimodal approach to control of postoperative pathophysiology and rehabilitation. *Br J Anaesth*, **78**(5), 606–17.

King, A. (1999) *King's Guide to TENS for Health Professionals.* King's Medical Physio-Med Services, Glossop, Derbyshire.

Kitson, A. (1994) Post-operative pain management: a literature review. *J Clin Nurs*, **3**(1), 7–18.

Klepstad, P. *et al.* (2005) Pain and pain treatments in European palliative care units. A cross sectional survey from the European Association for Palliative Care Research Network. *Palliat Med*, **19**(6), 477–84.

Knoerl, D.V., Faut-Calloahan, M. & Paice, J. (1999) Preoperative PCA teaching program to manage postoperative pain. *Medsurg Nurs*, **8**, 25–33 & 36.

Krishnasamy, M. (2001) Pain. In: *Cancer Nursing Care in Context* (eds J. Corner & C. Bailey). Blackwell Science, Oxford, pp. 339-350.

Lang, E. *et al.* (2000) Adjunctive non-pharmacological analgesia for invasive medical procedures: a randomised trial. *Lancet*, **355**(9214), 1486–90.

Lawler, K. (1997) Pain assessment. *Prof Nurs Study*, **13**(1, Suppl), S5–8.

Lewis, N.L. & Williams, J. (2005) Acute pain management in patients receiving opioids for chronic cancer pain. *Continuing Education in Anaesthesia, Critical Care and Pain*, **5**(4), 127–9.

Ling, J. (1997) The use of transdermal fentanyl in palliative care. *Int J Palliat Nurs*, **3**(2), 65–8.

Loveman, E. & Gale, A. (2000) Factors influencing nurses inferences about patient pain. *Br J Nurs*, **9**(6), 334–7.

Macintyre, P.E. & Jarvis, D.A. (1996) Age is the best predictor of postoperative morphione requirements. *Pain*, **64**, 357–64.

Macintyre, P.E. (2001) Safety and efficacy of patient-controlled analgesia. *Br J Anaesth*, **87**(1), 36–46.

Macintyre, P.E. & Ready, L. (2001) *Acute Pain Management. A Practical Guide.* W.B. Saunders, London.

Martyn, C. (1995) 'N = 1' cross-over trial using nabilone in a patient with multiple sclerosis. *Lancet*, **345**(8949), 579.

McCaffery M. (1968) *Nursing practice theories related to cognition, bodily pain and man environment.* Student store, UCLA, Los Angeles.

McCaffery, M. (1990) Nursing approaches to non-pharmacological pain control. *Int J Nurs Stud*, **27**(1), 1–5.

McCaffery, M. (2000) *Nursing Management of the Patient with Pain*, 3rd edn. Lippincott, Philadelphia.

McCaffery, M. & Beebe, A. (1989) Perspectives on pain. In: *Clinical Manual for Nursing Practice*, pp. 1–5. Mosby, St Louis.

McCaffery, M. & Ferrell, B.R. (1997) Nurses' knowledge of pain assessment and management: how much progress have we made? *J Pain Symp Manage*, **14**(3), 175–88.

MaCaffery, M. & Pasero, C. (2003) Breakthrough pain: it's common in patients with chronic pain. *Am J Nurs*, **103**(4), 83–6.

McCaffery, M. & Robinson, E.S. (2002) Your patient is in pain— here's how you respond. *Nursing*, **32**(10), 36–47.

McMillan, C. (2001) Breakthrough pain: assessment and management in cancer patients. *Br J Nurs*, **10**(13), 860–6.

McQuay, H. (1990) The logic of alternative routes. *J Pain Symp Manage*, **5**(2), 75–7.

McQuay, H. (1999) Opioids in pain management. *Lancet*, **353**, 2229–32.

McQuay, H. & Edwards, J. (2003) Meta-analysis of single dose oral tramadol plus acetaminophen in acute postoperative pain. *Eur J Anaesthesiol*, **28**(Suppl), 19–22.

McQuay, H. & Moore, A. (1998) Oral tramadol versus placebo, codeine and combination analgesics. In: *An Evidence Based Resource for Pain.* Oxford University Press, Oxford, pp. 138–46.

McQuay, H., Moore, A. & Justins, D. (1997) Treating acute pain in hospital. *Br Med J*, **314**(7093), 1531–5.

Mehta, V. & Langford, R.M. (2006) Acute pain management for opioid dependent patients. *Anaesthesia*, **61**, 269–76.

Melzack, R. (1975) The McGill Pain Questionnaire: major properties and scoring methods. *Pain*, **1**, 277–99.

Merskey, H. & Bogduk, N. (1994) *Classification of Chronic Pain.* 2nd edn. IASP Press, Seattle.

MHRA (2005) *Medical Device Alert.* Ref. MDA/2005/027. MHRA, London.

Mitchell, M. (1997) Patients' perceptions of pre-operative preparation for day surgery. *J Adv Nurs*, **26**(2), 356–63.

Morley, J.S. & Makin, M.K. (1998) The use of methadone in cancer pain poorly responsive to other opioids. *Pain Rev*, **5**, 51–8.

Mucci-LoRusso, P. *et al.* (1998) Controlled release oxycodone compared with controlled release morphine in the treatment of cancer pain: a randomised, double-blind, parallel group study. *Eur J Pain*, **2**, 239–49.

Nadler, S. *et al.* (2002) Continuous low-level heat wrap therapy provides more efficacy than ibuprofen and acetaminophen for acute low back pain. *Spine*, **27**(10), 1012–17.

NMC (2006) *A–Z Advice Sheet Consent.* www.nmc.org.

O'Connor, M. & Webb, R. (2002) Learning to rest when in pain. *Eur J Palliat Care*, **9**(2), 68–71.

Pargeon, K.L. & Hailey, B.J. (1999) Barriers to effective cancer pain management: a review. *J Pain Symp Manage*, **5**, 358–68.

Pasero, C. (1998) Pain control – is laughter the best medicine? *Am J Nurs*, **98**(12), 12–14.

Payne, R. (1995) *Relaxation Techniques: a Practical Handbook for Health Care Professionals.* Churchill Livingstone, Edinburgh.

Paz, S. & Seymour, J.E. (2004) Pain theories, evaluation and management. In: *Palliative Care Nursing* (eds S. Payne *et al.*). Open University Press, Berkshire, pp. 260–298.

Pease, N., Taylor, H. & Major, H. (2004) Strong painkillers and driving. *Palliat Med*, **18**, 663–8.

Perkins, F.M. & Kehlet, H. (2000) Chronic pain as an outcome of surgery. *Anasthesiology*, **93**, 1123–33.

Portenoy, R.K. & Lesage, P. (1999) Management of cancer pain. *Lancet*, **353**, 1695–1700.

Portenoy, R.K., Payne, R. & Coluzzi, P. (1999) Oral transmucosal fentanyl citrate (OTFC) for the treatment of breakthrough pain in cancer patients: a controlled dose titration study. *Pain*, **79**, 303–12.

Portenoy, R.K. *et al.* (2004) Difficult pain problems: an integrated approach. In: *Oxford Textbook of Palliative Medicine* (eds D. Doyle *et al.*). Oxford University Press, Oxford, pp. 316–36.

Poyhia, R. *et al.* (1993) Oxycodone an alternative to morphine for cancer pain. A review. *J Pain Symp Manage*, **8**, 63–7.

Quigley, C. (2004) Opioid switching to improve pain relief and drug tolerability. *Cochrane Database Syst Rev*, **3** CD004847.

Raiman J. (1986) Pain relief-a two way process. *Nursing Times*, **82**(15), 24–28.

Ready, L. & Edwards, W. (1992) *Management of Acute Pain: a Practical Guide.* IASP Publications, Seattle.

Reicin, A. *et al.* (2001) Efficacy of single-dose and multidose rofecoxib in the treatment of post orthopedic surgery pain. *Am J Orthoped*, **30**(1), 40–8.

Riley, J. *et al.* (2006) Opioids in palliative care. *Eur J Palliat Care*, **13**(6), 230–3.

Robinson, V.A. *et al.* (2002) Thermotherapy for treating rheumatoid arthritis. Cochrane Database of Systematic Review 2002, Issue 2, Article No. CD002826. Doi: 10: 1002/14651858.

Romsing, J., Moiniche, S. & Dahl, J.B. (2002) Rectal and parenteral paracetemol, and paracetemol in combination with NSAIDs for postoperative analgesia. *Br J Anaesth*, **88**, 215–26.

750

Rowbotham, D. (2000) Non-steroidal anti-inflammatory drugs and paracetamol. In: *Chronic Pain*. Martin Dunitz, London, pp. 19–26.

Saunders, C. & Sykes, N. (1993) *The Management of Terminal Malignant Disease*, 3rd edn. Hodder & Stoughton, Boston.

Schug, S.A. & Torrie, J.J. (1993) Safety assessment of postoperative pain management by an acute pain service. *Pain*, **55**, 387–91.

Scott, I. (1994) Effectiveness of documented assessment of post operative pain. *Br J Nurs*, **3**(10), 494–501.

Seers, K. (1996) The patients' experiences of their chronic nonmalignant pain. *J Adv Nurs*, **24**(6), 1160–8.

Seers, K. & Carroll, D. (1998) Relaxation techniques for acute pain management: a systematic review. *J Adv Nurs*, **27**(3), 466–75.

Sidebotham, D. *et al.* (1997) The safety and utilization of patient controlled analgesia. *J Pain Symp Manage*, **14**(4), 202–9.

Sindrup, S. & Jensen, T. (1999) Efficacy of pharmacological treatments of neuropathic pain: an update and effect related to mechanism of drug action. *Pain*, **83**, 389–400.

Sloman, R. *et al.* (1994) The use of relaxation for the promotion of comfort and pain relief in persons with advanced cancer. *Contemp Nurse*, **3**(1), 6–12.

Tasmuth, T., Estlandberg, A. & Kalso, E. (1996) Effect of present pain and memory of past post-operative pain in women treated with surgery for breast cancer. *Pain*, **68**(2–3), 343–7.

Taylor, H. (2001) Pain management supplement. The importance of providing good patient information. *Prof Nurse*, **17**(1), 34–6.

Trauger-Querry, B. & Haghighi, K. (1999) Balancing the focus: art and music therapy for pain and symptom management in hospice care. *Hospice J*, **14**(1), 25–37.

Turk, D.C. & Okifuji, A. (1999) Assessment of patients' reporting of pain: an integrated perspective. *Lancet*, **353**, 1784–9.

Twycross, R. & Wilcock, A. (2001) *Symptom Management in Advanced Cancer*, 3rd edn. Radcliffe Medical Press, Oxford.

Twycross, R., Harcourt, J. & Bergl, S. (1996) A survey of pain in patients with advanced cancer. *J Pain Symp Manage*, **12**(5), 273–82.

Tye, T. & Gell-Walker, V. (2000) Patient-controlled analgesia. *Nurs Times*, **96**(25), 38–9.

Vijayan, R. (1997) Subcutaneous morphine – a simple technique for postoperative analgesia. *Int J Acute Pain*, **1**(1), 21–6.

Walker, S.M., MacIntyre, P.E. & Visser, E. (2006) Acute pain management: current best practice evidence provides guide for improved practice. *Pain Med*, **7**(1), 3–5.

Walker, V.S. *et al.* (1987) Pain assessment charts in the management of chronic cancer pain. *Palliat Med*, **1**, 111–16.

Wall, J., Davis, S. & Ridgway, S. (2001) Cannabis: its therapeutic use. *Nurs Stand*, **16**(10), 39–44.

Walsh, D. (ed) (1997) Review of clinical studies on TENS. In: *TENS: Clinical Applications and Related Theory*. Churchill Livingstone, London, pp. 83–101.

Wheatley, R., Schug, S. & Watson, D. (2001) Safety and efficacy of postoperative epidural analgesia. *Br J Anaesth*, **87**(1), 47–61.

WHO (1996) *Cancer Pain Relief*. World Health Organization, Geneva.

Witt-Sherman, D. *et al.* (2004) Learning pain assessment and management. A goal of the end-of-life nursing education consortium. *J Contin Edu Nursing* **35**(3), 107–20.

Zarnegar, R. & Daniel, C. (2005) Pain management programmes. Continuing education in anaesthesia. *Crit Care Pain J*, **5**(3), 80–3.

Zaza, C. (2002) Cancer pain and psychosocial factors: a critical review of the literature. *J Pain Symptom Manage*, **24**(5), 526–40.

Zech, D., Lehmann, A. & Grond, S. (1994) A new treatment option for chronic cancer pain. *Eur J Palliat Care*, **1**(1), 26–30.

Multiple choice questions

1 Chronic pain is usually prolonged and defined as pain that exists for more than:

   a   1 week
   b   1 month
   c   3 months
   d   6 months

2 Fitzpatrick *et al.* (1998) state that it is important that pain assessment tools meet certain criteria. Which of these is NOT one of these criteria?

   a   Simplicity (ease of use)
   b   Feasibility/practicality (the degree of effort involved in using the tool)
   c   Reliability (results reproducible and consistent with other patients)
   d   Cultural sensitivity (acknowledging different cultures)

3 Co-analgesics are drugs that are used in conjunction with analgesics to treat specific pains. Which of the following may effectively be used in the treatment of muscular pain?

   a   Antibiotics
   b   Benzodiazepines
   c   Antispasmodics
   d   Non-steroidal anti-inflammatory drugs

4 **PCA is an effective means of delivering intravenous opioids. What does PCA stand for?**

a   Patient controlled analgesia
b   Patient controlled administration
c   Patient compliant analgesia
d   Patient centered administration

Answers to the multiple choice questions can be found in Appendix 3.

Chapter 21

Pain management: epidural and intrathecal analgesia

Definition

The spinal cord rests in a medium of cerebrospinal fluid (CSF), which is contained by the protective membrane of the dura mater. Analgesics applied outside the dura mater are termed epidural analgesia, and medications given into the CSF are termed intrathecal analgesia (Sloan 2004). The term 'spinal analgesia' refers to both the epidural and intrathecal route (Day 2001; Sloan 2004).

Epidural analgesia is the administration of analgesics (local anaesthetics and opioids with or without adjuvants such as corticosteroids and clonidine) into the epidural space via an indwelling catheter (ANZCA 2005). This technique enables analgesics to be injected close to the spinal cord and spinal nerves where they exert a powerful analgesic effect. It is one of the most effective techniques available for the management of acute pain (Macintyre & Ready 2001; Wheatley *et al.* 2001).

Intrathecal analgesia is the administration of analgesic drugs (as listed above) directly into the CSF in the intrathecal space (Urdan *et al.* 2006). Analgesic drugs given via this route are 10 times as potent as those given into the epidural space so doses given are much smaller. This method can use either an external infusion pump or can be part of a fully implantable reservoir system (Dickson 2004).

For cancer patients who do not obtain pain relief from treatment with opioids administered orally, rectally, by injection or continuous infusion, there is evidence that both epidural and intrathecal analgesia can be effective (Ballantyne & Carwood 2005).

Advantages

There are three main advantages in using epidural or intrathecal analgesia:

- It has the potential to provide effective dynamic pain relief for many patients (Wheatley *et al.* 2001).

- The combination of local anaesthetic agents with opioids has a synergistic action that allows the concentration of each drug to be reduced. This limits the unwanted side-effects of each drug (Fotiadis *et al.* 2004).
- There is also evidence that the use of epidural analgesia may reduce the stress response to surgery or trauma, thereby reducing morbidity, recovery time and hospital stay (Kehlet 1997).

Indications

- Provision of analgesia during labour.
- As an alternative to general anaesthesia, e.g. in severe respiratory disease or for patients with malignant hyperthermia.
- Provision of postoperative analgesia. Epidural analgesia has been used since the late 1940s as a method of controlling postoperative pain (Chapman & Day 2001).
- Provision of analgesia for pain resulting from trauma, e.g. fractured ribs, which may result in respiratory impairment due to pain on breathing.
- Management of chronic intractable pain in patients who experience the following:
    - Unacceptable side-effects with systemic opioids.
    - Unsuccessful treatment with opioids via other routes despite escalating doses.
    - Severe neuropathic pain due to tumour invasion or compression of nerves.
                    (Smitt *et al.* 1998; Mercadante 1999; Day 2001).
- To relieve muscle spasm and pain resulting from lumbar cord pressure due to disc protrusion or local oedema and inflammation.

Contraindications

These may be absolute or relative.

Absolute

- Patients with coagulation defects, which may result in haematoma formation and spinal cord compression, e.g. iatrogenic (anticoagulated patient) or congenital (haemophiliacs), or thrombocytopenia due to disease or as the result of anticancer treatment (Horlocker & Wedel 1998).
- Local sepsis at the site of proposed epidural or intrathecal injection; the result might be meningitis or epidural abscess formation.
- Proven allergy to the intended drug.
- Unstable spinal fracture.
- Patient refusal to consent to the procedure.

Relative

- Unstable cardiovascular system.
- Spinal deformity.
- Raised intracranial pressure (a risk of herniation if a dural tap occurs).
- Certain neurological conditions, for example multiple sclerosis, where an epidural may result in an exacerbation of the disease (Hall 2000).
- Unavailability of staff trained in the management of epidural or intrathecal analgesia (Macintyre & Ready 2001). Hall (2000) notes that staff managing patients with epidural or intrathecal analgesia should have undertaken a period of formal training to care for patients safely and competently.

Reference material

Anatomy of the epidural and intrathecal space (Figure 21.1)

The spinal cord is covered by the meninges; the *pia mater* is closely applied to the cord, and the *arachnoid mater* lies closely with the outer, tough covering of the *dura mater* (Day 2001).

The epidural space lies between the spinal dura and ligamentum flavum. The contents of the epidural space include a rich venous plexus, spinal arterioles, lymphatics and extradural fat.

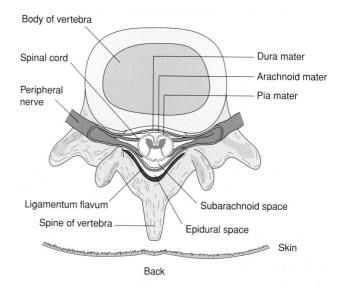

Figure 21.1   Diagram of the spinal spaces. (Courtesy of Day 2001.)

The intrathecal space (often also termed the subarachnoid space) lies between the arachnoid mater and pia mater and contains the CSF (Chapman & Day 2001).

There are 31 pairs of spinal nerves of varying size. These nerves pass out through the intervertebral foramina between each vertebra (Chapman & Day 2001). The two main groups of nerve fibres are:

- *Myelinated*. Myelin is a thin, fatty sheath which protects and insulates the nerve fibres and prevents impulses from being transmitted to adjacent fibres.
- *Unmyelinated*. Delicate fibres, more susceptible to hypoxia and toxins than myelinated fibres.

The spinal nerves are composed of a posterior and anterior root, which join to form a spinal nerve:

- *Posterior root*. Transmits ascending sensory impulses from the periphery to the spinal cord.
- *Anterior root*. Transmits descending motor impulses from the spinal cord to the periphery by means of its corresponding spinal nerve.

(Day 2001; Chapman & Day 2001; Urdan *et al.* 2006).

Specific skin surface areas are supplied/innervated by each of the spinal nerves. These skin areas are known as dermatomes (McCaffery & Pasero 1999) (Figure 21.2).

Classes of epidural and intrathecal drugs and mechanism of action

Three classes of drugs are commonly used to provide epidural or intrathecal analgesia: opioids, local anaesthetic agents and adjuvant drugs such as corticosteroids and clonidine.

Opioids

Whilst a number of different opioids have been used for epidural and intrathecal analgesia, two of the most commonly used are diamorphine and fentanyl (Cook *et al.* 1997; Romer & Russell 1998; Bannon *et al.* 2001). When either of these opioids is injected into the *epidural* space, part of the opioid dose:

- Crosses the dura and arachnoid membrane and enters the CSF. From the CSF a proportion of the drug is taken up into the spinal cord and reaches the opioid receptors in the spinal cord. Once bound to the opioid receptors, this results in blocking of pain impulses.
- Enters the systemic circulation and contributes to analgesia.
- Binds to the epidural fat and does not contribute to analgesia.

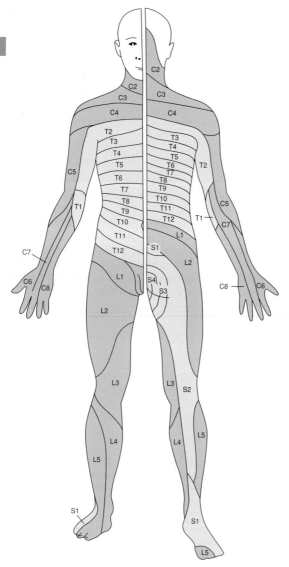

Figure 21.2   Dermatomes. (Redrawn with permission from Walsh 1997.)

When opioids are placed directly into the CSF in the *intrathecal* space they attach directly to the opioid spinal cord receptor sites (Urdan *et al.* 2006).

Fentanyl differs from diamorphine in that it is more lipid soluble. This means that it passes more easily into the CSF, gaining faster access to the opioid receptors and having a more rapid onset of action. Fentanyl also has a shorter duration of action (1–4 hours) as opposed to diamorphine (6–12 hours) (Macintyre & Ready 2001).

Local anaesthetic drugs

Commonly used local anaesthetic agents include bupivacaine, levobupivacaine and ropivacaine. These drugs gain access to the nerve roots and the spinal cord by crossing the dura and subarachnoid membranes (Macintyre & Ready 2001). They inhibit pain transmission by blocking sodium ion channels which are involved in the propagation of electrical impulses along the spinal nerves.

The dose of a local anaesthetic agent will also determine which nerves are blocked. Low concentrations of bupivacaine (e.g. 0.100–0.125%) preferentially block nerve impulses in the smallest diameter nerve fibres, which include the pain and temperature sensory fibres. As the larger diameter motor fibres are less likely to be blocked with concentrations of 0.100–0.125% bupivacaine, the incidence of leg weakness is reduced and the patient is able to mobilize.

Adjuvant drugs

Corticosteroids

Although not licensed for epidural or intrathecal use, corticosteroid injections are often used to relieve pain caused by inflammatory irritation of nerve roots (Papagelopoulos *et al.* 2001).

Clonidine

Clonidine is a mixed α-adrenergic agonist. Although its exact mechanism of action is unknown, clonidine is believed to enhance analgesia provided by spinal opioids and local anaesthetic drugs (Smith & Elliott 2001). Clonidine has a specific role in the management of neuropathic pain in patients with advanced cancer (Mercadante 1999).

Methods of administration

Continuous infusion

Continuous infusions of epidural drugs are the most effective way of providing dynamic pain relief after major surgical procedures (Kehlet & Holte 2001).

Continuous infusions of intrathecal analgesic drugs have been shown to be effective in the management of chronic intractable pain (Ballantyne & Carwood 2005). Continuous infusions can be given by either a syringe pump or a designated infusion pump system. The effectiveness of this method of administering drugs is dependent on a number of factors including the combination of drugs used, the position of the spinal catheter at a level appropriate to the site of surgery or pain (Weetman & Allison 2006) and the volume of the local anaesthetic agent infused (Hall 2000; Chapman & Day 2001).

Combination of drugs used

Epidural or intrathecal infusions of local anaesthetic and opioid combinations are commonly used in the UK (Wheatley *et al.* 2001; Baker *et al.* 2004). The rationale behind their combined use is based on the observation that better analgesia is achieved with lower doses of each drug, therefore minimizing drug-related side-effects produced by higher concentrations (Curatolo *et al.* 1998; Fotiadis *et al.* 2004). Although the solutions used will vary with the clinical situation, common solutions are bupivacaine 0.1–0.125% with 2–4 µg/ml of fentanyl.

Position of epidural or intrathecal catheter

Local anaesthetic drugs block nerve fibres at spinal segments adjacent to their site of administration. To ensure the local anaesthetic agent spreads to the dermatomes or nerves supplying the area of pain (e.g. the surgical site, or the pain location caused by a tumour), the tip of the spinal catheter should be placed within the mid-dermatomal distribution of the pain site (Table 21.1). This achieves optimal analgesia using the least amount of drugs. If the catheter is placed below the dermatomes supplying the pain site then analgesia is likely to be inadequate (Macintyre & Ready 2001).

Volume of infusion

As the volume of local anaesthetic agent influences the number of spinal nerves that are blocked, it is important to maintain the hourly infusion rate at a

Table 21.1 Optimal catheter location for different surgical sites.

Surgical site	Catheter location
Thoracic	T6–T9
Upper abdominal	T7–T10
Lower abdominal	T9–L1
Hip/knee	L1–L4

volume which keeps the appropriate nerves blocked (Hall 2000; Chapman & Day 2001).

Bolus injections

Bolus injections of opioids and local anaesthetic agents are used infrequently to manage postoperative pain but are more commonly used for managing labour pain (Grond *et al.* 2000).

Patient-controlled epidural analgesia

The use of patient-controlled epidural analgesia (PCEA) has gained popularity in recent years because it enables patients to control their analgesia. For patients with postoperative or chronic pain, PCEA is used more effectively in combination with a low-dose background infusion (Wheatley *et al.* 2001). This ensures a baseline level of analgesia which can then be supplemented by the patient when required.

Monitoring

When caring for a patient receiving epidural or intrathecal analgesia, it is important to monitor the patient for the following:

- Signs of drug-related side-effects.
- Pain intensity.
- Signs of complications due to the epidural or intrathecal procedure.

Drug-related side-effects

There are a number of drug-related side-effects associated with epidural/intrathecal opioids and local anaesthetic agents.

Opioids

- *Respiratory depression*: this is due to the action of opioids on the respiratory centre. Respiratory depression may occur at two different time intervals.
  - Early: usually within 2 hours of the opioid injection. This may occur if high blood levels of the opioid follow absorption from the epidural space into the systemic circulation (Macintyre & Ready 2001).
  - Late: this may not be seen for 6–12 hours after an opioid is given. It results from rostral migration of the drug in the CSF to the brainstem and respiratory centre (Macintyre & Ready 2001). This is less likely to occur with lipid-soluble opioids such as fentanyl.
- *Sedation*: although there may be many different causes of sedation, epidural/intrathecal opioids can cause sedation owing to their effect on the central

nervous system. Opioid-induced sedation is often an early warning sign of respiratory depression.

- *Nausea and vomiting*: nausea and vomiting is caused by the action of opioids on the vomiting centre in the brainstem and stimulation of the chemoreceptor trigger zone in the fourth ventricle of the brain.
- *Pruritus*: although the exact mechanism is unknown, pruritus is presumed to be centrally mediated and a consequence of activation of opioid receptors in the spinal cord (Sands *et al.* 1998).
- *Urinary retention*: this is due to opioid inhibition of the micturition reflex which is evoked by increases in bladder volume.

Local anaesthetic agents

- *Hypotension*: this can be caused by two mechanisms. Firstly, local anaesthetic agents can spread outside the epidural/intrathecal space, blocking the sympathetic nerves. This results in peripheral vasodilatation and hypotension. It is most likely to occur if a bolus dose of local anaesthetic agent (e.g. 10 ml of 0.25% bupivacaine) is given to improve pain control (Macintyre & Ready 2001). Secondly, if the local anaesthetic agent spreads above the T4 dermatome (nipple line) the cardio-accelerator nerves may become blocked, leading to bradycardia and hypotension (Macintyre & Ready 2001).
- *Motor blockade*: this will depend on the concentration and total dose of local anaesthetic agent used and the position of the epidural/intrathecal catheter (Hall 2000). Motor blockade occurs when the local anaesthetic agent blocks the larger diameter motor nerves. Leg weakness will occur if the motor nerves supplying the legs are blocked.
- *Urinary retention*: as with epidural/intrathecal opioids, blockade of the nerves supplying the bladder sphincter can cause urinary retention.

Routine monitoring of the patient for these side-effects must be carried out to facilitate early management. The patient's blood pressure, respiratory rate and peripheral tissue oxygenation should be monitored continuously initially and then according to local policy and as the patient's condition dictates.

For guidance on managing the side-effects associated with epidural/intrathecal opioids and local anaesthetic agents, see Problem solving: management of side-effects, p. 772.

Pain assessment

Pain should be assessed (at rest and on movement) at the same time that the patient's routine observations are carried out. Simple numerical (e.g. 0–10 where 0 is no pain and 10 is the worst pain imaginable) or verbal rating scales (e.g. none, mild, moderate, severe, or very severe) can be used.

Inadequate postoperative pain management can lead to physiological complications (respiratory, cardiovascular, gastrointestinal and endocrine systems) and adverse effects (behavioural, such as reduced mobility, and psychological, such as increased anxiety and reduced mood) (Macintyre & Ready 2001). Thus, when patients are assessed the practitioner should ensure the patient can take a deep breath and cough and mobilize with a minimal level of pain to reduce the impact of the physiological, behavioural and psychological effects of undertreated acute pain.

When used for chronic pain management the aim of epidural/intrathecal analgesia is to improve the overall quality of life of the patient. Although it is acceptable to use the above pain assessment rating scales, a more in-depth pain assessment scale may be used such as the Brief Pain Inventory (BPI) (Cleeland 1991).

If pain is not controlled and the infusion has already been titrated according to hospital guidelines, the pain/anaesthetic team should be contacted for advice after checking the following:

- The catheter is still in situ.
- The catheter is still connected to the bacterial filter.
- There are no leaks within the system.
- The height of the epidural/intrathecal block. This will indicate whether the block has fallen below the upper limit of the incision or pain site. To check the height of the block use a small piece of ice or cold solution (ethyl alcohol): start at the top of the chest above the patient's incision or pain site. Gently dab the ice (or apply the cold solution) down each side of the patient's body (one side and then the other). Use a dermatome map to assess the upper and lower limit where the sensation changes (see Figure 21.2).

If the height of the block has fallen below the upper limit of the incision or pain site, the pain/anaesthetic team may undertake the following: give the patient a bolus dose of local anaesthetic agent to re-establish the block; reposition the epidural catheter. If either of these fail, other methods of analgesia need to be considered.

Complications of epidural and intrathecal analgesia

As with any invasive technique, epidural/intrathecal analgesia results in potential complications, many of which are rare. They include the following.

Haematoma
An epidural haematoma can arise from trauma to an epidural blood vessel during catheter insertion or removal. Although the incidence of a haematoma occurring is extremely rare, particular care must be taken in patients receiving thromboprophylaxis (see Procedure guidelines: Epidural intrathecal catheter

removal, below). Initial symptoms include back pain and tenderness. As the haematoma expands to compress the nerve roots or the spinal cord, this proceeds to sensory/motor weakness (Chapman & Day 2001).

Abscess formation

Wheatley *et al.* (2001) note that infection can be introduced into the epidural space from an exogenous source via contaminated equipment or drugs or from an endogenous source, leading to bacteraemia which seeds to the insertion site or catheter tip. Alternatively the catheter can act as a wick through which the infection tracks down from the entry site on the skin to the epidural/intrathecal space. Symptoms include back pain and tenderness accompanied by redness with a purulent discharge from the catheter exit site (Day 2001).

Complications specific to epidural analgesia

Dural puncture

This usually occurs when the dura mater is inadvertently punctured during the placement of the epidural catheter. The incidence of a dural puncture arising during placement of the catheter is approximately 0.32–1.23% (Wheatley *et al.* 2001). The main symptom is a headache, which arises from leakage of CSF through the dura.

Catheter migration

Catheter migration is extremely rare, occurring in less than 0.2% of patients (Wheatley *et al.* 2001). The catheter may migrate into either a blood vessel or the CSF. If the catheter migrates into a blood vessel, opioid or local anaesthetic toxicity will occur. Opioid toxicity results in sedation and respiratory depression. Local anaesthetic toxicity results in circumoral tingling, numbness, twitching, convulsions and apnoea (Pasero & McCaffery 1999). If the catheter migrates into the CSF the epidural opioids and local anaesthetic agents may reach as high as the cranial subarachnoid space. If this occurs the respiratory muscles are paralysed together with the cranial nerves, resulting in apnoea, profound hypotension and unconsciousness (Macintyre & Ready 2001).

Complications specific to intrathecal analgesia

Meningitis is a rare complication of intrathecal analgesia. The epidural route is often considered safer as the intact dura serves as an effective barrier to the spread of infection to the subarachnoid space. In fact similar infection rates are reported with both intrathecal and epidural administration (Mercadante 1999). The incidence of major infections varies widely but is reported by Ballantyne and Carwood (2005) as zero and as approximately 5% by Sloan (2004) for epidural and intrathecal therapy with external pump systems.

Table 21.2   Epidural/intrathecal analgesia: safety checklist.

Checklist	Rationale
Check the prescription and rate of the epidural/intrathecal infusion	To ensure epidural/intrathecal drugs are being administered correctly
Check the epidural/intrathecal infusion/syringe pump extension set is connected to the epidural catheter and not to any other access device	To ensure drugs are administered via the correct route
Check the bacterial filter is securely attached to the epidural/intrathecal catheter	To prevent accidental disconnection of the catheter from the filter
Check that the dressing over the epidural/intrathecal catheter exit site is secure	To prevent catheter dislodgement and minimize the risk of contamination of the catheter site

If the patient presents with headaches, fever, neck stiffness or photophobia they must be reviewed as a matter of urgency by the medical/anaesthetic team, as if meningitis is suspected CSF samples can be obtained and sent to microbiology for analysis, and antiobiotic therapy initiated promptly (Day 2001; Baker *et al.* 2004).

Equipment and prescription safety checks

When a patient is receiving a continuous infusion of epidural/intrathecal analgesia it is advisable to carry out the safety checks given in Table 21.2 at least once per shift.

Procedure guidelines   Epidural/intrathecal catheter insertion

Note: patients undergoing epidural/intrathecal analgesia should always have a venous access device in situ before the procedure. This is because, although rare, a reaction to the opioid or local anaesthetic solution (e.g. respiratory depression or sympathetic blockade) may require immediate access to the venous system. The procedure should be performed in a clinical area with access to full resuscitation equipment.

Equipment

1 Chlorhexidine in 70% alcohol.
2 Local anaesthetic.
3 Selection of needles and syringes.
4 Sterile dressing pack.
5 Face mask.
6 Tuohy needle or assorted gauge lumbar puncture needles.

7 Epidural/intrathecal catheter.
8 Bacterial filter.
9 Moisture responsive transparent dressing and dressing tape to secure catheter (Cousins *et al.* 2003: E).

Procedure guidelines (*cont.*)

Procedure

Action	Rationale
1 Explain and discuss the procedure with the patient. If the intention is to provide postoperative analgesia then explanation and consent should have been discussed the day before surgery.	To ensure that the patient understands the procedure and gives his/her valid consent (NMC 2006b: C) and to ensure patient has time to assess information and ask questions (DH 2001: C).
2 Assist the patient into the required position: (a) Lying: Patient should be lying comfortably on a firm surface. Position pillow under patient's head. On side with knee drawn up to the abdomen and clasped by the hands. Support the patient in this position.	To allow identification of the spinal processes and intervertebral discs (Brown 1999: E).
(b) Sitting: Patient sits on firm surface with arms resting on a table, and with the head resting on the arms.	To ensure maximal widening of the intervertebral spaces which will provide easy access to the epidural/intrathecal space (Brown 1999: E).
3 Support, encourage and observe the patient throughout the procedure.	As the procedure takes place behind the patient, reassurance is very important (Chapman & Day 2001: E).
4 Assist the doctor as required. The doctor will proceed as follows: (a) Clean the skin with alcohol-based solution (e.g. chlorhexidine in 70% isopropyl alcohol).	To clean skin and minimize risk of contamination (Kinirons *et al.* 2001: R 1b; Hebl 2006: R 5).
(b) Identify the area to be punctured and inject the skin and subcutaneous layers with local anaesthetic.	To ensure the spinal catheter is inserted at the correct level to provide analgesia and numb the skin prior to insertion of the Tuohy needle (Brown 1999: E).
(c) Introduce Tuohy or spinal needles usually between the identified vertebrae.	To access the epidural or intrathecal space (Brown 1999: E).

(d) Ensure epidural/intrathecal space has been entered.	To prevent anaesthesia being given directly into spinal cord or intravenously by means of the dural veins (Brown 1999: E).
(e) Inject test dose of drug (may be performed).	To ensure the position of the needle (Brown 1999: E).
(f) Thread spinal catheter through barrel of Tuohy needle.	To facilitate intermittent topping-up of anaesthesia and to allow greater control (Brown 1999: E).
(g) Attach the bacterial filter.	To prevent injection of contaminants into spinal space (Brown 1999: E).
(h) Apply transparent occlusive dressing and tape to the catheter insertion site.	To prevent the catheter being dislodged, to aid visibility and minimize contamination of the site (Baker *et al.* 2004: E).
(i) Inject solution into epidural/intrathecal space via catheter.	To provide anaesthesia (Brown 1999: E).
5 Position the patient according to the doctor's instructions, tilting if appropriate.	To ensure spread of solution to provide optimum effect (Brown 1999: E).
6 Take vital signs observations of blood pressure, pulse, respiratory rate and sedation score as dictated by the anaesthetist in the immediate post-insertion period. After this refer to local guidelines for frequency of observations required.	To monitor for signs of hypotension and respiratory depression (Weetman & Allison 2006: E).
7 Make the patient comfortable. Usually the patient is nursed flat for the first 3–6 hours, then slowly elevated into a sitting position. Bedclothes should not constrict the feet.	To ensure that any CSF leak is minimized and to prevent the patient developing a headache. To prevent the development of footdrop due to motor and sensory alterations caused by local anaesthetics (E).
8 Assess pain regularly using a visual analogue scale or pain chart if appropriate. Observe the patient's movements and facial expressions. Discuss insufficient or ineffective analgesia with the anaesthetist.	To ensure optimal pain management and that the patient is involved in his/her pain management (Macintyre & Ready 2001: E).

Procedure guidelines   Epidural/intrathecal catheter for chronic pain management: post-insertion management

It should be noted that the monitoring required in this patient group is different from that required in the postoperative setting. In the chronic setting, patients have already been taking opioids and have not received a general anaesthetic and are therefore less likely to suffer respiratory depression or alterations to their blood pressure (De Leon-Casasola *et al.* 1993).

Respiratory and cardiac function assessment

Action	Rationale
1 Monitor the patient's respiratory and cardiovascular function whilst in a recovery or high dependency area for 1 hour post-insertion.	To monitor for signs of respiratory depression and hypotension and to allow for immediate intervention where indicated (E).
2 On return to the ward for a minimum of 4 hours perform hourly assessment of: respiratory rate and SaO_2, blood pressure and pulse.	To monitor for signs of respiratory depression and hypotension and to allow for intervention if indicated (E).
3 If patient is stable, 4-hourly observations of the above for 24 hours. After 24 hours if patient is stable, respiratory and cardiac monitoring should only be reintroduced if deemed necessary by the multidisciplinary team for the individual patient or as dictated by local policy. Monitoring will continue for temperature measurements and observation for signs of localized or systemic infection for the duration of the epidural or intrathecal analgesia therapy.	To monitor patient safety whilst minimizing invasive procedures in patients with chronic pain problems (E).

Pain assessment

Action	Rationale
1 Assess the patient for their comfort/freedom from pain at rest and on movement, utilizing the same tool as used preinsertion.	This allows the practitioner and the patient to make a valid comparison (JCAHO & NPC 2001: C).

2	Pain assessment should be performed by the practitioner and patient/family together.	To gain the patient's trust and to give the patient some control over their quality of life (Higginson 1998: E).
3	Pain assessment should be performed initially at least hourly and then a minimum of 4-hourly until the patient and clinician feel that an optimum target has been achieved.	To aid patient comfort and the adjustment of drug dosages (JCAHO & NPC 2001: C).
4	Document pain assessment.	To provide the patient/family with a visual record of achievement and to allow continuity of information for different clinicians (Higginson 1998: E).
5	Assess sensory and mobility quality.	Monitor for any loss of sensation, bladder function and motor function (E).

Procedure guidelines   Epidural/intrathecal exit site dressing change

The dressing over the epidural/intrathecal exit site needs to fulfil the following three functions:

1 To help secure the epidural/intrathecal catheter.
2 To minimize the risk of infection.
3 To allow observation of the site without disturbing the dressing.

A transparent moisture responsive occlusive dressing (e.g. Tegaderm™ or Opsite IV 3000™) fulfils these functions. Opsite IV 3000™ has been found to perform well as an epidural catheter fixation product (Lawler & Anderson 2002). The epidural/ intrathecal site should be inspected daily and the dressing changed at least once weekly or more frequently if there is any serous discharge from the site.

Equipment

1 Sterile dressing pack.
2 Skin cleaning agent, e.g. chlorhexidine in 70% alcohol.
3 Transparent occlusive dressing.

Procedure

Action	Rationale
1 Explain and discuss the procedure with the patient.	To ensure that the patient understands the procedure and gives his/her valid consent (DH 2001: C; NMC 2006b: C).

Procedure guidelines (*cont.*)

2 Wash hands with soap and water. Clean trolley (or plastic tray in the community) with chlorhexidine in 70% alcohol with a paper towel.	To minimize cross-infection (Preston 2005: C). To provide a clean working surface (Parker 2004: E).
3 Position the patient comfortably on their side or sitting forward so that the site is easily accessible without undue exposure of the patient.	To maintain the patient's dignity and comfort. This is especially important when carers are attending to an area that is not visible to the patient (Chapman & Day 2001: E).
4 Prepare trolley or tray with sterile field and cleaning solution.	To minimize risk of infection and ensure equipment available (Preston 2005: C).
5 Remove old dressing and place in disposable bag.	To prevent cross-infection (E).
6 Wash hands with bactericidal handrub.	To minimize the risk of microbial contamination (E).
7 Observe site for any signs of infection such as redness, swelling or purulent discharge. If any of these are present contact the hospital anaesthetic/pain team for advice.	To ensure careful monitoring of site to minimize the chance of any infection (Royal College of Anaesthetists 2004: C).
8 Clean site with skin-cleaning agent (chlorhexidine in 70% alcohol)	To minimize the risk of infection (Mimoz *et al* 1999: R 1b; Kinirons *et al*. 2001: R 1b; Hebl 2006: R 5).
9 Apply transparent occlusive dressing over the whole area.	To anchor the epidural/intrathecal catheter, minimize the risk of infection and allow observation of the epidural/intrathecal site (Burns *et al*. 2001: R 1b; Royce *et al*. 2006: E).
10 Ensure that the patient is comfortable.	
11 Dispose of all material in the clinical waste bag.	To prevent environmental contamination (Preston 2005: C).
12 Wash hands with soap and water.	To reduce the risk of cross-infection (Preston 2005: C).

Procedure guidelines   Epidural/intrathecal catheter removal

Note: before an epidural/intrathecal catheter is removed it is essential to consider the clotting status of the patient's blood. If the patient is fully anticoagulated a clotting profile must be performed and advice sought from the medical staff as to when the catheter can be removed. If the patient is receiving a prophylactic anticoagulant the following guidelines are recommended (Vandermeulen *et al.* 1994; Horlocker & Wedel 1998; Rowlingson & Hanson 2005).

■ Low-dose low molecular weight heparin. If this is given once daily the epidural/intrathecal catheter should be removed at least 12 hours after the last injection and several hours prior to the next dose (the timing will depend on the manufacturer's recommended guidelines, e.g. Tinzaparin [Leo Laboratories Ltd] recommend epidural or spinal catheters are removed a minimum of 4 hours before the subsequent dose).
■ Unfractionated heparin. The epidural/intrathecal catheter should be removed following local guidelines and the advice of the anaesthetic/pain management team.

Equipment

1 Dressing pack.
2 Skin cleaning agent, e.g. chlorhexidine in 70% alcohol.

3 Occlusive dressing.

Procedure

Action	Rationale
1 Explain and discuss the procedure with the patient.	To ensure the patient understands the procedure and gives his/her valid consent (DH 2001: C; NMC 2006b: C).
2 Wash hands with bactericidal soap and water or bactericidal alcohol handrub.	To minimize cross-infection (Preston 2005: C).
3 Open dressing pack.	
4 Wash hands and remove tape and dressing from catheter insertion site.	To minimize risk of cross-infection (Preston 2005: C).
5 Gently, in one swift movement, remove the catheter. Check that the catheter is intact. This can be done by observing that the tip of the catheter is marked blue and that the 1 cm marks along the length of the catheter are all intact. Add to document that catheter removed intact.	To ensure the catheter is removed intact with the minimum of discomfort to the patient (E).

Procedure guidelines (*cont.*)

6 Clean around the catheter exit site using skin cleaning agent.	To minimize contamination of site by micro-organisms (E).
7 Apply an occlusive dressing and leave in situ for 24 hours. The epidural/intrathecal tip may be sent for culture and sensitivity if infection is suspected, or according to local policy.	To prevent inadvertent access of micro-organisms along the tract (E).

Problem solving: Epidural/intrathecal infusions of local anaesthetic agents and opioids: management of side-effects

Problem	Cause	Suggested action
Respiratory depression.	*Increasing age.* Elderly patients are more susceptible to the side-effects of opioids due to age-related alterations in the distribution, metabolism and excretion of drugs.	If respiratory rate falls to 8 breaths a minute or below: (a) Stop the epidural/intrathecal infusion. (b) Summon emergency assistance. (c) Commence oxygen via face mask and encourage the patient to take deep breaths. (d) Review current analgesic prescription and consider reducing opioid and local anaesthetic doses before resuming the infusion (Macintyre *et al.* 2003).
	Concurrent use of systemic opioids or sedatives. Patients receiving opioids by epidural/intrathecal infusion should not be given opioids by any other route unless given in the palliative care setting for breakthrough pain.	1 Stop the epidural/intrathecal infusion. 2 Stay with the patient and monitor respiratory rate, sedation score and peripheral tissue oxygenation (using a pulse oximeter) continuously. 3 Commence oxygen therapy. 4 Consider giving naloxone if prescribed by anaesthetist or patient unrousable and naloxone already prescribed (when utilized for acute pain management). 5 Review analgesia: stop any other opioids prescribed and consider changing parameters of epidural/intrathecal infusion. (Pasero & McCaffery 1999: E.)

Problem	Cause	Suggested action
Sedation: 1 *Mild:* patient drowsy but easy to rouse. 2 *Severe:* patient difficult to rouse.	See under Respiratory depression, above	1 If patient has mild sedation, consider reducing the rate of the infusion or the dose of opioid or taking the opioid out of the infusion. 2 If patient is difficult to rouse and opioid toxicity/overdose is suspected, follow management for respiratory depression.
Hypotension.	Patients with hypovolaemia. Patients with a high thoracic epidural in whom the concentration of local anaesthetic agent and volume of infusion cause blockade of the cardio-accelerator nerves.	If blood pressure falls suddenly: (a) Stop the epidural/intrathecal infusion. (b) Summon emergency assistance. (c) Administer oxygen via face mask or nasal cannula. (d) Stay with the patient and monitor blood pressure at 5 minute intervals. (e) Ensure polyfusor of Haemacel or Gelofusine is readily available and use if prescribed by the anaesthetist. (f) Vasoconstrictor agents such as ephedrine or metaraminol may need to be given by the anaesthetic team if hypotension does not respond to a fluid challenge of Haemacel or Gelofusine. (Macintyre & Ready 2001.)
Motor blockade.	More likely to occur when higher concentrations of local anaesthetic agents are given by continuous infusion. If a high concentration of a local anaesthetic agent is administered via a low lumbar epidural/intrathecal catheter then the lumbar motor nerves are likely to be blocked, causing leg weakness.	Do not attempt to mobilize patient if leg weakness is evident. Contact pain or anaesthetic team for advice: reducing the concentration of the local anaesthetic agent or the rate of the epidural/intrathecal infusion may help to resolve this problem (Pasero & McCaffery 1999).

Problem solving *(cont.)*

Problem	Cause	Suggested action
Nausea and vomiting.	Previous episodes of nausea and vomiting with opioids. Exacerbated by low blood pressure.	Regular administration of antiemetics. Treat other causes, e.g. low blood pressure. Consider use of non-pharmacological methods (e.g. stimulation of the P6 acupressure point) (Lee & Done 2004).
Pruritus (usually more marked over the face, chest and abdomen).	Previous pruritus with opioids.	Administer an antihistamine such as chlorpheniramine (may be contraindicated in patients who are becoming increasingly sedated) or a small dose of naloxone (administer with caution as this can easily reverse analgesia). If pruritus does not resolve consider switching to another opioid or removing the opioid from the infusion (Pasero & McCaffery 1999).
Urinary retention.	More likely to occur if opioids and local anaesthetic agents are infused in combination.	Catheterize patient.

Problem solving: Epidural/intrathecal insertion: complications

Problem	Signs and symptoms	Suggested action
Dural puncture.	Headache.	Bedrest: headache will be less severe if patient lies flat. Replacement fluids either intravenously or orally to encourage formation of CSF. Administer analgesics for headache. If headache does not settle, contact the anaesthetic team who may consider an epidural blood patch to seal the puncture (Gaiser 2006).

Problem	Signs and symptoms	Suggested action
Catheter migration into an epidural blood vessel.	If catheter migrates into a blood vessel signs of opioid or local anaesthetic toxicity can occur: *opioid*: sedation and respiratory depression; *local anaesthetic*: circumoral tingling and numbness, twitching, convulsions and apnoea.	Stop epidural infusion. Contact pain/anaesthetic team or summon emergency assistance. Treat the patient for complications of opioid or local anaesthetic overdose. If necessary support ventilation (Chapman & Day 2001).
Catheter migration across the dura into the CSF (from the epidural space into the intrathecal space).	If an epidural catheter migrates into the CSF the analgesic solution may reach as high as the cranial subarachnoid space. If this occurs the respiratory muscles are paralysed together with the cranial nerves, resulting in apnoea, profound hypotension and unconsciousness. This is because intrathecal doses are calculated as one-tenth of the epidural dose and migration from the epidural space to the intrathecal space leads to a drug overdose.	Stop epidural infusion. Summon emergency assistance. Prepare emergency equipment to support respiration and ventilate lungs. Prepare emergency drugs and intravenous fluids and administer as directed. Prepare equipment for intubation.
Epidural haematoma.	Back pain and tenderness and nerve root pain with sensory and motor weakness.	Urgent neurological assessment. Computed tomography (CT) or magnetic resonance imaging (MRI) scan to accurately diagnose if there is nerve or spinal cord compression. If a haematoma is diagnosed prepare patient for urgent surgery. (Chapman & Day 2001). To avoid haematoma on removal of epidural in patients treated with prophylactic anticoagulants, see guidelines for timing of removal.

Problem solving *(cont.)*

Problem	Signs and symptoms	Suggested action
Epidural abscess.	Back pain and tenderness. May have redness and purulent discharge from catheter exit site. May also develop nerve root signs with neuropathic pain and sensory/motor weakness.	If the epidural catheter is still in situ, remove and send tip off for culture and sensitivity. Treat with antibiotics. Carry out CT or MRI scan and refer for urgent neurosurgery to prevent paraplegia (Chapman & Day 2001: E).
Meningitis.	Headaches, fever, neck stiffness, photophobia.	Assist anaesthetist/doctor to obtain CSF sample for microbiology analysis. Initiate antibiotic therapy as per hospital policy. Non pharmacological measures for symptom management, e.g. dim lights. If the infection does not respond to antibiotics it may be necessary to remove the catheter and convert back to systemic analgesia until meningitis has resolved (Mercadante 1999).
Intrathecal catheter granulona (an inflammatory mass that forms around the catheter tip).	Pain, parasthesia, numbness in lower extremeties that may progress to paresis.	MRI scan to diagnose the problem. Stop infusion (granulomas may resolve on their own once the infusion is stopped Du Pen (2005)).

Problem solving: Epidural/intrathecal catheter: issues with pump and site

The following can be used by nursing staff and then adapted for use by the patient/family.

Problem	Cause	Suggested action
Ambulatory pump auditory alarm.	Battery failure is most likely.	Stop pump, remove old and replace with new battery; ensure battery is fitted up snugly to connections. Turn on pump and ensure light indicator is flashing.

Problem	Cause	Suggested action
	Catheter occlusion.	Stop pump, draw up 0.9% sodium chloride and flush catheter. If catheter clears reattach pump, press start and ensure light indicator is flashing. If catheter is still obstructed and will not flush, phone cancer centre/general practitioner.
Sudden acute pain.	Catheter obstruction; catheter movement; change in pathology.	Check the catheter for any obvious problems which can be quickly resolved such as catheter disconnection. If the catheter has blocked or migrated outwards, stop the infusion pump and give the patient a breakthrough dose of analgesia orally or subcutaneously. Inform general practitioner and/or hospital anaesthetic/pain team as soon as possible. If the patient has had an exacerbation of pain due to disease progression, follow advice from hospital team (the infusion rate may require titrating or the concentration of drugs may need to be changed).
Disconnection of epidural/ intrathecal catheter from filter.	Patient movement: typically turning in bed at night.	Stop the pump. Wrap the disconnected end of the catheter in a piece of sterile gauze and contact the district nursing/hospital team for advice.

Suggested procedure for district nursing/hospital team (Langevin *et al.* 1996):
- Clean approximately 15 cm of the disconnected catheter with chlorhexidine in 70% alcohol. Allow to air dry completely.
- Using sterile scissors, cut the cleaned catheter 10 cm away from the contaminated end.
- Insert the cleaned end of catheter into a sterile screw connector and catheter filter.
- Change the epidural/intrathecal infusion extension set and recommence infusion. |

Problem solving *(cont.)*

Problem	Cause	Suggested action
Redness, swelling or leakage of discoloured fluid from site.	Infection *or* local irritation at site from skin interaction with the plastic catheter.	Contact general practitioner and hospital anaesthetic/pain team. If infection is suspected, the patient should be started on antibiotics to prevent spread of any infection into the epidural space. It may be necessary to remove the catheter if the patient has a temperature, there is pus at the exit site or if the patient has back pain.

References and further reading

ANZCA (2005) Epidural analgesia. In: *Acute Pain Management: Scientific Evidence*, 2nd edn. Australia and New Zealand College of Anaesthetics, Melbourne, Australia.

Baker, L. *et al.* (2004) Evolving spinal analgesia practice in palliative care. *Palliat Med*, **18**, 507–15.

Ballantyne, J.C. & Carwood, C.M. (2005) Comparative efficacy of epidural, subarachnoid and intracerebroventricular opioids in patients with pain due to cancer. *Cochrane Database Syst Rev*, **2**, CD005178.DOI:10.1002/14651858.

Bannon, L., Alexander-Williams, M. & Lutman, D. (2001) A national survey of epidural practice. *Anaesthesia*, **56**(10), 1021–2.

Brown, D.L. (1999) *Atlas of Regional Anaesthesia*, 2nd edn. W.B. Saunders Company, Philadelphia.

Burns, S.M. *et al.* (2001) Intrapartum epidural catheter migration: a comparative study of three dressing applications. *Br J Anaesth*, **86**(4), 565–7.

Chapman, S. & Day, R. (2001) Spinal anatomy and the use of epidurals. *Prof Nurs*, **16**(6), 1174–7.

Cleeland, C.S. (1991) The brief pain inventory. www.mdanderson.org/topics/paincontrol. Accessed 24/9/07.

Coniam, S. & Mendham, J. (2005) Management of acute pain: principles and practice. In: *Principles of Pain Management for Anaesthetists*. Hodder Arnold, London, pp. 74–5.

Cook, T., Eaton, J. & Goodwin, A. (1997) Epidural analgesia following upper abdominal surgery: United Kingdom practice. *Acta Anaesthesiol Scand*, **41**(1), 18–24.

Cousins, K. *et al.* (2003) Intrathecal catheters: developing consistency in filter use and dressings in Perth, Australia. *Int J Palliat Nurs*, **7**(9), 308–14.

Curatolo, M., Peterson-Felix, S., & Scaramozzino, P. (1998) Epidural fentanyl, adrenaline and clonidine as adjuvants to local anaesthetics for surgical anaesthesia: meta analysis of analgesia and side effects. *Acta Anaesthesiol Scand*, **42**, 910–20.

Day, R. (2001) The use of epidural and intrathecal analgesia in palliative care. *Int J Palliat Care*, **7**(8), 369–74.

De Cicco, M. *et al.* (1995) Time-dependent efficacy of bacterial filters and infection risk in long-term epidural catheterisation. *Anesthesiology*, **82**, 765–71.

De Leon-Casasola, O.A. *et al.* (1993) A comparison of post-operative epidural analgesia between patients with chronic cancer taking high doses of oral opioids versus opioid-naïve patients. *Anesth Analg*, **76**, 302–7.

Du Pen, A. (2005) Care and management of intrathecal and epidural catheters. *J Infusion Nursing*, **28**(6), 377–81.

DH (2001) Good practice in consent implementation guide: consent to examination or treatment. www.dh.gov.uk/en/Publicationsandstatistics/Publications/PublicationsPolicyAndGuidance/DH_4005762. Accessed 24/9/07.

Dickson, D. (2004) Risks and benefits of long term intrathecal analgesia. *Anaesthesia*, **59**, 633–5.

Fotiadis, R.J. *et al.* (2004) Epidural analgesia in gastrointestinal surgery. *Br J Surg*, **91**, 828–41.

Gaiser, R. (2006) Postdural puncture headache. *Curr Opin Anaesthesiol*, **19**, 249–53.

Grond, S. *et al.* (2000) Epidural analgesia for labour pain: a review of availability, current practices and influence on labour. *Int J Acute Pain Manage*, **3**(1), 31–43.

Hall, J. (2000) Epidural analgesia management. *Nurs Times*, **96**(28), 38–9.

Hebl, J.R. (2006) The importance and implications of aseptic techniques during regional anaesthesia. *Reg Anesth Pain Med*, **31**, 311–23.

Higginson, I. (1998) Can professionals improve their assessments? *J Pain Symptom Manage*, **15**(3), 149–50.

Horlocker, T. & Wedel, D. (1998) Spinal and epidural blockade and perioperative low molecular weight heparin: smooth sailing on the Titanic. *Anaesth Analg*, **8**, 1153–6.

JCAHO & NPC (2001) Pain: current understanding of assessment, management and treatments. www.jcaho.org. Accessed 8/06.

Kehlet, H. (1997) Multimodal approach to control postoperative pathophysiology and rehabilitation. *Br J Anaesth*, **78**(5), 606–17.

Kehlet, H. & Holte, K. (2001) Effect of postoperative analgesia on surgical outcome. *Br J Anaesth*, **87**(1), 62–72.

Kinirons, B. *et al.* (2001) Chlorhexadine versus povidine iodine in preventing colonisation of continuous epidural catheters in children. *Anaesthesiology*, **94**, 239–44.

Langevin, P. *et al.* (1996) Epidural catheter reconnection: safe and unsafe practice. *Anesthesiology*, **85**(4), 883–8.

Lawler, K. & Anderson, T. (2002) Regional trial of five epidural fixation products and a commonly used control. *Pain Network Newsletter*, Spring, pp. 6–8.

Lee, A. & Done, M.L. (2004) Stimulation of the wrist acupuncture point P6 for preventing post-operative nausea and vomiting. *Cochrane Database Syst Rev*, **3**, CD003281.DOI: 10.1002/14651858.

Leo Laboratories Ltd (2004) Tinzaparin sodium 10 000 IU/ml. Product information leaflet. www.emc.medicines.org.uk. Accessed 02/06.

Macintyre, P. & Ready, L. (2001) Epidural and intrathecal analgesia. In: *Acute Pain Management. A Practical Guide*, (eds P. Macintyre & L. Ready) 2nd edn. W.B. Saunders, London.

Macintyre, P., Upton, R. & Ludbrook, G.L. (2003) Pain in the elderly. In: *Clinical Pain Management: Acute Pain* (eds D.J. Rowbotham & P.E. Macintyre), pp. 157–58. Arnold, London.

Mackenzie, A.R. *et al.* (1998) Spinal epidural abscess: the importance of early diagnosis and treatment. *J Neurosurg Psychiatry*, **65**(2), 209–12.

McCaffery, M. & Pasero, C. (1999) *Pain: Clinical Manual*. Mosby, St. Louis, MO.

Mercadante, S. (1999) Problems of long-term spinal opioid treatment in advanced cancer patients. *Pain*, **79**(1), 1–13.

Mimoz, O., Karim, A. & Cosseron, M. (1999) Chlorhexidine compared with povidone-iodine as skin preparation before blood culture. A randomised controlled trial. *Ann Intern Med*, **131**(11), 834–7.

NMC (2005) *Guidelines for Records and Record Keeping*. Nursing and Midwifery Council, London.

NMC (2006a) *Medicines Management Advice Sheet*. Nursing and Midwifery Council, London.

NMC (2006b) *A–Z Advice Sheet Consent*. www.nmc.org.

Papagelopoulos, P. *et al.* (2001) Treatment of lumbosacral radicular pain with epidural steroid injections. *Orthopedics*, **24**(2), 145–9.

Parker, L.J. (2004) Decontamination of medical devices: legislation and compliance to practice. *Br J Nurs*, **13**(17), 1028–32.

Pasero, C. & McCaffery, M. (1999) Providing epidural analgesia. *Nursing*, **29**(8), 34–42.

Preston, R.M. (2005) Aseptic technique: evidence-based approach to patient safety. *Br J Nurs*, **14**(10), 540–5.

Richardson, J. (2001) Post-operative epidural analgesia: introducing evidence-based guidelines through an education and assessment process. *J Clin Nurs*, **10**(2), 238–45.

Romer, H. & Russell, G. (1998) A survey of the practice of thoracic epidural analgesia in the United Kingdom. *Anaesthesia*, **53**(10), 1016–22.

Rowlingson, J.C. & Hanson, P.B. (2005) Neuraxial anesthesia and low-molecular-weight heparin prophylaxis in major orthopedic surgery in the wake of the latest American Society of Regional Analgesia Guidelines. *Anesth Analg*, **100**, 1482–8.

Royal College of Anaesthetists (2004) *Good Practice in the Management of Continuous Epidural Analgesia in the Hospital Setting*. Royal College of Anaesthetists, London.

Royce, C.F., Hall, J. & Royce, A.G. (2006) The 'mesentery' dressing for epidural fixation. *Anaesthesia*, **61**, 713.

Sands, R., Yarussi, A. & de Leon-Casasola, D. (1998) Complications and side-effects associated with epidural bupivacaine/morphine analgesia. *Acute Pain*, **1**(2), 43–50.

Sloan, P.A. (2004) The evolving role of interventional pain management in oncology. *J Support Oncol*, **2**(6), 491–503.

Smith, H. & Elliott, J. (2001) Alpha2 receptors and agonists in pain management. *Curr Opin Anaesthesiol*, **14**, 513–18.

Smitt, P. *et al.* (1998) Outcome and complications of epidural analgesia in patients with chronic cancer pain. *Cancer*, **83**(9), 2015–22.

Stevens, R.A. & Ghazi, S.M. (2000) Routes of opioid analgesic therapy in the management of cancer pain. *Cancer Control*, **7**(2), 132–41.

Urdan, L.D., Stacy, K.M. & Lough, M.E. (2006) Pain and pain management. In: *Thelan's Critical Care Nursing Diagnosis and Management*. Mosby Elsevier, St Louis, MO.

Vandermeulen, E., Van Aken, H. & Vermylen, J. (1994) Anticoagulants and spinal-epidural anaesthesia. *Anaesth Analg*, **79**(6), 1165–77.

Wallace, M.S. (2002) Treatment options for refractory pain: the role of intrathecal therapy. *Neurology*, **59**(Suppl 2), S18–24.

Walsh, D. (1997) *TENS: Clinical Applications and Related Theory*. Churchill Livingstone, Edinburgh.

Weetman, C. & Allison W. (2006) Use of epidural analgesia in post-operative pain management. *Nursing Standard* Jul 12–18; **20**(44):54–64.

Wheatley, R., Schug, S. & Watson, D. (2001) Safety and efficacy of postoperative epidural analgesia. *Br J Anaesth*, **87**(1), 47–61.

Multiple choice questions

1 Epidural and intrathecal routes can be effective routes of analgesic administration. Drugs should not be administered by these routes if the patient has:

    a   An unstable spinal fracture
    b   Coagulation effects
    c   Local sepsis at proposed entry site
    d   All of the above

2 Following insertion of an epidural or intrathecal catheter the patient should lie flat to prevent the development of a headache from CSF leakage. How long should the patient lie flat for?

    a   1–3 hours
    b   3–6 hours
    c   6–9 hours
    d   9–12 hours

3 Patients receiving epidural or intrathecal analgesia must be cared for by:

    a   A registered nurse
    b   A student nurse under supervision
    c   A registered nurse who has undergone formal training
    d   A critical care nurse

Answers to the multiple choice questions can be found in Appendix 3.

Chapter 22

Perioperative care

Definition

Perioperative care refers to the nursing care delivered to a patient before (pre), during (intra) and after (post) surgery.

Preoperative care

Definition

Preoperative care is the assessment and preparation, physical and psychological, of a patient before surgery.

Objectives

Physical

- To assess the physical condition of the patient so that potential problems can be anticipated and prevented.
- To ensure that the patient understands the need to be in an optimum physical condition before surgery.
- To minimize postoperative complications, e.g. by teaching the patient deep breathing exercises, leg exercises and their importance to the individual's well-being postoperatively.

Psychological

- To ensure that the patient is fully informed and understands the nature of anaesthetic, surgery and possible complications.
- To minimize anxiety for the patient and help them to identify and implement useful coping mechanisms.

- To inform and ensure the patient understands what to expect postoperatively, e.g. presence of possible drains, catheters, pumps and monitors that may be necessary.

Reference material

Patient education and postoperative pain

Research has shown that preoperative patient education not only meets patients' information needs but also assists patients in reducing anxiety levels and promotes the patients' well being (Walker 2002). Patient information booklets can also help patients to have a greater understanding of surgery and what is expected of them.

Preoperative education can address some of the patients' concerns and fears. As pain and anaesthesia are patients' greatest worries, they need to be discussed in the preoperative period so that anxiety can be reduced (Mitchell 2000), which may result in patients requiring less analgesia (Beddows 1997). Preoperative visiting by recovery staff allows patients to ask questions, which could help them to manage their anxiety and provide baseline information about patients, which is important for effective management postoperatively, for example, of pain management. It also gives information to the surgical team to allow them to maintain continuity of care in the operating department (Beddows 1997).

The control of pain whilst the patient is still in the operating theatre and whilst recovering from his/her surgery is vital to further reduce anxiety and general well being. Use of patient-controlled analgesia (PCA) gives the patient a sense of autonomy, which may decrease anxiety and which will in turn influence the patient's pain perception (Field & Adams 2001). For further information see Chapter 20, Pain management and assessment.

Skin preparation

Traditionally patients had their operation site and surrounding area shaved the night before surgery in the belief that hair removal reduces the incidence of wound infection postoperatively. However, this method of hair removal can injure the skin and may increase the risk of infection by producing microscopic infected lacerations, so hair needs to be removed only from the area immediately around the site of incision. This should be done with depilatory cream the day before the operation. If this is not possible then shaving should take place in the anaesthetic room prior to surgery, using electric clippers. It should not be done in the operating room as this is a source of infection (Kjonniksen *et al.* 2002).

Preoperative fasting

General anaesthesia carries the risk of the patient inhaling gastric contents during induction, which could lead to serious complications and can even be fatal (Dean & Fawcett 2002). Ensuring that the patient understands the rationale for fasting is important in order to reduce anxiety. For elective surgery patients are kept 'nil by mouth' long enough to allow the stomach to empty. This means that patients can have water or clear fluids up to 3 hours before surgery and solid foods up to 6 hours provided this is light food (RCN 2005). However, gastric emptying can be delayed by anxiety or the action of some opiates, for example morphine (O'Callaghan 2002), so it is important to be aware of this when deciding when to commence patients 'nil by mouth'. Most patients prefer not to eat but would like to have a drink to keep their mouth moist before surgery and so are happy to comply with the 3 hours fasting for water and clear fluids.

Antiembolic stockings (graduated elastic compression stockings)

Patients should be assessed for the individual risk factors for venous thromboembolism (VTE), i.e. deep vein thrombosis (DVT) and pulmonary embolism (PE) when hospitalized in order to determine the most appropriate thromboprophylaxis (House of Commons Health Committee 2005; NICE 2007). Patients at higher risk include those with major illness e.g. acute cardiac or respiratory failure, major surgery, older patients, patients who are obese or with a previous history of DVT or PE (SIGN 2002; NICE 2007). All patients requiring an inpatient stay for surgery should have prophylactic treatment to reduce the risk of DVT, which may include anticoagulation and mechanical compression methods, for example antiembolic stockings and intermittent pneumatic compression methods (SIGN 2002; Roderick et al. 2005; NICE 2007). Patients should be given verbal and written information before surgery about the risks of VTE and the effectiveness of prophylaxis (NICE 2007). It is estimated that 20% of patients undergoing major surgery will develop a DVT with the risk increasing to 40% of patients undergoing major orthopaedic surgery (SIGN 2002). Mechanical compression methods reduce the risk of DVT by about two-thirds when used as monotherapy and by about half when added to pharmacological methods (Roderick et al. 2005). Graduated compression stockings (antiembolic) promote venous flow and reduce venous stasis not only in the legs but also in the pelvic veins and inferior vena cava (Hayes et al. 2002; Rashid et al. 2005; Roderick et al. 2005).

Thigh-length graduated compression/antiembolic stockings should be fitted from the time of admission to hospital unless contraindicated, for example peripheral arterial disease or diabetic neuropathy (NICE 2007, p. 121), and until the patient has returned to their usual level of mobility. Thigh-length stockings are difficult to put on and can roll down creating a tourniquet just above the knee restricting blood supply, so patient monitoring and/or assistance should take place to ensure that stockings are fitted smoothly, are not rolled down or the top band not folded down. If thigh-length stockings are inappropriate for a particular patient for reasons of compliance or fit, knee-length stockings may be used as a suitable alternative. It has been suggested that 15–20% of patients cannot effectively wear antiembolic stockings because of unusual limb size or shape (SIGN 2002). In reality, knee-high stockings have the advantage of simplicity, with greater patient compliance and economy (Byrne 2002; Barker & Hollingsworth 2004; Parnaby 2004). When applying the stockings, it is important that correct measurements are taken so that the appropriate stocking size is fitted for optimum effectiveness. The stocking compression profile should be equivalent to the Sigel profile, and approximately 18 mmHg at the ankle, 14 mmHg at the mid-calf and 8 mmHg at the upper thigh (NICE 2007, p. 52).

During surgery the use of heel supports which reduce the pressure on the calves on the operating table will also encourage venous return. The use of intermittent calf compression air boots that promote venous flow during surgery have also been reported to be effective (Davis & O'Neill 2002; NICE 2007). The intermittent calf compression boots can be used in conjunction with antiembolic stockings providing double protection. The only time this needs to be reviewed is when the patient is placed in Lloyd Davis position as there is a risk of developing compartment syndrome (see Positioning section, below). In this instance either the antiembolic stockings or the intermittent calf compression boots should be used: this decision will be made by the surgeon and the anaesthetist.

Assessment of latex allergy

Natural rubber latex is a durable flexible material composed of natural proteins and added chemicals. In the health care setting, natural rubber latex is present in gloves and other medical devices such as catheters and wound drains. Latex allergy results in a reaction to one or more of the components of natural rubber latex (AORN 2004).

As part of the patient's preoperative assessment, allergy status must be established. This information must be communicated to all members of the health care team and departments that the patient may visit including theatre, recovery, pathology and radiology. The assessment should cover the following known risk factors for latex allergy (AORN 2004):

- History of multiple surgeries beginning at an early age (e.g. spina bifida, urinary malformation).
- Known food allergies (avocado, chestnut or banana).
- History of an allergic reaction to latex.

Table 22.1 Symptoms of latex exposure and possible anaphylaxis.

The conscious patient	The unconscious patient
Itchy eyes	Facial oedema
Generalized pruritis	Urticaria/rash
Shortness of breath	Skin flushing
Sneezing/wheezing	Bronchospasm
Nausea	Laryngeal oedema
Oedema	Hypotension
Vomiting	Tachycardia
Abdominal cramp	Cardiac arrest
Diarrhoea	
Feeling faint	

- History of an allergic reaction during an operation.
- Past experience of itchy skin, skin rash or redness when in contact with rubber products.
- Past skin irritation from an examination by a doctor or dentist wearing rubber gloves.
- Past sneezing, wheezing or chest tightness when exposed to rubber.

Assessment and monitoring for symptoms of latex allergy in both the conscious and unconscious patient is required at all stages of perioperative care (Table 22.1).

Management of the patient with known latex allergy

Patients identified as having an allergy to natural latex rubber need to be treated in a latex-free environment following these recommendations:

- The theatre must be cleaned with latex-free gloves and equipment.
- All latex products removed or covered with plastics so that the rubber elements are not exposed.
- All health care staff must be made aware of the adverse reactions that could occur following the patient's exposure to natural rubber latex.
- All health care staff in direct contact with the patient must wear vinyl gloves during procedures and in the vicinity of the patient.
- The patient should be first on the operating list.
- Where a type I (immediate hypersensitivity reaction) allergy is suspected, suitable clinical management procedures must be ready for use in the event of the patient having a hypersensitivity reaction.

■ A latex-free contents box or trolley (this holds stock of all latex-free products that will be required during surgery and anaesthetic) should be ready in every theatre department and in recovery room. There should be a list of all latex-free equipment with the manufacturers listed available in the box or trolley.

788

Further guidance may be sought from the Association of Perioperative Registered Nurses (AORN) proposed latex guideline at www.aorn.org/proposed/latex.htm (accessed 16/2/06).

Procedure guidelines Antiembolic stockings: fitting and wearing

Note: antiembolic stockings are also known as graduated elastic compression stockings or thromboembolic deterrent stockings (TEDS).

Equipment

1 Tape measure.
2 Antiembolic stockings (calf or thigh length).

3 Apron.
4 Patient records/documentation.

Procedure

Action	Rationale
Patient assessment for antiembolic stockings	
1 Assess and record in the patient's documentation the patient's risk factors for venous thromboembolism (VTE), i.e. deep vein thrombosis (DVT) and pulmonary embolism (PE). Examples of risk factors: (a) patient undergoing major surgery or abdominal/pelvic surgery; (b) immobility, e.g. prolonged bedrest; (c) active cancer; (d) severe cardiac failure or recent myocardial infarction; (e) acute respiratory failure; (f) elderly; (g) previous history of DVT or PE; (h) acute infection/inflammation; (i) diabetes; (j) smoker;	All patients admitted to hospital should undergo a risk assessment for venous thromobosis to determine the most appropriate preventative measures, i.e. thromboprophylaxis (SIGN 2002: C; House of Commons Health Committee 2005: C; Roderick *et al.* 2005: C; NICE 2007: C). The higher the number of risk factors the greater the risk for VTE (SIGN 2002: C; NICE 2007: C).

(k) obesity;
(l) gross varicose veins;
(m) paralysis of lower limbs;
(n) clotting disorders;
(o) hormone replacement therapy;
(p) oral contraceptives;
(q) pregnancy;
(r) puerperium;
(s) anaesthesia.
(SIGN 2002; House of Commons Health Committee 2005; Rashid *et al.* 2005; NICE 2007)

2 Assess and record in the patient's documentation the patient's suitability for antiembolic stockings, identifying whether the patient has any contraindications for wearing antiembolic stockings. Contraindications: (a) Severe peripheral arterial disease (SIGN 2002). (b) Severe peripheral neuropathy (SIGN 2002). (c) Vascular disease resulting from congestive heart conditions (House of Commons Health Committee 2005). (d) Gangrene. (e) Pulmonary oedema or massive oedema of the legs (House of Commons Health Committee 2005). (f) Major leg deformity (SIGN 2002). (g) Certain types of skin disease, e.g. weeping skin lesions/dermatitis (SIGN 2002). (h) Recent skin graft (Rashid *et al.* 2005). (i) Cellulitis (Rashid *et al.* 2005). (j) Pressure sores to heels (NICE 2005; Rashid *et al.* 2005).	To comply with national guidelines and hospital policy/guidelines. To ensure that antiembolic stockings are fitted correctly and to reduce the complications associated with antiembolic stockings (SIGN 2002; NICE 2007: C). The stockings would hinder healing of local leg conditions, e.g. dermatitis (C). Pressure sores are a complication of antiembolic stockings and stockings should not be applied (NICE 2005: C).

Procedure guidelines *(cont.)*

3 Explain and discuss the procedure with the patient and provide written information as follows:

(a) Reasons for wearing antiembolic stockings.

(b) How to fit and wear stockings.

(c) What to report to the nurse, e.g. any feelings of pain or numbness or skin problems.

(d) Skin care, i.e. wash and dry legs daily.

(e) Reasons for early mobilization and adequate hydration.

(f) Reasons against crossing of legs or ankles.

(g) Length of time that the stockings should be worn, e.g. until they return to their usual level of mobility.

To ensure that the patient understands the procedure and gives his/her valid consent (NMC 2005: C; NMC 2006: C). To ensure that the patient understands how to fit and wear stockings including self-care measures and what to report to the nurse so as to detect complications early, e.g. pressure sores, circulation difficulties of wearing antiembolic stockings (SIGN 2002: C; NICE 2007: C).

Measuring for and fitting of antiembolic stockings

4 Perform hand hygiene and put on apron prior to the procedure.

To prevent cross-infection (Pratt *et al.* 2007).

5 Place the tape measure around the calf at the greatest point and measure the calf circumference (and leg measurements) according to the manuafacturer's instructions, recording the measurements in the patient's documentation.

To comply with the manufacturer's instructions (C).
Incorrect sizing causes swelling and bruising to ankles and can constrict blood supply leading to long term complications (C).

6 Check pedal pulses are intact.

To ensure the patient has good circulation to the feetx and antiembolic stockings are not contraindicated (SIGN 2002: C; NICE 2007: C).

Apply the antiembolic stocking to the legs according to the manufacturer's instructions. Refer to the Procedure guidelines: Compression garments (elastic): application of, Chapter 9, Professional edition.	To ensure correct size of stocking is fitted correctly (C).

Daily care of patient wearing antiembolic stockings

7 Remove stockings daily, observing for pain, skin damage, circulation difficulties which may arise as a result of wrinkling, etc. of stocking, but for no more than 30 minutes: confirm size is applicable (SIGN 2002).	To review calf and/or leg measurements to ensure stockings fit correctly (SIGN 2002: C; NICE 2005:C). Reported complications of wearing antiembolic stockings include pressure sores (NICE 2005:C) and circulation difficulties, e.g. arterial occlusion, thrombosis, gangrene (SIGN 2002: C). The circulation complications can be linked to the tourniquet effect of bunched-up stockings combined with swelling of the leg (SIGN 2002; House of Commons Health Committee 2005).
8 Where worn, ensure that antiembolic stockings are of the correct size and fit smoothly. Check the colour and tips of the toes. *Note*: top band of stockings must not be turned down.	To prevent a tourniquet effect if the stocking rolls down (C). To ensure the blood supply is not compromised (C).
9 Encourage early mobilization. For patients on bedrest, encourage deep breathing and exercises of the leg hourly; flexion/extension and rotation of the ankles.	To improve venous circulation (SIGN 2002: C; NICE 2007: C).
10 Encourage patient to sit with legs up when resting.	It is recognized that this will reduce limb swelling and promote venous return by its gravitational effect; however, there is little scientific data to clarify that this does reduce the risk of VTE. *Note*: care should be taken with patients with ischaemic legs (NICE 2007: C).

Procedure guidelines (cont.)

11 Monitor for signs of DVT or PE and report to medical staff immediately: (a) Complaints of calf or thigh pain. (b) Erythema, warmth, tenderness and abnormal swelling of the calf or thigh in the affected limb. (c) Numbness or tingling of the feet. (d) Dyspnoea, chest pain or signs of shock. (e) Pain in the chest, back or ribs which gets worse when the patient breathes in deeply. (f) Coughing up blood.	To monitor for signs of DVT and PE (Rashid *et al.* 2005: C; NICE 2007: C).
12 Monitor whether the patient has adequate hydration.	To ensure the patient is adequately hydrated (SIGN 2002: C; NICE 2007: C).
13 Record temperature daily.	To detect infection early and signs of inflammation associated with venous thrombosis (C).
14 Launder according to the manufacturer's instructions.	To reduce the risk of cross-infection and patient comfort (C).

Discharge care of patient with antiembolic stockings

15 On discharge from hosptial, check the patient understands the following: (a) Signs and symptoms of DVT. (b) Correct use of prophylaxis at home, e.g. how to wear antiemoblic stocking correctly. (c) Implications of not using prophylaxis correctly. (d) To continue to undertake leg exercises if immobile. (e) To avoid long periods of travel for 4 weeks after an operation.	To reduce the risks of developing a DVT or PE after an operation and to ensure that the patient reports any symptoms promptly to enable the early detection and management of DVT and/or PE (NICE 2007: C).

Procedure guidelines   Preoperative care

Equipment

1 Identification bracelets.
2 Allergy bands if necessary.
3 Theatre gown.
4 Cotton-based underwear or disposable pants can be worn if they do not interfere with surgery.
5 Antiembolic stockings if appropriate.
6 Labelled containers for dentures, glasses and/or hearing aid if necessary.

7 Hypoallergenic tape.
8 Patient records/documentation including medical records, consent form, X-ray films, blood test results, anaesthetic assessment, record and preoperative checklist.

Procedure

Action	Rationale
1 Assess the preoperative education received by the patient and ensure that it is complete and understood.	To ensure that the patient understands the nature and outcome of the surgery to reduce anxiety and possible postoperative complications (Walker 2002: R).
2 Check that the patient has undergone relevant investigative procedures, e.g. X-ray, electrocardiogram (ECG), blood test and that these are included with the patient's notes.	To ensure all relevant information is available to the nurses, anaesthetists and surgeons (AORN 2000: C).
3 (a) Check and confirm pregnancy status on all women of childbearing age. If a pregnancy test is required, ensure the result is known to all health care professionals involved in the operation.	To eliminate the possibility of unknown pregnancy prior to the planned surgical procedure.
(b) If appropriate, ask the patient if they are menstruating and ensure that they have a sanitary towel in place and not a tampon.	This is to prevent infection if the tampon is left in place for longer than 2 hours (www.tamponalert.org.uk: C).
4 Check the consent form is correctly completed, signed and dated.	To comply with legal requirements and hospital policy and to ensure that the patient has understood the surgical procedure (NMC 2006: C).

Procedure guidelines *(cont.)*

5 Check the operation site is marked correctly.	To ensure the patient undergoes the correct surgery for which he/she has consented (AORN 2000: C).
6 Check that the patient has undergone preanaesthetic assessment by the anaesthetist.	To ensure that the patient can be given the most suitable anaesthetic and any special requirements for anaesthetic have been highlighted (AORN 2000: C).
7 Record the patient's pulse, blood pressure, respirations, temperature and weight.	To provide baseline data for comparison intra and postoperatively. The weight is recorded so that the anaesthetist can calculate the correct dose of drugs to be administered (AORN 2000: C).
8 Instruct the patient to shower or bath as close to the planned time of the operation as possible and before a premedication is administered, if appropriate.	To minimize risk of postoperative wound infection and prevent patient accidents (Pratt *et al.* 2007: R).
9 Assist the patient to change into a theatre gown after having a shower/bath.	To reduce the risk of cross-infection, ease of access to operation site and soiling of patient's own clothes (Pratt *et al.* 2007: R).
10 Long hair should be held back with, for example, a non-metallic tie.	For safety to prevent hair getting caught in equipment and to reduce the risk of infection (E).
11 All jewellery, cosmetics, nail varnish and clothing, other than the theatre gown, are to be removed. Wedding rings may be left in situ, but must be covered and secured with hypoallergenic tape.	Metal jewellery may be accidentally lost or may cause harm to the patient, e.g. diathermy burns. Facial cosmetics make the patient's colour difficult to assess. Nail varnish makes the use of the pulse oximeter, used to monitor the patient's pulse and oxygen saturation levels, impossible and masks peripheral cyanosis (Vendovato *et al.* 2004: C).
12 Disposable or cotton underwear could be worn unless the patient is undergoing major urology or gynaecology procedure.	To maintain patient's dignity (NMC 2008: C).

13 Valuables should be placed in the hospital's custody and recorded according to the hospital policy.	To prevent loss of valuables (E).
14 Check whether patient micturated before premedication.	To prevent urinary incontinence when sedated and/or unconscious and possible contamination of sterile area (E).
15 Apply antiembolic stockings correctly.	To reduce the risk of postoperative deep vein thrombosis or pulmonary emboli (NICE 2007: C).
16 Ensure the patient is wearing an identification bracelet with the correct information.	To ensure correct identification and prevent possible patient misidentification (AORN 2000: C).
17 Ensure the patient is wearing an allergy alert band if appropriate.	To reduce allergic reactions to known causative agents and to alert all involved in the care of the patient in the operating theatre (AORN 2004: C).
18 Check when patient last had food or drink and ensure that it was at least 6 hours before planned operation time.	To reduce the risk of regurgitation and inhalation of stomach contents on induction of anaesthesia (Dean & Fawcett 2002: C).
19 Note whether the patient has dental crowns, bridge work or loose teeth.	The anaesthetist needs to be informed to prevent accidental damage. Loose teeth or a dental prosthesis could be inhaled by the patient when an endotracheal tube is inserted.
20 Ensure prosthesis, dentures and contact lenses are removed. Make a note of unremovable prosthesis (e.g. knee replacement) on the preoperative checklist.	To promote patient safety during surgery, e.g. dentures may obstruct airway, contact lenses can cause cornea abrasions.
21 Spectacles may be retained until the patient is in the anaesthetic room. Hearing aids may be retained until the patient has been anaesthetized. (These may be left in position if a local anaesthetic is being used.) Any prosthesis should then be labelled clearly and retained in the recovery room.	To allow the patient to communicate fully, thus reducing anxiety and enabling the patient to understand any procedures carried out (P).

Procedure guidelines *(cont.)*

22 Complete the preoperative checklist by asking the patient and checking records and notes before giving any premedication.	Questioning premedicated patients is not a reliable source of checking information as the patient may be drowsy and/or disorientated (AORN 2000: C).
23 Give the premedication, if prescribed, in accordance with the anaesthetist's instructions.	Different drugs may be prescribed to complement the anaesthetic to be given, e.g. Temazepam to reduce patient anxiety by inducing sleep and relaxation (C).
24 Advise the patient to remain in bed once the premedication has been given and to use the nurse call systems if assistance is needed.	To reduce the risk of accidental patient injury as the premedication may make the patient drowsy and disorientated (E).
25 Ensure the patient is supported fully on the canvas, especially the head, when transferred from the ward bed to the trolley.	To reduce the risk of injury to the neck, etc. during transfer from the ward to the operating theatre (AORN 2001: C).
26 Ensure that all relevant information, e.g. X-rays, notes, blood results, accompany the patient to the operating theatre.	To prevent delays which can increase the patient's anxiety and to ensure that the anaesthetist and surgeon have all the information they require for the safe treatment of the patient (C).
27 The patient should be accompanied to the theatre by a ward nurse who remains present until the patient has been checked by the anaesthetic assistant/nurse and/or anaesthetized.	To reduce patient anxiety and ensuring a safe environment during induction (C).
28 The ward nurse should give a full handover to the anaesthetic nurse or operating department practitioner on arrival in the anaesthetic room, using patient records and the preoperative checklist.	To ensure the patient has the correct operation. To ensure continuity of care and to maintain the safety of the patient by exchanging all relevant information (AORN 2000: C).

Intraoperative care

Definition

Intraoperative care is the physical and psychological care given to the patient in the anaesthetic room and theatre until transfer to the recovery room.

Objectives

- To ensure that the patient understands what is happening at all times in order to minimize anxiety.
- To ensure that the patient has the correct surgery for which the consent form was signed.
- To ensure patient safety at all times and minimize postoperative complications by:

  (a) Giving the required care for the unconscious patient.
  (b) Ensuring injury is not sustained from hazards associated with the use of swabs, needles, instruments, diathermy and power tools.
  (c) Minimizing postoperative problems associated with patient positioning, such as nerve or tissue damage.
  (d) Maintaining asepsis during surgical procedures to reduce the risk of postoperative wound infection in accordance with hospital policies on infection control.

Reference material

Diathermy

Diathermy is used routinely during operations to control haemorrhage by cauterizing blood vessels or cutting body tissues. Diathermy is potentially hazardous to the patient if used incorrectly. It is important that all theatre nurses know how to test and use all diathermy equipment in their department to prevent patient injury (Aigner *et al.* 1997; Wicker 2000; Molyneux 2001).

The main risk when using diathermy is of thermoelectrical burns. The most common cause is incorrect application of the patient plate or a break in the connecting lead (Vendovato *et al.* 2004) or if the patient is in contact with metal. The machine will automatically switch off if the neutral electrodes become loose from the patient or will alarm, but if the patient is in contact with metal this is a little harder to identify. To prevent these injuries only equipment fitted with adaptive neutral electrodes should be used.

Other causes of burns include skin preparation solutions or other liquids pooling around the plate site (Fong *et al.* 2000). With alcohol-based skin preparations especially, the skin should be allowed to dry before diathermy is used, as the alcohol can ignite (Fong *et al.* 2000). If the patient's position is changed during the operation the patient plate should be rechecked to ensure that it is still in contact and that the connecting clamp or lead is not causing pressure in the new position.

Use of diathermy and the plate position should be noted on the nursing care plan, and the patient's skin condition (plate site, pressure areas, and other areas where exposure to metal could have occurred) should be checked before the patient is transferred to the recovery unit.

The use of electrosurgical diathermy unit during surgical procedures results in a smoke by-product from the coagulation or cutting of tissue. This smoke plume can be harmful to the perioperative personnel because it can contain (Allen 2004):

- Toxic gases and vapors such as benzene, hydrogen cyanide and formaldehyde.
- Bioaerosols.
- Dead and live cellular material, including blood fragments.
- Viruses.

To reduce the risk for staff and patients, an efficient filtered evacuation system should be used, such as a smoke evacuation machine; piped hospital suction must not be used (Scott *et al.* 2004).

Patient positioning

The position of the patient on the operating table must be such as to facilitate access to the operation site(s) by the surgeon, and the patient's airway for the anaesthetist. It will also be dependent upon the type of surgery being performed, position of monitoring equipment and intravenous devices in situ. It should not compromise the patient's circulation, respiratory system or nerves. Preoperative assessment will identify patients with particular needs such as weight, nutritional state, age, skin condition and pre-existing disease which may necessitate extra precautions during positioning. Pre-existing conditions such as backache or sciatica can be exacerbated, particularly if the patient is in the lithotomy position as the sciatic nerve can be compressed against the poles (AORN 2001). Most postoperative palsies are due to improper positioning of the patient on the operating table (Ulrich *et al.* 1997). Consideration by and the co-operation of all theatre personnel can help prevent many of the postoperative complications related to intraoperative positioning and remains a team responsibility (McEwen 1996; AORN 2001).

All movements of the limbs of the unconscious patient should take into account the anatomy and natural planes of movement of that limb to avoid stretching and pressure on the related nerve planes (AORN 2001). Hyperabduction of the arm when placed on a board, for example, could stretch the brachial plexus, causing some postoperative loss of sensation and reduced movement of the forearm, wrist and fingers. The ulnar and radial nerves may be affected by direct pressure as a result of insufficient padding on arm supports.

Compartment syndrome is a life-threatening complication of the Lloyd Davies position and occurs when perfusion falls below tissue pressure in a closed anatomical space or compartment such as hand, forearm, buttocks, legs, upper arms and feet. It develops through a combination of prolonged ischaemia and reperfusion of muscle within a tight osseofascial compartment (Turnbull *et al.* 2002). Untreated it can lead to necrosis, functional impairment, possible renal failure and death (Callum & Bradbury 2000; Paula 2002).

If patients are placed in Lloyd Davies position and Trendelenburg tilt for longer than 4 hours, the legs should be removed from the support every 2 hours, or as close to 2 hours as possible, for a short period of time to prevent reperfusion injury (Raza *et al.* 2004).

The use of compression stockings and intermittent compression devices in the Lloyd Davies position need to be reviewed as this may contribute to compartment syndrome (Turnbull & Mills 2001). There is insufficient evidence to suggest use of one device over another will reduce the risk of compartment syndrome, nor is there enough evidence to recommend use of both devices at the same time because this will place pressure on the calf in the Lloyd Davies position. The use of devices will depend very much on the surgeon and anaesthetist and the patient's comorbidity.

All equipment that may be needed to support the patient during surgery, e.g. the table, arm supports, Lloyd Davies poles, lithotomy poles and securing straps, should be checked to ensure that they are in working order, clean and free from sharp edges. Metal parts that may come into contact with the patient should be covered as there is an increased risk of burns if diathermy is used (Vendovato *et al.* 2004). Pressure-relieving devices should be placed at the patient's elbows and heels, and pillows positioned between the legs if the patient is lying in a lateral position. Special consideration should also be given to vulnerable points or areas such as heels, elbows, ears, the head, back and sacrum where pressure-relieving devices, such as gel pads, should be used (AORN 2001).

When a patient is transferred between the trolley or bed and operating table, adequate personnel should be present to ensure patient and staff safety (AORN 2001). It is recommended that an approved rolling or sliding device is used to transfer patients from the trolley to operating table, in compliance with legislation on manual handling. Safe manual handling and the safety of the patient depend on the participation of the correct number of staff in the specified handling manoeuvre. There should be a minimum of four staff: one at either end of the patient to support the head and the feet and one on either side. Additional staff may be required if weight of the patient is over 90 kilos.

Control of infection and asepsis in operating theatres

The term asepsis means the absence of any infectious agents. The aseptic technique is the foundation on which contemporary surgery is built (Gruendemann & Meeker 1983). The aim of operating theatres is to provide an area free from infectious agents. Large quantities of bacteria are present in the nose, mouth, on the skin, hair and on the attire of personnel; therefore, people entering the operating theatres wear clean scrub suits and lint-free surgical hats to eliminate the possibility of these bacteria, hair or dandruff being shed into the environment (Tammelin *et al.* 2000). Sterile gowns and gloves are worn to prevent cross-infection. Well-fitting shoes with impervious soles should be worn and regularly cleaned to remove splashes of blood and body fluids (Woodhead *et al.* 2002). Face masks are worn to prevent droplets falling from the mouth into the operating field. The extent to which face masks are capable of preventing droplet spread is disputed (Lipp & Edwards 2002). It is, however, accepted that masks offer protection to the wearer from blood splashes and for safety reasons should be worn by the scrub team.

Presurgical hand washing is essential to the maintenance of asepsis in the operating theatre. New research has recommended a 1-minute hand wash with a non-antiseptic soap followed by hand rubbing with liquid aqueous alcoholic solution, prior to each surgeon's first procedure of the day. Before subsequent procedures the process should be repeated. This has been shown to be as effective as traditional hand scrubbing with antiseptic soap in preventing surgical site infections (Parienti *et al.* 2002). However, the traditional 3-minute first scrub of the day is recommended for all intermediate, major and complex cases.

Surgical gloves have a dual role, acting as a barrier for personal protection from the patient's blood and other exudate and preventing the bacterial transfer from the surgeon's hand to the operating site. It has been suggested that double gloving significantly reduces the number of perforations to the innermost glove in high-risk surgical patients, thus reducing infection rates during surgical procedures (Tanner & Parkinson 2002).

Universal precautions should be taken in theatres to minimize the risk of infection from blood and body fluids. These include the wearing of gloves, masks, barrier gowns and aprons. Protective eyewear or face shields should be worn during procedures likely to cause splashes or droplets of blood or generate bone chips (Tokars *et al.* 1995). Instruments must be handled carefully, and needle holders and forceps used to manipulate sutures to minimize the risk of needlestick or sharps injury.

The female patients of menstruating age also need to be made aware of the dangers of using tampons which can cause infection leading to toxic shock syndrome. At the time of admission it is important to ask the patients if they are menstruating and to highlight the dangers of using tampons during surgery. If these are left in situ for longer than 6 hours infection may develop (see www.tamponalert.org.uk/akta/tss, leaflet 2000 pdf, accessed 26/3/07).

Laparoscopic surgery

Laparoscopy has evolved from a diagnostic modality into a widespread surgical technique. Advantages for the patient include: a shorter stay in hospital, reduced postoperative pain and a shorter recovery period. However, this technique is not without its complications (O'Malley & Cunningham 2001). Laparoscopic surgery is now common in operating departments, and it is important that potential complications are identified and steps taken to minimize risk to the patient, both during surgery and in the recovery period. Patients should be prepared psychologically and physically for an open procedure, which may be undertaken under certain circumstances. Instruments and supplies for an open procedure must be readily available in the operating theatre.

Laparoscopy involves insufflation of the abdomen with carbon dioxide (CO_2). Prolonged insufflation can cause hypothermia since although the gas temperature in the hose equals room temperature, the temperature in the abdomen can decrease to 27.7°C due to high gas flow and the large amounts of gas used (Jacobs *et al.* 2000). Sharma *et al.* (1997) refer to the increased risk of hypercarbia and surgical emphysema during insufflation with CO_2. Careful monitoring and recording of the patient's vital signs, including oxygen saturation and expiratory gas levels, are therefore essential during laparoscopy.

Haemorrhage can occur during the procedure and may be difficult to detect because surgeons have a limited view of the area being operated upon. Electrosurgical injuries to organs may occur as a result of capacitive coupling (Wu *et al.* 2000) (capacitive coupling is the transfer of electrical currents from the active electrode through coupling of stray currents into other conductive surgical equipment). Theatre staff must be aware of potential complications and ensure that equipment is used safely and according to the manufacturer's instructions.

The equipment used for laparoscopic surgery is very specialized and can be daunting for theatre staff. AORN recommends that all equipment is regularly and competently maintained and a maintenance record kept in a log (AORN 2000; Wicker & O'Neill 2006). Policies and procedures should be developed for the checking procedure, and all staff thoroughly instructed in the operation of laparoscopic equipment.

Procedure guidelines Intraoperative care

Procedure

Action	Rationale
In the anaesthetic room	
1 Ensure all the equipment to be used is checked and in working order before the operating list commences, including suction, the anaesthetic machine, medical gases, monitoring equipment, diathermy and operating table.	To ensure all necessary equipment is present and to prevent accidental injury due to faulty equipment (C).
2 Greet the patient by name. Confirm with the ward nurse that it is the correct patient for the scheduled operation.	To reduce patient anxiety (P).
3 Identify the patient by checking the identification band (name and patient number) against the patient's notes and the operating list.	To safeguard against patient misidentification. Questioning the premedicated patient can be unreliable (AORN 2000: C).
4 Check and confirm the correct completion of the preoperative checklist.	To ensure that all of the listed measures have been completed and that any additional information has been recorded (E).
5 Check that the results of the investigative procedures, e.g. blood results, X-rays, etc., are included with the patient's notes.	To ensure that all of the required results are available for the theatre team's use (E).
6 Maintain a calm, quiet environment and explain all the procedures to the patient including the monitoring of blood pressure, pulse and oxygen saturation.	To reduce anxiety and enhance the smooth induction of anaesthesia (C).
7 When the patient is anaesthetized ensure that the eyes are closed and secured with hypoallergenic tape.	To prevent corneal damage due to eyes drying out or accidental abrasion.

In the operating room

8 Prior to transferring the patient from the trolley to the operating table check with the anaesthetist that the patient's airway is protected, patent and safe.

To prevent complications with breathing (E).

9 Ensure that there are adequate staff to transfer the patient onto the operating table. Ensure the brakes on the trolley and operating table have been applied. Ensure the patient's head and limbs are supported when transferring to the operating table.

To prevent patient injury during the transfer between trolley and operating table (AORN 2001: C).

10 When transferring the patient ensure all limbs are supported and secure on the table. Ensure adequate padding and cushioning of bony prominences. The patient's position will be dictated by the nature of the surgery but must take into account the requirements of the anaesthetist and the physical needs of the patient.

If the patient is unconscious and unable to maintain a safe environment, support is necessary to prevent injury. Nerve damage due to compression or stretching must be prevented. The patient is especially at risk from damage due to pressure and stretching, so measures to maintain the skin's integrity are vital (AORN 2001: C).

11 Ensure the patient is covered by the gown or blanket. These items should only be removed immediately before surgery.

To maintain the patient's dignity. To help prevent a reduction in body temperature or accidental hypothermia (E).

12 Use a warm air mattress on the operating table. Ensure all fluids used are warmed if possible.

To help maintain the patient's body temperature and prevent postoperative complications due to hypothermia (E).

13 Ensure diathermy patient plate is attached securely in accordance with the manufacturer's instructions and hospital policy.

To ensure that no injury is sustained from the use of diathermy during surgery (Molyneux 2001: C).

14 Follow hospital policy for the checking of swabs, needles and instruments.

To ensure that swabs, needles and instruments are accounted for at the end of the operation (C).

15 Follow hospital policy for the disposal of sharps and clinical waste.

To reduce the risk of injury to the patient and staff (Pratt *et al.* 2007: C).

Procedure guidelines (*cont.*)

In the recovery room

16 The scrub nurse accompanies the patient with the anaesthetist to the recovery area. A handover is given that includes:

To ensure continuity and effective communication of care for the patient. To ensure that the recovery nurse has all the information required to assess the patient's recovery needs (C).

(a) The surgical procedure performed.

The actual procedure performed may be different from the proposed procedure (E).

(b) Information including allergies or pre-existing medical conditions, e.g. diabetes mellitus.

To highlight specific potential postoperative complications to be assessed and monitored (E).

(c) The patient's cardiovascular state and pattern of anaesthesia used.

To maintain the patient's immediate postoperative safety with cardiovascular system and airway (E).

(d) The presence, position and nature of any drains, infusions or intravenous or arterial devices.

To ensure care and management of these drains is continued and the positioning of the patient is assessed to prevent any occlusion of drains or infusions (E).

(e) Information about any anxieties of the patient expressed before surgery, such as a fear of not waking after anaesthesia or fear about coping with pain.

To ensure appropriate action can be taken as the patient regains consciousness and to enable an assessment of the efficacy of nursing interventions used (E).

(f) Specific instructions from the anaesthetist for postoperative care.

To facilitate effective communication of the patient's care and treatment (C).

(g) All information is to be recorded in the perioperative nursing care plan.

Postanaesthetic recovery

Definition

Postanaesthetic recovery involves the short-term critical care required by patients during their immediate postoperative period within the recovery room, until they are stable, conscious, orientated and safe to transfer back to the ward environment.

Indication

All patients having undergone surgery and anaesthesia but not those who are transferred directly to the Critical Care Unit.

Reference material

The postanaesthetic recovery room is an area within the operating department specifically designed, equipped and staffed for the support, monitoring and assessment of patients through the reversing stages of anaesthesia.

The recovery period is potentially hazardous. Therefore, when the patient arrives in the postanaesthetic recovery room, individual nursing care is required until patients are able to maintain their own airway (AAGBI 2002). While the majority of patients can be expected to achieve uneventful recovery, 24% of all patients have complications (Hines *et al.* 1992). Although nausea and vomiting are high on the list of complications (Jolley 2001), the most notable are respiratory and circulatory complications. Obstruction of the upper airway is the most common respiratory complication in the immediate postoperative period (Dhara 2006). Close observation and appropriate action can prevent the sequence of respiratory obstruction resulting in hypoxia leading to cardiac arrest (Peskett 1999).

Layout of equipment

The need for speed, efficiency and economy of movement is essential when time becomes a critical factor in the ultimate safety of the patient in the recovery room. Thus, the basic equipment for monitoring airway maintenance, pulse oxymetry and non-invasive blood pressure monitoring and piped gases and suction must be available at the patient's head in each recovery bay. Equipment should be compatible between operating theatre and recovery room. This must be arranged for ease of access and always be clean and in full working order. Further support equipment, such as nerve stimulator, should be available centrally, whenever possible being stored on trolleys for ease of transportation (AAGBI 2002).

Assessment for discharge

The length of patient's stay in the recovery room is dependent on the patient's cardiovascular and respiratory condition and the rate at which that patient recovers physically and emotionally from the anaesthetic. A prior knowledge of the patient's cardiovascular and respiratory parameters as well as past medical history obtained through preoperative contact is of great value when assessing their return to normal state. It also has the advantage of helping the patient to orientate to time and place, as familiarity generates a degree of security and confidence.

The patients must meet the following criteria before they can be discharged from recovery room to the ward:

- The patient is fully conscious, able to maintain own airway, exhibits protective airway reflexes and is orientated.
- Respiratory function and good oxygenation is being maintained.
- The cardiovascular system is stable with no unexplained cardiac irregularity. The specific values of pulse and blood pressure are within normal preoperative limits on consecutive observation.
- There is no persistent or excessive bleeding from wound or drainage sites.
- Patients with urinary catheters have passed adequate amounts of urine (more than 0.5 ml/kg/hour) (Eltringham *et al.* 1989).
- Pain and emesis should be controlled and suitable analgesia and antiemetic regimes should be prescribed by the anaesthetist (AAGBI 2002).
- Body temperature is at least 36°C (Kean 2000).

Discharge from the recovery room is the responsibilty of the anaesthetist but the recovery staff are responsible for keeping the anaesthetist informed about any changes in the patient's condition that may arise during the recovery phase. This could be cardiovascular, respiratory or the level of consciousness. The recovery staff use the discharge criteria (Figure 22.1) as an assessment tool to determine whether the patient has achieved optimum recovery to enable them to return back to the ward safely. However, if there any changes in the patient's condition this needs to be discussed with the anaesthetist who should come and assess the patient before their return to the ward.

Local and regional anaesthesia

Patients having surgical procedures performed under local or spinal anaesthesia, whether intra- or extra- (epi) dural, will require a period of postoperative observation, although the priorities of their care will be geared towards different considerations, such as hypotension, headaches and dizziness (AAGBI 2002).

Summary

Postanaesthetic care can best be described and understood as a series of many nursing procedures performed in sequence and simultaneously on patients who are in an artificially induced and traumatized condition. These patients will display varying degrees of responsiveness and physical and emotional states. It is important to establish a rapport with each individual to gain the patient's confidence and co-operation and to aid assessment. It is also necessary to understand that when emerging from the final stage of anaesthesia, some patients can behave in an emotional and disinhibited fashion, at variance with their normal behaviour

Respiratory Function	Yes	No
1. Is the patient able to maintain their airway without assistance?		
2. Does the patient have a regular respiratory pattern and show no signs of cyanosis?		
3. Is the patient's respiratory rate > 10 and < 24 breaths per minute?		
4. Are oxygen saturation readings > 95% or the same as the patient's pre-operative oxygen saturation readings on air / prescribed oxygen?		
Cardiovascular Function		
5. Is the patient's pulse and blood pressure within pre-operative range? If not – is the anaesthetist satisfied with the patient's observations?		
6. Is the patient's temperature between 36°C and 37.5°C?		
7. Are drain(s) and wound(s) free from excessive bleeding i.e. < 50 ml blood / hour in drain or wound dressing requiring reinforcement/pressure?		
8. Are the drain(s) unclamped and vacuumed if appropriate? *State if not applicable*		
9. Is the patient free from neurovascular compromise? For example: check limb/flap observations, i.e. colour, warmth, blanching, sensation and movement, which are performed following limb reconstructive surgery. *State if not applicable*		
Level of Consciousness		
10. Is the patient conscious, orientated, able to lift head off pillow, can cough and take deep breath? (**Patient must have a minimum score of 8 on the SALIM score on discharge**) If patient is confused – was the patient confused pre-operatively?		
Fluid Administration & Management		
11. Is the patient's fluid balance satisfactory? For example: no signs of fluid overload – breathlessness, tachycardia, generalized oedema or dehydration – dry skin, poor urine output, bradycardia (refer to fluid balance chart if appropriate).		
12. Are the infusion sites satisfactory, i.e. patent and secured?		
13. Are all infusions and infusion administration sets appropriately labelled, e.g. Patient Controlled Analgesia, Epidural, Blood, Platelets, Insulin etc. and three-way taps removed?		
14. If catheterized, is the patient passing acceptable volumes of urine, i.e. 1–1.5 ml/kilogram/hour?		
Nausea & Vomiting		
15. Has the patient stated their nausea or vomiting is controlled (**see nausea & vomiting score**)? If not, state actions taken.		
16. Is the nasogastric tube correctly positioned, secured, patent and the drainage satisfactory, i.e. < 100 ml immediate post operation? *State if not applicable*		
Pain		
17. Has the patient stated their pain is controlled? (**Is the pain score < 5 on movement, whilst coughing or taking a deep breath?**)		
18. If nerve block or epidural analgesia – is the height of the nerve/epidural block recorded and the rate of the epidural analgesia recorded? *State if not applicable & delete as appropriate*		
Follow up care		
19. Are IV fluids, analgesia and anti-emetics prescribed for the next 24 hours if appropriate?		
20. Are the surgeon's post-operative written instructions clear and available?		
21. **Has the anaesthetist agreed the patient is fit for discharge from recovery?** NB If patient has had an adverse event or been in recovery > 2 hrs has the anaesthetist reviewed their condition?		
FOR INFORMATION ONLY		
22. Has the patient passed urine post-operatively? *State if not applicable*		
23. Is the patient's property accompanying them back to the ward area? *State if not applicable*		

	Signature	Full Name (PRINT)	Date	Time
Recovery Room Nurse / Operating Department Practitioner (ODP)				
Ward/Unit Nurse				

Time of Patient's Discharge from Recovery: ....(24 hr clock)

Figure 22.1   Recovery discharge criteria. Used with permission from The Royal Marsden NHS Foundation Trust (2007).

(Eckenhoff *et al*. 1961). These displays are always transient and fortunately patients seldom have any recollection of them. Most patients will have an uneventful recovery following surgery. However, recovery can be adversely affected by the extent and length of both surgery and anaesthesia.

Procedure guidelines   Postanaesthetic recovery

Equipment in the recovery room

1 Theatre trolley bed, which must incorporate the following features:
   (a) Oxygen supply.
   (b) Trendelenburg tilt mechanism.
   (c) Adjustable cot sides.
   (d) Adjustable back rest.
   (e) Brakes.
   (f) Radio translucency.

2 Basic equipment required for each patient:
   (a) Oxygen supply, preferably wall-mounted with tubing, face masks (with both fixed and variable settings), a T-piece system and full range of oropharyngeal and nasopharyngeal airways.
   (b) Suction: regulatable with tubing, and a range of nozzles and catheters.
   Note: spare oxygen cylinders with flowmeters and an electrically powered portable suction machine should always be available in case of pipeline failure.
   (c) Sphygmomanometer and stethoscope. Automatic blood pressure recorders are a valuable means of saving time and of minimizing disturbance to patients, especially those in pain or disorientated, and leaving the nurse's hands free to attend to other needs. However, such equipment can be non-functioning in certain cases, e.g. shivering or profoundly bradycardic patients, and is subject to electrical and mechanical failure. Therefore, manual equipment must always be available.
   (d) Pulse oximeter, whenever possible.
   (e) Miscellaneous items: receivers, tissues, disposable gloves, sharps container and waste receptacle.

3 Essential equipment centrally available for respiratory and cardiovascular support:
   (a) Self-inflating resuscitator bag, e.g. Ambu bag and/or Mapleson C circuit with face mask.
   (b) Full intubation equipment: laryngoscopes with spare bulbs and batteries, range of endotracheal tubes, bougies and Magill's forceps, syringe and catheter mount.
   (c) Anaesthetic machine and ventilator.
   (d) Wright respirometer.
   (e) Cricothyroid puncture set.
   (f) Range of tracheostomy tubes and tracheal dilator.
   (g) Intravenous infusion sets and cannulae, range of intravenous fluids.
   (h) Central venous cannulae and manometer.
   (i) Emergency drug box/trolley: contents in accordance with current hospital policy.
   (j) Defibrillator.

4 Standard equipment for routine nursing procedures such as dressing trolley.

Procedure

The following recommended actions are not necessarily listed in order of priority. Many will be carried out simultaneously and much will depend on the patient's condition, surgery and level of consciousness. All actions must be accompanied by commentary and explanation regardless of the apparent responsiveness, as the sense of hearing returns before the patient's ability to respond (Levinson 1965).

Action	Rationale
1 Assess the patency of the airway by feeling for movement of expired air.	To determine the presence of any respiratory depression or neuromuscular blockade. Observe chest and abdominal movement, respiratory rate, depth and pattern (Drummond 1991: C).
(a) Listen for inspiration and expiration. Apply suction if indicated. Observe any use of accessory muscles of respiration and check for tracheal tug.	To ensure airway is clear and laryngeal spasm is not present.
(b) If indicated, support the chin with the neck extended.	In the unconscious patient the tongue is liable to fall back and obstruct the airway, and protective reflexes are absent (E).
(c) Suction of the upper airway is indicated if gurgling sounds are present on respiration and if blood secretions or vomitus are evident or suspected, and the patient is unable to swallow or cough either at all or adequately. Suction must be applied with care to avoid damage to mucosal surfaces and further irritation or initiation of a gag reflex or laryngeal spasm.	Foreign matter can obstruct the airway or cause laryngeal spasm in light planes of anaesthesia. It can also be inhaled when protective laryngeal reflexes are absent (Dhara 2006: C).
(d) Endotracheal suction is performed following the same procedure as that for suction of tracheostomy tubes. (For further information see the procedure section in Chapter 29.)	To maintain the patency of the tube and remove secretions (Dhara 2006: C).

Procedure guidelines *(cont.)*

(e) Apply a face mask and administer oxygen at the rate prescribed by the anaesthetist. If an endotracheal tube or laryngeal mask is in position, check whether the cuff or mask is inflated and administer oxygen by means of a T-piece system.

To maintain adequate oxygenation. Oxygen should be administered to all patients in the recovery room (Nimmo *et al.* 1994: C).

(f) Observe skin colour and temperature. Check the colour of lips and conjunctiva, then peripheral colour and perfusion.

Central cyanosis indicates impaired gaseous exchange between the alveoli and pulmonary capillaries. Peripheral cyanosis indicates low cardiac output (Nimmo *et al.* 1994: C).

2 Feel and assess the pulse. The patient's position will probably mean that the head, carotid, facial or temporal arteries will offer the easiest access. Note the rate, rhythm and volume, and record.

To assess cardiovascular function and establish a postoperative baseline for future comparisons (Peskett 1999: C).

3 Obtain full information about:
■ Anaesthetic technique, potential problems and the patient's general medical condition.
■ Surgical procedure performed.
■ The presence of drains and packs.
■ Amount of blood loss.
■ Specific postoperative instructions.

To ensure effective communication of the patient's care and treatment and to aid the planning of subsequent care.

Note: the information gained from point 3 will be recorded within the patient's records, but an initial verbal handover will ensure that there is no delay in providing immediate care.

4 Perform and record blood pressure, pulse and respiratory rate measurements on reception and at a minimum of 5-minute intervals unless the patient's condition dictates otherwise.

To enable any fluctuations or gross abnormalities in cardiovascular and respiratory functions to be detected immediately (Peskett 1999: C).

5 Check the temperature of the patient, especially those who are at high risk of hypothermia, e.g. the elderly, children, those who have undergone long surgery or where large amounts of blood or fluid replacement therapy have been used. Temperature must be measured hourly or half hourly if hypothermic. Use Bairhugger blankets and extra blankets to warm the patient.

More than 70% of patients undergoing surgery experience some degree of postoperative hypothermia (Wagner 2003: C). The symptoms of hypothermia can mimic those of other postoperative complications, which may result in inappropriate treatment. Hypothermia interferes with the effective reversal of muscle relaxants, so monitor patients who are shivering, restless, confused or with respiratory depression (Bowers Feldman 1988: C). Shivering puts an increased demand on cardiopulmonary systems as oxygen consumption is increased (Bowers Feldman 1988: C; Frank *et al.* 1993: C). Other complications such as arrhythmias or myocardial infarct can result and the longer the duration of the postoperative hypothermia, the greater the patient mortality (Crayne *et al.* 1988: C; Frank *et al.* 1993: C).

6 Check and observe wound site(s),dressings and drains. Note and record leakage/drainage on the postoperative chart and also on the drain bottle/bag.

To assess and monitor for signs of haemorrhage (Eltringham *et al.* 1989: C).

7 Check intravenous infusions are running at the correct prescribed rate and the site of the venous device is satisfactory.

Care of venous devices/sites prevents complications and ensures fluid replacement and balance is achieved safely (E).

8 Check the prescription chart for medications to be administered during the immediate postoperative period, e.g. analgesia, antiemetic.

To treat symptoms swiftly and appropriately and to monitor their effectiveness (E).

Procedure guidelines *(cont.)*

9 Remain with the patient at all times. Assess level of consciousness during reversing stages of anaesthesia, observing for returning reflexes, i.e. swallowing, tear secretion and eyelash and lid reflexes and response to stimuli: both physical (*not* painful) and verbal (do not shout).	To monitor progress from unconscious state to rousable and orientated (AAGBI 2002: C).
10 Orientate the patient to time and place as frequently as is necessary.	To alleviate anxiety, provide reassurance, and gain the patient's confidence and co-operation. Premedication and anaesthesia can induce a degree of amnesia and disorientation (C).
11 Give mouth care. (For further information, see Procedure guidelines, Chapter 24.)	Preoperative fasting, drying gases and manipulation of lips, etc., leave mucosa vulnerable, sore and foul tasting (E).
12 After regional and/or spinal anaesthesia, assess the return of sensation and mobility of limbs. Check that the limbs are anatomically aligned.	To prevent inadvertent injury following sensory loss (AAGBI 2002: C).

Problem solving: Postanaesthetic recovery

Note: any concern/abnormality regarding the patient's condition requires a thorough holistic, individual assessment prior to any interventions. Liaise with appropriate medical colleagues accordingly.

Problem	Cause	Suggested action
Airway obstruction.	Tongue occluding the airway.	Support chin forward from the angle of the jaw. If necessary insert a Guedel airway. Use a nasopharyngeal airway if the teeth are clenched or crowned.
	Foreign material, blood, secretions, vomitus.	Apply suction. Always check for the presence of a throat pack.

Problem	Cause	Suggested action
	Laryngeal spasm.	Increase the rate of oxygen. Assist ventilation with an Ambu bag and face mask. If there is no improvement, inform anaesthetist and have intubation equipment ready. Offer the patient reassurance by talking to them and telling them what you are doing.
Hypoventilation.	Respiratory depression from medications, e.g. opiates, inhalations, barbiturates.	Inform the anaesthetist, keeping oxygen on and administer antagonist on instruction, e.g. naloxone (opiate antagonist), doxapram (respiratory stimulant). *Note*: if naloxone is given it can reverse the analgesic effects of opiates and has a duration of action of only 20–30 minutes. The patient must be observed for signs of returning hyperventilation (Nimmo *et al.* 1994).
	Decreased respiratory drive from a low partial pressure of carbon dioxide ($PaCO_2$), loss of hypoxic drive in patients with chronic pulmonary disease.	Administer oxygen using a Venturi mask with graded low concentrations (Atkinson *et al.* 1982).
	Neuromuscular blockade from continued action of non-depolarizing muscle relaxants, potentiation of relaxants caused by electrolyte imbalance, impaired excretion with renal or liver disease.	Inform the anaesthetist, have available neostigmine and glycopyrolate, or atropine potassium chloride and 10% calcium chloride. Often the degree of blockade is mild and will wear off in minutes without treatment, but it is extremely frightening and patients will need continuous reassurance that their condition is not unnoticed and is resolving and that they will not be left alone.

Problem solving (cont.)

Problem	Cause	Suggested action
Hypotension.	Hypovolaemia.	Take manual reading of the blood pressure. Take central venous pressure (CVP) readings if catheter is in place. Give oxygen. Lower the head of the trolley unless contraindicated, e.g. hiatus hernia, gross obesity. Check the record of anaesthetic agents used which might cause hypotension, e.g. enflurane, beta-blockers, nitroprusside, opiates, droperidol, sympathetic blockade following spinal anaesthesia. Check the peripheral perfusion. If the CVP is low, increase intravenous infusion unless contraindicated, e.g. congestive cardiac failure. Check drains and dressings for visible bleeding and haematoma. Inform the anaesthetist or surgeon.
Hypertension.	Pain, carbon dioxide retention. This may be due to retention during laparoscopic procedures.	Treat pain with prescribed analgesia and provide a quiet environment to enable them to rest/sleep. Pain from certain operation sites can also be alleviated by changing the patient's position.
	Fluid overload.	Check fluid balance sheet and the rate of intravenous infusion.
	Distended bladder.	Offer a bedpan or urinal and if necessary catheterize the patient.
	Some anaesthetic drugs given during reversal of anaesthetic.	Check the prescription chart for those patients on regular antihypertensive therapy. If the situation is not resolved inform the anaesthetist. Also check patient's past medical history.

Problem	Cause	Suggested action
Bradycardia.	Very fit patient, opiates, reversal agents, beta-blockers, pain, vagal stimulation, hypoxaemia from respiratory depression.	Connect the patient to the ECG monitor to exclude heart block and monitor cardiac activity. Ascertain pre operative cardiac function. Check the prescription chart and anaesthetic sheet for medication administered that may cause bradycardia. Inform and liaise with the anaesthetist.
Tachycardia.	Pain, hypovolaemia, some anaesthetic drugs, e.g. ephedrine, septicaemia, fear, fluid overload.	Assess patient's pain and provide analgesia. Check the anaesthetic chart to ascertain which anaesthetic drugs were used. Connect the patient to the ECG monitor to exclude ventricular tachycardia. Provide reassurance for the patient. Assess fluid balance.
Pain.	Surgical trauma, worsened by fear, anxiety and restlessness.	Provide prescribed analgesia and assess its efficacy. Reassure and orientate the patients, who can be unaware that surgery has been performed, in which case their pain is more frightening. Try positional changes where feasible, e.g. experience has shown that after breast surgery some relief can be obtained from raising the back support by 20–40°; patients with abdominal or gynaecological surgery can be more comfortable lying on their side; elevate limbs to reduce swelling where appropriate. Unless significant relief is obtained, inform the anaesthetist and the pain control specialist nurse.
Nausea and vomiting.	Anaesthetic agents, opiates, hypotension, abdominal surgery, pain; high-risk patients who have a history of postoperative nausea and vomiting.	Administer intravenous antiemetics and monitor effectiveness. Encourage slow, regular breathing. If the patient is unconscious, turn onto the side, tip the head down and suck out pharynx, give oxygen. Note: have wire-cutters available if the jaws are wired.

		Suggested action
	...sion of the ...gulating centre, ...latation, following ...inal surgery, large infusions of unwarmed blood and fluids.	Use extra blankets or a Bairhugger (Kumar *et al*. 2005). Monitor the patient's temperature. Administer warm intravenous fluids. In the event of bladder irrigation this should also be warmed but care has to be taken that the temperature of the warming cabinet is not too hot as this could burn the patient. The temperature should be the same as normal body temperature.
Shivering.	Some inhalational anaesthetics, hypothermia.	Give oxygen, reassure the patient and take patient's temperature. Provide a Bairhugger and warm blankets.
Hyperthermia.	Infection, blood transfusion reaction.	Give oxygen, use a fan or tepid sponging if this is warranted. Medical assessment of antibiotic therapy and obtaining blood cultures. Administer intravenous paracetamol if prescribed.
	Malignant hyperpyrexia (above 40°C).	Malignant hyperpyrexia is a medical emergency and a malignant hyperpyrexia pack with the necessary drugs should be readily available at a central point in theatre. All personnel must know its location.
Oliguria.	Mechanical obstruction of catheter, e.g. clots, kinking.	Check the patency of the catheter. Consider bladder irrigation. If clots present, inform surgeon.
	Inadequate renal perfusion, e.g. hypotension, systolic pressures under 60 mmHg, hypovolaemia, dehydration.	Take blood pressure and CVP if available. Increase intravenous fluids. Inform the anaesthetist.
	Renal damage, e.g. from blood transfusion, infection, drugs, surgical damage to the ureters.	Refer to the anaesthetist or surgeon.

Procedure guidelines   Postoperative recovery

Equipment

After discharge from the recovery room to the ward, the nursing care given during the postoperative period is directed towards the prevention of those potential complications resulting from surgery and anaesthesia which might be anticipated to develop over a longer period of time.

Consideration of the psychological and emotional aspects of recovery will of necessity be altered by the changed state of consciousness, awareness and knowledge of patients and their differing responses to surgery, diagnosis and treatment.

Potential respiratory complications

Action	Rationale
1 Observe respirations, noting rate and depth and any presence of dyspnoea or orthopnoea: (a) Observe chest movement for equal, bilateral expansion. (b) Observe colour and perfusion. (c) Position the patient to facilitate optimum lung expansion and reinforce preoperative teaching of deep breathing exercises and coughing.	Respiratory function postoperatively can be influenced by a number of factors: increased bronchial secretions from inhalation anaesthesia; decreased respiratory effort from opiate medication; pain or anticipation of pain from surgical wounds; surgical trauma to the phrenic nerve; pneumothorax as a result of surgical or anaesthetic procedures. All factors limiting the adequate expansion of the lung and the ejection of bronchial secretions will encourage the development of atelectasis and consolidation of the affected lung tissue (AAGBI 2002: C).
2 Change position of patients on bedrest every 2–3 hours.	To prevent and monitor formation of pressure sores and tissue viability (NICE 2007: R).
3 Provide adequate prescribed analgesia.	Patients in pain are more likely to be disorientated and show signs of high blood pressure and tachycardia (Nimmo *et al*. 1994: C).
4 Record temperature and pulse. If sputum produced, observe nature and quantity for culture.	If infection follows there may be a rise in temperature, pulse and respiratory rate (C).

Procedure guidelines *(cont.)*

Potential circulatory complications

Deep venous thrombosis and pulmonary embolus

Action	Rationale
1 Encourage early mobilization where patient's condition allows. For patients on bedrest, encourage deep breathing and exercises of the leg: flexion/extension and rotation of the ankles.	Patients are at increased risk of developing deep venous thrombosis as a result of muscular inactivity, postoperative respiratory and circulatory depression, abdominal and pelvic surgery, prolonged pressure on calves from lithotomy poles, etc., increased production of thromboplastin as a result of surgical trauma, pre-existing coronary artery disease (Rashid *et al.* 2005: C).
2 Where worn, ensure that antiembolic stockings are of the correct size and fit smoothly.	Incorrect sizing causes swelling and bruising to ankles and can constrict blood supply leading to long-term complications (NICE 2007: R).
3 Advise against crossing of legs or ankles.	To prevent constriction of blood supply and swelling.
4 Record temperature.	
5 Report any complaints of calf or thigh pain to medical staff.	To monitor for signs of DVT.
6 Observe for any dyspnoea, chest pain or signs of shock.	To monitor for signs of PE.

Haemorrhage

Action	Rationale
1 Observe dressings, drains and wound sites, and quantity and nature of drainage. Observe pulse, blood pressure, respirations and colour.	Early haemorrhage may occur as the patient's blood pressure rises. Record postoperatively re-establishing blood flow or blood as a result of the slipping of a ligature or the dislodging of a clot (Peskett 1999: C).
2 Observe wound for redness, tenderness and increased temperature.	Secondary haemorrhage may occur after a period of days as a result of infection (E).

Potential fluid and electrolyte imbalance and malnutrition

Action	Rationale
1 Maintain accurate records of intravenous infusions, oral fluids, wound and stoma drainage, nasogastric drainage, vomitus, urine and urological irrigation.	Preoperative fasting and dehydration, increased secretion of antidiuretic hormone, blood loss and paralytic ileus all contribute to potential fluid and electrolyte imbalance. Vomiting and stasis of intestinal fluid may lead to potassium depletion (Jolley 2001: C).
2 Observe nature and quantity of all drainage, aspirate, faeces, etc.	To monitor and replace fluid loss and to detect any abnormality as a result of surgery, e.g. a breakdown in anastomosis (E).
3 Give prescribed antiemetics if nausea or vomiting occur.	To make the patient comfortable (Jolley 2001: C).
4 Observe state of mouth for coating, furring and dryness.	To maintain oral hygiene and to assess for thrush and hydration (Jolley 2001: C).
5 Encourage oral fluids as soon as the patient is able to take them unless the nature of the surgery contraindicates this.	To encourage hydration, and promote diuresis and digestion. Also to maintain oral hygiene (Jolley 2001: C).
6 Encourage early resumption of diet.	Return to an adequate nutritional state is necessary for wound healing (see Chapter 34); it is particularly important that diabetic patients should return to their preoperative insulin/diet regime to avoid increased risk of metabolic disturbance (E).

Potential pain

Action	Rationale
1 Observe the patient, noting physiological signs indicative of pain, e.g. sweating, tachycardia, hypotension, pallor or flushed appearance.	These are the first indications of pain related to intraoperative trauma and postoperative complications (E).

Procedure guidelines *(cont.)*

2 Note restlessness, immobility and facial expressions.	Continuous severe pain can cause restlessness, anxiety, insomnia and anorexia, and may thus interfere with recovery by impeding deep breathing, mobilization and nutrition (E).
3 Listen to the patient and ascertain the location and nature of the pain. If necessary, use a pain scale chart (see Chapter 20).	Communication skills are necessary for the effective assessment and alleviation of pain as there may be multiple contributory factors, both physical and emotional in origin (C).
4 Administer prescribed analgesia and observe effect.	To relieve and control pain and if necessary to review pain relief available (E).
5 Try changing position of patient. Give attention, information and reassurance; assist with relaxation exercises.	To promote comfort and reduce anxiety due to pain (E).

References and further reading

AAGBI (2002) *Immediate Postanaesthetic Recovery*. Association of Anaesthetists of Great Britain and Ireland, London.

Aigner, N. *et al.* (1997) Complications in the use of diathermy. *Burns*, **23**, 256–64.

Allen, G. (2004) Smoke plume evacuation. *AORN J*, **79**(4), 866–70.

AORN (2000) Recommended practices for safety through identification of potential hazards in the perioperative environment. *AORN J*, **72**(4), 690–8.

AORN (2001) Recommended practices for positioning the patient in the perioperative practice setting. *AORN J*, **73**(1), 231–8.

AORN (2004) Latex guidelines, *AORN J*, **70**(3), 653–8, 660–4, 666, 668–72.

Atkinson, R.S. *et al.* (1982) *A Synopsis of Anaesthesia*, 9th edn. John Wright, Bristol.

Barker, S.G.E. & Hollingsworth S.J. (2004) Wearing graduated compression stockings: the reality of everyday deep vein thrombosis prophylaxis. *Phlebology*, **19**(1), 52–3.

Beddows, J. (1997) Alleviating pre-operative anxiety in patients: a study. *Nurs Stand*, **11**(37), 35–8.

Bowers Feldman, M.E. (1988) Inadvertent hypothermia, a threat to homeostasis in the postanaesthetic patient. *J Postanaesth Nurs*, **3**(2), 82–7.

Bryne, B. (2002) Deep vein thrombosis prophylaxis: the effectiveness and implications of using below knee or thigh length graduated compression stockings. *J Vasc Nurs*, **20**(2), 53–9.

Callum, K. & Bradbury, A (2000) ABC of arterial and venous disease: acute limb ischaemia. *BMJ*, **320**(7237), 764–7.

Crayne, H.E. *et al.* (1988) Thermoresuscitation for postoperative hypothermia using reflective blankets. *AORN J*, **47**(1), 222–3, 226–7.

Davis, P. & O'Neill, C. (2002) The potential benefits of intermittent pneumatic compression in the prevention of deep venous thrombosis. *J Orthopaed Nurs*, **6**(2), 95–100.

Dean, A. & Fawcett, T. (2002) Nurse's use of evidence in preoperative fasting. *Nurs Stand*, **17**(12), 33–37.

Dhara, S. (2006) Complications in the recovery room. *Singapore Med J*, 38(5), 190–1.

Drummond, G.B. (1991) Keep a clear airway. *Br J Anaesth*, **66**, 153–66.

Eckenhoff, J.E., Kneale, D.H. & Dripps, R.D. (1961) The incidence and aetiology of postanaesthetic excitement. *Anaesthesiology*, **22**, 667–73.

Eltringham, R. *et al.* (1989) *Post Anaesthetic Recovery. A Practical Approach*, 2nd edn. Springer, Berlin.

Field, L. & Adams, N. (2001) Pain management 2: the use of psychological approaches to pain. *Br J Nurs*, **10**(15), 971–4.

Fong, E.P., Tan, W.T. & Chye, L.T. (2000) Diathermy and alcohol skin preparations – a potential disastrous mix. *Burns*, **26**(7), 673–5.

Frank, S.M., Beattie, C. & Christopher, R. (1993) Unintentional hypothermia is associated with postoperative myocardial ischaemia *Anaesthesiology*, **78**, 468–76.

Gruendemann, B. & Meeker, H.M. (1983) *Alexander's Care of the Patient in Surgery*, 7th edn. Mosby, St. Louis, MO.

Hayes, C.A., Lehman, J.M. & Castonguay, P. (2002) Graduated compression stocking: updating practice, improving compliance. *Med Surg Nurs*, **11**(4), 163–7.

Hines, R. *et al.* (1992) Complications occurring in the postanaesthesia care unit: a survey. *Anaesth Analg*, **74**, 503–9.

House of Commons Health Committee (2005) *The Prevention of Venous Thromboembolism in Hospitalised Patients*. House of Commons Health Committee Second Report 2004–2005. The Stationary Office, London.

Hukushi, G. *et al.* (2007) Deep vein thrombosis prophylaxis methods. *AORN J*, **85**(2), 265–6.

Jacobs, V.R. *et al.* (2000) Intraoperative evaluation of laparoscopic insufflation technique for quality control in the OR. *J Soc Laparoendoscopic Surg*, **4**(3), 189–95.

Jolley, S. (2001) Managing post-operative nausea and vomiting. *Nurs Stand*, **15**(40), 47–52.

Juzo (2006) *Application of Compression Stockings*. Juzo UK Ltd, Dundee, Scotland.

Kean, M. (2000) Adult/elderly care nursing. A patient temperature audit within a theatre recovery unit. *Br J Nurs*, **9**(3), 150–6.

Kjonniksen, I. *et al.* (2002) Preoperative hair removal – a systematic literature review. *AORN J*, **75**(5), 928–34, 936, 938.

Kumar, S. *et al.* (2005) Effects of perioeprative hypothermia and warming in surgical practice. *Int Wound J*, **2**(3), 193–201.

Levinson, B.W. (1965) States of awareness during general anaesthesia. Preliminary communication. *Br J Anaesth*, **37**(7), 544–6.

Lipp, A. & Edwards, P. (2002) Disposable surgical face masks for preventing surgical wound infection in clean surgery. *Cochrane Database Syst Rev*, **1**: CD002929.

McEwen, D.R. (1996) Intra-operative positioning of surgical patients. *AORN J*, **63**(6), 1059–63, 1066–79, 1080–6.

Mitchell, M. (2000) Nursing interventions for pre-operative anxiety. *Nurs Stand*, **14**(37), 40–3.

Molyneux, C. (2001) Open forum. Electrosurgery policy, 'Electrosurgery in perioperative practice'. *Br J Periop Nurs*, **11**(10), 424.

NICE (2005) *The Prevention and Treatment of Pressure Ulcers*. National Institute for Health and Clinical Excellence, London.

NICE (2007) Venous thromboembolism: reducing the risk of venous thromboembolism (deep vein thrombosis and pulmonary embolism) in inpatients undergoing surgery. Full guidance. National Collaborating Centre for Acute Care, Royal College of Surgeons for England, London. www.guidance.nice.org. uk/CG/published/CG46. Accessed 30/4/07.

Nimmo, W.S. *et al.* (eds) (1994) *Anaesthesia*, 2nd edn. Blackwell Science, Oxford.

NMC (2005) *Records and Record Keeping*. Nursing and Midwifery Council, London.

NMC (2006) *A–Z Advice Sheet Consent*. www.nmc.org.

NMC (2008) *The Code: Standards of Conduct, Performance and Ethics for Nurses and Midwives*. Nursing and Midwifery Council, London.

O'Callaghan, N. (2002) Pre-operative fasting. *Nurs Stand*, **16**(36), 33–7.

O'Malley, C. & Cunningham, A.J. (2001) Physiologic changes during laparoscopy. *Anesthesiol Clin North Am*, **19**(1), 1–19.

Parienti, J.J. *et al.* (2002) Hand-rubbing with an aqueous alcoholic solution vs. traditional surgical hand-scrubbing and 30-day surgical site infection rates: a randomised equivalence study. *JAMA*, **288**(6), 722–7.

Parnaby, C. (2004) The new antiembolism stocking. *Br J Perioper Nurs*, **14**(7), 302–7.

Paula, R. (2002) Richard Paula Compartment Syndrome Extremity. www.emedicie.com/emerg/topic739.htm. Accessed 11/4/07.

Peskett, M.J. (1999) Clinical indicators and other complications in the recovery room or postanaesthetic care unit. *Anaesthesia*, **54**(12), 1143–9.

Pratt, R.J. *et al.* (2007) Epic 2: national evidence-based guidelines for preventing healthcare-associated infections in NHS hospitals in England. *J Hosp Infect*, **65**, S1–64.

Rashid, S.T. *et al.* (2005) Venous thromboprophylaxis in UK medical patients. *J R Soc Med*, **98**, 507–12.

Raza, A., Byrne, D. & Townell, N. (2004) Lower limb (well leg) compartment syndrome after urological pelvic surgery. *J Urol*, **171**(1), 5–11.

RCN (2005) *Perioperative Fasting in Adults and Children. A RCN Guideline for the Multidisciplinary Team*. Royal College of Nursing, London.

Roderick, P. *et al.* (2005) Towards evidence-based guidelines for the preventions of venous thromboembolism: systematic reviews of mechanical methods, oral anticoagulation, dextran and regional anaesthesia as thromboprophylaxis. *Health Technol Assess*, **9**(49), 1–78.

Scott, E., Beswick, A. & Wakefield, K. (2004) The hazards of diathermy plume. *Br J Perioper Nurs*, **14**(10), 453–6.

Sharma, K.C. *et al.* (1997) Laparoscopic surgery and its potential for medical complications. *Heart Lung: J Acute Crit Care*, **26**(1), 52–67.

SIGN (2002) *Prophylaxis of Venous Thromboembolism Guidelines*. Scottish Intercollegiate Guidelines Network, Edinburgh.

Tammelin, A., Domicel, P. & Hambraeus, A. (2000) Dispersal of methicillin-resistant *Staphylococcus epidermidis* by staff in an operating suite for thoracic and cardiovascular surgery: relation to skin carriage and clothing. *Hosp Infect*, **44**(2), 119–26.

Tanner, J. & Parkinson, H. (2002) Double gloving to reduce surgical cross-infection. *Cochrane Database Syst Rev*, **1**(3): CD003087.

Tokars, J.I. *et al.* (1995) Skin and mucous membrane contacts with blood during surgical procedures: risk and prevention. *Epidemiology*, **16**(12), 703–11.

Turnbull, D. & Mills, G. (2001) Compartment syndrome associated with the Lloyd Davies position. *Anaesthesia*, **56**(10), 980–7.

Turnbull, D. *et al.* (2002) Calf compartment pressures in the Lloyd Davies position, a cause for concern? *Anaesthesia*, **57**(9), 905–8.

Ulrich, W. *et al.* (1997) Damage due to patient positioning in anaesthesia and surgical medicine. *Anaesthesiol Intens Med Notfallmed Schmerzther*, **32**(1), 4–20.

Vendovato, J.W., Polvora, P. & Leonardi, D.F. (2004) *Burns as a Complication of the Use of Diathermy*. American Burn Association no. 0273 8481/2004. *J Burn Care Rehab*, **25**(1), 120–123.

Wagner, D.V. (2003) Impact of perioperative temperature management on patient safety. *SSM*, **9**(4), 38–43.

Walker, J.A. (2002) Emotional and psychological preoperative preparation in adults. *Br J Nurs*, **11**(8), 567–75.

Wicker, P. (2000) Back to basics. Electrosurgery in perioperative practice. *Br J Periop Nurs*, **10**(4), 221–6.

Wicker, P. & O'Neill, J. (2006) *Caring for the Perioperative Patient*. Blackwell Publishing, Oxford.

Woodhead, K., Taylor, E. & Bannister, G. (2002) Behaviours and rituals in the operating theatre: a report from the Hospital Infection Society Working Party on Infection Control in Operating Theatres. *Hosp Infect*, **51**(4), 241–55.

Wu, M.P. *et al.* (2000) Complications and recommended practices for electrosurgery in laparoscopy. *Am J Surg*, **179**(1), 67–73.

Multiple choice questions

1 Preoperative care involves removal of hair from immediately around the site of the incision. This should be performed with:

   a   An electric razor
   b   Scissors
   c   Depilatory cream
   d   Wet razor

2 It is important that patients understand the rationale to be 'nil by mouth' before elective surgery. This means:

   a   Nothing to eat or drink for 12 hours prior to surgery
   b   Nothing to eat for 6 hours and nothing to drink for 3 hours prior to surgery
   c   Nothing to eat or drink for 3 hours prior to surgery
   d   Nothing to eat or drink for 6 hours prior to surgery

3 When fitting antiembolic stockings prior to surgery you should:

   a   Wash your hands
   b   Wash hands, measure calf circumference
   c   Wash hands, measure calf circumference, check pedal pulses
   d   Wash hands, check pedal pulses

4 Diathermy is routinely used during operations to:

   a   Control hemorrhage
   b   Stop emboli
   c   Assist in pain control
   d   Reduce risk of infection

5 **Face masks are worn in theatre to:**

   a   Protect you against gases
   b   Protect you from unpleasant odours
   c   Prevent droplets from the mouth falling on the operating field
   d   Prevent you being splashed by blood

6 **Which is the most common complication in the immediate post-operative period?**

   a   Circulation difficulties
   b   Upper airway obstruction
   c   Nausea and vomiting
   d   Haemorrhage

Answers to the multiple choice questions can be found in Appendix 3.

Chapter 23

Personal hygiene: eye care

Definition

Eye care is the practice of assessing, cleaning or irrigating the eye and/or the instillation of prescribed ocular preparations (Stollery *et al.* 2005).

Indications

Eye care may be necessary under the following circumstances:

- To relieve pain and discomfort.
- To prevent or treat infection.
- To prevent or treat injury to the eye.
- To detect disease at an early stage.
- To detect drug-induced toxicity at an early stage.
- To prevent damage to the cornea in sedated or unconscious patients.
- To maintain contact lenses and care for false eye prostheses.
- Eye care may also include patient education and health and safety advice.
        (Cunningham & Gould 1998; Boyd-Monk 2005; Stollery *et al.* 2005)

Reference material

If able, and after appropriate instruction, patients should be encouraged to carry out many of the procedures involved in eye care themselves. However, in the case of postoperative, physically limited or unconscious patients, it is often the nurse who is responsible for eye care. A poor eye care technique may lead to the transmission of infection from one eye to the other or the development of irreversible damage to the eye (Ashurst 1997; Cunningham & Gould 1998). In some cases this can lead to loss of sight.

Anatomy and physiology

The eye consists of three main areas: the orbit, the globe (eyeball) and the extrinsic structures. The orbit, or socket, is formed by seven bones of the skull and is lined with fat; it supports and protects the globe and its accessory structures (blood vessels and nerves) and provides attachments for the ocular muscles (Stollery *et al.* 2005).

The globe is approximately 2.5 cm in diameter and can be divided into three layers (Figure 23.1):

- The outer layer or fibrous tunic, composed of the cornea and sclera.
- The middle layer or vascular tunic, composed of the choroid, ciliary body and iris.
- The inner layer or nervous tunic, composed of the retina.

The function of the outer layer is protective and gives shape to the eyeball. The middle layer contains the globe's vascular supply and is darkly pigmented. The inner layer, or retina, contains the light-sensitive cells known as the rods and cones and is also the site of the macula lutea (yellow spot), which contains the central

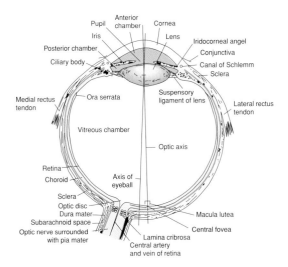

Figure 23.1   Horizontal section through eyeball at level of optic nerve. Optic axis and axis of eyeball are included.

fovea (the area of highest visual acuity). Extrinsic structures of the eye include the eyelids, eyelashes, eyebrows and lacrimal (tear) apparatus. These structures protect the globe from external injury (Stollery *et al.* 2005). The blood vessels inside the eye may be readily viewed with an ophthalmoscope and examined for changes due to systemic diseases, such as diabetes or hypertension, or local disease processes, such as senile macular degeneration (Tortora & Derrickson 2008).

828

The optic nerve which is responsible for vision (cranial nerve II) exits the eye to the side of the macula lutea at an area called the optic disc, sometimes called the anatomical blind spot. The optic nerve passes from the orbit, through the optic foramen and into the brain. The two separate optic nerves meet at the optic chiasma and some optic nerve fibres cross over here to the opposite side of the brain. The nerves then continue along the optic tracts and terminate in the thalamus. From there projections extend to the visual areas in the occipital lobe of the cerebral cortex (Tortora & Derrickson 2008) (Figure 23.2). An additional blind spot, or area of depressed vision called a scotoma, may be indicative of a brain tumour. For example, in pituitary gland tumours it is common to develop bilateral defects in the field of vision due to invasion of the optic chiasm (Goodman & Wickham 2005).

The inside of the globe is divided into two chambers by the lens: the anterior cavity, anterior to the lens, and the vitreous chamber, posterior to the lens. The anterior cavity is divided into the anterior chamber and the posterior chamber by the iris. It contains a clear, watery fluid called the aqueous humour. The vitreous chamber is filled with a jelly-like substance called the vitreous body or vitreous humour. Together these two fluid-filled cavities help maintain the shape of the eyeball and the intraocular pressure (Marieb 2001; Tortora & Derrickson 2008) (Figure 23.3).

The aqueous humour is continuously secreted by the ciliary process (a part of the ciliary body) located behind the iris. This fluid then permeates the posterior chamber, passing between the lens and the iris, and flows through the pupil into the anterior chamber. From the anterior chamber the aqueous humour drains into the scleral venous sinus (canal of Schlemm) and is absorbed back into the blood stream. The aqueous humour is the principal source of nutrients and waste removal for the lens and cornea, as these structures have no direct blood supply. If the outflow of aqueous humour is blocked, excessive intraocular pressure may develop, leading to the disease process known as glaucoma. This excess pressure can cause degeneration of the retina, which may result in blindness (Lee 2006). The vitreous humour is a clear gelatinous substance which fills the vitreous chamber, which unlike the aqueous humour, is produced during foetal development and is never replaced (Marieb 2001; Tortora & Derrickson 2008).

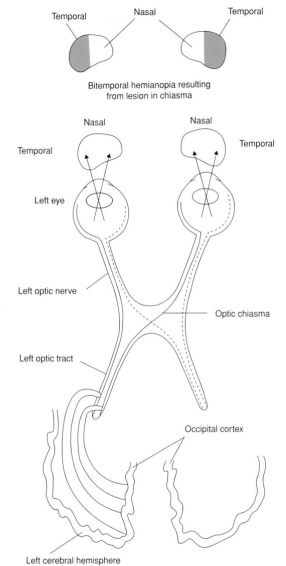

Figure 23.2   Visual pathways and visual fields.

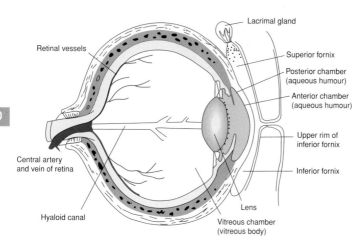

Figure 23.3 Anterior cavity in front of lens is incompletely divided into anterior chamber (anterior to iris) and posterior chamber (behind iris), which are continuous through pupil. Aqueous humour, which fills the cavity, is formed by ciliary processes and reabsorbed into venous blood by the canal of Schlemm.

Tears are produced in the lacrimal glands located at the upper, outer edge of the eye (Figure 23.4). They are excreted onto the upper surface of the globe and washed over the ocular surface by the action of blinking. The function of tears is to clean, moisten and lubricate the ocular surface and eyelids. Tears also provide antisepsis as they contain an enzyme called lysozyme that is able to rupture the cell membranes of some bacteria leading to their lysis and death (Forrester *et al.* 2002).

The tears collect in the nasal canthus (inner, medial aspect of the eye) where they drain into the upper and lower lacrimal puncti which drain into the lacrimal sac. From here the tears pass into the nasolacrimal duct and empty into the nasal cavity (Marieb 2001; Tortora & Derrickson 2008).

General principles of eye care

Aseptic technique is necessary only in certain circumstances, for example, when the eye is damaged or following ophthalmic surgery.

Position of patient

The patient should be sitting or lying with his or her head tilted backwards and chin pointing upwards. This allows for easy access to the eyes and is usually a good position for patient comfort and compliance (Stollery *et al.* 2005).

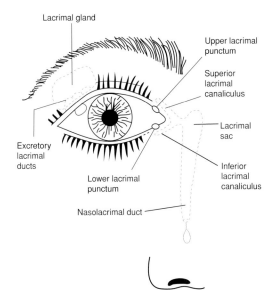

Lacrimal gland

Upper lacrimal punctum

Superior lacrimal canaliculus

Lacrimal sac

Excretory lacrimal ducts

Inferior lacrimal canaliculus

Lower lacrimal punctum

Nasolacrimal duct

Figure 23.4   Lacrimal apparatus.

Position of light source

A good light source is necessary prior to commencing eye care procedures to enable careful assessment of the eyes and to avoid damage to their delicate structures. The light source should be positioned above and behind the nurse. It should never be allowed to shine directly into the patient's eyes, as this will be extremely uncomfortable for the patient.

Instillation of drops

Most types of drops are instilled into the inferior fornix, the pocket formed by gently pulling on the lower eyelid (see Action figure 7 in Procedure guidelines: Eye drops instillation, below), as the conjunctiva in this area is less sensitive than that overlying the cornea. Administering medications into this area prevents immediate loss of the drops into the nasolacrimal drainage system. Exceptions to this instillation technique are as follows:

- *Drugs used to lubricate the cornea*: oil-based drops produce less corneal reaction than aqueous ones as they do not feel as cold to the cornea when administered. They may therefore be instilled directly into the inferior fornix.

- *Anaesthetic drops*: the first drop should be instilled into the inferior fornix for absorption and then directly onto the cornea one drop at a time until the patient is no longer able to feel the drops.
- *Drops used to treat the nasal passages*: these should be instilled at the nasal canthus end of the eye.
- The number of drops instilled depends on the type of solution used and its purpose. Usually, one drop only is ordered and will be sufficient if it is instilled in the correct manner. The exceptions to the 'one-drop' rule are:
- *Oil-based solutions*: these are used for lubricating the eyeball. Usually one drop is instilled and repeated as required.
- *Anaesthetic drops*: Used to anesthetize the eye, one drop should be instilled at a time. This is repeated until the drop cannot be felt on the eye.

If two different preparations are required at the same time an interval of 5 minutes should lapse before the second preparation is instilled to prevent dilution or overflow (BNF 2006).

The dropper should be held as close to the eye as possible without touching either the lids or the cornea (see Action figure 7 in Procedure guidelines: Eye drop instillation, below). This will avoid corneal damage and reduce the risk of cross-infection. If the drop falls from too great a height it is difficult to control and will also be uncomfortable for the patient. The eye should be closed for as long as possible after application, preferably for 1–2 minutes.

A variety of droppers and bottles are available for the instillation of eye preparations. These include pipettes, bottles incorporating pipettes, plastic bottles with a dropper attachment and single dose packs. Pipettes are easy to use but need to be dried and sterilized between doses. Plastic bottles can be squeezed and so avoid the need for a pipette and they are also cheaper than glass bottles with a dropper. Each patient should have their own individual eye drop container for each eye and single dose containers should be used for all patients in eye clinics or in accident and emergency departments (BNF 2006).

Instillation of ointments

Ointments are also applied to the upper rim of the inferior fornix using a similar technique to eye drops (see Action figure 7 in Procedure guidelines: Eye ointment instillation, below). A 2 cm line of ointment should be applied from the nasal canthus outwards. Similarly to the instillation of eye drops, the nozzle should be held approximately 2.5 cm above the eye to avoid contact with the cornea and eyelids.

Contact lenses and eye preparations

Contact lenses may affect the distribution and absorption of eye preparations. Some drugs and preservatives in eye preparations may accumulate in soft hydrogel lenses and induce a toxic reaction. For these reasons contact lenses should be removed prior to instillation of eye drops or ointments and not worn for the period of treatment (BNF 2006). Eye drops can be instilled over rigid contact lenses (BNF 2006).

Care of contact lenses

Contact lenses are thin, curved discs made of hard or soft plastic or a combination of both. Hard contact lenses are made of a rigid plastic that does not absorb water or saline solutions and can be worn for a maximum of 12–14 hours continuously. Soft contact lenses are more pliable, retain more water and so can be worn for up to 30 days and cleaned once weekly. Ill-fitting lenses may reduce the tear film between lens and cornea which may result in oxygen deprivation of the cornea leading to corneal oedema and blurred vision. Further damage to the corneal epithelial cells may lead to corneal abrasion and pain (Marsden & Spence 2006). Gas-permeable lenses are a combination of both hard and soft and permit oxygen to reach the cornea, providing greater comfort, and can be left in for several days (Olver & Cassidy 2005).

Most people look after their own contact lenses. Cleaning and storage solutions depend on the type of lenses used: manufacturers provide specific instructions for the care of their products. They should be stored in a container with slots for right (R) and left (L) eye, so they can be worn in the correct eye. Seriously ill patients should have their lenses removed and stored correctly until they can reinsert their own lenses. Contact lenses are stored in a sterile solution, usually sodium chloride, when they are not in the eye. This helps to lubricate the lens and enable the lens to glide over the cornea, reducing the risk of injury (Kozier *et al.* 1998).

Eye irrigation

Eye irrigation is most often perfomed to remove foreign bodies or caustic substances from the eye, e.g. domestic cleaning agents or medications, particularly cytotoxic material (Stollery *et al.* 2005). This should be done as soon as possible to minimize damage. The procedure is also used as a preoperative preparation or to remove infected material. The fluids most commonly used are sterile 0.9% sodium chloride, 'for irrigation', or sterile water, 'for irrigation'. However, using water may result in deeper corneal damage by corrosive chemicals due to water's hypotonic nature (Kuckelkorn *et al.* 2002). The volume used will vary depending on the degree of contamination; copious amounts are needed for corrosive chemicals and smaller volumes for removal of eye secretions. The solution may be directed to the area affected by using intravenous tubing. To avoid physical damage, the tubing should be held approximately 2.5 cm from the eye (Stollery *et al.* 2005).

Care of the insensitive eye

If the eye-blink reflex is absent the eye's surface will dry out, causing irreversible corneal damage. The cornea may become ulcerated or infected, leading to scarring and possibly loss of vision (Carlson 2002: E). This is a particular problem in the sedated, ventilated or unconscious patient. When the patient has lost this protective reflex, the nurse must initiate interventions to maintain eye moisture and corneal integrity. The surface of the eye and surrounding structures should be kept clean and moist by gentle cleaning with sterile 0.9% sodium chloride and, when necessary, the instillation of lubricating preparations. If there is no eye-blink reflex the eyelids should be kept closed by the use of hypoallergenic tape (Suresh *et al.* 2000). If the eyes become infected the relevant medication should be prescribed and administered.

With each of these measures care must be taken not to spread infection between the eyes. Any alteration to the appearance of the eye must be reported to the doctor.

Artificial eyes

These are made of glass or plastic; some are permanently implanted. Most people who have artificial eyes care for them themselves. If the patient is unconscious it is not necessary to remove the eye regularly for cleaning.

For all procedures which involve removal or insertion of contact lenses or prosthetic eyes the patient should be encouraged to remove/insert the lens/prosthetic themselves as they will have developed their own particular methods. However, the nurse must observe as the patient may still need education to improve upon their technique.

Eye medications

Drugs may be given either systemically or topically to exert an effect on the eye (BNF 2006). However, if given systemically the prescribing doctor needs to take account of the blood–aqueous barrier which exists within the eye. This barrier is selective in allowing drugs to pass into the intraocular fluids. The permeability of this barrier may increase during inflammatory conditions or following paracentesis, the removal of excess fluid with a needle or cannula (Andrew 2006).

Medications applied topically meet some resistance at the barrier presented by the lacrimal system (tear film barrier). A further barrier is the cornea which is selectively permeable and only allows the passage of water and not drugs. However, corneal resistance may alter if there is damage to the corneal epithelium (Kirkwood 2006). Many drugs will produce a similar effect on both the healthy and diseased eye. Drugs for use in the eye are usually classified according to their action.

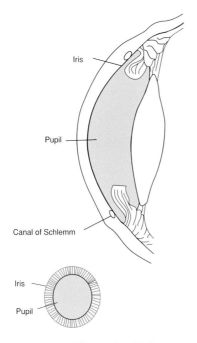

Figure 23.5   Effects of mydriatics.

Mydriatics and cycloplegics

These drugs cause pupil dilation and produce their effects by paralysing the ciliary muscle, stimulating the dilator muscle of the pupil (Figure 23.5) or by a combination of both (see Action figure 7 in Procedure guidelines: Eye drop instillation, below). They are used mainly for diagnostic purposes and most have an anticholinergic action. The most commonly used preparations are cyclopentolate hydrochloride, tropicamide and atropine (BNF 2006).

Miotics

These drugs produce their effects by contracting the ciliary muscle and constricting the pupil (Figure 23.6). Miotics help in the drainage of aqueous humour and are used primarily in the treatment of glaucoma. Examples are pilocarpine and carbachol (BNF 2006).

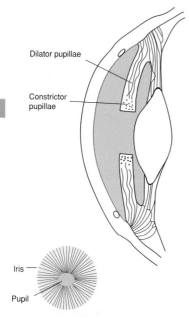

Figure 23.6 Effect of miotics.

Local anaesthetics

These render the eye and the inner surfaces of the lids insensitive. They are used before minor surgery, removal of foreign bodies and tonometry (measurement of intraocular pressure). The most widely used eye anaesthetics are oxybuprocaine and amethocaine (BNF 2006).

Anti-inflammatories

Anti-inflammatory drugs include steroids, antihistamines, lodoxamide and sodium cromoglycate. The most commonly used steroid preparations are dexamethasone, prednisolone and betamethasone (BNF 2006).

Corticosteroid eye drops should be used with caution as they can cause cataract formation or a gradual rise in intraocular pressure in a small percentage of people, particularly if they have a history of glaucoma (Forrester *et al.* 2002).

Antibacterials/antivirals/antifungals

Antibacterials and antivirals can be used for the active treatment of infections or as prophylactic treatment for eye surgery, after removal of a foreign body or following an eye injury. Antibiotic preparations in common use are chloramphenicol, neomycin and framycetin. Aciclovir is the only commonly used antiviral available as an eye preparation although Ganciclovir is licensed for the treatment of acute herpetic keratitis (BNF 2006). Antifungal preparations are not available so the patient needs to be referred to a specialist centre.

Artificial tears

Artificial tears are used when there is a deficiency in natural tear production. This can be due to a disease process, postradiotherapy treatment, as a side-effect of certain drugs or when the eye-blink reflex is absent. These artificial lubricants commonly contain hypromellose or hydroxyethylcellulose (BNF 2006). Additionally, pilocarpine can be given orally. The severity of the problem and the patient's choice will determine the treatment.

Toxic effects of some systemic drugs on the eye

As the eye may be the first place to show signs of systemic disease, so some systemic drugs may show their toxic effects in the eye; this is in part due to the small mass and the relatively high vasculature of the eye. The integrity, thus permeability of the blood–aqueous barrier may be a determining factor. These effects range from pruritis, irritation, redness, epiphora (excess tear production with overflow), photophobia and blepharoconjunctivitis (inflammation of the eyelids and conjunctiva), to disturbance of vision (Andrew 2006).

Particular effects of specific drugs are listed below:

- *Methotrexate and related antimetabolites*: these drugs may cause blepharoconjunctivitis. They may also induce photophobia, epiphora, periorbital oedema and conjunctival hyperaemia.
- *5-Fluorouracil (5-FU)*: 5-FU can cause canalicular fibrosis and oculomotor disturbances (probably secondary to a local neurotoxicity affecting the brain-stem).
- *Antihistamines*: these drugs decrease tear production and may lead to 'dry eye', especially in patients with Sjögren's syndrome (a wasting disease of the salivary glands), ocular pemphigus (rare, autoimmune disease of the skin), those who wear contact lenses and in the elderly.

- *Tamoxifen*: this drug can cause subepithelial whirl-like deposits in the cornea, and retinal lesions.
- *Indomethacin*: this can cause: blurred vision, corneal deposits and retinal pigmentary toxicity.
- *Oral contraceptives*: these can stimulate corneal steeping and intolerance to contact lenses.

- *Atropine, scopolamine and belladonna-like substances*: such drugs cause mydriasis (widening of the pupil) and cycloplegia (paralysis of the ciliary muscle that moves the iris).
- *Corticosteroids*: prolonged use of corticosteroids produces posterior subcapsular cataracts and can increase intraocular pressure.
- *Chloramphenicol*: chloramphenicol treatment can lead to optic neuritis.
- *Ethambutol*: this drug can cause damage to the optic nerve.
- *Rifampicin*: stains soft contact lenses and alters tear coloration.
- *Digoxin*: in overdose results in blurred vision and yellow/green vision.
- *Antidepressants*: may cause a rise in intraocular pressure causing acute glaucoma.
- *Amiodarone*: may increase corneal opacity.
- *Ciprofloxacin*: may deposit in the corneal epithelium.
- *Beta-blockers*: may affect lacrimation causing reduced tear secretion and dry eye.
- *Oxygen*: in neonates, high concentrations for a long period can cause retrolental fibroplasia (abnormal proliferation of fibrous tissue behind the lens causing blindness).

(Forrester *et al*. 2002; Abdollahi *et al*. 2004; Andrew 2006; BNF 2006)

Eye care of the comatose patient

The comatose patient may be unconscious due to injury or deliberate sedation in a critical care environment. The hygiene needs of these patients need to be addressed by nursing staff involved in their care (see Chapter 31). The loss of the physical and biological protective functions may result in damage to the eye. Muscle relaxants administered to sedated patients can reduce the contraction of the orbicularis oculi muscle thus inhibiting full eyelid closure, reduce the blink reflex and random eye movement resulting in diminished tear film coverage of the eye. This desiccation (drying) of the eye may result in exposure keratopathy or superficial corneal abrasions (Ashurst 1997; Cunningham & Gould 1998; Joyce & Evans 2006). To prevent drying of the eye regular interventions such as hygiene and/or administration of products are recommended. Paraffin preparations such as Lacri-Lube® have been shown to offer eye protection in the compromised eye (Ezra *et al*. 2005).

Eye swabbing

Equipment

1 Sterile dressing pack.
2 Sterile low linting swab.

3 Sterile 0.9% sodium chloride for irrigation or sterile water for irrigation.

Procedure

Action	Rationale
1 Explain and discuss the procedure with the patient.	To ensure that the patient understands the procedure and gives his/her valid consent (NMC 2006: C).
2 Assist the patient into the correct position: (a) Head well supported and tilted back. (b) Preferably the patient should be in bed or lying on a couch.	The patient needs to be discouraged from flinching or making unexpected movements and so should be in the most comfortable, pain free position possible at the start of the procedure (Shaw 2006: R 5).
3 Ensure an adequate light source, taking care not to dazzle the patient.	To enable maximum observation of the eyes without causing the patient harm or discomfort (Shaw 2006: R 5).
4 Wash hands thoroughly using bactericidal soap and water or bactericidal alcohol handrub, then dry hands.	To reduce the risk of cross-infection (DH 2005: C).
5 Always treat the uninfected or uninflamed eye first.	To reduce the risk of cross-infection (NT 2003: R 5).
6 Always bathe lids with the eyes closed first.	To reduce the risk of damaging the cornea and to remove any crusted discharge (E).

Procedure guidelines (cont.)

7	Using a slightly moistened low-linting swab, ask the patient to look up and gently swab the lower lid from the inner canthus outwards. Use an aseptic technique for the damaged or postoperative eye.	If the swab is too wet the solution will run down the patient's cheek. This increases the risk of cross-infection and causes the patient discomfort. Swabbing from the nasal corner outwards avoids the risk of swabbing discharge into the lacrimal punctum, or even across the bridge of the nose into the other eye. Aseptic technique reduces the risk of cross-infection (DH 2005: C).
8	Ensure that the edge of the swab is not above the lid margin.	To avoid touching the sensitive cornea (E).
9	Using a new swab each time, repeat the procedure until all the discharge has been removed.	To reduce risk of cross-infection (DH 2005: C).
10	Gently swab the upper lid by slightly everting the lid margin and asking the patient to look down. Swab from the nasal corner outwards and use a new swab each time until all discharge has been removed.	To effectively remove any foreign material from the eye (E). To reduce the risk of cross-infection (DH 2005: C).
11	Once both eyelids have been cleaned and dried, make the patient comfortable.	To ensure patient comfort (E).
12	Remove and dispose of equipment.	To keep area clean and reduce risk of cross-infection (DH 2005: C).
13	Wash hands.	To reduce the risk of cross-infection (DH 2005: C).
14	Record the procedure in the appropriate documents.	To monitor trends and fluctuations (NMC 2005: C).

Note: for information about obtaining an eye swab for pathological investigations, see Chapter 28.

Procedure guidelines   Contact lens care

Procedure

Removal of hard contact lenses

Action	Rationale
1 Explain and discuss the procedure with the patient.	To ensure that the patient understands the procedure and gives his/her consent (NMC 2006: C).
2 Wash hands thoroughly using bactericidal soap.	To reduce the risk of cross-infection (DH 2005: C).
3 Using thumb and forefinger separate the eyelids. Keeping the eyelid stationary, place the index finger on the lens. Gently move the lens to one side of the cornea and pull away (see Action figure 3).	To minimize corneal trauma (Stollery *et al.* 2005: R 5).
4 Store lenses in the appropriate solution as recommended by the manufacturers and ensure lenses are placed in the correct left and right storage pots.	To prevent deterioration and contamination (Stollery *et al.* 2005: R 5).
5 Refer to manufacturer's instructions for further storage information, particularly if patient will not be using the lenses for a lengthy period of time.	To prevent deterioration of lens and growth of organisms (C).

Removal of soft contact lenses

Action	Rationale
1 Explain and discuss the procedure with the patient.	To ensure that the patient understands the procedure and gives his/her consent (NMC 2006: C).
2 Wash hands thoroughly using bactericidal soap.	To reduce the risk of cross-infection (DH 2005: C).
3 Wearing gloves, gently pinch the lens between the thumb and index finger (see Action figure 3).	To encourage the lens to fold together, allowing air to enter underneath the lens for easy removal (C).

Procedure guidelines (*cont.*)

4 Store lenses in the appropriate solution as recommended by the manufacturers and ensure lenses are placed in the correct left and right storage pots.

To prevent deterioration and contamination (Stollery *et al.* 2005: E).

5 Refer to manufacturer's instructions for further storage information, particularly if patient will not be using the lenses for a lengthy period of time.

To prevent deterioration and growth of organisms (C).

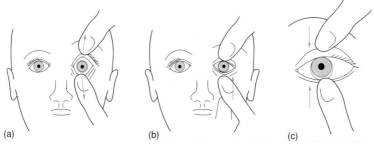

(a)   (b)   (c)

Action 3(a)   Removing hard contact lenses.

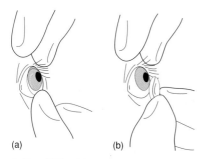

(a)   (b)

Action 3(b)   (a) Moving a soft lens down the interior part of the sclera. (b) Removing a soft lens by pinching it between the pads of the thumb and index finger.

Procedure guidelines   Eye drop instillation

Equipment

1 Sterile dressing pack.
2 Sterile 0.9% sodium chloride for irrigation or sterile water for irrigation.
3 Appropriate eye drops.
4 Low-linting swab.

Procedure

Action	Rationale
1 Explain and discuss the procedure with the patient.	To ensure that the patient understands the procedure and gives his/her valid consent (NMC 2006: C).
2 If there is any discharge, proceed as for eye swabbing.	To remove any infected material and thus ensure adequate absorption of the drops (C).
3 Consult the patient's prescription sheet, and ascertain the following: (a) Patient identification. (b) Drug. (c) Dose. (d) Date and time of administration. (e) Route and method of administration, including which eye the drops are prescribed for. (f) Expiry date on bottle. (g) Validity of prescription. (h) Signature of prescriber.	To ensure that the patient is given the correct drug in the prescribed dose in the correct eye, and that the drug has not expired (NMC 2008: C).
4 Assist the patient into the correct position, i.e. head well supported and tilted back.	To ensure that drops are instilled into the pocket of the inferior fornix and to avoid excess solution running down the patient's cheek (Stollery *et al.* 2005: E).
5 Wash hands thoroughly using bactericidal soap and water or bactericidal alcohol handrub, and dry them.	Asepsis is essential when the patient has a damaged eye or has just had an operation on the eye. Infection can lead to loss of an eye (DH 2005: C).

Procedure guidelines (cont.)

6 Place a wet low-linting swab on the lower lid against the lid margin and gently pull down to evert the lower eyelid.

To absorb any excess solution which may be irritating to the surrounding skin and open the inferior fornix (E).

7 Ask the patient to look up immediately before instilling the drop (see Action figure 7).

This opens the eye and allows the drop to be instilled into the upper rim of the inferior fornix. If drop instilled too soon, the patient may blink as the drop is instilled (E).

8 Ask the patient to close the eye for approximately 1 minute. Keep the wet low-linting swab on the lower lid.

To ensure adequate absorption of the fluid and to avoid excess running down the cheek (Stollery et al. 2005: E).

9 Make the patient comfortable.

10 Remove and dispose of equipment.

To keep area clean and reduce risk of cross infection (DH 2005: C).

11 Wash hands with bactericidal soap and water.

To reduce the risk of cross-infection (DH 2005: C).

12 Complete the patient's recording chart and other hospital and/or legally required documents.

To maintain accurate records. To provide a point of reference in the event of any queries. To prevent any duplication of treatment (NMC 2005: C).

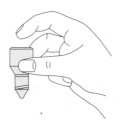
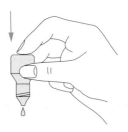
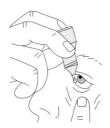

Action 7 How to instil eye drops.

Procedure guidelines   Eye ointment instillation

Equipment

1 Sterile dressing pack.
2 Sterile 0.9% sodium chloride for irrigation or sterile water for irrigation.
3 Appropriate eye ointment.
4 Low-linting swab.

Procedure

Action	Rationale
1 Explain and discuss the procedure with the patient.	To ensure that the patient understands the procedure and gives his/her valid consent (NMC 2006: C).
2 If there is any discharge, and to remove any previous application of ointment, proceed as for eye swabbing.	To remove any infected material and previous ointment to allow for absorption of ointment (C).
3 Consult the patient's prescription sheet, and ascertain the following: (a) Patient identification. (b) Drug. (c) Dose. (d) Date and time of administration. (e) Route and method of administration, including which eye the ointment is prescribed for. (f) Expiry date on bottle. (g) Validity of prescription. (h) Signature of prescriber.	To ensure that the patient is given the correct drug in the prescribed dose in the correct eye, and that the drug has not expired (NMC 2008: C).
4 Wash hands thoroughly using bactericidal soap and water or bactericidal alcohol handrub.	To reduce the risk of cross-infection (DH 2005: C).
5 Place a wet low-linting swab on the lower lid against the lid margin.	To absorb excess ointment which may be irritating to the surrounding skin (E).
6 Gently pull on the low-linting swab. Ask the patient to look up immediately before applying the ointment.	To allow the application to be made inside the lower lid into the lower fornix (E).

Procedure guidelines (cont.)

7 Apply the ointment by gently squeezing the tube and, with the nozzle 2.5 cm above the eye, drawing a line along the inner edge of the lower lid from the nasal corner outwards (see Action figure 7).

To reduce the risk of cross-infection, contamination of the tube and trauma to the eye (Stollery *et al.* 2005: E).

8 Ask the patient to close the eye and remove excess ointment with a new wet low-linting swab.

To avoid excess ointment irritating the surrounding skin (E).

9 Warn the patient that, when the eye is opened, vision will be a little blurred for a few minutes.

To prepare patient and to avoid anxiety (Stollery *et al.* 2005: E).

10 Make the patient comfortable.

11 Remove and dispose of equipment.

To keep area clean and reduce risk of cross infection (DH 2005: C).

12 Wash hands with bactericidal soap and water.

To reduce the risk of cross-infection (DH 2005: C).

13 Complete the patient's recording chart and other hospital and/or legally required documents.

To maintain accurate records. To provide a point of reference in the event of any queries. To prevent any duplication of treatment (NMC 2005: C).

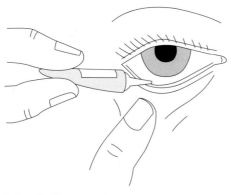

Action 7 How to instil eye ointment.

Procedure guidelines   Eye irrigation

Equipment

1 Sterile dressing pack.
2 Sterile 0.9% sodium chloride for irrigation or sterile water for irrigation (in an emergency tap water may be used).
3 Receiver.
4 Towel.
5 Plastic cape.
6 Irrigating flask.
7 Warm water in a bowl to warm irrigating fluid to tepid temperature.
8 Anaesthetic drops.

Procedure

Action	Rationale
1 Explain and discuss the procedure with the patient.	To ensure that the patient understands the procedure and gives his/her valid consent (NMC 2006: C).
2 Instil anaesthetic drops if required (proceed as for instillation of eye drops).	To avoid any discomfort (Marsden 2006: R 5).
3 Prepare the irrigation fluid to the appropriate temperature by placing in bowl of water until warmed.	Tepid fluid will be more comfortable for the patient. The solution should be poured across the inner aspect of the nurse's wrist to test the temperature (E).
4 Assist the patient into the appropriate position: (a) Head comfortably supported with chin almost horizontal. (b) Head inclined to the side of the eye to be treated.	To avoid the solution running either over the nose into the other eye to avoid cross-infection or out of the affected eye and down the side of the cheek (DH 2005: C). To reduce risk of cross-infection (DH 2005: C).
5 Wash hands using bactericidal soap and water or bactericidal alcohol handrub, and dry.	To prevent washing the discharge down the lacrimal duct or across the cheek (E).
6 If there is any discharge proceed as for eye swabbing.	
7 If possible remove any contact lens, proceed as for contact lens removal.	To ensure no reservoir of chemical remains in the eye (Marsden 2006: E).

Procedure guidelines (cont.)

8	Ask the patient to hold the receiver against the cheek below the eye being irrigated.	To collect irrigation fluid as it runs away from the eye (E).
9	Position the towel and plastic cape.	To protect the patient's clothing (E).
10	Hold the patient's eyelids apart, using your first and second fingers, against the orbital ridge.	The patient will be unable to hold the eye open once irrigation commences (E).
11	Do not press on the eyeball.	To avoid causing the patient discomfort or pain (E).
12	Warn the patient that the flow of solution is going to start and pour a little onto the cheek first.	To allow time to adjust to the feeling of water flow (E).
13	Direct the flow of the fluid from the nasal corner outwards (see Action figure 13).	To wash away from the lacrimal punctum and prevent contaminating other eye (E).
14	Ask the patient to look up, down and to either side while irrigating.	To ensure that the whole area including fornices are irrigated (Stollery *et al.* 2005: E).
15	Evert upper and lower lids whilst irrigating.	To ensure complete removal of any foreign body (E).
16	Keep the flow of irrigation fluid constant.	To ensure swift removal of any foreign body (Marsden 2006: E).
17	When the eye has been thoroughly irrigated, ask the patient to close the eyes and use a new swab to dry the lids.	For patient comfort (E).
18	Take the receiver from the patient and dry the cheek.	To prevent spillage of receiver contents and promote patient comfort (E).
19	Make the patient comfortable.	
20	Remove and dispose of equipment.	To keep area clean and reduce risk of cross-infection (DH 2005: C).

21	Wash hands with bactericidal soap and water.	To reduce the risk of cross-infection (DH 2005: C).
22	Complete the patient's recording chart and other hospital and/or legally required documents.	To maintain accurate records. To provide a point of reference in the event of any queries. To prevent any duplication of treatment (NMC 2005: C).

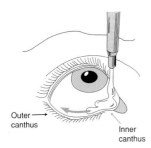

Outer canthus

Inner canthus

Action 13   Irrigation of eye from inner to outer canthus.

Procedure guidelines   Eyelid closure for comatose patients

If necessary clean and apply medication as outlined above.

Equipment

1 Sterile dressing pack.
2 Sterile 0.9% sodium chloride for irrigation or sterile water.

3 Hypoallergenic tape.

Procedure

Action	Rationale
1 Explain the procedure to the patient.	Hearing is often still present in unconscious patients so it is good practice to explain the procedure.
2 Wash hands thoroughly using bacterial soap and water or bactericidal alcohol handrub, then dry hands.	To reduce the risk of cross-infection (DH 2005: C).

Procedure guidelines (cont.)

3 Always treat and clean the uninfected or uninflamed eye first.	To reduce the risk of cross-infection (DH 2005: C).
4 Lubricate the eyelids (following procedure as outlined above for instillation of ointment).	To prevent corneal surface drying (Cunningham & Gould 1998: R 3a).
5 Gently hold down upper eyelid until it meets the lower lid.	To ensure there is no gap between eyelids (Joyce & Evans 2006: R 3a).
6 Place hypoallergenic tape across upper eyelid ensuring that there are no eyelashes caught underneath the tape.	To keep eyes closed and ensure patient does not feel pain when tape is removed (P).
7 Remove and dispose of equipment.	To keep area clean and reduce risk of cross-infection (DH 2005: C).
8 Wash hands.	To reduce the risk of cross-infection (DH 2005: C).
9 Record the procedure in the appropriate documents.	To monitor trends and fluctuation (NMC 2005: C).

References and further reading

Abdollahi, M. *et al.* (2004) Drug-induced toxic reactions in the eye. *J Infus Nurs*, **27**(6), 386–98.

Andrew, S. (2006) Pharmacology. In: *Ophthalmic Care* (ed. J. Marsden). Whurr, Chichester, pp. 42–65.

Ashurst, S. (1997) Nursing care of the mechanically ventilated patient in ITU: 1. *Br J Nurs*, **6**(8), 447–54.

BNF (2006) *British National Formulary No. 51*. British Medical Association, London.

Boyd-Monk, H. (2005). Bringing common eye emergencies into focus. *Nursing*, **35**(12), 46–51.

Carlson, B.A. (2002) Neurologic disorders. In: *Critical Care Nursing: Diagnosis and Management* (eds L. Urden, K. Stacy & M. Lough), 4th edn. Mosby, St. Louis, MO, pp. 671–700.

Char, D.H. (1993) Management of orbital tumours. *Mayo Clin Pract*, **68**, 1081–96.

Cunningham, C. & Gould, D. (1998) Eyecare for the sedated patient undergoing mechanical ventilation: the use of evidence-based care. *Int J Nurs Stud*, **35**, 32–40.

DH (2005) *Saving Lives: A Delivery Programme to Reduce Healthcare Associated Infection Including MRSA*. Department of Health, London.

Ezra, D. *et al.* (2005) Preventing exposure keratopathy in the critically ill: a prospective study comparing eye care regimes. *Br J Ophthalmol*, **89**, 1068–9.

Finger, P.T. (2000) Tumour location affects the incidence of cataract and retinopathy after ophthalmic plaque radiation therapy. *Br J Ophthalmol*, **84**(9), 1068–70.

Forrester, J. *et al.* (2002). *The Eye: Basic Science in Practice*, 2nd edn. Saunders, Edinburgh.

Foss, A.J.E. *et al.* (1999) Modelling uveal melanoma. *Br J Ophthalmol*, **83**, 588–94.

Goddard, A.G., Kingston, J.E. & Hungerford, J.L. (1999) Delay in diagnosis of retinoblastoma: risk factors and treatment outcome. *Br J Ophthalmol*, **83**(12), 1320–3.

Goodman, M. & Wickham, R. (2005) Endocrine malignancies. In: *Cancer Nursing: Principles and Practice* (eds C. Yarbo, M. Hansen Frogge & M. Goodman), 6th edn. Jones and Bartlett, Sudbury, MA, pp. 1215–43.

Joyce, N. & Evans, D. (2006) Eye care for patients in the ICU. *Am J Nurs*, **106**(1), 72AA–DD.

Kirkwood, B. (2006) The cornea. In: *Ophthalmic Care* (ed. J. Marsden). Whurr, Chichester, pp. 339–69.

Kozier, B. *et al.* (1998) Assisting with hygiene. In: *Fundamentals of Nursing: Concepts, Process, Practice*. Addison-Wesley, Menlo Park, CA, pp. 729–84.

Kuckelkorn, R. *et al.* (2002) Emergency treatment of chemical and thermal eye burns. *Acta Ophthalmol Scand*, **80**(1), 4–10.

Lee, A. (2006) The angle and aqueous. In: *Ophthalmic Care* (ed. J. Marsden). Whurr, Chichester, pp. 420–60.

Lindgren, G., Diffey, B.L. & Larko, O. (1998) Basal cell carcinoma of the eyelids and solar ultraviolet radiation exposure. *Br J Ophthalmol*, **82**(12), 1412–5.

Lund, V.J. (1987) The orbit. In: *Otolaryngology* (ed. A.G. Kerr), 5th edn. Butterworth, London.

Marieb, E.N. (2001) *Human Anatomy and Physiology*, 5th edn. Benjamin Cummings, San Francisco.

Marsden, J. (2006) The care of patients presenting with acute problems. In: *Ophthalmic Care* (ed. J. Marsden). Whurr, Chichester, pp. 209–52.

Marsden, J. & Spence, D. (2006) Optics. In: *Ophthalmic Care* (ed. J. Marsden). Whurr, Chichester, pp. 20–41.

McQueen, L. (2006) Eyelids and lacrimal drainage system. In: *Ophthalmic Care* (ed. J. Marsden). Whurr, Chichester, pp. 276–306.

Moeloek, N.F. (1993) Updates in orbital tumours. *Eye Sci*, **9**(1), 40–4.

NMC (2005) *Guidelines for Records and Record Keeping*. Nursing and Midwifery Council, London.

NMC (2006) *A–Z Advice Sheet Consent*. www.nmc.org.

NMC (2008) *Standards for Medicines Management*. Nursing and Midwifery Council, London.

NT (2003) NT skills update – eye care. *Nurs Times*, **99**(8), 28.

Olver, J. & Cassidy, L. (2005) *Ophthamology at a Glance*. Blackwell Science, Malden, MA.

Ryder, A. (2006) The orbit and extraocular muscles. In: *Ophthalmic Care* (ed. J. Marsden). Whurr, Chichester, pp. 510–53.

Shaw, M.E. (2006) Examination of the eye. In: *Ophthalmic Care* (ed. J. Marsden). Whurr, Chichester, pp. 66–84.

Souhami, R. & Tobias, J. (2005) *Cancer and its Management*, 5th edn. Blackwell Publishing, Oxford.

Stollery, R., Shaw, M. & Lee, A. (2005) *Ophthalmic Nursing*, 3rd edn. Blackwell Publishing, Oxford.

Suresh, P. *et al.* (2000) Eye care for the critically ill. *Intensive Care Med*, **26**, 162–6.

Tortora, G.J. & Derrickson, B. (2008) *Principles of Anatomy and Physiology*, 12th edn. John Wiley & Sons, Ltd, Chichester.

Ward, B., Raynel, S. & Catt, G. (2006) The uveal tract. In: *Ophthalmic Care* (ed. J. Marsden). Whurr, Chichester, pp. 396–420.

852

See page 891 for multiple choice questions covering this chapter.

Chapter 24

Personal hygiene: mouth care

Definition

Good mouth care (oral hygiene) is a vital part of nursing care and includes the careful assessment, correct care and the appropriate treatment of the oral cavity including the teeth and mouth (Roberts 2004). White (2004) states that while this is an essential part of nursing care it is an often overlooked aspect of patient care both in the community and hospital setting.

Oral hygiene has been given a much greater profile since its inclusion as one of the clinical benchmarks proposed in *The Essence of Care* (DH 2001). There is still a danger that with the increasing demands made on nursing time and lack of knowledge that oral care may be one of the first things to be set aside (Fitzpatrick 2000; Miller & Kearney 2001; Southern 2007). Damage to the oral cavity secondary to lack of care, disease or treatment may cause multiple problems to the patient and reduce their quality of life (White 2000; Miller & Kearney 2001; Borbasi *et al.* 2002; Sonis *et al.* 2004). The main aims of oral care are to (Cooley 2002):

- Keep the mucosa clean, soft, moist and intact and to prevent infection.
- Keep the lips clean, soft, moist and intact.
- Remove food debris as well as dental plaque without damaging the gingiva.
- Alleviate pain and discomfort and enhance oral intake.
- Prevent halitosis and freshen the mouth.

Reference material

Anatomy and physiology

The mouth is the oval cavity at the anterior end of the digestive tract (Marieb 2004). It consists of the mouth cavity (cavum oris proprium) and the vestibule (vestibulum oris), which is bounded by the lips containing the cheeks, gums, teeth, tongue, hard and soft palate (Thiobodeau & Patton 2007).

The oral cavity is lined with a mucous membrane consisting of three layers: top layer, sub-mucosa and basement layer, consisting of multiple layers of cells, including epithelial and connective tissue (Martini 2007). It is worth noting that damage to the oral mucosa may take place on any or on all of these layers, and while the oral cavity may look normal, damage may still be occurring (Sonis 2004). The oral mucosa is an area of rapid replication designed to meet the constant demands of activities such as chewing and talking, and it is thought that the epithelial layer of the oral mucosa is replaced every 7–14 days (Sonis 2004). The tongue forms the greater part of the floor of the oral cavity.

854

The mouth has three main functions: (i) to enable ingestion of food and fluids; (ii) to aid communication; and (iii) to support breathing (along with the nasal cavity) (Thiobodeau & Patton 2007).

The mouth is lubricated by secretions from the salivary glands: parotid, submandibular and sublingual. It is believed that as much as 1.5 litres of saliva are produced each day (Dickinson & Porter 2006). The functions of saliva are both protective (preventing infection) and digestive (supporting chewing and swallowing of food) in nature (Sreebny 2000).

Predisposing factors to poor oral health may include:

- Inability to take adequate fluids leading to dehydration and dryness of mucosa.
- Poor nutritional status leading to poor cellular repair and vitamin deficiencies.
- Insufficient saliva production leading to infection and dryness of the mucosa.
- Major intervention altering oral status; surgery, radiotherapy or chemotherapy causing structural changes.
- Lack of knowledge, ability or motivation towards maintaining oral hygiene.
- Other factors: pre-existing dental problems, co-morbidities, drug/oxygen therapy causing dryness, age (children and older adults), genetic factors, alcohol and tobacco use (Barasch & Peterson 2003; Beck 2004).

Oral complications

Oral complications may manifest as taste changes, pain, ulcers, infection, bone and dentition changes, bleeding and functional disorders affecting verbal and non-verbal communication, chewing and swallowing, and respiration (Porter 1994). Stomatitis (inflammation of the oral cavity) results from damage to the mucous membrane and may be induced by trauma, infection or by factors that decrease the proliferation rate of the cells (e.g. chemotherapy and radiotherapy). Oral mucositis is the term usually used to describe the inflammation and ulceration of the oral mucosa associated with chemotherapy and radiation (Dodds 2004). Although not fully understood, it is now clear that the mucosal damage related to cytotoxic treatment is a complex process and thought to consist of five simultaneous phases of mucosal damage consisting of: initiation, up-regulation, signalling and amplification, ulceration and healing (Sonis 2004). Many of the new and developing treatments for oral mucositis in the cancer care setting are aimed at preventing damage in these identified phases (Sonis 2004).

Xerostomia (oral dryness) is often but not always linked to salivary gland dysfunction; oral dryness can be caused by other factors including the continued use of oxygen therapy and inadequate hydration. Salivary gland dysfunction, which may be permanent or temporary, is an alteration in the production and composition of saliva and can be extremely distressing to patients (preventing sleep, causing difficulty in talking, eating and swallowing, and allowing oral pathogens to develop) (Torres *et al.* 2002; Davies 2005). While many patients may experience xerostomia and/or salivary dysfunction, some studies have shown that over 80% of dying patients may suffer from this condition (Chaushu *et al.* 2000; Davies *et al.* 2002). In the cancer setting salivary function can be affected by chemotherapy, radiotherapy and other drugs, including cyclizine and hyoscine (Cheng 2006). The production of saliva may be completely destroyed by radiation to the oral region as the salivary glands are highly sensitive to radiation (Shih *et al.* 2003). While a complex problem, good oral care can provide relief from this distressing symptom (Cheng 2006).

855

The oral cavity harbours a variety of endogenous bacteria which do not normally pose problems and serve to prevent other forms of pathogens from developing in the cavity (Sonis 2004). However, an inadequate functioning immune system secondary to disease and/or systemic treatments such as cytotoxic therapy (cancer setting), immunosuppression drugs (organ transplant setting) and antifungal therapies may increase the pathogenicity of these organisms leading to local infection. Common organisms include *Pseudomonas*, *Klebsiella*, *Escherichia coli* and *Candida* species (Porter 1994). Local infection may lead to a secondary infection or systemic infection (septicaemia), particularly when the mucosa barrier is damaged (Blijlevens *et al.* 2000).

Halitosis (oral offensive odour) may be very distressing for the patient and for family members (Shorthose & Davies 2005). It is thought that many people in the general population suffer from this condition (Loesche & Kazor 2002). The cause can be either physiological (food debris, epithelial cells, blood cells, saliva), or due to an underlying disease (infection, inflammation, malignancy) (Shorthose & Davies 2005). Careful brushing of the tongue to remove debris, advice on diet, smoking cessation, the use of mouthwashes and where possible treating the underlining cause can relieve this distressing symptom (Shorthose & Davies 2005).

Mouth care

Mouth care involves; patient education and support, regular oral assessment, appropriate frequency of care and the use of oral care equipment and agents. It is clear that nurses do not always feel they have the correct skills and knowledge to support patients with mouth care (Fitzpatrick 2000; Ohrn *et al*. 2000; Southern 2007). Cheng (2006) suggests that in order to achieve compliance, oral care should be realistic, simple and acceptable to patient and family members in hospital, hospice, nursing homes and home care settings.

Oral assessment

Thorough and correct oral assessment is required in planning effective care (Eilers 2004; Sonis *et al*. 2004; Jaroneski 2006; Quinn *et al*. 2007). Assessment of the oral cavity is required to: (i) provide baseline data; (ii) monitor and evaluate response to care and treatment; and (iii) identify new problems as they arise (Holmes & Mountain 1993).

A number of oral assessment tools have been developed including: World Health Organization (WHO) Mucositis Scale (WHO 1979), National Cancer Institute Common Toxicity Criteria (NCI-CTC) (National Institutes of Health 1987), Oral Mucositis Index (OMI) (Schubert *et al*. 1992) and Oral Assessment Guide (OAG; Eilers *et al*. 1988). While some of these assessment tools have been designed specifically for use in the oncology setting, their relevance and applicability to other settings is clear. The tools share much in common in that all include subjective and objective measures, and include the assessment of: the oral cavity, the presence or absence of erythema, ulcers, pain, saliva, and the ability to eat or drink. In most clinical situations it is essential that the patient is involved in the oral assessment process. In order to fully assess the oral cavity in the cancer setting, the eight areas most susceptible to cytotoxic damage must be inspected (Box 24.1).

Holmes and Mountain (1993) evaluated three oral assessment tools for reliability, validity and clinical usefulness. In their conclusion they showed a preference

---

Box 24.1 Areas of oral cavity most susceptible to cytotoxic damage

- Upper lip (labial mucosa)
- Lower lip (labial mucosa)
- Right buccal mucosa
- Left buccal mucosa
- Right lateral and ventral tongue
- Left lateral and ventral tongue
- Floor of mouth
- Soft palate
  (Sonis 2004)

for that developed by Eilers *et al.* (1988), but stressed that further work is required to develop a tool that is entirely satisfactory for use in clinical practice and future research. Andersson *et al.* (1999) found that Eilers' oral assessment guide with minor amendments for patients undergoing high-dose chemotherapy treatment was a reliable and clinically useful tool for assessing the oral cavity status and determining changes. Other studies have shown a preference for the NCI-CTC and WHO assessments because these simple scales enable the clinical team to consistently correctly assess the oral cavity (Sonis *et al.* 2004; Stone *et al.* 2007). The choice of assessment tool to be used should be decided on, after careful consideration of the clinical environment; however, the WHO scale is simple and easy to use in all clinical settings. Recognizing the need for guidance, a European group of nurses, physicians and dentists have developed recommendations that should be considered when assessing the oral cavity (Quinn *et al.* 2007).

Frequency of care

Dodd *et al.* (2000) concluded that the incidence of oral complications was reduced by the frequency of care rather than the agents employed. However, there has been little research to indicate the most effective frequency. Various suggested time intervals including 2-hourly, 4-hourly, after meals and before bed have been proposed (Beck 2004).

Following a review of earlier studies Krishnasamy (1995) recommends the following:

- Four-hourly care will reduce the potential for infection from micro-organisms.
- Two-hourly care will reduce mouth care problems and ensure patient comfort.
- One-hourly care is recommended for patients requiring oxygen therapy, those who are mouth breathing, who have an infected mouth or are unconscious (intubated and dying patients).

There is however a need for further research and frequency of care should be carefully considered in each particular clinical situation (McNeill 2000). Basic oral care should always include the removal of any debris to prevent infection and steps to keep the mucosa moist in order to provide comfort (Sonis 2004).

Oral care equipment

A variety of equipment that may be used in caring for the mouth has been reported in the literature, including toothbrush, foam-stick, dental floss and gauze. The most appropriate piece of equipment should be determined by its efficacy together with its potential to damage the gingiva. The use of the toothbrush is well supported by the literature and is the most effective tool at removing debris from the teeth and gums, including plaque (Clay 2000; Xavier 2000; Pearson &

Hutton 2002). The foamstick, however, can cause less trauma, particularly when oral care includes free surgical flaps and skin grafts (Hahn & Jones 2000) or oral bleeding occurs as a result of thrombocytopenia (Walton *et al.* 2002). Care must be taken to ensure that the toothbrush is kept free from infection as toothbrushes have been shown to harbour organisms such as group A beta-haemolytic strepto-cocci, staphylococci, *Candida* and *Pseudomonas* (Brook & Gober 1998). These organisms have been found to contribute to persistent oropharyngeal infections (Brook & Gober 1998; Taji & Rogers 1998). Borowski *et al.* (1994) demon-strated that good oral hygiene, such as brushing the gingiva and teeth, can help to decrease the incidence of septicaemia.

Maintaining good oral hygiene

In most clinical situations oral care should include tooth brushing and rinsing of the mouth to remove debris and reduce oral complications (Beck 2004). Nurses should:

- Encourage/support patient to clean teeth with toothpaste and toothbrush (removing debris) after meals. Toothpaste must be removed from the oral cavity through thorough rinsing as prolonged contact with teeth and mucosa of some agents (glycerine) can cause damage.
- Encourage/support the patient to keep mucosa and lips moist (sipping flu-ids/application of oral lubricant, such as petroleum gel, KY gel, Vaseline).
- Consider use of sodium chloride 0.9%, to be swilled in the mouth and dis-carded to help cleanse the mouth and remove any debris.
- Possible use of chlorhexidine gluconate 0.2% 5 ml, four times a day, which should be retained in the mouth for at least 1 minute before discarding.
- Consider use of other oral care agents and analgesia; glycerin, nystatin, parac-etamol, aspirin, opiates.
- Care should be delivered in a dignified and gentle manner (Sweeney 2005).

Oral care agents

The choice of an oral care agent will be dependent on the aim of care. The agent may be used to remove debris and plaque, prevent superimposed infection, alle-viate pain, provide comfort, stop bleeding, provide lubrication or treat specific problems (Dickinson & Porter 2006). A wide variety of agents are available and should be determined by the individual needs of the patient and the particular clinical situation together with a detailed nursing assessment. There is ongoing debate on the efficacy of the agents presently available and there remains in-sufficient evidence to clearly state the best agents to use in the clinical setting.

Most of the agents described below are included in *The Royal Marsden Hospital Prescribing Guidelines for Mouth Care* (Royal Marsden Hospital 2002).

Normal saline (sodium chloride 0.9%)

The use of normal saline is supported by a number of authors as part of a patient's oral care. This relatively cheap and generally well-tolerated solution can be rinsed in the mouth and then discarded. It helps to loosen and remove debris, moistens the mucosa, helps alleviate discomfort and promote healing (Madeya 1996; Cheng *et al.* 2001).

Chlorhexidine gluconate

Chlorhexidine is a compound with broad-spectrum antimicrobial activity that results in binding to and sustained release from mucosal surfaces (Ferretti *et al.* 1990). While chlorhexidine continues to be widely used in clinical settings its efficacy has been widely debated in certain clinical situations. Ferretti *et al.* (1990) in their study found that it had protected patients in their study group from infection and helped to resolve existing infections, reducing soft tissue disease and oral microbial burden. Likewise, Rawlins and Trueman (2001) believe that chlorhexidine can greatly reduce bacteria in seriously ill patients. However, some studies have shown that it is not effective as a prophylatic treatment in the cancer setting (Worthington *et al.* 2003). In one study of 222 outpatients, Dodd *et al.* (1996) found that chlorhexidine as a mouthwash was no more effective than water in preventing chemotherapy-induced mucositis. While Foote *et al.* (1994) showed that patients receiving chlorhexidine mouthwash while undergoing radiation therapy showed a trend to develop more mucositis than those receiving a placebo mouthwash, leading to the hypothesis that chlorhexidine may be detrimental in this clinical setting. Having reviewed the existing evidence, Barasch *et al.* (2006) advise against the use of chlorhexidine for chemotherapy-induced mucositis. It is clear that chlorhexidine should be used with caution and further research needs to be done within this area.

Antifungal treatment

Nystatin is the best known and most commonly used antifungal agent (Campbell 1995). It is an antifungal antibiotic that is used as an oral suspension (Finlay & Davies 2005). Barkvoll *et al.* (1989) showed in their in vitro study that combinations of nystatin and chlorhexidine gluconate were not effective against *Candida albicans* and recommended that the most efficient treatment plan must be restricted to the use of one of these drugs alone.

Fluconazole is an antifungal that has been demonstrated to be effective in the treatment of candidiasis of the oropharynx, oesophagus and a variety of deep tissue sites (Brammer 1990). Fluconazole can be administered as a capsule, suspension or as an intravenous infusion. Although most patients will not require fluconazole as a prophylactic measure, it may be given prophylactically in certain clinical settings when patients are severely immunocompromised (haemato-oncology/stem cell transplant setting). It is often the treatment of choice for suspected fungal infection (Finlay & Davies 2005). Other antifungal drugs may include: amphotericin, ketoconazole, miconazole and itraconazole (Finlay & Davies 2005).

860

Sucralfate

Sucralfate is a complex of aluminium hydroxide and sulphated sucrose which may be used to protect the oral mucosa. In one study, Barker *et al.* (1991) showed that consistent daily oral hygiene and use of a mouth-coating agent such as sucralfate in patients receiving radiotherapy results in less pain, may reduce weight loss and interruption of radiation therapy because of severe mucositis. However, Barasch *et al.* (2006) having reviewed the literature do not recommend the use of sucralfate for radiotherapy-induced mucositis. Some reduction in pain and increase in oral intake have been shown in patients with chemotherapy-induced ulcerating or erythematous mucositis taking oral sucralfate (Rattan *et al.* 1994). However, Chiara *et al.* (2001) performed a pilot study to assess the efficacy of sucralfate gel for the treatment of chemotherapy-induced mucositis and found that the suspension did not demonstrate any significant advantage over the placebo used. Further research is therefore needed. The administration of sucralfate and enteral feeds should be separated by 1 hour to avoid interactions and used with extreme caution in patients with renal impairment (Royal Pharmaceutical Society of Great Britain 2006).

Fluoride

Fluoride helps to prevent and arrest tooth decay, especially radiation caries, demineralization and decalcification. Following its use, no food or fluids should be taken for at least 30 minutes in order for it to work (Cooke 1996).

Artificial saliva

Saliva substitutes duplicate the properties of normal saliva (Kusler & Rambur 1992). They buffer the acidity of the mouth and lubricate the mucous membranes (Heals 1993).

Over-the-counter oral mouthwashes should be used with caution and the ingredients should be critically assessed before use as some ingredients, including alcohol, can cause further discomfort to an already damaged mucosa (Sonis 2004).

Problems

Fungal

Oral candidiasis is known to be the cause of most oral fungal infections. It usually occurs as a result of both host factors (immunosuppression, nutritional problems) and mucosal damage secondary to treatment (Finlay & Davies 2005).

Prophylaxis

Nystatin mouthwash 1 ml used four times a day. This should be rinsed around the mouth and retained for at least 1 minute before swallowing. Dentures must be removed prior to rinsing. One millimetre of nystatin oral suspension can be added to the water to soak acrylic dentures (Walton *et al.* 2002). If using chlorhexidine, a time interval of 15–30 minutes should be allowed between administration of chlorhexidine and nystatin to ensure efficacy.

Treatment

Surgical patients:

- First-line: nystatin 5 ml four times a day.
- Second-line: fluconazole 50 mg tablet or sugar-free suspension, daily for 7 days.

Radiotherapy/chemotherapy patients:

- First-line: fluconazole 50 mg orally, daily for 7 days. Use 100 mg intravenously daily if patients cannot tolerate oral therapy.
- Second-line: fluconazole 200–400 mg intravenously daily until able to tolerate oral therapy.

Viral infections

Many viral infections may not require any specific treatment. However, infections such as herpes simplex virus will require treatment with topical 5% aciclovir, while severely immunocompromised patients may require systemic treatment with aciclovir or other antiviral agents to prevent and treat infection (Bagg 2005b). Other viral infections will require careful treatment consideration.

Bacterial infections

Bacterial infections of the oral cavity may require treatment with antibiotics. Clinicians should liaise with the microbiology department about the most appropriate use of drug. Bacterial abscesses within the mouth may require drainage by a dental surgeon. While bacterial infections of the actual oral mucosa are generally rare in developed countries, nevertheless careful consideration should be given to patients who are immunosuppressed due to disease (malignancy, human immunodeficiency virus [HIV]) and/or treatment (Bagg 2005a).

Painful mouth

First-line

Aspirin mouthwash four times a day (1–2 × 300 mg soluble tablets) used as mouthwash for oral cavity or a gargle for the oropharynx, mixed with lemon or raspberry mucilage to aid adherence of aspirin to the mucosa when treating the hypopharynx. Paracetamol is an alternative if aspirin is contraindicated (e.g. in clotting disorders, thrombocytopaenia).

Second-line

Lidocaine (lignocaine) 2% gel: applied four times a day for pain relief of mucositis or ulceration. For extensive mucositis use lidocaine spray; however, this can cause a secondary numbing effect on the throat, producing an aspiration pneumonitis if patients are not informed of the delay required before recommencing diet and fluids (Beck 1992). Sucralfate suspension: 5 ml four times a day rinsed around the mouth and swallowed. Owing to its coating action, sucralfate must be used last in the oral care medication sequence otherwise it will block the effect of any topical agent (Toth *et al.* 1996). The sucralfate coating may mask mucosal infections (e.g. candidiasis) so there should be close monitoring for signs and symptoms of an infection during its use (Toth *et al.* 1996). Gelclair may also be useful in relieving discomfort from ulceration by protecting the ulcer site.

Third-line

Low-dose opiates by oral, transdermal, subcutaneous or intravenous route. A continuous infusion or the use of patient controlled analgesia to treat severe mucositis pain such as seen in the haemato-oncology/stem cell transplant setting may be beneficial (Barasch *et al.* 2006; Dickinson & Porter 2006).

Reduced salivary flow

Sodium fluoride (e.g. Fluorigard) mouthwash used after breakfast and subsequent cleaning of teeth. No other mouthwash should be used for at least 1 hour after use as its action may be affected. Fluoride gel (e.g. Gel-Kam) should be brushed on the teeth last thing at night.

Treatment of dry mouth

Encourage regular oral fluids, artificial saliva (e.g. Saliva Orthana), two or three sprays four times daily or as often as necessary.

Treatment of dry lips

Apply lubricants to prevent cracking of lips and promote comfort.

Taste changes

Taste changes may be due to a number of factors including disease, smoking, ageing, malnutrition, drug treatment, other treatment (radiotherapy) and infection. It is important to treat the underlying cause of the taste disturbance, give advice on experimenting and varying diet. In some situations zinc therapy may be of benefit (Ripamonti & Fulfaro 2005).

Advances in mouth care

The last few years have seen multiple advances in the management of oral complications. Much of the research has arisen from the dental literature and may need to be researched in the cancer arena.

Local delivery of antimicrobials

Periodontitis is a bacterial infection which often appears in local areas within the oral cavity. Local antimicrobial delivery systems such as tetracycline fibre, doxycycline polymer, chlorhexidine chip, minocycline ointment and metronidazole gel are now available and aim to deliver high concentrations of antimicrobials directly to the site of the infection (Killoy 1998). These systems are currently used predominantly in the treatment of chronic inflammatory periodontal diseases.

Autologous saliva

Sreebny et al. (1995) investigated the use of autologous saliva in patients undergoing radiation for head and neck cancer. Their study showed them that it was feasible to collect saliva from patients prior to receiving radiation, sterilize it and ensure that it retained its protective properties. Saliva could then be stored in a saliva bank for use in post-radiation xerostomia.

Growth factors

Studies have been carried out to determine the efficacy of colony stimulating factors such as granulocyte-colony stimulating factor (G-CSF) and granulocyte-macrophage colony stimulating factor (GM-CSF) as a local and systemic treatment on the incidence of oral mucositis. While some studies seem to suggest that treatment with these agents has reduced the incidence and severity of mucositis (Kannan et al. 1997; Nicolatou et al. 1998; Rovirosa et al. 1998), other studies appear to show no overall reduction in mucositis (Mascarin *et al.* 1999; Makkonen *et al.* 2000; Sprinzl *et al.* 2001). It has been shown that by giving transforming growth factor (TGF) – β3, a potent negative regulator of epithelial and haemopoietic stem cell growth, it is possible to temporarily arrest oral mucosal basal cell proliferation and provide a safe and effective intervention for patients who undergo aggressive regimens of cancer therapy (Spijkervet & Sonis 1998). Clearly further research is still required.

Chlorhexidine chewing gum

Smith *et al.* (1996) showed that the use of a chlorhexidine chewing gum was as effective to oral hygiene and gingival health as a 0.2% chlorhexidine mouthwash. Teeth staining, a common side-effect of chlorhexidine mouthwash, was less with the gum than with the mouthwash, although this was not statistically significant. The chewing action can also help stimulate saliva production (Davies 2005).

Pilocarpine

This has been shown to improve saliva production and relieve symptoms of xerostomia after radiation of head and neck cancer. As a cholinergic drug the minor side-effects associated with its use were limited to sweating (Johnson *et al.* 1993).

Cryotherapy

Two studies carried out by Cascinu *et al.* (1994) and Dose (1992) found that using ice chips within the oral cavity decreased the incidence of 5-fluorouracil (5-FU)-induced stomatitis. 5-FU has a relatively short half-life, so by reducing the blood supply to the oral mucosa by application of cold before, during and after systemic bolus administration of the drug, the amount of 5-FU taken up by the cells can be reduced, thereby reducing cellular damage.

Mahood *et al.* (1991) found that when patients received cryotherapy (ice chips) at the time of chemotherapy administration, mucositis toxicity scores were decreased. Worthington *et al.* (2003) summarize their review by suggesting that cryotherapy may reduce the frequency and grade of mucositis during cytotoxic treatment: further evaluations are required.

Other treatments

Other treatments may include: amifostine, prostaglandin E (protectants), chamomile, steroids (anti-inflammatory), capsaicin, morphine (topical agents), keratinocyte growth factor (palifermin), L-glutamine, benzdamine HCL, and

N-acetylcysteine (Sonis 2004). Palifermin has been recommended for use in the malignant haematology setting when high doses of cytoxic treatment may cause damage to the mucosa (Keefe *et al.* 2007). Although sodium bicarbonate rinses are still used in practice, the evidence suggests that this may not be appropriate as this leads to an alteration of the pH which can disturb mucosal healing (Feber 1996). Critical consideration of each clinical situation should be made before deciding on the use of an oral care agent.

Nutrition

The patient's nutritional intake may not only be compromised by oral problems and other disease and treatment factors but lack of nutrition can lead to the worsening of oral problems. Nurses and the team should not neglect the importance of nutritional advice and support. Nurses working with the team need to: support the patient to adapt their diet to compensate for oral changes including the presence of mouth ulcers and taste changes; advise on supplementary foods; and consider the use of supportive measures including nasogastric, nasojejunal, percutaneous feeding and total parenteral nutrition (Blijlevens *et al.* 2000).

Summary

It is essential that nurses working in collaboration with other multiprofessional colleagues in all care settings have the knowledge and skills to carry out good oral care. While there is ongoing debate as to the most appropriate treatment, nurses should give particular attention to educating the patient, accurate assessment and correct care of the oral cavity. Specific consideration is required for those patients at risk of potential isolation, social ostracism and prejudice if lesions are visible and if halitosis is evident (Grealy 1994; Shorthose & Davies 2005). Good oral hygiene will help to minimize complications related to taste changes, infection, foul odour, bleeding and pain. This in turn will facilitate patient comfort. Special attention should be given to patients who require oral prostheses. A comfortable mouth will not only assist with appetite and food intake but will also help the patient feel more sociable and confident (Xavier 2000). Sexual relationships can also be disrupted in this group of patients as the mouth plays an important role in oral stimulation and sexual expression. To achieve optimum oral status for each individual patient, it is vital that the nurse uses all resources available and involves members of the multidisciplinary team (clinical nurse specialist, physician, dentist, dental hygienist, maxillofacial prosthodontist, pharmacist, pain control team, speech and language therapist, and dietitian). Any oral regimen must be evaluated frequently for efficacy and the patients and their families should know how to access members of the team for advice and support in the inpatient, outpatient and community setting.

Procedure guidelines Mouth care

Equipment

1 Clean tray.
2 Plastic cups.
3 Mouthwash or clean solutions.
4 Appropriate equipment for cleaning.
5 Clean receiver or bowl.
6 Paper tissues/gauze.
7 Wooden spatula.
8 Small-headed, soft toothbrush.
9 Toothpaste.
10 Disposable gloves.
11 Denture pot.
12 Small torch.

Items 1–11 may be left in the patient's locker when appropriate, and should be cleaned, renewed or replenished daily.

Procedure

Action	Rationale
1 Explain and discuss the procedure with the patient. When possible encourage patient to carry out their own oral care.	To ensure that the patient understands the procedure and gives his/her valid consent (Kozier *et al*. 1998: E; NMC 2006: C). To enable patients to gain confidence in managing their own symptom management (Larson *et al*. 1998: E).
2 Wash hands with bactericidal soap and water/bactericidal alcohol handrub and dry with paper towel. Put on disposable gloves.	To reduce the risk of cross-infection (DH 2005: C, R).
3 Prepare solutions required.	Solutions must always be prepared immediately before use to maximize their efficacy and minimize the risk of microbial contamination (DH 2005: C, R).
4 If the patient cannot remove their own dentures, using a tissue or piece of gauze, grasp the upper plate at the front teeth with the thumb and second finger and move the denture up and down slightly. Lower the upper plate, remove and place in denture pot.	Removal of dentures is necessary for cleaning of underlying tissues. A tissue or topical swab provides a firmer grip of the dentures and prevents contact with the patient's saliva. The slight movement breaks the suction that secures the plate (Kozier *et al*. 2003: E).
5 Lift the lower plate, turning it so that one side is lower than the other, remove and place in denture pot.	Lifting the lower plate at an angle helps removal of the denture without stretching the lips (Kozier *et al*. 2003: E).

6 Remove a partial denture by exerting equal pressure on the border of each side of the denture.

Holding the clasps could result in damage or breakage (Kozier *et al.* 1998: E).

7 Carry out oral assessment using a reliable oral assessment tool.

Provides base line to enable monitoring of mucosal changes, and evaluate response to treatment and care (Sonis *et al.* 2004: R 5; Eilers *et al.* 1988: R 5).

8 Inspect the patient's mouth, including teeth, with the aid of a torch, spatula and gauze, paying special attention to the lips, buccal mucosa, lateral and ventral surfaces of the tongue, floor of the mouth and the soft palate. Ask the patient if they have any of the following: taste changes, change in saliva production and composition, oral discomfort or difficulty swallowing.

The mouth is examined for changes in condition with respect to moisture, cleanliness, infected or bleeding areas, ulcers, etc. These areas are known to be more susceptible to cytoxic damage (Sonis *et al.* 2004: R 5). To assess nutritional deficits, salivary changes and pain secondary to oral changes (Sonis 2004: R 5).

867

9 Using a soft, small toothbrush and toothpaste (or foamstick if the gingiva is damaged or susceptible to bleeding) brush the patient's natural teeth, gums and tongue.

To remove adherent materials from the teeth, tongue and gum surfaces (Beck 2004: E). Brushing stimulates gingival tissues to maintain tone and prevent circulatory stasis (Pearson & Hutton 2002: R 1b; Clay 2000: E). Foamstick reduces possibility of trauma (Walton *et al.* 2002: E).

10 Hold the brush against the teeth with the bristles at a 45° angle. The tips of the outer bristles should rest against and penetrate under the gingival sulcus. Then move the bristles back and forth using horizontal or circular strokes and a vibrating motion (bass sulcular technique), from the sulcus to the crowns of the teeth. Repeat until all teeth surfaces have been cleaned. Clean the biting surfaces by moving the toothbrush back and forth over them in short strokes and brush tongue to remove any debris.

Brushing loosens and removes debris trapped on and between the teeth and gums (Kozier *et al.* 1998: E). This reduces the growth medium for pathogenic organisms and minimizes the risk of plaque formation and dental caries (Clay 2000: E; Pearson & Hutton 2002: R 1b; Beck 2004: E). Foamsticks are ineffective for this (Beck 2004: E).

Procedure guidelines *(cont.)*

11 Give a beaker of water or mouthwash to the patient. Encourage patient to rinse the mouth vigorously with water, normal saline, then void contents into a receiver. Paper tissues should be to hand.	Rinsing removes loosened debris and toothpaste and makes the mouth taste fresher. The glycerine content of toothpaste will have a drying effect and an aftertaste if left in the mouth (Beck 2004: E).
12 If the patient is unable to rinse and void, use a rinsed toothbrush to clean the teeth and moistened foamsticks to wipe the gums and oral mucosa. Foamsticks should be used with a rotating action so that most of the surface is utilized.	To remove debris as effectively as possible (Sonis 2004: R 5; Beck 2004: E).
13 Apply artificial saliva to the tongue if appropriate and/or suitable lubricant to dry lips.	To increase the patient's feeling of comfort and well-being and prevent further tissue damage (Davies 2000: R 1b).
14 Clean the patient's dentures on all surfaces with a denture brush or toothbrush. Check the dentures for cracks, sharp edges and missing teeth. Rinse them well and return them to the patient.	Cleaning dentures removes accumulated food debris which could be broken down by salivary enzymes to products which irritate and cause inflammation of the adjacent mucosal tissue (Curzio & McCowan 2000: R 5, R 1a).
15 Dentures should be removed at night and placed in a suitable cleaning solution.	Some commercial denture cleaners may have an abrasive effect on the denture surface. This then attracts plaque and encourages bacterial growth (Sweeney *et al.* 1995: R 2b; Clay 2000: E).
16 Dentures should be soaked in diluted antifungal solution for 4–6 hours daily if oral *Candida* species are present.	Soaking in diluted antifungal reduces the risk of reinfecting the mouth with infected dentures (Walton *et al.* 2002: E.)

17 Floss teeth (unless contraindicated, e.g. clotting abnormality, thrombocytopaenia) once in 24 hours using lightly waxed floss. To floss the upper teeth, use your thumb and index finger to stretch the floss and wrap one end of floss around the third finger of each hand. Move the floss up and down between the teeth from the tops of the crowns to the gum and along the gum lines wherever possible. To floss the lower teeth, use the index fingers to stretch the floss.	Flossing helps to remove debris between teeth. Flossing when patient has abnormal clotting or low platelets may lead to bleeding and predispose the oral mucosa to infection (Larson *et al.* 1998: E; Clay 2000: E; Beck 2004: E).
18 Discard remaining mouthwash solutions.	To prevent infection (DH 2005: C, R).
19 Clean and thoroughly dry the toothbrush.	To prevent the risk of contamination (Brook & Gober 1998: R 2b).
20 Wash hands with soap and water or alcohol handrub and dry with paper towel.	To reduce the risk of cross-infection (DH 2005: C, R).

Problem solving: Mouth care

Problem	Cause	Suggested action
Xerostomia: dry mouth.	Inadequate hydration.	Monitor fluid balance and increase fluid intake where necessary.
	Impaired production of saliva, e.g. as a consequence of radiotherapy or chemotherapy, drug or oxygen therapy.	Encourage patient to take sips of fluid regularly. Give the patient ice cubes to suck. Apply artificial saliva to the oral cavity as required (Davies 2005: R 5).
	Presence of specific stressors, e.g. mouth breathing, oxygen therapy, no oral intake, intermittent oral suction.	Inspect the mouth frequently, e.g. half-hourly. Swab mucosa with water. Provide humidified oxygen.

Problem solving (*cont.*)

Problem	Cause	Suggested action
Dry lips.	As above.	Smear a thin layer of appropriate lubricant.
Thick mucus.	Postoperative closure of a tracheostomy. Radiotherapy. Poor swallowing mechanism.	Use sodium bicarbonate solution in the mouth care procedure. Rinse the mouth afterwards with water or 0.9% sodium chloride.
Patient unable to tolerate toothbrush.	Pain, e.g. postoperatively; stomatitis.	Use foamsticks to clean the patient's gums and mucosa; 0.9% sodium chloride is advisable as a cleaning agent. For severe pain use an anaesthetic mouth spray or mouthwash before giving mouth care. Consider oral opiates.
Toothbrush inappropriate or ineffective.	Infected stomatitis. Accumulation of dried mucus, new lesions, blood or debris.	As above and take a swab of any infected areas for culture before giving mouth care.

References and further reading

Andersson, P. *et al.* (1999) Testing an oral assessment guide during chemotherapy treatment in a Swedish care setting: a pilot study. *J Clin Nurs*, **8**, 150–8.

Bagg, J. (2005a) Bacterial infections. In: *Oral Care in Advanced Disease* (eds A. Davies & I. Finlay). Oxford University Press, Oxford, pp. 55–72.

Bagg, J. (2005b) Viral infections. In: *Oral Care in Advanced Disease* (eds A. Davies & I. Finlay). Oxford University Press, Oxford, pp. 87–96.

Barasch, A. & Peterson, D.E. (2003) Risk factors for ulcerative oral mucositis in cancer patients: unanswered questions. *Oral Oncol*, **39**, 91–100.

Barasch, A. *et al.* (2006) Antimicrobials, mucosal coating agents, anaesthetics, analgesics & nutritional supplements for alimentary tract mucositis. *Support Care Cancer*, **14**, 528–32.

Barker, G. *et al.* (1991) The effects of sucralfate suspension and diphenhydramine syrup plus kaolin-pectin on radiotherapy-induced mucositis. *Oral Surg Oral Med Oral Pathol*, **71**(3), 288–93.

Barkvoll, P. *et al.* (1989) Effect of nystatin and chlorhexidine digluconate on *Candida albicans*.*Oral Surg Oral Med Oral Pathol*, **67**, 279–81.

Beck, S. (1992) Prevention and management of oral complications in cancer patients. Current issues. *Cancer Nurs Pract Updates*, **1**, 1–12.

Beck, S.L. (2004) Mucositis. In: *Cancer Symptom Management* (eds C. Henke-Yarbro, M. Hansen-Frogge & M. Goodman), 3rd edn. Jones and Bartlett, Sudbury, MA, pp. 276–92.

Bellm, L.A. *et al.* (2000) Patient reports of complications of bone marrow transplantation. *Support Care Cancer*, **8**, 33–9.

Blijlevens, N.M.A, Donnelly, J.P. & De Pauw, B.E. (2000) Mucosal barrier injury: biology, pathology, clinical counterparts and consequences of intensive treatment for haematological malignancy: an overview. *Bone Marrow Transplant*, **25**(12), 1269–78.

Borbasi, S. *et al.* (2002) More than a sore mouth: patient's experience of oral mucositis. *Oncol Nurs Forum*, **29**(7), 1051–7.

Borowski, B. *et al.* (1994) Prevention of oral mucositis in patients treated with high dose chemotherapy and bone marrow transplantation: a randomised controlled trial comparing two protocols of dental care. *Eur J Cancer Oral Oncol*, **30B**(2), 93–7.

Brammer, K.W. (1990) Management of fungal infection in neutropenic patients. *Haematol Blood Transf*, **33**, 546–50.

Brook, I. & Gober, A.E. (1998) Persistence of group A beta-hemolytic streptococci in toothbrushes and removable orthodontic appliances following treatment of pharyngotonsillitis. *Arch Otolaryngol Head Neck Surg*, **124**(9), 993–5.

Campbell, S. (1995) Treating oral candidiasis. *Community Nurse*, **1**(5), 12–13.

Cascinu, S. *et al.* (1994) Oral cooling (cryotherapy) an effective treatment for the prevention of 5-fluorouracil induced stomatitis. *Eur J Cancer B Oral Oncol*, **30B**, 234–6.

Chaushu, G. *et al.* (2000) Salivary flow and its relation with oral symptoms in terminally ill patients. *Cancer*, **88**, 984–7.

Cheng, K.K.F. (2006) Oral complications in patients with cancer. In: *Nursing a Patient with Cancer: Principles and Practice* (eds N. Kearney & A. Richardson). Elsevier, Edinburgh, pp. 575–600.

Cheng, K.K.F. *et al.* (2001) Evaluation of an oral care protocol intervention in the prevention of chemotherapy induced oral mucositis in paediatric cancer patients. *Eur J Cancer*, **37**, 2056–63.

Chiara, S. *et al.* (2001) Sucralfate in the treatment of chemotherapy-induced stomatitis: a double-blind, placebo-controlled pilot study. *Anticancer Res*, **21**, 3707–10.

Clay, M. (2000) Oral health in older people. *Nurs Older People*, **12**(7), 21–5.

Cooke, C. (1996) Xerostomia: a review. *Palliat Med*, **10**, 284–92.

Cooley, C. (2002) Oral health: basic or essential care? *Canc Nurs Pract*, **1**(3), 33–9.

Curzio, J. & McCowan, M. (2000) Getting research into practice: developing oral hygiene standards. *Br J Nurs*, **9**(7), 434–8.

Davies, A.N. (2000) A comparison of artificial saliva and chewing gum in the management of xerostomia in patients with advanced cancer. *Palliat Med*, **14**, 197–203.

Davies, A.N. (2005) Salivary gland dysfunction. In: *Oral Care in Advanced Disease* (eds A. Davies & I. Finlay). Oxford University Press, Oxford, pp. 97–114.

Davies, A.N, Broadley, K. & Beighton, D. (2002) Salivary gland hypofunction in patients with advanced cancer. *Oral Oncol*, **38**, 680–5.

DH (2001) *The Essence of Care: Patient Focussed Benchmarking for Healthcare Professionals*. HMSO, London.

871

DH (2005) *Saving Lives: a Delivery Programme to Reduce Healthcare Associated Infections including MRSA: Skills for Implementation.* Department of Health, London.

Dickinson, L. & Porter, H. (2006) Oral care. In: *Nursing in Haematological Nursing* (ed. M. Grundy), 2nd edn. Balliere Tindall, Edinburgh, pp. 371–86.

Dodds, M.J. (2004) The pathogenesis and characterisation of oral mucositis associated with cancer therapy. *Oncol Nurs Forum*, **31**(4), 5–11.

Dodd, M.J. *et al.* (1996) Randomized clinical trial of chlorhexidine versus placebo for prevention of oral mucositis in patients receiving chemotherapy. *Oncol Nurs Forum*, **23**(6), 921–7.

Dodd, M.J. *et al.* (2000) Randomised clinical trial of the effectiveness of three commonly used mouthwashes to treat chemotherapy-induced mucositis. *Oral Surg Oral Med Oral Path*, **90**(1), 39–47.

Dose, A.M. (1992) Cryotherapy for prevention of 5-fluorouracil induced mucositis. Cancer nursing, changing frontiers. Proceedings of the 7th International Conference of Cancer Nursing. *Eur J Cancer Care*, **2**(1), 95–7.

Dudjak, L. (1987) Mouth care for mucositis due to radiation therapy. *Cancer Nurs*, **10**, 131–40.

Eilers, J. (2004) Nursing interventions and supportive care for the prevention and treatment of oral mucositis associated with cancer treatment. *Oncol Nurs Forum*, **31**(4), 13–23.

Eilers, J. *et al.* (1988) Development, testing and application of the oral assessment guide. *Oncol Nurs Forum*, **15**(3), 325–30.

Feber, T. (1996) Management of oral mucositis in oral irradiation. *Clin Oncol*, **8**, 106–11.

Ferretti, G.A. *et al.* (1990) Chlorhexidine prophylaxis for chemotherapy- and radiotherapy-induced stomatitis: a randomised double-blind trial. *Oral Surg Oral Med Oral Pathol*, **69**(3), 331–7.

Finlay, I. & Davies, A. (2005) Fungal infections. In: *Oral Care in Advanced Disease* (eds A. Davies & I. Finlay). Oxford University Press, Oxford, pp. 55–72.

Fitzpatrick, J. (2000) Oral health care needs of dependent older people: responsibilities of nurses and care staff. *J Adv Nurs*, **32**(6), 1325–32.

Foote, R.L. *et al.* (1994) Randomized trial of a chlorhexidine mouthwash for alleviation of radiation-induced mucositis. *J Clin Oncol*, **12**(12), 2630–3.

Grealy, L. (1994) *Autobiography of a Face.* Harperennial, New York.

Hahn, M.J. & Jones, A. (2000) Mouth care. In: *Head and Neck Nursing.* Churchill Livingstone, London, pp. 35–57.

Heals, D. (1993) A key to well being: oral hygiene in patients with advanced cancer. *Prof Nurse*, **8**(6), 391–8.

Holmes, S. (1990) *Cancer Chemotherapy.* Lisa Sainsbury Foundation. Austen Cornish, London, pp. 180–1.

Holmes, S. & Mountain, E. (1993) Assessment of oral status: evaluation of three oral assessment guides. *J Clin Nurs*, **2**, 35–40.

Howarth, H. (1977) Mouth care procedures for the very ill. *Nurs Times*, **73**, 354–5.

Jaroneski, L.A. (2006) The importance of assessment rating scales for chemotherapy-induced oral mucositis. *Oncol Nurs Forum*, **33**(6), 1085–93.

Johnson, J.T. *et al.* (1993) Oral pilocarpine for post irradiation xerostomia in patients with head and neck cancer. *N Engl J Med*, **329**(6), 390–5.

Jones, A.L. & Gore, M.E. (1995) Medical treatment of malignant tumours of the mouth, jaw and salivary glands. In: *Malignant Tumours of the Mouth, Jaws and Salivary Glands* (eds J.D. Langdon & J.M. Henk), 2nd edn. Edward Arnold, London, pp. 123–35.

Kannan, V. *et al.* (1997) Efficacy and safety of granulocyte macrophage-colony stimulating factor (GM-CSF) on the frequency and severity of radiation mucositis in patients with head and neck carcinoma. *Int J Radiat Oncol Biol Phys*, **37**(5), 1005–10.

Keefe, D.M. *et al.* (2007) Mucositis Study Section of the Multinational Association of Supportive Care in Cancer and the International Society for Oral Oncology. *Cancer,* **109**(5), 820–31.

Killoy, W.J. (1998) Chemical treatment of periodontitis: local delivery of antimicrobials. *Int Dent J*, **3**(Suppl), 305–15.

Kozier, B. *et al.* (2003) Hygiene. In: *Fundamentals of Nursing: Concepts, Process & Practice*. Pearson Education, New Jersy, pp. 695–755.

Krishnasamy, M. (1995) Oral problems in advanced cancer. *Eur J Cancer Care*, **4**, 173–7.

Kusler, D.L. & Rambur, B.A. (1992) Treatment for radiation-induced xerostomia: an innovative remedy. *Cancer Nurs*, **15**(3), 191–5.

Larson, P.J. *et al.* (1998) The PRO-SELF mouth aware programme: an effective approach for reducing chemotherapy-induced mucositis. *Cancer Nurs*, **21**(4), 263–8.

Lippold, A.J.C. & Winton, F.R. (1972) *Hearing and Speech Human Physiology*. Churchill Livingstone, Edinburgh, pp. 443–64.

Loesche, W.J. & Kazor, C. (2002) Microbiology and treatment of halitosis. *Periodontol 2000*, **28**, 256–79.

Madeya, M.L. (1996) Oral complications from cancer therapy. Part 2: nursing implications for assessment and treatment. *Oncol Nurs Forum*, **23**(5), 808–19.

Mahood, D.J. *et al.* (1991) Inhibition of fluorouracil-induced stomatitis by oral cryotherapy. *J Clin Oncol*, **9**(3), 449–52.

Makkonen, T.A. *et al.* (2000) Granulocyte macrophage-colony stimulating factor (GM-CSF) and sucralfate in prevention of radiation-induced mucositis: a prospective randomised study. *Int J Radiat Oncol Biol Phys*, **46**(3), 525–34.

Marieb, E.N. (2004) *Human Anatomy & Physiology*, 6th edn. Pearson, San Francisco.

Martini, F. (2007) *Fundamentals of Anatomy and Physiology*, 7th edn. Benjamin Cummings, San Francisco, CA.

Mascarin, M. *et al.* (1999) The effect of granulocyte colony-stimulating factor on oral mucositis in head and neck cancer patients treated with hyperfractionated radiotherapy. *Oral Oncol*, **35**, 203–8.

McGuire, D.B. *et al.* (2006) The role of basic oral care and good clinical practice principles in the management of oral mucositis. *Support Care Cancer*, **14**, 541–5.

McNeill, H.E. (2000) Biting back at poor oral hygiene. *Inten Crit Care Nurs*, **16**, 367–72.

Miller, M. & Kearney, N. (2001) Oral care for patients with cancer: a review of the literature. *Cancer Nurs*, **24**(4), 241–54.

National Institutes of Health (1987) *Consensus Development Conference Statement on Oral Complications of Cancer Therapies: Diagnosis, Prevention, and Treatment.* National Cancer Institute, 7(17), 1–11.

Nicolatou, O. *et al.* (1998) A pilot study of the effect of granulocyte-macrophage colony-stimulating factor on oral mucositis in head and neck cancer patients during X-radiation therapy. *Int J Radiat Oncol Biol Phys*, **42**(3), 551–6.

NMC (2006) *A–Z Advice Sheet Consent.* www.nmc.org.

Ohrn, K.E.O., Wahlin, Y.B. & Sjoden, P.O. (2000) Oral care in cancer nursing. *Eur J Cancer Care*, **9**, 22–9.

Pearson, L.S. (1996) A comparison of the ability of foam swabs and toothbrushes to remove dental plaque: implications for nursing practice. *J Adv Nurs*, **23**(1), 62–9.

Pearson, L.S. & Hutton, J.L. (2002) A controlled trial to compare the ability of foam swabs and toothbrushes to remove dental plaque. *J Adv Nurs*, **39**(5), 480–9.

Porter, H.J. (1994) Mouth care in cancer. *Nurs Times*, **90**(14), 27–9.

Porter, H.J. (2000) Oral care. In: *Nursing in Haematological Oncology* (ed. M. Grundy). Harcourt, London, pp. 371–85.

Quinn, B. *et al.* (2007) Ensuring accurate oral mucositis assessment in the European Group for Blood and Marrow Transplantation Prospective Oral Mucositis Audit. *Eur J Oncol Nurs*, **11**(Supp 1), 10–18.

Rattan, J. *et al.* (1994) Sucralfate suspension as a treatment of recurrent aphthous stomatitis. *J Intern Med*, **236**, 341–3.

Rawlins, C.A. & Trueman, J.W. (2001) Effective mouth care for seriously ill patients. *Prof Nurs*, **16**(14), 1025–8.

Ripamonti, C. & Fulfaro, F. (2005) Taste disturbance. In: *Oral Care in Advanced Disease* (eds A. Davies & I. Finlay). Oxford University Press, Oxford, pp. 115–24.

Roberts, J. (2004) Developing an oral assessment and intervention tool for older people. In: *Trends in Oral Health Care* (ed. R. White). Quay Books, Wiltshire, pp. 11–35.

Rovirosa, A., Ferre, J. & Biete, A. (1998) Granulocyte macrophage-colony stimulating factor mouthwashes heal oral ulcers during head and neck radiotherapy. *Int J Radiat Oncol Biol Phys*, **41**(4), 747–54.

Royal Marsden Hospital (2002) *The Royal Marsden Hospital Prescribing Guidelines for Mouth Care.* Drugs and Therapeutic Advisory Committee, September. The Royal Marsden Hospital, London.

Royal Pharmaceutical Society of Great Britain (2006) *British National Formulary.* RFS Publishing, Bedfordshire.

Rubenstein, E.B. *et al.* (2004) Clinical practice guidelines for the prevention and treatment of cancer therapy-induced oral and gastrointestinal mucositis. *Cancer*, **100**(9 Suppl), 2026–46.

Schubert, M.M. *et al.* (1992) Clinical assessment scale for rating of oral mucosal changes associated with bone marrow transplantation. *Cancer*, **69**, 2469–77.

Shih, A. *et al.* (2003) Mechanisms for radiation-induced oral mucositis and the consequences. *Cancer Nurs*, **26**(3), 222–9.

Shorthose, K. & Davies, A. (2005) Halitosis. In: *Oral Care in Advanced Disease* (eds A. Davies & I. Finlay). Oxford University Press, Oxford, pp. 125–32.

Smith, A.J. *et al.* (1996) The efficacy of an anti-gingivitis chewing gum. *J Clin Periodontol*, **23**(1), 19–23.

Sonis, S. (2004) The pathobiology of mucositis. *Nat Rev Cancer*, **4**(4), 277–84.

Sonis, S. *et al.* (2004) Perspectives on cancer therapy-induced mucosal injury: pathogenesis, measurement, epidemiology, and consequences for patients. *Cancer Suppl*, **100**(9), 1995–2025.

Southern, H. (2007) Oral care in cancer nursing: nurses' knowledge and education. *J Adv Nurs*, **57**(6), 631–8.

Spijkervet, F.K. & Sonis, S.T. (1998) New frontiers in the management of chemotherapy-induced mucositis. *Curr Opin Oncol*, **10**(Suppl 1), S23–7.

Sprinzl, G.M. *et al.* (2001) Local application of granulocyte-macrophage colony stimulating factor (GM-CSF) for the treatment or oral mucositis. *Eur J Cancer*, **37**, 2003–9.

Sreebny, L.M. (2000) Saliva in health and disease: an appraisal and update. *Int Dent J*, **50**, 140–61.

Sreebny, L.M., Zhu, W.X. & Meek, A.G. (1995) The preparation of an autologous saliva for use with patients undergoing therapeutic radiation for head and neck cancer. *J Oral Maxillofac Surg*, **53**(2), 131–9.

Stiff, P. (2001) Mucositis associated with stem cell transplantation: current status and innovative approaches to management. *Bone Marrow Transplant*, **27**, S3–11.

Stone, B. *et al.* (2005) Improving oral care: quality control of oral mucositis assessment in the EBMT prospective oral mucositis audit. *Bone Marrow Transplant*, **37**(1), S273–274.

Stone, R. *et al.* (2007) Management of oral mucositis at European transplantation centres. *Eur J Oncol Nurs*, **11**(Suppl 1), 3–9.

Sweeney, M.P. *et al.* (1995) Oral health in elderly patients. *Br J Nurs*, **4**(20), 1204–8.

Sweeney, P. (2005) Oral hygiene. In: *Oral Care in Advanced Disease* (eds A. Davies & I. Finlay). Oxford University Press, Oxford, pp. 21–36.

Taji, S.S. & Rogers, A.H. (1998) ADRF Trebitsch Scholarship. The microbial contamination of toothbrushes. A pilot study. *Aust Dent J*, **43**(2), 128–30.

Thiobodeau, G.A. & Patton, K.T. (2007) *Anatomy & Physiology*, 6th edn. Elsevier, St Louis, MO.

Torres, S.R. *et al.* (2002) Relationship between salivary flow rates and *Candida* counts in subjects with xerostomia. *Oral Surg Oral Med Oral Path*, **93**(2), 149–54.

Toth, B.B. & Frame, R.T. (1983) Dental oncology. *Curr Probl Cancer*, **10**, 7–35.

Toth, B.B., Chambers, M.S. & Fleming, T.C. (1996) Prevention and management of oral complications associated with cancer therapies: radiotherapy/chemotherapy. *Texas Dent J*, **113**(6), 23–9.

Walton, J.C., Miller, J. & Tordecilla, L. (2002) Elder oral assessment and care. *ORL Head Neck Nurs*, **20**(2), 12–19.

Waly, N.G. (1995) Local antifibrinolytic treatment with tranexamic acid in hemophiliac children undergoing dental extractions. *Egypt Dent J*, **41**(1), 961–8.

White, R. (2004) Oral health assessment: a review of current practice. In: *Trends in Oral Health Care* (ed. R. White). Quay Books, Wiltshire, pp. 1–10.

White, R.J. (2000) Nurse assessment of oral health: a review of practice and education. *Br J Nursing*, **9**(5), 260–6.

WHO (1979) *Handbook for Reporting Results of Cancer Treatment*. Offset Publications, Geneva, **48**, pp. 15–22.

Worthington, H.V., Clarkson, J.E. & Eden, O.B. (2003) Interventions for the prevention of oral mucositis for patients with cancer receiving treatments. *Cochrane Database Syst Rev*, **2**.

Xavier, G. (2000) The importance of mouth care in prevention. *Nurs Stand*, **14**(18), 47–51.

Yusef, Z.W. & Bakri, M.M. (1993) Severe progressive periodontal destruction due to radiation tissue injury. *J Periodontol*, **64**(12), 1253–8.

See page 891 for multiple choice questions covering this chapter.

Chapter 25

Personal hygiene: skin care

Definition

Personal hygiene is the physical act of cleaning the body to ensure that the skin, hair and nails are maintained in an optimum condition (DH 2001a). The prevention of infection is also pertinent and will be referred to within the text (see also Chapter 5).

Reference material

'Cleanliness is not a luxury in a highly developed country, it is ... a basic human right' (Young 1991, p. 54). When an individual becomes ill, he or she may depend on others to perform this elementary intervention. If this occurs, it is important that the nurse is able to appropriately observe and assess the patient.

Hygiene is a personal entity and everyone will have their own individual requirements and standards of cleanliness. In this way, 'nurses must take care not to impose their own norms on patients and clients and should respect their autonomy in decisions concerning care' (Spiller 1992, p. 431). When assessing personal considerations, the patient's religious and cultural beliefs should be taken into account. Personal hygiene is individual to that person and is also based on family influences, peer groups, economic and social factors (Cooper 1994). Various examples of this will be discussed in this chapter.

In Western culture, privacy is of the utmost importance and considered to be a basic human right. In some cultures, modesty is crucial, e.g. for Muslims, and can cause problems in the hospital setting (Neuberger 1987). Patients will feel a great deal of embarrassment having to depend on another person to help/assist them with this extremely private act and consideration should be given to their personal needs (Wagnild & Manning 1985; Spiller 1992). It is therefore surprising to find that such little reference is made to these elements in the literature. The nurse's role is continued provision of appropriate levels of cleanliness (Young 1991), which promotes 'comfort, safety and well-being' for the patient, and should be carried out with skill and knowledge (Whiting 1999, p. 339). Frequently, the time taken to attend to personal hygiene will provide ample opportunity for communication. Wilson states:

> … a bedbath facilitates listening and enables the nurse to pick up cues to a patient's anxieties and fears. It provides the time and opportunity for the nurse to offer support and encouragement when difficult situations have to be confronted, solutions sought and decisions made.
>
> (Wilson 1986, p. 81)

This also focuses on the nurse's ability to be with the patient as well as provide for the patient (Campbell 1984) and is part of the essence of nursing care (Kitson 1999). This derives from theorists such as Henderson (1966) and Nightingale (1969) focusing on the aspect of patient-centred care or holistic care. This is as essential when thinking of the personal hygiene of patients as it is about the uniqueness of patients, their needs and how they wish to be treated.

It is during the delivery of personal hygiene that the nurse is able to demonstrate a wide range of skills such as assessment, communication, observation and caring for the patient. This can be the most significant social interaction of the day for the patient, as the nurse develops a deeper understanding of the patient's personality and needs, providing a personal bond between the nurse and patient (Hector & Touhy 1997). Health care assistants with a recognized qualification such as a National Vocational Qualification (NVQ) can complement the role of the qualified nurse in the implementation of planned care. It is vital that health professionals share their knowledge and any changes identified during procedures; personal feedback and documentation are good vehicles for this.

Nursing models, which provide a conceptual framework for practice, all make some reference to meeting the patient's hygiene needs. Roper *et al.* (1981) adapted Henderson's original concept of nursing (Henderson 1966) to develop a model reflecting the activities of daily living. Another example was given by Orem (1980) who focused on the ability of the patient to self-care and refers to the universal self-care requisites of the skin, nail and hair condition and the patterns of standard hygiene. Gordon (1994) discusses formulation of nursing diagnosis. Following assessment, clusters of actual or potential health problems are established; specific diagnosis are used to describe these. Clinical knowledge is then applied, to provide problem solving activities to achieve a set outcome.

Benchmarking is a valid framework by which nurses can establish and share best practice throughout the work environment. Three benchmarks, hygiene, self-care and privacy and dignity cited in the *Essence of Care* (CH 2001a), are important to consider when reviewing patient hygiene, and the needs should be carried out to an uncompromising standard (Geraghty 2005):

- All patients are assessed to identify the advice and/or assistance required in maintaining and promoting their individual personal hygiene.

- Planned care is negotiated with patients and/or their carers and is based on assessment of their individual needs.
- Patients have access to an environment that is safe and acceptable to the individual.
- Patients are expected to supply their own toiletries but single-use toiletries are provided until they can supply their own.
- Patients have access to the level of assistance that they require to meet their individual personal hygiene (DH 2001a).

Areas of care

Skin care

A definition of healthy skin is that it is fulfilling all of its functions, so an individual's quality of life is not adversely affected (Penzer & Finch 2001). Being the largest organ of the body, maintaining its integrity is essential to the prevention of infection and the promotion of both physical and psychological health. The skin has several functions (Burr & Penzer 2005):

- Regulation of temperature.
- Physical protection and immunological protection.
- Excretion and preservation of water balance.
- Sensory perception.
- Psycho-social: how the individual is perceived.

It is made up of three layers: the epidermis, dermis and the deep subcutaneous layer.

The *epidermis* is the outer coating of the skin and contains no blood vessels or nerve endings. The cells on the surface are gradually shed from the surface and replaced by new cells which have developed from the deeper layers; this process takes approximately 28 days. The epidermis has hairs, sweat glands and the ducts of sebaceous glands passing through it. It provides an efficient natural barrier (Burr & Penzer 2005).

The *dermis* is the thicker layer which contains blood vessels, nerve fibres, sweat and sebaceous glands and lymph vessels. It is made up of white fibrous tissue and yellow elastic fibres which give the skin its toughness and elasticity. It provides the epidermis with structural and nutritional support (Holloway & Jones 2005).

The *subcutaneous layer* contains the deep fat cells (areolar and adipose tissue) and provides the heat regulation factor for the body. It is also the support structure for the outer layers of the skin (Ross & Wilson 2001). Maintaining the skin integrity, through good personal hygiene, will allow this complex process to provide the efficient natural barrier.

It is important to remember the skin is a changing organ, affected by internal and external factors, temperature, air humidity and age (Burr & Penzer 2005). It has a great ability to adapt to changes in the environment and stimuli; however, it will be affected by ill health and immobility (McLoughlin 2005). Its integrity, continuity and cleanliness are essential to maintain its physiological functions.

The ageing process can adversely affect the skin structure. Skin tissue becomes thin, less elastic and resistant to trauma and shearing forces. The blood supply is reduced as cells replace more slowly; affecting healing. Transmission from sensory receptors on stimuli slows and can lead to damage. The natural oils produced decline and can lead to dry skin which increases the risk of infection and tissue breakdown (Penzer & Finch 2001) (see Chapter 34). Hence extra care and vigilance should be taken when washing and drying elderly patients; nursing interventions can protect and restore the skin's natural barrier (Ersser *et al.* 2005).

An initial assessment using observational skills is essential to ascertain the skin's general condition, colour, texture, smell and temperature (Penzer & Finch 2001). To accurately observe and assess changes in the skin, an understanding of the structure and function and factors that cause disruption is essential, so as to identify those at increased risk (Ersser *et al.* 2005).

Several factors may influence the appearance of the tissue:

- Nutritional and hydration state: imbalances will cause loss of elasticity and drying of the skin. Oedema will cause stretching and thinning of the skin (Potter & Perry 1995).
- Incontinence: the presence of urine and faeces on the skin increase the normal pH of 4.0–5.5 and makes the skin wet. This rise of pH and excess moisture increase the risks of tissue breakdown and infection (Ersser *et al.* 2005).
- The individual's age, health and mobility status (Smoker 1999), e.g. presence of pressure ulcers (see Chapter 34).
- Treatment therapies, e.g. radiotherapy (skin may become moist and cracked), chemotherapy (some cytotoxic agents such as methotrexate can cause erythematous rashes) and continuous infusions of 5-fluorouracil (5-FU) can cause a condition called palmar–plantar erythrodysesthesia syndrome, which presents with cracking and epidermal sloughing of the palms and soles (Lokich & Moore 1984). A low platelet count can lead to an increased risk of bruising and a decrease in the white blood cells can influence the rate of healing. Steroids may cause the skin to become papery and fragile (see Chapters 35, Professional edition & 34).
- Any concurrent conditions, e.g. eczema, psoriasis, diabetes, or stress can affect the ability of skin to maintain its integrity (Holloway & Jones 2005).

Frailty and the presence of pressure ulcers, redness, abrasions, cuts, papery skin and open wounds should prompt the nurse to take extra care in the bathing procedure. Involving patients in their care plans ensures that correct and/or preferred lotions are used. Persistent use of some soaps can alter the pH of the skin and remove the natural oils, leading to drying and cracking (Smoker 1999), and provide an ideal environment for bacteria to multiply (Holloway & Jones 2005). According to Ersser *et al.* (2005), patients with dry skin have a 2.5-fold likelihood of skin break down. In addition, patients may like to use moisturizers and this should be respected and applied accordingly. Care should be taken with skin folds and crevices, paying particular attention to thorough drying of the areas and observing for any breaks in the skin. It is recommended that the skin is patted and not rubbed, to reduce damage caused by friction (Ersser *et al.* 2005).

A growing body of evidence is recommending a move away from traditional washing using soap and water, for some of the reasons mentioned previously. Penzer and Finch (2001) and Burr and Penzer (2005) recommend a soap substitute using emollient therapy, for washing and moisturizing to seal the skin. In a literature review of hygiene practices, the use of soap and water remains common practice; however several studies suggest skin cleansers, for example emollient creams, followed by moisturizing, may be less likely to disrupt the skin barrier and have a therapeutic benefit (Ersser *et al.* 2005). A different range of products are allowing the patient to play a more active role (Collins & Hampton 2003). Prepackaged clothes impregnated with cleanser and moisturizer are a cost-effective, evidence-based alternative (Sheppard & Brenner 2000). They require no rinsing and are as effective at cleansing and more skin preserving than soap and water (Byers *et al.* 1995).

Frequently, patients may have intravenous devices and wound drains inserted as part of their therapy and these should be handled with caution to prevent the hazards of introducing infection or of 'pulling' the tubes.

Patients who require assistance may be able to have a bath or shower depending on their level of dependence. Alternatively, assistance with care may occur by the bedside or in bed as 'bed bathing'. When practising bed bathing the nurse informs the patient of his/her plan of care, seeking consent from the patient or patient's family/carer, especially if hoists, slides or transfer sheets are to be used. The nurse must also respect cultural and religious factors, privacy and dignity at all times, e.g. some people prefer to sit under running water as opposed to sitting in a bath (Sampson 1982).

- Those following Islam must do ablution (Wudhu, to use the Islamic term) before the daily prayer, which is the formal washing of the face, hands and forearms, etc. One of the criteria for cleanliness is washing after the use of the lavatories. Any traces of urine or faeces must be eliminated by washing with water, at least. The use of toilet tissues for cleaning is not sufficient. With such emphasis on washing and personal hygiene, adhering to the practical teaching of Islam on washing would enhance personal hygiene for the individual and therefore reduce the chance of disease and sickness individually and sub-sequently for the whole society.

- Hindus also place importance on washing before prayer; they believe the left hand should dominate in this process and therefore do not eat with the left hand as it is deemed unclean.

- Sikhs place great importance on not shaving or cutting hair, choosing to comb their hair twice a day, wash regularly, and wear their hair underneath a turban in a sign of respect for God.

Perineal/perianal care

When the nurse is performing care for the perineal/ perianal area, the patient may be embarrassed or humiliated. Care should be taken to maintain privacy at all times. It is important that informed consent is sought. This requires the nurse and patient to engage in a two-way process: where agreement is given for the nurse to provide care (DH 2001b).

It is important to be meticulous with this area, especially for those people who may be prone to infection (see Chapter 13).

Problems arising from treatment therapy, for example radiotherapy, fistulae, diarrhoea, constipation and urinary tract infections, require additional vigilance with cleanliness and patients should be encouraged at every opportunity to per-form this themselves (see Chapter 35, Professional edition) (Haisfield Wolfe 1998).

Ideally, perineal hygiene should be attended to after the general bath or, at the very least, the water and wipes should be changed and cleaned once utilized (Gooch 1989; Gould 1994) due to the large colonies of bacteria that tend to live in or around this area (Gould 1994). It is generally acknowledged that soap and lotions administered improperly to the perineum/perianal area can cause irritation and infection (Ersser *et al*. 2005; Holloway & Jones 2005). Many nurses will use soap or a similar chemical derivative in order to promote and ensure thorough cleaning, but frequently lack of knowledge can lead to further problems and discomfort for the patients (Lindell & Olsson 1989). It is suggested that warm water alone be used to avoid irritating the mucous membranes which become sensitive during the ageing process.

Hair care

The way a person feels is often related to their appearance. Hair care can be complex: consideration should be given to the patient's personal preferences.

Washing of the hair can be difficult if a patient is bed-bound, but there are several ways to manage this. To wash a patient's hair, move the patient to the top of the bed and hang their head over the end. The patient's condition must be assessed before performing this task; for example, it would not be appropriate for patients with head and neck or spinal injuries. Shampooing frequency depends on the patient's well-being and his/her hair condition. Referral to a hairdresser may also be appropriate.

Grooming the hair provides an ideal opportunity to observe for dandruff, psoriasis, flaky skin and head lice. Head lice are extremely infectious so it is imperative to treat the hair with a medicated shampoo from the pharmacy as soon as possible. Hospital policy/protocol should be followed regarding the disposal of infected linen. Towel drying of hair should occur. Hairdryers can be used with the consent of the patient: use of a hairdryer may not be appropriate if patient has had recent alopecia due to chemotherapy. Hairdryers should be checked for safety by the hospital electrician.

A patient's cultural and religious beliefs should always be taken into consideration when attending to his/her hair. Some religions do not allow hair washing or brushing, while others may require the hair to be covered by a turban. Similarly, in some countries facial hair is significant and should never be removed without the patient's/relatives' consent. Always establish any preferences before beginning care.

In the oncology setting, chemotherapy is an established treatment and some cytotoxic drugs can cause alopecia (loss of hair). The patient's physical, psychological and social needs are affected by the loss of hair. Special care and skilled advice are required regarding the adjustment to hair loss. Referral to the hospital surgical appliance officer is appropriate to discuss the choice and fitting of a wig. A shampoo with a neutral pH is recommended for patients who are at risk of alopecia. Prevention of alopecia is discussed further in Chapter 39, Professional edition.

Care of the beard and moustache is also important. Excess food can often become lodged here so regular grooming is essential for hygiene and comfort purposes. Beard trimmers can be used as appropriate.

Care of the nails and feet

The feet and nails require special care in order to avoid pain and infection occurring. Nails should be trimmed correctly. Specialist advice from a chiropodist can be useful. Chronic diseases such as diabetes and the long-term use of steroids can result in problems such as pressure ulcers, breakdown of the skin integrity and delays in the healing process. Special attention should be paid to cleaning the feet and in between the toes to avoid any fungal infection (Geraghty 2005). Powders and creams are available that help with the treatment of infections and odour management, e.g. miconazole nitrate 2% for fungal infections.

Care of the ears and nose

Lack of attention to cleaning the ears and nose can lead to impairment of the senses. Usually these small organs require minimal care, but observation for a buildup of wax in the ears and deposits in the nose is essential to maintain patency.

Special care should be taken to avoid damage to the aural cavity or ear drum. Clean area with cotton wool or gauze and warm water.

Patients undergoing enteral feeding and oxygen therapy should have regular nasal care to avoid excessive drying and excoriating of the delicate air passages. Gentle cleaning of the nasal mucosa with wool/gauze and water is recommended and application of a thin coating of a water-based lubricant to prevent discomfort can be beneficial; this will remove debris and maintain a moist environment (Geraghty 2005).

Patients who have had piercing of the ears or nose will require cleaning of the holes to avoid the risk of infection. Gently cleaning around the piercing area, cotton wool/gauze and warm water should be used and the area towel dried. Observe for inflammation or oozing. If this occurs, inform the patient and doctor. Remove device on consent of the patient if inflammation or oozing occurs.

884

Eye care

Specific aspects of eye care, e.g. irrigation, are referred to in Chapter 23.

In general, the eye structure and delicate surface are protected by the tears that maintain the eye's moistness, but in a patient who is unconscious, drying of the eye may occur (Ross & Wilson 2001). Gentle cleaning with low-linting gauze and 0.9% sodium chloride will be sufficient to prevent infection and will keep the eyes moist. The eye is an important organ of communication and consideration should always be given to a patient's sight aids, e.g. glasses, contact lenses. Assistance may be required to help clean these aids and advice regarding the most appropriate method should be sought, preferably from the patient.

Some patients may have an artificial eye and care should be taken to ensure this remains clean. Advice regarding the ideal method of removal and insertion should be sought, from the local ophthalmology service or nursing team in ophthalmology unit.

Mouth care

Mouth care, e.g. cleaning and infection control, is referred to in Chapter 24.

Summary

Personal hygiene of patients is an integral part of the role of the nurse, creating a bond with the patient. In doing this, the nurse is able to spend time with his/her patient listening to issues, concerns or fears the patient may have regarding admission, treatment, discharge planning or prognosis. This may help to build a therapeutic relationship.

The nurse must recognize the uniqueness of the patient who may depend on others to assist them in times of ill health; respect and thought should be given to individual preferences (Whiting 1999). Comfort, cleanliness, availability of washing facilities, privacy and assistance from nurses were expressed as being important in providing hygiene care by patients in a recent ward audit (unpublished) at The Royal Marsden Hospital.

The world of nursing is ever changing, and there is a risk that activities such as attending to the personal hygiene of patients may become devalued or just another routine. The literature supports the enhanced quality of care to patients, when hygiene needs are attended to by qualified/experienced practitioners (Carr-Hill *et al.* 1992). Personal hygiene is considered part of the essence of care that nurses should never treat as ritualistic.

885

Procedure guidelines   **Bed bathing a patient**

Procedure

Prior to each part of the procedure, explain and obtain agreement from the patient. The procedure can provide the opportunity to build the nurse/patient relationship, during this time patients can discuss the issues troubling them. Planned care is negotiated with the patient and is based on assessment of their individual needs. Planned care should be documented and changed according to the patient's/carer's needs on a daily basis. Before commencing this procedure, read the patient's care plan, manual handling documentation and risk assessment to gain knowledge of safe practice.

Action	Rationale
1 Assess and plan care with the patient and family/friend if desired. Note personal preferences, addressing religious and cultural beliefs.	To plan care and encourage participation and independence (NMC 2008: E, C).
2 Clear area of any obstacles, ensure environment warm and draw curtains/close doors to guarantee privacy and dignity.	To maintain comfort, a safe environment and promote privacy and dignity (NMC 2008: C, E).
3 Offer patient urinal, bedpan or commode.	To reduce any disruption to procedure and prevent any discomfort (NMC 2008: C, E).

Procedure guidelines *(cont.)*

4 Collect all equipment by bedside:
  - Clean bed linen.
  - Bath towels.
  - Laundry skip, applying local guidelines for soiled and/or infected linen.
  - Flannels, preferably disposable.
  - Toiletries, as preferred by patient.
  - Clean clothes as desired.
  - Wash bowl and warm water; ensure bowl is cleaned with hot soapy water before use.
  - Comb/brush/razor/scissors/nail clippers.
  - Equipment for oral hygiene.
  - Any manual handling equipment.

To minimize time away from patient during procedure.
Disposable flannels are preferable as this reduces the risk of infection. To meet patient preference during procedure (NMC 2008: E, P, R).

5 Wash hands; use disposable gloves and aprons according to local guidelines.

To minimize risk of cross-infection (DH 2005: R).

6 Assist patient with removal of clothing, cover patient with bath towel or fleece and fold back bedclothes.

To maintain privacy and dignity and body temperature (NMC 2008: C, E).

7 Ask patient whether they use soap on the face, wash, rinse and dry face, neck and ears.

To promote cleanliness and independence (NMC 2008: C, E).

8 Assist male patients with facial shaving, apply chosen shaving foam/soap. Ensure skin is taut, begin shaving from cheeks down to neck in short strokes. Rinse razor as required. Change water and rinse face with clean water. Utilize electric shaver as desired.

To promote positive body image (C).

9 Wash, rinse and pat dry top half of body, starting with the side furthest away from you. Care needs to be taken not to wet drains/dressings and IV devices. Apply toiletries as required.

To promote patient well-being and cleanliness and reduce the risk of cross-infection (NMC 2008: C, E, R).

10 Change the water, and your disposable gloves. Inform the patient that you are going to wash around the genitalia, gain verbal consent from the patient or ask the patient if they wish to wash this area themselves. Using a separate flannel or wipe, wash around the area, then dry the area. Remove gloves, dispose as per hospital policy. If there is an indwelling catheter, put on your gloves and wash the tubing away from the genitalia area, dry tubing and remove gloves as per hospital policy. (Patients may prefer to do this themselves.) When washing this area, remember female patients wash from the front to back. Male patients should draw back the foreskin if uncircumcised when washing the penis.

To reduce risk of infection and to maintain a safe environment (NMC 2008: C, E, R).

11 Change water and gloves, ensuring patient has nurse call bell, and is covered.

To maintain cleanliness, preserving dignity and privacy (NMC 2008: C, E).

12 Wash, rinse and pat dry legs, starting with the side furthest away from you. Assess the need for possible chiropody referral. Roll patient, wash back, then using disposable flannel wash sacral area, observing pressure areas. Cover areas that are not being washed. Return patient onto their back, ensure they are covered. Apply toiletries as required.

To prevent and treat pressure ulcers, ensuring appropriate referrals are made (E).

13 Inspect finger and toenails, clean under nails using nail file. Cut or clip finger nails to top level of finger, edges can be shaped using an emery board. Toenails should be cut/clipped straight across. Note any areas of skin dryness, inflammation, callouses.

To enhance positive body image and patient comfort and reduce risk of infection (NMC 2008: C, E, R).

Procedure guidelines *(cont.)*

14 Replace clothes and change bottom sheet whilst patient is being turned, if they are to remain in bed. Ensure a minimum of two nurses are present during this procdure.	To reduce unnecessary activity for patient and nurse. To maintain safety of patient and safe manual handling, following risk assessment (NMC 2008: C, E).
15 Provide appropriate equipment and assist patient, if required, to brush teeth and/or rinse mouth.	To maintain good oral hygiene (E).
16 Dry and comb patient's hair as desired.	To enhance patient comfort, and to promote positive body image (NMC 2008: C, E).
17 Remake top bedclothes.	
18 Help patient to sit or lie in desired position.	To enhance patient comfort and reduce risk of pressure ulcers (NMC 2008: C, E).
19 Remove equipment from bedside; replace patient's possessions in their appropriate place. Place locker, bedside table and call bell within reach.	To maintain a safe environment and promote patient independence (NMC 2008: C, E).
20 Remove apron and gloves and dispose of them according to local rules.	To prevent cross-infection (Pratt *et al.* 2001: R).
21 Wash hands, use alcohol based hand wash.	
22 Document any changes in planned care.	To provide recorded documentation of care and aid in communication to the multiprofessional team (C, E, R).

888

References and further reading

Armstrong-Esther, C.A. (1981) Skin introduction. *Nursing*, **1** (26), 1115.

Burr, S. & Penzer, R. (2005) Promoting skin health. *Nurs Stand*, **19**(36), 57–65.

Byers, P.H. *et al.* (1995) Effects of incontinence care cleansing regimens on skin integrity. *J Wound Ostomy Continence Nurs*, **22**(4), 187–92.

Campbell, A. (1984) Nursing, nurturing and sexism. In: *Moderated Love: A Theology of Professional Care*. Society for Promoting Christian Knowledge, London.

Carr-Hill, R., Dixon, P. & Gibbs, I. (1992) *Skill Mix and the Effectiveness of Nursing Care*. Centre for Health Economics, York.

Clinical Skills (2003) Bed baths. *Nurs Times*, **99**(5), 29.

Collins, F. & Hampton S. (2003) The cost effective use of Bagbath: a new concept in patient hygiene. *Br J Nurs*, **12**(16), 985–90.

Cooper, C. (1994) Hygiene and the client. In: *Knowledge to Care* (eds C.A. McMahon & J. Harding). Blackwell Scientific, Oxford.

DH (2001a) *Essence of Care*. HMSO, London.

DH (2001b) *Reference Guide to Consent for Examination or Treatment*. Department of Health, London.

DH (2005) *Saving Lives: A Delivery Programme to Reduce Healthcare Associated Infection including MRSA*. Department of Health, London.

Ersser, S.J. *et al.* (2005) A critical review of the inter-relationship between skin vunerability and urinary incontinence and related nursing intervention. *Int J Nurs Stud*, **42**, 823–35.

Geraghty, M. (2005) Nursing the unconcious patient. *Nurs Stand*, **20**(1), 54–64.

Gooch, J. (1989) Skin hygiene. *Prof Nurse*, **5**(1), 13–17.

Gordon, M. (1994) *Nursing Diagnosis: Process and Application*, 3rd edn. Mosby, St Louis.

Gould, D. (1994) Helping the patient with personal hygiene. *Nurs Stand*, 8(34), 30–2.

Haisfield Wolfe, M.E. (1998) Providing effective perineal–rectal skin care to patients with cancer. *Oncol Nurs Forum*, **25**(3), 472.

Hector, L.M. & Touhy, T.A. (1997) The history of the bath: from art to task? Reflections for the future. *J Gerontol Nurs*, **23**(5), 7–15.

Henderson, V. (1966) *The Nature of Nursing*. Collier Macmillan, London.

Holloway, S. & Jones, V. (2005) The importance of skin care and assessment. *Br J Nurs*, **14**(22), 1172–6.

Kitson, A. (1999) The essence of nursing. *Nurs Stand*, **13**(23), 42–6.

Lindell, M. & Olsson, H. (1989) Lack of care givers' knowledge causes unnecessary suffering in elderly patients. *J Adv Nurs*, **14**, 976–9.

Lokich, J.J. & Moore, C. (1984) Chemotherapy associated palmar plantar erythrodysesthesia syndrome. *Ann Intern Med*, **101**, 798–800.

McLoughlin, C. (2005) A guide to wash creams. *Prof Nurse*, **20**(6), 46–7.

Neuberger, J. (1987) *Caring for Dying People of Different Faiths*, 2nd edn. Mosby, London.

Nightingale, F. (1969) *Notes on Nursing*. Dover Publications, New York.

NMC (2008) *The Code: Standards of Conduct, Performance and Ethics for Nurses and Midwives*. Nursing and Midwifery Council, London.

Orem, D. (1980) *Nursing – Concepts of Practice*, 2nd edn. McGraw Hill, New York.

Penzer, R. & Finch, M. (2001) Promoting healthy skin in older people. *Nurs Stand*, **15**(34), 46–52.

Potter, P.A. & Perry, G. (1995) *Basic Nursing Theory and Practice*. Mosby, London.

Pratt, R.J. *et al.* (2001) Guidelines for preventing infections associated with the insertion and maintenance of short-term indwelling urethral catheters in acute care. *J Hosp Infect*, **47**(Suppl), S39–46.

Roper, N. *et al.* (1981) *Learning to Use the Process of Nursing*. Churchill Livingstone, Edinburgh.

Ross, J. & Wilson, K. (2001) *Anatomy and Physiology in Health and Illness.* Churchill Livingstone, Edinburgh.

Sampson, C. (1982) *The Neglected Ethic; Religious and Cultural Factors in the Care of Patients.* McGraw-Hill, London, p. 36.

Sheppard, C.M. & Brenner, P.S. (2000) The effects of bathing and skin care practices on skin quality and satisfaction with an innovative product. *J Gerontol Nurs,* **26**(10), 36–45.

Smoker, A. (1999) Skin care in old age. *Nurs Stand,* **13**(48), 47–53.

Spiller, J. (1992) For whose sake – patient or nurse? *Prof Nurse,* **7**(7), 431–4.

Wagnild, G. & Manning, R.W. (1985) Convey respect during bathing procedures. *J Gerontol Nurse,* **11**(12), 6–10.

Whiting, L.S. (1999) Maintaining patient's personal hygiene. *Prof Nurse,* **14**(5), 338–40.

Wilson, M. (1986) Personal cleanliness. *Nursing,* **3**(2), 80–2.

Young, L. (1991) The clean fight. *Nurs Stand,* **5**(35), 54–5.

Multiple choice questions

1 To what temperature should the water/0.9% sodium chloride be heated to perform eye irrigation?

   a   It does not matter
   b   Chilled
   c   Tepid
   d   37°C

2 Skin has a number of functions. Which of the following is NOT a function of skin?

   a   Temperature regulation
   b   Preservation of water balance
   c   Energy production
   d   Expression of emotion

3 Personal hygiene is a significant issue in many religions. Which of the following statements is true?

   a   Hindus do not eat with their right hand
   b   Muslims wash their face, hands and feet before and after their daily prayers
   c   Sikhs must comb their hair at least three times a day
   d   Hindus deem their left hand to be unclean

4 Patients with poor swallowing reflexes or post-tracheotomy closure may experience unpleasant thick mucous in the oral cavity. What would you suggest to the patient as the most effective way to reduce this?

   a   Use sodium bicarbonate in the mouth care procedure
   b   Encourage the patient to suck ice cubes
   c   Apply artificial saliva to the oral cavity
   d   Advise a fluid-only diet

5 Which of the following is the recommended way to clean a patient's mouth (when the gingiva is intact)?

a   Finger
b   Foam sticks
c   Soft toothbrush
d   Gauze

Answers to the multiple choice questions can be found in Appendix 3.

Chapter 26

Positioning

Definition

The verb positioning is defined as 'a way in which someone or something is placed or arranged' (Pearsall 2001, p. 1116). In medical terms the word position relates to body position or posture. Positioning lies within the broader context of manual handling, which incorporates 'transporting or supporting a load (including lifting, putting down, pushing, pulling, carrying or moving) by hand or bodily force' (HSE 1992). In this chapter the principles of positioning will relate to the patient, but the practitioner needs to ensure that they consider their own position regarding the safety aspects of manual handling as advised by government and local policy and the manual handling advisor or the physiotherapist.

This chapter aims to provide guidance on various aspects of positioning patients acknowledging the need to be clinically effective and, where possible, evidence based.

The main objectives of the chapter are to:

1 Outline the general considerations of positioning.
2 Provide guidance on the principles of positioning whether the patient is in bed, sitting or mobilizing.
3 Review optimal positioning and modifications for patients requiring different clinical needs.
4 Provide suggestions for further reading.

Reference material

This chapter relates to conscious adults (for positioning of the unconscious patient see Chapter 31) and does not cover positioning in children or neonates.

Positioning is an important aspect in patient care because of its effect on the patient physically, physiologically and psychologically. It can have a major influence on patient recuperation and well being, addressing patients' impairments in order to optimize their function and participation in society. Although important, positioning must not be seen in isolation and is just one aspect of patient management within the context of preventative, rehabilitative, supportive and palliative rehabilitation models (Dietz 1981). Positioning is often used to provide a starting point to maximize the benefit of other interventions such as bed and breathing exercises, optimal rest, and rehabilitation to facilitate recovery.

It is essential to frequently evaluate the effect that positioning has on the individual and/or different pathologies to ensure that the intervention is helping to achieve the desired result or goal. This relates to considering whether the positioning procedure is being clinically effective and, where possible, is evidence based.

Points to consider regarding the clinical effectiveness of positioning are:

- Is the timing right to consider positioning? For example, is the pain relief adequate?
- Is it being carried out in the correct way? This relates to manual handling with regard to preventing trauma either to the patient or the practitioner.
- Is the required position taking into account all the pertinent needs of the patient? This emphasizes the need to consider the patient in a holistic manner.
- Is it achieving the desired or detrimental result?

Principles of positioning

Positioning is indicated for patients who are acutely ill or require bed rest when normal functioning is impaired. The aim of positioning is to reduce impairment, facilitate function, and alleviate symptomatic discomfort and to assist future rehabilitation where appropriate. The main principles underpinning all interventions regarding patient positioning focus on the short- and long-term goals of rehabilitation and management for each specific patient. It is imperative that a thorough assessment is carried out prior to any intervention in order to plan goals of treatment. Regular reassessment is required to allow for modification of plans to allow for changes in status. It may be necessary to compromise on one principle depending on the overall goal. For example, for the palliative patient, it may be that the primary aim of any intervention is to facilitate comfort at the cost of reducing function.

The principles of positioning are based on patterns of posture which maximize function with minimal amount of effort (Gardiner 1973) without causing damage to the body system (Pope 1996). These basic principles of positioning can be applied regardless of a patient's pathology.

To achieve a good position of the patient in bed the following points should be considered:

- wounds;
- pain;
- weakness;
- tonal changes;
- sensory changes;
- limitations of joint range;
- oedema;
- skin blistering;
- medical devices associated with treatment, e.g. catheter, intravenous infusion, venous access devices, drains;
- cardiovascular and respiratory status;
- cognitive state.

Medical considerations

Skin integrity should be assessed prior to positioning and vulnerable areas protected and placed so as to minimize harmful contact with other surfaces (see Chapter 34).

Patients may have complex symptoms that require control prior to moving or positioning. It is important to time the intervention to allow adequate time for medication to take effect or to ensure the patient is given a breakthrough dose before moving (see Chapter 20).

It is important to establish spinal stability before positioning or moving the patient. Suspected or confirmed spinal instability should be managed in accordance to local policy (see Chapter 41, Professional edition).

Caution should be taken in patients with known, possible pathological fracture(s) or pain. Before a lesion becomes apparent radiologically at least 50% of bone mass must be lost; so that pain may precede radiological changes (McGarvey 1990).

Fatigue can be a distressing symptom, so advice and help should be given to the patient to pace their everyday activities. Barsevick *et al.* (2002, p. 71) describe energy conservation as 'the deliberate planned management of one's personal energy resources in order to prevent their depletion'. Prioritizing activities may help to avoid engaging in tasks that are unnecessary or of little value (Cooper 2006). Sometimes it may be appropriate to assist with activities such as washing and dressing to help conserve energy for more meaningful or pleasurable activities.

Medical considerations for patient on bed rest

Patients with acute medical conditions and decreased mobility are at risk of secondary complications of bed rest such as pulmonary embolus (PE) (Reidel

2001), deep vein thrombosis (DVT) or respiratory infection (Convertino *et al.* 1995).

The severity of an illness may leave no choice except bed rest, but the rest itself is rarely beneficial. Historically patients complaining of pain, dyspnoea, neurological dysfunction and fatigue were advised to rest. However, inactivity may cause (Creditor 1993; Doyle *et al.* 2004):

- Deconditioning of many of the body's systems (particularly in cardiorespiratory and musculoskeletal systems).
- A worsening of symptoms.
- Fear of movement.
- Loss of independence.
- Social isolation.

Therefore, patients should be encouraged or assisted, to mobilize or change position, at frequent intervals. This so that deconditioning is minimized, unless their medical condition or fatigue makes this inappropriate. Early referral to therapy services is advantageous. If bed rest is unavoidable then the following factors should be taken into account:

- Patient comfort and adequate support.
- Avoidance of the complications of prolonged bed rest (see Chapter 25).
- Consideration regarding the optimal frequency of position change.

Patients on bed rest should be encouraged to practice regular deep breathing to maximize their respiratory function.

They should also be encouraged to practice active or passive movements, as advised by the physiotherapist, in order to (Adam & Forrest 1999):

- Maintain full joint range.
- Maintain full muscle length and extensibility.
- Assist venous return.
- Maintain sensation of normal movement.

Active ankle movements are to be encouraged to assist the circulation, as failure to exercise the calf muscle for prolonged periods may result in limited or poor blood circulation in the lower leg and increase the risk of DVT (O'Donovan *et al.* 2006).

Positioning in the bed

The body should be supported to maintain its natural contours, symmetry and alignment (Carter & Edwards 1996).

Procedure guidelines   **Positioning the patient supine**

Equipment

1 Pillows.
2 Towels.
3 Bed extension for tall patients.

Procedure

Action	Rationale
1 (a) Place one pillow squarely under the patient's head according to patient comfort.	To support the head in a neutral position and to compensate for the natural lordosis of the cervical spine (E).
For patients with a tracheostomy, endotracheal tube, soft tissue structural involvement or head and neck surgery take care not to occlude or displace tubes or increase pressure to vulnerable areas. Or:	To ensure the airway is patent (E). To increase patient support and comfort (E).
(b) Use two pillows in a 'butterfly' position so that two layers of pillow support the head and one layer of pillow under each shoulder. Or:	This may be necessary for the patient with pain, breathlessness (see Respiratory section, below) or an existing kyphosis (E).
(c) Use a folded towel if this provides natural spinal alignment (E).	To prevent excess neck flexion (E).
2 Ensure the patient lies centrally in the bed.	To ensure spinal and limb alignment (E).
3 Place pillows and/or towels under individual limbs to provide maximum support for patient with painful, weak or oedematous limbs.	To ensure patient comfort (E, P).
4 Ensure patient's feet are fully supported by the mattress. For taller patients use a bed extension if required.	To ensure patient comfort (E, P).

897

Procedure guidelines *(cont.)*

5 Place pillow at the end of the hospital bed to support ankle at 90° of flexion if the patient has weakness or is immobile. Refer to the occupational therapist or physiotherapist for orthosis/splinting if the patient is unable to actively flex their foot. Refer to the physiotherapist if the patient has a neurological pathology for advice regarding positioning to reduce altered tonal influences (R) (E).

To ensure patient comfort (E, P).
To prevent loss of ankle movement (E).

Procedure guidelines **Positioning the patient sitting in bed**

Patients should be encouraged to sit up in bed periodically if their medical condition prevents them from sitting out in the chair (Figure 26.1). If the patient is unable to participate fully in the procedure, manual handling equipment should be used to help achieve the desired position.

Attention should also be given to sitting posture. One of the most common causes of low back pain is poor posture and may frequently be brought on by sitting for a long time in a poor position (McKenzie 1985) as it causes an increase in pressure in the disc (Norris 1995).

Patients who have suspected or confirmed spinal instability should be nursed flat unless medical staff instruct otherwise. Patients should lie flat to prevent dural headache following lumbar puncture unless local policy states otherwise.

. . . .

Equipment

1 Pillows.
2 Manual handling equipment may be required, e.g. sliding sheets or a hoist depending on local policy.

. . . .

Procedure

Action

1 Ask the patient to sit up in bed. The angle at which the patient sits may be influenced by pain, fatigue, abdominal distension or level of confusion/agitation.

Rationale

To encourage haemodynamic stability (E).
To enable effective breathing pattern: maximizing basal expansion (Pryor & Webber 2002: R 4).

. . . .

2 Ask the patient to position their hips in line with the hinge of the automatic mattress elevator or backrest of the bed.

To ensure good postural alignment, i.e. flexing at the hip when sitting up in bed (E).
To prevent strain on the spine (E, R).

3 Place a pillow under the patient's knees or use the electrical control of the bed to slightly bend the patient's knees. Extra care should be taken if the patient has a femoral line or is on haemofiltration.

To reduce strain on the lumbar spine (E).
To maintain the position (E).

4 Place a pillow under individual or both upper limbs for patients with a chest drain, upper limb weakness, trunk weakness, surgery involving shoulder/upper limb/breast/thorax, fungating wounds involving axilla, breast and shoulder, upper limb /truncal lymphoedema or fractures involving ribs or upper limbs.

To provide upper limb support (E).
To maintain trunk alignment (E).
To encourage basal expansion (Pryor & Webber 2002: E, R 4).

899

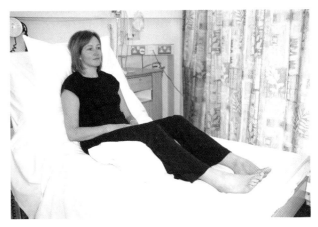

Figure 26.1 Sitting up in bed.

Procedure guidelines   Positioning the patient side lying

This can be a useful position for patients with:

1 Compromised venous return, e.g. pelvic/abdominal mass, pregnancy.
2 Global motor weakness.
3 Risk of developing pressure sores.
4 Unilateral pelvic or lower limb pain.
5 Altered tone (see Positioning the patient with neurological impairment section, below).
6 Fatigue.
7 Chest infection, for gravity-assisted drainage of secretions.
8 Lung pathology, to optimize ventilation and perfusion matching.
9 Abdominal distension, e.g. ascites, bulky disease, to optimize lung volume (for more information on the above three points (7, 8, 9) see Positioning of patients with cardiorespiratory compromise section, below).

See Figure 26.2

Equipment

1 Pillows.
2 Manual handling equipment may be required, e.g. sliding sheets or a hoist depending on local policy.

Procedure

Action	Rationale
1 Place one or two pillows in 'butterfly' position under the patient's head ensuring the airway remains patent. Extra care should be taken for those patients with a tracheostomy, central lines or recent head and neck surgery.	To support the head in mid-position (E). To support shoulder contours (E).
2 Ask/assist the patient to semiflex the underneath leg at the hip and the knee. Extra care should be taken with the degree of flexion for those patients who have hip or knee pain or loss of movement, fracture involving the femur or pelvis, leg oedema, femoral lines or other venous access devices.	To support the patient in a stable position and prevent rolling (E).
3 (a) Ask/assist the patient to semi-flex the uppermost leg at the hip and knee. Use a pillow to support under the leg placed on the bed. Or:	To prevent lumbar spine rotation (E). To support the pelvic girdle (E).
(b) Place a pillow between the patient's knees.	To aid pressure care (E).

4 Place the underneath arm in front with scapula protracted (this would not be appropriate for patients with shoulder pathology). Extra care should be taken with patients with low tone in the affected arm, lymphoedema or who have access lines in that arm.	To promote patient comfort (E, P). To promote shoulder alignment (E). To provide additional support and comfort (E, P).

Note: care should be taken in lying the patient directly over the greater trochanter as this increases pressure at this interface and the risk of developing pressure sores (Hawkins *et al.* 1999).

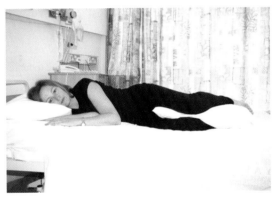

Figure 26.2 Side lying.

Guidance for assisting patients to move

This section covers general principles of assisting patients to move, enhancing their rehabilitation process by avoiding unnecessary debilitation. It serves as a guide only, is not prescriptive and does not attempt to cover mandatory local manual handling issues. Each situation should be risk assessed on an individual basis as part of standard nursing assessment.

Particular thought should be given to the patient's:

- Previous functional status.
- Consent and compliance to treatment or activity.
- Medical stability.
- Environmental safety.

- Level of consciousness.
- Symptom control.
- Muscle strength.
- Sensation.
- Co-ordination and balance.
- Cognitive function.
- Level of fatigue.
- Cardiovascular/respiratory status.

In order to assist recovery, postural alignment is essential to improve motor control. The term motor control is broadly defined as: 'the control of both movement and posture' (Shumway-Cook & Woollacott 1995, p. 3).

Postural alignment helps the patient develop an initial position that is (Shumway-Cook & Woollacott 1995, p. 224):

(a) appropriate for the task;
(b) efficient with respect to gravity, i.e. minimal muscle activity required to maintain the position; and
(c) maximizes stability, allowing postural control.

Procedure guidelines | **Moving from lying to sitting: assisting the patient**

See Figures 26.3–26.5.

Equipment

1 Manual handling equipment may be required, e.g. sliding sheets or a hoist depending on local policy.

Action	**Rationale**
1 Ask the patient to bend both knees and turn their head towards the direction they are moving. Abdominal wounds should be supported by the patient's hands. Extra care should be taken with patients who have joint pathology, oedema, ascites or positional vertigo.	To assist the patient to roll using their body weight (E).
2 Ask patient to reach toward the side of the bed with the uppermost arm and roll on to their side.	

3 Ask the patient to bend their knees and lower their feet over the edge of the bed.

4 Ask the patient to push through the underneath elbow and the upper arm on the bed to push up into sitting. As the patient sits up monitor changes in pain or dizziness which could indicate postural hypotension or vertigo. Be aware that the patient with neurological symptoms or weakness may not have safe sitting balance.

To help to lever the patient into a sitting position using the weight of their legs (E).

5 Achieve upright sitting position with appropriate alignment of body parts.

To ensure safe sitting position achieved.

903

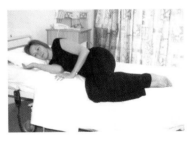

Figure 26.3 Lying to sitting (stage 1).

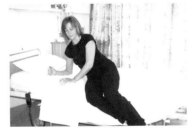

Figure 26.4 Lying to sitting (stage 2).

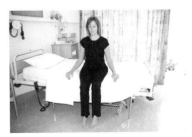

Figure 26.5 Lying to sitting (stage 3).

Procedure guidelines   Positioning the patient in a chair

Equipment

1 Upright chair with arms.
2 Manual handling equipment may be required, e.g. a hoist depending on local policy.
3 Pillows/rolled up towel.
4 Footstool if the patient has lower limb oedema.

Procedure

Action	Rationale
1 Ask the patient to sit well back in the chair. They should have a maximum 90° angle at their hips and knee joints. The patient may not be able to achieve this position if they have pain, abdominal distension or hip/back pain. It may be necessary to refer the patient to the occupational therapist for chair raises, a cushion or appropriate seating if a comfortable or safe position cannot be achieved.	To provide a stable base of support for balance (E). To ensure good body alignment (E). To achieve a safe sitting position (E).
2 Place a pillow or rolled up towel in the small of the patient's back as is comfortable for the patient.	To allow the patient's back to be supported in a good position (E).
3 Ensure the patient's feet are resting on the floor or supported surface. Use pillows or a rolled up towel to support under the feet if necessary.	To provide postural alignment and support the lumbar spine (E).
4 If the patient has a lower leg oedema use a foot stool placed under the patient's limb ensuring the whole leg and foot is supported and avoiding hyperextension at the knees.	To improve venous drainage.
5 Discourage the patient from crossing their legs.	To reduce risk of developing a DVT (O'Donovan *et al.* 2006: R 4).

Moving from sitting to standing: assisting the patient

If the patient stands from the side of a hospital bed, it is helpful to raise the bed slightly to reduce the work of standing for the patient to ensure that hips are level or higher than the knees with the feet in contact with the floor. A physiotherapy referral may be appropriate. See Figures 26.6 and 26.7.

Equipment

1 Walking aid if required (if previously issued by physiotherapist).
2 Suitable non-slip, well-fitting, supportive and flat footwear (if not available then bare feet are preferable to socks or stockings which may slip).

Procedure

Action	Rationale
1 Ask the patient to lean forward and move their bottom closer to the front of the chair or edge of the bed.	To bring the patient's weight over their feet (E).
2 Ask the patient to move their feet back so they are slightly tucked under them with their feet hip width apart.	To provide a stable base prior to moving (E).
3 Instruct the patient to lean forward from their trunk.	To help initiate movement (E). To facilitate a normal pattern of movement (E).
4 Instruct the patient to push through their hands on the arms of the chair or surface on which they are sitting as they stand. Encourage a forward and up motion whilst extending their hips and knees.	To minimize energy expenditure (E).
5 As the patient stands observe changes in pain or dizziness.	To be aware of postural hypotension (E).
6 Once standing, ask the patient to stand still for a moment to ensure balance is achieved before the patient attempts to walk.	To ensure safe static standing (E).

905

Procedure guidelines *(cont.)*

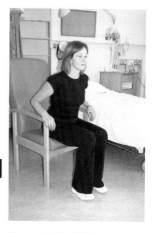

Figure 26.6 Sitting to standing (stage 1).

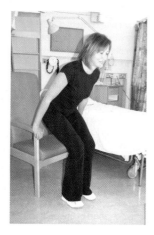

Figure 26.7 Sitting to standing (stage 2).

Walking

'Walking requires alternating support on one leg and then the other' (Gillis 1989, p.671). Successful walking is dependent on three specific functional tasks (Gillis 1989):

1 Weight acceptance.
2 Single limb support.
3 Limb advancement.

Patients may use a variety of different walking aids to help them mobilize. All aids are designed to improve balance and therefore reduce the risk of falls.

It is assumed that patients will take equal amounts of body weight through both legs, defined as being fully weight bearing (FWB). If a patient has to be non-weight bearing (NWB) or partially weight bearing (PWB) this will be due to bone or joint pathology, e.g. fracture, joint instability, inflammation or infection. Restrictions in weight bearing should always be clearly documented and communicated by the medical staff. Weight bearing will also be affected by pain, weakness, sensory changes and confidence. If the patient has difficulty mobilizing, appears unsafe or is at risk of falling for any reason refer for physiotherapy assessment.

A physiotherapist will assess and issue the patient with an appropriate walking aid. All patients should be given verbal and written instructions on their use. If they are unsure, please refer to the patient information sheets for instructions (Boxes 34.1–34.3).

Box 26.1 Using your walking sticks

Your physiotherapist has suggested that you would benefit from using a walking stick. This fact sheet is to remind you of the most important points that your physiotherapist has shown you. Your walking stick will help to give you more support when standing and walking. It can help you take weight off one leg if you have pain or weakness. It can also help with improving your balance.

Standing

- Use your arms to push up from the surface you are sitting on.
- Hold the stick in your stronger hand or the opposite hand to the painful or weak leg.

Walking

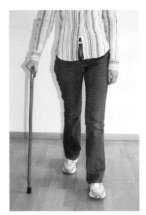

- Place the stick in front of you.
- Step forwards with your weaker leg so it is level with the stick.
- Lean on the stick and take a normal step with the other leg.
- Repeat this sequence always moving the stick forwards before or at the same time as the weaker leg as advised by your physiotherapist.
- It may take a bit of practice for you to get into a rhythm.

Sitting

- Always turn so you are backing towards the bed or chair.
- When you can feel the bed or chair on the backs of your legs, reach back with your hand to feel the arm of the chair or bed surface.
- Slowly sit down.

Continued on p. 908

907

Box 26.1 *(cont.)*

Stairs

Going up:

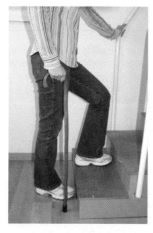

- Hold on to the banister with the stick in the other hand.
- Pushing down on the stick and banister, step up with the stronger leg.
- Bring the stick and weaker leg up to join the stronger leg on the same step.
- Repeat this sequence.

Going down:

- Hold on to the banister with the stick in the other hand.
- Place the stick on to the step below.
- Step down with the weaker leg.
- Lean on the stick and banister as you step down with the stronger leg on to the same stair.
- Repeat this sequence.

Take extra care using your stick where:

- There are loose rugs or carpet edges: try to remove or tape down.
- The floor is wet.
- The floor is rough or uneven.

Care and maintenance of your stick

You should wipe the stick down with warm soapy water and dry thoroughly with a soft cloth once a week or more frequently if necessary. Check the stick weekly for signs of wear and tear:

- Is the rubber tip worn or showing poor tread?
- Is the wood cracked or splintered?

©The Royal Marsden NHS Foundation Trust

Box 26.2 Using your elbow crutches

Your physiotherapist has suggested you use elbow crutches to help you walk. This fact sheet is to remind you of the most important points that your physiotherapist has shown you.

Your crutches will help to give you more support when standing and walking. They can help you take weight off one leg if you have pain or weakness. They can also help with improving your balance.

Standing
- Hold both crutches in one hand making an 'H' shape.
- Push up with the other hand from the surface you are sitting on. Don't put your arms through the rings until you are standing up.
- When you are standing, pass one crutch over to the other hand and put hands through the rings one at a time.
- Get your balance before beginning to walk.

Walking

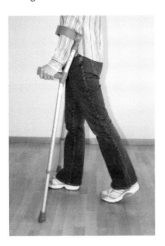

- Place the crutches in front of you.
- Step forwards with your weaker leg level with the crutches.
- Lean on the crutches and take a normal step with the other leg.
- Repeat this sequence always moving the crutches forwards before or at the same time as the weaker leg as advised by your physiotherapist.
- It may take a bit of practice for you to get into a rhythm.
- If your physiotherapist has shown you a different way to walk with crutches then follow the advice given to you.

Sitting

- When sitting down always turn so you are backing towards the bed or chair.
- When you can feel the bed or chair on the backs of your legs, pass one crutch over in to the other hand so you are holding both crutches in one hand.
- Take your hands out of the rings and make an 'H' shape with the crutches.
- Reach back with your free hand to feel the arm of the chair or bed surface.
- Slowly sit down.

Continued on p. 910

Box 26.2 (*cont.*)

Stairs

Going up:

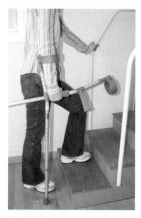

- Hold on to the banister with both crutches in the other hand as demonstrated by your physiotherapist. The second crutch should be held horizontally as demonstrated by your physiotherapist.
- Pushing down on the crutches and banister, step up with stronger leg.
- Bring the crutches and weaker leg up to join the strong leg on the same step.
- Repeat this sequence.

Going down:

- Hold on to the banister with both crutches in the other hand as demonstrated by your physiotherapist.
- Place the crutches on to the step below.
- Step down with the weaker leg.
- Lean on the crutch and banister as you step down with the strong leg on to the same stair.
- Repeat this sequence.
- Always remember to keep the crutches with the weak leg on the lower level.

Take extra care using your crutches where:

- There are loose rugs or carpet edges: try to remove or tape down.
- The floor is wet.
- The floor is rough or uneven.

Care and maintenance of your crutches

You should wipe the crutches down with warm soapy water and dry thoroughly with a soft cloth once a week or more frequently if necessary.
Check the crutches weekly for signs of wear and tear:

- Are the rubber tips worn and showing poor tread?
- Are the hand grips loose or cracked?
- Is the metal tubing cracked or damaged?

Box 26.3 Using your walking frame

Your physiotherapist has suggested that you would benefit from using a walking frame. This fact sheet is to remind you of the most important points that your physiotherapist has shown you. Your walking frame should help to give you more support when standing and walking. It can also help you take weight off one or both of your legs if you have pain or weakness. The walking frame can also help with improving your balance.

Your physiotherapist will have assessed the height of the frame when it was given to you.

There should be no need to adjust the height again.

Standing

- Always push up with your arms from the surface you are sitting on or from the arms of the chair.
- Shuffle to the edge of the chair or bed.
- Lean forwards and stand up pushing with your arms.
- Never put your hands on the frame until you are standing.
- Do not pull on the frame as it may tip back.

Walking

- Move the frame in front of you and lean on it.
- Step forwards into the middle of the frame. If you walk too far into the frame it may become unbalanced and tip backwards.
- If you have one leg that is weaker or painful step forward with that leg first.
- Always have both hands on the frame and do not try and carry anything while you are walking.

Sitting

- Always turn the frame using small steps, so you are backing towards the bed or chair.
- When you feel the bed or chair on the back of your legs, reach back with your hands one at a time, to hold the arms of the chair or surface of the bed.
- Slowly sit down.

Do not use your frame:

- Where there are loose rugs or carpet edges: always remove or tape down.
- Where the floor is wet.
- Where there is not enough space to turn the frame.
- Where there are stairs or steps.
- Where the floor is rough or uneven.
- Outside.

Continued on p. 912

Box 26.3 *(cont.)*

Care and maintenance of the frame

You should wash the frame down with warm soapy water and dry thoroughly with a soft cloth once a week or more frequently if necessary. Check the frame regularly for signs of wear and tear:

- Are the rubber tips worn and showing poor tread?
- Has the frame become wobbly or unstable?
- Are the hand grips loose or cracked?
- Is the metal tubing cracked or damaged?

©The Royal Marsden NHS Foundation Trust

912

Procedure guidelines   **Walking: assisting the patient**

Equipment

1 Walking aid (see above).
2 Suitable non-slip, well-fitting, supportive and flat footwear (if not available then bare feet is preferable to socks or stockings which may slip).

Action	Rationale
1 Stand next to and slightly behind the patient. If patient requires support place your arm nearest the patient lightly around their pelvis. Your other hand should hold the patient's hand closest to you. Observe changes in pain as the patient walks.	To give appropriate support (E). To increase patient's confidence (E, P).
2 Give verbal supervision/cueing as required to achieve safe walking.	To provide encouragement (E). To ensure patient safety (E).

Procedure guidelines   **Positioning to minimize the work of breathing**

The aim of any position is to restore a normal frequency (rate) and depth (tidal volume) of breathing in order to achieve efficient, adequate ventilation.

The positions will usually be used in conjunction with other interventions, e.g. breathing control and specific muscle relaxation, to achieve reduced work of breathing. These may include attention to symptom control (e.g. pain), environmental control (e.g. reducing unnecessary noise stressors).

Repositioning can cause a temporary fall in SaO_2 or a raised respiratory rate due to the work undertaken. If the fall is greater than 4% points or recovery time is protracted supplemental oxygen delivery may be required. If the clinical signs remain altered from normal then an alternative position may be indicated.

Procedure

Action

1 As shown in Action figure 1, the resting positions include:
   - High side lying (see Action figure 1a).
   - Forward lean sitting (see Action figure 1b).
   - Relaxed sitting (see Action figure 1c).
   - Forward lean standing (see Action figure 1d).
   - Relaxed standing (see Action figure 1e).

Rationale

These positions all serve to:
   - Support the body reducing the overall use of postural muscle and oxygen requirements.
   - Improve lung volumes.
   - Optimize the functional positions of the respiratory (thoracic and abdominal) muscles (Dean 1985: R 4, E, P).

913

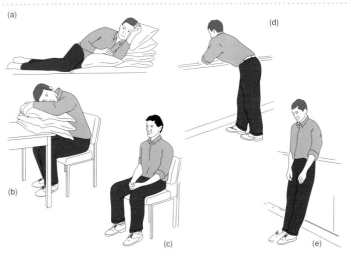

(a)   (d)   (b)   (c)   (e)

Action 1   (a–e) Positions to support breathing.

Procedure guidelines   **Positioning to maximize ventilation/ perfusion (V/Q) matching and oxygenation**

For optimal gaseous exchange to take place it is necessary to have an adequate perfusion of blood and a regular supply of inspired air (ventilation) in the same area of the lung. Ventilation and perfusion are not exactly matched even in the normal lung but can be changed by positional alteration to improve oxygenation and reduce the requirements for supplemental oxygenation (see Figures 26.8 and 26.9 and Chapter 27). In the presence of respiratory pathology, V/Q matching is better in the non-affected areas (Jones & Moffatt 2002). Where there is cardiac compromise, if there is an increase in heart rate or alteration in blood pressure, the head of the bed may need to be gradually raised until signs normalize.

The ideal positioning for V/Q matching will be determined by a number of factors:

- The cardiorespiratory pathophysiology.
- Co-existence of other pathophysiology.
- Auscultatory findings.
- X-ray or computed tomography (CT) findings.

In the spontaneously breathing patient

Action	Rationale
1 Supported side lying on the unaffected side for unilateral lung disease.	Maximizes V/Q in the unaffected lung as the ventilation and perfusion are both preferentially distributed to the dependent areas of the lungs (West *et al.*1964: R 4; Zach *et al.* 1974: R 4, E, P).
2 High supported sitting for bilateral lower lobe pathology or multi-lobe pathology.	Due to the effects of shunting in multi-lobe lung pathology perfusion may best match ventilation in supported high sitting (Dean 1985: R 4, E, P).

In patients receiving positive pressure ventilation

Each individual patient should be positioned according to their pathology and responses to the principles outlined below. Where positive pressure ventilation is delivered maximum ventilation will occur in the non-dependent regions, whilst the perfusion is still preferentially delivered to the dependent areas. This may vary again where there is respiratory pathology causing ventilatory shunt, whereby pulmonary venous blood re-enters the arterial circulation without being ventilated and hence not oxygenated (Wagner & West 2005).

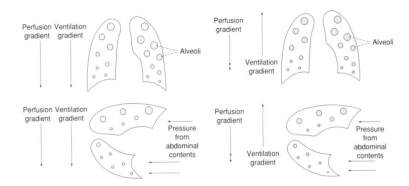

Figure 26.8 Effect of gravity on the distribution of ventilation and perfusion in the lung in the upright and lateral positions. From Hough (2001) with permission.

Figure 26.9 Effect of controlled mandatory ventilation on ventilation and perfusion gradients. In contrast to spontaneous respiration, the perfusion gradient increases downwards and the ventilation gradient is reversed. From Hough (2001) with permission.

Positioning of patients with cardiorespiratory compromise

The causes of cardiorespiratory compromise may be multifactorial and should be established before undertaking positioning interventions. Compromise may be due to medical intervention (e.g. surgery, side-effects of medication), metabolic, surgical or primary cardiorespiratory pathologies.

The guidelines regarding assisting patients to move are applicable to this group. However, particular observation is required regarding their response to the interventions and specific modifications may be required (e.g. increased assistance, paced activity or provision of supplemental oxygen) for the duration and recovery period following the procedure.

The main aim of positioning management of the patient with respiratory symptoms is to use gravity to:

- Minimize the work of breathing.
- Maximize the drainage of respiratory secretions.
- Maximize ventilation/perfusion (V/Q) matching and oxygenation.

In many instances positioning may combine the above aims to enhance medical management by the use of the effects of gravity upon the cardiovascular and respiratory systems. This may reduce the need for more invasive intervention (Jones & Moffatt 2002), i.e. assisted ventilation. As such, the most advantageous positioning should be integrated into the overall 24-hour plan, and positions that may have an adverse effect should be avoided (Brown *et al.* 1996).

It should be remembered that thoracic and abdominal muscles contribute to normal breathing patterns and that any compromise of the abdominal muscle activity (e.g. due to abdominal surgery, ascites or deconditioning) may lead to an alteration in the normal cardiorespiratory function and the ability to generate an effective cough (Hodges & Gandevia 2000).

Positioning to maximize the drainage of respiratory secretions

Sputum retention may lead to an increased bacterial load for the patient and may compromise respiratory functioning by causing airway obstruction leading to segmental atelectasis or lobar collapse increasing the mortality.

Optimal positioning for the gravity assisted positions to facilitate the drainage of respiratory secretions will be determined by a number of factors:

- The cardiorespiratory pathophysiology.
- Co-existence of other pathophysiology.
- Auscultatory findings.
- X-ray or CT findings.

Where secretions are found in a specific segment, the patient should be specifically positioned to place the bronchus of each bronchopulmonary segment perpendicular to gravity in order to be drained. Advice may be given by the physiotherapist on these positions.

The positions will usually be used in conjunction with other techniques to facilitate the clearing of respiratory secretions. These may be specific breathing and clearance techniques and/or other manual techniques.

If the respiratory muscles are ineffective the patient may not be able to clear secretions independently. Positions to reduce the work of breathing and optimize respiratory muscle function (see the above section) may enhance this. If clearance is still not effective then the physiotherapist may use or will advise the use of other techniques (Hough 2001; Jones & Moffatt 2002; Pryor & Webber 2002).

Positioning the patient with neurological impairment

For those with acute and long-standing neurological issues principles of positioning can be applied at any time along their treatment trajectory; those with rehabilitation potential; deteriorating function and those requiring palliative management for each of these clinical presentations. This relates to problems associated with abnormal tone, abnormal movement patterns, sensory and perceptual problems. The general principles of positioning discussed earlier can be applied for this group of patients. However, the complexity of these patients highlights the difficulty of a uniform approach to overall management. Therefore, this section will look at some of the variations in treatment of this patient group and suggest some principles to be considered when positioning these patients.

Disease or damage to the central or peripheral nervous system can lead to temporary or permanent complex physical, cognitive, psychological and psychosocial problems (Brada 1995; Lindsay & Bone 1997; Guererro 1998; Ellison & Love 2000; Kirschblum *et al.* 2001; Tookman *et al.* 2004). Their problems may include:

- Weakness: unilateral, bilateral or global.
- Sensory changes.
- Balance problems.
- Perceptual problems.
- Visual problems.
- Cognitive problems.
- Dysphagia.
- Dysphasia.
- Behavioural changes.

If a person with a neurological presentation is unable to move, they are deprived of the physical benefits of movement including:

- Sensory–motor appreciation.
- Posture and balance control.
- Maintenance of joint and soft tissue range of movement.
- Maximization of functional independence.
- Minimization of tonal changes such as spasticity (Hawkins *et al.* 1999).
- Cardiorespiratory fitness (Convertino *et al.* 1995).

This section will cover recommendations for assisting patients presenting with physical neurological symptoms affecting their central nervous systems (CNS) and peripheral nervous systems (PNS) as a consequence of their disease or treatment itself. These may include:

- Hemiparesis or monoparesis.
- Hemiaesthesia.
- Peripheral motor/sensory neuropathies.

Spinal cord compression will not be covered in this section (see Chapter 41, Professional edition).

Positioning can additionally offer control of positional influences of unwanted reflex activity for patients with altered tone (Davies 1985; Edwards 1996b;

Jackson 1998). Many positions advocated relate to the desire to avoid the development of abnormal patterns of movement associated with altered tone through minimizing the influence of primitive developmental reflexes (Bobath 1990). The three reflexes identified whose 'release' can be influenced are: (i) the tonic labyrinth reflex; (ii) the symmetrical tonic neck reflex; and (iii) the asymmetrical tonic neck reflex (Davies 1985; Jackson 1998 citing Carr & Kenney 1992; Davies 2000). Davies (2000) describes these primitive reflexes:

The tonic labyrinthine reflex is evoked by changes in the position of the head in space; originating at otolithic organs of the labyrinths and believed to be integrated at brainstem levels. In supine, extensor tone increases throughout the body with resultant extension of head, spine and limb extension and shoulder retraction. In prone lying, flexor tone increases throughout the body. This may only be seen as a reduction in extensor tone in a patient with severe spasticity. The influence of relative head position to body will also be noticed in sitting or standing and may affect functional movement or position.

The symmetrical tonic neck reflex is a proprioceptive reflex, elicited by stretching of the muscles and joints of the neck. When the head extends, extensor tone in the arms and flexor tone in the legs increases. When the head is flexed, the extensor tone in the lower limbs increases, with more flexor tone in arms. This position can be seen where the patient sits unsupported or is half lying in bed with their head flexed; their affected leg extends and affected arm flexes more. This can also be seen when a patient is sitting unsupported in a chair or wheelchair.

The asymmetrical tonic neck reflex is elicited as a proprioceptive response from the muscles of the joints and neck. Extensor tone increases in the limbs on the same side to which the head is turned. The limbs on the occipital side show an increase in flexor tone. Patients who have poor mobility requiring wheelchair dependence may have an increase in lower limb flexor tone on their weak side as well as affecting their arm. Here, a flexion contracture of the knee may develop requiring effective management strategies recommended by therapists following individual patient assessment.

Davies (1985, 2000) describes positioning for stroke patients and urges the avoidance of flat supine positioning due to its influence on the tonic neck and labyrinthine reflexes potentially resulting in an increase in inappropriate extensor activity throughout the body.

However, today there appears an overall lack of consensus in clinicians' actual practice regarding the key components of the positions necessary to limit the onset of spasticity and unwanted patterns of movement developing (Jackson 1998; Chatterton *et al.* 2001). A survey of physiotherapists specializing in treatment of stroke patients identified the most common aims of positioning for patients with neurological problems were: modulation of muscle tone (93%); prevention of damage to affected limbs (92%); and supporting and stabilizing body segments (91%) (Chatterton *et al.* 2001). These factors promote recovery in patients with neurological presentations where recovery is likely (Pope 1996; Edwards 1998;

Hawkins *et al.* 1999; Barnes 2001b). The evidence for positioning neurological patients is drawn from parallel literature for patients presenting with similar neurological symptoms and impairments affecting their function as a consequence of illness such as stroke and head injury (Davies 1985; Bobath 1990; Lynch & Grisogono 1991; Carter & Edwards 1996; Hawkins *et al.* 1999).

Joint protection

Positioning is suggested as a strategy to prevent hemiplegic shoulder pain and to prevent loss of range of movement (Kaplan 1995; Dean *et al.* 2000; Ada *et al.* 2005). This is a goal of rehabilitation to prevent the patient's functional deterioration (Gloag 1985). Dean *et al.* (2000) identified that these complications often prevent a patient's full participation in rehabilitation; contributing to poor upper limb functional outcome. Several factors were described for this:

919

- Glenohumeral subluxation due to lack of muscular activity around the shoulder.
- Trauma to the shoulder complex through unsuitable exercise.
- Trauma through inappropriate handling of the patient by staff during transfers.

Although their study failed to demonstrate significantly altered outcomes in pain and range through positioning the shoulder, Dean *et al.* (2000) acknowledged that consistency in education was essential for these common problems. Ada *et al.* (2005) recommended that patients with little upper limb function in the early stages post-stroke undergo a programme of positioning of the affected shoulder. This incorporated 45° shoulder abduction and comfortable external rotation for at least 30 minutes a day in addition to standard therapy. Their study showed statistical significance in maintaining shoulder range when compared with patients who received standard upper limb care of arm support and exercise only. Such specific joint positioning requires assessment by the physiotherapist for each individual patient.

Altered tone and abnormal patterns of movement

Tone is defined clinically as, 'the resistance that is encountered when the joint of a relaxed patient is moved passively' (Britton 1998, p. 57). Alterations in tone will affect functional recovery in patients with neurological problems and require careful management. This can be through positioning, splinting if required and oral and focal pharmacological intervention (Barnes 2001a).

Increased tone and spasticity are disorders of spinal proprioceptive reflexes. Spasticity is defined as:

a motor disorder characterised by a velocity dependent increase in tonic stretch reflexes (muscle tone) with exaggerated tendon jerks, resulting from hyper excitability of the stretch reflex, as one component on the upper motor neurone syndrome (Barnes 2001a, p. 1).

Abnormal movement patterns exist where there is interruption of the key components for normal movement. Normal movement is dependent on a neuromuscular system that can receive, integrate and respond appropriately to multiple intrinsic and extrinsic stimuli. Where this is altered through CNS or PNS disease, abnormal movement patterns will exist. Key components include:

- Normal postural tone.
- Reciprocal innervation of muscles.
- Sensory: motor feedback and feedforward.

Procedure guidelines   **Positioning the neurological patient with tonal problems**

Positional influences in the patient with neurological impairment may affect spinal, pelvic and shoulder girdle alignment with risk of soft tissue shortening due to potential:
- Flattened lumbar spine.
- Extended thoracic spine.
- Pelvis tilted backwards.
- Retracted hip.
- Elevated shoulder, retracted scapula.
- Feet tend toward plantar flexion.

Therefore, additional considerations should be applied for the neurological patient with severe tonal management issues. These should always be discussed with the physiotherapist. Appropriate seating is also advocated as an adjunct to management (Pope 1996; Kirkwood & Bardslay 2001). Referral to the occupational therapist and physiotherapist is essential for assessment where this is required.

Equipment

1 Pillows or towels (as guidance or basic positioning).
2 Foot resting splint if required.

Procedure

Action	Rationale
1 Follow basic positioning advice for positioning the patient in supine, side lying and sitting in bed as described in the above procedure guidelines for positioning patients.	To promote alignment of body segments for patients with high or low tone due to abnormal influences of primitive developmental reflexes resulting in asymmetrical posture in these patients (Davies 1985; Bobath 1990; Lynch & Grisogono 1991; Carter & Edwards 1996: R 4, E).

2 Consider and apply possible
  modifications as specified below:

(a) *Supine* (see Action figure 2a):

- Place pillow under hemiplegic hip for alignment.

  To control pelvic and spinal alignment (E).

- Place additional pillows or wedge under knees and/or head.

  To optimize patient comfort (E, P).

- Place pillow to support feet in neutral/plantargrade position.

  To maintain joint and soft tissue range (ACPIN 1998: C, E; Edwards 1998; Barnes 2001a: R 4).

- Apply foot resting splint (ankle foot orthosis [AFO]) to weak foot and ankle if recommended. NB. Ensure the splint is fitting correctly.

- Place pillow under weak arm.

(b) *Side lying* (see Action figure 2b):

- Place pillow under head and in front of trunk.

  To support the patient's affected shoulder and upper limb due to a risk of trauma, pain, muscle and soft tissue shortening (Dean *et al.* 2000; Ada *et al.* 2005: R 2b, E).
  To reduce the influence of primitive developmental reflexes and asymmetrical posturing of head and trunk in patients with high or low tone (E). May be effective in maintaining opposing trunk muscles (E).

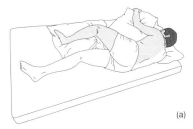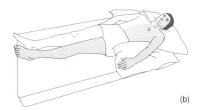

(a)   (b)

Action 2 Positioning the patient with neurological weakness. **(a)** Side lying: affected arm supported on pillow. **(b)** Supine: affected arm supported on pillow.

- Balance reactions (Edwards 1996a).
- Biomechanical properties of muscle (Edwards 1998).

The influence of altered tone and abnormal patterns of movement are key to therapeutic theories supporting treatment of recovery of motor control associated with patients with neurological problems. Patients attempt to perform functional skills as prerequisites of activities of daily living, but without appropriate background postural tone and normal properties of muscle, these movements will be performed in an abnormal way.

Soft tissue changes and contractures

Soft tissue changes and contractures occur through disuse in normal muscle (Jones & Moffatt 2002). With increased tone joint range and subsequent function is at risk. Restriction in the range of movement is not always simply through increased tone of the relevant muscles. The surrounding soft tissues, tendons, ligaments and the joints themselves can develop changes resulting in decreased compliance leading to an increased likelihood of them being maintained in a shortened position (Barnes 2001a). This creates a secondary biomechanical component of spasticity and is often seen in patients with functional mobility problems. Adaptation of the mechanical properties of muscle also contribute to increased tone in patients with hypertonia (O'Dwyer et al. 1996). It is possible, but not proven, that maintaining a joint through a full range of movement may prevent the longer term development of soft tissue contractures (Barnes 2001a).

Environment and positioning

Problems of perception are considered to be one of the main factors limiting functional motor recovery following stroke (Baer & Durward 2004). These can be applied to patients with disease or illness affecting their CNS. Here, the patient fails to respond appropriately to stimuli presented on their hemiplegic side, the contralateral side to the brain lesion; the left is more commonly affected following right parietal lesions (Lindsay & Bone 1997; Baer & Durward 2004). Environmental factors such as correct positioning are essential for ensuring optimal level of function for each individual (Edwards 1996b). Clinical management strategies include:

- Addressing the patient from the affected side.
- Deliberate placement of items such as drinks on that side.
- Advice to carers to position themselves on the patient's affected side whilst talking to them in order to orientate them to their affected side.
- Positioning the patient on their 'affected side' enabling function with their 'sound side'.

- Positioning the patient on their 'unaffected side', orientating the patient to their affected side.

Limited evidence exists to suggest the benefit of this (Baer & Durward 2004). However, it is recognized as a useful treatment adjunct for these patients by experienced occupational therapists and physiotherapists, through promotion of sensory awareness/appreciation, including perception and body image and enabling function (Davies 1985; Bobath 1990; Lynch & Grisogono 1991; Greive 1993; Carter & Edwards 1996).

Rehabilitation opportunity

Patients with neurological illness or disease present with an assortment of clinical symptoms. Positioning can assist in their holistic management and allow future opportunity for rehabilitation where their disease allows. Additional considerations for this patient group include the patient's:

923

- Respiratory function (see earlier section).
- Swallowing function; a referral to a speech and language therapist is recommended for any patient at risk.
- Cognitive function; a referral to occupational therapy or clinical psychology is recommended.

Procedure guidelines **Positioning the preoperative and postoperative amputee patient**

Equipment

1 Stump board (for below knee amputees sitting out in wheelchair).
2 Pillows.

Action	Rationale
Upper limb amputee	
1 Ensure patient is maintaining full range of motion of all joints of the upper limb.	To prevent contractures in case of possible prosthetic rehabilitation and functional use (E, P).

Procedure guidelines *(cont.)*

Positioning the below knee amputee

1 Maintain knee extension:

(a) **In bed**: do not place towel or pillow under knee unless supporting whole of stump, i.e. do not encourage the knee to be maintained in a flexed position.

To prevent knee flexion contracture (E).
To aid stump oedema management (E).
To promote healing (E).

(b) **In chair**: use stump board on wheelchair if one has been issued.

To support knee joint (E, P).
To prevent excessive knee flexion (E).
To aid stump oedema management (White 1992: R 4, E, P).
To protect the residual limb (E, P).

Positioning the above knee amputee

1 Maintain hip in a neutral position:

To maintain hip extension (E).

(a) **In bed**: ensure patient is periodically lying supine.
Or:

To prevent hip flexion contracture (E).

(b) Consider prone lying or side lying with hip in neutral position.

To avoid shortening of hip flexors and abductors (E).

(c) **In sitting**: ensure that patient does not place towel or pillow under stump.

To prevent excessive hip flexion (E).

Note: Following lower limb amputation patients should be mobilized with caution, particularly if a prosthetic assessment is planned. This is because standing for long periods or hopping can:

■ Negatively influence stump oedema and wound healing.
■ Overtire a patient particularly elderly patients or those who are physically de-conditioned prior to the amputation.
■ Encourage the patient to adopt poor gait patterns due to excessive weight bearing on the remaining limb leading to difficulty with prosthetic rehabilitation.

Appropriate management of these factors will influence the patient's future rehabilitation opportunity and will contribute to their recovery and/or management from an early stage. The latter are not covered in this book.

Positioning and amputee management

The main goal of positioning with regard to amputee management is the prevention of contractures (particularly if the patient's goal is prosthetic rehabilitation) and help controlling stump oedema in order to assist wound healing. Patients will need to be comprehensively assessed by the key professionals to identify realistic goals and ensure adequate pain management (BACPAR 2006). Where possible the process of positioning starts at the preoperative stage when the affected limb is often painful and therefore the patient may adopt positions of comfort that can lead to contractures. These positions are often maintained post-amputation due to comfort and habit but are also due to changes in muscle balance. For example, above knee amputees may adopt a flexed position of their stump due to an alteration in muscle balance and pain but this can lead to contracture over time if not corrected (Engstrom & Van de Ven 1999). Contractures can profoundly affect the potential for prosthetic rehabilitation so early correct positioning is paramount in this cohort of patients (Munin *et al.* 2001).

925

Amputation affecting either an upper or lower limb will alter the patient's centre of gravity resulting in decreased balance and likelihood to adopt poor postures. Although the guidelines regarding sitting or walking a patient outlined above are applicable to this client group, particular care needs to be taken with regard to body symmetry and posture when the patient is lying, sitting or mobilizing.

Conclusion

This chapter has discussed the aims and general principles of positioning in order to help optimize function for patients. These principles of positioning can apply to all patients regardless of their diagnosis. However, attention has been drawn to specific patient groups where additional considerations and/or modifications are required.

It is essential that maximum function and quality of life are achieved through early assessment and treatment including positioning, timely rehabilitation and provision of equipment. It highlights the need for early identification of problems and early referral to appropriate key health professionals for individual patient assessment. This helps to provide effective, patient-focused holistic management and care.

References and further reading

ACPIN (1998) *Clinical Practice Guidelines on splinting adults with neurological dysfunction.* Association of Physiotherapists Interested in Neurology, Chartered Society of Physiotherapy, London.

ACPOPC (1993) *Physiotherapy in Oncology and Palliative Care: Guidelines for Good Practice.* Association of Physiotherapists in Oncology and Palliative Care, Chartered Society of Physiotherapy, London.

Ada, L. *et al.* (2005) Thirty minutes of positioning reduces the development of shoulder external rotation contracture after stroke: a randomised controlled study. *Arch Phys Med Rehabil*, **86**, 230–4.

Adam, S. & Forrest, S. (1999) ABC of intensive care: other supportive care. *BMJ*, **319**, 175–8.

Anderson, F.A. & Spencer, F.A. (2003) Risk factors for venous thromboembolism. *Circulation*, **107**, 9–16.

BACPAR (2006) *Clinical Guidelines for the Pre and Post Operative Management of Adults with Lower Limb Amputation*. The Chartered Society of Physiotherapy, London.

Baer, G. & Durward, B. (2004) Stroke. In: *Physical Management in Neurological Rehabilitation* (ed M. Stokes), 2nd edn. Elsevier Mosby, Edinburgh, pp. 75–101.

Barnes, M.P. (2001a) An overview of the clinical management of spasticity. In: *Upper Motor Neurone Syndrome and Spasticity: Clinical Management and Neurophysiology* (eds M.P. Barnes & G.R. Johnson). Cambridge, Cambridge University Press, pp. 1–11.

Barnes, M.P. (2001b) Spasticity: a rehabilitation challenge in the elderly. *Gerontology*, **47**(6), 295–9.

Barsevick, A.M. *et al.* (2002) A pilot study examining energy conservation for cancer treatment-related fatigue. *Cancer Nurs*, **25**(5), 333–41.

Bausewein, C., Borasio, G.D. & Voltz, R. (2004) Brain tumours. In: *Oxford Textbook of Palliative Medicine* (eds D. Doyle *et al.*). Oxford University Press, Oxford, pp. 727–30.

Beck, L.A. (2003) Cancer rehabilitation: can it make a difference? *Rehab Nurs*, **28**(2), 42–7.

Bobath, B. (1990) *Adult Hemiplegia: Evaluation and Treatment*. Heinemann, Oxford.

Brada, M. (1995) Central nervous system tumours. In: *Oncology: A Multidisciplinary Textbook* (ed. A. Horwich). Chapman & Hall, London, pp. 395–416.

Britton, T.C. (1998) Abnormalities of muscle tone and movement. In: *Neurological Physiotherapy* (ed. M. Stokes). Mosby, London, pp. 57–65.

Brown, A. *et al.* (1996) *Physiotherapy Management of the Spontaneously Breathing, Acutely Breathless, Adult Patient – A Problem Solving Approach*. Association of Chartered Physiotherapists in Respiratory Care, London.

Carr, E.K. & Kenney, F. D. (1992) Positioning the stroke patient: a review of the literature. *Int J Nur Stud*, **29**, 335–6.

Carter, P. & Edwards, S. (1996) General principles of treatment. In: *Neurological Physiotherapy: A Problem Solving Approach* (ed S. Edwards). Churchill Livingstone, London, pp. 87–113.

Chatterton, H.J., Pomeroy, V.M. & Gratton J. (2001) Positioning for stroke patients: a survey of physiotherapists' aims and practices. *Disabil Rehabil*, **23**(10), 413–21.

Convertino, V.A., Bloomfield, S.A. & Greenleaf, J.E. (1995) An overview of the issues: physiological effects of bed rest and restricted physical activity. *Med Sci Sport Ex*, **29**(2), 187–90.

Cooper, J. (2006) *Occupational Therapy in Oncology and Palliative Care*. John Wiley & Sons, Ltd, Chichester.

Corcoran, P.J. (1991) Use it or lose it – the hazards of bed rest and immobility. *West J Med*, **154**(5), 536–8.

Creditor, M.C. (1993) Hazards of hospitalization of the elderly. *Ann Intern Med*, **118**(3), 219–23.

926

CSP (2002) Guidance on the manual handling for physiotherapists. www.csp.org.uk. Accessed 21/07/2003.

CSP (2003) CSP position statement: the role of physiotherapy for people with cancer. Chartered Society of Physiotherapy. www.csp.org.uk. Accessed 21/07/2003.

Davies, P.M. (1985) *Steps to Follow: a Guide to the Treatment of Adult Hemiplegia*. Springer-Verlag, Berlin.

Davies, P.M. (2000) *Steps to Follow: the Comprehensive Treatment of Adult Hemiplegia*, 2nd edn. Springer-Verlag, Berlin.

Dean, C.M., Makey, F.H. & Katrak, P. (2000) Examination of shoulder positioning after stroke: a randomised controlled pilot trial. *Aust J Physiother*, **46**, 35–40.

Dean, E. (1985) Effect of body positioning on pulmonary function. *Phys Ther*, **65**, 613–18.

DH (2000) The NHS cancer plan: a plan for investment, a plan for reform. www.doh.gov.org. Accessed 18/5/06.

Dietz, J.H. (1981) *Rehabilitation Oncology*. John Wiley & Sons, Inc., New York.

Doyle, D. *et al.* (2004) *Oxford Textbook of Palliative Medicine*, 3rd edn. Oxford University Press, Oxford.

Doyle, L., McClure, J. & Fisher, S. (2004) The contribution of physiotherapy to palliative medicine. In: *Oxford Textbook of Palliative Medicine* (eds D. Doyle *et al.*), 3rd edn. Oxford University Press, Oxford, pp. 1050–56.

Edwards, S. (1996a) An analysis of normal movement as the basis for development of treatment techniques. In: *Neurological Physiotherapy: a Problem Solving Approach*. Churchill Livingstone, London, pp. 15–40.

Edwards, S. (1996b) Abnormal tone and movement as a result of neurological impairment. In: *Neurological Physiotherapy: a Problem Solving Approach*. Churchill Livingstone, London, pp. 63–86.

Edwards, S. (1998) Physiotherapy management of established spasticity in spasticity rehabilitation. In: *Spasticity Management* (ed. G. Sheean). Churchill Communications Europe Ltd, London, pp. 71–90.

Ellison, D. & Love, S. (2000) Classification and general concepts of CNS neoplasms and astrocytic neoplasms. In: *Neuropathology: a Reference Text of CNS Pathology* (eds D. Ellison & S. Love). Mosby, London.

Engstrom, B. & Van de Ven, C. (1999) *Therapy for Amputees*, 3rd edn. Churchill, Harcourt Brace & Co, Edinburgh.

Fulton, C. (1994) Physiotherapy in cancer care: a framework for rehabilitation. *Physiotherapy*, **80**(12), 830–4.

Fyfe, N. *et al.* (1993) Orthoses, mobility and environmental control systems. In: *Neurological Rehabilitation* (eds R. Greenwood *et al.*). Churchill Livingstone, London, pp. 229–44.

Gardiner, M.D. (1973) *The Principles of Exercise Therapy*. Bell & Sons, London.

Gillis, M.K. (1989) Observational gait analysis. In: *Physical Therapy* (eds R.M. Scully & M.R. Barnes). Lippincott, Philadelphia, pp. 670–95.

Gloag, D. (1985) Rehabilitation after stroke: what's the potential? *Br Med J*, **290**, 699–701.

Greive, J. (1993) *Neuropsychology for Occupational Therapists: Assessment of Perception and Cognition*. Blackwell Publishing, London.

Guererro, D. (1998) *Neuro-oncology for Nurses*. Whurr, London.

927

Hawkins, S., Stone, K. & Plummer, L. (1999) An holistic approach to turning adults. *Nurs Stand*, **6**(14), 51–6.

Hodges, P.W. & Gandevia, S.C. (2000) Changes in intra-abdominal pressure during postural and respiratory activation of the human diaphragm. *J Appl Physiol*, **89**(3), 967–76.

Hough, A. (2001) *Physiotherapy in Respiratory Care: an Evidence-Based Approach to Respiratory and Cardiac Management*, 3rd edn. Nelson Thornes Ltd., Cheltenham.

HSE (1992) *Manual Handling Operations Regulations*. HMSO, London.

Jackson, J. (1998) Specific treatment techniques. In: *Neurological Physiotherapy* (ed. M. Stokes). Mosby, London, pp. 299–311.

Jones, M. & Moffatt, F. (2002) Deconditioning. In: *Cardiopulmonary Physiotherapy* (ed. A. Watts). BIOS Scientific Publishers Ltd, Oxford, pp. 129–38.

Kaplan, M.C. (1995) Hemiplegic shoulder pain – early prevention and rehabilitation. *Am J Phys Med Rehabil*, **162**(2), 151–152.

Kirkwood, C.A. & Bardslay, G.I. (2001) Seating and positioning in spasticity. In: *Upper Motor Neurone Syndrome and Spasticity: Clinical Management and Neurophysiology* (eds M.P. Barnes & G.R. Johnson). Cambridge University Press, Cambridge, pp. 122–141.

Kirschblum, S. *et al.* (2001) Rehabilitation of persons with central nervous system tumours. *Cancer*, **92**(54), 1029–38.

Lindsay, K.W. & Bone, I. (1997) *Neurology and Neurosurgery Illustrated*, 3rd edn. Churchill Livingstone, London.

Lynch, M. & Grisogono, V. (1991) *Strokes and Head Injuries: a Guide for Patients, Families, Friends and Carers*. John Murray, London.

McGarvey III, C.L. (1990) *Physical Therapy for the Cancer Patient*. Churchill Livingstone, New York.

McKenzie, R. (1985) *Treat Your Own Back*. Spinal Publications, New Zealand.

Munin, C. *et al.* (2001) Predictive factors for successful early prosthetic ambulation among lower limb amputees. *J Rehabil Res Dev*, **38**(4), 379–84.

National Council for Hospice and Specialist Palliative Care Services (NCHSPCS) (2000) *Fulfilling Lives: Rehabilitation in Palliative Care*. Land and Unwin, Northamptonshire.

NHSE (1995) A policy framework for commissioning cancer services: a report by the Expert Advisory Group on Cancer to the Chief Medical Officers of England and Wales (Calman–Hine Report). National Health and Safety Executive, Department of Health, London. Available from www.doh.gov.org. Accessed 21/03/2007.

NICE (2002) *Guidance on Cancer Services: Improving Outcomes in Breast Cancer*. National Institute for Health and Clinical Excellence, London.

NICE (2004) *Guidance on Cancer Services: Improving Supportive and Palliative Care for Patients with Cancer*. National Institute for Health and Clinical Excellence, London, pp. 134–147.

NICE (2005) *Guidance on Cancer Services: Improving Outcomes for People with Tumours of the Brain and Central Nervous System*. National Institute for Health and Clinical Excellence, London.

Norris, C.M. (1995) Spinal stabilisation 2. Limiting factors to end stage motion in the lumbar spine. *Physiotherapy*, **81**(2), 64–72.

O'Donovan K. *et al.* (2006) An investigation of recommended lower leg exercises for in-duced calf muscle activity. International Association of Science and Technology for Development. Proceedings of the 24th IASTED International Conference on Biomedical Engineering, Innsbrook.

O'Dwyer, N.J., Ada, L. & Neilson, P.D. (1996) Spasticity and muscle contracture following stroke. *Brain*, **119**, 1737–49.

Pearsall, J. (ed.) (2001) *The Concise English Dictionary*, 10th edn. Oxford University Press, Oxford.

Pope, P. (1996) Postural management and seating. In: *Neurological Physiotherapy: a Problem Solving Approach* (ed S. Edwards). Churchill Livingstone, London, pp. 135–60.

Pryor, J.A. & Webber, B.A. (2002) Physiotherapy techniques. In: *Physiotherapy for Respiratory and Cardiac Problems: Adults and Paediatrics* (eds J.A. Pryor & S.A. Prasad). Churchill Livingstone, Edinburgh, pp. 189–230.

Reidel, M. (2001) Acute pulmonary embolism 1: pathophysiology, clinical presentation, and diagnosis. *Heart*, **85**(2), 229–40.

Russell, L. (2004) Patient repositioning revisited. *J Wound Care*, **13**(8), 328–9.

Shumway-Cook, A. & Woollacott, M. (1995) *Motor Control: Theory and Practical Applications*. Williams and Wilkins, Baltimore.

Stokes, M. (2004) *Physical Management in Neurological Rehabilitation*, 2nd edn. Elsevier Mosby, Edinburgh.

Tookman, A.J., Hopkins, K. & Scharpen-von-Heusson, K. (2004) Rehabilitation in palliative medicine. In:*Oxford Textbook of Palliative Medicine* (ed. D. Doyle), 3rd edn. Oxford University Press, Oxford, pp. 1019–32.

Wagner, P.D. & West, J.B. (2005) Ventilation, blood flow and gas exchange. In: *Textbook of Respiratory Medicine* (eds R.J. Mason *et al.*), 4th edn. Elsevier Saunders, Philadelphia, pp. 51–85.

West, J.B., Dollery, C.T. & Naimark, A. (1964) Distribution of blood flow in isolated lung; relation to vascular and alveolar pressures. *J Appl Physiol*, **19**, 713–24.

White, E. (1992) Wheelchair stump boards and their use in lower limb amputees. *Br J Occupat Ther*, **55**(5), 174–8.

WHO (2001) International classification for functioning and health. World Health Organization. www3.who.int/icf/icftemplate.cfm. Accessed 9/2/07.

Zach, M.B., Pontoppidan, H. & Kazemi, H. (1974) The effect of lateral positions on gas exchange in pulmonary disease. *Am Rev Respir Dis*, **110**, 49–55.

Multiple choice questions

1 Traditionally, bed rest was seen as an effective means of managing certain conditions. Increasingly bed rest is seen as being detrimental to a patient's condition. Which of the following is not a consequence of inactivity?

   a Deconditioning of body systems
   b Fluid imbalance
   c Social isolation
   d Loss of independence

2 When sitting, patients should be discouraged from crossing their legs in order that they:

   a Reduce the risk of DVT
   b Reduce the risk of infection
   c Reduce the risk of foot drop
   d Reduce the risk of pathological fractures

3 Patients require sticks and walking aids for a variety of different reasons. How would you advise a patient with stick/walking aid to approach a chair or bed when wishing to sit from a standing position?

   a However the patient feels most confident
   b Forwards, letting the knees touch the bed or chair
   c Backwards, letting the back of the legs touch the bed or chair
   d Stand sideways to bed or chair, then pivot to seated position

4 When caring for patients following the amputation of a lower limb, which of the following is not true:

a Place a towel under the knee when sitting
b Periodically lie supine
c Periodically lie prone
d Encourage the use of a stump board

Answers to the multiple choice questions can be found in Appendix 3.

Chapter 27

Respiratory therapy

Definition

The principle of respiratory therapy is the application of pharmacological and non-pharmacological means to improve breathing and therefore improve gaseous exchange. This will include an assessment of the cause of the impaired breathing, reversal of causes where possible, and therapies to optimize respiratory function.

Indications

- Respiratory failure, of which there are two types, is characterized by problems with some or all of the four functions listed below:
  - *Type 1*, referred to as hypoxaemic respiratory failure (failure to oxygenate the tissues). The PaO_2 is <8 kPa (60 mmHg) while the carbon dioxide (PCO_2) is normal or low. Common causes include infectious conditions, pneumonia, pulmonary oedema and adult respiratory distress syndrome.
  - *Type 2*, referred to as hypercapnic (raised carbon dioxide) or respiratory pump failure. Alveolar ventilation is insufficient to excrete carbon dioxide accompanied by hypoxaemia (deficiency of oxygen in the arterial blood). The PCO_2 is >6 kPa (45 mmHg). Common causes include chronic obstructive pulmonary disease (COPD), chest wall deformities, drug overdose and chest injury.
- Acute myocardial infarction.
- Cardiac failure.
- Shock–haemorrhagic, bacteraemic and cardiogenic.
- Conditions in which there is a reduced ability to transport oxygen, e.g. anaemia.
- During anaesthesia.
- Postoperatively.
- Sleep apnoea.
- Severe pain.

- Asthma.
- Pulmonary embolus.
- Conditions that affect the neuromuscular control of breathing such as muscular dystrophy, Guillain Barré.
- Severe trauma affecting the diaphragm, ribs, lungs, or trachea.
- Tension pneumothorax.
- Pleural effusion.

Reference material

Physiology (see also Chapter 18)

The respiratory system is a complex system that is responsible for the efficient exchange of the respiratory gases primarily oxygen and carbon dioxide. The respiratory system is responsible for ensuring a continuous optimum supply of oxygen to the tissues and the elimination of carbon dioxide during expiration. Four separate functions are necessary to achieve optimal respiration (Marieb 2006):

1 Pulmonary ventilation: adequate breathing ensuring movement of air in and out of the lungs ensuring a fresh supply of oxygen to the alveoli;
2 External respiration: ensuring adequate gas exchange oxygen uptake and carbon dioxide unloading between the blood and the alveoli of the lungs.
3 Transport of respiratory gases: oxygen and carbon dioxide between the lungs and the body tissues. Transport is affected by the cardiovascular system and uses the blood as a carrying mechanism.
4 Cellular respiration: oxygen delivery and carbon dioxide uptake between the systemic blood and tissue cells.

The respiratory system is composed of the following structures:

- The two respiratory centres in the medulla oblongata and pons of the brain.
- The nose, mouth and connecting airways.
- The trachea, main bronchus, bronchioles and alveoli.
- The respiratory muscles: the diaphragm and the intercostal muscles.
- The respiratory nerves: the subphrenic nerve and the intercostal nerves.
- The bone structure of the thorax: the ribs, vertebrae and sternum.
- The lung parenchyma.
- The pleura.

Alteration, damage or blockage to any of the structures listed above may result in either respiratory impairment or respiratory failure. It is essential when considering respiratory function to remember the close association and dependence between the cardiovascular, neurological, musculoskeletal and respiratory system.

Tissue oxygenation

All the cells of the body require a continuous supply of oxygen to ensure growth and repair of tissues and optimum metabolism. Oxygen is drawn into the body through the nose and mouth; it then travels down the trachea and into the smaller airways and alveoli of the lungs. Once it has reached the alveoli oxygen in solution is able to transfer into the network of capillaries and from there travels via the venous network to all cells of the body. This tissue oxygenation is known as cellular oxygenation. Low oxygen levels are called hypoxia. In low oxygen conditions anaerobic cellular oxygenation will occur generating the waste product lactic acid. If the low oxygen state is allowed to continue lactic acid will accumulate leading to a metabolic acidosis and cell death (West 1995; Oh 1997; Berne & Levy 1998; Guyton 2000; Hess 2000; Pierson 2000; Kumar & Clark 2005; Marieb 2006; Tortora & Derrickson 2008).

There are three components to oxygenation: oxygen uptake, oxygen transportation and oxygen utilization. *Oxygen uptake* is the process of extracting oxygen from the environment. *Oxygen transportation* is the mechanism by which the uptake of oxygen results in the delivery of oxygen to the cells. *Oxygen utilization* is the metabolic need for molecular oxygen by the cells of the body.

In order for oxygenation to take place there needs to be an adequate cardiac output.

934

Oxygen uptake

The air that we breathe in during normal conditions from the atmosphere is composed of the following gases:

- oxygen 21%;
- carbon dioxide 0.03%;
- nitrogen 79%;
- rare gases 0.003%.

Inspired air at sea level has a total atmospheric pressure of 760 mmHg. According to Dalton's law, where there is a mixture of gases each gas exerts its own pressure as if there were no other gases present. The pressure of an individual gas in a mixture is called the partial pressure and is denoted as P, which is then followed by the type of gas so that the partial pressure of oxygen is written PO_2 (Tortora & Derrickson 2008):

- Oxygen $0.21 \times 760 = 159$ mmHg (21 kPa).
- Carbon dioxide $0.03 \times 760 = 22.8$ mmHg (3.0 kPa).
- Nitrogen $0.79 \times 760 = 600$ mmHg (80 kPa).

Table 27.1 Oxygen cascade. Pressure gradients for oxygen transfer from inspired gas to tissue cells.

	mmHg	kPa
Inspired air	150	20.0
Alveolar	103	13.7
Arterial	100	13.3
Capillary	51	6.8
Tissue	20	2.7
Mitochondrial	1–20	0.13–1.30

The partial pressure of gases controls the movement of oxygen and carbon dioxide through the body between the atmosphere and the lungs, the lungs and the blood and finally the blood and the cells. Movement of gases is by diffusion. Diffusion is the movement of gas molecules from an area of relatively high partial pressure to one of lower partial pressure.

Diffusion of oxygen takes place from the alveolus into the pulmonary capillaries and movement of carbon dioxide from the capillary into the alveolus. From the alveolus the oxygen diffuses from the capillaries into the tissues and mitochondria of the cells (Figure 27.1).

The alveolar oxygen partial pressure is higher than the arterial oxygen partial pressure in order to push the oxygen through the alveolar membrane into the interstitial spaces and from there into the pulmonary capillaries. Oxygen continues to diffuse from the capillaries into the tissues then to the mitochondria of the cells for metabolism (Carpenter 1991; Pierce 1995; Oh 1997; Berne & Levy 1998; Esmond 2000; Guyton 2000; Marieb 2006; Tortora & Derrickson 2008).

As inspired air enters the respiratory tract it encounters water vapour present in the upper airways which warms and humidifies it. Water vapour exerts its own partial pressure of 47 mmHg. The partial pressure of the water vapour must be subtracted from the total atmospheric pressure to give a corrected atmospheric pressure and partial pressure of each gas:

- Corrected total atmospheric $760 - 47 = 713$ mmHg.
- Oxygen $0.21 \times 713 = 150$ mmHg (20 kPa).
- Carbon dioxide $0.03 \times 713 = 21$ mmHg (2.8 kPa).

As oxygen continues to pass down the respiratory tract to the alveolus it encounters carbon dioxide leaving the respiratory tract which also exerts a partial pressure, equal to 40 mmHg. This in turn must be subtracted to determine the correct values. Oxygen has a corrected value of $150 - 40 = 110 - 100$ mmHg ($14.6 - 13.3$ kPa).

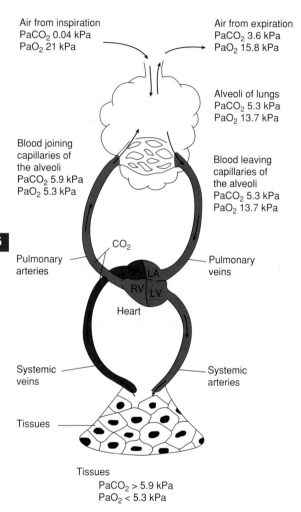

Air from inspiration
PaCO$_2$ 0.04 kPa
PaO$_2$ 21 kPa

Air from expiration
PaCO$_2$ 3.6 kPa
PaO$_2$ 15.8 kPa

Alveoli of lungs
PaCO$_2$ 5.3 kPa
PaO$_2$ 13.7 kPa

Blood joining
capillaries of
the alveoli
PaCO$_2$ 5.9 kPa
PaO$_2$ 5.3 kPa

Blood leaving
capillaries of
the alveoli
PaCO$_2$ 5.3 kPa
PaO$_2$ 13.7 kPa

CO$_2$

Pulmonary
arteries

RA   LA
RV   LV

Heart

Pulmonary
veins

Systemic
veins

Systemic
arteries

Tissues

Tissues
PaCO$_2$ > 5.9 kPa
PaO$_2$ < 5.3 kPa

Figure 27.1   Gas movement in the body is facilitated by partial pressure differences.
Top of figure illustrates pressure gradients that facilitate oxygen and carbon dioxide
exchange in the lungs. Bottom of figure shows pressure gradients that facilitate gas
movements from systemic capillaries to tissues.

936

Oxygen transportation

Oxygen is carried in the blood in two ways:

- *Dissolved in the plasma (serum)*: only 2–3% is carried in this way as oxygen is not very soluble (Aherns & Tucker 1999; Marieb 2006). This is measured as the PaO_2. There is 0.003 ml of blood for each 1 mmHg partial pressure oxygen. At 100 mmHg partial pressure, only 0.3 ml of oxygen would be carried per 100 ml of plasma.
- *Bound to haemoglobin in the red blood cells*: 95–98% of oxygen is carried in this way and is measured as the percentage of oxygen saturated (SaO_2). Each gram of haemoglobin can carry 1.34 ml of oxygen per 100 ml blood.

Haemoglobin is composed of haem (iron) and globulin (protein). Each haemoglobin molecule has four binding sites each able to carry one molecule of oxygen. A haemoglobin molecule is said to be fully saturated with oxygen when all four haem sites are attached to oxygen. When fewer than four attached the haemoglobin is said to be partially saturated.

937

The bond between haemoglobin and oxygen is affected by various physiological factors that shift the oxygen dissociation curve to the right or left (Figure 27.2).

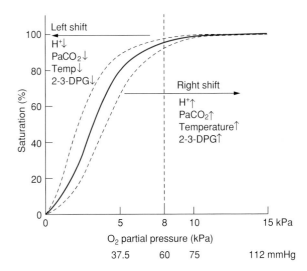

Figure 27.2 Oxyhaemoglobin dissociation curve. With a PaO_2 of 8 kPa and more, saturations will remain high (flat portion of curve). NB. The middle red line is the normal position of the curve.

Oxyhaemoglobin curve shift to the right

When a shift occurs to the right there is reduced binding of oxygen to haemoglobin and oxygen is given up more easily to the tissues. The saturation will be lower.

Factors that cause the curve to shift to the right are:

- Increase in body temperature due to infection, sepsis.
- Increase in hydrogen ion content (acidaemia), known as the Bohr effect due to infection, sepsis or other shock conditions.
- Increase in carbon dioxide due to sepsis, pulonary disease, postoperatively.
- Increase in 2-3-DPG (2-3-DPG is an enzyme found in the red blood cells that affects haemoglobin and oxygen binding).

Oxyhaemoglobin curve shift to the left

When a shift occurs to the left there is an increase in the binding of oxygen to the haemoglobin, oxygen is given less easily to the tissues and cellular hypoxia can occur.

Factors that cause the curve to shift to the left are:

- Decrease in body temperature due to exposure, near drowning, trauma.
- Decrease in hydrogen ion content (alkalaemia).
- Decrease in carbon dioxide.
- Decrease in 2-3-DPG.

Oxygen utilization

The relationship between the PaO_2 and the SaO_2 is represented as the oxygen dissociation curve. Oxygen uptake in the lungs is shown by the upper flat part of the curve. When the PaO_2 is between 8.0 and 13.3 kPa (60–100 mmHg) the haemoglobin is 90% or more saturated with oxygen. At this point of the curve, large changes in the PaO_2 lead to small changes in the SaO_2 of haemoglobin, because the haemoglobin is almost completely saturated. Release of oxygen to the tissues is shown by the lower part of the curve. There is easy removal of oxygen from the haemoglobin for use by the cells. It is at this part of the curve that small changes in the PaO_2 cause major changes in the SaO_2. This is important clinically.

A patient's oxygen level must be kept at 8.5 kPa or above (60 mmHg). Below this level desaturation can occur at a rapid rate, resulting in tissue hypoxia and cell death.

Oxygen consumption

At rest the normal oxygen consumption is approximately 200–250 ml/minute. As the available oxygen per minute in a normal man is about 700 ml, this means there is an oxygen reserve of 450–500 ml/minute. Factors that increase the above consumption of oxygen include fever, sepsis, shivering, restlessness and increased metabolism (Oh 1997). It is difficult to say at which absolute level oxygen therapy is necessary as each situation should be judged by the requirements for oxygen and the availability of oxygen. Therefore, all of the above information needs to be taken into account together with the measurement of the arterial blood gases.

Generally, additional oxygen will be required when the PaO_2 has fallen to 8.5 kPa (60 mmHg) or less (Oh 1997). Oxygen saturation level in the tissues can be measured using a pulse oximeter, which works by emitting narrow shafts of red and infrared light through the tissue of a finger, toe or earlobe. Different amounts of light rays are absorbed by the arterial blood depending on its saturation with oxygen. The final oxygen saturation (SaO_2) is then calculated by computer (Ehrhardt & Graham 1990).

Carbon dioxide excretion

The second function of the respiratory system is to excrete carbonic acid from the lungs during expiration. The normal level of carbon dioxide in the blood is 3.5–5.3 kPa. Carbon dioxide has a direct effect on the respiratory centres in the brain. As the carbon dioxide level rises and diffuses from the blood into the cerebrospinal fluid (CSF) it is hydrated and carbonic acid is formed. The acid then dissociates and hydrogen ions are liberated as there are no proteins in the CSF to buffer the hydrogen ions, the pH of the CSF falls which excites the central chemoreceptors, and the respiratory rate is increased (Marieb 2006).

Respiratory assessment

When assessing respiratory function it is essential to include all of the respiratory tree cited above in the evaluation. Having received information about the person's past medical history one of the most reliable and important assessments is to closely observe and talk to the patient. Normal respiration is effortless and almost unconscious, and the person can eat, drink and speak in full sentences without appearing breathless. Essential first steps in respiratory assessment are therefore to observe the person's breathing for the following:

- Ease and comfort.
- Rate.
- Pattern.
- Position the patient has adopted: for example does the patient need to sit at 90° upright to breathe effectively?
- Rate and ease of breathing during speaking or movement.
- General colour and appearance: is there any evidence of greyness, cyanosis, pallor, sweating?
- Additional audible breath sounds: wheezing or stridor?

Having rapidly made this assessment other essential assessments are a chest X-ray and arterial blood gas, and a computed tomography (CT) scan or ventilation/perfusion (V/Q) scan may also be necessary.

Having made a comprehensive assessment the immediate cause should be corrected where possible. It is important to recognize that this may result from interruption to any part of respiration; for example, the patient may be in severe pain and appropriate pain management may improve their respiratory function, or conversely an opioid overdose may result in decreased or absent respiration and the antidote to an opioid will then need to be given. There may be a mechanical obstruction to respiration such as an infective obstruction like epiglottitis and the treatment is therefore directed at treating the infection whilst also oxygenating the patient.

Respiratory therapy therefore covers a wide area and will include any manipulation or management of alteration to any part of the respiratory tree. It may include: pharmacological management including pain management, antidotes to drug toxicity, antimicrobials for infections of the respiratory tract, or respiratory stimulants; surgery to repair a ruptured diaphragm, to manage trauma, the insertion of a tracheostomy, the insertion of chest drains, or a thoraco-abdominal shunt for superior vena cava obstruction. Finally positioning and physiotherapy play a major role in improving respiratory function.

Any person who is unable to maintain tissue oxygenation will need to receive supplemental oxygen until they are able to manage again on room air. This oxygen may be delivered in different ways depending on the severity of the condition and the level of hypoxia.

General considerations

- Oxygen is an odourless, tasteless, colourless, transparent gas that is slightly heavier than air.
- Oxygen supports combustion; therefore, there is always a danger of fire when oxygen is being used. The following safety measures should be remembered:

  (a) Oil or grease around oxygen connections should be avoided.
  (b) Alcohol, ether and other inflammatory liquids should be used with caution in the vicinity of oxygen.
  (c) No electrical device must be used in or near an oxygen tent.
  (d) Oxygen cylinders should be kept secure in an upright position and away from heat.
  (e) There must be no smoking in the vicinity of oxygen.
  (f) A fire extinguisher should be readily available.
  (g) Care should be taken with high concentrations of oxygen when using the defibrillator in a cardiorespiratory arrest, or during elective cardioversion.

Equipment necessary to administer respiratory therapy

Any oxygen delivery system will include these basic components:

- Oxygen supply, from either a piped supply or a portable cylinder. All medical gas cylinders have to conform to a standardized colour coding: oxygen cylinders are black with a white shoulder and are labelled 'Oxygen' or 'O_2'. Since 2004, small portable oxygen cylinders have been in use: these are totally white and are a C-size cylinder.
- A reduction gauge: to reduce the pressure to that of atmospheric pressure.
- Flowmeter: a device that controls the flow of oxygen in litres per minute.
- Tubing: disposable tubing of varying diameter and length.
- Mechanism for delivery: a mask or nasal cannulae.
- Humidifier: to warm and moisten the oxygen before administration.
- Water trap if humidifier in use.

Oxygen delivery systems

Nasal cannulae catheter (Figure 27.3)

Nasal cannulae consist of two prongs that are inserted inside the anterior nares and supported on a light frame. Advantages to the patient are that they may seem

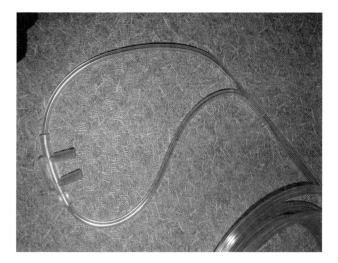

Figure 27.3 Nasal cannula.

Table 27.2 Oxygen flow rates for nasal cannulae.

Oxygen flow rate (l/min)	% Oxygen delivered
1	24
2	28
3	32
4	36
5	40
6	44

less claustrophobic and do not interfere with eating, drinking and communication. Nasal cannulae catheters provide an alternative to a mask, but can only be used where the patient only requires a low percentage of added oxygen. Nasal cannulae are usually used with flow rates of 1–4 litres of oxygen per minute and probably provide approximately 28–35% oxygen. Nasal cannulae cannot be attached satisfactorily to an external humidification device but in many cases the oxygen will be humidified as it passes through the nasal passages into the trachea (Table 27.2). Nasal cannulae are generally well tolerated and are useful postoperatively or where the patient requires minimal support. They are also used in the chronic setting where a patient at home requires long-term oxygen therapy.

Simple semi-rigid plastic masks (Figure 27.4)

Simple semi-rigid plastic masks are low-flow masks which entrain the air from the atmosphere and therefore are able to deliver a variable oxygen percentage (anything from 21 to 60%) (Table 27.3). Large discrepancies between the delivered fractional inspired oxygen (FiO_2) and the actual amount received by the patient will occur, dependent on the patient's rate and depth of breathing. These masks are useful for patients who need a higher percentage of oxygen temporarily whilst the cause for their hypoxia is treated. This type of mask may be worn for hours or several days, but they should be used in conjunction with a humidifier if used for more than 12 hours. If the patient requires 60% added oxygen or more this is the threshold for requiring more invasive respiratory support and expert help should be sought.

Fixed performance masks or high-flow masks (*Venturi-type masks*) (Figure 27.5)

With fixed performance masks it is possible to achieve an unvarying mixture of gases and a known concentration of oxygen using the high air flow oxygen

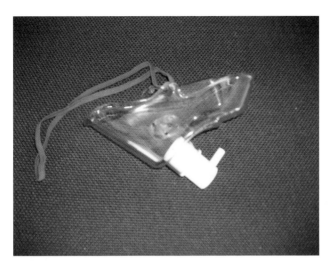

Figure 27.4 Semi-rigid plastic mask.

enrichment principle (Table 27.4). These masks derive their name from the Venturi barrel in which a relatively low-flow rate of oxygen is forced through a narrow jet. There are side holes in the barrel and this jet causes the air to be drawn in at a high rate. As the mixture of gas created is at a flow rate above that of inspiration, the mixture will be constant (Foss 1990). There are many Venturi-type masks available, but the larger-capacity masks are the most accurate and

Table 27.3 Approximate oxygen concentration related to flow rates of semi-rigid masks.

Oxygen flow rate (l/min)	% Oxygen delivered
2	24
4	35
6	50
8	55
10	60
12	65
15	70

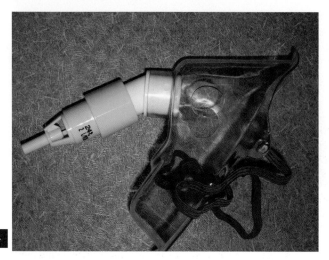

Figure 27.5   High-flow mask with venturi barrel.

therefore the safest when a known concentration of oxygen is required or when efficient elimination of carbon dioxide is essential, for example, to provide respiratory therapy for the patient with chronic respiratory disease (Fell & Boehm 1998).

Tracheostomy mask

Tracheostomy masks perform in a similar way to the simple semi-rigid plastic face mask, outlined above. The mask is placed over the tracheostomy tube or stoma (see also Chapter 29).

Table 27.4   Fixed performance mask oxygen flow rates.

Oxygen flow rate (l/min)	% Oxygen delivered
2	24
6	31
8	35
10	40
15	60

T-piece circuit

The T-piece circuit is a simple, large-bore, non-rebreathing circuit which is attached directly to an endotracheal or tracheostomy tube. Humidified oxygen is delivered through one part of the T, and expired gases leave through the other part. This device may be used as part of the weaning process when a patient has been ventilated previously by a mechanical ventilator (Oh 1997).

Domiciliary oxygen and portable oxygen

Some patients are so disabled by chronic respiratory disease that they require continual supplementary oxygen at home. Low-flow oxygen given over a period of time improves the prognosis of some patients (Benditt 2000).

Long-term oxygen may be prescribed for treatment of COPD, cystic fibrosis, interstitial lung disease, neuromuscular and skeletal disorders, pulmonary hypertension and palliation in lung cancer. Long-term oxygen may be provided in the form of cylinders. The problem with this supply is that the cylinders need changing frequently. Oxygen condensers (concentrators) are far more economical than cylinders. A condenser consists of a compressor powered by electricity. The condenser works by drawing in room air that is passed through a bacterial filter and a sieve bed. The sieve bed contains zeolite which has an affinity with nitrogen and when under pressure works by removing nitrogen and other gases, concentrating oxygen and delivering it through a meter at the front of the compressor.

The oxygen can be delivered to the patient by nasal cannulae or mask (Esmond 2000).

945

Liquid oxygen

The use of liquid oxygen in a portable cylinder has been developed for portable oxygen delivery. The patient is provided with a large tank in their own home from which smaller cylinders can be filled.

Continuous positive airway pressure

Definition

Continuous positive airway pressure (CPAP) therapy is the maintenance of a positive airway pressure greater than ambient pressure throughout inspiration and expiration. It can be delivered through a face mask, nasal mask or mouthpiece, or through an endotracheal or tracheostomy tube (Oh 1997).

Indications

- In acute respiratory failure in a spontaneously breathing patient who is able to maintain his or her own airway.
- As a method of weaning a patient from mechanical ventilation.

- After major surgery as a means of improving gaseous exchange.
- As a supportive measure in patients where intubation and mechanical ventilation are not considered appropriate (Greenbaum *et al.* 1976).
- Acute hypoxia with a normal $PaCO_2$.
- Acute respiratory distress syndrome (ARDS)
- Postoperatively (following major abdominal or thoracic surgery) prophylactically to prevent atelectasis.
- Pulmonary oedema.
- In patients with sleep apnoea.
- In neonates with respiratory distress syndrome/hyaline membrane disease.

Reference material

Use of the CPAP circuit dates back at least to 1912, when Bunnell used a primitive circuit during thoracic surgery. The first recorded use in intensive care was by Poulton and Oxon in 1936. In the 1940s increased interest in CPAP was prompted by research into respiratory support in high altitude flying. Further developments occurred in the 1950s and 1960s, and in 1976 Greenbaum *et al.* reported the use of CPAP with a face mask in ARDS. In 1972 Williamson & Modell successfully used CPAP for selected spontaneously breathing patients with acute respiratory failure.

The aim of CPAP therapy is to improve gas exchange (oxygen and carbon dioxide) within the lungs and improve the work of breathing. CPAP is able to do this by:

- Increasing the functional residual capacity (FRC), which is the amount of gas left in the lungs at the end of normal expiration available for pulmonary gas exchange. In acute lung injury where gaseous exchange is severely inhibited CPAP increases the FRC by improving ventilation in poorly or non-ventilated alveoli (Miller & Semple 1991).
- Improving the ventilation/perfusion ratio. Decreased intrapulmonary shunting with hypoxia could cause ventilation to the lungs to be reduced or blood flow to them impaired. Intrapulmonary shunting can then occur with under ventilation of the lungs. CPAP helps to decrease the intrapulmonary shunting by improving the ventilation to perfusion mismatch (Lenique *et al.* 1997).
- Improved lung compliance (elasticity) of the lungs. In respiratory failure the lungs become much stiffer and less compliant and breathing can become more difficult. Reduction in lung volume below a certain level results in airway collapse and under ventilation. The pressure required to overcome this can be achieved by CPAP.
- Increasing lung volume (alveolar volume) for gaseous exchange to take place. The factors above enable the work of breathing to be reduced plus a decrease in the percentage of oxygen that might be required.

Disadvantages of CPAP therapy

- With any circuit that includes the use of positive end expiratory pressure (PEEP) there is the possibility of reduction in cardiac output; however, spontaneous ventilation decreases both the incidence and severity of this complication (Oh 1997).
- There is a danger of vomiting and aspiration of gastric contents due to gastric insufflation, although this is minimized when used in awake patients, or by the insertion of an oro/nasogastric tube (Schumaker *et al.* 1996).
- Damage to skin integrity due to pressure from the tightly fitting face mask; the sites particularly vulnerable are the bridge of the nose and over the ears.

Non-invasive ventilation

Non-invasive ventilation refers to mechanical ventilatory support applied without an artificial airway (endotracheal tube or tracheostomy). It can be delivered to the patient via a nasal or face mask. The patient must be conscious and co-operative for this type of ventilation to be effective. It is particularly useful in patients with chronic respiratory disease:

- In restrictive pulmonary disease, e.g. muscular dystrophy.
- In progressive neuromuscular disease, e.g. motor neurone disease.
- In obstructive pulmonary disease, e.g. COPD, bronchiectasis, cystic fibrosis.
- In nocturnal hypoventilation.
- In patients with acute exacerbation of chronic respiratory disease.
- In patients where endotracheal intubation and ventilation may not be considered appropriate or where difficulties may be anticipated in weaning a patient from a ventilator.

Non-invasive ventilators generally fall into two categories (Esmond 2000):

- Pressure preset machines.
- Volume preset machines.

Mechanical ventilation

A mechanical ventilator is a device used to replace or assist breathing in order for satisfactory gas exchange to take place. The decision to ventilate a patient will be made after careful clinical examination including assessment of respiratory mechanics, oxygenation and ventilation.

Ventilators are able to control tidal volume, respiratory rate, time of inspiration against time of expiration, inspired flow rate and inspired oxygen concentration (Pierce 1995; West 1995; Hinds 1997; Bersten & Soni 2003).

Positive pressure ventilators

These devices provide a satisfactory gas exchange when inflating the lungs with a positive pressure via an endotracheal tube or tracheostomy.

Positive pressure ventilators have four main functions to perform during each respiratory cycle:

- Inflate the lungs.
- Cycle from inspiration to expiration.
- Allow expiration to take place.
- Cycle from expiration to inspiration.

They have a driving mechanism and can cycle from one phase of the respiratory cycle to another by a preset pressure, preset time or preset volume.

Varying modes of ventilation can be used:

- Intermittent mandatory ventilation (IMV).
- Pressure support.
- Pressure control.
- Simulated intermittent mandatory ventilation (SIMV).
- Continuous positive airway pressure (CPAP).

Humidification

Humidity is the amount of water vapour present in a gas. The terms used to define humidity are absolute humidity, maximum capacity and relative humidity. Absolute humidity is the mass of water vapour that a given volume of gas can carry at a set temperature. When a gas is at its maximum capacity it is said to be fully saturated. Relative humidity is the ratio of the absolute humidity to the maximum capacity.

The warmer the gas, the more vapour it can hold but if the temperature of the gas falls, water held as vapour will condense out of the gas into the surrounding atmosphere.

In normal health the nasal passages and upper airways are able to warm, moisten and filter the inspired gases very effectively. The process of humidification is necessary to compensate for the normal loss of water from the respiratory tract which, under resting conditions, is about 250 ml per day. This can increase in patients who are unwell.

Normal room air has an approximate temperature of $22°C$ with a relative humidity of 50% and a water content of 10 mg H_2O. For effective gas exchange to occur in the lungs, the air would need to be at a temperature of $37°C$ with 100% humidity and a water content of 44 mg H_2O per litre by the time it reaches the bifurcation in the trachea, which is referred to as the isothermic point.

When the temperature falls below 37°C and humidity falls below 100% several changes take place in the airways. The respiratory tract is lined with ciliated epithelial cells that secrete mucus. Each cell has about 200 hair-like structures known as cilia, whose role is to remove unwanted mucus and secretions. With a drop in temperature and humidity, the mucus that collects in the airways thickens and movement of the cilia is reduced. If there is no improvement the mucus will become thicker and immobile; the cilia will also lose their mobility so clearance of all secretions will stop and infection can set in.

If there is a continuing lack of humidity further damage occurs. The cilia can break off, causing damage to the mucosal lining of the respiratory tract. The isothermic point of saturation moves from the bifurcation of the trachea to a lower point in the lungs, resulting in further damage which can lead to collapse of the alveoli, decrease in lung function and hypoxaemia (Carroll 1997b; Fell & Boehm 1998; Ward & Park 2000).

Inhalation of oxygen used during respiratory therapy, which is a dry gas, can cause evaporation of water from the respiratory tract and lead to the consequences above if humidification is not provided.

In patients who are intubated or have a tracheostomy the natural pathway of humidification is bypassed.

Methods of humidification

Many devices can be used to supply humidification; the best of these will fulfil the following requirements:

- The inspired gas must be delivered to the trachea at a room temperature of 32–36°C with 100% humidity and should have a water content of 33–43 g/m^3 (Oh 1997).
- The set temperature should remain constant; humidification and temperature should not be affected by large ranges of flow.
- The device should have a safety and alarm system to guard against overheating, overhydration and electric shocks.
- It is important that the appliance should not increase resistance or affect the compliance of respiration.
- It is essential that whichever device is selected, wide-bore tubing (elephant tubing) is used to allow efficient formation of water vapour.

Devices for humidification (see Table 27.5)

- *Heat and moisture exchanger (HME)*. In this situation an HME performs the function of the nose and pharynx in conditioning the inspired air. It retains heat and moisture in the expired air and returns them to the patient in the next inspired breath. Many HMEs contain a bacterial filter.

Table 27.5 A comparison of devices for humidification.

Device	Advantages	Disadvantages
HME	Simple Cheap Short term	Inadequate humidity Risk of airway obstruction Can become waterlogged Infection risk
Cold water humidifier	Simple Cheap	Inadequate humidity Infection risk
Hot water humidifier	Delivers maximal humidification	Infection risk Overhumidification Risk of aspiration water/drowning Excessive condensation in circuit Overheating causing damage to trachea Resistance in circuit Restriction of gas flow

HME, heat and moisture exchanger.

The HME consists of spun, pleated, highly thermal conductive material. It can be used in a self-ventilating patient with a tracheostomy who is being weaned from oxygen (Figure 27.6a). It is also known as an artificial or 'Swedish' nose. It can also be used in ventilated patients, inserted between the patient's airway and the ventilator circuit (Figure 27.6b).

- *Cold water bubble humidifier.* This device delivers partially humidified oxygen at about 50% relative humidity. Gas is either forced across or bubbled through water at room temperature (Figure 27.6c). This method is not advised as it is so inefficient (Oh 1997).
- *Water bath humidifiers.* With these devices, inspired gas is forced over or through a heated reservoir of water (Figure 27.6d). To achieve an adequate humidity for the patient, the water bath must reach a set temperature. The gas will then cool as it moves down the breathing circuit to the patient, and a relative humidity of 100% will be reached. Hot water bath humidifiers are therefore very efficient and useful for humidification for the immobile patients particularly if they are receiving mechanical ventilatory support. However, they have four main disadvantages:

(a) Danger of overheating and causing damage to the trachea.
(b) Their efficiency can alter with changes in gas flow rate, surface area and the water temperature.

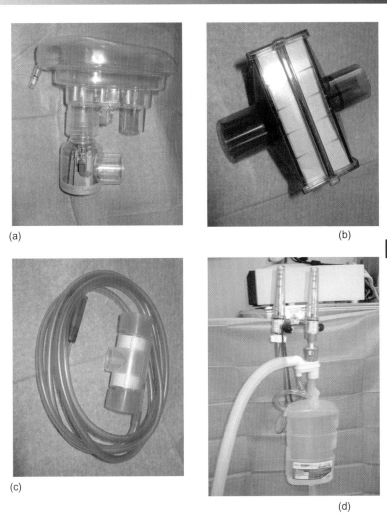

(a)

(b)

(c)

(d)

Figure 27.6 (a) Heat and moisture exchanger. (b) Cross-section of a heat and moisture exchanger (HME) used with a ventilator circuit. (c) Cold water bubble humidifier. (d) Hot water bath humidifier.

(c) Condensation and collection of water in the oxygen delivery tubes.
(d) The possibility of microcontamination of stagnant water (Tinker & Zapol 1992).

- *Aerosol generators.* These devices are not governed by temperature, but provide microdroplets of water suspended in the gas (Bersten & Soni 2003). The gas provided through aerosol devices can be very highly saturated with water. There are three main types of aerosol humidifier:

(a) Gas-drive nebulizer.
(b) Mechanical (spinning disc) nebulizer.
(c) Ultrasonic nebulizer.

These devices are useful for the spontaneously breathing patient with chronic chest disease.

Hazards of oxygen therapy

952

Carbon dioxide narcosis

Carbon dioxide is the chemical that most directly influences respiration by its direct effect on the efficiency of alveolar ventilation. The normal partial pressure of carbon dioxide in the blood is 4.0–6.0 kPa (30–45 mmHg). When this level rises, the pH of the CSF drops which in turn causes excitation of the central chemoreceptors, and hyperventilation occurs (Marieb 2006).

In people who always retain carbon dioxide, and are therefore usually hypercapnic because of chronic pulmonary disease such as chronic bronchitis, the chemoreceptors are no longer sensitive to a raised level of carbon dioxide. In these cases the falling PaO_2 becomes the principal respiratory stimulus (the hypoxic drive) (Marieb 2006). Therefore, if a high level of supplementary oxygen was delivered to such patients, severe respiratory depression would ensue and ultimately unconsciousness and death.

Oxygen toxicity

Pulmonary toxicity following prolonged higher percentages of oxygen therapy is recognized clinically, but there is still much to be learnt about the condition. The degree of injury is related to the length of time of exposure and percentage of oxygen to which the individual is exposed. The pattern is one of decreasing lung compliance as a result of a sequence of events, tracheal bronchial inflammation, haemorrhagic interstitial and intra-alveolar oedema, leading ultimately to fibrosis (Pierce 1995; Oh 1997; Pierson 2000).

Where possible, long periods (i.e. 24 hours or more) of oxygen therapy above 50% should be avoided.

Procedure guidelines   Humidification for respiratory therapy

Various humidifiers exist. Select the system most appropriate for the patient.

Procedure

Action	Rationale
1 Discuss with the team the choice of system to be used.	The most appropriate device is selected to meet the patient's needs (E).
2 Explain to patient the reason for use of the humidifier and how it works.	So patient understands what is happening and thus to help the patient tolerate the humidification (E).
3 Prepare the device to be used. (a) Some circuits are ready prepared with humidifier. (b) Prepare humidifier and circuit. (c) Humidifier/wide-bore oxygen tubing: ensure minimal length of tubing, water trap and mask.	
4 Once circuit is set up, run system to check it is functioning correctly and the circuit is intact.	To ensure that oxygen is being delivered through the circuit as set (E). To ensure the system is humidifying the oxygen and that no leaks exist (E).
5 If hot water system is in use check it is running within recommended temperature range.	To ensure no damage to the patient's lungs if temperature above range (E).
6 Ensure water is present in water source of system; do not allow to run dry.	Aid adequate delivery of humidity to the patient. Prevent damage to the humidifier (E).
7 Ensure circuit tubing is positioned below patient.	To ensure collection of humidity in the circuit is able to drain into the water trap or circuit rather than into the patient (E).
8 Ensure the patient finds the humidification comfortable.	
9 Continually check running of system.	To ensure the system is functioning adequately and delivering humidity (E).

Procedure guidelines *(cont.)*

10 Ensure the patient is well informed and continuously reassured. The patient may find the system noisy and may be distressed by excessive moisture in the circuit.

11 Change the humidification and circuit on a weekly basis.

Problem solving: Oxygen therapy by nasal cannulae or oxygen mask

Problem	Cause	Suggested action
Maintenance of airway.	Position of patient. Airway secretions.	Position patient preferably sitting up at an angle of greater than 45°. Encourage patient to cough and expectorate if able or remove secretions by suction if patient unable to do so (E).
Maintenance of adequate oxygenation.	Inadequate oxygen delivery, patient's condition deteriorating. More breathless. Oxygen saturation decreased. Deteriorating blood gases.	Assess level of oxygen support required by assessing previous medical history and current respiratory assessment. Increase oxygen delivery using the lowest percentage of oxygen to achieve the individual goal for the patient (E).
Dry mouth.	Oxygen therapy drying mouth.	Add humidification to the circuit (see Procedure guidelines: Humidification, above). Give regular mouth care (E).
Nasal cannulae or mask discomfort.	Position or use of cannulae and oxygen mask.	Ensure correct placement and that the patient is comfortable (E).
Development of pressure points on nose/ears.	Incorrect placement of cannulae support or mask headstrap.	Change position of cannulae or mask (E). Apply padding around headstrap or to bridge of nose to relieve pressure (E).

Problem	Cause	Suggested action
Intolerance of oxygen therapy.	Fear and anxiety. Confusion. Hypoxia.	Assess patient for change. Ensure continual reassurance given to patient. Ensure patient remains orientated to the environment and oxygen device. If intolerant of mask, nasal cannulae may be tolerated. If hypoxic, oxygen may need to be increased (E).
Communication.	Mask makes communication difficult; patient may not hear carer and nurse may not hear patient.	Assist patient to move around bed area if not able to go far. Mobilize patient with portable oxygen cylinder if appropriate (E).
Inability to maintain personal hygiene.	Immobility. On bedrest. Mask restricting independence.	Provide reassurance for patient to remain independent where able. Allow them to carry out their own hygiene if able or to help patient with hygiene if not (E).
Maintenance of safety.	Detachment of oxygen from flow meter. Kinked or looped oxygen tubing. Mask removed by patient.	Ensure oxygen attached to flow meter. Check patient regularly. Ensure no kinks or loops arise. Ensure patient is attached to oxygen.
Documentation.	Rapidly changing situation.	Ensure all changes to oxygen therapy or patient are documented in nursing care plan (E).

References and further reading

Aherns, T. & Tucker, K. (1999) Pulse oximetry. *Crit Care Clin North Am*, **11**(1), 87–97.

Allan, D. (1988) Making sense of oxygen delivery. *Nurs Times*, **83**(18), 40–2.

Allison, R.C. (1991) Initial treatment of pulmonary oedema: a physiological approach. *Am J Med Sci*, **302**(6), 385–91.

Ball, C. (1999) Optimising oxygen delivery: haemodynamic workshop, part 1. *Intensive Crit Care Nurs*, **15**, 371–3.

Ball, C. (2000a) Optimising oxygen delivery: haemodynamic workshop, part 2. *Intensive Crit Care Nurs*, **16**, 33–44.

Ball, C. (2000b) Optimising oxygen delivery: haemodynamic workshop, part 3. *Intensive Crit Care Nurs*, **16**, 84–7.

Beaumont, M. *et al.* (1997) Effects of chest wall counter pressure on lung mechanics under high level CPAP in humans. *J Physiol*, **83**(2), 591–8.

Benditt, J.W. (2000) Adverse effects of low flow oxygen therapy. *Respir Care*, **45**(1), 54–80.

Berne, R.M. & Levy, M.N. (1998) *Physiology*, 4th edn. Mosby, St. Louis, MO.

Bersten, A & Soni, N. (2003) *Oh's Intensive Care Manual*, 5th edn. Butterworth Heinemann, Sydney.

Byron Brow, C.W. & Dracup, K. (2000) Too much of a good thing. *Am J Crit Care*, **9**(5), 300–2.

Carpenter, D. (1991) Oxygen transport in the blood. *Crit Care Nurse*, **11**(9), 20–31.

Carroll, P. (1997a) Pulse oximetry at your fingertips. *RN Magazine*, **60**(2), 22–7.

Carroll, P. (1997b) When you want humidity. *RN Magazine*, **60**(5), 30–4.

Cooper, N. (2002) Oxygen therapy: myths and misconceptions. *Care Crit Ill*, **18**(3), 74–7.

Coull, A. (1992) Making sense of pulse oximetry. *Nurs Times*, **88**(32), 42–3.

Dunn, L. & Chrisholm, H. (1998) Oxygen therapy. *Nurs Stand*, **13**(7), 57–64.

Ehrhardt, B.S. & Graham, M. (1990) Pulse oximetry. An easy way to check oxygen saturation. *Nursing*, **20**(3), 50–4.

Esmond, G. (2000) *Respiratory Nursing*. Bailliere Tindall, London.

Fell, H. & Boehm, M. (1998) Easing the discomfort of oxygen therapy. *Nurs Times*, **94**(38), 56–8.

Foss, M.A. (1990) Oxygen therapy. *Prof Nurse*, January, **5**(4), 180–90.

Goldhill, D. (2001) Postoperative oxygen. *Care Crit Ill*, **17**(5), 154–5.

Greeg, R.W. *et al.* (1990) Continuous positive airway pressure by face mask in *Pneumocystis carinii* pneumonia. *Crit Care Med*, **18**(1), 21–4.

Greenbaum, D.M. *et al.* (1976) Continuous positive airways pressure without tracheal intubation in spontaneously breathing patients. *Chest*, **69**, 615–20.

Guyton, A. (2000) *A Textbook of Medical Physiology*, 10th edn. W.B. Saunders, Philadelphia.

Hess, D. (2000) Detection and monitoring of hypoxaemia and oxygen therapy. *Respir Care*, **45**(1), 65–80.

Hinds, C.J. (1997) *Intensive Care. A Concise Textbook*, 2nd edn. Bailliere Tindall, London.

Keen, A. (2000) Continuous positive airway pressure in the intensive care unit: uses and implications for nursing management. *Nurs Crit Care*, **5**(3), 137–41.

Keilty, S.E. & Bott, J. (1992) Continuously positive airway pressure. *Physiotherapy*, **78**(2), 90–2.

Kumar, P. & Clark, C. (2005) *Clinical Medicine*, 5th edn. W.B. Saunders, London.

Lenique, F. *et al.* (1997) Ventilatory and haemodynamic effects of continuous positive airway pressure in heart failure. *Am J Respir Crit Care Med*, **155**, 500–5.

Marieb, E.N. (2006) *Human Anatomy and Physiology and Brief Atlas of the Human Body*, 7th edn. Benjamin Cummings, New York.

Miller, R. & Semple, S. (1991) Continous positive airway pressure ventilation for respiratory failure associated with *Pneumocystis carinii* pneumonia. *Respir Med*, **85**, 133–8.

Oh, T.E. (1997) *Intensive Care Manual*. Butterworth-Heinemann, Sydney.

Petty, T.L. (2000) Historical highlights of long-term oxygen therapy. *Respir Care*, **45**(1), 29–38.

Pierce, L.N.B. (1995) *Guide to Mechanical Ventilation and Intensive Respiratory Care*. W.B. Saunders, London.

Pierson, D.J. (2000) Pathophysiology and clinical effects of chronic hypoxia. *Respir Care*, **45**(1), 39–51.

Place, B. (1998) Pulse oximetry in adults. *Nurs Times*, **94**(50), 48–9.

Romand, J.A. & Donald, E. (1995) Physiological effects of continuous positive airway pressure ventilation in the critically ill. *Care Crit Ill*, **11**(6), 239–42.

Schumaker, W.C. *et al.* (1996) *Textbook of Critical Care*. W.B. Saunders, Philadelphia, pp. 628–952.

Tinker, J. & Zapol, W. (1992) *Care of the Critically Ill Patient*. Springer, New York.

Tortora, G.J. & Derrickson, B.H. (2008) *Principles of Anatomy and Physiology*, 12th edn. John Wiley & Sons, Inc., New York.

Ward, B. & Park, G.R. (2000) Humidification of inspired gases in the critically ill. *Clin Intensive Care*, **11**(4), 169–76.

West, J.B. (1995) *Pulmonary Pathophysiology: The Essentials*. Williams and Wilkins, Baltimore.

Williamson, D.C. & Modell, J.H. (1972) Intermittent continuous airways pressure by mask – its use in the treatment of atelectasis. *Arch Surg*, **177**, 970–2.

Multiple choice questions

1 The air that we normally breathe is composed of which quantity of gases?

   a   Oxygen 21%, carbon dioxide 0.03%, nitrogen 79%, rare gases 0.003%

   b   Nitrogen 21%, carbon dioxide 0.03%, oxygen 79%, rare gases 0.003%

   c   Oxygen 21%, carbon dioxide 0.03%, nitrogen 79%, hydrogen 0.003%

   d   Oxygen 19%, carbon dioxide 0.03%, nitrogen 81%, hydrogen 0.003%

2 Nasal cannulae are usually used with flow rates of between 1 and 4 litres per minute. If the patient is receiving oxygen at a rate of 2 litres per minute what percentage of oxygen would be delivered?

   a   24%
   b   28%
   c   32%
   d   36%

3 CPAP is often used as a form of respiratory support. What does CPAP stand for?

   a   Continuous pressurised airway procedure
   b   Consistent positive airway pressure
   c   Continuous positive airway pressure
   d   Continuous pulmonary airway pressure

4   In normal health the nasal passages and upper airways are able to warm, moisten and filter the inspired gases very effectively. Sometimes this natural form of humidification is bypassed. Which of the following statements is true:

a   Humidified gas must be delivered at a temperature of 32–36°C, 100% humidification, via small bore tubing
b   Humidified gas must be delivered at a temperature of 32–36°C, 100% humidification, via wide bore tubing
c   Humidified gas must be delivered at a temperature of 30–34°C, 100% humidification, via small bore tubing
d   Humidified gas must be delivered at a temperature of 30–34°C, 100% humidification, via wide small bore tubing

Answers to the multiple choice questions can be found in Appendix 3.

Chapter 28

Specimen collection for microbiological analysis

Definition

Specimen collection is the collection of a required amount of tissue or fluid for laboratory examination, to allow for the isolation and identification of micro-organisms that cause disease, and to determine their antimicrobial sensitivity to guide the doctor with the selection of appropriate antimicrobial therapy (Mims *et al.* 2004).

Indications

Specimen collection is required when microbiological, biochemical or other laboratory investigations are indicated. Nursing staff should be able to identify the need for microbiological investigations and, if appropriate, initiate the taking of specimens (Papasian & Kragel 1997; Higgins 2007). Specimen collection is often a first crucial step in investigations that define the nature of the disease and determine diagnosis and the mode of treatment.

The clinical microbiology laboratory plays a fundamental role in the diagnosis of infection and an increasingly important role in reducing new antibiotic resistance (Peterson *et al.* 2001). Its importance increases in immunosuppressed and myelosuppressed cancer patients because the usual signs and symptoms of infection may be absent (Shelton 1999) and due to the significant associated morbidity and mortality (Sandin & Rinaldi 1996).

Reference material

General principles

Successful laboratory diagnosis depends on the collection of specimens at the appropriate time, using the correct technique and equipment and transporting them to the designated laboratory safely without delay. For this to be achieved, good liaison is essential between medical, nursing, portering and laboratory staff (Higgins 2007).

The first step in the accurate diagnosis of infectious disease is to recognize the need to obtain adequate specimens for microbiological examination. Signs of infection such as fever should trigger a careful clinical assessment to ensure unnecessary tests are avoided and the most useful laboratory samples are obtained to identify therapeutic options (O'Grady *et al.* 1998).

The nurse's role is:

- To identify the need for and importance of microbiological investigation.
- To initiate, if appropriate, the taking of a swab or specimen, e.g. during wound dressing it is usually the nurse who identifies signs of infection (Gilchrist 2000).
- To know the appropriate investigation to be undertaken so as to avoid indiscriminate specimen collection which wastes time and money.
- To collect the desired material in the correct container.
- To arrange prompt delivery to the laboratory.

Close communication between the doctor and the laboratory is important, especially when unusual infections are suspected or the patient is immunosuppressed, as the infection may be caused by unusual organisms whose identification requires special techniques (Thomson 2002).

Collection of specimens

If specimens of poor quality are sent to the microbiology department, then the results may be of little or no clinical utility (Wilson 1996; Higgins 2007). The greater the quantity of material sent for laboratory examination, the greater the chance of isolating a causative organism. Other considerations include the type of organisms and their growth requirements. Aerobic bacteria will grow in the presence of air (Gold & Eisenstein 2000). Anaerobic bacteria fail to grow in air, preferring an atmosphere reduced of oxygen. Facultative bacteria can grow in either the presence or absence of air. Fastidious bacteria require selective plating media to encourage growth (Finegold 2000), and may not survive prolonged storage or may be overgrown with less fastidious organisms, before cultures can be made (Gill *et al.* 2004). A delay in transporting a specimen to the laboratory can compromise the specimen integrity and cause a false negative or positive result (Peterson *et al.* 2001).

There are many types of specimen collection tools, for example, swabs and pots. Advice should be sought from the microbiology department with regard to the best type of container required for unusual specimens. It is essential that the specimen and its transport container are appropriate for the infection being investigated, to ensure that adequate quantity of material is obtained to allow complete microbiological examination. Material from skin and mucous membranes can be collected by a swab, which generally contains a transport medium. This is designed to preserve micro-organisms, while preventing the multiplication of rapidly growing organisms, which makes identification easier. Unfortunately only a limited amount of material can be collected by this means; therefore pus should be collected in a syringe which can be transferred to a sterile container (Wilson & Jenner 2006). Biopsy material, pus, fluid or tissue removed surgically provide ideal material in adequate quantities for appropriate microbiological smears and cultures (Gill *et al.* 2004).

Specimens are readily contaminated by poor technique. Cultures taken from such specimens often result in confusing or misleading results. Aseptic technique must be used when collecting specimens to avoid inadvertent contamination of the site of sample or the specimen (Macleod 1992). Specimens must be collected in sterile containers with close-fitting lids and swabs must never be removed from their sterile containers until everything is ready for taking the sample.

Ideally, samples should be collected before beginning any treatment, e.g. antibiotics or antiseptics. If the patient is receiving such treatment at the same time the specimen is collected, the laboratory staff must be informed. Both antibiotics and antiseptics may destroy organisms that are, in fact, active in the patient and will affect the outcome of the laboratory test. Specimens should also be obtained using safe technique and practices (Higgins 2007). For example, gloves should always be worn when handling all body fluids. Cross-infection precautionary measures should always be undertaken if an infection is suspected until a full microbiology report has been given and the causative agent confirmed (Wilson & Jenner 2001).

Documentation

Requests for microbiological investigations must include the following information:

- Patient's name, ward and/or department.
- Hospital number.
- Date specimen collected.
- Time specimen collected.
- Diagnosis.
- Relevant signs and symptoms.
- Relevant history, e.g. recent foreign travel.
- Any antimicrobial drug being taken by the patient.
- Type of specimen.
- Consultant's name.

- Name of the doctor who ordered the investigation, as it may be necessary to telephone the result before the typed report is dispatched.
- If the specimen is high risk, it should be labelled with a 'danger of infection' label (Health Services Advisory Committee 2003).

Without full information, it is impossible to examine a specimen adequately or to report it accurately. The most common reason for specimens to be rejected by the laboratory is improper labelling of the specimen (Malarkey & McMorrow 2005). Incorrectly or unlabelled specimens will normally be discarded (Health Services Advisory Committee 2003).

Transportation of specimens

Guidelines are now available on the labelling, transport and reception of specimens (Health Services Advisory Committee 2003). Specimens that need to be transported outside the hospital, e.g. by van, car, taxi or by post, must be transported in an adequate leak-proof primary container, a leak-proof secondary container and an outer box to comply with British Standards ISO 6710 (British Standards Institute 1995). Laboratory technicians will undertake this task, following local written instructions relating to containment, labelling and transport boxes (Health Services Advisory Committee 2003).

963

The sooner a specimen arrives in the laboratory, the greater is the chance of organisms present surviving and being identified. Delays will cause changes that may radically alter the result. The laboratory count of bacteria in a delayed specimen could be significantly different from that of the specimen when it was collected (Shanson 1999; Higgins 2007).

If specimens cannot be sent to a laboratory immediately, they should be stored as follows:

- Blood culture samples in a 37°C incubator (Higgins 2007).
- All other specimens in a specimen refrigerator at a temperature of 4°C, where the low temperature will slow the bacterial growth (Higgins 2007).

In diagnostic pathology it is likely that at any given time there will be a number of specimens that present a risk of infection. Every health authority, therefore, must ensure that medical, nursing, phlebotomy, laboratory, portering and any other staff involved in handling specimens are trained to do so (RCN 2005). The person collecting the specimen must ensure that the specimen container used is an appropriate one for the purpose, is properly closed and has not been externally contaminated by the contents (Health Services Advisory Committee 2003). Any accidental spillage must be cleaned up immediately by staff, who should wear gloves and other appropriate protective clothing to prevent contamination. Ideally, all specimens should be placed in a double self-sealing bag with one compartment containing the request form and the other the specimen. Specimens should be transported to the laboratory in boxes or deep-sided trays which are not used for any other purpose, are disinfected weekly and whenever contaminated (Health Services Advisory Committee 2003).

It is essential to remember that there will always be patients or specimens that have not been identified as presenting a particular risk of infection. If a specimen is suspected or known to present an infectious hazard, the person taking the specimen has the responsibility to ensure that the form and containers are correctly labelled with a biohazard label, to enable those handling the specimen to take appropriate precautions (Health Services Advisory Committee 2003).

Specimens from patients who have recently been treated with toxic therapy, i.e. gene therapy, drugs, radioactivity or active metabolites, need to be handled with caution. (See Chapter 19, Professional edition for further information related to gene therapy specimen collection). Local rules must be compiled, which will outline how such specimens should be labelled, bagged and transported to the laboratory. For example, in the case of gene therapy the specimen must be labelled with a biohazard label, double bagged and transported to the laboratory in a secure transport box with a fastenable lid. Each box must carry a warning label, and be made of smooth impervious material such as plastic or metal which will retain liquid and can be easily disinfected and cleaned in the event of leakage of the specimen (Health Services Advisory Committee 2003). (See Chapter 36, Professional edition for further information related to unsealed sources and specimen collection.)

Types of investigation

Bacterial

A wide range of methods are available for obtaining cultures and identifying organisms from a specimen or swab. To employ all these tests would be time consuming and costly. Testing, therefore, tends to be selective. It is at this stage that the laboratory request form plays a particularly important part. A faecal specimen, for example, from a patient with diarrhoea who also has a recent history of foreign travel, would be investigated for organisms not normally looked for in faecal specimens from patients without such a history.

The majority of specimens undergo microscopic investigation. This is valuable as an early indication of the causative organisms in an infection. The specimen is often cultured for 24–48 hours longer in the case of blood cultures. Prolonged incubation (up to 21 days) may be required for growth of some organisms, e.g. *Brucella* species (Mims *et al.* 2004). This is followed by antibiotic sensitivity testing on any pathogenic organisms that are isolated. This involves the application of paper discs impregnated with antibiotics onto the agar plates. After overnight incubation during which time the growth of bacteria may be inhibited by the antibiotic disc, the zones of inhibition can be observed for the degree of sensitivity of the organism (Mims *et al*. 2004).

Viral

In order to interpret positive viral specimens, the choice of specimen and time of collection in relation to the onset of the patient's illness and transportation to the laboratory are all of prime importance (Baker *et al*. 1998). The collection of specimens for virology investigations should ideally be discussed with the microbiology laboratory beforehand (Shanson 1999). There are three main laboratory techniques available for the diagnosis of viral infections (Baker *et al*. 1998):

- Direct microscopy.
- Culture (isolation of growth in living cell systems).
- Serology.

For culture specimens the use of viral transport media and speed of delivery to the laboratory are important as viruses do not survive well outside the body. With good liaison, the nurses should obtain the specimen when the laboratory staff have the transport ready to take it to the virus laboratories. If delays occur, the specimen should be refrigerated at a temperature of $4°C$, but never frozen in normal refrigerator freezers, where the temperature is around $-20°C$, as viruses may die rapidly at this temperature (Shanson 1999).

The time at which specimens are collected for viral investigations is important. Many viral illnesses have a prodromal phase during which the multiplication and shedding of the virus are at a peak and the patient is most infectious (Mims *et al*. 2004). Immunocompromised patients are particularly susceptible to viral respiratory tract infections. When an upper respiratory specimen is collected it is important to ensure the recovery of respiratory epithelial cells from the lining of the upper part of the nasal passage. To obtain an adequate number of cells nasopharyngeal swabs, aspirates and washes need to be undertaken correctly (Buller 2000).

Serological

Serological testing for the presence of antigens and antibodies is used when it is not possible to isolate the organism easily from the patient's tissue. By demonstrating serum antibodies to suspected organisms it is inferred that the patient is, or has been, infected with the organism. Despite the disdavantage of the test being performed retrospectively, antibody testing is the main method of diagnosing viral infections (Mims *et al*. 2004). A single test is inadequate as if the titres (the concentration of the substance being measured) are raised it is impossible to determine whether this is due to past or present infection. Two tests need to be carried out, both of which involve the collection of 10 ml of blood once at the beginning of the illness and again 10–14 days later. If a rising titre level is demonstrated it suggests the patient's infection is current (Mims *et al.* 2004).

Mycosis

Although many pathogenic fungi will grow on ordinary bacteriological culture media, they grow better and with less risk of bacterial overgrowth on special mycological media. The presence of fungi in clinical specimens is difficult to interpret, as *Candida albicans*, for example, is commonly present in the upper respiratory, alimentary and female genital tract and on the skin of healthy people. However in people where immune function has been affected by disease or treatment, such as cancer, this fungi can lead to systemic disease (Baker *et al.* 1998).

Mycobacteriological

For further information, please refer to the procedure on tuberculosis (see Chapter 6, Professional edition).

Protozoa

Most protozoa do not cause disease, but those that do, e.g. malaria, make a formidable contribution to human illness (Armitage & King 2000). Laboratory investigations depend on direct microscopy which necessitates specimens being delivered to the laboratory as quickly as possible, while the protozoa are mobile and therefore visible.

Blood

Blood specimens are obtained for several reasons (Weinstein 2007):

- To indicate relatively common disorders.
- To make a diagnosis.
- To follow the course of a disease.
- To regulate therapy and drug dosage.

Wherever possible, blood should be obtained peripherally (see Chapter 32). Blood samples can be obtained from central venous access devices (CVADs); however, the first sample must be discarded to ensure accurate results and the device must then be flushed directly after obtaining the blood sample to avoid an occlusion (Gabriel 2008) (see Chapter 45, Professional edition).

Blood cultures

Bacteraemia and fungaemia are frequent complications in immunocompromised and critically ill patients; the accurate and timely detection of these remains one on the most important functions of clinical microbiology (Wilson 1996). Intravenous antibiotic therapy needs to be started within the first hour of recognition of severe sepsis after cultures have been obtained (Dellinger *et al.* 2004). Accurate and speedy microbiological detection of infection using blood cultures is of paramount importance to determine the cause and guide the treatment (see Chapter 5). Success in gaining information from blood cultures relies on the accurate timing of the specimen and obtaining the correct volume of blood. The volume is critial to ensure the optimum blood to broth ratio, so the manufacturer's instructions should be followed as to the total volume required for each bottle. However the potential to cause anemia also needs to be considered, so a smaller volume (1–5 ml) for infants and small children should be obtained from each venepuncture site (Wilson 1996; Gill *et al.* 2004). As there are a number of systems in use it is essential that maufacturers' guidelines are followed. Most bacteraemias are intermittent, so blood cultures should be taken when the signs of infection are present (Gill *et al.* 2004). These may include fever, chills, rigors, changes in mental status and lethargy (Shelton 1999).

Blood for culture should be sampled before administration or modification of antibiotic therapy, as antibiotics may delay or prevent bacterial growth, causing false negative results (Engervall & Bjorkholm 1996; Higgins 2007).

One of the most important aspects of identifying a causative agent using blood cultures is the level of contamination of the blood samples which remains a common problem with rates varying from 2 to 10% (Madeo *et al.* 2003; DH 2007). Failure to use aseptic technique when obtaining blood cultures can result in diagnosis of a pseudobacteraemia, due to contamination of the culture by bacteria originating outside the patient's bloodstream. As the majority of this contamination comes from endogenous microbial flora on the skin, preparation is very important in reducing the number of false positive blood cultures (Traunter *et al.* 2002; DH 2007). This could result in inappropriate antibiotic therapy being administered and a significant waste of health care resources (Jumaa & Chattopadhyay 1994).

The use of needles to decant into the bottles is now largely redundant due to the common use of vacuumed blood collection systems to acquire blood samples (Rushing 2004). However, if a needle is used then it must be changed prior to decanting the blood into the blood culture bottle, as studies have indicated an increase in contamination rates when the needle is not changed (Spitalnic *et al.* 1995).

Catheter-related sepsis is the main risk factor when using central venous catheters and has an incidence of between 4 and 14% (Theaker 2005). CVAD-related infection and its morbidity and mortality associated with sepsis are often underestimated in clinical practice (Moller *et al.* 2005). Studies have found that between 16 and 44% of bone marrow transplant patients with CVAD experience catheter-related infections (Zitella 2003). When it is suspected that the CVAD is the source of infection, a blood culture sample must be obtained from all lumens of the device and a peripheral vein (Gabriel 2008; Dellinger *et al.* 2004; DH 2007). If there are signs of infection, e.g. redness and/or discharge around the site of insertion, a swab should also be taken for microbiological culture but at the same time the patient should be assessed for any other source of infection. Controversy continues about the sensitivity and specificity between catheter-drawn and peripheral blood cultures; some studies suggest that peripheral cultures are more reliable when the results of paired cultures are different (McBryde *et al.* 2005; Safdar *et al.* 2005), whereas others conclude the sensitivity from either route is not adequate to eliminate the need to take samples from the other site (Beutz *et al.* 2003).

Urine

The correct collection of urine specimens is very important as urinary tract infections are considered to be the most common bacterial infection (Foxman 2002). Urinary catheter associated infections are the most common type of noscomial infection (Godfrey & Evans 2000), and have been associated with both morbidity and mortality (Wazait *et al.* 2003). Urine is normally sterile, while the distal urethra of both men and women is normally colonized with a large number of bacteria (Gill *et al.* 2004; Higgins 2007) and even a carefully taken urine specimen may contain a number of bacteria. As urine is such a good culture medium, any bacteria present at the time of collection will continue to multiply in the specimen container, resulting in a falsely raised bacteriuria (Higgins 2007), which will then result in misleading information (Gill *et al.* 2004).

It was thought that cleaning of the area around the urinary meatus prior to the collection of a midstream specimen of urine makes no difference to contamination rates (Holliday *et al.* 1991), although perineal and penile cleaning was potentially beneficial to those patients whose personal hygiene was poor (Holliday *et al.* 1991). Higgins (2007) now suggests that to collect a specimen uncontaminated by bacteria, which may be present on the skin, peri-anal region, external genital tract or distal third of the urethra, patients should be encouraged to wash their hands prior to collecting a 'clean catch' midstream urine specimen and to clean around the urinary meatus prior to sample collection. Female patients should also be instructed to part the labia while passing urine to avoid possible contamination (Graham & Galloway 2001; Higgins 2007).

The principle for obtaining midstream collection of urine is that any bacteria present in the urethra are washed away in the first portion of urine voided (Higgins 2007).

Procedure guidelines   Specimen collection: section swabs

Procedure

Action	Rationale
1 Explain and discuss the procedure with the patient and ensure privacy while the procedure is being carried out.	To ensure that the patient understands the procedure and gives his/her valid consent (NMC 2006: C; NMC 2008: C).
2 Wash hands using bactericidal soap and water or bactericidal alcoholic handrub before and after obtaining specimen.	Hand washing greatly reduces the risk of infection transfer (DH 2005: C).
3 On completion of procedure, place specimens and swabs in the appropriate, correctly labelled containers.	To ensure that only organisms for investigation are preserved (Health Services Advisory Committee 2003: C).
4 Dispatch specimens promptly to the laboratory with the completed request form.	To ensure the best possible conditions for any laboratory examinations (Baker *et al.* 1998: R 5; Higgins 2007: E).

Ear swab

Action	Rationale
1 No antibiotics or other chemotherapeutic agents should have been used in the aural region 3 hours before taking the swab.	To prevent collection of traces of such therapeutic agents (Mims *et al.* 2004: E).
2 Place the swab into the outer ear as shown in Action figure 2. Rotate the swab gently.	To avoid trauma to the ear. To collect any secretions (Mims *et al.* 2004: E).

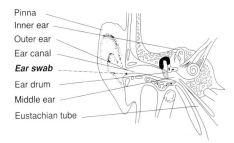

Pinna
Inner ear
Outer ear
Ear canal
Ear swab
Ear drum
Middle ear
Eustachian tube

Action 2   Area to be swabbed when sampling the outer ear.

Procedure guidelines *(cont.)*

Eye swab

Action	Rationale
1 Seek advice from microbiology about what type of culture medium and swab is required.	Different culture media and swabs are required for bacteria, viruses and chlamydia (Stollery *et al.* 2005: E).
2 Using a cotton wool swab, hold the swab parallel to the cornea and gently rub the conjunctiva in the lower eyelid from the nasal side outwards.	To ensure that a swab of the correct site is taken. To avoid contamination by touching the eyelid (Buller 2000: E; Marsden & Shaw 2003: E; Stollery *et al.* 2005: E).
3 If both eyes are to be swabbed, ensure the specimens are labelled 'right' and 'left'.	To prevent cross-infection (Stollery *et al.* 2005: C).

Nose swab

Action	Rationale
1 Moisten the swab beforehand with sterile water.	To prevent discomfort to the patient. The healthy nose is virtually dry and a dry swab may cause discomfort (Tortora & Derrickson 2006: C).
2 Move the swab from the anterior nares and direct it upwards into the tip of the nose (see Action figure 2).	To swab the correct site and to obtain the required sample (E).
3 Gently rotate the swab.	

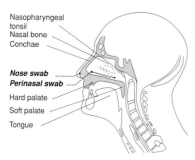

Nasopharyngeal tonsil
Nasal bone
Conchae
Nose swab
Perinasal swab
Hard palate
Soft palate
Tongue

Action 2 Area to be swabbed when sampling the nose.

Penile swab

Action	Rationale
1 Retract prepuce.	To obtain maximum visibility of area to be swabbed (E).
2 Rotate swab gently in the urethral meatus.	To collect any secretions (Malarkey & McMorrow 2005: E).

Rectal swab

Action	Rationale
1 Pass the swab, with care, through the anus into the rectum.	To avoid trauma. To ensure that a rectal and not an anal sample is obtained (E).
2 Rotate gently.	To avoid trauma (E).
3 In patients suspected of suffering from threadworms, take the swab from the perianal region.	Threadworms lay their ova on the perianal skin (Mims *et al*. 2004: E).

971

Throat swab

Action	Rationale
1 Ask the patient to sit in such a position that he/she is facing a strong light source. Depress the patient's tongue with a spatula.	To ensure maximum visibility of the area to be swabbed. The procedure is one that is likely to cause the patient to gag and the tongue will move to the roof of the mouth, contaminating the specimen (Parini 2000: E).
2 Quickly, but gently, rub the swab over the prescribed area, usually the tonsillar fossa or any area with a lesion or visible exudate (see Action figure 2).	To obtain the required sample (Parini 2000: E).
3 Avoid touching any other area of the mouth or tongue with the swab.	To prevent contamination by other organisms (Mims *et al*. 2004: E).

Procedure guidelines *(cont.)*

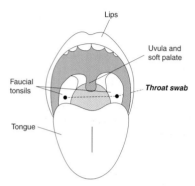

Labels:
Lips
Uvula and soft palate
Faucial tonsils
Throat swab
Tongue

Action 2   Area to be swabbed when sampling the throat.

Vaginal swab

Action	Rationale
1 Introduce a speculum into the vagina to separate the vaginal walls. Take the swab as high as possible in the vaginal vault.	To ensure maximum visibility of the area to be swabbed. To ensure that the swab is taken from the best site (Malarkey & McMorrow 2005: E). If infection by *Trichomonas* species is suspected, a charcoal-impregnated swab is recommended as this organism survives longer in this medium (Mims *et al.* 2004: E).

Wound swab

Action	Rationale
1 Take any swabs required before cleaning procedure begins.	To collect the maximum number of micro-organisms and to prevent collection of any therapeutic agents that may be employed in the dressing procedure (Gilchrist 2000: E).
2 Rotate the swab gently.	To collect samples. It is preferable to send samples of purulent discharge instead of swabs (Parini 2000: E).

Note: the use of disposable gloves is recommended in the following procedures in order to prevent cross-infection.

Procedure guidelines   Specimen collection: body fluid

Faecal collection

Action	Rationale
1 Ask the patient to defecate into a clinically clean bedpan.	To avoid unnecessary contamination from other organisms (Parini 2000: E).
2 Scoop enough material to fill a third of the specimen container using a spatula or a spoon, often incorporated in the specimen container.	To obtain a usable amount of specimen. To prevent contamination (Malarkey & McMorrow 2005: E).
3 Examine the specimen for such features as colour, consistency and odour, and record your observations.	To monitor any fluctuations and trends (Gill 1999: E).
4 Segments of tapeworm are seen easily in faeces and any such segments should be sent to the laboratory for identification.	Unless the head is dislodged, the tapeworm will continue to grow. Laboratory confirmation of the presence of the head is essential (Gill 1999: E).
5 Patients suspected of suffering from amoebic dysentery should have any stool specimens dispatched to the laboratory immediately.	The parasite causing amoebic dysentery exists in a free-living non-motile cyst. Both are characteristic in their fresh state but are difficult to identify when dead (Baker *et al.* 1998: E).
6 Patients with diarrhoea and especially in the presence of a fever should have samples taken to the laboratory immediately.	Due to the risk of *Clostridium difficile* (Poutanen & Simor 2004: R 2a).

Sputum collection

Action	Rationale
1 Use a sterile specimen container with a leakproof top.	Sputum is never free from organisms since material originating in the bronchi and alveoli has to pass through the pharynx and mouth, areas that have a normal commensal population of bacteria (Thomson 2002: E).

Procedure guidelines (cont.)

2 Care should be taken to ensure that the material sent for investigations is sputum, not saliva.	To obtain the required sample (Health Services Advisory Committee 2003: C).
3 Encourage patients who have difficulty producing sputum to cough deeply first thing in the morning. Alternatively, a physiotherapist should be called to assist.	To facilitate expectoration (E).
4 Send any sputum specimen to the laboratory within 1 hour.	The bacterial population alters rapidly and rapid dispatch should ensure accurate results (Thomson 2002: R 5).

Urine specimen

Action	Rationale
1 Specimens of urine should be collected as soon as possible after the patient wakes in the morning and at the same time each morning if more than one specimen is required.	The bladder will be full of concentrated urine which has accumulated overnight (Malarkey & McMorrow 2005: E). If specimens are taken at other times, the urine may be diluted (E).
2 Dispatch all specimens to the laboratory as soon after collection as possible.	Urine specimens should be examined within 2 hours of collection or 24 hours if kept refrigerated at a temperature of 4°C. At room temperature overgrowth will occur and lead to misinterpretation (Buller 2000: E).

Midstream specimen of urine (MSU): male

Action	Rationale
1 Retract the prepuce and clean the skin surrounding the urethral meatus with soap and water, 0.9% sodium chloride solution or a solution that does not contain a disinfectant.	To prevent other organisms contaminating the specimen. Disinfectants may irritate or be painful to the urethral mucous membrane (Malarkey & McMorrow 2005: E; Higgins 2007: E).
2 Ask the patient to direct the first and last part of his stream into a urinal or toilet but to collect the middle part of his stream into a sterile container.	To avoid contamination of the specimen with organisms normally present on the skin (Parini 2000: E; Higgins 2007: E).

Midstream specimen of urine (MSU): female

Action	Rationale
1 Part the labia, clean the urethral meatus with soap and water, 0.9% sodium chloride solution or a solution that does not contain a disinfectant.	To prevent other organisms contaminating the specimen (Parini 2000: E). Disinfectants may irritate or be painful to the urethral mucous membrane (Malarkey & McMorrow 2005: E).
2 (a) If using a cotton swab, use a separate cotton-wool swab for each wipe.	To prevent cross-infection (Parini 2000: E).
(b) Wipe in a downwards motion from the front to the back encourage the patient to still separate the labia with one hand while micturating.	To prevent perianal contamination (Parini 2000: E). To avoid contamination of the specimen with organisms normally present on the skin (Higgins 2007: E; Graham & Galloway 2001: E).
3 Place sterile receiver or a wide-mouthed sterile container under the stream of urine and remove before micturation finishes.	To prevent contamination of specimen (Parini 2000: E).
4 Transfer the specimen into a sterile universal container and screw the cap on immediately. Care should be taken not to touch inside of cap or rim of the universal container.	To prevent contamination with bacteria in the environment (Higgins 2007: E).

Specimen of urine from an ileal conduit

For further information see the relevant section in the procedure on stoma care (see Chapter 12).

Catheter specimen of urine

For further information see the relevant section in the procedure on urinary catheterization (see Chapter 13).

Twenty-four-hour urine collection

Action	Rationale
1 Request the patient to void the bladder at the time appointed to begin this procedure. Discard this specimen.	To ensure the urine collected is that produced in the 24 hours stated (Malarkey & McMorrow 2005: E).

975

Procedure guidelines *(cont.)*

2 All urine passed in the next 24 hours is collected in a large specimen bottle. The final specimen is collected at exactly the same time the bladder was voided 24 hours earlier.	Body chemistry alters constantly. A 24-hour collection will accommodate all the variables within a representative period (Thomson 2002: E).
3 Care must be taken to ensure the patient understands the procedure in order to eliminate the risk of an incomplete collection.	A 24-hour collection will not be obtained if one sample is lost, and the results will be invalid (Malarkey & McMorrow 2005: E).

References and further reading

Armitage, K.B. & King, C.H. (2000) Malaria. In: *Principles and Practice of Infectious Diseases* (eds G. Mandell, J. Bennett & R. Dolin). Churchill Livingstone, Philadelphia, pp. 2817–31.

Baker, F.J., Silverton, R.E. & Pallister, C.J. (1998) Microbiology. In: *Introduction to Medical Laboratory Technology*. Butterworth Heinemann, Oxford, pp. 251–325.

Beutz, M. *et al.* (2003) Clinical utility of blood cultures drawn from central vein catheters and peripheral venipuncture in critically ill medical patients. *Chest*, **123**, 854–61.

Bille, J. (2000) Microbiologic diagnostic procedures. In: *Management of Infection in Immunocompromised Patients* (eds M. Glauser & P. Pizzo). W.B. Saunders, London, pp. 230–65.

British Standards Institute (1995) *BS ISO 6710. Single-use Containers for Venous Blood Specimen Collection*. British Standards Institute, London.

Buller, R. (2000) Specimen collection and transport. In: *Diagnostic Virology* (ed. G.A. Storch). Churchill Livingstone, New York, pp. 25–36.

Cunningham, R. *et al.* (2007) Effect on MRSA transmission of rapid PCR testing of patients admitted to critical care. *J Hosp Infect*, 65 (1), 24–8.

Dellinger, R.P. *et al.* (2004) Surviving sepsis campaign guidelines for management of severe sepsis and septic shock. *Intens Care Med*, **30**, 536–55.

DH (2005a) *Saving Lives: A Delivery Programme to Reduce Healthcare Associated Infection including MRSA: Skills for Implantation*. Department of Health, London.

DH (2005b) *Hazardous Waste (England) Regulations*. Department of Health, London.

DH (2007) *Saving Lives: a Delivery Programme to Reduce Healthcare Associated Infection Including MRSA: Taking Blood Cultures – a Strategy for NHS Trusts, a Summary of Best Practice*. Department of Health, London.

Downie, G., Mackenzie, J. & Williams, A. (2000) Drug treatment of infections. In: *Pharmacology and Drug Management for Nurses*. Churchill Livingstone, Edinburgh, pp. 189–206.

Durnell Schuiling, K. & Likis, F.E. (2006) *Women's Gynecologic Health*. Jones and Bartlett Publishers, Sudbury, MA.

Engervall, P. & Bjorkholm, M. (1996) Infections in neutropenic patients II: management. *Med Oncol*, **13**(1), 63–9.

Finegold, S.M. (2000) Anaerobic bacteria: general concepts. In: *Principles and Practice of Infectious Diseases* (eds G. Mandell, J. Bennett & R. Dolin). Churchill Livingstone, Philadelphia, pp. 1805–62.

Foxman, B. (2002) Epidemiology of urinary tract infections: incidence, morbidity, and economic costs. *Am J Med*, **113**(1, Suppl 1), 5–13.

Gabriel, J. (2008) Long-term central venous access. In: *Intravenous Therapy in Nursing Practice* (eds L. Dougherty & J. Lamb), 2nd edn, Blackwell Publishing, Oxford.

Gilchrist, B. (2000) Taking a wound swab. *Nurs Times*, **96**(4), 2.

Gill, D. (1999) Stool specimen part 1. *Nurs Times*, **95**(25), 1–2.

Gill, V.J., Fedorko, D.P. & Witebsky, F.G. (2004) The clinician and the microbiology laboratory. In: *Principles and Practice of Infectious Diseases* (eds G. Mandell, J. Bennett & R. Dolin). Churchill Livingstone, Philadelphia, pp. 203–41.

Godfrey, H. & Evans, A. (2000) Catherization and urinary tract infections: microbiology. *Br J Nurs*, **9**(11), 682–4.

Gold, H.S. & Eisenstein, B.I. (2000) Introduction to bacterial diseases. In: *Principles and Practice of Infectious Diseases* (eds G. Mandell, J. Bennett & R. Dolin). Churchill Livingstone, Philadelphia, pp. 2065–9.

Graham, J.C. & Galloway, A. (2001) The laboratory diagnosis of urinary tract infections. *J Clin Pathol*, **54**, 911–19.

Hazardous Waste (England and Wales) Regulations (2005) HMSO, London.

Health Services Advisory Committee (2003) *Safe Working and the Prevention of Infection in Clinical Laboratories and Similar Facilities*. HMSO, London.

Henderson, D.K. (2000) Bacteraemia due to percutaneous intravenous devices. In: *Principles and Practice of Infectious Diseases* (eds G. Mandell, J. Bennett & R. Dolin). Churchill Livingstone, Philadelphia, pp. 3005–3020.

Henker, R. (2000) Infection control. Use of blood cultures in critically ill patients. *Crit Care Nurs*, **20**(1), 45–9.

Higgins, C. (2007) *Understanding Laboratory Investigations for Nurses and Health Professionals*, 2nd edn. Blackwell Publishing, Oxford.

Himberger, J.R. & Himberger, L.C. (2001) Acuracy of drawing blood through infusing intravenous lines. *Heart Lung*, **30**(1), 66–73.

Holliday, G., Strike, P.N. & Masterton, R.G. (1991) Perineal cleansing and midstream urine specimen in ambulatory women. *J Hosp Infect*, **18**(1), 71–5.

Ismail, R. *et al.* (1997) Therapeutic drug monitoring of gentamicin: a 6-year follow-up audit. *J Clin Pharm Ther*, **22**(1), 21–5.

Jumaa, P.A. & Chattopadhyay, B. (1994) Pseudobacteraemia. *J Hosp Infect*, **27**(3), 167–77.

Karnon, J. *et al.* (2004) Liquid-based cytology in cervical screening: an updated rapid and systematic review and economic analysis. Executive summary. *Health Technol Assess*, **8**(20).

Leong, C.L. *et al.* (2006) Providing guidelines and education is not enough: an audit of gentamicin use at The Royal Melbourne Hospital. *Intern Med J*, **36**(1), 37–42.

Macleod, J.A. (1992) Collecting specimens for the laboratory tests. *Nurs Stand*, **6**(20), 36–7.

Madeo, M. *et al.* (2003) Reduction in the contamination rate of blood cultures collected by medical staff in the accident and emergency department. *Clinical Effectiveness in Nursing*, **7**, 30–2.

Magadia, R.R. & Weinstein, M.P. (2001) Laboratory diagnosis of bacteremia and fungemia. *Infect Dis Clin North Am*, **15**(4), 1009–24.

Malarkey, L.M. & McMorrow, M.E. (2005) *Saunders Nursing Guide to Laboratory and Diagnostic Tests*. Elsevier Saunders, St Louis, MO.

Marsden, J. & Shaw, M. (2003) Correct administration of topical eye treatment. *Nurs Stand*, **17**(30), 42–4.

McBryde, E.S. *et al.* (2005) Comparison of contamination rates of catheter-drawn and peripheral blood cultures. *J Hosp Infect*, **60**, 118–21.

Mead, M. (1999) High vaginal swab. *Practice Nurse*, **17**(9), 642.

Mims, C. *et al.* (2004) *Medical Microbiology*, 3rd edn. Elsevier Mosby, Edinburgh.

Moller, T. *et al.* (2005) Patient education – a strategy for prevention of infections caused by permanent central venous catheters in patients with haematological malignancies: a randomized clinical trial. *J Hosp Infect*, **61**, 330–41.

National Collaborating Centre for Women's and Children's Health (2004) *Fertility: Assessment and Treatment for People with Fertility Problems. Clinical Guidelines*. Royal College of Obstetricians and Gynaecologists (RCOG) Press, London.

NHS Cancer Screening Programmes (2003) *Inequalities of Access to Cancer Screening: a Literature Review*. Series No 1. NHS Cancer Screening Programmes Publication, Sheffield.

NHS Cancer Screening Programmes (2004) *Colposcopy and Programme Management Guidelines for the NHS Cervical Screening Programmes*. No. 20. NHS Cancer Screening Programmes Publication, Sheffield.

NHS Cancer Screening Programmes (2006) *An Easy Guide to Cervical Screening*. NHS Cancer Screening Programmes Publication, Sheffield.

NHS Screening Programmes (2004) *Training in Taking Samples for Liquid Based Cytology*. Implementation Guide No 4, Version 1. National Health Service Screening Programmes Publication, Sheffield.

NHS Screening Programmes (2006) *Taking Samples for Cervical Screening: a Resource Pack for Trainers*. No 23 April. National Health Service Screening Programmes Publication, Sheffield.

NICE (2004) *Referral for Suspected Cancer: NICE Guideline*. National Institute for Health and Clinical Excellence, London.

NMC (2006) *A–Z Advice Sheet Consent*. www.nmc.org.

NMC (2008) *The Code: Standards of Conduct, Performance and Ethics for Nurses and Midwives*. Nursing and Midwifery Council, London.

O'Grady, N.P. *et al.* (1998) Practice guidelines for evaluating new fever in critically ill adult patients. *Clin Infect Dis*, **26**(5), 1042–59.

Papasian, C.J. & Kragel, P.J. (1997) The microbiology laboratory's role in life-threatening infections. *Crit Care Nurse*, **20**(3), 44–59.

Parini, S. (2000) How to collect specimens. *Nursing*, **30**(5), 66–7.

Peterson, L.R. *et al.* (2001) Role of clinical microbiology laboratories in the management and control of infectious diseases and the delivery of health care. *Clin Infect Dis*, **32**, 605–11.

Poutanen, S.M. & Simor, A.E. (2004) *Clostridium difficile*-associated diarrhoea in adults. *Can Med Assoc J*, **171**(1), 51–68.

RCN (2005) *Good Practice in Infection Prevention and Control – Guidance for Nursing Staff*. Royal College of Nursing, London.

Rushing, J. (2004) Drawing blood with vacuum tubes. *Nursing*, **34**(1), 26.

Safdar, N. *et al.* (2005) Meta-analysis: methods for diagnosing intravascular devise-related bloodstream infection. *Ann Intern Med*, **142**(6), 451–66.

Sandin, R.L. & Rinaldi, M. (1996) Special consideration for the clinical microbiology laboratory in the diagnosis of infections in the cancer patient. *Infect Dis Clin North Am*, **10**(2), 413–30.

Shanson, D.C. (1999) Use of the microbiology laboratory – general principles. In: *Microbiology in Clinical Practice*. Butterworth-Heinemann, Oxford, pp. 24–36.

Shelton, B.K. (1999) Sepsis. *Semin Oncol Nurs*, **15**(3), 209–21.

Shirrel, D.J. *et al.* (1999) Understanding therapeutic drug monitoring. *Am J Nurs*, **99**(1), 42–4.

Shulman, R.J. *et al.* (1998) Central venous catheter versus peripheral veins for sampling blood levels of commonly used drugs. *J Parenteral Enteral Nutr*, **22**(4), 234–7.

Spitalnic, S.J., Woolard, R.H. & Mermel, L.A. (1995) The significance of changing needles when inoculating blood cultures: a meta-analysis. *Clin Infect Dis*, **21**(5), 1103–6.

Stollery, R., Shaw, M. & Lee, A. (2005) *Ophthalmic Nursing*. Blackwell Publishing, Oxford, p. 27.

Tam, V.H. *et al.* (1999) Vancomycin peak serum concentration monitoring. *J Intraven Nurs*, **22**(6), 336–42.

Theaker, C. (2005) Infection control issues in central venous catheter care. *Intensive Crit Care Nurs*, **21**, 99–109.

Thomas, L.C. *et al.* (2007) Development of a real-time *Staphylococcus aureus* and MRSA (SAM) PCR for routine blood culture. *J Microbiol Methods*, **68**(2), 296–302.

Thomson, R.B. (2002) Use of microbiology laboratory tests in the diagnosis of infectious diseases. In: *Expert Guide to Infectious Diseases* (ed. J. Tan). American College of Physicians, Philadelphia, pp. 1–41.

Tobin, C.M. (2002) Vancomycin therapeutic drug monitoring: is there a consensus view? The results of a UK National External Quality Assessment Scheme (UK NEQAS) for antibiotic assays questionnaire. *J Antimicrob Chemother*, **50**(5), 713–18.

Tortora, G.J. & Derrickson, B.H. (2006) *Introduction to the Human Body: the Essentials of Anatomy and Physiology*, 7th edn. John Wiley & Sons, New Jersey, pp. 900–52.

Traunter, W.B. *et al.* (2002) Skin antisepsis kits containing alcohol and chlorhexidinegluconate or tincture of iodine are associated with low rates of blood culture contamination. *Infect Control Hosp Epidemiol*, **23**, 397–401.

Wazait, H.D. *et al.* (2003) Catheter-associated urinary tract infections: prevalence of uropathogens and pattern of antimicrobial resistance in a UK hospital (1996–2001). *Br J Urol*, **91**(9), 806–9.

Weinstein, S.M. (2007) Laboratory tests. In: *Plumer's Principles and Practice of Intravenous Therapy*. J.B. Lippincott, Philadelphia, pp. 63–93.

Wilson, J. & Jenner, E.A. (2006) Understanding the microbiology laboratory. In: *Infection Control in Clinical Practice*. Bailliere Tindall, Edinburgh, pp. 19–33.

Wilson, M.L. (1996) General principles of specimen collection. *Clin Infect Dis*, **22**(5), 766–77.

WHO (2006) *Comprehensive Cervical Cancer Control: a Guide to Essential Practice*. World Health Organization Press, Switzerland.

Zitella, L. (2003) Central venous cathether care for blood and marrow transplant recipients. *Clin J Oncol Nurs*, **7**(3), 289–97.

Multiple choice questions

1 Aerobic bacteria grow in the presence of:

   a   Moisture
   b   Air
   c   Dirt
   d   Reduced oxygen

2 Anaerobic bacteria grow in the presence of:

   a   Air
   b   Reduced oxygen
   c   Dirt
   d   Moisture

3 Ideally microbiological samples should be collected:

   a   In the morning
   b   Before the patient begins any treatment, e.g. antiseptics or antibiotics
   c   After treatment begins
   d   By laboratory staff

4 If blood cultures cannot be transported to the laboratory immediately they should be stored:

   a   In a locked cupboard
   b   In the fridge
   c   In a 37°C incubator
   d   In the clinical room

5 **Prior to obtaining a midstream specimen of urine patients should be asked to:**

   a   Wash their hands
   b   Put on gloves
   c   Empty their bladder
   d   Wash their hands and the urethral meatus

6 **What do you need to do prior to obtaining a nose swab?**

   a   Moisten the swab with sterile water
   b   Ask patient to blow their nose
   c   Moisten swab with tap water
   d   Nothing

Answers to the multiple choice questions can be found in Appendix 3.

Chapter 29

Tracheostomy care and laryngectomy care

Tracheostomy and laryngectomy care

Definition

A tracheostomy (or tracheotomy) is the surgical creation of an opening into the trachea through the neck (Figure 29.1a) (Serra 2000). Once formed the tracheostomy opening is kept patent with a tube (Serra 2000) which is curved to accommodate the anatomy of the trachea.

Indications

Tracheostomy may be carried out:

- To enable the aspiration of tracheobronchial secretions.
- To bypass any upper respiratory tract obstruction.
- To aid in weaning patients from ventilatory support (Serra 2000; Woodrow 2002).

Reference material

Types of tracheostomy

Temporary

A temporary tracheostomy (Figure 29.1b) is performed for patients as an elective procedure, e.g. at the time of major surgery such as a total glossectomy (Prior & Russell 2004).

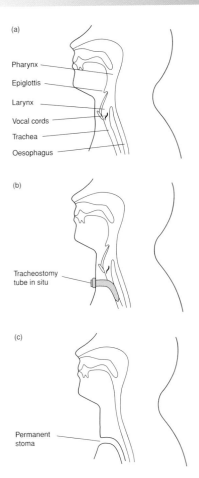

Figure 29.1   (a) Anatomy of the head and neck. (b) Temporary tracheostomy. (c) Permanent tracheostomy (total laryngectomy).

Permanent

A permanent tracheostomy is the creation of a tracheostomy following a total laryngectomy (Prior & Russell 2004) (Figure 29.1c). The larynx is removed and the trachea is sutured in position to form a permanent structure known as a laryngectomy stoma (Clotworthy *et al*. 2006a). The patient will breathe through this stoma for the remainder of his/her life. As a result, there is no connection between the nasal passages and the trachea (Edgtton-Winn & Wright 2005).

Emergency

A tracheostomy may be performed as an emergency procedure when a patient has an obstructed airway. Among the more common conditions causing obstruction are trauma to the airway or neck, poisoning, infections or neoplasms.

Percutaneous

This technique enables the pretracheal tissues to be incised under local anaesthesia. A sheath is inserted into the trachea between the cricoid and the first tracheal ring or between the first and second rings. The trachea is dilated with forceps or a conical dilator, which is then slipped over a guidewire, ready for a tracheostomy tube to be inserted. Frequently performed in the critical care setting, the procedure takes less time and requires fewer resources, such as theatres and surgeons, resulting in fewer costs than a surgical tracheostomy (Patel & Matta 2004). Another potential benefit of percutaneous tracheostomy is more rapid stomal closure and smaller scar formation once the tracheostomy tube has been removed (Patel & Matta 2004).

984

Surgical

This procedure is often performed under a general anaesthetic, although it can be carried out using local anaesthetic. A horizontal incision is made halfway between the sternal notch and the cricoid cartilage (Price 2004a). The thyroid isthmus is divided enabling the trachea to be exposed and the tracheal cartilages to be counted. The tracheostomy should be sited over the second and third or third and fourth tracheal cartilages (Price 2004a).

Mini-tracheostomy

Unlike the previous two techniques, which enable oxygen therapy and mechanical ventilation to be given, this method is used only when frequent tracheal suctioning is required. The procedure is also referred to as a cricothyroidotomy or a laryngotomy (Price 2004b). The cricothyroid ligament is incised enabling a small endotracheal tube or a minitracheostomy tube to be inserted (Price 2004b). The mini-tracheostomy tube has a small internal diameter, of often only 4 mm.

Types of tracheostomy tube

Tracheostomy tubes are available in different designs. Some have both an outer and an inner tube. The outer tube maintains the patency of the airway, while the inner tube, which fits snugly inside the outer tube, can be removed for cleaning without disturbing the stoma site. Disposable inner tubes are now available; these single-use items are quicker to use (Dropkin 1996) and minimize cross-infection as no cleaning is required.

The majority of tracheostomy tubes are manufactured from plastic. Some also have a high volume, low pressure cuff. This type of cuff distributes the pressure evenly on the tracheal wall and aims to reduce the incidence of tracheal ulceration, necrosis and/or stenosis at the cuff site (Russell 2004a).

The cuff when inflated provides a seal between the tube and tracheal wall enabling effective ventilation and protection from aspiration (Russell 2004a). The size and style of the tube chosen will depend upon the size of the trachea and the needs of the individual patient (Serra 2000; Bond *et al.* 2003; Lewarski 2005).

A selection of tubes is described below.

Portex cuffed tracheostomy tube

This is a disposable plastic tracheostomy tube constructed of siliconized polyvinyl chloride with an introducer and inflatable cuff which gives an airtight seal (Figure 29.2). It is a softer and more pliable tube and is often used when percutaneous tracheostomy is performed in the critical care setting to aid weaning from me-

985

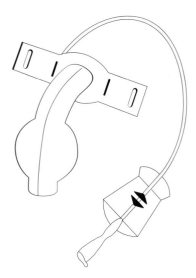

Figure 29.2   Portex cuffed tube.

chanical ventilation. Once the stoma is well-formed, after about 7–10 days and depending on the patient's specific weaning needs, the Portex tube may be replaced by a more suitable, sturdier tube such as a Shiley fenestrated tube (Hess 2005).

Shiley cuffless tracheostomy tube (Figure 29.3a)

This is a plastic tube with an introducer and two inner tubes. One inner tube has an extension known as a 15 mm hub or adaptor at its upper aspect. The majority of tracheostomy tubes used in the hospital setting have the universally sized 15 mm hub to allow attachment to ventilators, speaking valves and other equipment (Russell 2004a). The other tube has no 15 mm hub extension and is less obtrusive and suitable for those patients not requiring attachment to other equipment (Russell 2004a).

This tube is usually used for the following reasons:

- To keep the tracheostomy tract patent if the patient is going to have further surgery.
- In place of a metal tracheostomy tube if the patient is going to have radiotherapy to the neck area when a metal tube would cause tissue reaction (Holmes 1996). This is because the metal can interfere with the radiotherapy beam and cause an increased dose to be given to the underlying stoma and surrounding skin (Prior & Russell 2004).
- For a laryngectomy patient who has a benign or malignant stenosis of the trachea and requires a longer tube than the regular length laryngectomy tube to keep the stenosis patent.

Shiley cuffed tracheostomy tube (Figure 29.3b)

This is a plastic tube with an introducer and one inner tube. The inner tube has the universal 15 mm extension at its upper aspect to facilitate connection to other equipment. The outer tube has an inflatable cuff to give an airtight seal. The cuff prevents secretions from reaching the lungs. The seal facilitates ventilation.

This is often used for the immediate postoperative phase, i.e. 24–72 hours. For those patients who require a cuffed tracheostomy tube for lengthy periods, a cuff manometer should be used to check cuff pressure. In order to prevent tracheal tissue necrosis, stenosis and/or fistula formation (Mol *et al.* 2004; Russell 2004a) cuff pressure should not exceed 18 mmHg (Russell 2004b; Edgtton-Winn & Wright 2005; Clotworthy *et al.* 2006b).

Cuff pressure should be checked every shift (Clotworthy *et al.* 2006b) and each time the cuff is re-inflated (Woodrow 2002).

Shiley fenestrated tube (Figure 29.3c)

This is a plastic tube with an introducer and three inner tubes. One inner tube has no hub jutting out, is less obtrusive and is suitable for those patients not requiring

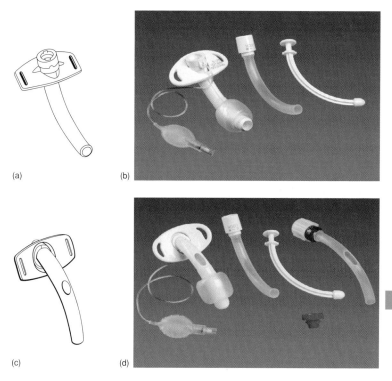

(a)

(b)

(c)

(d)

987

Figure 29.3   Shiley's tracheostomy tubes. (a) Shiley plain tube. (b) Shiley cuffed tube (courtesy of Tyco Healthcare). (c) Shiley plain fenestrated tube. (d) Shiley cuffed fenestrated tube (courtesy of Tyco Healthcare).

attachment to other equipment (Russell 2004a). The other two inner tubes have the universal 15 mm extension at the upper aspect to facilitate connection to other apparatus, and one of these (with a green coloured hub) also has a fenestration midway down the tube. This is to encourage the passage of air and secretions into the oral and nasal passages. It is useful when attempting to encourage a return to normal function following long-term use of a temporary tracheostomy, e.g. enabling the patient to communicate verbally.

The fenestrations enable this type of tube to be most suitable for the weaning method. A cap is inserted onto the tube, occluding the artificial airway. This enables the patient to become used to breathing via the oral and nasal passages again. The cap can be left in situ for certain periods of time until the patient can tolerate the tube occluded for a full uninterrupted 24 hours. Only then can removal of the entire tube, known as decannulation, be considered (Serra 2000; Harkin 2004). The decannulation procedure should take place in the morning, during the week to ensure that a specialist assessment can be sought in the unlikely event that the patient requires tracheostomy tube reinsertion (Harkin 2004).

Shiley cuffed fenestrated tube (Figure 29.3d)

This is a plastic tube with an introducer and two inner tubes. Both inner tubes have the universal 15 mm extension at the upper aspect to facilitate connection to other apparatus, and one of these (with a green coloured hub) also has a fenestration midway down the tube. The fenestrated tube can also be occluded with a cap, to assess the patient's oral and nasal airway, first ensuring that the cuff has been completely deflated and that the fenestrated inner tube is in situ. The outer tube has a fenestration in the middle of the cannula, again to encourage a return to normal function. The outer tube also has an inflatable cuff to give an airtight seal. The cuff prevents secretions from reaching the lungs. This tube is particularly useful for patients who require both periods of cuff inflation (to protect the airway) and cuff deflation (to enable a speaking valve to be used) (Russell 2004a).

Jackson's silver tracheostomy tube

This is a silver tube with an introducer and inner tube (Figure 29.4a). The inner tube is locked in position by a small catch on the outer tube and may be removed and cleaned as necessary without disturbing the outer tube.

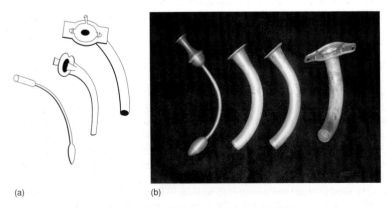

(a)   (b)

Figure 29.4 (a) Jackson's silver tube. (b) Negus's silver tube.

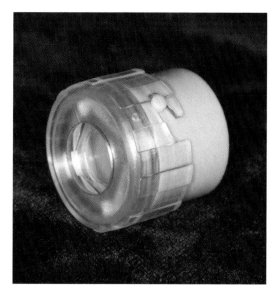

Figure 29.5 Rusch speaking valve.

Negus's silver tracheostomy tube

This is a silver tracheostomy tube with an introducer and a choice of inner tubes, with and without speaking valves (Figure 29.4b). The outer tube does not have a safety catch; consequently the inner tube may be coughed out inadvertently.

Speaking valve

This is a plastic device with a two-way valve which fits onto the 15 mm hub of the fenestrated inner tube (Figure 29.5). Distinction should be made between open and closed position valves:

The open position speaking valve (e.g. *Rusch* valve) is open by default and closes with positive pressure (expiration) which diverts air through the upper airways past the vocal cords, therefore allowing production of a voice. The closed position speaking valve (e.g. *Passy Muir* valve) is closed by default and requires negative pressure (patient's inspiratory effort) to open; as soon as expiration starts it closes which causes air to be diverted as described above. This type of valve can be used in ventilator circuits for patients who are mechanically ventilated.

If a non-fenestrated cuffed tube is in situ, the cuff should always be deflated before a speaking valve is fitted as the patient will not be able to exhale

(Clotworthy *et al.* 2006b). Ordinarily, practitioners will also consider changing a non-fenestrated tube for a fenestrated tube (double lumen, with fenestrated inner tube). This will allow air to be diverted through the fenestrations of the tube in addition to air already diverted past the cuff to the upper airways. If a non-fenestrated tube is in situ, depending on the size of the tracheostomy tube and the diameter of the patient's trachea, sufficient air may not be diverted past the cuff. This will result in pressure building up because the patient will not be able to breathe out and the valve will not be tolerated. In this case it will be necessary for a complete outer tube change to a fenestrated tube.

However, anecdotal evidence from practice would suggest that in some instances cuff deflation alone (without changing a non-fenestrated tube for a fenestrated tube) may be sufficient to allow air diversion past the cuff through the upper airways as described above. It is important that each individual case is considered carefully and that practitioners weigh up the potential discomfort and distress a complete tracheostomy tube change may cause against the potential risks of fitting a speaking valve on a non-fenestrated tube. It is therefore imperative that when a speaking valve is used for the first time, the patient is carefully monitored for any signs of respiratory distress.

Kapitex Tracoetwist fenestrated tube

This is a plastic tube with an introducer and two inner tubes (Figure 29.6a). One of these inner tubes has an extension at its upper end to facilitate connection to

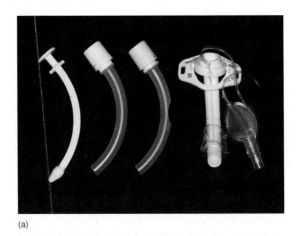

(a)   (b)

Figure 29.6 **(a)** Kapitex Tracoetwist cuffed fenestrated tube. **(b)** Decannulation plug.

other apparatus. The other inner tube has a fenestration midway down the tube. The outer tube also has a fenestration consisting of a series of small holes. This helps to reduce the risk of granulation tissue growing through the fenestration. The neck plate or flange moves in a vertical and horizontal direction enabling the plate to move as the patient moves. An inner tube with integrated speaking valve can be ordered separately.

A variety of other tubes are available in this series, including both cuffed and plain tracheostomy tubes.

Decannulation plug

This is a small plastic plug which fits into the outer fenestrated tube (Figure 29.6b). It is used to encourage patients to breathe via the oral and nasal air passages before removal of the tracheostomy tube. Alternatively, a small plastic plug (Kapitex) or a blind hub (Shiley) can be fitted into or over the inner fenestrated tube. This is particularly useful for patients who are still producing tenacious secretions as the plug or hub can be removed to enable the inner tube to be cleaned (Harkin 2004).

Colledge silver laryngectomy tube

This is a silver laryngectomy tube with an introducer (Figure 29.7a). It is often used to dilate a laryngectomy stoma which has stenosed. These tubes can be cleaned, autoclaved and reused.

Shiley laryngectomy tube

This is a plastic tube with an introducer and inner tube (Figure 29.7b). The inner tube has the universal 15 mm hub enabling the attachment to other equipment. It is shorter in length than a tracheostomy tube, thereby conforming to the slightly shorter trachea in the patient who has undergone a total laryngectomy. The inner tube may be removed and cleaned frequently without disturbing the outer tube. It is sometimes worn postoperatively while the stoma is healing to help facilitate a good shaped stoma.

Shaw's silver laryngectomy tube

This is a silver laryngectomy tube with an introducer and an inner tube beyond both lower and upper aspects of the outer tube (Figure 29.7c). Thus pressure dressings may be secured without occluding the stoma. The silver catch on the outer tube keeps the inner tube in position.

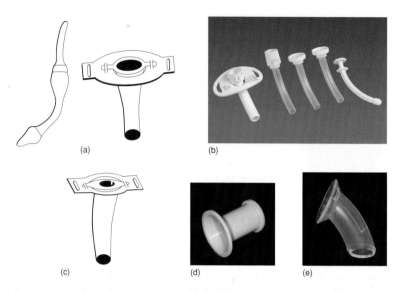

(a)

(b)

(c)

(d)

(e)

Figure 29.7 Tubes for permanent tracheostomies. (a) Colledge silver tube. (b) Shiley laryngectomy tube. (c) Shaw's laryngectomy tube. (d) Stoma button. (e) Laryngectomy tube.

Stoma button

This is a soft Silastic 'button' (Figure 29.7d). It may be used in place of a laryngectomy tube. It is very light and comfortable to wear and can be used in conjunction with a Blom–Singer speaking valve. In order to facilitate the use of the Blom–Singer speaking valve a diamond-shape is cut out of the Silastic (see Laryngectomy voice rehabilitation section, Chapter 42, Professional edition, for specific information on surgical voice restoration).

Laryngectomy tube

This is a slightly opaque Silastic tube which is longer in length in comparison to the stoma button. These tubes are 36 and 55 mm in length and are available in a variety of different sizes (Figure 29.7e). This tube is most suitable for patients who experience a degree of stenosis further down the trachea (see Stoma buttons and vents, in Laryngectomy voice rehabilitation section, Chapter 42, Professional edition).

Heat and moisture exchange filters

Following a tracheostomy or a laryngectomy, patients lose normal nasal airway functions. The air they breathe is no longer warmed, humidified and filtered by the nasal passages as they now breathe directly in and out of the tracheostomy. Drying of the airway impairs mucous and cilia function resulting in thickened airway secretions (Woodrow 2002). The amount of secretions produced will vary from patient to patient but is greater in the immediate and early postoperative period and gradually improves over the ensuing months. Patients find that any sharp change in temperature stimulates excessive mucus production (Mathieson 2001).

Prior to the development of heat and moisture exchange (HME) filters, patients coped with this by spraying the tracheostomal area with water, using a Roger's spray or equivalent and wearing either a small foam pad, a 'bib' or specially designed cravat or scarf over the stoma. HME filters are now widely available on prescription in many different styles enabling the patient and/or the nurse to decide on the appropriate method of humidification, depending on the individual patient's circumstances (Billau 2004). The importance of systemic hydration of the patient via a feeding tube, intravenous fluids or oral fluids must not be overlooked (Clotworthy *et al.* 2006c) as this can impact on the tenacity of secretions.

HME filters for laryngectomy use consist of a self-adhesive baseplate, which is placed around the stoma and a specially treated foam filter which is clipped into the centre. This enables the patient to breathe more easily while the air is warmed, humidified and filtered by the foam. For a minority of patients who cannot tolerate the baseplate on the skin or maintain a good seal, the filter section can also be clipped into a flexible Silastic laryngectomy tube, vent or stoma button. It is the role of the speech and language therapist and/or clinical nurse specialist and/or physiotherapist to assess and fit the HME filter in the initial stages of care (Pathways in Cancer Care 2001).

HME filters for tracheostomy use follow the same rationale as those for laryngectomy use. The filter is attached directly onto the tracheostomy tube and some have an integral speaking valve and enable suctioning to be performed and/or oxygen to be administered whilst still in situ, e.g. trachphone (Figure 29.8).

Communication for the patient with a tracheostomy

The presence of a cuffed tracheostomy tube can impair verbal communication as air can no longer flow over the vocal cords. Loss of speech can be both frustrating and frightening (Serra 2000) and it is essential for the nurse to encourage both the patient and family to use other forms of communication during this time. The ultimate goal is to restore the patient's ability to communicate verbally, consistently and effectively (Hales 2004a). The call bell must be within reach at all times and pen and paper or a magic slate should be provided. The latter enables

993

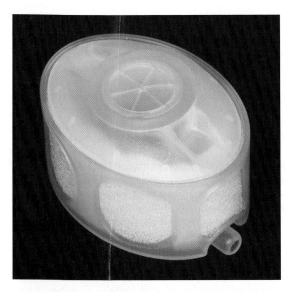

Figure 29.8 A trachphone.

the patient to erase previous conversations enabling some confidentiality to be maintained. For those patients unable to read or write and/or understand written English a picture board or alphabet board combined with phrases can be useful. This is where laminate A4 sheets displaying the alphabet in large letters, or simple pictures depicting basic activities (e.g. drink, toilet) supplemented with useful phrases are used (Clotworthy *et al.* 2006d). Those proficient at using a keyboard can communicate using a laptop or an electronic communication aid. The latter enables the individual to type in a phrase to obtain an automated voice repeating the phrase. The importance of a thorough nursing assessment on admission to hospital and the provision of patient information cannot be overestimated as this will help to identify communication issues early as well as patient and family concerns regarding the tracheostomy (Serra 2000).

Extra attention should be given to non-verbal communication, such as facial expression, hand and body positions and movement (Serra 2000). Lip reading may be appropriate for some patients. The patient is encouraged to exaggerate lip movements and use short but complete sentences in order to make the message clearer (Clotworthy *et al.* 2006d). Whichever communication method is utilized by the patient it is essential that all recipients (hospital staff, friends or relatives) allow the patient time to express him or herself.

Communication for the patient with a laryngectomy

The same strategies for effective communication can also be used for the patient who has undergone a total laryngectomy. This is particularly important in the early postoperative days and for those patients who have not undergone surgical voice restoration (see Laryngectomy voice rehabilitation section, Chapter 42, Professional edition, for specific information on surgical voice restoration). An electro-larynx can be used in the short- and long-term period. This device vibrates the air in the airway (in place of the vocal cords) creating a sound which can be shaped into speech sounds by the palate, tongue, cheeks, teeth and lips (Hales 2004a). Some patients prefer to use oesophageal speech. This is produced by inhaling or injecting air into the pharynx and upper oesophagus and then releasing it in a controlled fashion through the pharynx into the mouth (Rhys Evans & Blom 2003). All patients who have undergone total laryngectomy require immense support and encouragement to persevere with communication whichever method is chosen to enable them to achieve intelligible speech (Hahn & Jones 2000).

Swallowing for the patient with a tracheostomy

The presence of a tracheostomy tube can impair swallowing and consequently compromise the patient's nutritional status (Bond *et al.* 2003). The presence of a tracheostomy tube can cause tethering of the larynx, hindering the normal swallowing mechanism, particularly movement of the epiglottis over the airway to prevent aspiration (Hales 2004b). Assessment by a speech and language therapist is an essential part of these patients' care (Serra 2000). It is now recommended that patients should be nil by mouth when the cuff is inflated on the tracheostomy tube (Hales 2004b). There are two reasons for this: firstly, the inflated cuff does not offer complete protection from aspiration and can potentially disguise obvious signs of aspiration; and secondly, the cuff puts additional pressure on the larynx reducing laryngeal elevation needed for the normal swallowing mechanism (Hales 2004b).

Swallowing for the patient with a laryngectomy

Following the total laryngectomy procedure the patient is usually nil by mouth for 7 days if no previous radiotherapy has been given (Rhys Evans & Blom 2003) to enable healing in the pharynx. Once oral diet and fluids commences, the patient's stoma site should be observed closely for any evidence of leaking which might indicate a pharyngocutaneous fistula. Patients who have undergone previous radiotherapy are nil by mouth for 10 days and commence oral diet following a satisfactory barium swallow (Rhys Evans & Blom 2003). Patients who have a tracheo-oesophageal puncture as a primary procedure for the fitting of a voice valve may be fed immediately postoperatively via a catheter inserted through the puncture site (Shaw 2003) (see Laryngectomy voice rehabilitation section, Chapter 42, Professional edition, for specific information on surgical voice restoration). A nasogastric, gastrostomy or jejenostomy tube will be used to provide nutrition to those without a tracheo-oesophageal puncture (see Chapter 17 for specific information).

At times a speaking valve may leak or fall out (see Laryngectomy voice rehabilitation section, Chapter 42, Professional edition, for specific information on surgical voice restoration). A leaking valve can usually be replaced fairly quickly by a speech and language therapist or surgical doctor or a nurse who has undergone training. It may be necessary to insert a cuffed tracheostomy tube to prevent the patient aspirating diet/fluids and/or saliva until the valve is replaced. If a valve has fallen out, it is essential to check clinically and if necessary with a chest X ray that this has not fallen into the trachea or bronchus, and a temporary catheter should be inserted into the tracheo-oesophageal puncture promptly to ensure that the tract remains patent and to ensure that food and fluids do not leak into the stoma causing aspiration. Some patients are capable of effectively coughing the prosthesis out, while others require endoscopic retrieval (Singer & Deschler 1998).

General care of tracheostomy patients

■ When caring for a tracheostomy patient the following should always be at the bedside or accessible if the patient is self-caring or ambulant:

(a) Humidified oxygen with tracheostomy mask.

(b) Suction machine with a selection of suction catheters.

(c) Sterile water (Serra 2000) can be used to help clear suction tubing of secretions after suctioning has been performed.

(d) Clean disposable gloves and individually packaged, sterile, disposable gloves (Edgtton-Winn & Wright 2005).

(e) Disposable plastic apron and goggles (Day *et al.* 2002).

(f) Two cuffed tracheostomy tubes, one the same size as the patient is wearing, the other a size smaller, in the event of an emergency tracheostomy tube change (Serra 2000; Tamburri 2000).

(g) One 10 ml syringe to inflate cuff on tracheostomy tube.

(h) Tracheal dilators, in the event of tracheostomy tube falling out or being removed and inability to insert another tube. Tracheal dilators can be used to keep stomal opening patent until medical assistance arrives.

(i) Cuff pressure manometer (Serra 2000).

■ Outer tube changes are mostly dependent on the type of secretions the patient has, for example, a patient with copious, tenacious secretions will need a daily tube change, sometimes twice a day, as this will be the only way of ensuring that the stoma and tube are free from any accumulation of secretions. If the patient has minimal secretions then the necessity to change the tube decreases until some patients need to have their tube changed only weekly. Sometimes if the patient has a wound area up to the stoma edge, the entire tracheostomy tube has to be removed to gain access for cleaning the wound and observing its general status.

■ The frequency of inner tube changes depends on the volume, tenacity and viscosity of secretions and the comfort of the patient. In the immediate postoperative phase it may be necessary to change the inner tube half hourly. Any nurse starting a span of duty should perform a baseline assessment of the airway and tube to check on the type and amount of secretions and the need for humidification (Rhys Evans 2003).

The tracheostomy dressing can be renewed without removing the tube which should be done twice a day or more frequently if necessary (Serra 2000). Changing the dressing will ensure that the surrounding skin remains clean, dry and free from irritation and infection (Edgtton-Winn & Wright 2005).

General care of patients with a total laryngectomy

■ When caring for the patient who has undergone a total laryngectomy, the following should always be at the bedside or accessible if the patient is self-caring or ambulant:

(a) Humidified oxygen with tracheostomy mask.

(b) Suction machine with a selection of suction catheters.

(c) Sterile water (Serra 2000) can be used to help clear suction tubing of secretions after suctioning has been performed.

(d) Clean disposable gloves and individually packaged, sterile, disposable gloves (Edgtton-Winn & Wright 2005).

(e) Disposable plastic apron and goggles (Day *et al.* 2002).

(f) Two cuffed tracheostomy tubes, one the same size as the patient is wearing, the other a size smaller, in the event of an emergency tube change (Serra 2000; Tamburri 2000).

(g) One 10 ml syringe to inflate cuff on tracheostomy tube.

(h) Tilley's forceps: these are angled forceps that can be used to remove crusts or plugs of mucous from in and around the stoma.

(i) Pen torch (or access to a light source).

(j) Micropore or Elastoplast tape for those with a tracheo-oesophageal puncture, to ensure that the catheter keeping the puncture patent is secured firmly with tape or a suture (see Laryngectomy voice rehabilitation section, Chapter 42, Professional edition, for specific information on surgical voice restoration).

■ Patients who have undergone a total laryngectomy may require a cuffed tracheostomy tube for the first 24–48 hours. The tube stents the often oedematous stoma and the inflated cuff prevents blood-stained secretions from entering the lungs. The frequency of inner tube changes depends on the volume, tenacity and viscosity of secretions and the comfort of the patient. In the immediate postoperative phase it may be necessary to change the inner tube half hourly. Any nurse starting a span of duty should perform a baseline assessment of the airway and tube to check on the type and amount of secretions and the need for humidification (Rhys Evans 2003).

■ The dressing around the tracheostomy tube can be renewed without removing the tube which should be done twice a day or more frequently if necessary (Serra 2000). Changing the dressing will ensure that the surrounding skin remains clean, dry and free from irritation and infection (Edgtton-Winn & Wright 2005).

■ During the immediate postoperative phase the decision on whether a tube is required and which type is required is made by the surgeon (Clotworthy *et al.* 2006a). For those patients with no tube in situ, the nurse must be extremely vigilant, assessing the bare stoma frequently to ensure that the stoma is not at risk of stenosis. A stenosed stoma will restrict the patient's breathing, hinder the removal of secretions and prevent the insertion of a cuffed tube in an emergency situation. Stoma size should be sufficiently large, ideally 20–25 mm in diameter (Rhys Evans & Blom 2003) in order to insert a size 6 or above Shiley tracheostomy tube or equivalent. In the longer term, many patients no longer require a tube of any type in situ.

■ Stoma sutures are removed on day 7. If the patient has previously received external beam radiotherapy to the neck, stoma sutures are removed on day 10.

■ A moisturizing cream, such as E45, can be applied twice daily to the stoma once the tracheostomy tube and associated dressing is removed. For those patients with secretions that tend to accumulate around the stoma, a Cavilon wand can be used to prevent the skin becoming red and excoriated (Hampton 1998).

Suctioning via a tracheostomy or a laryngectomy

Patients with a tracheostomy or a laryngectomy will often require suctioning due to their impaired ability to clear tracheo-bronchial secretions. The function of the upper airways is to filter, warm and humidify inspired air. When a patient breathes through a tracheostome the upper airways are bypassed and cold, unfiltered and unhumidified air reaches the tracheo-bronchial tree. This is thought to impair the normal beating action of the cilia on the mucosal lining of the trachea which under normal circumstances causes an upward stream of mucous and foreign bodies (Pilbeam 1998). Furthermore, patients with a tracheostomy may have a reduced ability to generate a forceful cough and, in addition may experience an increased production of bronchial secretions due to irritation of the trachea

998

caused by the tracheostomy tube (Hooper 1996). These factors all contribute to the potential for the patient with a tracheostomy to develop sputum retention which could be detrimental and result in an increased risk of infection and impaired gas exchange, due to the plugging of airways and airflow limitation.

Indications for suctioning

The use of routine suctioning should be avoided and careful assessment of the patient's respiratory function should be carried out instead. Inspection, auscultation, percussion and palpation will help to determine the following (Pryor & Prasad 2001; Hough 2001):

- Patient's ability to clear his or her own secretions.
- Location of any secretions.
- Whether these secretions could be reached by the catheter.
- How detrimental these secretions might be for the patient.

Despite the benefits of suctioning, this action can also be hazardous for the patient:

- *Hypoxia*: the act of suctioning reduces vital lung volume from the lungs and upper airways. Each suctioning procedure should last no longer than 10–15 seconds to decrease the risk of trauma, hypoxia and other side-effects (The Joanna Briggs Institute 2000; Day 2000). Ventilator disconnection or the removal of the oxygen supply will also add to the risk of hypoxia prior to suctioning. Within a critical care setting this risk can be avoided by hyper-oxygenating the lungs with 100% oxygen, either manually or via a ventilator (Glass & Grap 1995; Hough 2001).
- *Mucosal trauma*: an incorrect choice of catheter, poor technique and the use of an excessively high suction pressure may all lead to mucosal trauma. The recommended suction pressure is 80–150 mmHg or 11–20 kPa for adults (Day 2000; Day *et al.* 2002).
- *Cardiac arrhythmias*: arrhythmias may be brought about by the onset of hypoxaemia or a vagal reflex instigated by tracheal stimulation by the catheter (MacIntyre & Branson 2001).
- *Raised intracranial pressure*: this may occur if the suction catheter causes excessive tracheal stimulation and result in coughing and an increase in the patient's intrathoracic pressure, both of which compromise cerebral venous drainage (Pryor & Prasad 2001).
- *Infection risk*: both care giver and patient are at risk of infection when suctioning is performed. In order to minimize this, examination gloves should be worn and an aseptic technique should be used, decontaminating hands with an alcoholic handrub before and after the suction procedure (DH 2005).

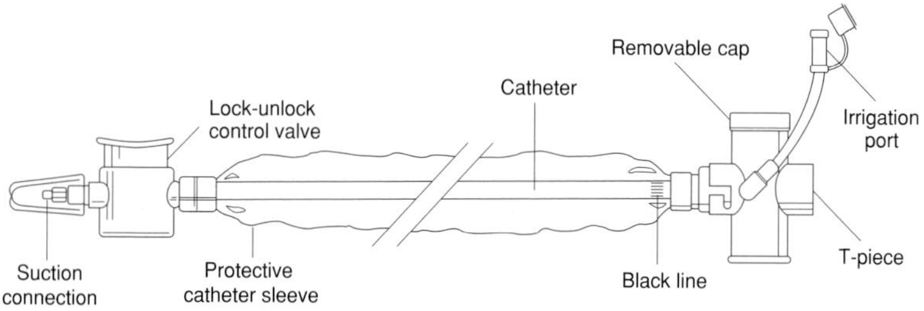

Figure 29.9   Components of a closed-circuit catheter. The control valve locks the vacuum on or off. The catheter is protected inside an airtight sleeve. A T-piece connects the device to the tracheal tube. The irrigation port allows saline instillation for irrigating the patient's airway or for cleaning the catheter (Hough 2001).

Suction catheters

Choosing the correct suction catheter size depends on the size of the tracheostomy tube. As a guide, the diameter of the suction catheter should not exceed one-half of the internal diameter of the tracheostomy tube (Griggs 1998; Hough 2001). The following formula can be used to determine the correct size catheter: divide the internal diameter of the tracheostomy tube by two and multiply this by three to obtain the French gauge of the suction catheter (Billau 2004).

Within a critical care setting, a closed-circuit suction system is an alternative method to the open suction system for patients being mechanically ventilated. This closed system has the catheter sealed in a protective plastic sleeve, which is connected permanently into a standard ventilator circuit thus preventing the catheter becoming contaminated (Figure 29.9). This also reduces the number of times the patient is disconnected from the ventilator, avoiding further hypoxia and cross-infection. Other patient groups who may benefit from its use include those who are immunosuppressed, actively infectious patients or those who require high levels of positive end expiratory pressure (PEEP) (Billau 2004).

Resuscitation

In the event of a patient with a tracheostomy needing resuscitation, the nurse should ensure that the tracheostomy is clear then connect an artificial ventilation device (for example, an Ambu bag with a connector or catheter mount attached) to the tracheostomy tube in order to perform manual ventilation. The cuff of the tracheostomy tube must be inflated to prevent air leakage, thus ensuring adequate oxygenation and ventilation.

Procedure guidelines   Tracheostomy dressing change

Equipment

1 Sterile dressing pack.
2 Tracheostomy dressing or a keyhole dressing.
3 Cleaning solution, such as 0.9% sodium chloride.

4 Tracheostomy tape.
5 Bactericidal alcohol handrub.

Procedure

Action	Rationale
1 Explain and discuss the procedure with the patient.	To ensure that the patient understands the procedure and gives his/her valid consent (DH 2001: C).
2 Screen the bed or cubicle.	To ensure the patient's privacy (E).
3 Wash hands using bactericidal soap and water or bactericidal alcohol handrub, and prepare the dressing tray or trolley.	To minimize the risk of infection (DH 2005: C).
4 Perform the procedure using aseptic technique.	To minimize the risk of infection (E).
5 Remove the soiled dressing from around the tube, clean around the stoma with 0.9% sodium chloride using low-linting gauze.	To reduce the risk of dressing fragments entering the altered airway (Russell 2005: E) and to remove secretions and any crusts.
6 Replace with a tracheostomy dressing or a comfortable keyhole dressing.	To ensure the patient's comfort (E). To avoid pressure from the tube (Scase 2004: E).
7 Renew tracheostomy tapes, checking that 1–2 fingers can be placed between the tapes and neck.	To secure the tube (E). To ensure that the tapes are not too tight (Woodrow 2002: E; Scase 2004: E) or too loose, thus decreasing the chance of necrosis caused by excessive pressure from the tapes (Serra 2000: E).

Procedure guidelines Tracheostomy suction

Equipment

1 Suction source (wall or portable), collection container and tubing, changed every 24 hours to prevent growth of bacteria (Billau 2004).

2 Sterile suction catheters (assorted sizes; see Action 7).

3 A selection of non-sterile, clean boxed gloves.

4 Sterile bottled water (labelled 'suction' with opening date), changed every 24 hours to prevent the growth of bacteria (Billau 2004).

5 Disposable plastic apron.

6 Eye protection, e.g. goggles.

7 Bactericidal alcohol handrub.

Procedure

Action	Rationale
1 If secretions are tenacious, consider using, as prescribed, 2 hourly or more frequently 0.9% sterile sodium chloride nebulizers or other mucolytic agents such as acetylcisteine.	Suctioning may not be as effective if the secretions become too tenacious or dry. Anecdotal evidence through practice suggests that frequent 0.9% sterile sodium chloride or acetylcisteine nebulizers may assist in loosening dry and thick secretions (E).
2 Explain procedure to patient and ensure upright position if possible. If the patient is able to perform his/her own suction, self-suction should be taught.	To obtain the patient's co-operation and to help him or her relax (E). The procedure is unpleasant and can be frightening for the patient (Billau 2004: E). Reassurance is vital (E). Selfcontrol of the patient's suction is preferable if the patient is able to manage it (E).
3 If a patient has a fenestrated outer tube, ensure that a plain inner tube is in situ, rather than a fenestrated inner tube (Russell 2005).	Suction via a fenestrated inner tube allows a catheter to pass through the fenestration and cause trauma to the tracheal wall (Billau 2004: E).
4 Wash hands with bactericidal soap and water or bactericidal alcohol handrub, and put on a disposable plastic apron, disposable gloves and eye protection.	To minimize the risk of cross-infection (E). Some patients may accidently cough directly ahead at the nurse; standing to one side with tissues at the patient's tracheostomy minimizes this risk (E).
5 If patient is oxygen dependent, hyperoxygenate for a period of 3 minutes.	To minimize the risk of acute hypoxia (Billau 2004: E).

6 Check that the suction pressure is set to the appropriate level.

Recommended suction pressure is 80–150 mmHg or 11–20 kPa for adults (Day 2000: E; Day *et al.* 2002: C).

7 Select the correct size catheter. As a guide, the diameter of the suction catheter should not exceed one-half of the internal diameter of the tracheostomy tube (Griggs 1998; Hough 2001). To ensure the correct catheter size use the formula: divide the internal diameter of the tracheostomy tube by two and multiply by three (Billau 2004).

This ensures that hypoxia does not occur while suctioning: the larger the volume, the greater the bore of the tube (E).

8 Open the end of the suction catheter pack and use the pack to attach the catheter to the suction tubing. Keep the rest of the catheter in the sterile packet.

To reduce the risk of transferring infection from hands to the catheter and to keep the catheter as clean as possible (E).

9 For new surgically formed tracheostomy and laryngectomy stomas, use an individually packaged, sterile disposable glove on the hand manipulating the catheter (Ward *et al.* 1997). For subsequent admissions use clean, disposable gloves on both hands. To facilitate easy disposal of the suction catheter after suction, an additional clean, disposable glove can be used on the dominant hand.

Gloves minimize the risk of infection transfer to the catheter or from the sputum to the nurse's hands (DH 2005: C).

1003

10 Remove the catheter from the sleeve and introduce the catheter to about one-third of its length, until the resistance of the carina is felt or until the patient coughs. If resistance is felt, withdraw catheter approximately 1 cm before applying suction by placing the thumb over the suction port control and withdraw the remainder of the catheter gently (Dean 1997; Wood 1998).

Gentleness is essential; damage to the tracheal mucosa can lead to trauma and respiratory infection (E). The catheter should go no further than the carina to prevent trauma (E). The catheter is inserted with the suction off to reduce the risk of trauma (Clotworthy *et al.* 2006e: C).

Procedure guidelines *(cont.)*

11	Do not suction the patient for more than one breath cycle, 10–15 seconds (MacIntyre & Branson 2001).	Prolonged suctioning may result in acute hypoxia, cardiac arrhythmias (Day *et al.* 2002: C), mucosal trauma, infection and the patient experiencing a feeling of choking.
12	Wrap catheter around dominant hand, then pull back glove over soiled catheter, thus containing catheter glove, then discard.	Catheters are used only once to reduce the risk of introducing infection (E).
13	If the patient is oxygen dependent, reapply oxygen immediately.	To prevent hypoxia (E).
14	Rinse the suction tubing by dipping its end into the sterile water bottle and applying suction until the solution has rinsed the tubing through.	To loosen secretions that have adhered to the inside of the tube (E).
15	If the patient requires further suction, repeat the above actions using new gloves and a new catheter. Allow the patient sufficient time to recover between each suction (Billau 2004), particularly if oxygen saturation is low or if patient coughs several times during the procedure. The patient should be observed throughout the procedure.	To ensure general condition is stable.
16	Repeat the suction until the airway is clear. No more than three suction passes should be made during any one suction episode (Glass & Grap 1995; Day 2000) unless an emergency such as tube occlusion (Nelson 1999).	To minimize the risk of hypoxaemia (Day 2000: E).
17	Where appropriate, reconnect the patient to oxygen.	To minimize the risk of hypoxaemia within 10 seconds post-suctioning (Day 2000: E).

Humidification

Definition

Humidification can be defined as increasing water content, the moisture or dampness in the atmosphere or a gas (Hough 2001; Pryor & Prasad 2001). In health, inspired air is filtered, warmed and moistened by the ciliated lining, and mucus is produced in the upper respiratory pathways. Because the upper respiratory pathways are bypassed in patients with a tracheostomy, they need artificial humidification to ensure that these pathways remain moist (Pryor & Prasad 2001).

Procedure guidelines   Humidification of patient with tracheostomy

Procedure

Action	Rationale
1 **For patients requiring oxygen therapy** fill a suitable nebulizer with sterile water and attach it to the oxygen supply, then set the gas rate for the liquid to form into humidification droplets.	Constant humidification is required while the new stoma adapts to the outside environment. Humidification also prevents the formation of crusts which are liable to obstruct the airway. The use of sterile water reduces the risk of infection (Hough 2001: E). Any liquid remaining after 24 hours should be replaced.

1005

Subsequent care

Action	Rationale
1 **For patients no longer requiring oxygen therapy** give humidification as required. Usually, patients need about 10–15 minutes of humidification every 4 hours. This may be adapted according to the patient's needs, e.g. throughout the night, according to time.	Patients begin to adapt to breathing through their tracheostomy after the first 24–48 hours. Some humidification is required according to individual needs and to prevent crust formation in the airway (E).
2 Provide laryngeal stoma protectors, e.g. Laryngofoam, Buchanan bib, Romet or heat and moisture exchangers.	To protect and humidify the airway (E).

Problem solving: Tracheostomy

Problem	Cause	Suggested action
Profuse tracheal secretions.	Local reaction to tracheostomy tube.	Suction frequently, e.g. every 1–2 hours.
Lumen of tracheostomy tube occluded.	Tenacious mucus in tube.	Change the inner tube. Use 0.9% sodium chloride nebulizers, heat and moisture exchangers and suction.Continue to change the inner tube regularly, e.g. 1–3-hourly.
	Dried blood and mucus in the tube, especially in the postoperative period.	Provide humidified air. (For further information, see Procedure guidelines: Humidification, administering air if there is no need for oxygen.)
Tracheostomy tube dislodged accidentally.	Tapes not secured adequately.	Put in spare tube. This should be clean and ready at the bedside (Serra 2000). *Note*: tracheal dilators must be kept at the bedside of patients with tracheostomies (Serra 2000).
Unable to insert clean tracheostomy tube.	Unpredicted shape or angle of stoma.	Remain calm since an outward appearance of distress may cause the patient to panic and lose confidence. Lubricate the tube well and attempt to reinsert at various angles. If unsuccessful, attempt to insert a smaller-size tracheostomy tube. If this is impossible, keep the tracheostomy tract open using tracheal dilators and inform the doctor.
	Tracheal stenosis due to patient coughing, patient being very anxious or because the tube has been left out too long.	Insert a smaller-size tracheostomy tube. If insertion still proves difficult, do not leave the patient but ask for a tube to be brought to the bed. Keep the tracheostomy patent with tracheal dilators if stenosis is pronounced until the tube is reinserted.

1006

Problem	Cause	Suggested action
Tracheal bleeding following or during change of the tube.	Trauma due to suction or to the tube being changed. Presence of tumour. Granulation tissue forming in fenestration of tube.	Change the tube as planned if bleeding is minimal. For profuse bleeding, insert a cuffed tube and inflate the cuff (Clotworthy *et al.* 2006f). Inform the doctor. Perform tracheal suction to remove the blood from the trachea.
Infected sputum.	Nature of surgery and condition of patient often predispose to infection.	Encourage the patient to cough up secretions and/or suction regularly. Change the tube and clean the stoma area frequently, e.g. 4-hourly. Protect permanent stomas with a bib or gauze. Following result of sputum specimen, commence appropriate antibiotics as needed.

References and further reading

Billau, C. (2004) Suctioning. In: *Tracheostomy. A Multiprofessional Handbook* (eds C. Russell & B. Matta). Greenwich Medical, London, pp. 157–71.

Blom, E.D. (1998) Evolution of tracheo-oesophageal voice prosthesis. In: *Tracheoesophageal Voice Restoration Following Total Laryngectomy* (eds E.D. Blom, M.I. Singer & R.C. Hamaker). Singular Publishing Group, San Diego, pp. 1–8.

Bond, P. *et al.* (2003) Best practice in the care of patients with a tracheostomy. *Nurs Times*, 90(30), 24–5.

Brown, I. (1982) Trach care? Take care – infection on the prowl. *Nursing*, 6, 70–1.

Clotworthy, N. *et al.* (2006a) Post-operative care of the patient following a laryngectomy. In: *Guidelines for the Care of Patients with Tracheostomy Tubes*. St George's Healthcare NHS Trust. Smiths Medical International Limited, Watford, pp. 15–16.

Clotworthy, N. *et al.* (2006b) Tracheostomy tubes. In: *Guidelines for the Care of Patients with Tracheostomy Tubes*. St George's Healthcare NHS Trust. Smiths Medical International Limited, Watford, pp. 9–14.

Clotworthy, N. *et al.* (2006c) Humidification. In: *Guidelines for the Care of Patients with Tracheostomy Tubes*. St George's Healthcare NHS Trust. Smiths Medical International Limited, Watford, pp. 17–18.

Clotworthy, N. *et al.* (2006d) Communication. In: *Guidelines for the Care of Patients with Tracheostomy Tubes*. St George's Healthcare NHS Trust. Smiths Medical International Limited, Watford, pp. 27–32.

Clotworthy, N. *et al.* (2006e) Suctioning. In: *Guidelines for the Care of Patients with Tracheostomy Tubes*. St George's Healthcare NHS Trust. Smiths Medical International Limited, Watford, pp. 23–6.

Clotworthy, N. *et al.* (2006f) Tube changes. In: *Guidelines for the Care of Patients with Tracheostomy Tubes*. St George's Healthcare NHS Trust. Smiths Medical International Limited, Watford, pp. 39–42.

Day, T. (2000) Tracheal suctioning: when, why and how. *Nurs Times*, **96**(20), 13–15.

Day, T., Farnell, S. & Wilson-Barnett, J. (2002) Suctioning: a review of current research recommendations. *Intens Crit Care Nurs*, **18**, 79–89.

Dean, B. (1997) Evidence based suction management in accident and emergency: a vital component of airway care. *Accid Emerg Nurs*, **5**(2), 92–8.

Delassus Gress, C. & Singer, M.I. (2005) Tracheoesophageal voice restoration. In: *Contemporary Considerations in the Treatment and Rehabilitation of Head and Neck Cancer. Voice, Speech and Swallowing* (eds P.C. Doyle & R.L. Keith) PRO-ED Incorporated, Austin, Texas, pp. 431–52.

DH (2001) *Good Practice in Consent Implementation Guide: Consent to Examination or Treatment.* www.dh.gov.uk. Accessed 24/9/07.

DH (2005) *Saving Lives: A Delivery Programme to Reduce Healthcare Associated Infection including MRSA.* Department of Health, London.

Dropkin M. (1996) Nursing Research. SOHN's 20 year experience. *ORL Head and Neck Nursing*, **14**(3), 14–16.

Edgtton Winn, M. & Wright, K. (2005) Tracheostomy: a guide to nursing care. *Aust Nurs J*,**13**(5), 17–20.

Gibson, I.M. (1983) Tracheostomy management. *Nursing*, **2**(18), 538.

Glass, C. & Grap, M. (1995) Ten tips for safe suctioning. *Am J Nurs*, **5**(5), 51–3.

Griggs, A. (1998) Tracheostomy: suctioning and humidification. *Nurs Stand*, **13**(2), 49–56.

Hahn, M.J. & Jones A. (2000) Psychosocial problems. In: *Head and Neck Nursing* (eds M.J. Hahn & A. Jones). Churchill Livingstone, London, pp. 137–42.

Hales, P. (2004a) Communication. In: *Tracheostomy. A Multiprofessional Handbook* (eds C. Russell & B. Matta). Greenwich Medical, London, pp. 211–34.

Hales, P. (2004b) Swallowing. In: *Tracheostomy. A Multiprofessional Handbook* (eds C. Russell & B. Matta). Greenwich Medical, London, pp. 187–208.

Hampton, S. (1998) Film subjects win the day. *Nurs Times*, **94**(24), 80–2.

Harkin, H. (2004) Decannulation. In: *Tracheostomy. A Multiprofessional Handbook* (eds C. Russell & B. Matta). Greenwich Medical, London, pp. 255–69.

Hess, D.R. (2005) Tracheostomy tubes and related appliances. *Respir Care*, **50**(4), 497–510.

Holmes, S. (1996) *Radiotherapy. Radiation Induced Side Effects.* Austin Cornish, London, pp. 67–78.

Hooper, M. (1996) Nursing care of the patient with a tracheostomy. *Nurs Stand*, **10**(340), 40–3.

Hough, A. (2001) *Physiotherapy in Respiratory Care. An Evidence-Based Approach to Respiratory and Cardiac Management*, 3rd edn. Nelson Thornes, Cheltenham.

Leder, S.B. & Blom, E.D. (1998) Tracheoesophageal voice prosthesis fitting and training. In: *Tracheoesophageal Voice Restoration Following Total Laryngectomy* (eds E.D. Blom, M.I. Singer & R.C. Hamaker). Singular Publishing Group, San Diego, pp. 57–65.

Lewarski, J.S. (2005) Long-term care of the patient with a tracheostomy. *Respir Care*, **50**(4), 535–7.

Lewin, J.S. (1998) Maximising tracheo-oesophageal voice and speech. In: *Tracheoe-sophageal Voice Restoration Following Total Laryngectomy* (eds E.D. Blom, M.I. Singer & R.C. Hamaker). Singular Publishing Group, San Diego, pp. 67–72.

MacIntyre, N.R. & Branson, R.D. (2001) *Mechanical Ventilation*. W.B. Saunders, Philadelphia.

Mathieson, L. (2001) Physiological effects of laryngectomy. In: *The Voice and its Disorders* (ed. L. Mathieson). Whurr, London, pp. 597–600.

Mol, D.A. *et al.* (2004) Use and care of an endotracheal/tracheostomy tube cuff – are intensive care unit staff adequately informed? *SAJS*, **42**(1), 14–16.

Nelson, L. (1999) Points of friction. *Nurs Times*, **95**(34), 72–5.

Patel, J. & Matta, B. (2004) Percutaneous dilatational tracheostomy. In: *Tracheostomy. A Multiprofessional Handbook* (eds C. Russell & B. Matta). Greenwich Medical, London, pp. 59–68.

Pathways in Cancer Care (2001) *Head and Neck Cancer Care Pathway*. NHS Executive Northwest. SC Research, London.

Pilbeam, S.B. (1998) Physiological effects and complications of positive pressure ventilation. In: *Mechanical Ventilation: Physiological and Clinical Applications*, 3rd edn (ed. S.B. Pilbeam). Mosby, St Louis, pp. 161–2.

Price, P. (2004a) Surgical tracheostomy. In: *Tracheostomy. A Multiprofessional Handbook* (eds C. Russell & B. Matta). Greenwich Medical, London, pp. 35–58.

Price, P. (2004b) What is a tracheostomy? In: *Tracheostomy. A Multiprofessional Handbook* (eds C. Russell & B. Matta). Greenwich Medical, London, pp. 29–34.

Prior, T. & Russell, S. (2004) Tracheostomy and head and neck cancer. In: *Tracheostomy. A Multiprofessional Handbook* (eds C. Russell & B. Matta). Greenwich Medical, London, pp. 269–83.

Pryor, J.A. & Prasad, S.A. (2001) *Physiotherapy for Respiratory and Cardiac Problems: Adult and Paediatric*, 3rd edn. Churchill Livingstone, Edinburgh.

Rhys Evans, F. (2003) Nursing care of head and neck cancer patients. In: *Principles and Practice of Head and Neck Oncology* (eds P.H. Rhys Evans, P.Q. Montgomery & P.J. Gullane). Taylor & Francis, London, pp. 115–26.

Rhys Evans, P.H. & Blom, E.D. (2003) Functional restoration of speech. In: *Principles and Practice of Head and Neck Oncology* (eds P.H. Rhys Evans, P.Q. Montgomery & P.J. Gullane) Taylor & Francis, London, pp. 571–602.

Rossoff, L.J. *et al.* (1993) Is the use of boxed gloves in an intensive care unit safe? *Am J Med*, **94**(6), 602–7.

Russell, C. (2004a) Tracheostomy tubes. In: *Tracheostomy. A Multiprofessional Handbook* (eds C. Russell & B. Matta). Greenwich Medical, London, pp. 85–114.

Russell, C. (2004b) Tracheostomy tube changes. In: *Tracheostomy. A Multiprofessional Handbook* (eds C. Russell & B. Matta). Greenwich Medical, London, pp. 235–54.

Russell, C. (2005) Providing the nurse with a guide to tracheostomy care and management. *Br J Nurs*, **14**(8), 428–33.

Scanlan, C.L., Wilkins, R.L. & Stoller, J.K. (1999) *Fundamentals of Respiratory Care*, 7th edn. Mosby, St. Louis, MO.

Scase, C. (2004) Wound care. In: *Tracheostomy. A Multiprofessional Handbook* (eds C. Russell & B. Matta). Greenwich Medical, London, pp. 173–87.

Seay, S.J., Gay, S.L. & Strauss, M. (2002) Tracheostomy emergencies correcting accidental decannulation or displaced tracheostomy tube. *Am J Nurs*, **102**(3), 59–63.

Serra, A. (2000) Tracheostomy care. *Nurs Stand*, **14**(42), 45–52.

Shaw, C. (2003) Nutritional support of head and neck cancer patients. In: *Principles and Practice of Head and Neck Oncology* (eds P.H. Rhys Evans, P.Q. Montgomery & P.J. Gullane). Taylor & Francis, London, pp. 127–35.

Singer, M.I. & Deschler, D.G. (1998) Complications of primary and secondary tracheo-oesophageal voice restoration. In: *Tracheo-esophageal Voice Restoration Following Total Laryngectomy* (eds E.D. Blom, M.I. Singer & R.C. Hamaker). Singular Publishing Group, San Diego, pp. 51–5.

Tamburri, L.M. (2000) Care of the patient with a tracheostomy. *Orthop Nurs*, **19**(2), 49–60.

The Joanna Briggs Institute (2000) Tracheal suctioning of adults with an artificial airway. *Best Practice*, **4**(4), 1–6.

Ward, V. *et al.* (1997) *Supplement to Hospital Acquired Infection: Surveillance, Policies and Practice. Preventing Hospital-Acquired Infection. Clinical Guidelines.* Public Health Laboratory Service, London.

Wood, C.J. (1998) Endotracheal suctioning: a literature review. *Intens Crit Care Nurs*, **14**, 124–36.

Woodrow, P. (2002) Managing patients with a tracheostomy in acute care. *Nurs Stand*, **16**(44), 39–48.

Multiple choice questions

1 A tracheostomy is the surgical opening into the trachea through the neck. Which of the following statements is not true?

   a A permanent tracheostomy is always created following a total glossectomy

   b A permanent tracheostomy is created following a total laryngectomy

   c A tracheostomy may be performed under local or general anaesthetic

   d A tracheostomy may be formed to enable aspiration of secretions

2 What should always be kept at the bed side of a patient with a tracheostomy?

   a Humidified oxygen with nasal cannulae mask, apron and goggles, tracheal dilators

   b Humidified oxygen with tracheostomy mask, apron and goggles, tracheal dilators

   c Resuscitation trolley, apron and goggles, tracheal dilators

   d Suction machine, preloaded syringe containing adrenaline, humidified oxygen with tracheostomy mask, apron and goggles, tracheal dilators

3 Patients with a tracheostomy or laryngectomy will often require suctioning. Which of the following statements is not true?

   a Excessive coughing as a result of excessive tracheal stimulation can lead to raised intracranial pressure

   b Each suctioning procedure should last no longer than 60 seconds

   c Both patient and care giver are at risk of infection when suction is performed

   d The diameter of the suction tube should not exceed one half of the internal diameter of the tracheostomy tube

4 **When changing a tracheostomy dressing what cleaning fluid is recommended?**

a   Chlorhexidine
b   None, the stoma should be kept completely dry
c   0.9% sodium chloride
d   Dilute hydrogen peroxide

Answers to the multiple choice questions can be found in Appendix 3.

Chapter 30

Transfusion of blood and blood products

Definition

The administration of whole blood or any of its components into the bloodstream to correct or treat a clinical abnormality (Anderson *et al*. 1994).

Reference material

Blood safety and quality in the UK

Approximately 3.4 million blood products are administered in the UK every year (Gray & Illingworth 2006). The transfusion of blood and its components is usually safe and uneventful; however, there are associated risks and there have been significant developments over recent years to improve the quality and safety of transfusion practice in the UK. The Blood Safety and Quality Regulations came into effect in February 2005 and were fully implemented on 8 November 2005. These regulations cover the collecting, testing, processing, storing and distributing of blood and blood components (Crown 2005). The official government agency with jurisdiction for these regulations is the Medicines and Healthcare Products Regulatory Agency (MHRA) who are the competent authority.

The principal requirements of these regulations in relation to transfusion practice are:

(a) *Traceability* whereby hospitals must have a system to record and retain information on the fate of each unit of blood/blood component for a period of 30 years.

(b) *Haemovigilance*, an organized surveillance procedure relating to serious adverse or unexpected events or reactions. The reporting of such events can be done via the on-line Serious Adverse Blood Reactions and Events (SABRE) reporting system which is maintained by the medical device adverse incident reporting centre. This will usually be done by a designated member of laboratory staff and therefore clinical staff must ensure all incident reporting is conducted in line with hospital policy.

The MHRA define such events as follows:

A **serious adverse event** is defined as an unintended occurrence associated with the collection, testing, processing, storage and distribution of blood or blood components that might lead to death or life threatening, disabling or incapacitating conditions for patients or which results in, or prolongs, hospitalisation or morbidity.

A **serious adverse reaction** is defined as an unintended response in a donor or in a patient associated with the collection or transfusion of blood components that is fatal, life-threatening, disabling or incapacitating, or which results in or prolongs hospitalisation or morbidity.

(MHRA 2006)

Prior to these regulations, Better Blood Transfusion initiatives aimed to ensure that such guidance became an integral part of National Health Service (NHS) care making blood transfusion safer, ensuring that all blood used in clinical practice is necessary and improve the information both patients and the public receive about blood transfusion (DH 2002). Therefore it is a key requirement that all staff involved in the process of transfusion maintain their awareness of all appropriate guidance.

1014 *Blood donation and testing*

All blood donated in the UK is given voluntarily. The successful selection of a donor must protect them from any harm that may be caused by the donation process and also protect the possible recipient of products derived from the donor's blood. Donors of blood for therapeutic use should be in good health; if there is any doubt about their suitability the donation should be deferred and they should be fully assessed by a designated medical officer. All donors of blood or its components (via apherisis) should be assessed in accordance with the Joint UKBTS/NIBSC Professional Advisory Committee (JPAC) donor selection guidelines (JPAC 2005). The assessment of fitness to donate includes a questionnaire relating to general health, lifestyle, past medical history and medication. Donation may be temporarily or permanently deferred for a variety of reasons including cardiovascular disease, central nervous system diseases, malignancy and some infectious diseases, all of which are detailed in the JPAC (2005) guidelines. Donors are also screened for risk of exposure to transmissible infectious diseases, and specific guidance is provided for donors receiving therapeutic drugs. Prevention of transmission of infection is determined by donor selection criteria and laboratory testing. In the UK, all blood donations are tested for infections which could be passed on to the recipient. However, concern about transfusion-related variant

Creutzfeldt–Jakob disease (vCJD) transmission is now supported by clinical evidence (Ludlam & Turner 2006) and, despite continuing research, a screening test for preclinical human infection has yet to be developed (Brown 2005). Therefore, donor exclusion criteria remain an ever important precautionary measure (Cervenakova & Brown 2004; Brown & Cervenakova 2004). When a donor has been successfully screened, they must validate the information they have provided and record that they have given consent to proceed.

Autologous donation

Since the 1980s there has been interest in autologous donation. This has largely been attributed to high profile infection risks; human immunodeficiency virus (HIV), hepatitis C and more recently vCJD (James & Harrison 2002). However, autologous donation is not risk free and is contraindicated in certain circumstances. Furthermore, there has been significant concern about the efficacy of some methods (Henry *et al.* 2001; Carless *et al.* 2004). Three principal methods of autologous donation exist:

Preoperative autologous donation (PAD)

This requires the patients to donate up to 4 units of blood whilst simultaneously taking iron supplements in the month preceding surgery. However, the efficacy of this method has been questioned by systematic review (Henry *et al.* 2001) and is only indicated in very specific circumstances such as patients with very rare blood types, patients donating bone marrow, and fit patients who have a significant fear of receiving allogeneic blood products such that it is preventing them from seeking necessary surgery (James 2004).

Acute normovolaemic haemodilution (ANH)

This involves the donation of up to 3 units of blood immediately prior to surgery. The patient is then given crystalloids to dilute the circulating volume. This method is only indicated for surgery where considerable blood loss is expected on the principle that the number of red cells lost will be reduced and the patient's autologous whole blood can be returned after surgery; however, little evidence exists to support the efficacy of ANH (Harrison 2004).

Intra-operative cell salvage (ICS)

Blood loss during surgery is collected, anticoagulated, filtered and held in a sterile reservoir. The collected blood is then processed, washed and suspended in saline for return. Although ICS is not without risks such as embolism, bacterial contamination and enhanced inflammatory responses through reinfusion of inflammatory mediators (Harrison 2004), it has been recommended as the most effective form

1015

Table 30.1   Blood group compatability.

Group	Antigens	IgM antibodies	Compatible donor for	Compatible recipient of
A	A	Anti B	A AB	A O
B	B	Anti A	B AB	B O
AB	A & B	None	AB	A B AB O
O	None	Anti A Anti B	A B AB O	O

of autologous transfusion to assist in the conservation of blood supplies (James 2004). However, it is not currently recommended in surgery for malignant disease, gastrointestinal surgery or postpartum haemorrhage (Harrison 2004).

Blood component donation

Donors of blood components by automated apherisis are subject to the same selection criteria used for donating whole blood and any exception to this must be decided by a designated medical officer. Apherisis can be used to collect plasma, red cells and platelets. Leukapheresis procedures are used for the collection of granulocytes, lymphocytes and peripheral blood progenerator cells (James 2005).

ABO blood groups and rhesus types

In 1901, Landsteiner discovered that human blood groups existed and developed the ABO system which marked the start of safe blood transfusion (Bishop 2008). There are four principal blood groups: A, B, AB and O. Each group relates to the presence or absence of surface antigens on the red blood cells and antibodies in the serum which dictate blood compatibility (Table 30.1).

People with the blood group **AB** have red cells with A and B surface antigens, but they do not have any anti-A or anti-B immunoglobulin M (IgM) antibodies in their serum. Therefore they are able to receive blood from any group, but can only donate to other people from group AB.

People with group **O** red cells do not have either A or B surface antigens, however they do have anti-A and anti-B IgM antibodies in their serum. They are only able to receive blood from group **O**, but can donate to A, B, O and AB groups.

People with group **A** red cells have type A surface antigens, and they have anti-B IgM antibodies in their serum. They are only able to receive blood from groups **A** or **O** and can only donate blood to people from A and AB groups.

People with group **B** red cells have type B surface antigens and they have anti-A IgM antibodies in their serum. They are therefore only able to receive blood from groups **B** or **O** and can only donate blood to people from B and AB groups.

In addition to the ABO system described above the rhesus (Rh) system was discovered in 1940; again these are surface antigens and they are another essential system used in transfusion therapy (Mollison *et al.* 1997). The Rh D antigen is the most immunogenic of the Rh antigens (Porth 2005). However, many other red cell antigens exist and exposure to them may stimulate the development of corresponding antibodies (McClelland 2007).

Blood group incompatibility

The transfusion of ABO incompatible red cells can lead to intravascular haemolysis where the recipient's IgM antibodies bind to the corresponding surface antigens of the transfused cells (McClelland 2007). Complement activation results in lysis of the transfused cells and the haemoglobin that is released precipitates renal failure with the fragments of the lysed cells activating the clotting pathways, which in turn leads to the development of disseminated intravascular coagulation (DIC) (Mollison *et al.* 1997). Transfusion of rhesus positive cells to a rhesus negative individual will result in immunization and the appearance of anti-D antibodies (Hoffbrand *et al.* 2001). However, on any subsequent exposure extravascular haemolysis occurs when rhesus antibody coated red cells are destroyed by macrophages in the liver and spleen (McClelland 2007). A patient's rhesus status is of particular note in pregnancy as haemolytic disease of the newborn (HDN) can occur when the mother is rhesus negative and the developing foetus is rhesus positive as exposure to foetal blood can stimulate anti-D activation in the mother which in turn can cross the placenta causing haemolysis (McClelland 2007).

Blood groups in haemopoietic stem cell transplantation

The human leucocyte antigen (HLA) is used to determine compatibility for organ transplantation including bone marrow and peripheral blood stem cells. However, because ABO blood groups and HLA tissue types are determined genetically, it is not uncommon to find a suitable HLA donor who is ABO and/or rhesus incompatible with the recipient. In such circumstances, major transfusion reactions can be avoided by red cell and/or plasma depletion of the donor cells in the laboratory before reinfusion (Mollison *et al.* 1997). Occasionally, if the recipient has a very high titre of anti-A or anti-B lytic antibody and the donor marrow or peripheral blood stem cells are blood group A, B or AB, then plasmapheresis of the recipient may be performed to lower the titre of this antibody to safe limits. This is necessary because it is not possible to remove all the red cells from the donor product and those remaining may cause a major transfusion reaction in this situation (Mollison *et al.* 1997).

Appropriate use of blood and blood products

The impetus from recent publications and legislation has created greater awareness of the need to continue to improve transfusion practice in many ways. Blood and blood products are no longer regarded as safe unlimited resources. There are risks that are inherent to transfusion practice and therefore unnecessary exposure to blood products should be avoided. This is of particular importance for patients who may only have one transfusion in their lifetime, such as surgical patients. Therefore, these patients should only receive a transfusion when it is absolutely necessary. Furthermore the appropriate use of products is essential for the conservation of blood supplies. Regularly updated guidance on the safe appropriate use of blood and blood products is now available online at www.transfusionguidelines.org.uk and these should be consulted in collaboration with local hospital and blood transfusion service guidelines.

Infusion of cryopreserved bone marrow and peripheral blood stem cells

Stem cells from either the bone marrow or peripheral blood are cryopreserved between collection (harvesting) and reinfusion. Stem cells can be either administered/used as an autologous or an allogeneic transfusion. Thawing of the cells is carried out using a large-volume water bath. Care should be taken as heating may cause cellular damage. As there is an increased risk of bacterial contamination, aseptic techniques should be adopted during administration to reduce any possibility of contamination (McClelland 2007) in a recipient group that is already immunocompromised.

Indications

Blood and blood products have varying shelf lives and storage requirements. The range of products currently available, indications for use and recommendations for administration are listed in Table 30.2.

Table 30.2   Blood and blood products used for transfusion.

Type	Description	Indications	Cross-matching	Shelf life	Average infusion time	Technique	Special considerations
Red cells in optimal additive solutions (SAGM)*	Red cells with plasma removed: 100 ml additive fluid used as replacement to give optimal red cell preservation; haematocrit 60–65% Leucodepleted	Correction of anaemia	ABO and Rh compatible (not necessarily identical)	35 days at 2–6°C	1–2 hours/ unit	Give via a blood administration set	If more than half blood volume is replaced with red cells in SAGM, use of FFP should be considered to replace clotting factors
Washed red blood cells	Red cells centrifuged and resuspended twice in 0.9% sodium chloride Leucodepleted	Correction of anaemia where patient may react to plasma components. For example in IgA deficiency	As above	Prepared by non-sterile process, therefore to be used within 24 hours	1–2 hours/ unit	As above	—
Frozen red blood cells	Red cells of very rare phenotype Leucodepleted	To treat patients with very rare antibody	As above	Stored frozen cells: 3 years. Use within 12 hours of thawing	2–3 hours/ unit	As above	—

(continued)

Table 30.2 (continued)

Type	Description	Indications	Cross-matching	Shelf life	Average infusion time	Technique	Special considerations
White blood cells (buffy coat or apheresed granulocytes)¹	Mainly granulocytes obtained by leucophoresis or by 'creaming' off the white blood cell layer from fresh blood	To treat patients with life-threatening granulocytopenia	As above	24 hours after preparation. Stored at room temperature	60–90 minutes/unit	Administer via a blood administration set	White blood cell infusion induces fever, may cause hypotension, rigors and confusion. Treat symptoms and reassure patient. Preparation is always irradiated to prevent initiation of transfusion-associated graft-versus-host disease (TA-GVHD). *Do not* give to patients receiving amphotericin B. Indications for granulocyte transfusions should be when possible benefits are thought to outweigh considerable hazards of the treatment option (Brozovis *et al.* 1998)
Platelets*	Platelets in 200–300 ml plasma. May be pooled from 5 donors or apheresed from a single donor. Leucodepleted	To treat thrombocytopenia	No cross-matching necessary	Up to 7 days after collection. Storage is at 22°C, with continuous gentle agitation	20–30 minutes/unit	Administration using a platelet administration set. Use a new set for each transfusion. Do not use micro-aggregate filters	General guide to use: 1 Count less than 10×10^9/l 2 Count $10–20 \times 10^9$/l with haemorrhage and/or persistent pyrexia 3 Count $20–50 \times 10^9$/l in special cases or pre-invasive procedure

Product	Description	Indication	Crossmatching	Storage	Time	Administration	Notes
Fresh frozen plasma (FFP)	Citrated plasma separated from whole blood	To treat a deficiency in clotting factors due to dilution effects, consumption (in disseminated intravascular coagulation [DIC]), liver failure or overdose of coumarin anticoagulant	No crossmatching necessary	2 years at −30°C. Once thawed, kept at 4°C, to be used as soon as possible but within 24 hours	15–45 minutes/unit (approx. 250 ml)	Administer rapidly via a blood administration set	FFP should be considered if patient has received more than half their blood volume in red cells, to prevent dilutional hypocoagulability
Albumin 4.5% (HAS)	Solution of albumin from pooled plasma in a buffered, stabilized 0.9% sodium chloride diluent. Supplied in 250 ml or 500 ml bottle	To treat hypovolaemic shock or hypoproteinaemia due to burns, trauma, surgery or infection Sourced outside UK to reduce risk of transmission of variant Creutzfeldt–Jakob disease (vCJD)	Unnecessary. Not blood group specific	5 years at room temperature Kept in dark	30–60 minutes/unit	Administer via a standard solution administration set	The solution should be crystal clear with no deposits

(continued)

1021

Table 30.2 (*continued*)

Type	Description	Indications	Cross-matching	Shelf life	Average infusion time	Technique	Special considerations
Albumin 20% (HAS)	Heat-treated, aqueous, chemically processed fraction of pooled plasma	To treat hypovolaemic shock or hypoproteinaemia due to burns, trauma, surgery or infection. To maintain appropriate electrolyte balance	Unnecessary	5 years at room temperature Kept in dark	30–60 minutes/unit	Administer via a blood administration set undiluted or diluted with 0.9% sodium chloride or 5% glucose solution. Slower administration is advised if a cardiac disorder is present to avoid gross fluid shift	The solution should be crystal clear with no deposits

(continued)

Cryoprecipitate	Cold-insoluble portion of plasma recovered from FFP: rich in factor VIII, von Willebrand's disease and fibrinogen. Available as single packs (20–40 ml) or 5 units pooled (120–140 ml)	To control bleeding disorders due to lack of factor VIII or fibrinogen, e.g. haemophilia, von Willebrand's disease, DIC	No crossmatchng necessary	2 years at −30°C. Use immediately after thawing.	15–30 minutes via infusion, 10–15 minutes via intravenous push	Administer rapidly via syringe or blood administration set
Cryo-depleted plasma	FFP with cryoprecipitate removed	Useful in treating thrombotic thrombocytopenic purpura: patients are plasma-exchanged daily to reduce circulating von Willebrand's disease	No crossmatching necessary	2 years at −30°C. Once thawed, kept at 4°C, to be used as soon as possible but within 24 hours	Time varies on machine average ±2.5 hours	Via apheresis machine

*Most commonly used blood products.
†See leucocyte depletion.

The process of transfusion

Errors made in the process of transfusion present a significant risk to patients. Although there is little evidence to support the efficacy for set procedures to manage this risk, current professional opinion has been provided by the British Committee for Standards in Haematology (BCSH) in collaboration with The Royal College of Nursing (RCN) and the Royal College of Surgeons for England (RCS) (BCSH 1999; Gray & Illingworth 2006). As a result of this guidance every hospital should have a policy in place for the administration of blood and blood components including identification of the patient, blood sampling, special blood requirement requests, processing of blood samples, the storage, collection and transportation of blood products, administration of blood products and the care and monitoring of the transfused patient. Furthermore, hospitals are also required to manage and report any adverse event or near misses with a statutory requirement to hold a record of every step of the transfusion process including the final fate of each blood product for 30 years (James 2005). Only staff authorized to do so should be involved at any stage in the transfusion process.

Caring for the patient receiving a blood transfusion

Patients who are to receive a transfusion of blood products must always wear an identity wristband with their full name, date of birth and unique hospital number clearly written or printed. The nurse caring for the patient should clearly explain the procedure ensuring that the patient fully understands the information they have been given. The patient should be asked to inform a member of staff if they complain of any symptoms which may indicate a transfusion-related adverse event such as complaining of feeling anxious, rigors (shivering), flushing, pain or shortness of breath. The patient should be cared for where they can be visually observed and the patient should be shown how to use the nurse call system. The patient should have vital signs monitored as indicated in the procedure guidelines below; however, it may be necessary to take additional observations if clinically indicated, such as if the patient complains of feeling unwell or they develop signs of a transfusion reaction (Gray & Illingworth 2006). As many drugs may cause a pyretic hypersensitivity reaction (Mehta 2006), nurses caring for patients receiving the transfusion of blood and blood products should ensure that they do not simultaneously administer drugs such as antifungals or first- or second-course antibiotics.

Jehovah's Witnesses and blood transfusion

The role of blood in Jehovah's Witnesses' spiritual belief is based on scripture and followers are usually well informed both of their beliefs and their rights. Many Jehovah's Witnesses carry information with them regarding any objection and therefore the need to ensure informed consent is very important. Staff caring for patients must ensure that decisions to consent to or refuse treatment are respected and recorded appropriately (McClelland 2007). Furthermore, in individual circumstances, practitioners should endeavour to consider non-blood or autologous methods described above where appropriate (McClelland 2007).

Transfusion reactions and complications

In November 1996 the Serious Hazards of Transfusion (SHOT) scheme was launched. This voluntary and anonymized reporting scheme collected data from participating hospitals across the UK and Ireland. The purpose of SHOT is to collect data on the serious morbidity related to the transfusion of blood and blood products. These data have since been utilized to inform education programmes, policy development, guideline development, ultimately improving hospital transfusion practice (SNBTS 2004). Although the Blood Safety and Quality Regulations have now made the reporting of such events via SABRE mandatory (see above), the SHOT scheme remains active and important and has presented yearly retrospective reports of data collected since its inception. These data demonstrate improved performance in recognizing reporting of transfusion-related incidents and continue to generate key recommendations to improve all transfusion practice (SNBTS 2004). Despite significant improvement in the reduction of risk from transfusion transmitted infection, human error which results in the Incorrect Blood Component Transfused (IBCT) remains the greatest risk to patients (SNBTS 2004). An IBCT is the transfusion of a blood product that is not suitable for or not intended for the recipient. Most IBCT incidents are the result of one or more errors in the transfusion pathway (SHOT 2005).

Managing adverse transfusion events

The prompt management of any adverse transfusion reaction can reduce associated morbidity and can be life saving. Therefore staff caring for patients receiving transfused products must be fully familiar with the immediate management of any suspected reaction. However, specialist advice should always be sought for the diagnosis and ongoing management of transfusion reactions, such as haemolytic, anaphylactic and septic reactions (SNBTS 2004; McClelland 2007).

Minor transfusion reactions

It should always be remembered that the symptoms of a 'minor' transfusion reaction may be the prelude to a major, life-threatening reaction. It is essential that staff take any transfusion reaction seriously. Symptomatic patients should have their vital signs monitored closely and they should be clearly observable. Patients with persistent or deteriorating symptoms should always be managed as a major reaction and urgent medical and specialist support should be sought (SNBTS 2004; McClelland 2007).

Symptoms of minor reactions include: a temperature rise of up to 1.5°C, rash without systemic disturbance and moderate tachycardia without hypotension (SNBTS 2004). Such reactions may be caused by an immunological reaction to components of the blood product. Whilst it may be possible to manage such symptoms and continue with the transfusion the following action should always be taken (Contreras & Mollison 1998):

- Stop the transfusion and inform the responsible medical team.
- Confirm the patient's identity and re-check their details against the product compatibility label.
- Antihistamines should be considered for skin rashes or urticarial itch.
- Antipyretic agents can be considered for mild fever.

It may be possible to continue with the transfusion at a reduced rate once the patient's symptoms are controlled; however, it may be necessary to increase the frequency of observations until the transfusion is completed. Some patients who have regular transfusions may experience recurrent febrile reactions and may benefit from an antipyretic pre-medication. *Note*: aspirin and other non-steroidal anti-inflammatory drugs (NSAIDs) are contraindicated in patients with a thrombocytopenia or coagulopathy (Mehta 2006).

Major transfusion reactions

1026

Major transfusion reactions include anaphylaxis, haemolysis and sepsis and may present as a fever of >38.5°C, tachycardia ± hypotension. In such circumstances a severe reaction should always be considered and the transfusion should be stopped until a specialist assessment has been conducted (Box 30.1).

Care should be taken when returning the blood product to the laboratory, to ensuring that the product does not leak and that no needles remain attached. Any further products being held locally for the patient should also be returned to the hospital transfusion laboratory for assessment. The events surrounding the reaction should be clearly documented and reported in the following ways:

- Record the adverse event in the patient's clinical record.
- Complete a detailed incident form as per local policy.
- Follow local, regional and national criteria for reporting via SABRE and SHOT.

Reactions and complications

Acute haemolytic reactions

These are usually directly related to ABO incompatibilities due to an IBCT where antigen/antibody reactions occur when the recipient's antibodies react with

---

Box 30.1 Initial management of a suspected transfusion reaction

- Stop the transfusion and seek urgent medical help.
- Initiate appropriate emergency procedures, e.g. call resuscitation team.
- Depending on venous access withdraw the contents of the lumen being used and disconnect the blood product.
- Keep venous access patent.
- Confirm the patient's identity and re-check their details against the product compatibility label.
- Keep the patient and relative informed of all progress and reassure as indicated.
- Initiate close and frequent observations of temperature, pulse, blood pressure, fluid balance.
- Inform the transfusion laboratory and seek the urgent advice of the haematologist for further management.
- Return the transfused product to the laboratory with new blood samples (10 ml clotted and 5 ml ethylenediamine tetraacetic acid (EDTA)) from the patient's opposite arm (SNBTS 2004) with a completed transfusion reaction notification form (if available) or note the patient's details, the nature and timing of the reaction and details of the component transfused.

---

surface antigens on the donor red cells. This reaction causes a cascade of events within the recipient as described above. Such reaction can present with chills/rigor, facial flushing, pain/oozing at cannula site, burning along the vein, chest pain, lumbar or flank pain, or shock (Gillespie & Hillyer 2001; McClelland 2007). Patients may express a feeling of anxiety or doom, which may be associated with cytokine activity. Haemolytic shock can occur after only a few millilitres of blood has been infused. Treatment is often vigorous to reverse hypotension, aid adequate renal perfusion and renal flow to reduce potential damage to renal tubules, and appropriate therapy for DIC reactions (Provan *et al.* 1998). It is important to remember that most acute haemolytic reactions are preventable as they are usually caused by clerical or checking errors at the bedside, and as this is the final check before administration it presents the last opportunity to identify and avert an error, thus emphasizing the importance of the final check before transfusion (McClelland 2007) (Figure 30.1).

Acute anaphylactic reactions

These are rare and usually occur after only a few millilitres of blood or plasma has been infused (Weinstein 2007) and present with bronchial spasm, respiratory distress, abdominal cramps, shock and potential loss of consciousness.

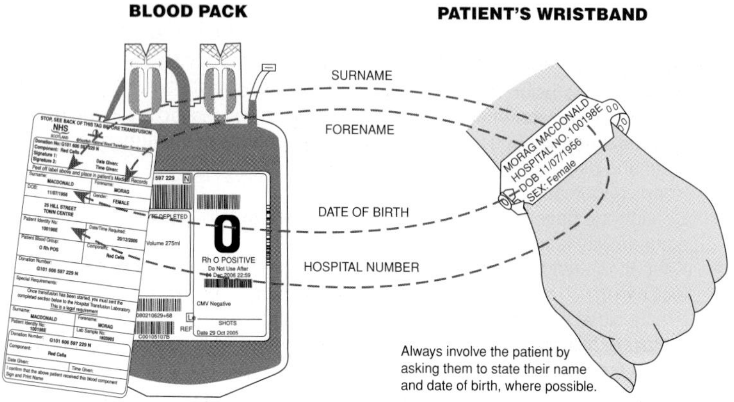

Figure 30.1 Check the compatability label or tie-on-tag against the patient's wrist-band.

Air embolism

Air embolism is a risk with any intravenous therapy (Shamash 2002) and care should be taken throughout the transfusion process.

Circulatory overload (transfusion-associated circulatory overload [TACO])

Circulatory overload can occur when blood or any of its components are infused rapidly or administered to a patient with an increased plasma volume, causing hypervolaemia. Patients at risk are those with renal or cardiac deficiencies, the young and elderly (Weinstein 2007). Patients with signs of cardiac failure should receive their transfusion slowly with diuretic support (McClelland 2007). The need for concomitant drugs such as diuretics should always be assessed before commencing treatment (SNBTS 2004).

Febrile non-haemolytic reactions

These reactions are due to an immunological response to the transfusion of cellular components such as donor leucocytes. Specific patient groups are at risk of greater sensitization to leucocytes, for example, critically ill patients, those receiving anticancer therapies or patients requiring multiple transfusion therapy (Williamson *et al.* 1998). Such reactions present with a mild fever (up to 1.5°C), rash without systemic disturbance and moderate tachycardia without hypotension (SNBTS 2004).

Hypothermia

Infusing large quantities of cold blood rapidly can cause hypothermia. Patients likely to suffer from this reaction are those who have suffered massive blood loss due to trauma, haemorrhage, clotting disorders or thrombocytopenia (McClelland 2007). Such reactions present with alteration in vital signs, and development of pallor and chills.

Blood warming devices

The warming of blood and blood products is generally not recommended as it is of limited benefit and can be dangerous. Blood warmers are only indicated when:

- Massive, rapid transfusion could result in cooling of cardiac tissue, causing potentially fatal dysrythmia (McClelland 2007). If the rate of transfusion is greater than 100 ml per minute blood warming devices should be used (McClelland 2007).
- Transfusion is required by patients with cold agglutination disease (Gray & Illingworth 2006).
- Exchange transfusion is indicated in the newborn (Weinstein 2007).
- Thawing of cryopreserved stem cells prior to transfusion (blood or marrow).

Both water baths and dry heat blood warmers are available. However, whichever device is chosen the temperature should be maintained below 38°C. Warming in excess of this can cause haemolysis of red cells and can denature proteins and increase the risk of bacterial infection. Blood warmers must always be used and maintained according to the manufacturer's guidelines. Blood products must **never** be warmed by improvisation, such as putting the pack into hot water, in a microwave or on a radiator, as uncontrolled heating can damage the contents of the pack (Gray & Illingworth 2006; McClelland 2007). The use of water baths also increases the risk of bacterial contamination. Therefore certain safety measures must be adhered to:

- Water baths must be drained after each use and must be stored dry and empty.
- The blood warmer should be drained after each use and must be stored dry and empty.
- When needed, they should be refilled with sterile water.
- A protective sterile over-bag to thaw blood and blood products reduces the entry of contaminants through microscopic punctures or breaks in the seal.
- The product should be used immediately after it has been thawed.

All devices should be serviced as per hospital health and safety policies, Medicines and Healthcare Products Regulatory Agency (MHRA) and manufacturers' guidelines.

Sepsis

Sepsis occurs when bacteria enter the blood or blood product that is to be infused. Bacteria can enter at any point from the time of collection, during storage through to administration to the patient. Organisms implicated in transfusion-related sepsis include Gram-negative *Pseudomonas*, *Yersinia* and *Flavobacterium* (Provan *et al.* 1998). Septic reactions usually present with a fever, tachycardia and/or hypotension, and can lead rapidly to systemic inflammatory response syndrome (SIRS) (Porth 2005). This is a serious life-threatening condition, sometimes referred to as septic shock, and requires urgent medical attention.

Transfusion-related acute lung injury (TRALI)

TRALI is usually caused by anti-leucocyte antibodies reacting against donor leucocytes. This reaction can result in 'leucoagglutination'. Leucoagglutinins can in turn become trapped in the pulmonary microvasculature, causing severe respiratory distress without evidence of circulatory overload or cardiac failure (Contreras & Mollison 1998). TRALI presents with a rapid onset of breathlessness, a non-productive cough, distress, chills or fever, cyanosis, hypotension and coma. A chest X-ray will show bilateral nodular infiltrates in a characteristic 'bat wing' presentation (McClelland 2007). TRALI is usually treated as any adult respiratory distress syndrome (ARDS) and therefore patients that develop TRALI may require ventilatory support (SNBTS 2004) and should be treated as an emergency. As TRALI is donor related it is essential that cases are reported to the blood transfusion services so that donors can be contacted and removed from the donor panel (McClelland 2007).

Urticaria

This uncommon reaction is caused by the recipient reacting to protein in the donor plasma (Davies & Williamson 1998). Urticaria is characterized by localized oedematous plaques, hives and itching and is usually mediated by histamines (Porth 2005). Therefore urticarial reactions usually respond well to antihistamines and they should be administered once the patient has been assessed and antihistamine therapy has been prescribed (SNBTS 2004). The infusion can then be recommenced; however, if symptoms return, the infusion should be discontinued.

Delayed effects

These reactions may occur days, months or even years after transfusion.

Delayed haemolytic reactions

These reactions are caused when immune antibodies react to a foreign antigen. Reactions are classified as primary or secondary. A *primary* reaction is often mild, occurring days or weeks after initial transfusion, and may be indicated by no clinical alteration in haemoglobin following transfusion therapy (Cook 1997a). *Secondary* reactions occur with re-exposure to the same antigen, and on rare occasions may be associated with ABO incompatibilities (Cook 1997a). The patient may present with a fever, mild jaundice and unexplained decrease in haemoglobin value and may require antiglobulin testing (McClelland 2007).

Hyperkalaemia

Hyperkalaemia is a rare complication associated with trauma and the subsequent infusion of large quantities of blood. Potassium is known to leak out of red cells during storage, thereby increasing circulatory levels in recipients receiving blood products (Cook 1997b). The process is exacerbated if products are kept too long at room temperature or gamma irradiated (Davies & Williamson 1998). From starting the infusion to completion, the infusion should take a maximum of 4 hours (McClelland 2007). The patient may present with irritability, anxiety, abdominal cramps, diarrhoea and weakness in the extremities (Cook 1997b). The patient's medical team should be contacted to assess the patient.

Iron overload

1031

Patients who are dependent on frequent transfusion, such as those with thalasemic, sickle cell and other transfusion-dependent disorders can become overloaded with iron (McClelland 2007). A unit of red blood cells contains 250 mg iron, which the body is unable to excrete, and as a result patients receiving large volumes of blood are at risk of iron overload (Davies & Williamson 1998). This can result in poor growth, pigment changes, hepatic cirrhosis, hypoparathyroidism, diabetes, arrhythmia, cardiac failure and death. Chelation therapy through the use of desferrioxamine, which induces iron excretion, is used to minimize the accumulation of iron (Mehta 2006).

Transfusion-associated graft-versus-host disease (TA-GVHD)

Although rare, TA-GVHD is a serious complication for recipients and is often fatal. TA-GVHD is usually caused by an IBCT incident where non-irritated blood components containing immunocompetent T lymphocytes are given to severely immunocompromised recipients. The donor T lymphocytes engraft and multiply, reacting against the recipient's 'foreign' tissue causing a graft-versus-host reaction (Davies & Williamson 1998). It is not commonly associated with fresh frozen plasma (FFP) or cryoprecipitate. Onset occurs 1–2 weeks after transfusion and the condition is predominantly fatal (McClelland 2007). Irradiation (25 gray) of blood and blood products, to inactivate T lymphocytes (McClelland 2007) is essential in the prevention of TA-GVHD and is especially important in the following recipients:

- Foetuses receiving intrauterine transfusions.
- Patients undergoing or who have undergone blood or bone marrow progenitor cell transplantation.
- Immunocompromised recipients.

Infectious complications of blood products

Bacterial infections

Contamination of blood and blood products can occur during donation, collection, processing, storage and administration. Despite strict guidelines and procedures, the risk of contamination remains. Most common contaminating organisms are skin contaminants such as staphylococci, diphtheroids and micrococci, which enter the blood at the time of venesection (Barbara & Contreras 1998; Provan *et al.* 1998). Bacterial contamination can lead to severe septic reaction as discussed above.

Viral infections

Viruses transmissible via blood transfusions can be either plasma borne or cell associated (Barbara & Contreras 1998; Williamson *et al.* 1998). Plasma-borne viruses include hepatitis B, hepatitis C, hepatitis A (rarely), serum parvovirus B19, and human immunodeficiency viruses (HIV-1 and HIV-2). Cell-associated viruses include cytomegalovirus (CMV), Epstein–Barr virus, human T-cell leukaemia/lymphoma viruses (HTLV-1/HTLV-2) and HIV-1/HIV-2.

Human T-leukaemia/lymphoma virus type 1 (HTLV-1)

HTLV-1 is an oncogenic retrovirus, associated with the white cells that cause adult T-cell leukaemia, and is connected with several degenerative neuromuscular syndromes. The enzyme-linked immunosorbent assay (ELISA) has been recommended because of concerns relating to the transmission of the virus via blood transfusion, and the associated long incubation period of adult T-cell leukaemia. In the UK all blood is tested for HTLV (JPAC 2005).

Cytomegalovirus (CMV)

CMV is classified as part of the herpes family and hence has the ability to establish latent infection with reactivation during periods of immunosuppression

(Barnes 1992; Barbara & Contreras 1998). Approximately 50% of the population in the UK has antibodies to CMV. Therefore it is recognized that the virus may be transmitted by transfusion. Although it poses little threat to immunologically competent recipients, CMV infection in vulnerable patient groups can cause significant morbidity and mortality. For example, CMV pneumonitis carries an 85% mortality rate in blood and bone marrow transplant recipients (Mollison *et al.* 1997). Screening of donors and the use of CMV-seronegative or leucocyte-depleted blood and blood products are seen as essential for neonates and immunocompromised recipients who have tested negative to CMV (Prentice *et al.* 1998).

Hepatitis B virus (HBV)

Screening for hepatitis B surface antigen (HBsAg) in donor blood is mandatory as it is estimated that approximately 180 000 people in the UK currently suffer from chronic hepatitis B (Foundation for Liver Research 2004).

Hepatitis C virus (HCV)

Screening for hepatitis C using the ELISA is mandatory in the UK. Hepatitis C is transmitted primarily via contact with blood or blood products (Friedman 2001).

Human immunodeficiency virus (HIV-1 and HIV-2)

HIV is a retrovirus that infects and kills helper T cells, also known as CD4-positive lymphocytes. Transmission of the virus can be via most blood products including red cells, platelets, FFP, and factor VIII and IX concentrates. These viruses are not known to be transmitted in albumin, immunoglobulins or antithrombin III products (Barbara & Contreras 1998). The retrovirus invades cells and slowly destroys the immune system, rendering the individual susceptible to opportunistic infections. Since 1983, when it was recognized that the virus could be transmitted via transfusion, actions were developed to safeguard blood supplies from transmitting the virus that caused acquired immune deficiency syndrome (AIDS). These include the careful screening of donors and the testing of donated blood.

Other infective agents

Parasites

Plasmodium falciparum is the most dangerous of the human malarial parasites (Barbara & Contreras 1998). Prevention is maintained by questioning donors about foreign travel, in particular those who have visited areas where the disease is prevalent (Bishop 2008).

Prion diseases

Known as transmissible spongiform encephalopathies (TSEs), these are a rare group of conditions which cause progressive neurodegeneration in humans and some animal species. Prion diseases are believed to be caused by the presence of an abnormal form of a cellular protein (Aguzzi & Collinge 1997; Barbara & Contreras 1998; Vamvakas 1999). These abnormal proteins have an altered cellular shape, and become infectious and multiply by converting normal cellular protein to the irregular form. This irregular form is resistant to digestion and breakdown, and, once accumulation occurs, can result in the formation of plaque in brain tissue. Transmission is thought to be by direct contact with infected brain or lymphoreticular tissue (Aguzzi & Collinge 1997; Barbara & Contreras 1998; Vamvakas 1999).

1 Prion diseases in animal species:
   (a) Scrapie, a disease of sheep.
   (b) Bovine spongiform encephalopathy (BSE).
   (c) Feline spongiform encephalopathy (FSE).
   (d) Chronic wasting disease of deer, mule and elk.
2 Prion diseases in humans:
   (a) Sporadic: classic Creutzfeldt–Jakob disease (CJD).
   (b) Inherited: CJD, Gerstmann–Sträussler–Scheinker disease, fatal familial insomnia (FFI).
   (c) Acquired: kuru, variant Creutzfeldt–Jakob disease (vCJD).

1034

There is evidence to suggest that in TSEs, of which vCJD is one, leucocytes, particularly lymphocytes, are the key cells in the transportation of the putative infectious agent to the brain (Aguzzi & Collinge 1997; Bradley 1999). Leucodepletion of all blood and blood components is viewed as a sensible yet precautionary action to reduce any risk of blood-borne infection. All products in the UK are now leucodepleted at source. Currently, all plasma products are brought in from the USA, except FFP and cryoprecipitate which are leucodepleted at source in the UK.

Procedure

The transfusion of any blood product carries with it the potential of reaction and risk (SHOT 2005). All staff involved in the process of the transfusion of blood and/or blood products must have the knowledge and skills to ensure the process is completed safely. Therefore the nurse caring for those receiving transfusion therapy must do so within his or her sphere of competence, always acting to minimize risk to the patient (NMC 2008). A guide to the necessary elements of blood pack labelling is shown in Figure 30.2.

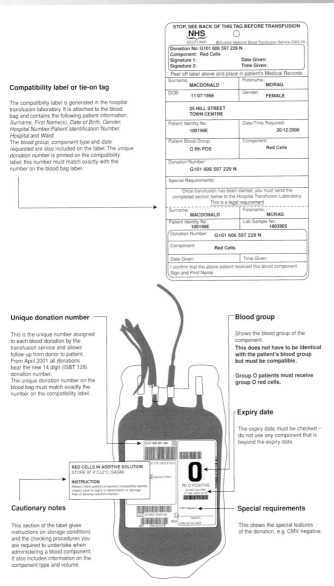

STOP, SEE BACK OF THIS TAG BEFORE TRANSFUSION

NHS
SCOTLAND   ©Scottish National Blood Transfusion Service 2005 V9

Donation No: G101 606 597 229 N
Component: Red Cells
Signature 1:   Date Given:
Signature 2:   Time Given:

Peel off label above and place in patient's Medical Records

Surname: MACDONALD	Forename: MORAG
DOB: 11/07/1956	Gender: FEMALE

25 HILL STREET
TOWN CENTRE

Patient Identity No: 100198E	Date/Time Required: 20/12/2006
Patient Blood Group: O Rh POS	Component: Red Cells

Donation Number:
G101 606 597 229 N

Special Requirements:

Once transfusion has been started, you must send the
completed section below to the Hospital Transfusion Laboratory.
This is a legal requirement

Surname: MACDONALD	Forename: MORAG
Patient Identity No: 100198E	Lab Sample No: 1803905

Donation Number: G101 606 597 229 N

Component: Red Cells	
Date Given:	Time Given:

I confirm that the above patient received this blood component
Sign and Print Name

Compatibility label or tie-on tag

The compatibility label is generated in the hospital transfusion laboratory. It is attached to the blood bag and contains the following patient information; *Surname, First Name(s), Date of Birth, Gender, Hospital Number/Patient Identification Number, Hospital* and *Ward*.
The *blood group, component type* and *date requested* are also included on the label. The *unique donation number* is printed on the compatibility label; this number must match exactly with the number on the blood bag label.

Unique donation number

This is the unique number assigned to each blood donation by the transfusion service and allows follow-up from donor to patient. From April 2001 all donations bear the new 14 digit (ISBT 128) donation number.
The unique donation number on the blood bag must match exactly the number on the compatibility label.

Blood group

Shows the blood group of the component.
This does not have to be identical with the patient's blood group but must be compatible.

Group O patients must receive group O red cells.

Expiry date

The expiry date must be checked – do not use any component that is beyond the expiry date.

RED CELLS IN ADDITIVE SOLUTION
STORE AT 4°C±2°C (SAGM)

INSTRUCTION
Always check patient/component compatibility/identify
Inspect pack for signs of deterioration or damage
Risk of adverse reaction/infection

G101 606 597 229 N
LEUCOCYTE DEPLETED
Volume 275ml
O
Rh O POSITIVE
Do Not Use After
31 Dec 2006 22:59
CMV Negative
LOT B1060310629-88
REF C001051078
SHOT5
REF Date 29 Oct 2005

Cautionary notes

This section of the label gives instructions on storage conditions and the checking procedures you are required to undertake when administering a blood component. It also includes information on the component type and volume.

Special requirements

This shows the special features of the donation, e.g. CMV negative.

Figure 30.2   Blood pack labelling.

Procedure guidelines   Transfusion of blood components

Blood administration sets should be changed at least every 12 hours or after every second unit for a continuing transfusion (Gray & Illingworth 2006). Platelet transfusions may be administered using a standard blood administration set or a dedicated platelet administration set (McClelland 2007). Platelets should not be administered through an administration set that has been used for red cells or other blood components as this may cause aggregation and retention of platelets in the set/device (McClelland 2007).

Equipment

1 Blood administration giving set with 170–200 µm macroaggregate filter.
2 Equipment for patient's intravenous access requirements (if necessary).

3 Blood product to be transfused.
Note: all blood products that require leucocyte depletion are leucodepleted at source by the blood transfusion service (SNBTS 2004).

Procedure

Action	Rationale
Pre-administration check:	
1 Ensure that the component has been correctly prescribed, including any special requirements such as irradiated or CMV-negative blood and if the patient requires any other medications, e.g. diuretic, pre-medication.	Prevention of Incorrect Blood Component Transfused (IBCT) error: ABO incompatibility or non-irradiated CMV-positive products may cause a fatal reaction if transfused (McClelland 2007: C). Negative and positive status should always be written in full and not as + or − as they may get defaced and be incorrectly processed (E).
2 Record the patient's baseline vital signs, temperature, pulse, blood pressure and respirations.	To ensure that any transfusion reaction can be immediately identified and managed appropriately (SNBTS 2004: C) due to changes in baseline (E).
3 Check the expiry date of the component to be used.	To prevent the administration of expired blood products (E).
4 Conduct a visual inspection of the component to be used for signs of clumping, discoloration damage or leaks. ***Note*: if there are any discrepancies at this point do not proceed until they have been resolved.**	Expired or damaged products must not be used (E). To ensure an Incorrect Blood Component Transfused (IBCT) event does not occur (E).

5 Positively identify the patient by asking him/her to state the following information:
   (a) First name.
   (b) Surname.
   (c) Date of birth.

This is the final check of identity prior to transfusion and is absolutely vital in minimizing the risk of Incorrect Blood Component Transfused (IBCT) errors (SNBTS 2004: C).

6 Check the details given against the patient's name band and the patient details on the blood product.

To minimize the risk of error (SNBTS 2004: C).

7 Check that the information on the compatibility label matches the details on the blood component.
Note: if there are any discrepancies at this point do not proceed until they have been resolved.

To minimize the risk of error (SNBTS 2004: C).

8 Where necessary obtain venous access (see Chapter 32).

To enable transfusion to be administered (E).

9 No agent other than 0.9% saline should be administered through the same lumen as a blood product.

Other agents may damage the product components and precipitate transfusion complications (SNBTS 2004: C).

10 Prime the blood administration set with the required product.

It is not necesarry to prime the device with saline unless there is a concern about device patency.
Dextrose should never be used to prime a set or flush the blood administration set following a transfusion as this can cause haemolysis (SNBTS 2004: C).

11 Set up infusion via a volumetric infusion pump if appropriate.

Some older infusion pumps can damage the red cells. Blood administration sets for specific infusion pumps must always be used. If none are available the standard blood administration set should be used via gravity and the rate monitored as necessary (E).

12 Set the desired infusion rate as indicated by the blood product being used and the patient's condition:

1037

Procedure guidelines (cont.)

(a) Red-cell administration can range from 5–10 minutes in acute blood loss to the maximum time of 4 hours in elderly patients (SNBTS 2004).

The rate of administration is indicated by the patient's clinical condition (SNBTS 2004: C; Weinstein 2007: E). Dictated by current guidelines (SNBTS 2004: C).

(b) Platelets, fresh frozen plasma and cryoprecipitate should be transfused over 30–60 minutes and must be completed within 4 hours of puncturing the blood component.

---

13 Take and record the patient's temperature and pulse 15 minutes after commencing each unit.

Adverse reactions will often occur during the first 15 minutes of transfusion (Gray & Illingworth 2006 : C). Complaints of serious anxiety, transfusion site pain, loin pain, backache, fever, skin flushing or urticaria could be indicative of a serious transfusion reaction (McClelland 2007: C). In such cases the transfusion should be stopped immediately and urgent medical advice sought (SNBTS 2004: C).

---

14 Record the start and finish times of each unit. All units must be completed within 4 hours of commencing.

Continuation of a transfusion beyond 4 hours increases the risk of transfusion reaction and complications (E).

---

15 Take and record the patient's vital signs on completion of each unit.

This forms a record of the patient's progress and acts as a baseline for subsequent units (E).

---

16 Record the volume of the product transfused on the patient's fluid balance chart.

Monitoring of fluid balance can demonstrate fluid overload in at-risk patients (Weinstein 2007: E).

---

17 Carefully file all transfusion documentation in the patient's clinical record. In line with local policy return information on the final fate of each blood product to the hospital laboratory manager.

To maintain the clinical record for patient safety.
To comply with *Statutory Instrument 2005 No. 50*.
The Blood Safety and Quality Regulations 2005 where the final fate of all blood products must be held for a duration of 30 years (Crown 2005: C).

18 Return any unused blood products to the laboratory promptly.	Unused products may be re-allocated if returned in time. Refer to local guidelines (E).	
19 Keep all empty blood component bags in the clinical area until the transfusion is completed. Once the transfusion is completed, dispose of in clinical waste.	Access to transfused bags is generally only useful for acute reactions (SNBTS 2004: C).	
20 For patients receiving ongoing transfusion support the blood administration set should be changed every 12 hours.	Minimize risk from macroaggregates and bacterial contamination (SNBTS 2004:C).	

Problem solving: Transfusion of blood components

Problem	Cause	Suggested action
Unable to obtain verbal confirmation.	Patient unconscious.	Confirm identity with a relative or use unique patient identifier as above.
	Patient unable to verbally communicate.	Confirm identity with a relative or second member of staff (SNBTS 2004). Always follow local policy and never use secondary identifiers such as bed numbers, notes or request forms that the patient may be carrying (BCSH 1999).
Patient does not have a name band.	Name band has been removed or is no longer legible. Patient is in an outpatient setting.	All inpatients are required to wear a name band. Therefore replace name band and reconfirm identity as above. Follow local hospital policy.
Infusion slows or stops.	Venous spasm due to cold infusion.	Apply warm compress to dilate the vein and increase the blood flow.

Problem solving (cont.)

Problem	Cause	Suggested action
	Occlusion.	Flush gently with 0.9% sodium chloride and resume infusion. If occlusion persists consider resiting canula.
Elevation in temperature after commencing a unit of blood with no other symptoms. Temperature falls if the blood is slowed/stopped.	Pyrogenic reaction.	Observe the patient's temperature, pulse and blood pressure during the transfusion as indicated. If the patient has received multiple transfusions or previous history ensure that appropriate medication is prescribed before commencing transfusions.
Complaints of serious anxiety, transfusion site pain, loin pain, backache, fever, skin flushing or urticaria.	Adverse reaction to transfusion/ transfusion error.	Stop infusion immediately and seek urgent medical advice.

1040

References and further reading

Aguzzi, A. & Collinge, J. (1997) Post exposure prophylaxis after accidental prion inoculation. *Lancet*, 350, 1519–20.

Anderson, K.N., Anderson, L.E. & Glanze, W.D. (eds) (1994) *Mosby's Medical, Nursing, and Allied Health Dictionary*, 4th edn. Mosby, St. Louis, MO.

Barbara, J.A.J. & Contreras, M. (1998) Infectious complications of blood transfusion: bacteria and parasites. In: *ABC of Transfusion* (ed. M. Contreras), 3rd edn. British Medical Journal Publishing, London, pp. 58–61.

Barnes, R. (1992) Infections following bone marrow transplantation. In: *Bone Marrow Transplantation in Practice* (eds J. Treleavan & J. Barrett). Churchill Livingstone, Edinburgh, pp. 281–8.

BCSH (1999) Guidelines on the administration of blood components and the management of transfused patients. Blood Transfusion Task Force. *Transfus Med*, 9, 227–38.

Bishop, E. (2008) Blood transfusion therapy. In: *Intravenous Therapy in Nursing Practice* (eds L. Dougherty & J. Lamb), 2nd edn. Blackwell Publishing, Oxford.

Bradley, R. (1999) BSE transmission studies with particular reference to blood. *Dev Biol Stand*, 99, 35–40.

Brown, P. (2005) Blood infectivity, processing and screening tests in transmissible spongiform encephalopathy. *Vox Sanguinous*, 89(2), 63–70.

Brown, P. & Cervenakova, L. (2004) The modern landscape of transfusion-related iatrogenic Creutzfeldt–Jakob disease and blood screening tests. *Curr Opin Hematol*, **11**(5), 351–6.

Brozovic, B., Hows, J. & Contreras, M. (1998) Platelet and granulocyte transfusion. In: *ABC of Transfusion* (ed. M. Contreras), 3rd edn. British Medical Journal Publishing, London, pp. 17–23.

Carless, P. *et al.* (2004) Autologous transfusion techniques: a systematic review of their efficacy. *Transfus Med*, **14**(2), 123–44.

Cervenakova, L. & Brown, P. (2004) Advances in screening test development for transmissible spongiform encephalopathies. *Expert Review in Anti-infective Therapy*, **2**(6), 873–80.

Contreras, M. & Mollison, P.L. (1998) Immunological complications of transfusion. In: *ABC of Transfusion* (ed. M. Contreras), 3rd edn. British Medical Journal Publishing, London, pp. 53–7.

Cook, L.S. (1997a) Blood transfusion reactions involving an immune response. *J Intraven Nurs*, **20**(1), 5–14.

Cook, L.S. (1997b) Non-immune transfusion reactions: when type and crossmatch aren't enough. *J Intraven Nurs*, **20**(1), 15–22.

Crown (2005) *The Blood Safety and Quality Regulations 2005*. HMSO, London. Available at www. opsi.gov.uk.

Davies, S.C. & Williamson, L.M. (1998) Transfusion of red cells. In: *ABC of Transfusion* (ed. M. Contreras), 3rd edn. British Medical Journal Publishing, London, pp. 10–17.

DH (2002) *Better Blood Transfusion: Appropriate Use of Blood, HSC 2002/009*. Department of Health, London. Available at www.transfusionguidelines.org.uk.

Friedman, D. (2001) Hepatitis. In: *Handbook of Transfusion Medicine*. Academic Press, New York, pp. 275–84.

Foundation for Liver Research (2004) *Hepatitis B: Out of the Shadows, a Report into the Impact of Hepatitis B on the Nation's Health*. Foundation for Liver Research, London.

Gillespie, T. W. & Hillyer, D. (2001) Granulocytes. In: *Handbook of Transfusion Medicine*. Academic Press, New York, pp. 63–8.

Gray, A. & Illingworth, J. (2006) *Right blood, Right Patient, Right Time.RCN Guidance for Improving Transfusion Practice*. Royal College of Nursing, London.

Harrison, J. (2004) Getting your own back – an update on autologous transfusion. *Blood Matters*, **16**, 7–9.

Henry, D.A. *et al.* (2001) Pre-operative autologous donation for minimising perioperative allogeneic blood transfusion. *Cochrane Database Syst Rev*, **4**, CD003602. DOI: 10.1002/14651858.CD003602.

Hewitt, P.E. & Wagstaff, W. (1998) The blood donor and tests on donor blood. In: *ABC of Transfusion* (ed. M. Contreras), 3rd edn. British Medical Journal Publishing, London, pp. 1–5.

Hoffbrand, A.V., Pettit, J.E. & Moss, P.A.H. (2001) *Essential Haematology*. Blackwell Science, Oxford.

James, V. (2004) *A National Blood Conservation Strategy for NBTC and NBS: Report from the Working Party on Alternatives to Transfusion*. National Blood Service, London.

James, V. (ed.) (2005) *Guidelines for the Blood Transfusion Services in the United Kingdom*, 7th edn. HMSO, London.

James, V. & Harrison, J. (2002) The pros and cons of predeposit autologous donation & transfusion (PAD). *Blood Matters*, **11**, 4–5.

JPAC (Joint UKBTS/NIBSC Professional Advisory Committee) (2005) JPAC Donor Selection Guidelines, available at www.transfusionguidelines.org.uk.

Ludlam, C.A. & Turner, M. (2006) Managing the risk of transmission of variant Creutzfeldt Jakob disease by blood products. *Br J Haematol*, **132**(1), 13–24.

MacLennan, S. (2003) Transfusion related acute lung injury (TRALI). NBS Transfusion Medicine Clinical Policies Group. www.blood.co.uk/hospitals/library/pdf/TRALI.pdf. Accessed 06/08/06.

McClelland, D.B.L. (ed) (2007) *Handbook of Transfusion Medicine*. HMSO, London.

Mehta, D. (2006) *British National Formulary*, V.51. BMJ Publishing, London.

MHRA (2006) Haemovigilance – how we monitor the safety of blood and blood components. www.mhra.gov.uk/home/idcplg?IdcService=SS_GET_PAGE&nodeId=282. Accessed 30/7/06.

Mollison, P.L., Engelfriet, C.P. & Contreras, M. (1997) *Blood Transfusion in Clinical Medicine*. Blackwell Science, London.

NMC (2008) *The Code: Standards of Conduct, Performance and Ethics for Nurses and Midwives*. Nursing and Midwifery Council, London.

Porth, C.M. (2005) *Pathophysiology: Concepts of Altered Health States*, 7th edn. Lippincott, Williams & Wilkins, Philadelphia.

Prentice, G., Grundy, J.E. & Kho, P. (1998) Cytomegalovirus. In: *The Clinical Practice of Stem Cell Transplantation* (eds J. Barrett & J. Treleaven). Isis Medical Media, Oxford, pp. 697–708.

Provan, D. *et al.* (1998) *Oxford Handbook of Clinical Haematology*. Oxford University Press, Oxford.

Shamash, J. (2002) Blood counts. *Nurs Times*, **98**(45), 23–6.

SHOT (2005) *Annual Report 2004*. Serious Hazards of Transfusion, London.

SNBTS (2004) Better blood transfusion level 1 safe transfusion practice. self-directed learning pack. Effective Use of Blood Group, Scottish National Blood Transfusion Service. www.learnbloodtransfusion.org.uk/Level_1_SDL.pdf. Accessed 06/08/06.

Vamvakas, E.C. (1999) Risk of transmission of Creutzfeldt–Jakob disease by transfusion of blood, plasma, and plasma derivatives. *J Clin Apher*, **14**(3), 135–43.

Weinstein, S. (2007) *Plumer's Principles and Practices of Intravenous Therapy*, 8th edn. Lippincott, Philadelphia.

Williamson, L.M. *et al.* (1998) *Serious Hazards of Transfusion (SHOT). Summary of Annual Report 1996–97*. Serious Hazards of Transfusion Office, Manchester.

Multiple choice questions

1 The official government agency with jurisdiction over the administration of blood products is?

   a   MRSA
   b   MJRA
   c   MHRA
   d   MNRA

2 People with blood group AB:

   a   Are able to receive blood of any blood group
   b   Are able to donate blood to any blood group
   c   Are unable to donate blood
   d   Can only donate platelets

3 People with blood group O:

   a   Are able to donate blood to any blood group
   b   Are able to receive blood from any blood group
   c   Are unable to donate blood
   d   Can only donate platelets

4 If you suspect that a patient is having a reaction to a blood transfusion you should initially:

   a   Inform the doctor
   b   Stop the transfusion
   c   Stop the transfusion and seek urgent medical help
   d   Give them some paracetamol

5 **Blood administration sets should be changed:**

    a   Every 24 hours
    b   Every 12 hours or after administration of every second unit
    c   After every unit
    d   Every 6 hours

6 **Prior to commencing the administration of a blood product, which of the following checks should be made?**

    a   Positive identification of the patient
    b   Correct prescription of blood product
    c   Compatibility label and details on blood component match
    d   All of the above

Answers to the multiple choice questions can be found in Appendix 3.

Chapter 31

The unconscious patient

Definition

Consciousness is a state of awareness of self, environment and one's response to that environment. To be fully conscious means that the individual appropriately responds to the external stimuli. An altered level of consciousness represents a decrease in this full state of awareness and response to environmental stimuli (Boss 1998).

Unconsciousness is a physiological state in which the patient is unresponsive to sensory stimuli and lacks awareness of self and the environment (Hickey 2003a). There are many central nervous system conditions that can result in the patient being in an unconscious state. The depth and duration of unconsciousness span a broad spectrum of presentations from fainting, with a momentary loss of consciousness, to prolonged coma lasting several weeks, months or even years. If a patient is unconscious and in the terminal phase of an illness, the focus will be on the general care of any person who is dying. Care of the dying encompasses an integrated model of care between health care professionals, the patient and family (Seymour & Ingleton 2004).

In the critically ill patient sedation is an essential part of the management. Sedation helps to minimize anxiety, promote sleep and keep the patient comfortable. It facilitates mechanical ventilation, helps to control physiological reactions to stress such as hypertension, tachycardia and raised intracranial pressure (Adam & Osborne 2005). A sedation scoring system such as the Riker scale should be used to achieve a therapeutic sedation level. This scale is a numerical scale from one to seven with one equivalent to unrousable and seven equivalent to dangerously agitated (Janz *et al.* 2005).

The nurse often cares for those who are unconscious for prolonged periods of time. In addition to managing the primary neurological problem, the nurse must also incorporate a rehabilitation framework to maintain intact function, prevent complications and disabilities, and restore lost function to the maximum that is possible. Total care of the patient involves communicating with families and

friends on a regular basis to ensure they are supported and are able to participate in patient care if they wish to, and if this is appropriate (Geraghty 2005).
There is evidence that unconscious patients are aware of what is happening to
them and can hear conversations around them (Lawrence 1995; Jacobson 2000).
Being aware of what the unconscious patient may be experiencing will add to the
ongoing holistic approach to the needs of the patient physically, psychologically
and spiritually.

Reference material

Assessment of level of consciousness

There are many methods available to measure a patient's level of consciousness.
The most commonly used and universally accepted tool is the Glasgow Coma
Scale (GCS) (Hickey 2003a; Geraghty 2005). A detailed explanation of examination techniques and correct evaluation of this tool is vital to ensure accuracy of
rating of the GCS by nurses (Heron *et al.*, 2001; Geraghty 2005). However, the
use of the GCS to assess the sedated and intubated patient is thought to be inappropriate. Sedation influences the patient's level of consciousness and is likely to
impede the patient's eye opening and motor responses whereas the presence of an
endotracheal tube will hinder assessment of the patient's verbal response (Price
et al. 2000) (see Chapter 19). The unconscious patient is a medical emergency.
Assessment of the patient's airway, breathing and circulation is vital (Geraghty
2005) (see Chapter 6).

1046 *Physiological changes in the unconscious patient*

The physiological changes that occur in unconscious patients will depend on
the cause of unconsciousness, on the length of immobility while unconscious,
outcome and quality of care. It is not only being unconscious that will have a
deleterious effect on the body but also drugs, e.g. some muscle relaxants such as
those used in intensive care, can contribute to muscle weakness, raised intraocular
and intracranial pressure, electrolyte imbalances and airway tone (Booij 1996).
Unconsciousness can lead to changes and problems for the patient which have
implications for nursing interventions. The discussion below is not exhaustive
but offers an insight into the effects of unconsciousness on the main systems of
the body.

Immobility

The human body is designed for physical activity and movement. Therefore any
lack of exercise, regardless of reason, can result in multisystem deconditioning, anatomical and physiological changes. Involvement of a physiotherapist for

passive exercises early in the period of unconsciousness may help in the prevention of further complications.

- *Decreased muscle strength*: the degree of loss varies with the particular muscle groups and the degree of immobility. The antigravitational muscles of the legs lose strength twice as quickly as the arm muscles and recovery takes longer.
- *Muscle atrophy*: this alludes to loss of muscle mass. When the muscle is relaxed, it atrophies about twice as rapidly as in a stretched position. As increased muscle tone prevents complete atrophy, patients with upper motor neurone disease lose less muscle mass than those with lower motor neurone disease (Hickey 2003b).

Gastrointestinal function

Bowel action is likely to become irregular in the unconscious patient, thus monitoring and observation are a priority (Geraghty 2005). Gastric complications can develop in the unconscious patient for a variety of reasons. Gastric ulcers, bleeding, constipation and faecal impaction can be identified as causing symptomatic problems. Nutrition is commonly provided by enteral tube feeding (see Chapter 17) which does not generally stimulate peristalsis. Loose stool can be a result of poorly tolerated enteral feeding or antibiotics. In contrast to this, some pharmacological interventions can lead to constipation. It is imperative that a diagnosis is made to differentiate between true diarrhoea and faecal impaction as they can occasionally be misinterpreted as being one and the same thing (see Chapter 11).

Genitourinary function

An unconscious state can induce urinary incontinence or retention of urine. The unconscious patient is at risk of two problems: urinary tract infections and kidney or bladder stones. On admission an unconscious patient will usually have an indwelling catheter (see Chapter 13). This is necessary for accurate fluid monitoring and to prevent skin breakdown.

Respiratory function

Due to the immobile nature of the unconscious patient, there is an increased threat of developing respiratory complications such as, atelectasis, pneumonia, aspiration and airway obstruction. If the patient is intubated with an endotracheal tube they are at increased risk of developing nosocomial infections (Hickey 2003b).

Respiratory assessment should include checking patency of the airway, monitoring the rate, pattern and work of breathing, pulse oximetry to check oxygen saturations and blood gases to assess adequacy of gaseous exchange. If the patient

1047

is intubated and ventilated then lung volumes and respiratory mechanics should be continuously monitored (Hickey 2003b).

Cardiovascular function

Immobility can cause changes in cardiovascular function, for example increased cardiac workload, decreased cardiac output and decreased blood pressure. In addition, the positioning of the unconscious patient causes central fluid shift, from the legs to the thorax and head, so the head of the unconscious patient with raised intracranial pressure may need to be elevated to 30° (Hickey 2003b).

Changes in cardiovascular function may be secondary to neurological changes; therefore the patient's neurological function should be monitored. Hypovolaemia, sepsis or cardiogenic shock are other factors that should be considered as they will cause cardiovascular instability and should be treated accordingly (Geraghty 2005).

The risk of deep vein thrombosis and pulmonary embolism is increased in the unconscious patient. This is due to several factors: blood pooling in the legs, hypercoagulability and prolonged pressure from immobility in bed (Hickey 2003b).

Impaired tissue integrity

Skin

Direct pressure to the skin and friction during movement of patients are two of the most common causes of injury to the skin that can result in pressure ulcers. Correct moving and handling of the patient will minimize the risk of pressure ulcer formation (see Chapter 34). Other contributing factors include incontinence, profuse perspiration, poor nutrition and obesity (Hickey 2003b). Use of special beds may be required depending on individual assessment. Skin integrity should be assessed using the Waterlow Scale (see Chapter 34).

Eyes

The blink reflex is absent in the unconscious patient and tear production may be reduced (Carpenito 2002). Assessment of the eyes for signs of oedema, irritation, corneal drying or abrasions is essential. Application of an eye patch may protect the eye from injury (Hickey 2003b) (see Chapter 23).

Mouth

The lips, oral mucosa and tongue must be assessed for signs of dryness, irritation and infection (see Chapter 24).

Self-care

The fluid unconscious patient will require nursing care for all self-care needs. The nurse's role is to ensure that the patient's hygiene needs are met and that the patient is clean and comfortable (see Chapter 25)

Fluid/electrolyte imbalance

The fluid volume and electrolyte composition within the extracellular and intra-cellular compartments in the healthy patient are generally static. Different states may bring about changes in fluid volume or electrolye composition within the compartments (Kumar & Clark 2001). Therefore, serum electrolytes will require regular monitoring in the acute period of unconsciousness. Monitoring of fluid balance is important and correct fluid balance will assist in the prevention of deep vein thrombosis, pulmonary embolism, pressure ulcers and constipation.

Ethical considerations

There are many ethical considerations when nursing the unconscious patient, e.g. consent, organ donation, advance directives and termination of life support. It is not within the scope of this manual to discuss these in detail. However, consenting adults who lack capacity, e.g. unconscious patients, can be given treatment under the doctrine of necessity under common law (Leung 2002).

Advance directives enable people to document their wishes regarding refusal of medical treatment in the event of their being unable to make decisions about their medical and nursing care (UK Clinical Ethics Network 2003). These are legally binding documents; nevertheless, in practice these may be difficult to interpret and of little value in the acute setting (Travis *et al*. 2001; Leung 2002).

1049

Procedure guidelines   **Unconscious patient care**

Equipment

1 Airway of correct size.
2 Suction.
3 Oxygen mask.
4 Intravenous infusion equipment.
5 Personal hygiene equipment (measures for eye, oral and catheter care).

6 Cotsides (to be assessed on an individual basis, according to hospital policy).
7 Observation charts (neurological, fluid balance).
8 Feeding equipment.
9 Pen torch.

Procedure guidelines (cont.)

Procedure

Action	Rationale
1 Introduce yourself. Call the patient by their preferred name, as discussed with family/carer. Explain each procedure before starting.	Hearing often remains intact and recognition of a familiar word may assist in orientation of the unconscious patient (Elliott & Wright 1999: R 4; Leigh 2001: R 5).
2 Orientate the patient to day, date, time and place.	To promote orientation (Elliott & Wright 1999: R 4; Leigh 2001: R 5).
3 Remove dentures, note any loose teeth caps or crowns. Insert oropharyngeal or nasopharyngeal airway if appropriate. Monitor rate, rhythm and pattern of breathing.	To obtain and maintain a patent airway. To assess condition of the mouth and teeth. To assess breathing pattern and note changes (Geraghty 2005: E).
4 Monitor and document the patient's vital signs. Monitor electrolytes and full blood count as appropriate. Administer intravenous fluids as required. Monitor fluid balance.	To detect any changes in the patient's condition and manage as required. To detect potential fluid or electrolyte imbalances (Geraghty 2005: E).
5 Positioning of the unconscious patient: (a) Head: maintain proper alignment of head and neck; support with pillow, towel roll or soft collar.	Helps to maintain a patent airway (P).
(b) Elevate the head of the bed by 30°.	Helps reduce the risk of nosocomial pneumonia (Drakulovic et al. 1999: R 1b). It facilitates the drainage of secretions from the oropharynx, minimizes the risk of aspiration, assists the maintenance of adequate cerebral perfusion pressure and promotes an effective breathing pattern (Hickey 2003b: E).
(c) Body: position in alignment with spine (utilize towels and pillows).	This helps to maintain proper alignment of the body and helps minimize complications such as contractures and helps maintain musculoskeletal function (Geraghty 2005: E).
(d) Limbs: *Upper*. Support arms and wrists on pillows and flex the arms at the elbow.	To prevent shoulder drag and wrist drop (Geraghty 2005: E).

	Lower. Place a pillow between the knees, use pillows or splints to flex the ankles parallel to the feet, align the hips with the head.	To prevent skin breakdown and footdrop (Geraghty 2005: E). To prevent internal rotation of the upper leg (Hickey 2003b: E).
(e)	Fit antiembolic stockings on the patient if appropriate.	Helps reduce the risk of venous thromboembolism (Geraghty 2005:E).
(f)	Liaise with the physiotherapist about positioning/exercises for the patient. Monitor colour, temperature and pulses of the limbs.	To enhance pulmonary function, prevent atelectasis and hypostatic pneumonia (Geraghty 2005: E) and to help preserve musculoskeletal function and prevent deep vein thrombosis (Hickey 2003b: E).
6	Perform neurological assessment as frequently as patient condition dictates using Glasgow Coma Scale or appropriate tool (see Chapter 19).	To note changes in patient's condition and respond appropriately (NICE 2003: R 1a).
7	Assess skin integrity using Waterlow Scale or appropriate tool. Change position every 2 hours or sooner if condition indicates (see Chapter 34)	To prevent and monitor for signs of pressure ulcers (Waterlow 1998: C).
8	Carry out oral care as frequently as patient's condition indicates (see Chapter 24).	To maintain a clean and healthy mouth and to promote comfort.
9	Carry out eye care as frequently as patient's condition indicates. Place eye patch if appropriate (see Chapter 23).	To prevent corneal scratches, dryness or ulceration, which can lead to blindness.
10	Assess bowel pattern as per hospital policy (colour, frequency, consistency and size).	To prevent diarrhoea, constipation, abdominal discomfort, bloating and to promote comfort (Klaschik *et al.* 2003: R 5).
11	Catheterize as per hospital policy (see Chapter 13).	To promote comfort and prevent stasis of urine, infection and renal calculi (Geraghty 2005: R 5).
12	Move patient as indicated by their condition. Choose type of pressure-relieving mattress according to the patient needs. Passive exercises as discussed with physiotherapist.	To prevent complications associated with bedrest, e.g. pressure sores, deep vein thrombosis. To prevent muscle wasting and contractures (Cullum *et al.* 2004: R 1a).

Conclusion

For the nurse there are physical, psychological and ethical considerations when caring for the unconscious patient. The preservation of life and avoidance of further disabilities are priorities of care, but the psychological effects on the patient's family and carers also require sensitivity and open communication. Patients' psychological needs should be addressed and Leigh (2001) suggests that these can be met through communication about their environment and through touch. Nursing this group of patients can be complex and challenging; however, being proactive to the needs of the unconscious patient can result in positive outcomes for the patient, family and health care professional.

References and further reading

Adam, S.K. & Osborne, S. (2005) *Critical Care Nursing: Science and Practice*, 2nd edn. Oxford University Press, Oxford.

Booij, L. (1996) Muscle relaxants and concurrent diseases. In: *Neuromuscular Transmission* (eds L. Booij *et al.*). BMJ Books, London, pp. 124–59.

Boss, B.J. (1998) Nursing management of adults with common neurologic problems. In: *Adult Health Nursing*, 3rd edn (eds P. Gauntlett Beare & J.L. Myers). Mosby, St. Louis, MO, pp. 904–47.

Carpenito, L.J. (2002) *Nursing Diagnosis: Application to Clinical Practice*, 9th edn. Lippincott, Philadelphia.

Cullum, N. *et al.* (2004) Support surfaces for pressure ulcer prevention. *Cochrane Database Syst Rev*, **3**, CD001735. DOI: 10.1002/14651858.CD001735.pub2.

Drakulovic, M.B. *et al.* (1999) Supine body positions as a risk factor for nosocomial pneumonia in mechanically ventilated patients: a randomised trial. *Lancet*, **354**, 1851–8.

Elliott, R. & Wright, L. (1999) Verbal communication: what do critical care nurses say to their unconscious or sedated patients? *J Adv Nurs*, **29**(6), 1412–20.

Geraghty, M. (2005) Nursing the unconscious patient. *Nurs Stand*, **20**(1), 54–66.

Heron, R. *et al.* (2001) Interrater reliability of the Glasgow Coma Scale scoring among nurses in subspecialities of critical care. *Aust J Crit Care*, **14**(3), 100–5.

Hickey, J.V. (2003a) Neurological assessment. In: *The Clinical Practice of Neurological and Neurosurgical Nursing*, 5th edn. Lippincott, Williams & Wilkins, Philadelphia, pp. 159–84.

Hickey, J.V. (2003b) Management of the unconscious neurological patient. In: *The Clinical Practice of Neurological and Neurosurgical Nursing*, 5th edn. Lippincott, Williams and Wilkins, Philadelphia, pp. 345–57.

Jacobson, A.F. (2000) Caring for unconscious patients. *Am J Nurs*, **100**(1), 69.

Janz B.A. *et al.* (2005) *A Multivariable Analysis of Sedation, Activity and Agitation in Critically Ill Patients Using the Riker Scale, ECG, Blood Pressure, and Respiratory Rate.* Harvard–MIT Division of Health Sciences and Technology, Cambridge MA.

Klaschik, E., Nauck, F. & Ostgathe, C. (2003) Constipation – modern laxative therapy. *Support Care Cancer*, **11**, 679–85.

Kumar, P. & Clark, M. (2001) *Clinical Medicine*, 4th edn. W.B. Saunders, Edinburgh.

Lawrence, M. (1995) The unconscious experience. *Am J Crit Care*, **4**(3), 227–32.

Leigh, K. (2001) Communicating with unconscious patients. *Nurs Times*, **97**(48), 35–6.

Leung, W.C. (2002) Consent to treatment in the A&E department. *Accident Emerg Nurs*, **10**, 17–25.

NICE (2003)*Head Injury, Triage, Assessment, Investigation and Early Management of Head Injury in Infants, Children and Adults*. National Institute for Health and Clinical Excellence, London.

Price, T., Miller, L. & Descissa, M. (2000) The Glasgow Coma Scale in intensive care: a study. *Crit Care Nurs*, **5**(4), 170–3.

Seymour, J. & Ingleton, C. (2004) Transitions into the terminal phase: overview. In: *Palliative Care Nursing: Principles and Evidence for Practice* (eds S. Payne, J. Seymour & C. Ingleton). Open University Press, Milton Keynes, Berks, pp. 187–9.

Travis, S. *et al.* (2001) Guidelines in respect of advance directives. *Int J Palliat Nurs*, **7**(10), 493–500.

UK Clinical Ethics Network (2003) Advance directives (online version). www.ethics-network.org.uk/Ethics/eendlife.htm#advance. Accessed 29/6/06.

Waterlow, J. (1998) The treatment and use of the Waterlow Card. *Nurs Times*, **94**(7), 63–7.

Multiple choice questions

1 What is the recommended position in which to nurse an unconscious patient?

   a   Prone
   b   Supine
   c   Bed head elevated to 30 degrees
   d   Bed head elevated to 45 degrees

2 There are many methods available to measure a patient's level of consciousness. The most commonly used is which of the following?

   a   Glasgow Coma Scale
   b   Glasgow Consciousness Scale
   c   Generalized Consciousness Score
   d   Glasgow Coma Score

3 There are many ethical considerations when caring for an unconscious patient. Some patients may have an advance directive documenting their wishes. Which of the following is true about an advance directive?

   a   Legally binding, but can be difficult to enforce in acute settings
   b   Not legally binding
   c   At the consultant's discretion
   d   Not worth the paper it is written on

4 Which sense is thought to remain intact for the longest time?

   a   Sight
   b   Touch
   c   Hearing
   d   Smell

Answers to the multiple choice questions can be found in Appendix 3.

Chapter 32

Venepuncture

Definition

Venepuncture is the procedure of entering a vein with a needle.

Indications

Venepuncture is carried out for two reasons:

- To obtain a blood sample for diagnostic purposes.
- To monitor levels of blood components.

Reference material

Venepuncture is one of the most commonly performed invasive procedures (Castledine 1996) and is now routinely being undertaken by nurses (Ernst 2005). In order to perform venepuncture safely the nurse must have basic knowledge of the following:

- The relevant anatomy and physiology.
- The criteria for choosing both the vein and device to use.
- The potential problems which may be encountered, how to prevent them and necessary interventions.
- The health and safety/risk management of the procedure, as well as the correct disposal of equipment (RCN 2005).

Certain principles, such as adherence to an aseptic technique, must be applied throughout (see Chapter 4). The circulation is a closed sterile system and a venepuncture, however quickly completed, is a breach of this system providing a means of entry for bacteria.

The nurse must be aware of the physical and psychological comfort of the patient (Hoeltke 2006). He or she must appreciate the value of adequate explanation and simple measures to prevent the complications of venepuncture, such as haematoma formation, when it is neither a natural nor acceptable consequence of the procedure (Hoeltke 2006).

Anatomy and physiology

The superficial veins of the upper limb are most commonly chosen for venepuncture. These veins are numerous and accessible, ensuring that the procedure can be performed safely and with minimum discomfort (Ernst 2005). In adults veins located on the dorsal portion of the foot may be selected but there is an increased risk of deep vein thrombosis (Garza & Becan McBride 2005) or tissue necrosis in diabetics (Ernst 2005). Therefore, veins in the lower limbs should be avoided where possible.

The veins commonly used for venepuncture are those found in the antecubital fossa because they are sizeable veins capable of providing copious and repeated blood specimens (Weinstein 2007). However, the venous anatomy of each individual may differ. The main veins of choice are (Figure 32.1a):

- The median cubital veins.
- The cephalic vein.
- The basilic vein.
- The metacarpal veins (used only when the others are not accessible) (Figure 32.1b).

The median cubital vein may not always be visible, but its size and location make it easy to palpate. It is also well supported by subcutaneous tissue, which prevents it from rolling under the needle.

On the lateral aspect of the wrist, the cephalic vein rises from the dorsal veins and flows upwards along the radial border of the forearm as the median cephalic, crossing the antecubital fossa as the median cubital vein. Care must be taken to avoid accidental arterial puncture, as this vein crosses the brachial artery. It is also in close proximity to the radial nerve (Masoorli 2002; Dougherty 2008).

The basilic vein is often overlooked as a site for venepuncture and has its origins in the ulnar border of the hand and forearm (Waugh & Grant 2006). It may well be prominent but is not well supported by subcutaneous tissue, making it roll easily, which can result in difficult venepuncture. Owing to its position, a haematoma may occur if the patient flexes the arm on removal of the needle, as this squeezes blood from the vein into the surrounding tissues (McCall & Tankersley 2003; Weinstein 2007). Care must also be taken to avoid accidental puncture of the median nerve and brachial artery (Garza & Becan McBride 2005).

(a)

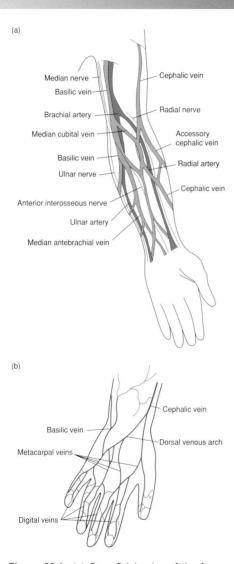

Median nerve
Basilic vein
Brachial artery
Median cubital vein
Basilic vein
Ulnar nerve
Anterior interosseous nerve
Ulnar artery
Median antebrachial vein

Cephalic vein
Radial nerve
Accessory cephalic vein
Radial artery
Cephalic vein

(b)

Basilic vein
Metacarpal veins
Digital veins

Cephalic vein
Dorsal venous arch

Figure 32.1 (a) Superficial veins of the forearm. (b) Superficial veins of dorsal aspect of the hand. (Reproduced with permission from Becton Dickinson and Company.)

The metacarpal veins are easily visualized and palpated. However, the use of these veins is contraindicated in the elderly where skin turgor and subcutaneous tissue are diminished (Weinstein 2007).

Veins consist of three layers: the tunica intima is a smooth endothelial lining, which allows the passage of blood cells. If it becomes damaged, the lining may become roughened and there is an increased risk of thrombus formation (Weinstein 2007). Within this layer are folds of endothelium called valves, which keep blood moving towards the heart by preventing back flow of blood. Valves are present in larger vessels and at points of branching and are present as noticeable bulges in the veins (Weinstein 2007). However, when suction is applied during venepuncture, the valve can compress and close the lumen of the vein, thus preventing the withdrawal of blood (Weinstein 2007). Therefore, if detected, venepuncture should be performed above the valve in order to facilitate collection of the sample (Weinstein 2007).

The tunica media, the middle layer of the vein wall, is composed of muscular tissue and nerve fibres, both vasoconstrictors and vasodilators, which can stimulate the vein to contract or relax. This layer is not as strong or stiff as an artery and therefore veins can distend or collapse as the pressure rises or falls (Waugh & Grant 2006; Weinstein 2007). Stimulation of this layer by a change in temperature, mechanical or chemical stimulation can produce venous spasm, which can make a venepuncture more difficult.

The tunica adventitia is the outer layer and consists of connective tissue, which surrounds and supports the vessel.

Arteries tend to be placed more deeply than veins and can be distinguished by the thicker walls, which do not collapse, the presence of a pulse and the blood is bright red. It should be noted that aberrant arteries may be present. These are arteries that are located superficially in an unusual place (Weinstein 2007).

1058

Choosing a vein

The choice of vein must be that which is best for the individual patient. The most prominent vein is not necessarily the most suitable vein for venepuncture (Weinstein 2007). There are two stages to locating a vein:

1   Visual inspection.
2   Palpation.

Visual inspection is the scrutiny of the veins in both arms and is essential prior to choosing a vein. Veins adjacent to foci of infection, bruising and phlebitis should not be considered, owing to the risk of causing more local tissue damage or systemic infection (Dougherty 2008). An oedematous limb should be avoided as there is danger of stasis of lymph, predisposing to such complications as phlebitis and cellulitis (Smith 1998; Hoeltke 2006). Areas of previous venepuncture should be avoided as a build-up of scar tissue can cause difficulty in accessing the vein and can result in pain due to repeated trauma (Hoeltke 2006).

Palpation is an important assessment technique, as it determines the location and condition of the vein, distinguishes veins from arteries and tendons, identifies the presence of valves and detects deeper veins (Dougherty 2008). The nurse should use the same fingers for palpation as this will increase the sensitivity and ability of the nurse to know what she or he is feeling. The less dominant hand should be used for palpation so that in the event of a missed vein the nurse can repalpate and realign the needle (Hoeltke 2006). The thumb should not be used as it is not as sensitive and has a pulse, which may lead to confusion in distinguishing veins from arteries in the patient (Weinstein 2007).

Thrombosed veins feel hard and cord-like, and should be avoided along with tortuous, sclerosed, fibrosed, inflamed or fragile veins, which may be unable to accommodate the device to be used and will result in pain and repeated venepunctures (Dougherty 2008). Use of veins which cross over joints or bony prominences and those with little skin or subcutaneous cover, e.g. the inner aspect of the wrist, will also subject the patient to more discomfort (Dougherty 2008). Therefore, preference should be given to a vessel that is unused, easily detected by inspection and palpation, patent and healthy. These veins feel soft and bouncy and will refill when depressed (Weinstein 2007).

Influencing factors

- Injury, disease or treatment may prevent the use of a limb for venepuncture thereby reducing the venous access, e.g. amputation, fracture and cerebrovascular accident. Use of a limb may be contraindicated because of an operation on one side of the body, for example mastectomy and axillary node dissection, as this can lead to impairment of lymphatic drainage, which can influence venous flow regardless of whether there is obvious lymphoedema (Ernst 2005; Hoeltke 2006).

- The age and weight of the patient will also influence choice. Young children have short fine veins, and the elderly have prominent but fragile veins. Care must be taken with fragile veins and the largest vein should be chosen along with the smallest gauge device to reduce the amount of trauma to the vessel. Malnourished patients will often present with friable veins.

- If the patient is in shock or dehydrated there will be poor superficial peripheral access. It may be necessary to take blood after the patient is rehydrated as this will promote venous filling and blood will be obtained more easily.

- Medications can influence the choice of vein in that patients on anticoagulants or steroids or those who are thrombocytopenic tend to have more fragile veins and will be at greater risk of bruising both during venepuncture and on removal of the needle. Therefore choice may be limited by areas of bruising present or the inability to access the vessel without causing bruising.

- The temperature of the environment will influence venous dilatation. If the patient is cold, no veins may be evident on first inspection. Application of heat, e.g. in the form of a warm compress or soaking the arm in warm water, will increase the size and visibility of the veins, thus increasing the likelihood of a successful first attempt (Lenhardt *et al.* 2002; Weinstein 2007).

- Venepuncture itself may cause the vein to collapse or go into a spasm. This will produce discomfort and a reduction in blood flow. Careful preparation and choice of vein will reduce the likelihood of this and stroking the vein or applying heat will help resolve it.

- Patient anxiety about the procedure may result in vasoconstriction. The nurse's manner and approach will also have a direct bearing on the patient's experience (Garza & Becan McBride 2005). Approaching the patient with a confident manner and giving an adequate explanation of the procedure may reduce anxiety. Careful preparation and an unhurried approach will help to relax the patient and this in turn will increase vasodilatation (Weinstein 2007; Dougherty 2008). It is important to remember that patients may dread venepuncture (Ernst 2005; Lavery & Ingram 2005) and if a patient is particularly anxious, or for venepuncture in children, the use of a topical local anaesthetic cream may be appropriate (Ernst 2005; Weinstein 2007). Involving patients in the choice of vein, even if it is simply to choose the non-dominant arm, can increase a feeling of control which in turn helps to relieve anxiety (Hudek 1986).

Improving venous access

There are a number of methods of improving venous access:

- Application of a tourniquet: this promotes venous distension. The tourniquet should be tight enough to impede venous return but not restrict arterial flow. The tourniquet should be placed about 7–8 cm above the venepuncture site. It may be more comfortable for the patient to position it over a sleeve or paper towel to prevent pinching the skin. The tourniquet should not be left on for longer than 1 minute as it may result in haemoconcentration or pooling of the blood, leading to inaccurate blood results (Hoeltke 2006).
  There are several types of tourniquet available. A good-quality, buckle closure, single hand release type is most effective but the choice will depend on availability and operator. Consideration should be given to the type of material and the ability to decontaminate the tourniquet (Golder 2000; RCN 2005).

- The patient may be asked to clench the fist and encourage venous distension but should avoid 'pumping' as this action may affect certain blood results, e.g. potassium (Ernst 2005; Garza & Becan McBride 2005).
- Lowering the arm below heart level also increases blood supply to the veins.
- Light tapping of the vein may be useful but can be painful and may result in the formation of a haematoma in patients with fragile veins, e.g. thrombocytopenic patients (Dougherty 2008).
- The use of heat in the form of a warm pack or by immersing the arm in a bowl of warm water for 10 minutes helps to encourage venodilatation and venous filling (Lenhardt *et al.* 2002).
- Ointment or patches containing small amounts of glyceryl trinitrate have been used to improve local vasodilatation to aid venepuncture (Weinstein 2007).

Choice of device

The intravenous devices commonly used to perform a venepuncture for blood sampling are a straight steel needle and a steel winged infusion device. The optimum gauge to use is 21 swg (standard wire gauge), which measures internal diameter: the smaller the gauge size, the larger the diameter. Standard wire gauge measurement is determined by how many cannulae fit into a tube with an inner diameter of 1 inch (2.5 cm), and uses consecutive numbers from 13 to 24. This enables blood to be withdrawn at a reasonable speed without undue discomfort to the patient or possible damage to the blood cells.

Equipment available will depend on local policy (Table 32.1), but with increasing concern about the possibility of contamination to the practitioner, blood collection systems with integrated safety devices are now readily available and should be used wherever possible (Infection Control Nurses Association 2003). However, the nurse must always select the device after assessing the condition and accessibility of the vein.

1061

Skin preparation

Asepsis is vital when performing a venepuncture as the skin is breached and a foreign device is introduced into a sterile circulatory system. The two major sources of microbial contamination are:

- Cross-infection from practitioner to patient.
- Skin flora of the patient.

Good hand washing and drying techniques are essential on the part of the nurse; gloves should be changed between patients (see Chapter 4).

Table 32.1 Choice of intravenous device.

Device	g	Advantages	Disadvantages	Use
Needle	21	Cheaper than winged infusion devices. Easy to use with large veins	Rigid. Difficult to manipulate with smaller veins in less conventional sites. May cause more discomfort. Venous access only confirmed when sample tube attached	Large, accessible veins in the antecubital fossa. When small quantities of blood are to be drawn
Winged infusion device with or without safety shield	21	Flexible due to small needle shaft. Easy to manipulate and insert at any site. Increases the success rate of venepuncture and causes less discomfort (Hefler et al. 2004) Usually shows a 'flashback' of blood to indicate a successful venepuncture	More expensive than steel needles The 12–30 cm length of tubing on the device may be caught and dislodge the needle	Veins in sites other than the antecubital fossa When quantities of blood greater than 20 ml are required from any site
	23	Flexible due to small needle shaft. Easy to manipulate and insert at any site. Causes less discomfort. Smaller swg and therefore useful with fragile veins	More expensive than steel needles, plus there can be damage to cells which can cause inaccurate measurements in certain blood samples, e.g. potassium	Small veins in more painful sites, e.g. inner aspect of the wrist, especially if measurements are related to plasma and not cellular components

To remove the risk presented by the patient's skin flora, firm and prolonged rubbing with an alcohol-based solution, such as chlorhexidine 0.5% in 70% alcohol, is advised (Walther *et al.* 2001). This cleaning should continue for about 30 seconds, although some authors state a minimum of 1 minute or longer (Weinstein 2007). The area that has been cleaned should then be allowed to dry to: (i) facilitate coagulation of the organisms, thus ensuring disinfection; and (ii) prevent a stinging pain on insertion of the needle due to the alcohol on the end of the needle. The skin must not be touched or the vein repalpated prior to venepuncture.

Skin cleaning is a controversial subject and it is acknowledged that a cursory wipe with an alcohol swab does more harm than no cleaning at all as it disturbs the skin flora.

Safety of the practitioner

It is recommended that well-fitting gloves are worn during any procedure that involves handling blood and body fluids, particularly venepuncture and cannulation (Infection Control Nurses Association 2003; NHS Employers 2007; RCN 2005). This is to prevent contamination of the practitioner from potential blood spills. Whilst it is recognized that gloves will not prevent a needle-stick injury, the wiping effect of a glove on a needle may reduce the volume of blood to which the hand is exposed, thereby reducing the volume inoculated and the risk of infection (Mitchell Higgs 2002; Infection Control Nurses Association 2003; National Audit Office 2003). However, there is no substitute for good technique and practitioners must always work carefully when performing venepuncture.

A range of safety devices are now available for venepuncture which can reduce the risk of occupational percutaneous injuries among health care workers, in particular vacuum blood collection systems (CDC 1997). A vacuum system consists of a plastic holder which contains or is attached to a double-ended needle or adaptor. It is important to use the correct Luer adaptor to ensure a good connection and avoid blood leakage (Garza & Becan McBride 2005). The blood tube is vacuumed in order that the exact amount of blood required is withdrawn, when the tube is pushed into the holder. Filling ceases once the tube is full which removes the need for decanting blood and also reduces blood wastage. The system can also be attached to winged infusion devices (Dougherty 2008).

Used needles should always be discarded directly into an approved sharps container, without being resheathed (Infection Control Nurses Association 2003; RCN 2005). Specimens from patients with known or suspected infections such as hepatitis or human immunodeficiency virus (HIV) should have a biohazard label attached. The accompanying request forms should be kept separately from the

1063

specimen to avoid contamination (Health Service Advisory Committee 2003). All other non-sharp disposables should be placed in a universal clinical waste bag.

Removal of the device

It is important to ensure that the needle is removed correctly on completion of blood sampling and that the risk of haematoma formation is minimized. Pressure should be applied as the needle is removed from the skin. If pressure is applied too early, it causes the tip of the needle to drag along the intima of the vein, resulting in sharp pain and damage to the lining of the vessel.

The practitioner should ensure that firm pressure is maintained until bleeding has stopped. The patient should also be instructed to keep his or her arm straight and not bend it as this also results in an increased risk of bruising (Ernst 2005). A longer period of pressure may be necessary where the patient's blood may take longer to clot, for example, if the patient is receiving anticoagulants or is thrombocytopenic. The practitioner may choose to apply the tourniquet over the venepuncture site to ensure even and constant pressure on the area (Perdue 2001). Alternatively they can elevate the arm slightly above the heart to decrease venous pressure (Garza & Becan McBride 2005).

The practitioner should inspect the site carefully for bleeding or bruising before applying a dressing to the site, and the patient leaving the department. If bruising has occurred the patient should be informed of why this has happened and given instructions for what to do to reduce the bruising and any associated pain. Initially the application of an ice pack may help to soothe and decrease bruising. The application of Hirudoid cream, which is used for the treatment of thrombophlebitis, may be helpful (BMA & RPS 2008).

1064 ## Summary

In order to perform a safe and successful venepuncture, it is important that the practitioner:

- Considers carefully the choice of vein and device.
- Applies the principles of asepsis.
- Adheres to and understands safe technique and practices.

Recently there has been an increase in the number of cases of litigation involving injuries, which have occurred as a result of venepuncture (Garza & Becan McBride 2005). It is therefore vital that nurses receive accredited and appropriate training, supervision and assessment by an experienced member of staff (RCN 2005). The nurse is then accountable and responsible for ensuring that his or her skills and competence are maintained and his or her knowledge is kept up to date, in order to fulfil the criteria set out in the *The Code* (NMC 2008).

Procedure guidelines **Venepuncture**

Equipment

1 Clean tray or receiver.
2 Tourniquet or sphygmomanometer and cuff.
3 21 swg multiple sample needle or 21 swg winged infusion device and multiple sample Luer adaptor.
4 Plastic tube holder, standard or for blood cultures.
5 Appropriate vacuumed specimen tubes.
6 Swab saturated with chlorhexidine in 70% alcohol, or isopropyl alcohol 70%.
7 Low-linting swabs.
8 Sterile adhesive plaster or hypoallergenic tape.
9 Specimen request forms.
10 Non-sterile well-fitting gloves.
11 Plastic apron (optional).
12 Sharps bin.

A number of vacuum systems are available that can be used for taking blood samples. These are simple to use and cost effective. The manufacturer's instructions should be followed if one of these systems is used. Vacuum systems reduce the risk of health care workers being contaminated, because they offer a completely closed system during the process of blood withdrawal and there is no necessity to decant blood into bottles (Dougherty 2008). This makes them the safest method for collecting blood samples using venepuncture. If not available, the following items replace the vacuum system:

1 21 swg needle or 21 swg winged infusion device.
2 Syringe(s) of appropriate size.
3 Appropriate blood specimen bottle(s).

Procedure

Action	Rationale
1 Approach the patient in a confident manner and explain and discuss the procedure with the patient.	To ensure that the patient understands the procedure and gives his/her valid consent (DH 2001: C; NMC 2008: C).
2 Allow the patient to ask questions and discuss any problems which have arisen previously.	Anxiety results in vasoconstriction; therefore, a patient who is relaxed will have dilated veins, making access easier (E).
3 Consult the patient as to any preferences and problems that may have been experienced at previous venepunctures.	To involve the patient in the treatment. To acquaint the nurse fully with the patient's previous venous history and identify any changes in clinical status, e.g. mastectomy, as both may influence vein choice (Dougherty 2008: E).

Procedure guidelines (*cont.*)

4 Check the identity of the patient matches the details on the request form by asking for their full name and date of birth and checking their identification bracelet.

To ensure the sample is taken from the correct patient (E).

5 Assemble the equipment necessary for venepuncture.

To ensure that time is not wasted and that the procedure goes smoothly without unnecessary interruptions (E).

6 Carefully wash hands using bactericidal soap and water or bactericidal alcohol handrub, and dry before commencement.

To minimize risk of infection (DH 2005: C).

7 Check hands for any visibly broken skin, and cover with a waterproof dressing.

To minimize the risk of contamination to the practitioner (DH 2005a: C).

8 Check all packaging before opening and preparing the equipment on the chosen clean receptacle.

To maintain asepsis throughout and check that no equipment is damaged (E).

9 Take all the equipment to the patient, exhibiting a competent manner.

To help the patient feel more at ease with the procedure (E).

10 In both an inpatient and an outpatient situation, lighting, ventilation, privacy and positioning must be checked.

To ensure that both patient and operator are comfortable and that adequate light is available to illuminate this procedure (E).

11 Support the chosen limb on a pillow.

To ensure the patient's comfort and facilitate venous access (E).

12 (a) Apply a tourniquet to the upper arm on the chosen side, making sure it does not obstruct arterial flow. If the radial pulse cannot be palpated then the tourniquet is too tight (Weinstein 2007). The position of the tourniquet may be varied, e.g. if a vein in the hand is to be used it may be placed on the forearm. A sphygmomanometer cuff may be used as an alternative.

To dilate the veins by obstructing the venous return (Dougherty 2008: E).

(b) The arm may be placed in a dependent position. The patient may be asked to clench their fist.

To Increase the prominence of the veins (E).

(c) The veins may be tapped gently or stroked.

(d) If all these measures are unsuccessful, remove the tourniquet and apply moist heat, e.g. a warm compress, soak limb in warm water or, with medical prescription, apply glyceryl trinitrate ointment/patch.

To promote blood flow and therefore distend the veins (Lenhardt *et al*. 2002: R 3; E).

13 Select the vein using the aforementioned criteria (see Action figure 13).

To prevent haemocentration and pooling of the blood (Hoeltke 2006: E).

14 Release the tourniquet.

To ensure patient comfort (E).

15 Select the device, based on vein size, site, etc.

To reduce damage or trauma to the vein (RCN 2005: C; Dougherty 2008: E).

16 Wash hands with bactericidal soap and water or bactericidal alcohol handrub.

To maintain asepsis, and minimize the risk of infection (DH 2005a: C).

17 Reapply the tourniquet.

To dilate the veins by obstructing the venous return (Dougherty 2008: E).

18 Put on gloves.

To prevent possible contamination of the practitioner (NHS Employers 2007: C).

19 Clean the patient's skin carefully for 30 seconds using an appropriate preparation, e.g. chlorhexidine in 70% alcohol, and allow to dry. Do not repalpate or touch the skin (see Action figure 19).

To maintain asepsis and minimize the risk of infection (DH 2005a: C). To prevent pain on insertion (DH 2005a: C; RCN 2005: C; Dougherty 2008: E).

20 Remove the cover from the needle and inspect the device carefully.

To detect faulty equipment, e.g. bent or barbed needles. If these are present place them in a safe container, record batch details and return to manufacturer (MHRA 2005: C; RCN 2005: C).

Procedure guidelines (*cont.*)

21 Anchor the vein by applying manual traction on the skin a few centimetres below the proposed insertion site (see Action figure 21).	To immobilize the vein. To provide countertension to the vein which will facilitate a smoother needle entry (Dougherty 2008: E).
22 Insert the needle smoothly at an angle of approximately 30°. However, this will depend on size and depth of the vein (also see Action figure 21).	To facilitate a successful, pain-free venepuncture (E).
23 Reduce the angle of descent of the needle as soon as a flashback of blood is seen in the tubing of a winged infusion device or when puncture of the vein wall is felt. If you are using a needle and syringe, pull the plunger back slightly prior to venepuncture and a flashback of blood will be seen in the barrel on vein entry.	To prevent advancing too far through vein wall and causing damage to the vessel (E).
24 Slightly advance the needle into the vein, if possible.	To stabilize the device within the vein and prevent it becoming dislodged during withdrawal of blood (E).
25 Do not exert any pressure on the needle.	To prevent a puncture occurring through the vein wall (E).
26 Withdraw the required amount of blood using a vacuumed blood collection system or syringes (see Action figure 26). Collect blood samples in the following order: ■ Blood culture. ■ Coagulation. ■ Serum tube with or without clot activator or gel separator. (Glass, non-additive tubes can be filled before the coagulation tube.) ■ Additive tubes such as: (a) gel separator tubes (may contain clot activator or heparin); (b) heparin tubes; (c) EDTA. ■ All other tubes (National Committee for Clinical Laboratory Standards 2003 cited in Garza & Becan McBride 2005, pp. 277–8).	To minimize the risk of transferring additives from one tube to another and bacterial contamination of blood cultures (Manufacturer's guidelines: C).

27 Release the tourniquet. In some instances this may be necessary at the beginning of sampling as inaccurate measurements may be caused by haemostasis, e.g. when taking blood to assess calcium levels.	To decrease the pressure within the vein (E).
Remove tube from plastic tube holder.	To prevent blood spillage caused by vacuum in the tube (Campbell *et al.* 1999: E).
28 If using a needle and syringe withdraw a small amount of blood into the syringe.	To reduce the amount of static blood in the vein and therefore the likelihood of leakage at the venepuncture site on removal of the needle (E).
29 Pick up a low-linting swab and place it over the puncture point.	To apply pressure (E).
30 Remove the needle, but do not apply pressure until the needle has been fully removed.	To prevent pain on removal and damage to the intima of the vein (E).
31 Activate safety device, if applicable, and then discard the needle immediately in sharps bin.	To reduce the risk of accidental needlestick injury (NHS Employers 2007: C).
32 Apply digital pressure directly over the puncture site. Pressure should be applied until bleeding has ceased; approximately 1 minute or longer may be required if current disease or treatment interferes with clotting mechanisms.	To stop leakage and haematoma formation. To preserve vein by preventing bruising or haematoma formation (E).
33 The patient may apply pressure with the finger but should be discouraged from bending the arm if a vein in the antecubital fossa is used.	To prevent leakage and haematoma formation (Ernst 2005: E).
34 Where a syringe has been used, transfer the blood to appropriate specimen bottles as soon as possible, making sure that the correct quantity is placed in each container.	To prevent clotting in the syringe. To ensure that an adequate amount is available for each test (E).

1069

Procedure guidelines (*cont.*)

35 Gently invert tube at least six times.	To prevent damage to blood cells and to mix with additives (Manufacturer's guidelines: C).
36 Label the bottles with the relevant details.	To ensure that the specimens from the right patient are delivered to the laboratory, the requested tests are performed and the results returned to the correct patient's records (E).
37 Inspect the puncture point before applying a dressing.	To check that the puncture point has sealed (E).
38 Ascertain whether the patient is allergic to adhesive plaster.	To prevent an allergic skin reaction (E).
39 Apply an adhesive plaster or alternative dressing.	To cover the puncture and prevent leakage or contamination (E).
40 Ensure that the patient is comfortable.	To ascertain whether patient wishes to rest before leaving (if an outpatient) or whether any other measures need to be taken (E).
41 Remove gloves and discard waste, making sure it is placed in the correct containers, e.g. sharps into a designated receptacle.	To ensure safe disposal and avoid laceration or other injury of staff. (DH 2005b: C). To prevent reuse of equipment. (MDA 2000: C).
42 Follow hospital procedure for collection and transportation of specimens to the laboratory.	To make sure that specimens reach their intended destination (E).

1070

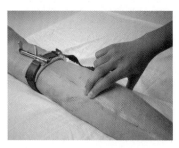

Action 13 Palpating the vein.

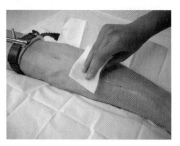

Action 19 Cleaning the skin.

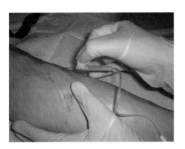

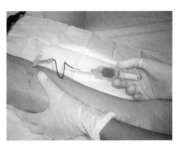

Action 21   Anchoring the skin.

Action 26   Attach sample bottle to holder.

Problem solving: Venepuncture

Problem	Cause	Prevention	Suggested action
Pain.	Puncturing an artery.	Knowledge of location of an artery. Palpate vessel for pulse.	Remove device immediately and apply pressure until bleeding stops. Explain to patient what has happened. Inform patient to contact doctor if pain continues or there is increasing swelling or bruising. Document in the patient's notes. Provide information leaflet.
	Touching a nerve (sharp, shooting pain along arm and fingers).	Knowledge of location of nerves. Avoid excessive or blind probing after needle has been inserted.	Remove the needle immediately and apply pressure. Explain to the patient what has happened and that the pain or numbness may last a few hours. Document in the patient's notes. Inform patient to contact doctor if pain continues or becomes worse. Provide information leaflet.
	Anxiety.	(See below.)	(See below.)
	Use of vein in sensitive area (e.g. wrist).	Avoid using veins in sensitive areas wherever possible. Use local anaesthetic cream.	Complete procedure as quickly as possible.

Problem solving *(cont.)*

Problem	Cause	Prevention	Suggested action
Anxiety.	Previous trauma.	Minimize the risk of a traumatic venepuncture. Use all methods available to ensure successful venepuncture.	Approach patient in a calm and confident manner. Listen to the patient's fears and explain what the procedure involves. Offer patient opportunity to lie down. Suggest use of local anaesthetic cream (Lavery & Ingram 2005).
	Fear of needles.		All of the above and perhaps referral to a psychologist if fear is of phobic proportions.
Limited venous access.	Repeated use of same veins.	Use alternative sites if possible.	Do not attempt the procedure unless experienced.
	Peripheral shutdown.	Ensure the room is not cold.	Put patient's arm in warm water. Apply glycerol trinitrate patch.
	Dehydration.		May be necessary to rehydrate patient prior to venepuncture.
	Hardened veins (due to scarring and thrombosis).		Do not use these veins as venepuncture will be unsuccessful.
Bruising and/or haematoma.	Needle has punctured the posterior wall of the vein. Inadequate pressure on removal of needle.	Lower angle of insertion. The practitioner should apply pressure.	Remove the needle and apply pressure at the venepuncture site until bleeding stops. The following actions apply regardless of cause: (a) Elevate the limb. (b) Apply ice pack if necessary. (c) Apply Hirudoid cream or arnica cream (as per instructions) with pressure dressing.

Problem	Cause	Prevention	Suggested action
	Forgetting to remove the tourniquet before removing the needle.		Explain to patient what has happened. Inform patient to contact doctor if area becomes more painful as haematoma may be pressing on a nerve. Do not reapply tourniquet to affected limb. Provide information leaflet. Document.
	Poor technique/ choice of vein or device.	Ensure correct device and technique are used.	
Infection at the venepuncture site.	Poor aseptic technique.	Ensure good hand washing and adequate skin cleaning.	Report to doctor as patient may require systemic or local antibiotics.
Vasovagal reaction.	Fear of needles. Pain.	Spend time listening to patient's fears in a calm, confident manner.	Place patient's head between his/her legs if patient is feeling faint. Encourage patient to lie down. Call for assistance. It may be appropriate to secure the device (short term) in case it is required for the administration of medication.
	Warm environment.	Ensure environment is comfortable temperature.	Open a window or door.
Needle inoculation of or contamination to practitioner.	Unsafe practice. Incorrect disposal of sharps.	Maintain safe practice. Activate safety device if applicable. Ensure sharps are disposed of immediately and safely.	Follow accident procedure for sharps injury, e.g. make site bleed and apply a waterproof dressing. Report and document. An injection of hepatitis B immunoglobulin or triple therapy may be required.

1073

Problem solving (cont.)

Problem	Cause	Prevention	Suggested action
Accidental blood spillage.	Damaged/faulty equipment.	Check equipment prior to use.	Report within hospital and/or MHRA.
	Reverse vacuum.	Use vacuumed plastic blood collection system. Remove blood tube from plastic tube holder before removing needle.	Ensure blood is handled and transported correctly.
Missed vein.	Inadequate anchoring. Poor vein selection. Wrong positioning. Lack of concentration. Poor lighting.	Ensure that only properly trained staff perform venepuncture or that those who are training are supervised. Ensure the environment is well lit.	Withdraw the needle slightly and realign it, providing the patient is not feeling any discomfort. Ensure all learners are supervised. If the patient is feeling pain, then the needle should be removed immediately.
	Difficult venous access.		Ask experienced colleague to perform the procedure.
Spurt of blood on entry.	Bevel tip of needle enters the vein before entire bevel is under the skin; usually occurs when the vein is very superficial.		Reassure the patient. Wipe blood away on removal of needle.

Problem	Cause	Prevention	Suggested action
Blood stops flowing.	Through puncture: needle inserted too far.	Correct angle.	Draw back the needle, but if bruising is evident, then remove the needle immediately and apply pressure.
	Contact with valves.	Palpate to locate.	Withdraw needle slightly to move tip away from valve.
	Venous spasm.	Results from mechanical irritation and cannot be prevented.	Gently massage above the vein or apply heat.
	Vein collapse.	Use veins with large lumen. Use a smaller device.	Release tourniquet, allow veins to refill and retighten tourniquet.
	Small vein.	Avoid use of small veins wherever possible.	May require another venepuncture.
	Poor blood flow.	Use veins with large lumens.	Apply heat above vein.

References and further reading

BMA & RPS (2008) *British National Formulary*. British Medical Association and Royal Pharmaceutical Society of Great Britain, London.

Campbell, H., Carrington, M. & Limber, C. (1999) A practice guide to venepuncture and management of complications. *Br J Nurs*, 8(7), 426–31.

Castledine, G. (1996) Nurses' role in peripheral venous cannulation. *Br J Nurs*, 5(20), 1274.

CDC (1997) Evaluation of safety devices for preventing percutaneous injuries among health care workers during phlebotomy procedures. *JAMA*, 277(6), 449–50.

DH (2001) *Good Practice in Consent Implementation Guide: Consent to Examination or Treatment*. www.dh.gov.uk. Accessed 24/9/07.

DH (2005a) *Saving Lives: A Delivery Programme to Reduce Healthcare Associated Infection including MRSA*. Department of Health, London.

DH (2005b) *Hazardous Waste (England) Regulations*. Department of Health, London.

Dougherty, L. (2008) Obtaining vascular access. In: *IV Therapy in Practice* (eds L. Dougherty & J. Lamb), 2nd edn. Blackwell Publishing, Oxford.

Ernst, D. & Ernst, C. (2001) *Phlebotomy for Nurses and Nursing Personnel*. Health Star Press, Indiana.

Ernst, D.J. (2005) *Applied Phlebotomy*. Lippincott, Williams & Wilkins, Baltimore.

Garza, D. & Becan McBride, K. (2005) *Phlebotomy Handbook: Blood Collection Essentials*. Prentice Hall, New Jersey.

Golder, M. (2000) Potential risk of cross infection during peripheral venous access by contamination of tourniquets. *Lancet*, **355**, 44.

Health Service Advisory Committee (2003) *Safe Working and the Prevention of Infection in Clinical Laboratories and Similar Facilities.* HMSO, London.

Hefler, L. *et al.* (2004) To butterfly or to needle: the pilot phase. *Ann Intern Med*, **140**(11), 935–6.

Hoeltke, L.B. (2006) *The Complete Textbook of Phlebotomy*, 3rd edn. Thomson Delmar Learning, New York.

Hudek, K. (1986) Compliance in IV therapy. *J Can Intraven Nurs Assoc*, **2**(3), 3–8.

Hyde, L. (2008) Legal and professional aspects of IV therapy. In: *IV Therapy in Practice* (eds L. Dougherty & J. Lamb). Churchill Livingstone, Edinburgh.

Infection Control Nurses Association (2003) *Reducing Sharps Injury – Prevention and Risk Management.* Infection Control Nurses Association, London.

Intravenous Nursing Society (2006) *Standards for Infusion Therapy.* Intravenous Nursing Society & Becton Dickinson and Company, New York.

Lavery, I. & Ingram, P. (2005) Venepuncture: best practice. *Nurs Stand*, **19**(49), 55–65.

Lenhardt, R. *et al.* (2002) Active hand warming eases peripheral intravenous catheter insertion. *BMJ*, **325**, 409–12.

Masoorli, S. (2002) Catheter related nerve injury: inherent risk or avoidable outcome? *J Vasc Access Devices*, **7**(4), 49.

McCall, R.E. & Tankersley, C.M. (2003) Blood collection variables and procedural errors. In: *Phlebotomy Essentials*, 3rd edn. Lippincott, Williams & Wilkins, Philadelphia.

Medical Devices Agency (MDA) (REFA) (2000) Single-use medical devices: implications and consequences of reuse. In: *Device Bulletin 2000, 04.* Department of Health, London.

MHRA (2005) *Alert MDA 2005/01 and Device Bulletin DB 2005 (01), Reporting Adverse Incidents and Disseminating Medical Device Alerts.* Medicines and Healthcare Products Agency, London.

Mitchell Higgs, N. (2002) Personal protective equipment – improving compliance. All Points Conference, Safer Needles Network, London, May.

National Audit Office (2003) *A Safer Place to Work – Management of Health and Safety Risks in Trusts.* National Audit Office, London.

NHS Employers (2007) Needlestick injury. In: *The Healthy Workplaces Handbook.* National Health Service, London, Chapter 19.

NMC (2008) *The Code: Standards of Conduct, Performance and Ethics for Nurses and Midwives.* Nursing and Midwifery Council, London.

Perdue, M.B. (2001) Intravenous complications. In: *Infusion Therapy in Clinical Practice* (eds J. Hankin *et al.*), 2nd edn. W.B. Saunders, Philadelphia, pp. 418–45.

RCN (1995) *Universal Precautions.* Royal College of Nursing, London.

RCN (2005) *Standards for Infusion Therapy.* Royal College of Nursing, London.

Smith, J. (1998) The practice of venepuncture in lymphoedema. *Eur J Cancer Care*, **7**, 97–8.

Walther, K. *et al.* (2001) IV therapy in the older adult. In: *Infusion Therapy in Clinical Practice* (eds J. Hankin *et al.*), 2nd edn. W.B. Saunders, Philadelphia, pp. 592–603.

Waugh, A. & Grant, A. (2006) The cardiovascular system. In: *Anatomy and Physiology in Health and Illness*, 10th edn. Churchill Livingstone, Edinburgh, p. 101.

Weinstein, S.M. (2007) *Plumer's Principles and Practice of Intravenous Therapy*, 8th edn. Lippincott, Williams & Wilkins, Philadelphia.

Multiple choice questions

1 Venepuncture should always be performed as:

    a   A clean procedure
    b   A quick procedure
    c   An aseptic procedure
    d   An alcoholic procedure

2 The main veins that should be used for venepuncture are:

    a   Median cubital and cephalic
    b   Cephalic
    c   Median cubital, cephalic, basilic and metarcapal
    d   Metarcarpal and cephalic

3 What methods could be used to improve access to a vein?

    a   Application of a tourniquet
    b   Use of heat
    c   Light tapping of the vein
    d   All of the above

4 Skin cleansing is important prior to venepuncture. The recommended skin cleansing solution is:

    a   0.9% sodium chloride
    b   Sterile water
    c   Chlorohexidine 0.5% in 70% alcohol
    d   Alcohol swab

5 Following venepuncture, used needles should be:

 a Discarded when the patient is comfortable
 b Discarded into a sharps container without being resheathed
 c Discard into a sharps container
 d Discard into a sharps container resheathed

6 Following removal of needle you should:

 a Immediately cover site with a plaster
 b Apply pressure to insertion site until bleeding stops
 c Apply an op-site dressing
 d Immediately apply gauze dressing

Answers to the multiple choice questions can be found in Appendix 3.

Chapter 33

Violence: prevention and management

Definition

Violence is endemic in our health care system and is, for many staff working in certain areas, an almost daily occurrence (NMC 2002). Violence at work can be defined as:

> Any incident in which a health care employee is verbally abused, threatened or assaulted by a patient or member of the public in the circumstances of their employment.
>
> (HSE 2000: 1)

The Royal College of Nursing (RCN) recommends the following definition of violence orientated towards staff members:

> Any incident in which a health professional experiences abuse, threat, fear or the application of force arising out of the course of their work, whether or not they are on duty.
>
> (RCN 1998: 3)

However, as violence is also directed towards other individuals and objects, the local policy should encompass these aspects. The Nursing and Midwifery Council (NMC) advises nurses to be aware of their individual organizational policies on assessment and management of violence. This should extend to being aware of what support is available should an incident occur.

It can therefore be concluded from the above definitions that violence is an act or type of behaviour that may take the form of aggression, abuse, threat or assault (with or without injury).

Reference material

Prevalence

In 1999, the government developed the National Health Service (NHS) 'Zero Tolerance' Campaign in England with the aim of tackling the issue of violence and intimidation against NHS staff. The target was to reduce incidents of violence in all trusts by 30% by 2003. However, violent crime in the UK is steadily increasing and nearly 650 000 workers had experienced at least one violent incident during 1997 (Mahar 2002). In 1999 there were 65 000 reported violent incidents in British hospitals. By 2001 the number had increased by 30% to 85 000 (DH 2001). In April 2003 the NHS Security Management Service was set up to work with the Crown Prosecution Service taking legal action against those who assault health care workers. Donnelly (2006) described the figures released, showing 51 prosecutions in 2002/03 compared to 759 in 2004/05. With improved reporting systems there has been a 15-fold increase in the number of prosecutions (DH 2006). Official figures for 2005 showed 60 385 NHS staff physically assaulted, i.e. one assault for every 22 NHS staff (DH 2006). The RCN's Working Well Survey (RCN 2005) showed 79% of Accident and Emergency (A&E) nurses reported being victims of violent attack during 2005/06 compared to ward (52%) and care home (48%) nurses.

Moreover, there is evidence to suggest that acts of violence against NHS staff, for a variety of reasons, are still underreported (Arnetz & Arnetz 2000; Rippon 2000; Beech 2001; Paterson *et al.* 2001; Fern 2006). Nonetheless, assaults in the UK are now the third most common type of reported accident after slips, falls and needle accidents. Nurses, ambulance and A&E staff, and those caring for psychologically disturbed patients, are particularly vulnerable (Dobson 1999). Incidents range from threats and abuse to permanently disabling injuries and, rarely, loss of life. Wells and Bowers (2002) carried out a systematic literature search focusing on data of the prevalence of violence towards nurses in general hospitals in the UK; they concluded a majority of assaults occur outside the A&E, citing Whittington *et al.* (1996). They also identified differences in definition of violence and suggested a three category classification; namely, abuse, threats and assaults (with or without injury). The issue of underreporting was also highlighted.

This chapter aims to consider assessment and management of violence in non-psychiatric hospital settings. It is set out following the National Institute for Health and Clinical Excellence (NICE) guideline on violence (NICE 2005) considering: prediction, prevention, intervention and post-incident review. Firstly, a reference to legislation.

1080

Legislation

The law on health and safety at work applies to risks from violence, just as it does to other risks at work. Key points are summarized as follows.

1 *Health and Safety at Work Act* (Department of Employment 1974):
Employers must:
 (a) Protect the health and safety at work of their employees
 (b) Protect the health and safety of others who might be affected, such as visitors, contractors, students and patients.

2 *Management of Health and Safety at Work Regulations* (HSE 1999):
  Employers must:
  (a) Assess the risks to the health and safety of their employees
  (b) Identify the precautions needed to reduce the risks of violence
  (c) Make arrangements for the effective management of risks
  (d) Appoint competent people to advise them on health and safety
  (e) Provide information and training to employees.

3 *The Reporting of Injuries, Diseases and Dangerous Occurrences Regulations* (HSE 1995):
  These Regulations state that employers must report cases in which employees have been off work for 3 days or more following an assault which has resulted in physical injury. This should be in conjunction with the local incident policy in which any psychological injury is also documented.

4 *The Safety Representatives and Safety Committees Regulations 1977 and The Health and Safety (Consultation with Employees) Regulations 1996* (HSE 1996):
  Employers must consult with safety representatives and employees on health and safety matters (Health Services Advisory Committee 1997).

5 *Employment Rights Act (1996)* (Department of Employment 1996):
  Outlines staff member's right to withdraw from his/her care environment if he/she feels seriously under threat.

6 In 2003, the NHS Security Management Service
  instigated a new reporting system based on clear definitions of violence. Special investigators and NHS legal protection units work now with the Crown Prosecution Service.

Policy formation

NHS Trusts must establish targets for reducing violence against their staff. In addition, NHS Trusts will be expected to have systems in place to monitor and record violence against staff and have published strategies in place to achieve a reduction in such incidents (Dobson 1999).

In forming a policy for managing aggression or violence, the following aspects need to be considered:

- Anticipation and prevention of violence.
- Environmental and organizational factors.
- Action following an incident.

Prediction

The NICE guidance for the short-term management of violence (NICE 2005) refers to a list of risk factors to predict potential violent behaviour. The risks are divided into the following categories: demographic or personal history; clinical variables; situational variables; antecedents and warning signs:

Demographic/personal history

- History of violent behaviour.
- History of substance/alcohol misuse.
- Previous expression of violent intent.
- Known personal triggers.
- Verbal threats of violence.
- Recent severe stress.

Clinical variables

- Active symptoms, e.g. hallucinations, agitation.
- Substance misuse.
- Poor collaboration with treatment.
- Antisocial, impulsive personality traits.
- Organic dysfunction.

Situation variables

- Extent of social support.
- Availability of weapon.
- Relationship to potential victim especially if previous difficulties known.
- Access to potential victim.
- Limit settings.
- Staff attitudes.

Antecedents/warning signs

- Tense angry facial signs.
- Increased restlessness.
- General overarousal of body systems (increased heart rate, breathing, muscle twitching, dilating pupils).
- Increased volume of speech.
- Prolonged eye contact.
- Discontentment, refusal to communicate, fear.
- Unclear thought process.
- Delusions or hallucinations.
- Verbal threats.

- Similar behaviour to previous incidents of violence.
- Reporting angry feelings.
- Blocking escape routes.

Prediction of violence may also be understood in terms of factors that may combine to explain or produce a violent act. These are reviewed by Harrington (1972) and Gunn (1973). Generally, theories of violence may be classified as biological (Lorenz 1966; Gray 1971; Montague 1979), psychological (Freud 1955; Dollard & Miller 1961) or sociocultural (Bandura & Walters 1963; Wertham 1968; Gelles 1972). Although the latter of these cannot be completely divorced from organic or biological predisposition, certain factors may increase the risk of violent or aggressive behaviour. Glasser (1998) also discusses the psychoanalytical perspective of violent acts which may be characterized as one of two types: self-preservation violence or sado-masochistic violence. Self-preservation violence is given as an instinctive, primitive response to danger or threat, whereas sado-masochistic violence is premeditated, usually sustained and pleasure is derived from the suffering of the object (Glasser 1998). In the hospital setting where reactions to stress, illness and treatment are prevalent, prediction, assessment and prevention will help to manage potentially violent situations.

It is important to realize that each visitor, contractor, outpatient or relative visiting the hospital will have individual needs, anxieties and expectations. Tension may be released in terms of anger, and on occasions violence, towards other members of their family or staff that they encounter. Factors such as poor sign-posting, failure to find a parking space, long waiting times for an appointment, inadequate welfare facilities, perceived queue-jumping and inadequate information can all increase the risk of conflict and aggression (Royal Marsden Hospital 2002).

Under certain circumstances patients may have little or no ability to exercise control over their aggression. In these instances aggression may be related to pathological physiology. Internal stressors may include endocrine imbalance such as hyperthyroidism and hyperglycaemia. Krakowski and Czobor (1994) confirmed an association between persistent violence and neurological impairment, e.g. convulsive disorders, human immunodeficiency virus (HIV), encephalopathy, dementia and brain tumours. The effects of alcohol and substance abuse should also be considered. One study showed that rates for people with schizophrenia perpetrating violent acts were four times those of populations without mental disorders. For the so-called dual diagnosis populations (with co-existing mental illness and drug/alcohol misuse), rates were four times higher than for people with schizophrenia, i.e. 16 times higher than the general population (NMC 2002). Among the physiological causes given by Kerr and Taylor (1997) are pain, side-effects of medication (including neuroleptic-induced akathisia) and childhood disorders such as autism and mental retardation.

1083

Common antecedents include patients' boredom, inadequate staffing levels, lack of opportunity for patients to participate in therapy and social groups, and staff attitudes, including physical abuse, racism, ridicule of service users and matters of confidentiality (NMC 2002).

Incidents of verbal or physical abuse are more likely to happen in long-term care and emergency areas and may be directed towards nurses and nursing assistants rather than doctors. In the UK, of all health care professions and grades, student nurses were at the greatest risk of being the victim of a work-related violent incident (Beech 1999). Furthermore, male staff were more involved in actual recorded incidents than expected in the given population (Vanderslott 1998). Violence may be viewed as behaviour influenced by various factors including personality, environment and social culture. Each perspective may add to the development of a body of knowledge about the problem of violence in the hospital setting.

Risk assessment

The purpose of risk assessment of violence is to identify how and why conflict can occur and consider what measures can be taken to reduce the risks of such events within the workplace. The risk assessment process for the identification and control of violence can be separated into the following steps: environmental; organizational; situational and attitudinal (NICE 2005).

It is helpful if there is an assessment form for the risks that are being assessed which can be completed in discussion with staff within the department. A review of past incidents will provide an opportunity to identify potential sources of conflict, potential aggressors and likely risk factors. For example, the assessment should consider whether any particular areas present a higher risk of violence such as:

- Front-line reception areas.
- Inpatient clinical areas.
- Outpatient clinical areas.
- Communal areas.
- Community.
- Lone working, e.g. interview rooms, isolated offices.

Regular and comprehensive risk assessments will ensure the clinical environment remains safe. Assessments can also highlight specific interventions which may be required in the management of an ongoing violent situation.

Structured and sensitive interviews ascertaining the patient's view and their level of awareness in relation to their trigger factors and early warning signs.

Multidisciplinary involvement appropriate to the clinical setting should also be reflected in the assessment.

Cultural awareness is important specifically in relation to behaviours which may be misinterpreted as being aggressive.

Following assessment, if the risk of violent behaviour is identified intervention and management strategies should be recorded within a care plan and in the medical records. High risk assessments may necessitate searching the person identified as a risk. This must only happen according to local policy.

Prevention

Preventing situations of violent and aggressive behaviour include consideration of the following factors:

- Use of communication skills including de-escalation techniques.
- Training.
- Formulating a care plan.
- Deciding upon the appropriate level of observation.
- Environmental and organizational.

Signs of high arousal (boisterousness), irritability, confusion and anger (threats or attacks on inanimate objects) are reliable predictors of imminent assaults on staff (Whittington 1997). Responding to these cues to violence with an appropriate verbal interaction and non-verbal behaviour can prevent the escalation of an incident (NMC 2002).

Sheffield University has developed a model for de-escalation called 'CASE', the acronym standing for Calming, Accessing and Self Enabling, which takes into account the internal (thoughts and feelings) and external (behaviour) communication factors for both the nurse and the patient (Walker 2002). The nurse uses verbal and non-verbal skills to calm the situation down and access his or her own thoughts and feelings whilst encouraging the patient to do the same. For example, the nurse asks the angry patient if he would like to sit down and talk about what is upsetting him. This enables the nurse to assess not only the patient's level of emotion but also his cognitive ability to help resolve the conflict. When the patient sits down as offered and is ready to engage in conversation, the enabling phase comes into effect. There may be more negotiating language in the communication which gives an indication that the anger is subsiding to a level where he is more able to think and behave rationally (Walker 2002).

Knowledge of the propensities of individual patients will enable a nurse to recognize many of the signs of impending violence, thus allowing steps to be taken to help patients find alternative outlets for their aggressive feelings. These can be documented in the patient's care plan.

1085

The way in which staff are deployed influences the likelihood and outcome of any violent incident. Teaching sessions on the management of violence should be held on a regular basis so that staff benefit from controlled practice of the required techniques for avoiding or containing violence. Topics may include assessment and prediction of risk factors, the do's and don'ts of verbal and non-verbal interaction and breakaway skills training (Beech 1999).

The NICE guidance for the short-term management of violence (2005) describes four different levels of observation: general; intermittent; within eyesight; and within arm's length. The least intrusive level should be adopted as appropriate.

Hospital environments can be stressful places and so certain design features can help to maximize a tranquil ambience. Calming features include creating a perception of space, ensuring there is natural daylight and fresh air and noise levels are controlled, providing smoking and non-smoking areas and ensuring privacy in toilet and bathroom areas. In creating a secure environment (in psychiatric settings) there must be a safe room for severely disturbed people. This list is not exhaustive and many other features are possible when considering environmental factors (Royal College of Psychiatrists 1998).

The response of staff to aggressive situations may be influenced by factors such as workload, stress, illness, confidence and experience. When long hours are worked, or a heavy workload is undertaken, staff may feel under increased stress. Misunderstandings, failure to clarify task requirements or requests can lead to verbal abuse or aggression. It should not be seen as a weakness of staff if they try to avoid violence. The level of training provided for staff (in terms of undertaking the work required, customer care skills, dealing with aggression, how to diffuse awkward situations, etc.) can also influence the degree of risk (Royal Marsden Hospital 2002).

Once the hazards and risks have been identified, the next step required is a review of the procedures already in place to reduce the risks. Any additional precautions, procedures or control measures required can then be implemented:

1086

- Providing comfortable seating.
- Providing access to refreshment.
- Providing appropriate facilities for the disabled.
- Improving communication systems and multilingual notices and signposts.
- Reducing waiting times.
- Providing staff training.
- Increasing personal security systems, such as closed-circuit television.
- Providing staff support.
- Introducing an incident reporting system.

Intervention

Agreement within the policy should be considered concerning what criteria are used before calling the police to attend an incident. This will depend on the severity of the situation and persons or property at risk (RCN 1998). The involvement of the police and the criminal justice system is discussed at greater length in the NMC (2002) document. To summarize:

- Summoning police assistance generally means that the police will assume responsibility for the control of the violent incident, rather than seeing themselves as assisting nursing staff. The police will then deal with the situation as they see fit.
- The police are obliged to take action after any crime, which may take the form of a warning, a caution or a charge.
- The victim may be asked if they wish to take part in proceedings but does not have the responsibility, as is often thought, of 'pressing charges'.

Taking police action is often thought of as a last resort because of staff feeling that they have failed to manage the incident effectively or that the patient's medical or mental health needs will be overlooked, or fearing that a police presence will inflame the situation. However, there may be several benefits: it would increase the likelihood of the incident being recorded in the medical notes; it may lead to more appropriate future treatment; it may also communicate and enforce a firm message that violence will not be tolerated and that the patient is to be held responsible for his or her behaviour (NMC 2002).

Perhaps the most significant advance in the management of violence in recent years is the documentation on physical restraint. This has been comprehensively reviewed by Wright (1999) and is recognized as being a controversial and emotive topic. Since the mid-1980s, staff in health care and local authority settings have received training in methods for physically managing violence and aggression, termed 'control and restraint' (C&R). The use of this procedure has expanded to such an extent that in a survey of inpatient care in inner London (Gournay *et al.* 1998, cited in Wright 1999), only one of 11 inner London trusts surveyed did not routinely train acute nursing staff in C&R. However, there are safety, ethical and legal implications to be considered before embarking on these methods. There have been instances of accidental death of patients resulting from restraint procedures being inappropriately or incorrectly applied (Wright 1999). This is particularly relevant when working with patients who are elderly, infirm or sedated. It is also worth noting that while physical restraint may be seen as potentially damaging to a patient's physical or mental well-being, the consequences of not restraining a patient who is attempting to harm themselves or others may be even more damaging to the patient's self-esteem and may preserve life and/or minimize harm in the short term (Wright 1999). Whatever physical restraint method is employed, it is vital to apply it uniformly and it should only be conducted by appropriately trained and accredited staff. If there is an incident team in the hospital that is expected to respond to urgent situations where there is violence or the threat of violence, then each member of that team should have received training commensurate with their role and contact with patients (NMC 2002).

Once violence has occurred, the following may be regarded as important management decisions that need to be implemented:

- Medical personnel should be informed immediately because medication may be required as part of the management of the situation.
- Some nurses must be delegated to attend to the needs of the remaining patients, to telephone for help and to prepare any required medication.
- If immobilization is needed, the agreed local policy for seclusion of the patient, physical intervention of a patient or rapid tranquillization must be implemented.

Post-incident review

The law regarding assault and self-defence is complicated and often inconsistent. There is further complication in that, while certain responses to violence may be permissible under the law, the actions of health care staff are also regulated by codes of professional practice (Wright 1999). At all times *The NMC Code* must be adhered to (NMC 2008). This is discussed in further detail in *Dealing with Violence against Nursing Staff* (RCN 1998) but Point 5.3 on confidentiality and information disclosure and Point 8 on identifying and minimizing risk are particularly pertinent. If legal advice needs to be obtained in a particular case, such as financial compensation or prosecution following personal injury or damage to property, this should be obtained from a solicitor, barrister, health and safety representative and/or trade union representative.

Following the incident, staff should be given an opportunity to discuss their feelings about the aggressor(s), other members of staff involved and the way the incident was managed. This should happen as soon as possible after the incident has resolved and with as many of the staff concerned as possible. There should be discussion on:

- What happened during the incident.
- Any trigger factors.
- Roles of the people involved in the incident.
- How they feel now and may feel in the near future.

- What can be done to address concerns.
- Any measures that can be taken to avoid a repeat of the situation (RCN 1998).

Emotional debriefing aims to recognize potential stress, acknowledge it as a normal response and provide a supportive and structured setting to allow people to cope more effectively. Discussion should not be focused on any person's performance but address the effects on them as individuals (Health Services Advisory Committee 1997). In addition to the debriefing procedure, the physical and psychological well-being of the staff involved and the team as a whole need to be addressed. Staff injured as a result of their involvement in the incident may be entitled to industrial injuries benefit or a payment under the criminal injuries compensation scheme and will need to be informed of their rights by the appropriate body (RCN 1998). Consideration must be given to the risk of infection in cases where injury has occurred; for example, bites or needlestick injuries. Staff must receive continued support when returning to work after a violent incident (RCN 1998). Debriefing can be supplemented by making confidential counselling available through in-house counsellors, occupational health departments or independent external bodies (Health Services Advisory Committee 1997).

Some staff view reporting of incidents as admission of failure, especially if violence is rare in the area in which they work, therefore debriefing becomes particularly relevant in order to promote reporting of incidents (Rippon 2000; Paterson *et al.* 2001; NMC 2002).

All documentation required by law (such as the reporting of staff off work for 3 days or more following an assault) or hospital policy (such as completing an incident form) should be completed and forwarded to the appropriate departments. Specific and accurate written records will aid recall if it is required, perhaps years later (RCN 1998).

Summary

Violent incidents often arise from a patient feeling vulnerable and attack may become the preferred means of defence. The manner in which a patient is approached may be crucial in determining whether the patient will feel secure enough to cease the behaviour or to continue to feel threatened, perhaps leading on to violent behaviour. The need for rapid tranquillization, seclusion or physical intervention should be seen as the application of the appropriate technique in a particular situation and not as a failure of other methods. Protection against any administrative or legal problems lies in following the appropriate guidelines and applying them in good faith and with due restraint.

Procedure guidelines   **Violence: prevention and management**

This guideline is based on the NICE guideline, *Violence. The Short-Term Management of Disturbed/Violent Behaviour in Psychiatric In-Patient Settings and Emergency Departments* (NICE 2005). This evidence is graded C, E.

Prediction of violence

Procedure

Action	Rationale
Multidisciplinary team assessment for:	To reduce risk of a violent situation developing. If risk identified, steps should be taken to avoid violence arising.
1 Demographic/personal history:	

1 Demographic/personal history:
- History of violent/disturbed behaviour.
- Misuse of substances.
- Evidence of social restlessness.
- Known personal triggers.
- Verbal threats of violence.
- Recent severe stress especially loss.

2 Clinical variables:
- Organic dysfunction, e.g. endocrine imbalance, convulsive disorders, dementia, neurological impairment, encephalopathy.
- Drug toxicity.
- Alcohol and substance misuse.
- Psychiatric factors, e.g. personality disorder, symptoms of schizophrenia, antisocial impulsive behaviour.

3 Situational variables:
- Staff attitudes.
- Extent of social support.
- Limit settings.

4 Antecedents/warning signs:
- Tense angry facial signs.
- Increased restlessness.
- General overarousal of body systems (increased heart rate, breathing, muscle twitching, dilating pupils).
- Increased volume of speech.
- Prolonged eye contact.
- Discontentment, refusal to communicate, fear.
- Unclear thought process.
- Delusions or hallucinations.
- Verbal threats.
- Similar behaviour to previous incidents of violence.
- Reporting angry feelings.
- Blocking escape routes.

5 Process of risk assessment considering:
- Environmental.
- Organizational.
- Situational.
- Attitudinal.

To identify why and how conflict can occur.

Prevention of violence

Procedure

Action

Consideration of the following factors:
1 Environmental/organizational:
- Perception of space.
- Natural daylight.
- Noise levels.
- Provide smoking and non-smoking areas.
- Privacy in toilet/bathroom and changing room areas.

Rationale

To maintain a safe environment for all patients, staff and visitors present and to avoid aggravating the situation further.

2 Use of communication skills:
- Respond to cues with measured and reasonable action.
- Consider appropriate de-escalation technique.
- Avoid provocation.
- Develop staff and patient awareness of triggers and document in care plan.

3 Observation:
- Consider level of observation according to local policy.

1091

Procedure guidelines (*cont.*)

Intervention and management of violence

Procedure

Action	Rationale
1 A staff member should assume control and consider the need for further personnel to assist with the management of the situation.	To effectively manage the situation and inform staff and distressed individual who is taking responsibility for resolving the issues.
2 Remove other patients and relatives from area.	To minimize the risk of physical injury to patients and others.
3 Staff should ensure their non-verbal communication is non-threatening and non-provocative.	To de-escalate the risk of violence.
4 Use appropriate alarm to enlist help and contact patient's medical team.	To ensure the patient is given the appropriate treatment if required.
5 Consider contacting police if local policy indicates.	To maintain safe environment and contain violence if occurring.
6 If necessary apply physical intervention, seclusion, consider rapid tranquillization.	Physical and/or medical restraint may be required in the management of the patient.

Post-violent-incident review

Procedure

Action	Rationale
1 Attend to patients and staff injured during the incident.	To provide care and support to those involved.
2 A post-incident review should occur within 72 hours to address psychological concerns of patients and staff.	To comply with legal obligations and hospital policy.
3 Document incident.	
4 Identify risk factors and/or triggers.	To prevent a repeat of the incident.

References and further reading

Arnetz, J.E. & Arnetz, B.B. (2000) Implementation and evaluation of a practical intervention programme for dealing with violence towards health care workers. *J Adv Nurs*, **31**(3), 668–80.

Bandura, A. & Walters, R. (1963) *Social Learning and Personality Development*. Holt, Rinehart & Winston, New York.

Beech, B. (1999) Sign of the times or the shape of things to come? A 3-day unit of instruction on 'aggression and violence in health settings for all students during pre-registration nurse training'. *Nurse Educ Today*, **19**(8), 610–16.

Beech, B. (2001) Zero tolerance of violence against health care staff. *Nurs Stand*, **15**(16), 39–41.

Briant, A. (2003) Developing a risk assessment policy. *Prim Health Care*, **13**(4), 39–41.

Brockmann, M. (2002) New perspectives on violence in social care. *J Soc Work*, **2**(1), 29–44.

Cembrowicz, S. (1989) Dealing with difficult patients: what goes wrong? *Practitioner*, **233**(5), 486–9.

Department of Employment (1974) *Health and Safety at Work Act*. www.hse.gov.uk/legislation/hswa.pdf. Accessed 30/11/07.

Department of Employment (1996) *Employment Rights Act*. www.opsi.gov.uk/acts/1996/1996018.htm.

DH (2001) *Withholding Treatment from Violent and Abusive Patients in NHS Trusts: NHS Zero Tolerance Zone*. HSC 2001/18. HMSO, London.

DH (2006) *Bullies Who Threaten NHS Staff are Shown Red Card as New Figures Reveal 1 in 22 NHS Workers Suffer Violence*. Press Release, ref. 2006/0214, HMSO, London.

Dobson, F. (1999) *Dobson Steps Up Major Drive to Protect NHS Staff from Assaults: Violence and Security*. Memorandum from NHS Executive. Press Release, 15 April. Stationery Office, London.

Dollard, J. & Miller, N.E. (1961) *Frustration and Aggression*. Yale University Press, New Haven.

Donnelly, C. (2006) Tackling violence head on. *Emerg Nurse*, **13**(10), 5.

Fern, T. (2006) Underreporting of violent incidents against nursing staff. *Nurs Stand*, **20**(40), 41–5.

Freud, S. (1955) *The Complete Psychological Works of Sigmund Freud*, Vol. 18. Hogarth Press, London.

Gelles, R.J. (1972) *The Violent Home*. Sage, Beverly Hills.

Glasser, M. (1998) On violence: a preliminary communication. *Int J Psycho-Analysis*, **79**(5), 887–902.

Gray, J.A. (1971) Sex differences in emotional behaviour in mammals including man: endocrine basis. *Acta Psychol*, **35**, 29–44.

Gunn, J. (1973) *Violence*. David & Charles, Newton Abbot.

Harrington, J.A. (1972) Violence: a clinical viewpoint. *Br Med J*, **1**, 228–31.

Health Services Advisory Committee (1997) *Violence and Aggression to Staff in Health Services: Guidance on Assessment and Management*, 2nd edn. Health and Saftey Executive Books, Suffolk.

HSE (1995) *A Guide to the Reporting of Injuries, Diseases and Dangerous Occurrences Regulations 1995 (RIDDOR)*. L73. HMSO, London.

HSE (1996) *A Guide to the Health and Safety (Consultation with Employees) Regulations 1996*. Guidance on Regulations L95. HMSO, London.

HSE (1999) *Management of Health and Safety at Work Regulations* 1999. Approved Code of Practice L21. HMSO, London.

HSE (2000) *Violence at Work*. LAC 88/1. HMSO, London.

Kerr, I.B. & Taylor, D. (1997) Acute disturbed or violent behaviour: principles of treatment. *J Psychopharmacol*, **11**(3), 271–7.

Krakowski, M. & Czobor, P. (1994) Clinical symptoms, neurological impairment, and prediction of violence in psychiatric inpatients. *Hosp Commun Psychiatry*, **45**(7), 711–13.

Leather, P. *et al.* (2005) Weighing up the benefits of training programmes. *Prof Nurse*, **20**(5), 6–7.

Lorenz, K. (1966) *On Aggression*. Harcourt, Brace & World, New York.

Montague, M.C. (1979) Physiology of aggressive behaviour. *J Neurosurg Nurs*, **11**, 10–15.

Morgan, S. (2001) The problems of aggression and violence for health-care staff. *Prof Nurse*, **17**(2), 107–8.

Mulholland, H. (2003) Analysis. Why are nurses still being attacked? *Nurs Times*, **99**(14), 10–11.

NICE (2005) *Violence. The Short-Term Management of Disturbed/Violent Behaviour in Psychiatric In-Patient Settings and Emergency Departments*. National Institute for Health and Clinical Excellence, London.

NMC (2002) *The recognition, prevention and therapeutic management of violence in mental health care*. Nursing and Midwifery Council. www.nmc-uk.org. Accessed 8/10/03.

NMC (2008) *The Code: Standards of Conduct, Performance and Ethics for Nurses and Midwives*. Nursing and Midwifery Council, London.

Paterson, B., Leadbetter, D. & Bowie, V. (2001) Zero in on violence. *Nurs Manage*, **8**(1), 16–22.

Paterson, B., Leadbetter, D. & Miller, G. (2005) Workplace health. Beyond zero tolerance: a varied approach to workplace violence. *Br J Nurs*, **14**(15), 810–15.

Pinker, S. (2002) The killer instinct. *The Times*, T2, 3 September; Suppl, pp. 2–3.

RCN (1998) *Dealing with Violence against Nursing Staff: an RCN Guide for Nurses and Managers*. Royal College of Nursing, London.

RCN (2005) *At Breaking Point? A Survey of the Well-Being and Working Lives of Nurses in 2005*. Royal College of Nursing, London.

Reilly, P. *et al.* (1994) Anger management and temper control: critical components of post traumatic stress disorder and substance abuse treatment. *J Psychoactive Drugs*, **26**(4), 401–7.

Rew, M. & Ferns, T. (2005) Conflict management. A balanced approach to dealing with violence and aggression at work. *Br J Nurs*, **14**(4), 227–32.

Rippon, T.J. (2000) Aggression and violence in health care professions. *J Adv Nurs*, **31**(2), 452–60.

Robinson, L. (1983) *Psychiatric Nursing as a Human Experience*. W.B. Saunders, Philadelphia.

Royal College of Psychiatrists (1998) *Management of Imminent Violence – Clinical Practice Guidelines: Quick Reference Guide*. Royal College of Psychiatrists, London.

Royal Marsden Hospital (2002) *The Violence at Work Policy*. Royal Marsden Hospital, London.

Strachan-Bennett, S. (2005) Managing violent patients. *Nurs Times*, **101**(13), 18–20.

Vanderslott, J. (1998) A study of incidents of violence towards staff by patients in an NHS trust hospital. *J Psychiatr Mental Health Nurs*, **5**, 291–8.

Walker, J. (2002) Safety first. *Nurs Times*, **98**(9), 20–1.

Wells, J. & Bowers, L. (2002) How prevalent is violence towards nurses working in general hospitals in the UK? *J Adv Nurs*, **39**(3), 230–40.

Wertham, D.J. (1968) *A Sign for Cain*. Hale, New York.

Whittington, R. (1997) Violence to nurses: prevalence and risk factors. *Nurs Stand*, **12**(5), 49–56.

Whittington, R., Shuttleworth, S. & Hill, L. (1996) Violence to staff in a general hospital setting. *J Adv Nurs*, **24**, 326–33.

Worthington, K. (2000) Violence in the health care workplace. *Am J Nurs*, **100**(11), 69–70.

Wright, S. (1999) Physical restraint in the management of violence and aggression in in-patient settings: a review of issues. *J Mental Health*, **8**(5), 459–72.

Multiple choice questions

1 Where is violent behaviour more likely to occur?

   a Front-line reception areas
   b Outpatient clinical areas
   c Inpatient clinical areas
   d All of the above

2 Which of these signs are reliable predictions of imminent violent episodes?

   a Irritability and confusion
   b Boisterous behaviour, irritability, confusion and anger
   c Anger and confusion
   d Confusion

3 NICE Guidelines to short term management of violence (2005) describe different levels of observation. The levels are:

   a Watch, restrict
   b General, intermittent, within eyesight, within arm's length
   c General, close contact, restrictive
   d General, occasional, intermittent, within eyesight

4 Following an incident staff should be given an opportunity to:

   a Go home
   b Discuss their feelings about the aggressor(s), other members of staff involved and the way the incident was managed
   c Have a tea break and chat with colleagues about the incident
   d Write an incident report

Answers to the multiple choice questions can be found in Appendix 3.

Chapter 34

Wound management

Definition of a wound

A wound can be defined as an injury to the body that involves a break in the continuity of tissues or of body structures (Martin 2002). Wounds can be divided into six basic categories:

1 contusion (bruise);
2 abrasion (graze);
3 laceration (tear);
4 incision (cut);
5 puncture (stab);
6 burn.

Both external and internal factors can contribute to the formation of a wound. These may include:

- *External*: mechanical (friction, shear, surgery); chemical, electrical, temperature extremes (burns); radiation; micro-organisms.
- *Internal*: circulatory system failure (venous, arterial, lymphatic); endocrine (diabetes); neuropathy; haematological (porphyria cutanea tarda, mycosis fungoides); malignancy (fungating wound, Marjolin's ulcer) (Naylor *et al.* 2001).

Wound healing and management

Reference material

Classification of wounds

There are many different wound classification systems available and choice depends on the type of information required. A wound may be classified simply according to the method of healing, for example primary, secondary or tertiary intention (Miller & Dyson 1996), but this does not provide any information about the wound's characteristics. Further simple classification systems include whether the wound is acute (of short duration), chronic (of long duration) or according to the amount of tissue loss (Dealey 2005). A classification system that contains an appraisal of tissue loss is considered most useful (Flanagan 1996). Superficial, partial-thickness wounds are usually traumatic and painful, but retain the hair follicles or sweat glands and part of the dermis, and are usually considered **acute wounds,** whilst full-thickness wounds destroy the dermis and some deeper layers may also be involved (Dealey 2005). Full thickness wounds take longer to heal and can be life threatening if necrosis or infection complicate healing (Hampton & Collins 2004) and are therefore **chronic wounds.**

Wound healing

Wound healing is the process by which tissues damaged or destroyed by injury or disease are restored to normal function. Healing may occur by first, second or third intention. Healing by **first intention** involves the union of the edges of a wound under aseptic conditions without visible granulation, for example, a laceration or an incision that is closed with sutures, clips or skin adhesive (Miller & Dyson 1996; Dealey 2005).

Healing by **secondary intention** occurs when the wound's edges cannot be brought together. In this case the wound is left open and must fill with new tissue (granulate) until the level of intact epidermis is reached. When this is achieved epithelial cells will begin to migrate over the wound surface to restore integrity of the skin (Flanagan 1998). Wounds that heal by secondary intention include surgical or traumatic wounds where a large amount of tissue has been lost, heavily infected wounds, chronic wounds (leg or pressure ulcers) or, in some cases, where a better cosmetic or functional result will be achieved (Miller & Dyson 1996; Calvin 1998).

Healing by **tertiary intention** (sometimes referred to as delayed primary intention) may be employed when there is considerable infection or contamination of the wound. The wound is left open until it is clean or free of infection and then the edges are brought together, as with primary intention healing (Sussman 1998).

Phases of wound healing

Wound healing is a complex series of physiological events which occur in a predictable sequence (Flanagan 1999). These descriptive phases are dynamic, highly complex, dependent upon each other and overlap (Dealey 2005; Timmons 2006). It is important to support a wound healing environment that encourages progression from one phase to the next without bacterial contamination, which increases slough and necrosis (Hampton & Collins 2004).

The generally accepted stages of healing are:

1 Haemostasis.
2 Inflammatory phase.
3 Proliferation or reconstructive phase.
4 Maturation or remodelling phase.
   (Miller & Dyson 1996; Calvin 1998; Moore & Foster 1998; Ehrlich 1999;
                                                              Flanagan 2000)

There are a number of internal and external factors that may have an influence
on normal wound healing and cause a delay in progress through these stages
(Table 34.1). Growth factors are involved throughout these phases and are listed
in Table 34.2.

Haemostasis (minutes)

Vasoconstriction occurs within a few seconds of tissue injury and damaged blood
vessels constrict to stem the blood flow. When platelets come into contact with
exposed collagen from damaged blood vessels they release chemical messengers
that stimulate a 'clotting cascade' (Flanagan 2000; Hampton & Collins 2004;
Timmons 2006). Platelets adhere to vessel walls and edges and are stabilized
by a network of fibrin to form a clot. Bleeding ceases when the blood vessels
thrombose, usually within 5–10 minutes of injury (Hampton & Collins 2004).

Inflammatory phase (1–5 days)

With the activation of clotting factors comes the release of histamine and vasodilatation begins (Flanagan 1996, Dowsett 2002). The liberation of histamine also
increases the permeability of the capillary walls, and plasma proteins, leucocytes,
antibodies and electrolytes exude into the surrounding tissues. The wound becomes red, swollen and hot. These signs are accompanied by pain and tenderness
at the wound site, last for 1–3 days and can be mistaken for wound infection
(Hampton & Collins 2004).

1099

Polymorphonuclear leucocytes (neutrophils) and macrophages are chemotac-
tically attracted to the wound to defend against infection and begin the process of
repair (Hart 2002). The macrophage is also known as the 'director cell' of wound
healing (Silver 1994). If the number and function of macrophages is reduced, as
may occur in disease, e.g. diabetes (Springett 2002), or due to treatment, e.g.
chemotherapy in cancer patients (Souhami & Tobias 1998), healing is seriously
affected.

Neutrophils and macrophages combine to destroy and ingest bacteria, debris
and devitalized tissue. This involves a great deal of cellular activity which requires

Table 34.1   Factors that may delay wound healing. (From Hampton & Collins 2004; Convatec Wound Therapeutics 2005; Bale & Jones 2006.)

Extrinsic factor	Action	Intrinsic factor	Action
Cold	Any drop in temperature delays healing by up to 4 hours (Lock 1979)	Age	Elderly have a gradual thinning of the dermis and underlying structural support for the wound (i.e. less moisture and subcutaneous fat) and the metabolic process and circulation also slows with age
Excessive heat	Temperature over 30°C reduces tensile strength and causes vasoconstriction	Medical and general health conditions	Diabetes, cardiopulmonary disease, hypovolaemic shock, rheumatoid arthritis, anaemia, obesity
Chronic excessive exudate	Wounds should not be too wet or too dry (see moisture balance section in Table 34.3)	Malnutrition or protein–energy malnutrition	Poor healing, decreased tensile strength and higher risk of wound dehiscence and infection Low serum albumin causes oedema
Poor dressing application and techniques	If dressings are too tight or compression therapy is inadequate, adherence of dressings to wound bed, etc.	Psycho-social factors	Alcohol and smoking (carbon monoxide affects the blood vessels and circulation of oxygen), poor mobility, stress, isolation, anxiety and altered body image
Poor surgical technique	Prolonged operating time, inappropriate use of diathermy and drains can lead to 'dead space' haematomas and infection	Drugs	Steroids and non-steroidal anti-inflammatories, anti-inflammatories, immunosuppressives, cytotoxic chemotherapy

1100

up to 20 times the normal resting rate of oxygen of phagocytic cells (Timmons 2006). Patients with hypoxic wounds are, therefore, more susceptible to wound infection. The degradation of unwanted material causes an increased osmolarity within the area, resulting in further swelling.

Table 34.2 Growth factors involved in wound healing. (From Timmons 2006; Hampton & Collins 2004.)

Growth factor	Actions
Epidermal growth factor (EGF)	Influences the rate of epithelialization
Fibroblast growth factor 2 (FGF-2)	Promotes angiogenesis, stimulates proliferation of epithelial cells and fibroblasts
Transforming growth factor (TGF-β)	Sustains fibrotic process that leads to scar formation
Insulin-like growth factor 1 (IGF-1)	Presence of these low molecular peptides predicts presence of underlying conditions and nutritional status.
Platelet derived growth factor (PDGF)	Triggers clotting cascade and promotes cell migration and repair at the injured site
Vascular endothelial growth factor (VGF)	Stimulates angiosentesis (formation of new cells)
Nerve growth factor (NGF)	Accelerates healing and is produced by fibroblasts and epithelial cells
Keratinoctye growth factor (KGF)	Stimulates keratinoctye proliferation and migration through the extra cellular matrix (during re-epithelialization)

This phase of wound healing requires energy and good nutrition and complications or infection will both delay the process and can be debilitating for the patient (Dealey 2005). A chronic wound can get stuck in this phase of wound healing (Collier 2002) with prolonged healing, tendency to infection and high levels of exudate (Timmons 2006).

Proliferative phase (3–24 days)

Acute wounds will start to granulate within 3 days, but the inflammatory and proliferative phases can overlap with both granulation and sloughy tissue present (Timmons 2006). The macrophage secretes a fibroblast-stimulating factor known as vascular endothelial growth factor (VEGF) which, in the presence of a platelet derived growth factor released by the dead platelets, causes the fibroplast to migrate into the wound soon after damage has occurred (Silver 1994; Calvin 1998).

The fibroblasts are activated to divide and produce collagen by processes initiated by the macrophages (Timmons 2006). This develops a network of poorly organized collagen which increases the strength and elasticity of the wound. Newly synthesized collagen creates a 'healing ridge' below an intact suture line, thus giving an indication of how wound healing is progressing. This mechanism is dependent on the presence of iron, vitamin C and oxygen. Vitamin C (ascorbic acid) and lactate are stimulants for fibroblast activity (Hampton & Collins 2004). Fibroblasts are also dependent on the local oxygen supply (Dealey 2005).The wound surface and the oxygen tension within encourages the macrophages to instigate the process of angiogenesis; forming new blood cell vessels (Hampton & Collins 2004; Dealey 2005). These vessels branch and join other vessels forming loops. The fragile capillary loops are held within a framework of collagen. This complex is known as granulation tissue. At this stage the wound will appear pink and moist with raised red bumps (Hampton & Collins 2004).

The process of wound contraction can significantly reduce the size of the wound and the area that new tissue must cover. It is extremely important, and only observable, in open wounds healing by secondary intention. There is debate about the exact method by which wound contraction occurs (Tejero-Trujeque 2001). The cell contraction theory proposes that an altered fibroblast, called a myofibroblast (which has similar properties to a smooth muscle cell), has the ability to contract and pull collagen fibrils towards itself, thereby reducing the size of the wound (Flanagan 1996; Calvin 1998).

Re-epithelialization of the wound usually begins within 24 hours of injury (Garrett 1997; Calvin 1998). Macrophages produce a number of growth factors including keratinocyte growth factor (KGF) which stimulates a proliferation of cells within the wound bed (Timmons 2006). Epithelial cells (keratinocytes) may migrate from hair follicles and sweat glands within the wound or from the perimeter of the wound (Moore & Foster 1998). The migration of epithelial cells across the wound surface may occur via single cell migration or 'leap-frogging' where a cell moves forward and stops while other cells move over the top of it (Calvin 1998). Epithelial cells will burrow under contaminated debris and unwanted material (Waldorf & Fewkes 1995) while also secreting an enzyme that separates the scab from underlying tissue. Dissolving dry eschar requires nearly 50% of the cell's metabolic energy (Messer 1989; Dealey 2005). Through a mechanism called contact inhibition epithelial cells will cease migrating when they come into contact with other epithelial cells (Garrett 1997).

The ability of the epithelium to cover the wound surface is limited to approximately 2 cm^2. This means that the process of contraction is of vital importance to healing wounds (Messer 1989). Epithelialization (migration, mitosis and differentiation) occurs at an increased rate in a moist wound environment, as do the synthesis of collagen and formation of new capillaries (Winter 1972; Eaglstein 1985; Dyson *et al.* 1988; Miller 1998a; Flanagan 1999). A hypoxic (low oxygen) environment has also been shown to increase the motility of epidermal cells (O'Toole *et al.* 1997). The rate of epithelialization is also influenced by growth factors (Timmons 2006). However, little is known about the reality of growth factor activity in chronic wounds (Hampton & Collins 2004).

Maturation phase (21 days onward)

This stage begins at around 21 days following the initial injury. Maturation or remodelling of the healed wound may last for more than a year. Collagen is re-organized, the fibres becoming enlarged and orientated along the lines of tension in the wound (at right angles to the wound margin) (Silver 1994). This occurs via a process of lysis and resynthesis. Intermolecular cross-linking aids the tensile strength of the wound. The reorganization of collagen may result in further contraction of the wound, which may potentiate contraction deformities (Silver 1994; Moore & Foster 1998). During this phase the number of blood vessels within the scar is reduced. Maximum strength is reached in approximately 3 months, although the scar will only achieve about 70–80% of normal skin strength (Calvin 1998; Ehrlich 1999). At the end of the maturation phase the delicate granulation tissue of the wound will have been replaced by stronger avascular scar tissue.

For acute wounds these phases flow relatively smoothly, however chronic wounds may get stuck in one phase or heal very slowly. It is necessary to bring a chronic wound back into the acute phase for it to heal. This process is termed 'wound bed preparation' (S. Hampton, pers. comm., October 2006).

Wound bed preparation

Wound bed preparation (WBP) focuses on controlling and optimizing the wound environment for healing (Falanga 2000). It provides a means of bringing together a cohesive plan of both patient and wound care (Vowden & Vowden 2002).

Doctors have always applied the principles of wound bed preparation, even before it was given a name as, when they debrided a wound, they would cut through to healthy bleeding tissues. This would initiate the clotting cascade and the wound would become acute. Today, there are improved methods of achieving the same end through assessment and appropriate dressing selection (S. Hampton, pers. comm., October 2006).

In order to provide a method of assessment and a simplistic selection of appropriate dressings, an international group of wound care experts developed this concept using 'TIME' (tissue, infection, moisture and edge advancement) as an acronym to identify the key barriers to healing (Dowsett & Ayello 2004). See Table 34.3 for overview of TIME principles.

Tissue factors affecting wound healing

The rate of wound healing varies depending on the general health of the individual, the location of the wound, the degree of damage and the treatment applied.

Table 34.3 TIME principles for wound bed preparation. (Adapted from Schultz *et al.* 2003; permission granted by Smith & Nephew.)

TIME	Status	Problem	Solution
Tissue	Tissue not viable	Defective matrix Cell debris impairing healing	Debridement
Inflammation and infection	Colonized → infection continuum	Wound healing delayed	Topical antimicrobials dependent on bacterial load
Moisture balance	Dry → excessive moisture	Maceration potential	Restore moisture balance Prevent maceration to peri-wound margins May require compression/drug therapy
Edge of wound	Non-migrating keratinocytes	Wound not closing	Reassess cause Removal of callus

Factors that may delay healing include systemic variables such as disease, poor nutritional state and infection. Other influences involve the local microenvironment of the wound, including temperature, pH, humidity, air gas composition, oxygen tension, blood supply and inflammation (Dyson *et al.* 1988; Cutting 1994; Benbow 1995; Collier 1996; Thomson 1998). Whether this influence is positive or negative may depend on the stage of wound healing that has been reached. Other important considerations are external variables such as continuing trauma, possibly caused by treatment or the presence of foreign bodies.

It is necessary when treating a wound to appraise all potential detrimental factors and minimize them, where possible, in order to provide the optimum systemic, local and external conditions for healing. Factors known to affect wound healing are listed in Table 34.1.

Nutrition and wound healing

Nutrition regulates wound healing as an extrinsic factor via two concepts: firstly that wound-related complications are more likely in the malnourished, and secondly, nutritional supplements can accelerate healing (Mandal 2006). A dietitian's assessment is advisable to set specific goals (Dealey 2005). Patients are considered 'at risk' for wound healing if they have lost 20% or more of their body weight within the previous 6 months or 10% in the previous 2 months (Messer 1989).

These patients should be screened holistically and offered interventions to prevent wound failure postoperatively, as most wounds heal adequately despite preoperative fasting (Dealey 2005; Mandal 2006). Patient's age, debilitating disease, current medications, usual diet and methods of cooking and preparing food are all considerations (Dealey 2005).

Many concurrent conditions affect diet, and both protein and calorie malnutrition are possible in patients with chronic or acute malabsorption. This includes diabetes, Crohn's disease, alcohol abuse, gastrointestinal surgery, liver disease and long-term steroid therapy. Malignancy, major trauma, fever, inflammatory disease, smoking, drug use, stress and iatrogenic starvation are associated with deficient intake or high energy demands (Lewis 1996; Casey 1998).

Patients who are elderly, malnourished, have severe diabetes or rheumatoid arthritis or who have suffered significant injury (especially burns) or surgery may be deficient in vitamin A (Messer 1989; Hamilton 1995; Ferguson *et al.* 2000). Therefore vitamin A supplementation may be beneficial as a means of speeding wound healing in these patient groups. Vitamin A has also been shown to reduce the adverse effects of corticosteroids (slowed wound healing, increased rate of infection and weaker scars), when given orally or applied topically to the wound (Ehrlich & Hunt 1968; Smith *et al.* 1986; Hamilton 1995).

Vitamin C is necessary for collagen synthesis during the proliferative stage of the wound healing process. Deficiency of vitamin C is also associated with lowered resistance to infection (Lewis 1996; Casey 1998; Russell 2001). Patients with poor nutritional status may benefit from zinc supplements because of the role of zinc in DNA synthesis and the immune response (Wells 1994; Lewis 1996).

Promotion of wound healing

Wound care begins with the care of the patient. The psychological care of the patient is important to ensure acceptance of the wound and reduction in stress. It is also imperative to assess and treat pain. Apart from the obvious unpleasantness for the patient, this will also lead to stress which will then delay wound healing (Kiecolt-Glaser *et al.* 1995; Moore & Foster 1998). A holistic assessment is very important (Collier 2002; Hampton 2004).

1105

Achieving a well-vascularized wound bed

Improving the blood flow to the wound bed will increase the availability of nutrients, oxygen, active cells and growth factors within the wound environment (Collier 2002). This may be achieved through the use of compression therapy, topical negative pressure therapy or wound management products that exert an osmotic pull on the wound bed, increasing capillary growth, e.g. Vacutex (Collier 2002).

Principles of wound cleaning

The aim of wound cleaning is to help create the optimum local conditions for wound healing by removal of excess debris, exudate, foreign and necrotic material, toxic components, bacteria and other micro-organisms.

If the wound is clean and little exudate is present, repeated cleaning is contraindicated since it may damage new tissue, decrease the temperature of the wound unnecessarily and remove exudate (Morison 1989). A fall in the temperature of the wound of 12°C is possible if the procedure is prolonged or the lotions are cold. It can take 3 hours or longer for the wound to return to normal temperature, during which time the cellular activity is reduced and therefore the healing process slowed (Collier 1996).

Sodium chloride (0.9%) is a physiologically balanced solution that has a similar osmotic pressure to that already present in living cells and is therefore compatible with human tissue (Lawrence 1997). Used at body temperature, it is the safest and best cleaning solution for non-contaminated wounds (Miller & Dyson 1996; Fletcher 1997). Although sodium chloride has no antiseptic properties it dilutes bacteria and is non-toxic to tissue (Morgan 2000). Tap water is also advocated for cleaning chronic wounds (Riyat & Quinton 1997). A study demonstrated that, in comparison with sterile 0.9% sodium chloride, lower rates of infection were found in the group where tap water was used (Angeras *et al.* 1992).

A number of other solutions have been used traditionally to clean wounds, some of which need to be used with caution (Table 34.4).

Debridement of devitalized tissue

Surgical debridement is the most effective method of removing necrotic tissue (debridement) (Hampton 1999). It is performed by a surgeon and usually involves excision of extensive or deep areas of necrosis. This is usually performed to the point of bleeding viable tissue to 'kickstart' healing (Hampton & Collins 2004). While this option is very effective it carries the risks associated with general anaesthesia. An alternative method of rapid debridement is 'sharp' debridement, which may be utilized for the removal of loose, devitalized, superficial tissue only (Vowden & Vowden 1999). Sharp debridement can be performed at the patient's bedside by an experienced health care professional with relevant training (Poston 1996). However, this can be a dangerous practice in inexperienced hands and is controversial (Fairbairn *et al.* 2002). Potentially ligaments may be severed as they can have the appearance of sloughy tissue or vascular damage could occur (Hampton & Collins 2004). Guidelines for sharp debridement have been drawn up and presented but have not been adopted yet (Davies 2004). It is also acknowledged that informed patient consent is required as this is an invasive procedure with potential risks and complications (Fairbairn *et al.* 2002).

Table 34.4 Suitability of products used on wounds. (From Miller & Dyson 1996; Lawrence 1997; Hampton 1999; Morgan 2000; Royal Marsden Wound Management Guidelines 2000; Hess 2005; BNF 2006.)

Product type	Suitability	Caution
Normal saline solution (sodium chloride 0.9%)	All types of wounds and sterile for aseptic technique on acute wounds	Should be warmed to avoid cooling wound surface and for comfort
Tap water	Chronic wounds. A shower may be used to remove old dressings, or affected limb soaked in a bucket of water	Ensure water is correct temperature and patient is suitable
Antiseptic solutions (i.e. chlorhexidine, hydrogen peroxide, acetic acid, povidone iodine, proflavin)	Not ideal as can cause sensitization, irritation and delay healing Proflavin cream may be used as second line treatment for moist desquamation in radiotherapy induced skin reactions	Hydrogen peroxide can cause an air embolism and is only used to clean very dirty wounds (i.e. road traffic accidents, or those contaminated by foreign matter) Iodine and proflavin stain clothing and are not for prolonged use
Topical antibiotics		
■ Fusidic acid	Penicillin-resistant staphylococci	Not recommended on open wounds
■ Metronidazole	Antibacterial (anaerobes), odour	Nausea when used systemically
■ Mupirocin (Bactroban)	For MRSA treatment, seek advice first after positive wound swab	Can burn or itch (consult microbiologist before use)

Autolytic debridement is recommended as a less invasive technique which utilizes the body's natural debriding mechanism. This process involves the removal of necrotic tissue by neutrophils and macrophages. This effect is enhanced in a moist wound environment, which can be achieved through the use of hydrogel dressings or semi-occlusive dressings that maintain moisture at the wound surface (Bale 1991; Hofman 1996; Freedline 1999) (Table 34.5). A holistic wound assessment is needed to decide appropriate methods of debriding devitalized tissue (Davies 2004).

The National Institute for Health and Clinical Excellence (NICE) guidance (NICE 2001) suggests that less robust studies favour autolytic debridement or bio-surgical interventions (sterile maggots) which are more comfortable and

1107

Table 34.5 Dressing groups. Please refer to manufacturer's recommendations with regard to individual products (Dealey 2005; Hess 2005).

Dressings	Description	Advantages	Disadvantages
Activated charcoal	Contain a layer of activated charcoal that traps odour-causing molecules thereby reducing/removing wound odour	Easy to apply as either primary or secondary dressing; work immediately to reduce odour	Need to obtain a good seal to prevent leakage of odour; some dressings lose effectiveness when wet
Adhesive island	Consist of a low adherent absorbent pad located centrally on an adhesive backing	Quick and easy to apply; one-piece design negates need for multiple product use; protect the suture line from contamination and absorb exudate/blood	Only suitable for light exudate; some can cause skin damage (excoriation, blistering) if applied incorrectly
Alginates	A textile fibre dressing made from the calcium salt of an alginic acid polymer derived from brown seaweed; contain mannuronic and guluronic acids in varying amounts; available as a sheet, ribbon or packing	Provide a moist wound environment; suitable for moderate to heavy exudate; can be used on infected wounds; useful for sinus and fistula drainage; have haemostatic properties; can be irrigated out of wound with sodium chloride (0.9%)	Cannot be used on dry wounds or wound with hard necrotic tissue (eschar); sometimes a mild burning or 'drawing' sensation is reported on application; secondary dressing required
Antimicrobials	These topical dressings can be used as primary or secondary dressings and are available as alginates, hydrocolloids, alginates, charcoal impregnated and creams	Suitable for chronic wounds with heavy exudate that need protection from bacterial contamination by providing a broad range of antimicrobial activity; can reduce or prevent infection	Cannot be used during radiotherapy, sometimes sensitivity occurs with the use of silver and some skin staining can occur; instructions vary with products and dressings are expensive

Table 34.5 (*continued*)

Dressings	Description	Advantages	Disadvantages
Capillary wound dressings	Composed of 100% polyester filament outer layers and a 65% polyester and 35% cotton woven inner layer; outer layer draws exudate, interstitial fluid and necrotic tissue into the inner layer via a capillary action Example: 'Vacutex'	Suitable for light to heavy exudate; debride necrotic tissue; protect and insulate the wound; maintain a moist environment and prevent maceration; encourage development of granulation tissue; can be cut to any shape and are available in large rolls; can be used as a wick to drain sinus and cavity wounds	Can be hard to cut and are quite stiff to fit into wounds; cannot be used on malignant wounds or where there is the risk of bleeding due to the 'drawing' action and resultant increase in blood flow to the wound bed
Collagens	This protein is fibrous and insoluble and produced by fibroblasts. Collagen encourages collagen fibres into the granulation tissue. It is available in sheets/gels	Conforms well to wound surface, maintains a moist environment, suitable for most wounds to accelerate healing (example: Promogran). Supports ECM	Requires a secondary dressing and not recommended for necrotic wounds
Cadexomer bead dressings	Consist of hydophilic beads which contain iodine in powder or paste form, which swell and form a gel on contact with exudate	Useful in the treatment of infected, sloughy and necrotic wounds	Require retaining dressing; may be difficult to apply, caution in using products containing iodine. Should only be used for 3 months at a time. Not suitable for people with thyroid disorders
Foams	Produced in a variety of forms, most being constructed of polyurethane foam and may have one or more layers; foam cavity dressings are also available	Suitable for use with open, exuding wounds; highly absorbent, non-adherent and provide a moist, thermally insulated wound environment	May be difficult to use in wounds with deep tracts

1109

(*continued*)

Table 34.5 (*continued*)

Dressings	Description	Advantages	Disadvantages
Honey	Available as impregnated dressing pads or tubes of liquid honey; most widely used is Manuka honey	Suitable for acute and chronic infected, necrotic or sloughy wounds; provide a moist wound environment; non-adherent; antibacterial; assist with wound debridement; eliminate wound malodour; have an anti-inflammatory effect	Can be messy to use and cause leakage if excess exudate is present; caution in diabetes due to absorption of glucose and fructose
Hydrocolloids	Usually consist of a base material containing gelatin, pectin and carboxymethylcellulose combined with adhesives and polymers; base material may be bonded to either a semi-permeable film or a film plus polyurethane foam; some have an adhesive border	Suitable for acute and chronic wounds with low to no exudate; provide a moist wound environment; promote wound debridement; provide thermal insulation; waterproof and barrier to micro-organisms; easy to use	May release degradation products into the wound; strong odour produced as dressing interacts with exudate; some hydrocolloids cannot be used on infected wounds
Hydrogels	Contain 17.5–90% water depending on the product, plus various other components to form a gel or solid sheet	Suitable for light exudate wounds; absorb small amounts of exudate; donate fluid to dry necrotic tissue; reduce pain and are cooling; low trauma at dressing changes; can be used as carrier for drugs	Cool the wound surface; use with caution in infected wounds; can cause skin maceration due to leakage if too much gel is applied or the wound has moderate to heavy exudate

Table 34.5 (*continued*)

Dressings	Description	Advantages	Disadvantages
Hydrofibre	A soft, non-woven dressing composed of 100% hydrocolloid fibres (sodium carboxymethylcellulose); available as sheet or ribbon	Suitable for highly exuding wounds (able to absorb up to 30 times its weight in fluid); holds exudate within its structure and keeps it away from surrounding skin; very easy to remove, gels more easily than alginates	Requires a secondary dressing
Semi-permeable films	Polyurethane film with a hypoallergenic acrylic adhesive; have a variety of application methods often consisting of a plastic or cardboard carrier	Only suitable for shallow superficial wounds; prophylactic use against friction damage; useful as retention dressing; allow passage of water vapour; allow monitoring of the wound	Possibility of adhesive trauma if removed incorrectly; do not contain exudate and can macerate, slip or leak
Skin barrier films	Alcohol-free liquid polymer that forms a protective film on the skin	Non-cytotoxic; do not sting if applied to raw areas of skin; high wash-off resistance; protect the skin from body fluids (including urine, diarrhoea, saliva and wound exudate), friction and shear and the effects of adhesive products	Require good manual dexterity to apply; may cause skin warming on application

1111

acceptable methods for patients. The sterile larvae (maggots) are applied to and retained at the wound bed and are used generally in chronic wounds (Hinshaw 2000). The larvae move over the surface of the wound, secreting a powerful mixture of proteolytic enzymes which break down necrotic tissue. They remove devitalized tissue by this method (the enzymes are neutralized by live tissue) while at the same time ingesting and destroying bacteria.

This action may cause a significant increase in exudate production due to the rapid debridement of necrotic tissue. It has been proposed that the larval secretions may also change the wound pH and may stimulate healing (Hinshaw 2000). Maggots are also obtainable in 'tea bag' form where they are encased and unable to escape. This method is often more acceptable to nurses (S. Hampton, pers. comm., October 2006). Patient compliance is also an important consideration and a detailed explanation is required (Jones & Thomas 2000; Thomas *et al.* 2001).

Indications for sterile larvae use include:

- Gangrenous or necrotic tissue (the necrotic tissue needs to be softened before applying therapy [S. Hampton, pers. comm., October 2006]).
- Infected diabetic foot ulceration.
- Arterial leg ulceration.
- Traumatic infected ulcers.
- Chronic wounds with underlying co-morbidities (Steenvoorde *et al.* 2005).

In a study by Kitching (2004) participants were positive about the effects of using the larvae and had been previously disillusioned by the failure of other treatments. Pain management was also an issue as the larvae grew and patients were controlled on durogesic plasters (Steenvoorde *et al.* 2005). Both studies reported good rates of debridement, reduction in malodour and exudate (Kitching 2004; Steenvoorde *et al.* 2005).

Inflammation and infection (or bacterial burden)

It is generally agreed that all chronic wounds harbour a variety of bacteria to some degree and this can range from contamination through colonization to infection. There is also a stage between colonization and infection called 'critical colonization' where the bacterial load has reached a level just below clinical infection (Collier 2002). When a wound becomes infected it will display the characteristic signs of heat, redness, swelling, pain, heavy exudate and malodour. The patient may also develop generalized pyrexia. However, immunosuppressed patients, diabetic patients or those on systemic steroid therapy may not present with the classic signs of infection. Instead they may experience delayed healing, breakdown of the wound, presence of friable granulation tissue that bleeds easily, formation of an epithelial tissue bridge over the wound, increased production of exudate and malodour, and increased pain (Miller & Dyson 1996; Cutting 1998; Miller 1998b; Gilchrist 1999). Careful wound assessment is essential to identify potential sites for infection, although routine swabbing of the area is not considered to be beneficial (Donovan 1998). Methods available for the management of wound infection or to decrease the bacterial burden in the wound include debridement, antimicrobial dressings, e.g. those containing iodine or silver, topical negative pressure therapy and antibiotic therapy. Honey and essential oils have also been used and there is a growing body of literature to this effect. Appropriate antibiotic treatment of the infection should be determined from a positive wound swab(s).

Moisture balance

Wound exudate usually performs a useful function of cleaning the wound and providing nutrients to the healing wound bed. However, in the presence of excess exudate the process of wound healing can be adversely affected. This is especially so in chronic wounds where wound fluid may actually prevent the proliferation of cells vital to wound healing, such as fibroblasts, keratinocytes and endothelial cells (Phillips *et al.* 1998; White 2001; Vowden & Vowden 2002).

The control of oedema or lymphoedema and lessening the bacterial burden on the wound will undoubtedly help in the reduction of wound exudate. However, if the methods for achieving these goals are unsuccessful or contraindicated then exudate must be managed through the use of wound management products. These include such products as absorbent wound dressings (e.g. alginates, hydrofibre, foams), non-adherent wound contact layers with a secondary absorbent pad, wound manager bags and topical negative pressure therapy (White 2001). Immunosuppressive drugs or steroids may be indicated in the treatment of inflammatory exudate produced by wounds such as pyoderma gangrenosum or rheumatoid ulcers (Vowden & Vowden 2002). It is also vital to protect the skin surrounding the wound from maceration by excess exudate and excoriation from corrosive exudate. Useful products for skin protection include ointments/pastes (e.g. zinc oxide BP), alcohol-free skin barrier films and thin hydrocolloid sheets used to 'frame' the wound.

Principles of dressing a wound

With the exception of wounds where the main aim is to ameliorate symptoms **1113** such as malignant wounds, an ideal wound dressing must be capable of fulfilling the following functions:

- Removes excess exudate and toxic components.
- Maintains a high humidity at the wound–dressing interface.
- Allows gaseous exchange.
- Provides thermal insulation.
- Be impermeable to bacteria.
- Be free from particulate or toxic components.
- Allows change without trauma.

- Be acceptable to the patient.
- Be highly absorbent (for heavily exuding wounds).
- Be cost-effective.
- Provide mechanical protection.
- Be conformable and mouldable.
- Be able to be sterilized.

(Field & Kerstein 1994; Hampton 1999; Morgan 2000)

In addition, the dressing should minimize pain, odour and bleeding and be comfortable when in place.

Occlusive dressings achieve many of these criteria. They affect the wound and healing in several ways. Occlusive dressings have the ability to maintain hydration and prevent the formation of an eschar.

A moist wound environment has been shown to affect a wound in the following ways. It:

- Increases rate of epithelial migration.
- Reduces the lag phase between epithelial cell proliferation and differentiation.
- Encourages synthesis of collagen and ground substance.
- Promotes formation of capillary loops.
- Decreases length of inflammatory phase.
- Reduces pain and trauma due to dressing adherence.
- Promotes breakdown of necrotic tissue.
- Speeds wound contraction.

(Miller & Dyson 1996; Garrett 1997; Flanagan 1998;
Williams & Young 1998)

Dry dressings (such as gauze) do not provide most of the criteria for an ideal dressing and should not be used as a primary contact layer (Dealey 2005). This depends on the definition of 'dry' dressing as Aquacel, alginates, etc. can be considered dry. The wound itself has the ability to produce moisture and make the dressings into 'wet' dressings. Wet dressings, such as first generation amorphous hydrogels, can make a wound too wet if used inappropriately. Compare the 'wetness' of first generation hydrogel with second generation hydrogel (such as ActiFormCool). The amorphous gels do not absorb and donate fluid to already wet wounds. This means they could be responsible for maceration if used inappropriately. Second generation hydrogel (ActiFormCool) is in a sheet and absorbs large amounts. First generation hydrogel should be used on dry eschar to soften. Second generation hydrogel can be used on wet and dry wounds (S. Hampton, pers. comm., October 2006).

Care should be taken with wounds that are difficult shapes to treat. These include long, narrow cavities which require a dressing that can be comfortably inserted into the space but removed easily without leaving any fibres behind and without trauma (Bale 1991). (See Table 34.5 for details of groups of dressings.)

Edge non-advancement

The clearest sign that the wound is failing to heal is when the epidermal edge is not advancing over time (Dowsett & Ayello 2004). In this case a thorough assessment should recommence using the TIME principles and interventions.

Wound assessment

The wound should be evaluated each time a dressing is applied or if it gives rise for concern. The aim of evaluating the wound is to assess healing and to establish which treatment will best provide the ideal environment for healing. The surface area or volume of the wound should be measured. This can be carried out using a number of methods; for example, planimetry measurements using a ruler, tracing the wound onto grid paper or Vistrak, a box similar to a child's Etch a Sketch but one that converts the tracing into measurement of surface area or through the use of a computer mapping program (S. Hampton, pers. comm., October 2006). Photography also provides a useful record of wound progression (Vowden 1995). The amount and type of drainage are also important, in both traumatic and surgical wounds, but difficult to assess (S. Hampton, pers. comm., October 2006).

A simple method is to use dressing change. Change dressings daily exudates. Change alternate days to every 3rd day medium exudates. Change weekly low exudates (S. Hampton, pers. comm., October 2006).

A list of variables that require regular assessment is shown in Table 34.3. Figure 34.1 is an example of a wound assessment chart. Teare & Barrett (2002) recommend that the underlying cause of the wound should also be assessed, with the primary focus on details such as size and depth as well as the stage of healing. Links can then be made between the wound dressing and the optimal healing environment. The use of this type of documentation to assist in the assessment process is recommended to:

- Facilitate continuity of care by providing a central reference point for wound progression.
- Facilitate appropriate evaluation of all relevant parameters.
- Fulfil legal and professional requirements (Teare & Barrett 2002).

Other treatments

Other treatments for wounds include the use of hyperbaric oxygen therapy, topical negative pressure therapy (TNP), bio-engineered skin substitutes, topical wound treatments and complementary therapies.

THE ROYAL MARSDEN WOUND ASSESSMENT CHART Complete one chart for each wound						
Patient name:						
Hospital number:						
Date of assessment (weekly)						
Wound dimensions						
Max length (cm)						
Max width (cm)						
Max depth (cm)						
Wound bed – approximate % cover (enter %)						
Necrotic (BLACK)						
Slough (YELLOW)						
Granulating (RED)						
Epithelializing (PINK)						
Skin around wound						
Intact						
Healthy						
Fragile						
Dry						
Scaly						
Erythema						
Maceration						
Oedema						
Eczema						
Skin nodules						
Skin stripping						
Dressing allergy						
Tape allergy						
Other (please state)						
Exudate level						
None						
Low						
Moderate						
High						
Amount increasing						
Amount decreasing						
Odour (see over for rating scale)						
None						
Slight						
Moderate						
Strong						
Bleeding						
None						
Slight						
Moderate						
Heavy						
At dressing change						
Pain from wound (see over for rating scale)						
Level (0–10)						
Continuous						
At specific times (specify)						
Wound infection suspected						
Swab taken (Y/N)						
Swab result						
Treatment						
Assessment review date						
Initials of Assessor						

Figure 34.1 Wound assessment chart. (Courtesy of The Royal Marsden Hospital.)

Location (mark diagram):	Visual Analogue Scale (VAS) for Patient's Rating of Pain.

Right	Left	Left	Right

Visual Analogue Scale (VAS) for Patient's Rating of Pain.

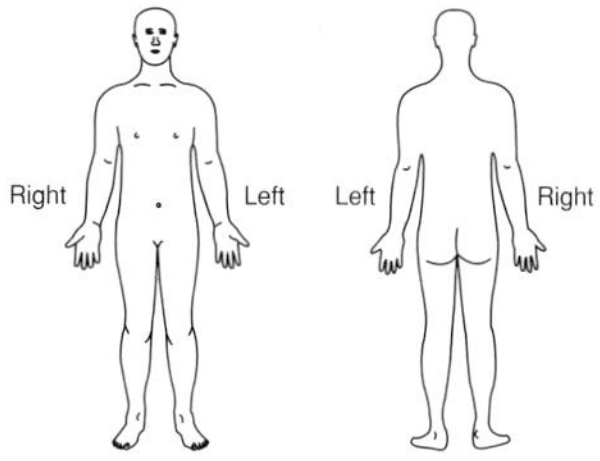

0 1 2 3 4 5 6 7 8 9 10
No pain — Worst pain imaginable

Rating Scale for Odour

Score	Assessment
None	No odour evident, even when at the patient's bedside with the dressing removed.
Slight	Wound odour is evident at close proximity to the patient when the dressing is removed.
Moderate	Wound odour is evident upon entering the room (1.5 to 3 metres from patient) with the dressing removed.
Strong	Wound odour is evident upon entering the room (1.5 to 3 metres from patient) with the dressing intact.

Diagram of wound if appropriate (or attach tracing/photograph):

Date: _____	Date: _____
Date: _____	Date: _____
Date: _____	Date: _____

1117

Notes on use
Use one chart per wound.
Complete a wound assessment at least once a week.
Measure the wound at its widest points using a clean ruler, use a sterile wound swab or blunt probe to measure wound depth.
For the 'skin around wound' assessment more than one box may be ticked.
Odour and pain should be assessed using the scales at the top of page 2.
Following the assessment a wound management care plan should be written and updated if necessary after each reassessment.

Figure 34.1 (*continued*)

Hyperbaric oxygen therapy

Wound hypoxia is common in patients with chronic wounds and may be exacerbated by diabetes, venous stasis, vascular insufficiency, cardiopulmonary disease or smoking (Messer 1989). Hyperbaric oxygen therapy has been used successfully in healing these wounds (Barr *et al*. 1990). Treatment involves the patient breathing 100% oxygen while in a chamber where the pressure is elevated above atmospheric pressure, thus increasing the amount of oxygen in solution and therefore the quantity of oxygen reaching the wound bed (Simmons 1999). Topical hyperbaric oxygen can also be used (S. Hampton, pers. comm., October 2006).

Topical negative pressure therapy

Topical negative pressure therapy (TNP) is the application of a uniform negative pressure across the wound bed. The benefits of TNP therapy are recognized as promotion of healing, improved exudates management, reduction of odour and bacteria.

This technique involves sealing a sterile foam or gauze dressing into the wound cavity and applying a controlled sub-atmospheric pressure. The negative pressure is achieved through a closed system, removing fluid from open wounds through sealed tubing which is connected to a container. Pressures are set at the level best suited to the wound type and can be set on continuous or intermittent according to the therapy required (Benbow 2006). Maintaining the vacuum seal is essential in providing this therapy (Kaufman & Pahl 2003). It has proven to be cost efficient, safe and effective as a treatment modality for wound care.

TNP therapy is indicated for:

- Chronic wounds.
- Diabetic foot ulcers.
- Pressure ulcers.
- Dehisced wounds and incisions.
- Partial thickness burns.
- Flaps and grafts.

(Kaufman & Pahl 2003; KCI International 2004)

1118

This therapy is contraindicated in grossly contaminated wounds, malignant wounds, untreated osteomyelitis, non-enteric and unexplored fistula or necrotic tissue with eschar present (KCI International 2004).

Precautions should be exercised when there is active bleeding in the wound, difficult haemostasis or when the patient is taking anticoagulants (Benbow 2006). Careful assessment of the wound site must be made to ensure that TNP therapy is indeed the appropriate treatment modality (Kaufman & Pahl 2003).

Bio-engineered skin substitutes

Bio-engineered skin substitutes have arisen from a need to find an alternative to skin grafts (autograft, allograft or xenograft) and dressings in the management of extensive burns (Boyce *et al.* 2002; Harding *et al.* 2002; Pouliot *et al.* 2002). Original cultures of human epidermis have been replaced by new skin-equivalent products that contain living cells, predominantly keratinocytes and fibroblasts, within natural or synthetic scaffolding. Examples of these products are:

- Apligraf (Graftskin): a cultured human skin equivalent containing viable dermal and epidermal cells (Morgan 2000; Harding *et al.* 2002).
- Dermagraft: a bio-absorbable mesh containing living neonatal fibroblasts, which produce normal dermal proteins and cytokines (Gentzkow *et al.* 1996).

Topical wound treatment dressings

Currently there are several dressing products, Hyalofill and Promogran, Catrix, Cadesorb and Prisma, which are classified as 'topical treatments' although they are not classed as medicines (S. Hampton, pers. comm., October 2006). Hyalofill is a soft conformable fleece composed entirely of HYAFF, an ester of hyaluronic acid (Edmonds & Foster 2000; Baxter & Ballard 2001). It has been shown to increase angiogenesis and the phagocytic response of macrophages; when used as a wound dressing, it promotes granulation and contraction (Chen & Abatangelo 1999; Hollander *et al.* 2000).

Proteases have an important role in regulating the balance between tissue synthesis and degradation. However, in chronic wounds, this regulation may be defective and healing problems will result (Derbyshire 2003) and, if their activity becomes uncontrolled, proteases can mediate devastating tissue damage and consequently have been implicated in chronic wound pathophysiology (Cullen *et al.* 2002). Collagen can inactivate potentially harmful factors such as proteases, oxygen free radicals and excess metal ions present in chronic wound fluid (Cullen *et al.* 2002). Collagen dressings bind excess proteases and other inflammatory proteins to its structure and lower the wound pH to around pH5 which, in turn, helps to reduce the harmful protease activity (S. Hampton, pers. comm., October 2006).

Collagen is the most abundant protein in the human body and its synthesis plays a very important role in the early phases of the process of healing and formation of granulation tissues, which afterwards will form a healing tissue. Inside this process the collagen formation is due to the action of cytokines and the interaction between extra cellular mould and fibroblasts (Torra I Bou *et al.* 2001). The macrophages control the liberation of collagen by fibroblasts by means of so-called growth factors: platelet derived growth factor (PDGF), epidermal growth

1119

factor (EGF), fibroblast growth factor (FGF) and transforming growth factor (TGF-β) (Torra I Bou et al. 2001).

Catrix is designed to reduce protease levels in wound fluids by providing a competitive substrate (collagen) for the proteases. It thereby reduces proteolytic destruction of essential extracellular matrix ECM components and platelet-derived growth factors (S. Hampton, pers. comm., October 2006).

Cadesorb is a protease modulating ointment, which contains an absorbent starch based polymer, polythene Glycol and poloxamer. In the presence of exudate, Cadesorb transforms into a soft moist gel to promote an ideal wound-healing environment. The ointment has been designed specifically for non-healing wounds to rebalance the levels of protease activity in the wound and by removing excess exudate and slough from the wound bed.

Promogran is a matrix of freeze-dried collagen (55%) and oxidized regenerated cellulose (45%) (Morgan 2002; Thomas 2002). It forms a gel on contact with wound exudate and interacts with products found in wound exudate that impair healing, specifically binding to and inactivating metalloproteases that degrade growth factors. Promogran also binds to and protects growth factors, which are released back into the wound as the dressing is absorbed (Morgan 2002). Prisma has a similar makeup but has the addition of silver (S. Hampton, pers. comm., October 2006).

Complementary therapies

The use of complementary therapies in wound management is based very much on anecdotal evidence. However, there have been trials using essential oils in wound care, in particular for the relief of pain and wound odour (Price & Price 1995; Baker 1998). Complementary therapies such as relaxation, massage, visualization, imagery and distraction may be very useful in the reduction of wound pain, especially that associated with procedures such as dressing changes (Naylor 2001). Other complementary therapies that may be useful in the management of wound pain include acupuncture, acupressure, autogenic therapy, biofeedback and hypnosis (Rankin-Box 2001).

Complementary therapies should only be administered by health care professionals with the relevant training and qualifications (Stone 2001). When used alongside conventional management treatments, these therapies can be extremely beneficial in reducing pain or the response to pain.

Pressure ulcers or decubitus ulcers

Definition

Pressure ulcers (decubitus ulcers) are areas of localized tissue damage caused by excess pressure, shearing or friction forces (Benbow 2006). The extent of this damage can range from persistent erythema to necrotic ulceration involving muscle, tendon and bone (Reid & Morison 1994).

Pressure ulcers are a serious problem in health care systems, and are associated with pain, prolonged hospital stay, and if not prevented, can result in fatalilty (Schoonhoven *et al.* 2002). Clark (2002) discusses the significant reduction in quality of life for patients with pressure ulcers. He acknowledged that factors such as social isolation, pain and limitations on activity can have detrimental effects on patients and their families.

The Nursing and Midwifery Council's (NMC's) *The Code* states that nurses must act without delay if the patient is put at risk (NMC 2008). It was suggested that the focus of attention for pressure ulcers should be on prevention of initial tissue damage, prevention of progression of an ulcer to a more severe grade and prevention of infection (Bennett *et al.* 2004). There is a need to monitor and treat pressure ulcers effectively because they are generally avoidable, and this will prevent unnecessary pain and suffering for the patient (Grewal *et al.* 1999). It must be emphasized that the prevention of pressure ulceration is a multidisciplinary responsibility, and not solely for nursing staff (Beldon 2006).

Reference material

Prevalence

Pressure ulcers represent a significant financial burden on health care systems (Benbow 2006). Approximately 412 000 individuals will develop a new pressure ulcer annually in the UK: one in every 150 in the general population and one in 23 of the population over 65 years of age (Bennett *et al.* 2004). While the total cost of presssure ulcer care in the UK between 1999 and 2000 was £1.4–2.1 billion, 90% of this cost is nurse time (Bennett *et al.* 2004). The National Service Framework for Older People (DH 2001a) has identified the need to reduce the risk of pressure damage in older persons in both community and inpatient settings, and highlighted the importance of specialist care for this vulnerable group of people.

1121

Aetiology

The three major extrinsic factors that were identified as being significant contributory factors in the development of pressure ulcers include pressure, shearing and friction. These factors should be removed or diminished to prevent injury (NICE 2003).

■ *Pressure*. The blood pressure at the arterial end of the capillaries is approximately 35 mmHg, while at the venous end this drops to around 16 mmHg (the average mean capillary pressure equals about 17 mmHg) (Guyton & Hall 2000; Tortora & Grabowski 2008). Any external pressures exceeding this will cause capillary obstruction as the capillaries close when the pressure between the bed surface and the bony prominence exceeds the 16–32 mmHg (Landis 1930; S. Hampton, pers. comm., October 2006). Tissues that are dependent on these capillaries are deprived of their blood supply. Eventually, the ischaemic tissues will die (Bridel-Nixon 1999; Tong 1999). The pressure as it approaches the bony prominences can be up to five times greater and is known as the 'cone of pressure': it explains why a surface redness can hide extensive tissue damage nearer the bone. It also explains why a small ulcer can open into a large, undetermined ulcer with overhanging edges and sinus formation (S. Hampton, pers. comm., October 2006). Bliss (1993) identifies that the formation of undermined tissues and sinuses are not due to infection but are produced by lysis of necrotic tissue produced during the original ischaemic episode (S. Hampton, pers. comm., October 2006).

- *Shearing.* This may occur when the patient slips down the bed or is dragged up the bed. As the skeleton moves over the underlying tissue the microcirculation is destroyed and the tissue dies of anoxia. In more serious cases, lymphatic vessels and muscle fibres may also become torn, resulting in a deep pressure ulcer (Simpson *et al.* 1996; Collier 1999; Clay 2000).
- *Friction.* This is a component of shearing, which causes stripping of the stratum corneum, leading to superficial ulceration (Waterlow 1988; Johnson 1989). Poor lifting and moving techniques may be a major contributory factor (NICE 2001).

The most common sites for pressure ulcer development are areas where soft tissue is compressed between a prominence (such as the sacrum) and an external surface (such as a mattress or seat of a chair) (Hess 2005).

Identifying at-risk patients

Assessing a patient's risk of developing pressure ulcers should involve both informal and formal assessment procedures (NICE 2003). A patient's risk of developing a pressure ulcer should be assessed either on admission to hospital or in the community when the patient first comes into contact with health services. The NICE guidelines suggest that this should take place within 6 hours of the start of admission to the episode of care (NICE 2003). The European Pressure Ulcer Advisory Panel (EPUAP 2003) pointed out that assessment should be ongoing and frequency of reassessment should be dependent on change in the patient's condition with the environment.

Many predisposing factors are involved in the development of pressure ulcers. An individual's potential to develop pressure ulcers may be influenced by the following intrinsic factors (NICE 2003):

- Reduced mobility or immobility.
- Acute illness.

- Level of consciousness.
- Extremes of age.
- Vascular disease.
- Severe, chronic or terminal illness.
- Previous history of pressure damage.
- Malnutrition and dehydration.

Skin inspection should occur regularly and frequency must be established according to the patient's medical condition (NICE 2003). Patients who are willing to be involved should be taught and encouraged to inspect their own skin. A mirror can be provided for patients to inspect areas that they cannot see easily.

Grades of pressure ulcers

If a pressure ulcer develops then classification of the wound may assist in determining the most appropriate treatment. These are valuable in describing the state of the ulcer and the most pertinent care required by the patient.

The EPUAP (2003) outlined four grades for risk of tissue damage:

- *Grade 1*: non-blanchable erythema of intact skin.
- *Grade 2*: presents clinically as an abrasion or blister.
- *Grade 3*: superficial lesions.
- *Grade 4*: deep lesions, extensive destruction, tissue necrosis, or damage to muscle, bone or supporting structures.

Assessment tools

There are several risk assessment tools in pressure ulcer development such as those developed by Norton, Braden and Waterlow (Norton *et al.* 1985; Braden & Bergstrom 1987; Waterlow 1991; Waterlow1998). Deeks (1996) suggested that no single tool is considered reliable and valid for universal use. It has become common for particular areas of care to construct their own hybrid assessment tool as a result of professional discussion and tailoring to specific patient needs (Birtwistle 1994; Chaplin 2000; Lindgren *et al.* 2002). NICE (2001) cautions professionals to use risk assessment tools as an *aide mémoire* and recommends their use in conjunction with clinical judgment (Chaplin 2000; RCN 2001).

Some of the most commonly used tools include the following:

Norton scale

With the Norton scale (Table 34.6) patients with a score of 14 or below are considered to be at greatest risk of pressure ulcer development. A score of 14–18 is not considered at risk but will require reassessment and a score of 18–20 indicates minimal risk.

Table 34.6 The Norton scale (From Norton *et al.* 1985 and Braden & Bergstrom 1996).

Physical condition	Score	Mental condition	Score	Activity	Score	Mobility	Score	Incontinent	Score
Good	4	Alert	4	Ambulant	4	Full	4	Not	4
Fair	3	Apathetic	3	Walk/help	3	Slightly limited	3	Occasionally	3
Poor	2	Confused	2	Chairbound	2	Very limited	2	Usually/urine	2
Very bad	1	Stuporous	1	Bedfast	1	Immobile	1	Doubly	1

The 'cut off' point for 'at risk' patients was later raised to 15 or 16 by Norton (Norton *et al.* 1985; Papanikolaou *et al.* 2006). Norton acknowledged that the tool was not intended as a universal tool, otherwise age and nutrition would have formed part of the criteria (Waterlow 2005).

Waterlow scale

The Waterlow scale (Figure 34.2) defines a score of 11–15 as being 'at risk', 16–20 as 'high risk' and over 20 as 'very high risk' (Waterlow 2005). In a study of the Norton and Waterlow scales, 75.7% of patients identified as 'at risk' by the Waterlow scale developed a pressure ulcer, whereas 62% of those with a score of 16 or less on the Norton scale developed ulcers (Smith *et al.* 1986). This suggests that the Waterlow scale may give a more accurate prediction of patient risk.

Braden scale

The Braden scale (Table 34.7) consists of six subscores (sensory perception, activity, moisture, nutrition, mobility, and friction and shearing) which are scored from 1 to 4 depending on the severity of the condition (with the exception of friction and shearing which is scored 1–3). The total score is then added up with a range possible from 6 to 23. The lower the score, the higher the risk of developing a pressure ulcer. Hospital patients are considered to be at risk if their score is 16 or below. It has been tested in a variety of settings and validated by expert opinion (Bergstrom *et al.* 1987; Bergstrom & Braden 1992).

The Braden scale was originally designed as a pressure ulcer predictor, unlike the Norton and Waterlow scales which assess risk (Waterlow 2005). This distinction is important to note when tools are used, or compared. Targeted interventions are likely to differ; for instance, Braden, although used widely in the USA, has been criticized for being difficult to use in a working environment (RCN 2003; Waterlow 2005).

Name: _____ Hospital No: _____

Instruction for use:
1. Score on admission and update weekly or if significant change in patient's condition
2. Add scores together and insert total score
3. Document actions taken in the evaluation section
4. If total score is 10+ initiate core care plan At Risk of Pressure Damage/Pressure Ulcer Formation

10+ AT RISK   **15+ HIGH RISK**   **20+ VERY HIGH RISK**

	Date (Day/Month/Year)								
	Time								
GENDER	Male	1							
	Female	2							
AGE	14–49	1							
	50–64	2							
	65–74	3							
	75–80	4							
	81+	5							
BUILD	Average	0							
	Above average	1							
	Obese	2							
	Below average	3							
APPETITE (select one option ONLY)	Average	0							
	Poor	1							
	NG Tube/fluids only	2							
	NBM/anorexic	3							
VISUAL ASSESSMENT OF AT RISK SKIN AREA (may select one or more options)	Healthy	0							
	Thin and fragile	1							
	Dry	1							
	Oedematous	1							
	Clammy (Temp↑)	1							
	Previous pressure sore or scarring	2							
	Discoloured	2							
	Broken	3							

Figure 34.2 Waterlow pressure ulcer risk assessment. (Adapted from the Waterlow Pressure Sore/Ulcer Risk Assessment Scoring System [available from www.judywaterlow.fsnet.co.uk] with permission and acknowledgement of the copyright holder, J. Waterlow 1991, revised 1995, 1998 & 2005.)

MOBILITY (select one option ONLY)	Fully	0							
	Restless/fidgety	1							
	Apathetic	2							
	Restricted	3							
	Inert (due to ↓ consciousness/traction)	4							
	Chairbound	5							
CONTINENCE (select one option ONLY)	Continent/catheterized	0							
	Occasional incontinence	1							
	Incontinent of urine	2							
	Incontinent of faeces	2							
	Doubly incontinent	3							
TISSUE MALNUTRITION (may select one or more options)	Smoking	2							
	Anaemia	2							
	Peripheral vascular disease	5							
	Cardiac failure	5							
	Cachexia	8							
NEUROLOGICAL DEFICIT (score depends on severity)	Diabetes, CVA, MS, motor/sensory paraplegia epidural	4–6							
MAJOR SURGERY TRAUMA (up to 48 hours post surgery)	Above waist	2							
	Orthopaedic, below waist, spinal > 2 hours on theatre table	5							
MEDICATION	Cytotoxics, high dose steroids, anti-inflammatory	4							
TOTAL SCORE									
NURSE SIGNATURE									

Figure 34.2 (*continued*)

Table 34.7 Braden scale for predicting pressure sore risk. (Copyright B. Braden and N. Bergstrom 1988. [available from www.bradenscale.com].)

				Date of assessment
Sensory perception Ability to respond meaningfully to pressure related discomfort	**1.** *Completely limited:* Unresponsive (does not moan, flinch or grasp) to painful stimuli, due to diminished level of consciousness or sedation *or* limited ability to feel pain over most of body surface	**2.** *Very limited:* Responds only to painful stimuli. Cannot communicate discomfort except by moaning or restlessness *or* has a sensory impairment that limits the ability to feel pain or discomfort over half of the body	**3.** *Slightly limited:* Responds to verbal commands, but cannot always communicate discomfort or need to be turned *or* has some sensory impairment that limits ability to feel pain or discomfort in 1 or 2 extremities	**4.** *No impairment:* Responds to verbal commands. Has no sensory deficit that would limit ability to feel or voice pain or discomfort
Moisture Degree to which skin is exposed to moisture	**1.** *Constantly moist:* Skin is kept moist almost constantly by perspiration, urine etc. Dampness is detected every time patient is moved or turned	**2.** *Very moist:* Skin is often, but not always moist. Linen must be changed at least once a shift	**3.** *Occasionally moist:* Skin is occasionally moist, requiring an extra linen change approximately once a day	**4.** *Rarely moist:* Skin is usually dry, linen only requires changing at routine intervals
Activity Degree of physical activity	**1.** *Bedfast:* Confined to bed	**2.** *Chairfast:* Ability to walk severely limited or non-existent Cannot bear own weight and/or must be assisted into chair or wheelchair	**3.** *Walks occasionally:* Walks occasionally during day, but for very short distances, with or without assistance. Spends majority of each shift in bed or chair	**4.** *Walks frequently:* Walks outside the room at least twice a day and inside room at least once every 2 hours during waking hours
Mobility Ability to change and control body position	**1.** *Completely immobile:* Does not make even slight changes in body or extremity position without assistance	**2.** *Very limited:* Makes occasional slight changes in body or extremity position but unable to make frequent or significant changes independently	**3.** *Slightly limited:* Makes frequent though slight changes in body or extremity position independently	**4.** *No limitations:* Makes major and frequent changes in position without assistance

(continued)

	1. Very poor:	2. Probably inadequate:	3. Adequate:	Date of assessment
				4. Excellent:

Nutrition
Usual food intake pattern:
1 NBM: nothing by mouth
2 IV: intravenously
3 TPN: total parenteral nutrition

1. Very poor: Never eats a complete meal. Rarely eats more than 1/3 of any food offered. Eats 2 servings or less of protein (meat or dairy products) per day. Takes fluids poorly. Does not take a liquid dietary supplement
or
is NBM 1 and/or maintained on clear fluids or IV 2 for more than 5 days

2. Probably inadequate: Rarely eats a complete meal and generally eats only about 1/2 of any food offered. Protein intake includes only 3 servings of meat or dairy products per day. Occasionally will take a dietary supplement
or
receives less than the optimum amount of liquid diet or tube feeding

3. Adequate: Eats over half of most meals. Eats a total of 4 servings of protein (meats, dairy products) each day Occasionally will refuse a meal, but will usually take a supplement if offered
or
is on a tube feeding or TPN 3 regimen that probably meets most of nutritional needs

4. Excellent: Eats most of every meal. Never refuses a meal Usually eats a total of 4 or more servings of meat and dairy products. Occasionally eats between meals. Does not require supplementation

Friction and shear

1. Problem: Requires moderate to maximum assistance in moving. Complete lifting without sliding against sheets is impossible. Frequently slides down in bed or chair, requiring frequent repositioning with maximum assistance. Spasticity, contractures or agitation lead to almost constant friction

2. Potential problem: Moves feebly or requires minimum assistance. During a move skin probably slides to some extent against sheets, chair, restraints, or other devices. Maintains relatively good position in chair or bed most of the time but occasionally slides down

3. No apparent problem: Moves in bed and in chair independently and has sufficient muscle strength to lift up completely during move. Maintains good position in bed or chair at all times

Total score   Total score of 12 or less represents **high risk**
Assess   Date   Evaluator/signature/title   Assess   Date   Evaluator/signature/title
1   / /   3   / /
2   / /   4   / /
Name: last, first, middle   Attending physician   ID number

High risk: Total score <12 Moderate risk: Total score 13–14 Low risk: Total score 15–16 if under 75 years old or 15–18 if over 75 years old.

Table 34.7 *(continued)*

Treatment and prevention

Treatment of pressure ulcers is the same as for any other wound. The aetiology and underlying or related pathology, as well as the wound itself, must be assessed in order to provide the most appropriate treatment. Care should be aimed at relief of pressure, the minimization of symptoms from predisposing factors and the provision of the ideal microenvironment for wound healing.

When positioning patients, it must be ensured that prolonged pressure on bony prominences is minimized. An awareness of interface pressures, e.g. creased bed linen and night clothing, is also important to avoid increased friction and further skin breakdown. Repositioning is recommended by the NICE (2003) but with taking into consideration other factors such as patient's medical condition, comfort, overall plan of care and the support surface. NICE (2003) also suggested that a repositioning schedule must be available. This must be agreed with the patient and recorded. If patients are able, they should be taught the underlying principles of pressure relief and enabled to manage repositioning themselves (NICE 2001) (see Chapter 26). It has also been suggested that consideration must be given to whether sitting time should be restricted to less than 2 hours per session (NICE 2003). It is important to seek specialist advice for assessment for positioning, aids and equipment to use.

It was suggested that nurses should possess a basic level of knowledge relating to the underlying principles of pressure ulcer prevention, healing and treatment in order to reduce unnecessary occurrence and discomfort (Mockridge & Anthony 1999).

Devices used for relief of pressure

A wide variety of devices are available to help relieve pressure over susceptible areas, e.g. cushions, overlays, static/dynamic mattresses and replacement beds. These devices differ in function and complexity, and choice must be based on meeting the patient's individual need, sound criteria for decision-making and effective use of available resources (Table 34.8). NICE (2003) emphasized that the quality of data currently available to evaluate the clinical effectiveness of pressure-relieving devices is variable.

The following are recommendations from NICE (2001):

- Patients with pressure ulcers should have access to pressure-relieving support surfaces and strategies, for example mattresses and cushions, 24 hours a day and this applies to all support surfaces.
- All individuals assessed as having a grade 1–2 pressure ulcer should, as a minimum provision, be placed on a high-specification foam mattress or cushion with pressure-reducing properties. Observation of skin changes,

Table 34.8 A selection of mechanical methods for relieving pressure. It is important to remember the risk of cross-infection with the use of special beds. Most companies provide adequate cleaning/sterilizing of their equipment. Sheepskin is not a pressure relieving device and can become hard and matted with washing although it has been commended for helping with shearing in the past. (Hampton & Collins 2004; NICE 2005 Guidelines: www.nice.org.uk/page.aspx?o=cg029fullguideline.)

Aid	Use	Advantages	Disadvantages
Silicone-filled mattress pad/cushion (e.g. Transoft)	Waterlow 10 or patients on prolonged bedrest, able to move spontaneously	Relieves pressure by distributing it over a greater area. Comfortable. Machine (industrial) washable. Acceptable in community settings as well as in hospital. Can be used for incontinent patients. Relatively cheap purchase price. Plastic protective covers available	If the patient is very incontinent of urine, even if the plastic side is uppermost, there is seepage into the core material. Stitching comes undone after several launderings. Not recommended for routine use in pressure ulcer prevention
Roho air-filled mattress/ cushions	High–medium-risk patients, Waterlow 10–15	Interlinked air cells transfer air with movement. Patient can be nursed sitting or recumbent. Non-mechanical. Washable	Can be punctured and is expensive to repair. Often incorrectly inflated due to lack of understanding and education. Can be mechanically cleaned in sterile supply department
Alternating pressure beds	High–medium-risk patients, Waterlow 15 r	Mechanical alteration of pressure. Reduce the frequency of (but not need for) repositioning. Available on hire at short notice	Must be checked and maintained. May increase pressures in very thin patients. Punctures possible. Patients may complain of nausea due to movement of cells
Pressure redistributing foam mattress	Moderate-risk as above	Two-way multi-stretch foam and flexible covers, less expensive than beds	Should be audited 6 monthly for cross-infection risk. Should be placed on meshed mattress board, not solid, and turned monthly
Dynamic air mattress or low air loss bed	Moderate–high-risk patients, Waterlow 15–20	Equalizes pressure and weight and can be programmed to adjust air support to give optimal pressure redistribution. Warm	Expensive to buy, but can be hired. Makes some patients feel 'sea-sick'. Reduces self-motivated movement. Cells can become quite hard
Air fluidized bed	High-risk patients, Waterlow 20, or indicated because of medical condition	As near to levitation as possible. Warm, sterile air produces a beneficial environment for healing wounds. One nurse can manage even a very heavy or debilitated patient on his/her own. Can be used for incontinent patients or those with heavy wound exudate. May help to alleviate severe pain	Expensive to hire. Need to reinforce floors before it can be installed. Minimizes self-motivation. Can be difficult for the patient to get in and out of bed even with help. Available on hire basis only

documentation of positioning and repositioning scheme must be combined in the patient's care.

- If there is any potential or actual deterioration of affected areas or further pressure ulcer development, an alternating pressure (AP) (replacement or overlay) or sophisticated continuous low pressure (CLP) system (e.g. low air loss, air fluidized, air flotation, viscous fluid) should be used.
- For patients who require bed rails, AP overlay mattresses should be placed on a reduced-depth foam mattress to maintain their safety.
- Depending on the location of ulcer, individuals assessed as having grade 3–4 pressure ulcers (including intact eschar where depth, and therefore grade, cannot be assessed) should be, as a minimum provision, placed on an AP mattress or sophisticated CLP system.
- If AP equipment is required, the first choice should be an overlay system. However, circumstances such as patient weight or patient safety indicate the need for a replacement system.
- Create the optimum wound healing environment by using modern dressings (e.g. hydrocolloids, hydrogels, hydrofibres, foams, films, alginates, soft silicones) in preference to basic dressing types such as gauze, paraffin gauze and simple dressing pads.

In 2005, NICE in collaboration with the Royal College of Nursing (RCN) created a clinical guideline in pressure ulcer management (NICE 2005; RCN 2005). This included data looking at evidence-based practice, cost-effectiveness and economic evaluations in the different devices, drugs, procedures, among others in the management of pressure ulcers (see Table 34.8).

Plastic surgery wounds

Definition

Plastic surgery is the collective term that refers to surgical procedures that are performed to restore function and assist in the healing of exposed or nonunion fractures, soft tissue defects or to improve natural contours. Patients whose lives have changed following excision of a cancerous tumour or other misfortunes can be reconstructed and made whole again (Dinman 1999). This is achieved by using flaps and skin grafts for reconstruction purposes, in addition to using the natural elasticity and mobility of the skin. A surgical flap is a strip of tissue, usually consisting of skin, underlying fat, fascia, muscle and/or bone, which is transferred from one part of the body (known as the donor site) to another (known as the recipient site) (Edwards 1994; Brown *et al.* 1998).

A skin graft is living, but devascularized (separated from its blood supply), tissue consisting of all or some of the layers of the skin which is removed from one area of the body and applied to a wound on another area of the body. The three types of skin graft are full-thickness skin graft (FTSG), in which the entire epidermis and dermis is removed, split-thickness or split skin graft (SSG), which consists of the epidermis and the upper part of the dermis only (Francis 1998; Young & Fowler 1998), and pinch grafting, which can be undertaken by a nurse educated in the procedure (S. Hampton, pers. comm., October 2006).

Reference material

Aetiology

Surgical reconstruction is often required following extensive surgery for cancers of the breast, head and neck, skin (melanoma), soft tissue (sarcomas) and genitourinary system. The aim is to perform the simplest procedure that will provide the best aesthetic and functional outcome (Clamon & Netscher 1994). Each patient will require individually planned, and therefore unique, surgery. Reconstructive surgery of this type often results in altered anatomy, in both appearance and function, which may impact upon the psychological and physical well-being of the patient.

Assessment

Preoperative patient assessment must be as detailed as possible; this should include information on past and present medical conditions that may delay wound healing (see Wound assessment and Tissue factors affecting wound healing sections, above). For certain patient groups, e.g. those with recurrence of head and neck cancer, anatomy may already have been altered, through previous surgery, thereby narrowing down the possible options for reconstruction.

Postoperative observation of the wound sites, dressings and drains is crucial as deterioration of a wound can occur suddenly, e.g. fluid-filled seromas, necessitating the need for prompt nursing action. The main aim following flap reconstruction is to allow easy access for observation and to ensure circulation and overall care is monitored efficiently during the crucial first 72 hours. Figure 34.3 shows a flap observation chart.

Associated problems

Split skin graft donor site

The two most common problems associated with a split skin graft donor site are slipping of dressing and infection.

Name: .... Hospital No: .... Ward: ....

THE ROYAL MARSDEN

Flap Observation Chart

Instructions	Criteria for Assessment	Normal	Arterial Insufficiency	Venous Congestion
1. **Confirm with the surgeon the frequency of flap observations (see medical notes / nursing care plan)** Suggested immediate post-op assessment frequency: • every 15 minutes for first 4 hours, • every 30 minutes for the next 4 hours, • hourly for 24–36 hours, • then 2–4 hourly thereafter 2. **If signs of venous or arterial occlusion seek immediate help** 3. **At each handover, confirm flap status/observations at the bedside**	**Colour** • If it is an external flap then check with the donor site or original colour • If it is an internal flap then monitor for extremes of colour	Usual skin tone	Paler than usual skin tone	Blue / Purple / Mottled
	Temperature • An external or internal flap should always feel warm to touch • If the flap feels cool or has increased warmth, ***seek medical assessment immediately*** • A warmer flap may be due to an abnormal inflammatory response, e.g. infection	Warm	Cold	Increased warmth
	Turgidity (Texture) • The flap should usually feel soft (spongy), not hard or flaccid • Hard or swollen flap indicates possible oedema or haematoma	Soft	Flaccid	Turgid (hard)
	Capillary Refill (Blanching) • If possible this should be timed (in seconds) • If timing not possible and an alteration in perfusion is suspected, ***seek medical assessment immediately***	2–3 seconds	Absent / Sluggish > 6 seconds	Brisk < 3 seconds
	Specific Monitoring Instructions (*e.g. Monitor the tension on the flap and check for kinking*)			

Type & Location of Flap: .... **Donor Area (if appropriate):** ....

....

Timing		Colour (*tick one*)			Temperature (*tick one*)			Turgidity (Texture) (*tick one*)			Capillary Refill (Blanching) (*tick one*)			Specific Instructions (specify):	Signature and Print Name
Date	Time	Usual skin tone	Paler than usual skin tone	Blue / purple / mottled	Warm	Cold	Increased warmth	Soft	Flaccid	Turgid (hard)	2–3 seconds	Absent / sluggish > 6 seconds	Brisk < 3 seconds		

Title: Flap Observation Chart | Version No: 2 Issue Date: March 2005 Unique Identification Number: NR027 | Document Type: Clinical Record - Chart

Department: Nursing & Rehabilitation – Nursing | Page 1 of 2 |

Figure 34.3 Flap observation chart.

1134

Timing		Colour (tick one)			Temperature (tick one)			Turgidity (Texture) (tick one)			Capillary Refill (Blanching) (tick one)			Specific Instructions (specify):	Signature and Print Name
Date	Time	Usual skin tone	Paler than usual skin tone	Blue / purple / mottled	Warm	Cold	Increased warmth	Soft	Flaccid	Turgid (hard)	2–3 seconds	Absent / sluggish > 6 seconds	Brisk < 3 seconds		

Title: Flap Observation Chart

Department: Nursing & Rehabilitation – Nursing

Version No: 2 Issue Date: March 2005 Unique Identification Number: NR027

Page 2 of 2

Document Type: Clinical Record - Chart

© 2005 The Royal Marsden Hospital

Figure 34.3 *(continued)*

Slipping of dressing, resulting in pain and discomfort

The donor sites chosen for SSG harvesting are usually the upper thigh, upper arm or upper buttock. Less conspicuous areas of the body are chosen wherever possible. The excision of the thin layer of skin leaves nerve endings exposed, resulting in pain at the donor site (Wilkinson 1997). Traditionally paraffin gauze combined with an absorbent layer of gauze padding and a bandage have been applied to donor sites in theatre and left intact for 10 days. However, adherence to the wound bed, complicated by slipping of the secondary dressing once heavy with exudate, commonly occurs causing pain and delaying healing. Beldon (2003) observed four different dressings on donor sites in a sample of 40 patients and found healing and comfort were improved in the alginate combined with a semi-permeable film group. (The comparison groups used a film alone, paraffin gauze or alginate as a primary dressing and padding with a bandage as a secondary dressing [Beldon 2003].)

Infection

A high amount of exudate on the dressing, evident by new and excessive strikethrough, can indicate the presence of infection (Beldon 2003). The entire dressing should be soaked off in order to assess the wound site, and the site should be swabbed for microbial culture and sensitivity. While infected, the wound site should be dressed daily. *Pseudomonas aeruginosa* is a common infecting organism of donor sites and is often evidenced by a strong musty smell and bright blue–green exudate.

Flamazine (silver sulphadiazine) is usually an effective treatment for *Pseudomonas* when applied topically to the donor site and covered with a non-adherent dressing (Hamilton-Miller *et al.* 1993), but this is not commonly used today as there is a dearth of dressings containing silver which are used instead of creams. There are also products, such as Cadesorb, which modulate the pH of a wound and drop the pH from >8 to <6. *Pseudomonas aeruginosa* survives in a pH of 8.4 but not in an acidic pH (S. Hampton, pers. comm., October 2006).

If the patient experiences a raised temperature, increased pain or appears unwell, this may indicate the presence of a systemic infection and they will require a course of antibiotics (Wilkinson 1997).

Split skin recipient site (flap donor site)

When a flap is transferred from its original site or a tumour is widely excised, it leaves a deficit of tissue. Split skin is applied to this site, as primary closure is not usually possible. The most common problem with SSG recipient sites is fluid-filled seromas.

Fluid-filled seromas

On removing the dressing after 5 days, the SSG should be smooth and pink or red in colour. Any seromas, characterized by blisters containing air and haemoserous fluid, must be expelled. Without performing this, the graft will not 'take'. A sterile needle is used to evacuate the fluid, enabling the graft to be carefully rolled from the centre outwards (Coull 1991). This can be performed by using a cotton bud and enables the graft to adhere to the underlying tissue. A tulle dressing, low-linting gauze and a bandage, or a tapeless dressing are then applied. The pressure from the dressing assists in expelling the blisters (Coull 1991).

Scarring

Definition

A scar is defined as the mark left after a wound has healed with the formation of connective tissue, giving rise to an altered appearance of the skin (Davis *et al.* 1993; Eisenbeiss *et al.* 1998). Initially the scar is red and raised; then over a period of 6–12 months this matures to produce a hypopigmented, flat scar (Davies 1985).

Hypertrophic and keloid scars

Occasionally the scar continues to become increasingly red, raised and itchy, defined as hypertrophic. If these symptoms continue, with the scar tissue invading surrounding unaffected tissue as well as increasing in height, a keloid scar is formed (Williams 1996; Eisenbeiss *et al.* 1998). The areas that are most susceptible are the upper back, shoulders, anterior chest, presternal area and the upper arms (Munro 1995a; Beldon 2000). Darker skinned people have a greater susceptibility to developing keloid scars than those who are lighter skinned (Eisenbeiss *et al.* 1998).

Reference material

Aetiology

There are a number of possible predisposing factors (Munro 1995a):

- Increased skin tension can contribute to the formation of keloid and hypertrophic scars; however, earlobes, which are free of tension, can also develop keloid scars.

- These scars appear to have a genetic basis. In addition to this, keloid formation is more common in females (3 : 1 female : male ratio).
- There is thought to be a relationship between endocrine changes and keloid formation, e.g. keloids have been known to occur after a thyroidectomy and with increased hypothalamic activity.
- The production of hypertrophic and keloid scars may have an immunological basis.
- Biochemical differences between healthy scars, keloid and hypertrophic scars have been found, indicating that collagen synthesis is altered.
- Growth factors may have a role in keloid formation. During the inflammatory stage several growth factors (collagenase, gelatinase and stromelysin) migrate into the wound and affect the collagen fibre formation of a matrix which enhances the strength of the wound. When they are overactive or these processes are interrupted, abnormal scarring can occur (Smith 2005).

Management

Patients may be offered a number of treatments to help prevent or improve an abnormal scar:

- *Finger massage* can improve the condition of the scar. A non-perfumed moisturizing cream should be used to prevent friction between the finger and scar. Finger massage can begin when the wound has completely healed and all bruising has subsided. Massage should be performed for 10 minutes, six times each day using firm pressure in a tight circular motion over the scar.
- *Pressure treatment* with individually tailored elastic garments may be used for both keloid and hypertrophic scars. This treatment is used to prevent secondary contractures and to restore flatness and smoothness to scars. Pressure must be applied continuously for at least 12 months and any break in pressure should not exceed 30 minutes per day (Munro 1995b; Puzey 2001). Enhancement of cosmetic appearance and an increased rate of scar maturation are promoted by compression (Smith 2005). Pressure must be applied continuously for at least 12 months and any break in pressure should not exceed 30 minutes per day (Munro 1995b; Puzey 2001).
- *Intralesional corticosteroid injections* may help reduce scar tissue deposition and to soften and flatten keloid scars (Munro 1995b). There is a risk of scar recurrence with this treatment and it is only suitable for small scars (Eisenbeiss *et al*. 1998).
- *Silicone gel sheeting* will soften, flatten and blanch keloid and hypertrophic scars (Carney *et al*. 1994; Williams 1996).

- *Glycerine-based hydrogel sheet* (Novogel) may be effective in the prevention and treatment of hypertrophic and keloid scars. It can soften, flatten and relieve itching, redness and burning of scars (Baum & Busuito 1998). CicaC is a recognized treatment for scar tissue (S. Hampton, pers. comm., October 2006).

- *Surgical excision* may be considered to release scar contractures; for example, a 'W' or 'Z' plasty to release a scar contracture by cutting it in the line of relaxed skin tension (Allsworth 1985; Beldon 2000). In the case of larger scars, surgical excision with or without skin grafting may be performed but there is a high rate of scar recurrence especially with keloid scars. Postoperative radiotherapy may reduce the recurrence rate by up to 70% (Eisenbeiss *et al.* 1998).

- *Cosmetic camouflage*, utilizing specialist cosmetic products, can be used to hide scarring; this is most successful in patients with atrophic (indented) and hypertrophic scars. This service is provided by appropriately trained professionals who also provide advice and education to enable patients to perform their own camouflage make-up.

Methods of wound closure

There are four main methods of wound closure:

(a)   Sutures.
(b)   Adhesive skin closure strips.
(c)   Tissue adhesive.
(d)   Metal clips and staples.

See Table 34.9 for advantages and disadvantages of each method.

Wounds may vary and therefore careful assessment is required before the method of closure is selected and attempted (Richardson 2007). Richardson (2007) lists the following guiding principles to assist with decision making:

1   What is the aim of the wound closure: e.g. eliminating dead space where a haematoma can develop, realigning tissue correctly, or holding aligned tissues until healing has occurred.

2   What is the history of the wound: this informs the practitioner about the depth of the wound and likelihood of infection.

3   What is the wound site pattern: this and biomechanical properties may rule out some methods of closure.

Table 34.9 Advantages and disadvantages of methods of wound closure. (From Jay 1999; Elkin *et al.* 2004; Richardson 2007.)

Method:	Disadvantages
Sutures: Non-absorbable sutures are more widely used for skin closure where the material causes little reaction or rejection. A monofilament nylon is a strong single stranded nylon providing continued strength; silk is a braided strand and fairly easy to handle. Interrupted sutures are separate sutures each with its own knot and are used on the majority of wounds because they are the most versatile. They are not recommended for fragile skin. A continuous suture is one long thread that spirals along the entire suture line at evenly spaced intervals Absorbable sutures degrade rapidly and thus allow the deep tissues within a wound to be closed successfully. They are also useful for patients who may not remember they have had sutures or will not attend for follow up Sutures can be removed once healing has occurred normally 5–10 days after injury	Suturing must be performed by an experienced practitioner Requires local anaesthetic Suture material is a foreign body in the wound and thus increases the risk of infection Sutures tied too tightly can damage tissues Sutures too loose may delay healing If skin layers are not aligned then patients can be left with a scar Forceps used to lift skin may crush the tissue
Adhesive skin closure strips: Available in a variety of widths Useful for superficial wounds that are not subject to tension Strips are cheap and easy to use and remove No local anaesthetic required and tissue damage is minimal	Strips do not adhere to sweaty or hairy skin If there is tissue oedema it makes it difficult to achieve good apposition of the wound edges May be suitable over some joints but where skin is taut or subject to movement they do not provide optimum closure
Tissue adhesive: Surgical 'superglues' are now popular for emergency settings Good cosmetic results Less painful than suturing Wound complication rates are low	It is expensive Not suitable over joints and areas of high tension Need second person to assist in getting skin edges aligned
Metal clips and staples: Staples are made of stainless steel wire Provide greatest tensile strength Quick method and offers low level of tissue reactivity and better resistance to infection than sutures Can be performed without local anaesthetic	Staples are more expensive than sutures and may be confined to wounds where needlestick injury is a high risk Must be inserted by an experienced practitioner Failure to align tissue edges may cause scar deformity Only useful for superficial skin layers

Procedure guidelines   **Wound dressings change for acute and surgical wounds**

Equipment

1 As for Procedure guidelines: Aseptic technique (see Chapter 4).

2 Cleaning fluid for irrigation (see Table 34.4).

3 Appropriate dressing (see Table 34.5).

Procedure

See Procedure guidelines: Aseptic technique (see Chapter 4) up to and including step 11, then loosen the dressing.

Action	Rationale
12 Where appropriate, loosen the old dressing.	The dressing can then be lifted off without causing trauma (E).
13 Clean hands with a bactericidal alcohol handrub.	Hands may become contaminated by handling outer packets, dressing, etc. (DH 2005: C).
14 Using the plastic bag in the pack, arrange the sterile field. Pour cleaning solution into gallipots or an indented plastic tray.	The time the wound is exposed should be kept to a minimum to reduce the risk of contamination. To prevent contamination of the environment. To minimize risk of contamination of cleaning solution (E).
15 Remove dressing by placing a hand in the plastic bag, lifting the dressing off and inverting the plastic bag so that the dressing is now inside the bag. Thereafter use this as the 'dirty' bag.	To reduce the risk of cross-infection. To prevent contamination of the environment (E).
16 Attach the bag with the dressing to the side of the trolley below the top shelf.	Contaminated material should be below the level of the sterile field (E).
17 Assess wound healing with reference to volume, amount of granulation tissue and epithelialization, signs of infection, underlying pathology, etc. (see Table 34.3/Figure 34.1). (Record assessment in relevant documentation at the end of the procedure.)	To evaluate wound care (Hampton & Collins 2004: E; Dealey 2005: E; Hess 2005: E).

18 Put on gloves.	To reduce the risk of infection to the wound and contamination of the nurse. Gloves provide greater sensitivity than forceps and are less likely to traumatize the wound or the patient's skin (E).
19 If necessary, gently clean the wound with a gloved hand using 0.9% sodium chloride, unless another solution is indicated (see Table 34.3). If appropriate, irrigate by flushing with water or 0.9% sodium chloride.	To reduce the possibility of physical and chemical trauma to granulation and epithelial tissue (Hess 2005: E).
20 Apply the dressing that is most suitable for the wound using the criteria for dressings (see Table 34.5).	To promote healing and/or reduce symptoms (E).
21 Remove gloves; fasten dressing as appropriate with hypoallergenic tape/Netelast/bandage/tapeless retention dressing.	To prevent irritation of skin and to avoid trauma to wound (E).
22 Make sure the patient is comfortable and the dressing is secure.	A dressing may slip or feel uncomfortable as the patient changes position (E)

Continue with steps 18–21 from the Procedure guidelines: Aseptic technique (see Chapter 4).

Procedure guidelines **Sutures, clips or staples removal**

Equipment

1 As for Procedure guidelines: Aseptic technique (see Chapter 4).

2 Sterile scissors, stitch cutter, staple remover (E).

3 Sterile adhesive sutures (E).

Procedure

Action

1 Explain and discuss the procedure with the patient.

Rationale

To ensure that the patient understands the procedure and gives his/her valid consent (E; DH 2001b: C).

Procedure guidelines *(cont.)*

2 Perform procedure using aseptic technique.	To prevent infection (for further information see Procedure guidelines: Aseptic technique, see Chapter 4) (DH 2005: C).
3 Clean the wound with an appropriate sterile solution such as 0.9% sodium chloride (see Table 34.4).	To prevent infection (E).

For removal of sutures

4 Lift knot of suture with metal forceps. Snip stitch close to the skin. Pull suture out gently.	Plastic forceps tend to slip against nylon sutures (E). To prevent infection by drawing exposed suture through the tissue (E).
5 Use tips of scissors slightly open or the side of the stitch cutter to gently press the skin when the suture is being drawn out.	To minimize pain by counteracting the adhesion between the suture and surrounding tissue (E).

For removal of clips

6 Squeeze wings of clips together with forceps to release from skin.	To release clips atraumatically from the wound (E).
7 If the wound gapes use adhesive sutures to oppose the wound edges.	To improve the cosmetic effect (E).
8 When necessary, cover the wound with an appropriate dressing (see Table 34.5).	To provide the best possible environment for wound healing to take place. To reduce the risk of infection. To prevent the suture line from rubbing against clothing (E).

1142

For removal of staples

9 Slide the lower bar of the staple remover with the V-shaped groove under the staple at an angle of 90°. Squeeze the handles of the staple removers together to open the staple.	To release the staple atraumatically from the wound. If the angle of the staple remover is not correct, the staple will not come out freely (E).
If the suture line is under tension, use free hand to gently squeeze the skin either side of the suture line.	To reduce tension of skin around suture line and lessen pain on removal of staple (E).

10 If the wound gapes use adhesive sutures to oppose the wound edges.	To improve the cosmetic effect (E).

For all suture lines

11 Record condition of suture line and surrounding skin (amount of exudate, pus, inflammation, pain, etc.; see Table 34.3).	To document care and enable evaluation of the wound (Dealey 2005: E; NMC 2005: C; Bale & Jones 2006: E).

Procedure guidelines   **Wound drain dressing (Redivac: closed drainage systems)**

Equipment

1 As for Procedure guidelines: Aseptic technique (see Chapter 4).	**2** Non-adherent, absorbent dressing.

Procedure

Action	**Rationale**
1 Explain and discuss the procedure with the patient.	To ensure that the patient understands the procedure and gives his/her valid consent (DH 2001b: C).
2 Perform procedure using aseptic technique.	To prevent infection (for further information on asepsis, see Procedure guidelines: Aseptic technique, see Chapter 4) (DH 2005: C).
3 Clean the surrounding skin with an appropriate sterile solution such as 0.9% sodium chloride (see Table 34.4).	To prevent infection and remove excess debris (E).
4 Check condition of surrounding skin.	To assess for any excoriation of the skin (E).
5 Ensure that the skin suture holding the drain site in position is intact.	To prevent the drain from leaving the wound (E).

1143

Procedure guidelines *(cont.)*

6 Cover the drain site with a non-adherent, absorbent dressing.	To protect the drain site, prevent infection entering the wound and absorb exudate (E).
7 Tape securely.	To prevent drain coming loose (E).
8 Ensure that the drain is primed or that the suction pump is in working order.	To ensure continuity of drainage (E). Ineffective drainage can result in oedema/haematoma (Hess 2005: E).

Procedure guidelines   **Change of vacuum drainage system**

(See also Chapter 20, Professional edition.)

Equipment

1 Sterile topical swab.   2 Dressing pack.

Procedure

Action	Rationale
1 Explain and discuss the procedure with the patient.	To ensure that the patient understands the procedure and gives his/her valid consent (DH 2001b: C).
2 Perform procedure using aseptic technique.	To prevent infection (see Procedure guidelines: Aseptic technique, see Chapter 4) (DH 2005: C).
3 Wash hands using bactericidal soap and water or bactericidal alcohol handrub.	To minimize the risk of infection (DH 2005: C).
4 Ensure sterile drainage system is readily available.	To ensure sterility during change of system (E).
5 Measure the contents of the bottle to be changed and record this in the appropriate documents.	To maintain an accurate record of drainage from the wound and enable evaluation of state of wound (E).

6 Clamp the tube with the tubing clamps on the drainage tube and bottle connector and remove the bottle.	To prevent air and contamination entering the wound via the drain (E).
7 Clean the end of the tube and attach it to the sterile bottle.	To maintain sterility (E).
8 Unclamp the tubing clamps.	To re-establish the drainage system (E).
9 Place used vacuum drainage system into the clinical waste bag.	To safely dispose of used system (E).

Procedure guidelines   **Wound drain removal (Yeates vacuum drainage system)**

Equipment

1 As for Procedure guidelines: Aseptic technique (see Chapter 4).

2 Sterile scissors or suture cutter.

Procedure

Action	**Rationale**
1 Check the patient's operation notes.	To establish the number and site(s) of internal and external sutures (E).
2 Explain and discuss the procedure with the patient.	To ensure that the patient understands the procedure and gives his/her valid consent (DH 2001b: C).
3 If appropriate (in closed drainage systems) release vacuum.	To prevent pulling at wound tissue, causing pain and tissue damage (E).
4 Perform the procedure using aseptic technique.	To minimize the risk of infection (DH 2005: C). (For further information on asepsis, see Chapter 4.)

1145

Procedure guidelines *(cont.)*

5 Where the wound is covered with an occlusive dressing (e.g. following lumpectomy in the breast), lift and snip the dressing from around the drain. Do not remove it from the entire wound.

To prevent disturbing the incision or contaminating the wound (E).

6 Only clean the wound if necessary, using an appropriate sterile solution, such as 0.9% sodium chloride (see Table 34.4).

To reduce risk of infection (E).

7 Hold the knot of the suture with metal forceps and gently lift upwards.

Plastic forceps tend to slip against nylon sutures. To allow space for the scissors or stitch cutter to be placed underneath (E).

8 Cut the shortest end of the suture as close to the skin as possible.

To prevent infection by allowing the suture to be liberated from the drain without drawing the exposed part through tissue (E).

9 Remove drain gently. If there is resistance, place free gloved hand against the tissue to oppose the tugging of the drain being removed. If the resistance is felt to be excessive, nitrous oxide (e.g. Entonox) may be required.

To minimize pain and reduce trauma (E).

10 Cover the drain site with a sterile dressing and tape securely.

To prevent infection entering the drain site (E).

1146

11 Measure and record the contents of the drainage bottle in the appropriate documents.

To maintain an accurate record of drainage from the wound and enable evaluation of state of wound (NMC 2005: C).

12 Dispose of used drainage system in clinical waste bag.

To ensure safe disposal (E).

Wound drain shortening (Penrose: open drainage systems)

Procedure

Action	Rationale
1 Follow steps 1–8 above (removal of drain), i.e. to the stage where the suture has been cut.	
2 Using gloved hand, gently ease the drain out of wound to the length requested by surgeons (usually 3–5 cm).	To allow healing to take place from base of wound (E).
3 Using gloved hand, place a sterile safety pin through the drain as close to the skin as possible, taking great care not to stab either the nurse or patient.	To prevent retraction into the wound and minimize the risk of cross-infection and sharps injury (E).
4 Cut same amount of tubing from distal end of drain as withdrawn from wound.	So there is a convenient length of tubing to drain into the bag. To ensure patient comfort (E).
5 Place a sterile, suitably sized drainage bag over the drain site.	To allow effluent to drain into the bag. To prevent excoriation of the skin. To contain any odour (E).
6 Check bag is secure and comfortable for the patient.	For patient comfort (E).
7 Record by how much the drainage tube was shortened.	To ensure the length remaining in the wound is known (NMC 2005: C).

1147

Topical negative pressure (TNP) therapy

Equipment

1 1 TNP therapy unit.
2 1 TNP dressing pack.
3 1 TNP canister and tubing.
4 Sterile scissors.
5 Sterile gloves.
6 Apron.

7 Dressing procedure pack.
8 Sterile 0.9% sodium chloride for irrigation (warmed to approx. 37°C in a jug of warm water).
9 Clamp (Spencer Wells forceps).

Procedure guidelines *(cont.)*

Additional materials as required (follow manufacturer's instructions as there are several systems)

- Extra semi-permeable film dressings to seal any leaks.
- Non-adherent wound contact layer to prevent foam adhering to wound bed.
- Alcohol-free skin barrier film to protect any fragile or macerated skin around the wound *or* thin hydrocolloid sheet to 'frame' the wound.

Procedure

Action	Rationale
1 Explain and discuss the procedure with the patient. Agree a time limit for the procedure. The nurse should have completed supervised practice in advance of TNP commencement.	To ensure the patient understands the procedure and other options available and gives his/her valid consent (DH 2001b: C). Ensure competency and correct complementary dressings are used in the wound bed (Beldon 2006: C).
2 Provide routine analgesia prior to dressing procedure.	To prevent unnecessary procedural pain (E).
3 Ensure there is adequate lighting and the patient is comfortable and in a position where the wound can be accessed and viewed easily. Assemble all necessary equipment (Beldon 2006: C).	To allow access to area for dressing change. Dressing application can be complicated and take a long time so the patient should be in a comfortable position for the procedure (E).
4 Perform steps 2–15 of the Procedure guidelines: Aseptic technique (see Chapter 4).	To reduce the risk of cross-infection and reduce the amount of time the wound is exposed (DH 2005: C; E).

TNP dressing removal

Action	Rationale
5 Put on a pair of non-sterile gloves.	To reduce the risk of cross-infection (E).
6 Clamp the dressing tubing and disconnect it from the canister tubing. Allow any fluid in the canister tubing to be sucked into the canister. Switch off the pump and clamp the canister tubing.	To prevent spillage of body fluid waste from the tubing or canister (E).
7 Remove and discard the canister (if full or at least weekly).	To prevent pump alarming and for infection control (E).

8 Carefully remove the occlusive film drape by gently lifting one edge and then stretching the drape horizontally and slowly pulling up from the skin.	To prevent damage to the peri-wound skin (E).
9 Carefully remove the foam dressing from the wound bed.	To prevent damage to newly formed tissue within the wound bed and prevent pain (E).
10 Clean the wound with an appropriate sterile solution such as 0.9% sodium chloride (see Table 34.4).	To prevent infection and remove surface debris/necrotic tissue (Dealey 2005: E).
11 Debride the wound if applicable.	To remove loose necrotic tissue that may be a focus for infection (Vowden & Vowden 2002: C).

TNP dressing application

12 Apply semi-permeable film over the outer foam dressing and cut a small hole for the drainage tubing prior to applying the suction device and tubing (Beldon 2006).	To prevent skin damage and ensure a good seal (Beldon 2006: E).
13 Cut the TNP foam to fit the size and shape of the wound, including tunnelling and undermined areas.	The foam should fit the wound exactly to ensure full benefit of the negative pressure therapy (KCI International 2004: C; Beldon 2006: E).
14 Avoid cutting the foam over the wound bed.	To prevent loose particles of foam falling into the wound (E).
15 Place the foam into the wound cavity. (*Note*: if the wound is bigger than the largest foam dressing, more than one piece of foam may be used as long as the edges of the foam are in contact with each other.)	The whole wound bed must be covered with foam. If the foam is touching it will transfer the negative pressure to the next piece (E).
16 Cut the occlusive film drape to size and apply over the top of the foam, ensuring a 3–5 cm border onto intact skin, TNP gel strip or hydrocolloid. (*Note*: do not compress the foam into the wound.)	To obtain a good seal around the wound edges (E).

1149

Procedure guidelines *(cont.)*

17 Choose a location on the sealed occlusive film drape to apply the tubing where the tubing will not rub or cause pressure. Cut a hole through the film, approximately 2 cm in diameter, leaving the foam intact.	To reduce the risk of pressure injury to skin (E).
18 Place the TRAC pad on the film with the hole in the centre of the elbow joint directly over the hole in the film drape. Gently press around the TRAC pad (KCI International 2004).	To ensure correct position and seal of the pad. (NB. TRAC is for the vacuum-assisted closure [VAC] system; follow manufacturer's individual instructions: C.)

Commencing TNP therapy

20 Insert the canister into the pump until it clicks into place.	Indicates the canister is positioned correctly and is secure (Beldon 2006: E).
21 Connect the dressing tubing to the canister tubing and open clamps.	The pump will alarm if the tubing is clamped or not connected (E).
22 Press POWER button and follow the on-screen instructions to set the level and type of pressure required according to instructions from the patient's medical/surgical team.	To ensure the therapy is set to the individual requirements of the patient (E).
23 Start the pump by pressing THERAPY ON/OFF: the foam should contract into the wound.	Any small air leak will prevent the foam dressing from contracting and reassessment is required (E).

References and further reading

Allsworth, J. (1985) *Skin Camouflage. A Guide to Remedial Techniques.* Arnould–Taylor, Cheltenham.

Angeras, M.H. *et al.* (1992) Comparison between sterile saline and tap water for the cleaning of acute traumatic soft tissue wounds. *Eur J Surg*, **58**, 347–50.

Archambeau, J.O., Pezner, R. & Wasserman, T. (1995) Pathophysiology of irradiated skin and breast. *Int J Radiat Oncol Biol Phys*, **31**(15), 1171–85.

Back, I.N. & Finlay, I. (1995) Analgesic effect of topical opioids on painful skin ulcers. *J Pain Symptom Manage*, **10**(7), 493.

Baker, J. (1998) Essential oils: a complementary therapy in wound management. *J Wound Care*, **7**(7), 355–7.

Bale, S. (1991) A holistic approach and the ideal dressing. *Prof Nurse*, **6**(6), 316–23.

Bale, S. & Jones, V. (2006) *Wound Care Nursing: a Patient Centred Approach*, 2nd edn. Mosby Elsevier, Edinburgh.

Barr, P.O. *et al.* (1990) Hyperbaric oxygen and problem wounds. *Care Sci Pract*, **8**(1), 3–6.

Baum, T.M. & Busuito, M.J. (1998) Use of a glycerin-based gel sheeting in scar management. *Adv Wound Care*, **11**(1), 40–3.

Baxter, H. & Ballard, K. (2001) A novel wound dressing containing HYAFF an ester of hyaluronic acid for the treatment of recalcitrant wounds. Poster presentation: Tissue Viability Society. 31st UK Conference. September 16-17, 1998.

Beldon, P. (2000) Abnormal scar formation in wound healing. *Nurs Times*, **96**(10), 44–5.

Beldon, P. (2003) Comparison of four different dressings on donor site wounds. *Br J Nurs*, **13**(6)(Tissue Viability Suppl), S38–45.

Beldon, P. (2006) Topical negative pressure dressings and vacuum-assisted closure. *Wound Essentials*, **1**, 110–14.

Benbow, M. (1995) Parameters of wound assessment. *Br J Nurs*, **4**(11), 647–51.

Benbow, M. (2006) An update on VAC therapy. *J Community Nurs*, **20**(4), 28–32.

Bennett, G. & Moody, M. (1995) *Wound Care for Health Professionals*. Chapman & Hall, London.

Bennett, G., Dealey, C. & Posnett, J. (2004) The cost of pressure ulcers in the UK. *Age Aging*, **33**(3), 230–5.

Bergstrom, N. & Braden, B. (1992) A prospective study of pressure sore risk among institutionalized elderly. *J Am Geriatr Soc*, **40**(8), 747–58.

Bergstrom, N. *et al.* (1987) The Braden Scale for Predicting Pressure Sore Risk. *Nurs Res*, **36**(4), 205–10.

Bird, C. (2000) Supporting patients with fungating breast wounds. *Prof Nurse*, **15**(10), 649–52.

Birtwistle, J. (1994) Pressure sore formation and risk assessment in intensive care. *Care Crit Ill*, **10**(4), 154–5, 157–9.

Blackmar, A. (1997) Focus on wound care: radiation-induced skin alterations. *Medsurg Nurs*, **6**(3), 172–5.

Bliss, M. (1993) Aetiology of pressure sores. *Rev Clin Gerontol*, **3**, 379–97.

BNF (2006) *British National Formulary*. British Medical Association and Royal Pharmaceutical Association, London.

Boots-Vickers, M. & Eaton, K. (1999) Skin care for patients receiving radiotherapy. *Prof Nurse*, **14**(10), 706–8.

Bower, M. *et al.* (1992) A double-blind study of the efficacy of metronidazole gel in the treatment of malodorous fungating tumours. *Eur J Cancer*, **28**(4/5), 888–9.

Boyce, S.T. *et al.* (2002) Cultured skin substitutes reduce donor skin harvesting for closure of excised, full-thickness burns. *Ann Surg*, **235**(2), 269–79.

Braden, B.J. & Bergstrom, N. (1987) A conceptual schema for the study of aetiology of pressure sores. *Rehabil Nurs*, **12**(1), 8–12.

Braden, B.J. & Bergstrom, N. (1996) Risk assessment and risk based programs of prevention in various settings. *Ostomy Wound Manage*, **42**, 65–125.

Bridel-Nixon, J. (1999) Pressure sores. In: *Nursing Management of Chronic Wounds*, 2nd edn (eds M. Morison, C. Moffatt, J. Bridel-Nixon & S. Bale). Mosby, London.

Brown, A.S. *et al.* (1998) *Essentials for Students – Plastic and Reconstructive Surgery*, 5th edn. Plastic Surgery Information Service: www.plasticsurgery.org/profinfo/essen/essentia.htm. Accessed 17/12/01.

Calvin, M. (1998) Cutaneous wound repair. *Wounds*, **10**(1), 12–32.

Campbell, J. & Lane, C. (1996) Developing a skin-care protocol in radiotherapy. *Prof Nurse*, **12**(2), 105–8.

Carney, S.A. *et al.* (1994) Cica-care gel sheeting in the management of hypertrophic scarring. *Burns*, **20**(2), 163–7.

Carson, C.F., Hammer, K.A. & Riley, T.V. (2006) Melaleuca alternifolia (Tea Tree) oil: a review of antimicrobial and other medicinal properties. *Clin Microbiol Rev*, **19**(1), 50–62.

Casey, G. (1998) The importance of nutrition in wound healing. *Nurs Stand*, **13**(3), 51–6.

Castille, K. (1998) Suturing. *Nurs Stand*, **12**(41), 41–8.

Chaplin, J. (2000) Pressure sore risk assessment in palliative care. *J Tissue Viability*, **10**(1), 27–31.

Chen, W.Y. & Abatangelo, G. (1999) Functions of hyaluronan in wound repair. *Wound Repair Regen*, **7**, 79–89.

Clamon, J. & Netscher, D.T. (1994) General principles of flap reconstruction: goals for aesthetic and functional outcome. *Plastic Surg Nurs*, **14**(1), 9–14.

Clark, M. (2002) Pressure ulcers and quality of life. *Nurs Stand*, **13**(16), 74–80.

Clay, M. (2000) Pressure sore prevention in nursing homes. *Nurs Stand*, **14**(44), 45–50.

Collier, M. (1996) The principles of optimum wound management. *Nurs Stand*, **10**(43), 47–52.

Collier, M. (1999) Pressure ulcer development and principles for prevention. In: *Wound Management: Theory and Practice* (eds M. Miller & D. Glover). Nursing Times Books, London.

Collier, M. (2002) Wound care. Wound-bed preparation. *Nurs Times*, **98**(2), 55–7.

Collinson, G. (1992) Improving quality of life in patients with malignant fungating wounds. *Proceedings of the Second European Conference on Wound Management*. Macmillan, London.

Cornwall, J.V., Dore, C.J. & Lewis, J.D. (1986) Leg ulcers: epidemiology and aetiology. *Br J Surg*, **73**(9), 693–6.

Coull, A. (1991) Making sense of split skin grafts. *Nurs Times*, **87**(27), 54–55.

Cullen, B. *et al.* (2002) The role of oxidised regenerated cellulose/collagen in chronic wound repair and its potential mechanism of action. *Int J Biochem Cell Biol*, **34**(12), 1544–56.

Cutting, K. (1994) Factors influencing wound healing. *Nurs Stand*, **8**(50), 33–7.

Cutting, K.F. (1998) *Wounds and Infection*. Wound Care Society, Huntingdon.

D'Haese, S. *et al.* (2005) Management of skin reactions during radiotherapy: a study of nursing practice. *Eur J Cancer Care*, **14**, 28–42.

Davies, D.M. (1985) Plastic and reconstructive surgery. *Br Med J*, **290**, 1056–8.

Davies, P. (2004) Current thinking on the management of necrotic and sloughy wounds. *Prof Nurse*, **19**(10), 34–6.

Davis, M.H. *et al.* (1993) *The Wound Handbook*. Centre for Medical Education, Dundee, and Perspective, London.

Dealey, C. (2005) *The Care of Wounds: a Guide for Nurses*, 3rd edn. Blackwell Science, Oxford.

Dean, A. & Tuffin, P. (1997) Fibrinolytic inhibitors for cancer-associated bleeding problems. *J Pain Symptom Manage*, **13**(1), 20–4.

Deeks, J.J. (1996) Pressure sore prevention: using and evaluating risk assessment tools. *Br J Nurs*, **5**(5), 313–20.

Derbyshire, A. (2003) A case study to demonstrate the role of proteases in wound healing. *Prof Nurse*, **19**(2), 108–11.

DH (2001a) *National Service Framework for Older People*. Department of Health, London.

DH (2001b) *Good Practice in Consent Implementation Guide: Consent to Examination and Treatment*. www.dh.gov.uk. Accessed 24/9/07.

DH (2005) *Saving Lives: a Delivery Programme to Reduce Healthcare Associated Infection Including MRSA*. Department of Health, London.

Dinman, S. (1999) Flaps and grafts revisited: cross-leg and thigh flaps for lower extremity wounds. *Plast Surg Nurs*, **19**(2), 62–5.

Donovan, S. (1998) Wound infection and wound swabbing. *Prof Nurse*, **13**(11), 757–9.

Dowsett, C. (2002) The role of the nurse in wound bed preparation. *Nurs Stand*, **16**(44), 69–76.

Dowsett, C. & Ayello, E. (2004) TIME principles of chronic wound bed preparation and management. *Br J Nurs*, **13**(15), S16–22.

Dunford, C. (2000) The use of honey in wound management. *Nurs Stand*, **15**(11), 63–8.

Dyson, M. *et al.* (1988) Comparison of the effects of moist and dry conditions on dermal repair. *J Invest Dermatol*, **91**(5), 434–9.

Eaglstein, W.H. (1985) The effect of occlusive dressings on collagen synthesis and re-epithelialisation in superficial wounds. In: *An Environment for Healing: The Role of Occlusion* (ed. T.J. Ryan). Royal Society of Medicine, London.

Edmonds, M. & Foster, A. (2000) Hyalofill: a new product for chronic wound management. *Diabetic Foot*, **3**(1), 29–30.

Edwards, M. (1994) The reliability and validity of the Waterlow pressure sore risk scale when used within district nursing to assess elders nursed in a domiciliary setting. MSc dissertation, University of London, London.

Ehrlich, H.P. (1999) The physiology of wound healing: a summary of normal and abnormal wound healing processes. *Adv Wound Care*, **11**(7), 326–8.

Ehrlich, H.P. & Hunt, T.K. (1968) Effects of cortisone and vitamin A on wound healing. *Ann Surg*, **167**(3), 324–8.

Eisenbeiss, W. *et al.* (1998) Hypertrophic scars and keloids. *J Wound Care*, **7**(5), 255–7.

Elkin, M.K., Perry, A.G. & Potter, P.A. (2004) Skill 22.3 removing staples and sutures. In: *Nursing Interventions and Clinical Skills*, 3rd edn. Mosby, St Louis. Missouri.

EPUAP (2003) Pressure ulcer prevention guidelines. www.epuap.org.uk. Accessed 11/05.

Fairbairn, K. (1993) Towards better care for women. *Prof Nurse*, **9**(3), 204–12.

Fairbairn, K. (1994) A challenge that requires further research: management of fungating breast lesions. *Prof Nurse*, **9**(4), 272–7.

Fairbairn, K. *et al.* (2002) A sharp debridement procedure devised by specialist nurses. *J Wound Care*, **11**(10), 371–5.

Falanga, V. (2000) Classifications for wound bed preparation and stimulation of chronic wounds. *Wound Repair Regen*, **8**(5), 347–52.

Ferguson, M. *et al.* (2000) Pressure ulcer management: the importance of nutrition. *Medsurg Nurs*, **9**(4), 163–75.

Field, C.K. & Kerstein, M.D. (1994) Overview of wound healing in a moist environment. *Am J Surg*, **167**(Suppl 1a), S2–6.

Finlay, I. *et al.* (1996) The effect of 0.75% metronidazole gel on malodorous cutaneous ulcers. *J Pain Symptom Manage*, **11**(3), 158–62.

Fisher, J. *et al.* (2000) Randomized phase III study comparing best supportive care to Biafine as a prophylactic agent for radiation-induced skin toxicity for women undergoing breast irradiation: Radiation Therapy Oncology Group (RTOG). *Int J Radiat Oncol Biol Phys*, **48**, 1307–10.

Flanagan, M. (1996) A practical framework for wound assessment 1: physiology. *Br J Nurs*, **5**(22), 1391–7.

Flanagan, M. (1998) The characteristics and formation of granulation tissue. *J Wound Care*, **7**(10), 508–10.

Flanagan, M. (1999) The physiology of wound healing. In: *Wound Management: Theory and Practice* (eds M. Miller & D. Glover). Nursing Times Books, London, pp. 14–22.

Flanagan, M. (2000) The physiology of wound healing. *J Wound Care*, **9**(6), 299–300.

Fletcher, J. (1997) Update: wound cleansing. *Prof Nurse*, **12**(11), 793–6.

Francis, A. (1998) Nursing management of skin graft sites. *Nurs Stand*, **12**(33), 41–4.

Freedline, A. (1999) Types of wound debridement. Wound Care Information Network. www.medicaledu.com/debridhp.htm. Accessed 8/10/99.

Garrett, B. (1997) The proliferation and movement of cells during re-epithelialisation. *J Wound Care*, **6**(4), 174–7.

Gentzkow, G.D. *et al.* (1996) Use of Dermagraft, a cultured human dermis, to treat diabetic foot ulcers. *Diabetes Care*, **19**(4), 350–4.

Gilchrist, B. (1999) Wound infection. In: *Wound Management: Theory and Practice* (eds M. Miller & D. Glover). Nursing Times Books, London, pp. 96–107.

Glean, E. *et al.* (2001) Intervention for acute radiotherapy induced skin reactions in cancer patients: the development of clinical practice guidelines recommended for use by the College of Radiographers. *J Radiother Pract*, **2**(2), 75–84.

Grewal, P.S. *et al.* (1999) Pressure sore prevention in hospital patients: a clinical audit. *J Wound Care*, **8**(3), 129–31.

Grocott, P. (2000a) Palliative management of fungating malignant wounds. *J Wound Care*, **9**(1), 4–9.

Grocott, P. (2000b) Palliative management of fungating malignant wounds. *J Commun Nurs*, **14**(3), 31–2, 35–6, 38.

Guyton, A.C. & Hall, J.E. (2000) *Textbook of Medical Physiology*, 10th edn. W.B. Saunders, Philadelphia.

Haisfield-Wolfe, M.E. & Rund, C. (1997) Malignant cutaneous wounds: a management protocol. *Ostomy Wound Manage*, **43**(1), 56–66.

Hallett, A. (1995) Fungating wounds. *Nurs Times*, **91**(47), 81–3.

Hamilton, K. (1995) Wound healing and nutrition – a review. *J Aust Coll Nutr Environ Med*, **14**(2), 15.

Hamilton-Miller, J.M.T., Shah, S. & Smith, C. (1993) Silver sulphadiazine: a comprehensive *in vitro* reassessment. *Chemotherapy*, **39**, 405–9.

Hampton, S. (2004) Holistic Wound Care. Journal of Community Nurs, **18**(8), 12–7.

Hampton, S. (1999) Choosing the right dressing. In: *Wound Management: Theory and Practice* (eds M. Miller & D. Glover). Nursing Times Books, London pp. 14–22.

Hampton, S. & Collins, F. (2004) *Tissue Viability: The Prevention, Treatment and Management of Wounds*. Whurr Publishers, London.

Harding, K.G., Morris, H.L. & Patel, G.K. (2002) Healing chronic wounds. *BMJ*, **324**(7330), 160–3.

Hart, J. (2002) Inflammation 1: its role in the healing of acute wounds. *J Wound Care*, **11**(6), 205–9.

Heggie, S. *et al.* (2002) A phase III study on the efficacy of topical aloe vera gel on irradiated breast tissue. *Cancer Nurs*, **25**(6), 442–51.

Hess, C.T. (2005) Pressure ulcers. In: *Wound Care Clinical Guide*, 5th edn. Lippincott, Williams & Wilkins, Philadelphia, pp. 79–93.

Hinshaw, J. (2000) Larval therapy: a review of clinical human and veterinary studies. *World Wide Wounds*: www.worldwidewounds. com/2000/oct/Janet-Hinshaw/Larval-Therapy-Human-and-Veterinary. html. Accessed 20/12/02.

Hofman, D. (1996) Know how: a guide to wound debridement. *Nurs Times*, **92**(32), 22–3.

Hollander, D., Schmandra, T. & Windolf, J. (2000) Using an esterified hyaluronan fleece to promote healing in difficult-to-treat wounds. *J Wound Care*, **9**(10), 463–6.

Hollinworth, H. (1997) Less pain, more gain. *Nurs Times*, **93**(46), 89–91.

Ivetic, O. & Lyne, P.A. (1990) Fungating and ulcerating malignant lesions: a review of the literature. *J Adv Nurs*, **15**, 83–8.

Jay, R. (1999) Suturing in A&E. *Prof Nurse*, **14**(6), 412–15.

Johnson, A. (1989) Granuflex wafers as a prophylactic pressure sore dressing. *Care Sci Pract*, **7**(2), 55–8.

Jones, M. & Thomas, S. (2000) Larval therapy. *Nurs Stand*, **14**(20), 47–51.

Kaufman, M. & Pahl, D. (2003) Vacuum-assisted closure therapy: wound care and nursing implications. *Dermatol Nurs*, **15**(4), 317–20, 323–25.

KCI International (2004) *VAC Recommended Guidelines for Use: Physician and Caregiver Reference Manual*. KCI International, Oxfordshire.

Kelly, N. (2002) Malodorous fungating wounds: a review of current literature. *Prof Nurse*, **17**(5), 323–6.

Kiecolt-Glaser, J.K. *et al.* (1995) Slowing of wound healing by psychological stress. *Lancet*, **346**(4), 1194–6.

Kitching, M. (2004) Patients' perceptions and experiences of larval therapy. *J Wound Care*, **13**(1), 25–9.

Krajnik, M. & Zylicz, Z. (1997) Topical morphine for cutaneous cancer pain. *Palliat Med*, **11**(4), 326–30.

Landis, E.M. (1930) Micro-injection studies of capillary blood pressure in human skin. *Heart*, **15**, 209–28.

Laverty, D. (2003) Fungating wounds: informing practice through knowledge/theory. *Br J Nurs*, **12**(15), S29–S40.

Laverty, D., Mallett, J. & Mulholland, J. (1997) Protocols and guidelines for managing wounds. *Prof Nurse*, **13**(2), 79–81.

Laverty, D. *et al.* (2000) *Wound Management Guidelines*. Royal Marsden Foundation Trust, London.

Lavery, B.A. (1995) Skin care during radiotherapy: a survey of UK practice. *Clin Oncol*, **7**(3), 184–7.

Lawrence, J.C. (1997) Wound irrigation. *J Wound Care*, **6**(1), 23–6.

Lewis, B. (1996) Zinc and vitamin C in the aetiology of pressure sores. *J Wound Care*, **5**(10), 483–4.

Lindgren, M. *et al.* (2002) A risk assessment scale for the prediction of pressure sore development: reliability and validity. *J Adv Nurs*, **38**(2), 190–9.

Lund-Nielsen, B., Muller, K. & Adamsen, L. (2005) Malignant wounds in women with breast cancer: feminine and sexual perspectives. *J Clin Nurs*, **14**(1), 56–64.

Maddocks-Jennings, W., Wilkinson, J.M. & Shillington, D. (2005) Novel approaches to radiotherapy-induced skin reactions: a literature review. *Complement Ther Clin Pract*, **11**(4), 224–31.

Maher, K.E. (2005) Radiation therapy: toxicities and management. In: *Cancer Nursing: Principles and Practice* (eds C. Henke Yarbro *et al.*), 6th edn. Jones and Barlett, Boston, pp. 283–314.

Mallett, J. *et al.* (1999) An integrated approach to wound management. *Int J Palliat Nurs*, **5**(3), 124–32.

Mandal, A. (2006) Do malnutrition and nutritional supplementation have an effect on the wound healing process? *J Wound Care*, **15**(6), 254–7.

Margolin, S.G. *et al.* (1990) Management of radiation-induced moist skin desquamation using hydrocolloid dressing. *Cancer Nurs*, **13**(2), 71–80.

Martin, E.A. (2002) *Concise Colour Medical Dictionary*. Oxford University Press, Oxford.

Messer, M.S. (1989) Wound care. *Crit Care Nurs Q*, **11**(4), 17–27.

Middleton, K. (1990) Sugar pastes in wound management. *Dressings Times*, **3**(2): www.smtl.co.uk/WMPRC/DressingsTimes/vol3.2.txt. Accessed 27/6/00.

Miller, M. (1998a) Moist wound healing: the evidence. *Nurs Times*, **94**(45), 74–6.

Miller, M. (1998b) How do I diagnose and treat wound infection? *Br J Nurs*, **7**(6), 335–8.

Miller, M. & Dyson, M. (1996) *Principles of Wound Care*. Macmillan, London.

Mockridge, J. & Anthony, D. (1999) Nurses' knowledge about pressure sore treatment and healing. *Nurs Stand*, **13**(29), 66–72.

Moore, P. & Foster, L. (1998) Acute surgical wound care 2: the wound healing process. *Br J Nurs*, **7**(19), 1183–7.

Morgan, D.A. (2000) *Formulary of Wound Management Products: a Guide for Healthcare Staff*, 8th edn. Euromed Communications, Haslemere.

Morgan, D.A. (2002) Formulary of wound management products: a guide for healthcare staff, 8th edn (Internet update). Euromed Communications. www.euromed.uk.com/formulary6update.htm. Accessed 20/12/02.

Morison, M.J. (1989) Wound cleansing – which solution? *Prof Nurse*, **4**, 220–5.

Moss, A. (1989) Treatment of terminal breast cancer. *Br Med J*, **298**(6670): 388.

Munro, K.J.G. (1995a) Hypertrophic and keloid scars. *J Wound Care*, **4**(3), 143–8.

Munro, K.J.G. (1995b) Treatment of hypertrophic and keloid scars. *J Wound Care*, **4**(5), 243–5.

Naylor, W. (2001) Assessment and management of pain in fungating wounds. *Br J Nurs*, **10**(22 Suppl), S33–56.

Naylor, W. (2002) Malignant wounds: aetiology and principles of management. *Nurs Stand*, **16**(52), 45–53.

Naylor, W., Laverty, D. & Mallett, J. (2001) *The Royal Marsden Hospital Handbook of Wound Management in Cancer Care*. Blackwell Science, Oxford.

Newman, V. *et al.* (1989) The use of metronidazole gel to control the smell of malodorous lesions. *Palliat Med*, **3**, 303–5.

NHS Employers (2005) *The Management of Health, Safety and Welfare Issues for NHS Staff*. National Health Service Employers, London.

NICE (2001) Technology appraisal guidance 24. Wound care – debriding agents. Guidance on the use of debriding agents and specialist wound care clinics for difficult to heal surgical wounds. April 2001, updated March 2004. National Institute for Health and Clinical Excellence, London. www.nice.org.uk/page.aspx?o=TA024guidance. Accessed 09/2006.

NICE (2003) Pressure ulcer risk assessment and prevention. National Institute for Health and Clinical Excellence. www.nice.org.uk. Accessed 11/11/06.

NMC (2005) *Guidelines for Records and Record Keeping*. Nursing and Midwifery Council, London.

NMC (2006) *A–Z Advice Sheet Consent*. www.nmc.org.

NMC (2008) *The Code: Standards of Conduct, Performance and Ethics for Nurses and Midwives*. Nursing and Midwifery Council, London.

Noble-Adams, R. (1999) Radiation-induced skin reactions 2: development of a measurement tool. *Br J Nurs*, **8**(18), 1208–11.

Norton, D. *et al.* (1985) *An Investigation of Geriatric Nursing Problems in Hospital*. Churchill Livingstone, Edinburgh.

Nystedt, K.E. *et al.* (2005) The standardization of radiation skin care in British Columbia: a collaborative approach. *Oncol Nurs Forum*, **32**(6), 1199–1206.

O'Toole, E.A., Marinkovich, M.P., Peavey, C.L. *et al.* (1997) Hypoxia increases human keratinocyte motility on connective tissue. *J Clin Invest*, **100**(11), 288–91.

Papanikolaou, P., Lyne, P. & Anthony, D. (2006) Risk assessment scales for pressure ulcers: A methodological review. *International Journal of Nursing Studies*, **44**(2), 285–96.

Patawardhan, A., Sharma, V. & Dinshaw, K.A. (2002) Duoderm CGF vs Gentian violet 1% dressing in the treatment of radiation induced ulcers. *World Council of Enterostomal Therapists Journal*, **22**(2), 32–8.

Phillips, T.J., Al-Amoudi, H.O., Leverkus, M. & Park, H.y. (1998) Effect of chronic wound fluid on fibroblasts. *J Wound Care*, **7**(10), 527–32.

Pickering, D. & Warland, S. (1992) The management of desquamative radiation skin reactions. *Dressing Times*, **5**(1): www.smtl.co.uk/WMPRC/DressingsTimes/vol5.1.txt. Accessed 11/10/06.

Pickworth, J.J. & De Sousa, N. (1988) Differential wound angiogenesis: quantitation by immunohistological staining for factor Vlll-related antigen. In: *Beyond Occlusion: Wound Care Proceedings* (ed. T.J. Ryan). Royal Society of Medicine, London.

Porock, D. & Kristjanson, L. (1999) Skin reactions during radiotherapy for breast cancer: the use and impact of topical agents and dressings. *Eur J Cancer Care*, **8**, 143–53.

Porock, D. *et al.* (1998) Predicting the severity of radiation skin reactions in women with breast cancer. *Oncol Nurs Forum*, **25**(6), 1019–29.

Porock, D., Nikcoletti, S. & Cameron, F. (2004) The relationship between factors that impair wound healing and the severity of acute radiation skin and mucosal toxicities in head and neck cancer. *Cancer Nurs*, **27**(1), 71–8.

Poston, J. (1996) Sharp debridement of devitalised tissue: the nurse's role. *Br J Nurs*, **5**(11), 655–62.

Pouliot, R. *et al.* (2002) Reconstructed human skin produced *in vitro* and grafted on athymic mice. *Transplantation*, **73**(11), 1751–7.

Price, S. & Price, L. (1995) *Aromatherapy for Health Professionals*. Churchill Livingstone, New York.

Pudner, R. (1998) The management of patients with a fungating or malignant wound. *J Commun Nurs*, **12**(9), 30–4.

Pudner, R. (2001) Low/non-adherent dressings in wound management. *J Commun Nurs*, **15**(8), 12, 15–17.

Puzey, G. (2001) The use of pressure garments on hypertrophic scars. *J Tissue Viability*, **12**(1), 11–15.

Rankin-Box, D. (2001) *The Nurse's Handbook of Complementary Therapies*, 2nd edn. Bailliere Tindall, London.

Reid, J. & Morison, M. (1994) Towards a consensus classification of pressure sores. *J Wound Care*, **3**(3), 157–9.

Reynolds, T.M. (2000) The future of nutrition and wound healing. *J Tissue Viability*, **11**(1), 5–13.

Rice, A.M. (1997) An introduction to radiotherapy. *Nurs Stand*, **12**(3), 49–54.

Richardson, M. (2007) Exploring various methods for closing traumatic wounds. *Nurs Times*, **103**(5), 30–1.

Rigter, B., Clendon, H. & Kettle, S. (1994) Dermatology. Skin reactions due to radiotherapy. *New Zealand Pract Nurse*, September 17–19, 21–2.

Riyat, M.S. & Quinton, D.N. (1997) Tap water as a wound cleansing agent in accident and emergency. *J Accid Emerg*, **14**, 165–6.

Robinson, B.J. (2000) The use of a hydrofibre dressing in wound management. *J Wound Care*, **9**(1), 32–4.

Rollins, H. (1997) Special focus: tissue viability – nutrition and wound healing. *Nurs Stand*, **11**(51), 49–52.

Roy, L., Fortin, A. & Larochelle, M. (2001) The impact of skin washing with water and soap during breast irradiation: a randomised study. *Radiother Oncol*, **58**, 333–9.

RCN (2001) *Pressure Sore Prevention*. Royal College of Nursing, London. Accessed via National Institute for Health and Clinical Excellence: www.nice.org.uk. Accessed 17/03/07.

RCN (2003) *Pressure Ulcer Risk Assessment and Prevention*. Royal College of Nursing, London.

RCN (2005) The management of pressure ulcers in primary and secondary care: a clinical practice guideline. www.nice.org.uk/ page.aspx?o=cg029fullguideline. Accessed 24/11/06.

Royal Marsden Hospital (1999) *Radiotherapy: Your Questions Answered*. Royal Marsden Hospital, London.

Russell, L. (2001) The importance of patients' nutritional status in wound healing. *Br J Nurs*, **10**(6 Suppl), S44–9.

Scholl, D. & Langkamp-Henken, B. (2001) Nutrient recommendations for wound healing. *J Intraven Nurs*, **24**(2), 124–32.

Schoonhoven, L., Defloor, T. & Grypdonck, M.H.F. (2002) Incidence of pressure ulcers due to surgery. *J Clin Nurs*, **11**(4), 479–87.

Schultz, G.S. *et al.* (2003) Wound bed preparation: systematic approach to wound management. *Wound ep Reg*, **11**, 1–28. wound.smith-nephew.com/ca_en/Standard.asp?NodeId=3077. Accessed 17/10/06.

Silver, I.A. (1994) The physiology of wound healing. *J Wound Care*, **3**(2), 106–9.

Simmons, S. (1999) Hyperbaric therapy. In: *Wound Management: Theory and Practice* (eds M. Miller & D. Glover). Nursing Times Books, London.

Simonen, P. *et al.* (1998) Do inflammatory processes contribute to radiation-induced erythema observed in the skin of humans? *Radiother Oncol*, **46**(1), 73–82.

Simpson, A., Bowers, K. & Weir-Hughes, D. (1996) *Clinical Care: Pressure Sore Prevention.* Whurr, London.

Smith, F.R. (2005) Causes of and treatment options for abnormal scar tissue. *J Wound Care*, **14**(2), 49–52.

Smith, K.P., Zardiackas, L.D. & Didlake, R.H. (1986) Cortisone, vitamin A, and wound healing: the importance of measuring wound surface area. *J Surg Res*, **40**(2), 120–5.

Souhami, R. & Tobias, J. (1998) *Cancer and Its Management.* Blackwell Science, Oxford.

Sparrow, G. *et al.* (1980) Metronidazole in smelly tumours. *Lancet*, **1**(8179), 1185.

Springett, K. (2002) The impact of diabetes on wound management. *Nurs Stand*, **10**(1), 72–4.

Steenvoorde, P., Budding, T. & Oskam, J. (2005) Determining pain levels in patients treated with maggot debridement therapy. *J Wound Care*, **14**(10), 485–8.

Stein, C. (1995) The control of pain in peripheral tissue by opioids. *N Engl J Med*, **332**(25), 1685–90.

Stone, J. (2001) Ethical and legal issues. In: *The Nurse's Handbook of Complementary Therapies* (ed. D. Rankin-Box), 2nd edn. Bailliere Tindall, London, pp. 51–56.

Sussman, C. (1998) Wound healing biology and chronic wound healing. In: *Wound Care: A Collaborative Practice Manual for Physical Therapists and Nurses* (eds C. Sussman & B.M. Bate-Jensen). Aspen Publishers, MD, pp. 31–47.

Teare, J. & Barrett, C. (2002) Using quality of life assessment in wound care. *Nurs Stand*, **17**(6), 59–68.

Tejero-Trujeque, R. (2001) How do fibroblasts interact with the extracellular matrix in wound contraction? *J Wound Care*, **10**(6), 237–42.

Thomas, S. (1992) *Current Practices in the Management of Fungating Lesions and Radiation Damaged Skin.* Surgical Materials Testing Laboratory, Bridgend.

Thomas, S. (2002) SMTL Dressings Datacard: Promogran. Surgical Materials Testing Laboratory, Bridgend. www.dressings.org/Dressings/promogran.html. Accessed 25/7/02.

Thomas, S. & Hay, N. (1991) The antimicrobial properties of 2 metronidazole-mediated dressings used to treat malodorous wounds. *Pharm J*, **246**(6625), 264–66.

Thomas, T. *et al.* (2001) The current status of maggot therapy in wound healing. *Br J Nurs*, **10**(22 Suppl), S5–12.

Thomson, P. (1998) The microbiology of wounds. *J Wound Care*, **7**(9), 477–8.

Timmons, J. (2006) Skin function and wound healing physiology. *Wound Essentials*, **1**, 8–14.

Tong, A. (1999) Back to basics wound care. *Nurs Times Nurs Homes*, **1**(1), 20–3.

Topham, J. (2000) Sugar for wounds. *J Tissue Viability*, **10**(3), 86–9.

Torra I Bou, J.E. *et al.* (2001) Clinical evaluation of the effect of a collagen dressing in the treatment of pressure ulcers. In: *Final Abstracts from the Fifth EPUAP Open Meeting. Le Mans, France, 2001.* European Pressure Ulcer Advisory Panel Review, **4**(1).

Tortora, G.J. & Grabowski, S.R. (2008) *Principles of Anatomy and Physiology*, 12th edn. John Wiley & Sons, Chichester.

Twillman, R.K. *et al.* (1999) Treatment of painful skin ulcers with topical opioids. *J Pain Symptom Manage*, **17**(4), 288–92.

Vowden, K. (1995) Common problems in wound care: wound and ulcer measurement. *Br J Nurs*, **4**(13), 775–9.

Vowden, K. & Vowden, P. (1999) Wound debridement, part 2: sharp techniques. *J Wound Care*, **8**(6), 291–4.

Vowden, K. & Vowden, P. (2002) Wound bed preparation. *World Wide Wounds*: www.worldwidewounds.com/2002/april/Vowden/Wound-Bed-Preparation.html. Accessed 20/12/02.

Waldorf, H. & Fewkes, J. (1995) Advances in dermatology. *J Wound Heal*, **10**, 77–97.

Warnke, P.H. *et al.* (2004) Tumour smell reduction with antibacterial essential oils. *Cancer*, **100**(4), 879–80.

Warnke, P.H. *et al.* (2005) Antibacterial essential oils reduce tumor smell and inflammation in cancer patients. *J Clin Oncol*, **23**(7), 158–9.

Warnke, P.H. *et al.* (2006) Antibacterial essential oils in malodorous cancer patients: clinical observations in 30 patients. *Phytomedicine*, **13**(7), 463–7.

Waterlow, J. (1988) Prevention is cheaper than cure. *Nurs Times*, **84**(25), 69–70.

Waterlow, J. (1991) A policy that protects. *Prof Nurse*, **6**(5), 258–64.

Waterlow, J. (1998) The treatment and use of the Waterlow card. *Nurs Times*, **94**(7), 63–7.

Waterlow, J. (2005) From costly treatment to cost-effective prevention: using Waterlow. *Wound Care*, **10**(9 Suppl), S25–30.

Wells, L. (1994) At the front line of care, the importance of nutrition in wound management. *Prof Nurse*, **9**(8), 525–30.

Wells, M. & MacBride, S. (2003) Radiation skin reactions. In: *Supportive Care in Radiotherapy* (eds S. Faithfull & M. Wells). Churchill Livingstone, Edinburgh, pp. 135–39.

Westbury, C. *et al.* (2000) Advice on hair and scalp care during cranial radiotherapy: a prospective randomised trial. *Radiother Oncol*, **54**, 109–16.

White, R. (2001) Managing exudate. *Nurs Times*, **97**(14), 59–60.

White, R.J. (2000) *The Management of Exuding Wounds*. Wound Care Society, Huntingdon.

Wickline, M.M. (2004) Prevention and treatment of acute radiation dermatitis: A literature review. *Oncol Nurs Forum*, **31**, 237–47.

Wilkinson, B. (1997) Hard graft. *Nurs Times*, **93**(16), 63–4, 66, 68.

Wilkes, L. *et al.* (2001) Malignant wound management: what dressings do nurses use? *J Wound Care*, **10**(3), 65–70.

Williams, C. (1996) Product focus. Cica-care: adhesive gel sheet. *Br J Nurs*, **5**(14), 875–6.

Williams, C. (1999) Product focus: an investigation of the benefits of Aquacel Hydrofibre wound dressing. *Br J Nurs*, **8**(10), 676–80.

Williams, C. & Young, T. (1998) *Myth and Reality in Wound Care*. Mark Allen, Dinton.

Williams, L. (2002) Assessing patients' nutritional needs in the wound-healing process. *J Wound Care*, **11**(6), 225–8.

Wilson, V. (2005) Assessment and management of fungating wounds: a review. *Br J Cancer Nurs* (Wound Care Suppl), **10**(3), 528–34.

Winter, G.D. (1972) Epidermal regeneration studied in the domestic pig. In: *Epidermal Wound Healing* (eds H.I. Maibach & D.T. Rovee). Year Book Medical Publishers, Chicago, pp. 71–112.

Young, T. & Fowler, A. (1998) Nursing management of skin grafts and donor sites. *Br J Nurs*, **7**(6), 324, 326, 328, 330, 332–4.

Multiple choice questions

1 There are four phases of wound healing: inflammatory phase, proliferation phase, reconstructive phase and what else?

   a   Haemostasis
   b   Haemopoesis
   c   Incision phase
   d   contamination phase

2 Elderly patients are at greater risk of delayed wound healing. Which of the following is NOT a contributing factor?

   a   Comorbidities
   b   Thinning of the dermis
   c   Slower metabolic processes and circulation
   d   Obesity

3 Malnutrition can be a major factor in delaying wound healing. Patients are considered 'at risk' if they have lost:

   a   30% body weight in 6 months or 10% in 2 months
   b   20% body weight in 6 months or 10% in 2 months
   c   15% body weight in 6 months
   d   5% body weight in 2 months

4 What is 'debridement'?

   a   Mechanism of wound healing
   b   Managing a wound to avoid scarring
   c   Deep cleansing of a wound
   d   Removal of necrotic tissue

5 Which of the following are thought to be major contributing factors in the development of pressure ulcers?

  a Pressure, shearing and friction
  b Pressure, neglect and malnutrition
  c Pressure, shearing and malnutrition
  d Pressure, neglect and friction

6 A number of scales are available to assess the risk of developing pressure ulcers. Which of these is not such a scale?

  a Waterlow scale
  b Braden scale
  c Lister scale
  d Norton scale

7 When changing a dressing the wound should be exposed for the minimum period of time so that:

  a The wound is kept wet
  b Risk of contamination is reduce
  c The wound is kept at the optimum temperature
  d The development of MRSA is prevented

8 When removing a vacuum drain the vacuum should first be released to avoid:

  a Infection
  b Pain and tissue damage
  c Seroma development
  d Haematoma development

Answers to the multiple choice questions can be found in Appendix 3.

The Code

Standards of conduct, performance and ethics for nurses and midwives

Reproduced with permission from the Nursing and Midwifery Council, London

The people in your care must be able to trust you with their health and wellbeing.

To justify that trust, you must

- make the care of people your first concern, treating them as individuals and respecting their dignity
- work with others to protect and promote the health and wellbeing of those in your care, their families and carers, and the wider community
- provide a high standard of practice and care at all times
- be open and honest, act with integrity and uphold the reputation of your profession

As a professional, you are personally accountable for actions and omissions in your practice and must always be able to justify your decisions.

You must always act lawfully, whether those laws relate to your professional practice or personal life.

Failure to comply with this Code may bring your fitness to practise into question and endanger your registration.

This Code should be considered together with the Nursing and Midwifery Council's rules, standards, guidance and advice available from www.nmc-uk.org.

Make the care of people your first concern, treating them as individuals and respecting their dignity

Treat people as individuals

- You must treat people as individuals and respect their dignity
- You must not discriminate in any way against those in your care
- You must treat people kindly and considerately
- You must act as an advocate for those in your care, helping them to access relevant health and social care, information and support

Respect people's confidentiality

- You must respect people's right to confidentiality
- You must ensure people are informed about how and why information is shared by those who will be providing their care
- You must disclose information if you believe someone may be at risk of harm, in line with the law of the country in which you are practising

Collaborate with those in your care

- You must listen to the people in your care and respond to their concerns and preferences
- You must support people in caring for themselves to improve and maintain their health
- You must recognise and respect the contribution that people make to their own care and wellbeing
- You must make arrangements to meet people's language and communication needs
- You must share with people, in a way they can understand, the information they want or need to know about their health

Ensure you gain consent

- You must ensure that you gain consent before you begin any treatment or care
- You must respect and support people's rights to accept or decline treatment and care
- You must uphold people's rights to be fully involved in decisions about their care
- You must be aware of the legislation regarding mental capacity, ensuring that people who lack capacity remain at the centre of decision making and are fully safeguarded

1165

- You must be able to demonstrate that you have acted in someone's best interests if you have provided care in an emergency

Maintain clear professional boundaries

- You must refuse any gifts, favours or hospitality that might be interpreted as an attempt to gain preferential treatment
- You must not ask for or accept loans from anyone in your care or anyone close to them
- You must establish and actively maintain clear sexual boundaries at all times with people in your care, their families and carers

Work with others to protect and promote the health and wellbeing of those in your care, their families and carers, and the wider community

Share information with your colleagues

- You must keep your colleagues informed when you are sharing the care of others
- You must work with colleagues to monitor the quality of your work and maintain the safety of those in your care
- You must facilitate students and others to develop their competence

Work effectively as part of a team

- You must work cooperatively within teams and respect the skills, expertise and contributions of your colleagues
- You must be willing to share your skills and experience for the benefit of your colleagues
- You must consult and take advice from colleagues when appropriate
- You must treat your colleagues fairly and without discrimination
- You must make a referral to another practitioner when it is in the best interests of someone in your care

Delegate effectively

- You must establish that anyone you delegate to is able to carry out your instructions
- You must confirm that the outcome of any delegated task meets required standards
- You must make sure that everyone you are responsible for is supervised and supported

Manage risk

- You must act without delay if you believe that you, a colleague or anyone else may be putting someone at risk
- You must inform someone in authority if you experience problems that prevent you working within this Code or other nationally agreed standards
- You must report your concerns in writing if problems in the environment of care are putting people at risk

1167

Provide a high standard of practice and care at all times

Use the best available evidence

- You must deliver care based on the best available evidence or best practice.
- You must ensure any advice you give is evidence based if you are suggesting healthcare products or services
- You must ensure that the use of complementary or alternative therapies is safe and in the best interests of those in your care

Keep your skills and knowledge up to date

- You must have the knowledge and skills for safe and effective practice when working without direct supervision
- You must recognise and work within the limits of your competence
- You must keep your knowledge and skills up to date throughout your working life
- You must take part in appropriate learning and practice activities that maintain and develop your competence and performance

Keep clear and accurate records

- You must keep clear and accurate records of the discussions you have, the assessments you make, the treatment and medicines you give and how effective these have been
- You must complete records as soon as possible after an event has occurred
- You must not tamper with original records in any way
- You must ensure any entries you make in someone's paper records are clearly and legibly signed, dated and timed
- You must ensure any entries you make in someone's electronic records are clearly attributable to you
- You must ensure all records are kept confidentially and securely

Be open and honest, act with integrity and uphold the reputation of your profession

Act with integrity

- You must demonstrate a personal and professional commitment to equality and diversity
- You must adhere to the laws of the country in which you are practising
- You must inform the NMC if you have been cautioned, charged or found guilty of a criminal offence
- You must inform any employers you work for if your fitness to practise is impaired or is called into question

Deal with problems

- You must give a constructive and honest response to anyone who complains about the care they have received
- You must not allow someone's complaint to prejudice the care you provide for them
- You must act immediately to put matters right if someone in your care has suffered harm for any reason
- You must explain fully and promptly to the person affected what has happened and the likely effects
- You must cooperate with internal and external investigations

Be impartial

- You must not abuse your privileged position for your own ends
- You must ensure that your professional judgment is not influenced by any commercial considerations

Uphold the reputation of your profession

- You must not use your professional status to promote causes that are not related to health
- You must cooperate with the media only when you can confidently protect the confidential information and dignity of those in your care
- You must uphold the reputation of your profession at all times

Information about indemnity insurance

The NMC recommends that a registered nurse, midwife or specialist community public health nurse, in advising, treating and caring for patients/clients, has professional indemnity insurance. This is in the interests of clients, patients and registrants in the event of claims of professional negligence.

Whilst employers have vicarious liability for the negligent acts and/or omissions of their employees, such cover does not normally extend to activities undertaken outside the registrant's employment. Independent practice would not be covered by vicarious liability. It is the individual registrant's responsibility to establish their insurance status and take appropriate action.

In situations where an employer does not have vicarious liability, the NMC recommends that registrants obtain adequate professional indemnity insurance. If unable to secure professional indemnity insurance, a registrant will need to demonstrate that all their clients/patients are fully informed of this fact and the implications this might have in the event of a claim for professional negligence.

Contributors to previous editions

First edition edited by

A. Phylip Pritchard
Research Assistant, Department of Nursing Research

Valerie-Anne Walker
Research Assistant, Department of Nursing Research

Second edition edited by

A. Phylip Pritchard
Assistant to the Director of In-Patient Services/Chief Nursing Officer

Jill A. David
Director of Nursing Research

Third edition edited by

A. Phylip Pritchard
Formerly Co-ordinator of European Educational Initiatives
The Royal Marsden Hospital
and
Executive Secretary, European Oncology Nursing Society
Jane Mallett
Research and Practice Development Co-ordinator

Fourth edition edited by

Jane Mallett
Research and Practice Development Manager

Christopher Bailey
Macmillan Research Practitioner, Macmillan Practice Development Unit, Centre for Cancer and Palliative Care Studies, Institute of Cancer Research

Fifth edition edited by

Jane Mallett
Research and Practice Development Manager The Royal Marsden Hospital

Lisa Dougherty
Clinical Nurse Specialist Intravenous Services, The Royal Marsden Hospital

Sixth edition edited by

Lisa Dougherty
Nurse Consultant Intravenous Therapy, The Royal Marsden Hospital

Sara E. Lister
Assistant Chief Nurse/Head of School, The Royal Marsden Hospital School of Cancer Nursing & Rehabilitation

Contributors

Emma Allum, Senior Staff Nurse (Wiltshaw Ward)

Sarah Aylott, formerly Practice Development Facilitator

Caroline Badger, formerly Senior Nurse (Lymphoedema)

Christopher Bailey, Macmillan Research Practitioner Institute of Cancer Research

Sophie Baty, Sister (Recovery Theatre)

Rachel Bennett, formerly Ward Sister (Wilson Ward)

Chris Berry, formerly Back Care Advisor

Judith Bibbings, formerly Sister (Gastro-intestinal/Genito-urinary)

Peter Blake, Consultant Clinical Oncologist

Yannette Booth, formerly Lecturer in Cancer Nursing

Derryn Borley, formerly Assistant Director of Nursing Services

David Brighton, Professional Development Facilitator (IT)

Monica Burchall, formerly Sister (High Dependency)

Nancy Burnett, Senior Nurse Manager

Susannah Button, formerly Ward Sister (Ellis Ward)

Antoinette Byrne, formerly Dietitian

Jill Carter, formerly Clinical Nurse Specialist (Palliative Care)

Neve Carter, Senior Staff Nurse (Horder Ward) and Practice Development Facilitator

Patrick Casey, formerly Clinical Nurse Specialist/Unit Manager (Gastro-intestinal/Genito-urinary)

Anne Chandler, Clinical Nurse Specialist in Pain Management

Belinda Crawford, Matron (Neurointensive Care), Atkinson Morley Hospital

Gay Curling, Clinical Nurse Specialist (Breast Diagnostic Unit)

Lisa Curtis, formerly Macmillan Lecturer, Institute of Cancer Research

Tonia Dawson, Clinical Nurse Specialist (Pelvic Cancer)

Barbara Dicks, Director of Patient Services/Chief Nursing Officer

Emma Dilnutt, formerly Clinical Nurse Specialist (Palliative Care)

Anne Doherty, formerly Staff Nurse (Operating Theatres)

Nuala Durkin, formerly Clinical Nurse Specialist/Unit Manager (High Dependency)

Jean Edwards, Senior Nurse Manager/Private Patient Co-ordinator

Stephen Evans, Radiation Protection Adviser (Physics Department)

Sarah Faithfull, CRC Nursing Fellow, Institute of Cancer Research

Deborah Fenlon, formerly Group Clinical Nurse Specialist (Breast Care Services)

Emma Foulds, Lecturer Practitioner, The Royal Marsden Hospital School of Cancer Nursing & Rehabilitation

Tracey Gibson, Senior Staff Nurse (Critical Care Unit)

Aileen Grant, Staff Nurse (Children's Unit)

Jacqueline Green, Senior Dietitian

Douglas Guerrero, Clinical Nurse Specialist (Neuro-oncology)

Rachel Hair, formerly Senior Nurse (Neuro-oncology)

Shujina Haq, Specialist Registrar (Occupational Health)

Cathryn Havard, formerly Senior Nurse (Gastro-intestinal/Genito-urinary)

Pauline Hill, Clinical Nurse Specialist (Community Liaison)

Sian Horn, formerly Sister (High Dependency)

Elizabeth Houlton, formerly Senior Nurse (Community Liaison/Self-Care Unit)

Nest Howells, formerly Information Officer, CancerLink

Jennifer Hunt, Director, Nursing Research Initiative for Scotland

Maureen Hunter, Rehabilitation Services Manager

Elizabeth Janes, formerly Dietitian

Margareta Johnstone, formerly Clinical Nurse Specialist (High Dependency Unit)

Penelope A. Jones, formerly Clinical Nurse Specialist (Community Liaison Palliative Care)

Danny Kelly, formerly Lecturer in Cancer Nursing, Institute of Cancer Research

Betti Kirkman, formerly Clinical Nurse Specialist (Breast Diagnostic Unit)

Glynis Knowles, Senior Staff, Breast Care (OPD Sutton)

Diane Laverty, Clinical Nurse Specialist (Palliative Care)

Susan J. Lee, formerly Occupational Health Manager

Annie Leggett, formerly Clinical Nurse Specialist (Intravenous Therapy)

Anne Lister, formerly Clinical Nurse Specialist/Unit Manager (Palliative Care)

Philippa A. Lloyd, Senior Staff Nurse (Wiltshaw Ward)

Nicholas Lodge, Clinical Group Research Nurse (Gynaecology)

E. Lopez-Verdugo, Senior Technician/Theatre Manager

Jane Machin, Specialist Speech and Language Therapist

Hazel Mack, formerly Acting Ward Sister (Horder Ward)

Elizabeth MacKenzie, Sister (Critical Care Unit)

Jean Maguire, Ward Sister/Specialist Sister for Lung Cancer

Jane Mallett, Research and Practice Development Manager

Glynis Markham, formerly Director of Nursing Services

Lisa Mercer, Senior Dietitian

Catherine Miller, formerly Senior Nurse (Continuing Care)

Marion Morgan, formerly Research Sister (Gynaecology)

Wayne Naylor, Clinical Nurse Specialist, Wellington Cancer Centre, New Zealand, formerly Wound Management Research Nurse, The Royal Marsden Hospital

Katrina Neal, formerly Clinical Nurse Specialist/Unit Manager (Palliative Care)

Liz O'Brien, Clinical Team Leader, District Nursing Croydon Primary Care Trust

Emma Osenton, Ward Sister (Wiltshaw Ward)

Evelyn Otunbade, Backcare Adviser

Buddy Joe Paris, Staff Nurse (Critical Care Unit)

Rachelle Pearce, formerly Sister (Medical Day Unit)

Emma Pennery, formerly Senior Clinical Nurse Specialist/Honorary Clinical Research Fellow

Helen Jayne Porter, formerly Clinical Nurse Specialist (High Dose Chemotherapy)

Joanne Preece, formerly Head of Risk Management

Judith Pretty, formerly Clinical Nurse Specialist (Head and Neck)

Ffion M. Read, Senior Staff Nurse (Medical Day Unit)

Elizabeth Rees, formerly Research Nurse Palliative Care

Francis Regan, formerly Senior Staff Nurse (Burdett Coutts Ward)

Frances Rhys-Evans, formerly Clinical Nurse Specialist/Ward Manager (Head & Neck and Thyroid Cancer)

Jean Maurice Robert, Staff Nurse (Critical Care Unit)

Helen Roberts, formerly Senior Nurse (Head and Neck)

Tim Root, Chief Pharmacist

Corinne Rowbotham, Senior Staff Nurse (IV Services)

Ray Rowden, formerly Director of Nursing Services

Miriam Rushton, formerly Senior Nurse (Gynaecology)

Patricia Ryan, Senior Sister (Haemato-oncology Unit)

Lena Salter, formerly Patient Services Manager

Kate Scott, Clinical Nurse Specialist (Psychological Care)

James Smith, formerly Chaplain

Val Speechley, Patient Information Officer

Moira Stephens, Clinical Nurse Specialist (Haemato-oncology)

Mavis Stork, formerly Theatre Services Manager

June Toovey, formerly Sister (Intravenous Therapy Team)

Anne Topping, formerly Senior Nurse (Gastro-intestinal/Genito-urinary)

Jennie Treleaven, Consultant Haematologist

Robert Tunmore, formerly Clinical Nurse Specialist (Psychological Support)

Beverley van der Molen, formerly Clinical Nurse Specialist/Unit Manager (General Oncology)

Rebecca Verity, formerly Senior Staff Nurse (Bud Flanagan Ward)

Chris Viner, Clinical Nurse Specialist (Ambulatory Chemotherapy)

Clare Webb, Specialist Sister in Psychological Care

Richard Wells, formerly Rehabilitation Services Manager

Isabel White, Head of Undergraduate Cancer Care Studies

Jane Wilson, formerly Group Theatre Manager

Karen Wright, formerly Research Assistant Nursing Research Unit

Karen Young, formerly Physiological Measurement Technician

Appendix 3

Multiple choice answers

Chapter 2, Assessment and the process of care

1   The correct answer is c, Emotional, psychological, spiritual, physical, cultural and social (page 28).

2   The correct answer is d, Patient focused (page 28).

3   The correct answer is b, Provide an effective framework for patient assessment.

4   The correct answer is b, Simple, acceptable, reliable and valid with an interpretable scoring system.

5   The correct answer is b, Nurses making clinical judgements about an individual's response to health and illness.

6   The correct answer is c, Provide information to other health care workers.

Chapter 3, Communication

1   The correct answer is a, Squarely, Open posture, Leaning slightly forward, Eye contact, Relaxed (Page 62).

2   The correct answer is d, Empathy (page 66).

3   The correct answer is b, Clarifying (page 65).

4   The correct answer is d, All of the above (page 72).

Chapter 4, Aseptic technique

1   The correct answer is a, Urinary (page 84).

2   The correct answer is c, Backs of thumbs and fingertips (page 89).

3   The correct answer is d, Yellow (page 96).

4   The correct answer is d, 70% in spirit.

Chapter 5, Barrier nursing

1   The correct answer is **d, Strict source isolation, cohort source isolation, protective isolation, source isolation** (page 117) DH 1998a.

2   The correct answer is **b, Self-infection** (page 119).

3   The correct answer is **c, Food, environment, hospital staff, patients, visitors** (page 120) Ayliffe *et al.* 2000.

4   The correct answer is **c, *Clostridium difficile, Staphylococcus aureus,* Vancomycin-resistant enterococci** (page 127) Perry *et al.* 2001.

5   The correct answer is **d, 60 days** (page 130) Gastmeier *et al.* 2006.

6   The correct answer is **b, Red alginate bag tied shut and put in a red linen bag** (page 132) DH (1995a).

7   The correct answer is **b, Widespread use of antibiotics** (page 142) Chen *et al.* 2004.

8   The correct answer is **c, Gut** (page 143).

9   The correct answer is **b, Skin and mucous** (page 144) Ayliffe *et al.* 2000.

10 The correct answer is **c, Vaccination and use of universal precautions** (page 161) Talaat *et al.* 2003.

Chapter 6, Cardiopulmonary resuscitation

1   The correct answer is **b, 3–4 minutes** (page 206) Docherty & Hall 2002.

2   The correct answer is **d, Asystole, pulseless electrical activity, ventricular tachycardia, ventricular fibrillation** (page 205).

3   The correct answer is **c, Tongue** (page 208).

4   The correct answer is **d, Head tilt/chin lift** (page 208) Simmons 2002.

5   The correct answer is **c, 30** (page 211) RCUK 2005.

6 The correct answer is **d, Epinephrine 1 mg** (page 216) RCUK 2005.

Chapter 7, Discharge planning

1 The correct answer is **a, Hospital medical staff** (page 249).

2 The correct answer is **d, All of the above** (page 236).

3 The correct answer is **b, Minimum 48 hours** (page 248).

4 The correct answer is **c, Production of a centrally held summary of care resulting in an individual care plan** (page 240).

Chapter 8, Drug administration: general principles

1 The correct answer is **d, Patient group direction** (page 257) NMC 2008a.

2 The correct answer is **c, Misuse of Drugs Act 1971** (page 256).

3 The correct answer is **d, Naloxone** (page 261).

4 The correct answer is **c, A registered nurse** (page 268).

5 The correct answer is **d, Beneath the epidermis into fat and connective tissue** (page 276).

6 The correct answer is **c, What you need, divided by what you have got, multiplied by volume of stock solution** (page 285).

Chapter 9, Drug administration delivery

1 The correct answer is **c, Will alter the rate of flow of the infusion, increasing in speed as it becomes higher above the infusion site.**

2 The correct answer is **d, Syringe drivers can be used to give small volumes of intravenous fluids slowly.**

3 The correct answer is **b, Syringe driver.**

Chapter 10, Elimination: bladder lavage and irrigation

1 The correct answer is **b, To clear an obstructed catheter or remove potential sources of obstruction** (page 375).

2 The correct answer is **c, After prostatic surgery and on rare occasions to remove material from a heavily diseased bladder** (page 376).

3 The correct answer is **b, Over 90% of patients within 4 weeks of catheterization** (page 377).

4 The correct answer is **b, Sterile low-linting gauze and an antiseptic solution** (page 384).

Chapter 11, Elimination: bowel care

1 The correct answer is **d, Sudden onset lasting less than 2 weeks** (page 405).

2 The correct answer is **b, Bowel disease, e.g. ulcerative colitis, Crohn's disease** (page 405).

3 The correct answer is **b, A side room with access to a toilet** (page 408).

4 The correct answer is **d, Inadequate diet, poor fluid intake, lifestyle change, ignoring the urge to defecate.**

5 The correct answer is **d, 2–2.5 litres** (page 413).

6 The correct answer is **d, Blunt end first.**

Chapter 12, Elimination: Stoma care

1 The correct answer is **b, Large bowel** (page 433).

2 The correct answer is **d, All of the above** (page 438) Qin & Bao-Min 2001.

3 The correct answer is **c, Colour, size, general appearance, state of peristomal skin, stoma/skin margin** (page 442) Black 2000b.

4 The correct answer is **c, Lifestyle, site of stoma, type of effluent, condition of peristomal skin, manual dexterity, cognitive ability, type of stoma, patient preference** (page 445).

5 The correct answer is **c, Mild soap and water** (page 447).

6 The correct answer is **c, Free from local chemist, free home delivery or direct from manufacturer.**

Chapter 13, Elimination: Urinary

1 The correct answer is **c, 5–10 ml** (page 462).

2 The correct answer is **b, Sterile water** (page 463).

3 The correct answer is **d, All of the above** (page 467).

4 The correct answer is **d, 0.9% sodium chloride or antiseptic solution** (page 477).

5 The correct answer is **d, Take a catheter specimen of urine, clean the area, check the volume of water in the catheter and deflate** (page 482–3).

6 The correct answer is **c, If leaking, when catheter is changed or at times recommended by manufacturer's directions.**

Chapter 14, Intrapleural drainage

1 The correct answer is **d, All of the above.**

2 The correct answer is **b, Air in the pleural cavity.**

3 The correct answer is **c, Chest X-ray.**

4 The correct answer is **b, Bubbling or swinging of the water that reduces over time.**

Chapter 15, Last offices

1 The correct answer is **c, Washing and grooming the deceased, understanding of the legal issues around death, removing unnecessary equipment, correctly labelling the body** (page 525).

2 The correct answer is **b, If the death is referred to the coroner** (page 535).

3 The correct answer is **b, A senior nurse if there is an agreed local policy, a registered medical practitioner** (page 528).

4 The correct answer is **c, By a nurse in the presence of another nurse** (page 532).

Chapter 16, Lumbar puncture

1 The correct answer is **d, All of the above.**

2   The correct answer is **b, Manometer.**

3   The correct answer is **c, 3.**

4   The correct answer is **b, On side with knees drawn up to abdomen and clasped hands.**

5   The correct answer is **c, 4 hours.**

6   The correct answer is **d, All of the above.**

Chapter 17, Nutritional support

1   The correct answer is **b, Allow hot food to cool before eating** (page 578).

2   The correct answer is **a, Parenteral nutrition** (page 583).

3   The correct answer is **d, Body mass index.**

4   The correct answer is **b, BMI less than 22 kg/m^2** (page 568).

5   The correct answer is **c, Infection** (page 585).

6   The correct answer is **a, Semi-upright** (page 595).

Chapter 18, Observations

1   The correct answer is **b, Radial** (page 611).

2   The correct answer is **a, Sinoatrial** (page 615).

3   The correct answer is **b, 30%** (page 624).

4   The correct answer is **c, Hypothalamus gland** (page 656).

5   The correct answer is **a, Slightly acidic** (page 669).

6   The correct answer is **b, Wash hands** (page 681).

7   The correct answer is **b, Ensure upper arm is supported and positioned at heart level** (page 632).

8   The correct answer is **c, Observing the number of breaths taken over a minute** (page 635).

9   The correct answer is **b, Tympanic membrane** (page 661).

10 The correct answer is **d, Heart rate slower than 60 beats per minute** (page 614).

Chapter 19, Observations: neurological

1 The correct answer is **c, Cheyne–Stokes breathing** (page 702).

2 The correct answer is **c, Less than 8** (NICE 2003).

3 The correct answer is **a, Eye opening, verbal response, motor response.**

4 The correct answer is **d, III.**

5 The correct answer is **d, All of the above.**

Chapter 20, Pain management and assessment

1 The correct answer is **c, 3 months** (page 715).

2 The correct answer is **d, Cultural sensitivity (acknowledging different cultures)** (page 719).

3 The correct answer is **d, Non-steroidal anti-inflammatory drugs** (page 724).

4 The correct answer is **a, Patient controlled analgesia** (page 726).

Chapter 21, Pain management: epidural and intrathecal analgesia

1 The correct answer is **d, All of the above** (page 755–6).

2 The correct answer is **b, 3–6 hours** (page 767).

3 The correct answer is **c, A registered nurse who has undergone formal training** (page 756).

Chapter 22, Perioperative care

1 The correct answer is **c, Depilatory cream** (page 784).

2 The correct answer is **b, Nothing to eat for 6 hours and nothing to drink for 3 hours prior to surgery** (page 785).

3 The correct answer is **c, Wash hands, measure calf circumference, check pedal pulses** (page 790).

4 The correct answer is **a, Control haemorrhage** (page 797).

5 The correct answer is **d, Prevent you being splashed by blood** (page 800).

6 The correct answer is **b, Upper airway obstruction** (page 805) Dhara 2006.

Chapters 23, 24, 25, Personal hygiene

1 The correct answer is **c, Tepid** (page 847).

2 The correct answer is **c, Energy production** (page 879).

3 The correct answer is **d, Hindus deem their left hand to be unclean** (page 882).

4 The correct answer is **a, Use sodium bicarbonate in the mouth care procedure** (page 870).

5 The correct answer is **c, Soft toothbrush** (page 867).

Chapter 26, Positioning

1 The correct answer is **b, Fluid imbalance** (page 896).

2 The correct answer is **a, Reduce the risk of DVT** (page 904).

3 The correct answer is **c, Backwards, letting the back of the legs touch the bed or chair** (page 908).

4 The correct answer is **a, Place a towel under the knee when sitting** (page 924).

Chapter 27, Respiratory therapy

1 The correct answer is **a, Oxygen 21%, carbon dioxide 0.03%, nitrogen 79%, rare gases 0.003%** (page 934).

2 The correct answer is **b, 28%** (page 942).

3 The correct answer is **c, Continuous positive airway pressure** (page 945).

4 The correct answer is **b, Humidified gas must be delivered at a temperature of 32–36°C, 100% humidification, via wide bore tubing** (page 949).

Chapter 28, Specimen collection for microbiological analysis

1 The correct answer is **b, Air** (page 961).

2 The correct answer is **b, Reduced oxygen** (page 961).

3 The correct answer is **b, Before the patient begins any treatment, e.g. antiseptics or antibiotics** (page 962).

4 The correct answer is **c, In a 37°C incubator** (page 967).

5 The correct answer is **d, Wash their hands and the urethral meatus** (page 968).

6 The correct answer is **a, Moisten the swab with sterile water** (page 970).

Chapter 29, Tracheostomy care and laryngectomy care

1 The correct answer is **a, A permanent tracheostomy is always created following a total glossectomy** (page 982).

2 The correct answer is **b, Humidified oxygen with tracheostomy mask, apron and goggles, tracheal dilators** (page 996).

3 The correct answer is **b, Each suctioning procedure should last no longer than 60 seconds** (page 1004).

4 The correct answer is **c, 0.9% sodium chloride** (page 1001).

Chapter 30, Transfusion of blood and blood productions

1 The correct answer is **c, MHRA.**

2 The correct answer is **a, Are able to receive blood of any blood group.**

3 The correct answer is **a, Are able to donate blood to any blood group.**

4 The correct answer is **c, Stop the transfusion and seek urgent medical help.**

5 The correct answer is **b, Every 12 hours or after administration of every second unit.**

6 The correct answer is **d, All of the above.**

Chapter 31, The unconscious patient

1 The correct answer is **c, Bed head elevated to 30 degrees** (page 1052).

2 The correct answer is **a, Glasgow Coma Scale** (page 1046).

3 The correct answer is **a, Legally binding, but can be difficult to enforce in acute settings** (page 1049).

4 The correct answer is **c, Hearing** (page 1050).

Chapter 32, Venepuncture

1 The correct answer is **c, An aseptic procedure.**

2 The correct answer is **c, Median cubital, cephalic, basilic and metarcapal** (page 1056).

3 The correct answer is **d, All of the above** (page 1060–1).

4 The correct answer is **c, Chlorohexidine 0.5% in 70% alcohol** (page 1063) Walther *et al.* 2001.

5 The correct answer is **b, Discarded into a sharps container without being resheathed.**

6 The correct answer is **b, Apply pressure to insertion site until bleeding stops** (page 1064) Ernst 2005.

Chapter 33, Violence: prevention and management

1 The correct answer is **d, All of the above** (page 1084).

2 The correct answer is **b, Boisterous behaviour, irritability, confusion and anger** (page 1085) Whittington 1997.

3 The correct answer is **b, General, intermittent, within eyesight, within arm's length** (page 1086).

4 The correct answer is **b, Discuss their feelings about the aggressor(s), other members of staff involved and the way the incident was managed** (page 1088).

Chapter 34, Wound management

1 The correct answer is **a, Haemostasis** (page 1099).

2 The correct answer is **d, Obesity** (page 1100).

3 The correct answer is **b, 20% body weight in 6 months or 10% in 2 months** (page 1104).

4 The correct answer is **d, Removal of necrotic tissue** (page 1106).

5 The correct answer is **a, Pressure, shearing and friction** (page 1120).

6 The correct answer is **c, Lister scale** (page 1123).

7 The correct answer is **b, Risk of contamination is reduce** (page 1140).

8 The correct answer is **b, Pain and tissue damage** (page 1145).

Index

Page numbers in *italics* refer to figures and those in **bold** to tables and boxes.

ABC of resuscitation 206–11, *207*
abdominal distension
    during bladder lavage/irrigation 392,
        393
    enterally fed patients **584**
ABO blood groups **1016**, 1016–17
ABO incompatibility 1017–18,
        1026–7
abscess, epidural 764, 776
accidents *see* incidents; spillages
aciclovir (acyclovir) 837, 861
Acinetobacter, antibiotic resistant
        143
acquired immune deficiency syndrome
        (AIDS) 1033
activated charcoal dressings **1108**
acupuncture 732
acute lung injury, transfusion-related
        (TRALI) 1030
acute normovolaemic haemodilution
        (ANH) 1015
acute pain 714–15
    assessment tools 718–21, *720*
    management 725–33
    need for effective control 721
    see also postoperative pain
acyclovir *see* aciclovir
Adapt ring Convex inserts 450
adefovir dipivoxil 163
adenosine 221
adhesive, tissue **1139**
adhesive island dressings **1108**

adhesive skin closure strips **1139**
adjuvant analgesics **724**, 739
    epidural/intrathecal 759
administration of drugs *see* drug
        administration
administration sets
    blood *see* blood administration sets
    enteral feeding 580
    gravity flow 359–60
    infusion flow rates 351
    intravenous infusion 284–5,
        288
    parenteral nutrition 285, 586
    volumetric infusion pumps 360–1
adrenaline (epinephrine)
    blood glucose regulation 675
    cardiopulmonary resuscitation 216,
        221
advance directives 1049
advanced beginner nurse 10–11
advanced life support (ALS) 206, 209,
        211, 216–18
advanced practice 12–13
aerosol containers, storage 262
aerosol generators, humidification
        952
aerosolization 266
affirming 63
ageing, skin 880
aggression *see* violence
AIDS (acquired immune deficiency
        syndrome) 1033

air
  embolism 335, 1028
  inspired 934, 948
  leaks, chest drainage systems 505–6,
    520
air conditioning and ventilation systems
  negative pressure 121–2, 125
  positive pressure 121, 125
air fluidized beds **1130**
air-in-line detectors 358
airborne infection 96, 121–2
  Clostridium difficile 153
  extra precautions **128**
  MRSA 147
airway
  assessment, postanaesthetic recovery
    809–10
  basic life support 208, *208*
  defence mechanisms 645
  evaluation of ability to protect 703
  functions 635
  maintenance, during oxygen therapy
    954
  resistance 641
  secretions *see* respiratory secretions
airway management
  cardiopulmonary resuscitation 208,
    221, 222–3
  postanaesthetic recovery 809–10,
    812–13
  unconscious patients 1050
airway obstruction
  emergency tracheostomy 984
  postoperative 805, 812–13
Aitken report (1958) 257–60
albumin
  plasma 571–2, **588**
  solutions, human (HAS) **1021–2**
alcohol consumption, and violence 1083
alcohol solutions/swabs, injection site
    preparation 281–2, 304, 306
alcoholic handrubs 90, 121
  procedure guidelines 104–5
aldosterone 622, 668
alfentanil 737–8
alginate wound dressings **1108**
allergic reactions, intravenous infusions
    333, 336

allodynia 734
alopecia 883
ALS *see* advanced life support
alternating pressure (AP) system **1130**,
    1131
alveoli 642–4, **644**
  gaseous exchange 935, *936*
Ambu bag and mask ventilation 209,
    223
ambulatory blood pressure monitoring
    630
ambulatory infusion devices 363–7
amino acids, parenteral nutrition
    solutions 585
amiodarone 216, 221, 838
ammonia, catheter encrustation and 379
amoebic dysentery 973
amputees, positioning 923–5
anaemia 644–5
  in malnutrition 572
  oxygen saturation 649
anaesthesia
  pain management interventions 740–1
  preoperative fasting 785
  pumps 363
  recovery after *see* postanaesthetic
    recovery
  see also local anaesthesia; spinal
    anaesthesia/analgesia; topical
    anaesthesia
anaesthetic room, procedure guidelines
    802
anaesthetist 806
analgesia
  acute/postoperative pain 725–9
  around the clock (ATC) 723
  breakthrough *see* breakthrough
    analgesia
  epidural *see* epidural analgesia
  inhalation (Entonox) 729
  intrapleural drainage 506–7
  intrathecal *see* intrathecal analgesia
  oral mucositis 862
  see also pain management
analgesic ladder 723, *723*, 733–8
analgesics
  acute/postoperative pain 725–9
  adjuvant (co-analgesics) **724**, 739

chronic pain 733–8
epidural/intrathecal use 757–9
non-opioid 728–9, 733
opioid *see* opioid analgesics
anaphylactic reactions, blood
transfusions 1027
anesthesia *see* anaesthesia
angiogenesis 1102
angiotensin 622
animals, carrying/transmitting infections
122–3
anorexia, dietary advice **578**
antecubital fossa, veins for venepuncture
1056, *1057*
anti-inflammatory drugs, eye 846
antibacterial eye preparations 837
antibacterial surfaces and materials 131
antibiotics
bladder lavage solutions 377
Clostridium difficile infection and
153, 154
local oral delivery 863
oral infections 861–2
pain management **724**
resistance 142–51
sensitivity testing 964–5
specimen collection and 962, 967
topical, wound management **1107,
1108**
antibody testing 965–6
anticoagulants
epidural catheter removal 771
intrapleural drainage and 502
lumbar puncture risks 552
anticonvulsants, pain management **724**
antidepressants 838
antidiuretic hormone (ADH) 668, 669
antiembolic stockings 785–6
contraindications 789
daily care 791–2
discharge care 792
fitting 786, 790–1
Lloyd Davies position and 786, 799
postoperative use 818
procedure guidelines 788–92
antifungal agents
eye preparations 837
oral infections 859–60, 861

antihistamines, eye toxicity 837
antihypertensive drug therapy 624
antimetabolites 837
antimicrobial agents *see* antibiotics
antimicrobial resistance 142
antimicrobial-resistant organisms
142–51
antimotility drugs 408
antipyretic agents 660–1
antiseptics
bladder lavage 376, 377
specimen collection and 962
wound cleaning **1107**
see also chlorhexidine
antispasmodics **724**
antiviral therapy
eye preparations 837
hepatitis B 163
anxiety 69–70
effects on pain 715
infected patients in isolation
133–4
during venepuncture 1060, 1072
aperients 414
aphasic patients, communicating with
74–5
apheresis, donor 1016
Apligraf 1119
apnoeustic respiration 648, **702**
Appeal wipes and spray 450
aprons, plastic 93–4
barrier nursing 128, 136
procedure guidelines 96–8, 98–9
aqueous humour 828, *830*
arachis oil enema 418
arachnoid mater 756, *756*
arachnoiditis 557
arginine 582
argyria 466
arm *see* upper limb
arousability 693
arrhythmias 615–16
causing cardiac arrest 205
ECG features *617*
tracheal suctioning-induced 999
art therapy 730–1
arterial blood gases, severe asthma
652–3

arteries 1058
  accidental puncture 1071
  blood pressure monitoring 624
arterioles 620
ascorbic acid (vitamin C) **674**, 679,
  1102, 1105
asepsis 83
aseptic technique 83–116
  airborne contamination 96
  compliance with 86, 87
  defined 83
  dressing trolley 93
  environmental cleanliness 95
  hand washing 88–91
  inanimate objects 91–2
  indications 83–4
  intravenous drug administration
    284–5
  medical or clean 83
  microbiological specimen collection
    962, 967
  multiple choice questions 116, 1176
  non touch technique 91
  operating theatre 800–1
  patient hygiene 95–6
  personal protective equipment 93–5
  principles 87–96
  procedure guidelines 99–102
  surgical or sterile 83
  urinary catheterization 472–9
  venepuncture 1055
aspiration, gastric contents
  to check enteral tube position 577–9,
    596
  complicating enteral feeding **584**
  during CPAP 947
aspirin **674**, 733, 862
assessment 27–36
  comprehensive **31**
  discharge planning 246–7
  documentation 43–4
  focused **31**
  guidance and recommendations 44–5
  interviews 32–4, **33–4**
  methods 32–6
  multiple choice questions 52–3, 1176
  ongoing **31**
  principles 28–9

  self- 36, **36**
  single 240–4
  structure 29–32
  tools 34–6, **35**
  types **31**
Association for the Advancement of
  Medical Instrumentation (AAMI)
  626
Association of Perioperative Registered
  Nurses (AORN) 788, 801
asthma 652–4, **654**
asymmetrical tonic neck reflex 918
asystole 205, 216
ataxic breathing **702**
atelectasis 639
athletes, heart rate 614
atmosphere 643–4, **644**
atrial fibrillation 616
atrioventricular (AV) block, Mobitz type
  2 *617*
atrioventricular (AV) bundle (bundle of
  His) *615*
atrioventricular (AV) node *615*
atropine 216, 221, 838
audit, resuscitation 219
autologous blood donation 1015–16
autolytic wound debridement 1107
automated external defibrillators (AEDs)
  218
awareness, conscious 693–4
axillary temperature 662–3
azotaemia, parenteral nutrition 590

B/P. sphyg. *see* sphygmomanometers
Babinski response 701, 708
back pain (backache)
  intraoperative positioning and 798
  post-lumbar puncture 557, 561,
    562
bacteraemia 664
  blood cultures 967
  Gram-negative 144
bacteria
  aerobic 961
  anaerobic 961
  facultative 961
  fastidious 961
  oral cavity 855

specimen collection 964–5
wound colonization 1112
bacterial infections
antibiotic-resistant 142–51
oral 861–2
transfusion-transmitted 1030
see also specific infections
bacteriuria 669, *670*
bad news, breaking 72
Bahai faith, last offices 538
balloon catheters *see* Foley catheters
barrier nursing 117–204
cohort 117, 126, 147
defined 117
indications 117
multiple choice questions 202–4, 1177
principles 126–34
reverse (protective isolation) 117, 124
sources of infection 119–20
standard and extra precautions 127,
127
types 123–4
see also isolation rooms; source
isolation
basic life support (BLS) 206–11, *207*
basilic vein 1056, *1057*
basins, hand 102, 121
bathing 95–6, 881–2
barrier-nursed patients 131–2, 138
preoperative 794
see also bed bathing; showering
baths, cleaning 132
battery-operated infusion devices 364–5
bed(s)
linen *see* linen/laundry
positioning in 896–901
amputees 924
neurological patients 920–1
side lying 900–1, *901*
sitting up 898–9, *899*
supine 897–8
pressure-relieving devices 1129–31,
1130
bed bathing 132, 881
procedure guidelines 885–8
bed rest 895–6
bedpans 399–401, 413
belladonna-like substances 838

benchmarks
food and nutrition 573, **574–5**
personal and oral hygiene 131, 853,
878–9
Benner's model of skill acquisition 10,
13
benzodiazepines **724**
beta-blockers 838
Better Hospital Food programme 573
bio-engineered skin substitutes 1119
biochemical tests
nutritional status 571–2
parenteral nutrition **588–9**
bioelectrical impedance analysis (BIA)
570
biofilms 149, 377–8
biohazard labels 964
Biot's respiration 648
bisacodyl 416, 423
bisphosphonates **724**, 739
bladder, empty, catheterized patients 484
bladder irrigation (continuous) 375–97
catheters for 381, *382*
defined 375
indications 375–6
multiple choice questions 397, 1178–9
patient assessment 380–1
problem solving 392–3
procedure guidelines 388–90
recording chart 390–1, *391*
solutions 376–7
bladder lavage 375–97
defined 375
indications 375–6
multiple choice questions 397,
1178–9
patient assessment 380–1
problem solving 392–3
procedure guidelines 382–5
solutions 376 7
bleeding/haemorrhage
cardiopulmonary arrest 213–14
hepatitis B-infected patients 166–7,
167
lumbar puncture-associated 557
postoperative care 818
blind patients, communication with
72–3

blink reflex 700, 708
  absent, eye care 834
blocking behaviour 67–8
Blom–Singer speaking valve 992
blood
  accidental spillage 1074
  clots, bladder irrigation 381, 390
  hepatitis B-infected 165, 166
  pH 644
  spurting, during venepuncture 1074
  testing, donors 1014–15
  traceability 1013
  viscosity 620
  warming devices 1029
blood administration sets
  changing 285, 1039
  transfusion procedure 1036, 1037
blood borne infections 122
  blood donor selection and 1014–15
  hepatitis B 160, 165–7
blood cells, in CSF 556
blood components/products
  donation 1016
  traceability 1013
  used for transfusion **1019–23**
blood cultures 963, 967–8
blood donation 1014–16
  autologous 1015–16
blood flow 620
  problems during venepuncture
    1075
  resistance to 620, *621*
  wound bed, improving 1105
blood gases, arterial, severe asthma
    652–3
blood glucose *see* glucose, blood
blood groups 1016–18
  haemopoietic stem cell
    transplantation 1017–18
  incompatibility 1017
blood pack labelling *1035*
blood pressure (BP) 620–34
  ambulatory monitoring 630
  continuous arterial monitoring 624
  defined 620
  diastolic 622
  factors affecting 622, *623*
  measurement

auscultatory method 624–6, *625,
    628*
  clinical aspects 630–1
  indications 620
  methods and equipment 624–9
  neurological patients 703, 707
  postanaesthetic recovery 810
  practical aspects 629–30
  procedure guidelines 632–4, *634*
  top tips **631**
  see also sphygmomanometers
  normal 622
  regulation 620–2, *621*
  systolic 622
  see also hypertension; hypotension
blood products *see* blood
    components/products
Blood Safety and Quality Regulations
    2005 1013–14
blood sampling 966–8
  blood cultures 967–8
  blood glucose monitoring 678, 681
  order of collection 1068
  via CVADs 966, 968
  via intravenous devices 1061, **1062**
  see also venepuncture
blood transfusion *see* transfusion
blood vessels, resistance to blood flow
    620
blood warmers 1029
bloodstream infections, health care
    acquired 118
body, care after death *see* last offices
body bag 528, 529, 533, 535
body composition, measurement 570
body fluids
  hepatitis B transmission 159–60
  specimen collection 973–6
body mass index (BMI) 569
body weight 569–70
  loss 569–70
    percentage 568, 569
  measuring, procedure guidelines
    591–2
Bohr effect 938
bone marrow transplantation (BMT)
  blood cultures 968
  cryopreserved cells 1018

see also neutropenia; stem cell
    transplantation
bovine spongiform encephalopathy
    (BSE) 1034
bowel
  anatomy and physiology 403–5
  function, unconscious patients 1047
bowel care 398–431
  bedpans 399–401
  commodes 401–3
  enemas 416–22
  multiple choice questions 430–1, 1179
  suppositories 422–5
  unconscious patients 1051
bowel habit
  factors affecting 411
  history taking 412
  normal 411
  see also constipation; diarrhoea
BP *see* blood pressure
brachial artery, blood pressure recording
    624, 629, 633
Braden scale 1124, **1127–8**
bradycardia 614, 815
bradypnoea 647
brainstem
  damage 699, *699*
  herniation, after lumbar puncture
    557, 562
breaking bad news 72
breakthrough analgesia 734–5, 738–9
breakthrough pain 715, 738
breast surgery, blood pressure
    measurement after 630
breathing
  agonal 208
  cardiopulmonary resuscitation 208–9,
    210
  positioning to minimize work of 913,
    913
  see also respiration
breathlessness 647
Brief Pain Inventory (BPI) 721
Bristol Stool Form Chart *407*, 412
British Committee for Standards in
    Haematology (BCSH) 1024
British Humanist Association 539
British Hypertension Society 623–4, 626

British Medical Association (BMA), do
    not attempt resuscitation
    guidance 219–20
British Thoracic Society, intrapleural
    drainage guidelines 503
bronchitis, chronic 636, 952
Broviac (skin-tunnelled) catheters,
    parenteral nutrition 585
bruising, after venepuncture 1064,
    1072–3
BSE (bovine spongiform
    encephalopathy) 1034
buccal tablets 263, 294
Buddhism, last offices 538
Buddhist Hospice Trust 538
buffy coat **1020**
bundle of His (AV bundle) *615*
bupivacaine, epidural/intrathecal 759
buprenorphine 738
Burial Society of the United Synagogue
    542
burns, diathermy 797–8
butterfly devices *see* winged infusion
    devices

C-reactive protein (CRP) 572, **589**
Cadesorb 1119, 1120, 1135
Cadexomer bead dressings **1109**
calcium, plasma **588**
calcium chloride 216–17, 221
calf compression boots, intermittent
    786, 799
Campylobacter food poisoning 122
cancer
  communication 55, 69–72
  dietary modification 577, **578**
  health care acquired infections 118
  mouth care 859
  nutritional assessment 570, 571
  oral assessment 856
  oral complications 854–5
  patient assessment 30, **35**, 35–6,
    36
  personal hygiene 131–2
  plastic surgery 1132
  skin complications 880
  specimen collection for
    microbiological analysis 960

Cancer Action Team, assessment
  guidance 30
cancer pain 717
  assessment 717, **718**, 722
  management 733–41
  pain chart 721, *722*, 743–4
  spinal analgesia 754, 755
  see also chronic pain
candidiasis *(Candida albicans* infections*)*
  oral 859–60, 861
  specimen collection 966
cannabis 738
capillary wound dressings **1109**
capsules 263
  administration guidelines 292–5
  opening 263
  storage 262
carbohydrates
  parenteral nutrition solutions 585
  supplements 576
carbon dioxide
  control of respiration 636
  excretion 939
  narcosis 952
  pulmonary exchange 642–4, **644**,
    935, *936*
  transport *643*, 644
carbon dioxide partial pressure (PCO₂)
  934–5
  in blood (PaCO₂) 644, 952
carbon monoxide (CO) poisoning 649
cardiac arrest 205
  agonal breathing 208
  arrhythmias causing 205
  assessment 206
  management *see* cardiopulmonary
    resuscitation
  post-resuscitation care 225–7
  potentially reversible causes 212–16
  team 218, 223
cardiac arrhythmias *see* arrhythmias
cardiac massage *see* chest compressions
cardiac output (CO) 613
cardiac tamponade 215
cardiopulmonary arrest *see* cardiac
  arrest
cardiopulmonary resuscitation (CPR)
  205–31

advanced life support (ALS) 206, 209,
  211, 216–18
  assessment 206, *207*
  basic life support 206–11, *207*
  decision making 219–20
  defibrillation 217–18
  drugs 216–17, 221
  equipment 218, 221
  ethics 219
  in-hospital algorithm *207*
  indications 205
  multiple choice questions 230–1,
    1177–8
  post-procedure care 225–7
  potentially reversible causes of arrest
    212–16
  principles 206
  procedure guidelines 221–7
  standards and training 218–19
  tracheostomy patients 1000
cardiovascular disease
  positioning patients with 915–16
  pulse monitoring 618
cardiovascular function
  epidural/intrathecal analgesia 768
  postanaesthetic assessment 806, *807*,
    810
  unconscious patients 1048
care 39–46
  communicating (handover) 46
  documentation 42–3, **43–4**
  evaluating 42
  implementing 39–41
  multiple choice questions 53, 1176
  planning 39–41, **43–4**
care homes, discharge to 244–5
care of body after death *see* last offices
carers, informal
  discharge planning and 236, 251–2
  see also family
carotid pulse, checking 209–10, *212*
carpets 140
CASE method, prevention of violence
  1085
cathartics 414
catheter-associated infections, urinary
  see urinary catheter-associated
    infections

catheter specimen of urine (CSU)
477–80, *481*
catheters
defined 460
intrapleural drainage 503
tracheal suctioning 1000, *1000*
urinary *see* urinary catheters
Catrix 1119, 1120
Cavilon barrier film 448
CDs *see* controlled drugs
CE mark
gloves 94, 107, 130
medical devices 92
cell salvage, intra-operative (ICS)
1015–16
cellulitis, intravenous infusion-related
332
central lines *see* central venous catheters
central venous access devices (CVAD)
blood sampling 966, 968
occlusion 330
central venous catheters (CVCs)
infections related to 967–8
parenteral nutrition 585
Centre for Evidence Based Nursing
16
Centre for Reviews and Dissemination,
York 16
cephalic vein 1056, *1057*
cerebral oedema 699
cerebrospinal fluid (CSF) 554–5, 754
abnormalities 555–6
investigations 551, 556
leakage from lumbar puncture site
561, 562
pressure 555
sampling 551, 555
cervical spine injuries, assessment
206
chair
positioning in 904
standing up from 905, *906*
chapters, structure of **11**
charcoal dressings **1108**
charrière (ch) 463
charting by exception (CBE) 42
chemical irritation, intravenous
infusions 331

chemotherapy
cancer pain management 739–40
see also cytotoxic drugs
chest compressions
cardiopulmonary resuscitation
210–11, *213*, 223
intubated patients 224
chest drains *see* intrapleural drains
chest X-rays
enteral tube feeding 577, 596
post-CPR 226
Cheyne–Stokes respiration 648, **702**
Chief Nursing Officer's '10 key roles' for
nurses 13
children *see* paediatric patients
Chiron barrier cream 448
chloramphenicol 838
chlorhexidine
bladder lavage 376, 377
chewing gum 864
mouthwash 859
MRSA eradication 145
Christianity, last offices 539
chronic obstructive pulmonary disease
(COPD) 636, 652, 952
see also emphysema
chronic pain 715
assessment 717–21, **718**
epidural analgesia *see under* epidural
analgesia
intrathecal analgesia *see under*
intrathecal analgesia
management 723–4, 733–41
non-pharmacological techniques
729–33
pain chart 721, *722*, 743–4
procedure guidelines 743–4
see also cancer pain
chronic wasting disease 1034
Church of Jesus Christ of the Latter Day
Saints, last offices 542
chylothorax 501
ciprofloxacin 838
circulation
cardiopulmonary resuscitation
209–11, *212*, *213*
postanaesthetic recovery 810
postoperative monitoring 818

circulatory (fluid) overload
  bladder irrigation 376–7
  blood pressure monitoring 631
  blood transfusion 1028
  intravenous infusions 334, 352–3, **354**
  parenteral nutrition 587
  see also overinfusion
citric acid 3.23% and magnesium oxide
    solution (Suby G) 376, 379
citric acid 6% solution (solution R) 376,
    379
CJD *see* Creutzfeldt–Jakob disease
clamps, infusion devices 351
clarifying 64–5
cleaning
  baths 132
  environmental 95, 121, 130–1
    Clostridium difficile infections 154
    hepatitis B 165
    isolation rooms 134, 139–40
    MRSA 146–7
    see also domestic staff
  skin *see* skin preparation
  stoma 447
  wounds 1106, **1107**, 1141
cleanliness, environmental 95, 121
clients *see* patients
clinical experience/expertise 18, 20
clinical governance 15
clinical nurse specialists 13
clips, metal **1139**
  removal 1141–2
clonidine, epidural/intrathecal 759
Clostridium difficile 151–4
  diagnosis 152
  nursing care 154
  prevention of spread/management
    153–4
  transmission 153
clothing
  deceased patient 527, 532
  protective *see* protective clothing
cluster breathing **702**
co-analgesics **724**, 739
coagulopathies
  lumbar puncture 552
  spinal analgesia 755
cockroaches 122–3

Code, NMC 5, 10, 1088, 1121,
    1163–70
codeine phosphate 408, 440, 734
coffee 413
cohort barrier nursing 117, 126
  MRSA-infected patients 147
cold therapy (cryotherapy) 733, 864
colectomy, total 434
collaboration, with patients 1165
collagen 1101–2, 1103, 1119
  dressings **1109**, 1119–20
Colledge silver laryngectomy tube 991,
    992
collusion 70–2
colon 404
colonic conduits 434
colonization, wound 1112
colony stimulating factors 863–4
colostomy 432–3
  defunctioning or loop 432–3, *434*
  end or terminal 432, *433*
  indications 435–6
  irrigation 441
  plugs 440, 447
  postoperative care 441–2
  postoperative function 440
  pouches 445–7, *446*
  problem solving 453–4
  see also stoma(s)
comatose patients *see* unconscious
    patients
Comfeel wafers 448
comfort measures, pain management
    731
Committee on Medical Aspects of Food
    Policy (COMA) report 573
commodes 401–3
communication 54–80
  aids 62–3
  aphasic patients 74–5
  during assessment 32
  barriers to effective 56–7
  blind and partially sighted 72–3
  breaking bad news 72
  de-escalation of violence 1085
  deaf and hard of hearing 73–4
  defined 54
  discharge planning and 238–40, **239**

guidelines 57–9
intershift (handover) 46
language and cultural issues 68
laryngectomy patients 995
multiple choice questions 79–80, 1176
non-verbal 62–3
oxygen therapy and 955
recognizing own agenda 59–60
skills 61–6
specific problems 67–75
specific therapeutic 4
tracheostomy patients 993–4
training 67
verbal 62
community care
home enteral feeding 583
MRSA-infected patients 148
Community Care (Delayed Discharges)
Act 234, **239**
community nurses, discharge planning
241–3, 248–9
compartment syndrome 799
competence
Benner's model of acquisition 10
definition 10
to give consent 7
nursing staff 9–12
competent nurses 9–12
complaints, dealing with 1169
complementary therapies, wound
management 1120
Complex Discharge Coordinator **236**,
240, **241–3**
compliance
aseptic technique 86, 87
hand washing 89, 90, 120
self-administration of medicines 268
compression, intermittent pneumatic
786, 799
compression stockings, graduated elastic
see antiembolic stockings
computed tomography (CT) 552
conduction system, heart *615*
confidentiality, respect for 1165
conformable catheters 465–6
Conformité Europèene mark *see* CE
mark
confusion, evaluation **695**, 697

consciousness 693–8
arousability 693
assessment 694–8, 1046
cardiopulmonary arrest 206, *207*,
226
postanaesthetic recovery 806, *807*,
812
procedure guidelines 705–6
see also Glasgow coma scale
awareness 693–4
defined 1045
level 694
Conseal plugs 440
consent 6–9, 1165–6
components of valid 7
documentation 7–9
forms 7, 9
implied **8**
verbal 6, **8**
written 7–9, **8**
constipation 409–16
assessment 411–12
causes 409, *410*, 412
defined 398
enterally fed patients **584**
management 412–16, **414**
multiple choice questions 430–1,
1179
opioid-induced 735
Rome diagnostic criteria 409–11
contact lenses 832–3
care of 833, 841–2, *842*
eye preparations and 832–3
surgical patients 795
contact transmission of infection 91–2,
120–1
extra precautions **128**
hepatitis B 159
containers
medicine 261–2
specimen 961–2, 963
context
as evidence source 18–19, 20
nursing 3–22
continuous intravenous infusions *see*
intravenous infusions, continuous
continuous low pressure (CLP) system
1131

continuous positive airway pressure
(CPAP) 945–7
contractures 922, 924–5
control and restraint (C&R) 1087
Control of Substances Hazardous to
Health (COSHH) regulations 130
controlled drugs (CDs) 257–61
legal requirements 257, **258–9**
procedure guidelines 295–6
register 260
safe practice guidance 260–1
controlled-release tablets 263
conveens *see* penile sheaths
cooling, in pyrexia 661
COPD *see* chronic obstructive
pulmonary disease
coping mechanisms 70–1
coring, multidose vials 302, *303*
corneal (blink) reflex 700, 708
corticosteroids (steroids)
as analgesics **724**
epidural/intrathecal 759
eye drops 836
intra-articular injections 275
intralesional, hypertrophic and keloid
scars 1137
toxic effects on eye 838
cortisol 675
COSHH (Control of Substances
Hazardous to Health) regulations
130
cosmetic camouflage, scars 1138
cost effectiveness 14–16
costs, health care-acquired infections 84,
85, 86, 118
cough **646**
counselling
after violent incidents 1089
before stoma surgery 436–7
see also psychological support
covert drug administration 269–70
CPAP (continuous positive airway
pressure) 945–7
CPR *see* cardiopulmonary resuscitation
creams 262, 264
creatinine **588**, 668
Creutzfeldt–Jakob disease (CJD)
transmission in blood 1015, 1034

variant (vCJD) 1034
cricothyroidotomy 984
critical care, last offices 533–5
critical colonization, wounds 1112
critical thinking 27–8
critically ill patients
blood pressure measurement 631
pulse monitoring 618
respiratory monitoring 648
sedation 1045
temperature monitoring 664
crockery/cutlery
hepatitis A-infected patients 158
source barrier nursing 133, 137
cross-infection 120
prevention *see* infection control
crutches, elbow **909–10**
cryo-depleted plasma **1023**
cryoprecipitate **1023**
cryopreservation, bone
marrow/peripheral blood stem
cells 1018
cryotherapy (cold therapy) 733, 864
CSF *see* cerebrospinal fluid
CSU (catheter specimen of urine)
479–80, *481*
cues, non-verbal 59, 61
cuff, sphygmomanometer 627, 632–3
cultural issues
communication 68
last offices 526–7, 538–44
personal hygiene 877, 881–2
Cushing reflex 703
cushions, pressure-relieving 1129–31,
1130
cutlery *see* crockery/cutlery
CVAD *see* central venous access devices
cyanosis 645
cyclizine 279
cycloplegics 835
cylinders, oxygen 940, 941, 945
cytology, CSF 556
cytomegalovirus (CMV),
transfusion-related infection
1032–3
cytotoxic drugs
eye toxicity 837
hair loss 883

oral damage 854–5, 856, **856**, 865
skin complications 880

Dansac washers 449
danthron 416
dead space, anatomical 642
deaf patients, communication with 73–4
death
    confirmation 528
    hepatitis B 163, 168
    last offices 525–50
debridement, wound 1106–12
debriefing, after violent incidents
        1088–9
decannulation plug, tracheostomy *990*,
        991
decision making 36–9
decubitus ulcers *see* pressure ulcers
deep vein thrombosis (DVT)
    postoperative care 818
    prophylaxis *see* thromboprophylaxis
    risk factors 785, 788–9
    signs 792
    see also venous thromboembolism
defecation 404–5
    advice for patients 413
    assisting, procedure guidelines
        399–403
defibrillation *211*, 217–18, 225
    placement of paddles/electrodes 218
    safe practice 217
defibrillators 218
dehydration
    blood glucose testing 679
    in diarrhoea 405–6
    dysphagia and 602
    infusion-related 353, **354**
    venepuncture in 1059
delegation, effective 1167
delta (hepatitis D) virus **155**
deltoid muscle injections 280, *280*
denial 70–2
dental crowns/bridges 795
dentures
    procedure guidelines 866–7, 868
    surgical patients 795
    unconscious patients 1050
deodorizers, stoma 446, 451

depression 69, 133–4
Dermagraft 1119
dermatomes 757, *758*
dermis 879
detergent, bactericidal 90, 105–6, 120–1
dexamethasone, subcutaneous infusions
        279
diabetes mellitus 674, 675
    blood glucose monitoring 678–80
    consequences of hyperglycaemia
        676–8, 677
    foot care 883
    odour of urine 669
diabetic ketoacidosis 647, 676–8, 677
diagnosis, nursing 36–9
    concept 37–8, **38**
    example **39**
    process 37
dialysis, blood glucose testing 679
diamorphine
    acute/postoperative pain 725–6, 727
    chronic pain 737
    epidural/intrathecal 757–9
    nasal spray 737
    safer practice guidance 260–1
diarrhoea 405–9
    assessment 406–8
    causes 405
    Clostridium difficile 152
    defined 398
    enterally fed patients **584**
    management 408–9
    multiple choice questions 430, 1179
    specimen collection 964, 973
    stoma patients 406, 440
    vancomycin-resistant enterococci 150
diastolic blood pressure 622
    measurement 629, 634
diathermy 797–8
diclofenac 728
diet
    constipation management 412–13
    in dysphagia 604
    history 568–9
    modification 567, 577, **578**
    stoma patients 443–4
    see also food; nutrition
dietary reference values 573

dietary supplements 567, 575–7
diffusion 935
digital rectal examination (DRE) 412
digital veins, hand *1057*
dignity, respect for 5–6
digoxin 838
dihydrocodeine 734
2, 3-diphosphoglycerate (2,3-DPG) 938
dipstick (reagent) tests, urine 671–2,
    672, **674**
discharge
  to a care home 244–5
  complex 240, **241–3**
  delay monitoring form *235*
  delays 234, **239**, 245
  hepatitis B 167–8
  intermediate care 244
  against medical advice 234–6, **236**
  NHS Continuing Healthcare 245
  nurse-led 240
  patients with particular care needs
    233
  postanaesthetic recovery 805–6, *807*
  source isolation 141
  thromboembolism prophylaxis 792
  urgent, for palliative care at home
    236, *237–8*
Discharge Coordinators **236**, 240,
  241–3, 248
discharge planning 232–54
  aims 233
  communication and 238–40, **239**
  complex cases 240, **241–3**
  defined 232
  multiple choice questions 254, 1178
  principles 233–4
  procedure guidelines 246–52
  process 234–6
  role of informal carers 236
  single assessment process 240–4
  stoma patients 443
dishwashing
  source barrier nursing 133, 137
  see also crockery/cutlery
disseminated intravascular coagulation
  (DIC) 1017, 1027
district nurses, discharge planning
  241–3, 248–9

do not attempt resuscitation (DNAR)
  219–20
doctors
  discharge against advice **236**
  white coats 129
documentation
  blood transfusion 1038
  consent 7–9
  controlled drugs **258**
  CPR decisions 220
  NMC *Code* 1168
  nursing care 42–3, **43–4**
  refusals 59
  specimen collection 962–3
  violent incidents 1089
docusate sodium (dioctyl sodium
    sulphosuccinate)
  enema 418
  laxative 415
domestic staff
  barrier nursing 134, 139–40
  see also cleaning
L-dopa **674**
dorsogluteal intramuscular injections
  280, 280–1
double gloving 130, 800
2, 3-DPG (2,3-diphosphoglycerate) 938
drainage
  intrapleural *see* intrapleural drainage
  vacuum, changing, procedure
    guidelines 1144–5
  see also urine drainage bags
drains *see* wound drains
dressing trolley 93
dressings
  barrier-nursed patients 138
  changing
    acute and surgical wounds 1140–1
    aseptic technique 92
    epidural/intrathecal exit site 769–70
    total laryngectomy 998
    tracheostomy 997, 1001
  chest drain insertion site 506
  poor application/techniques **1100**
  see also wound dressings
drinks
  assisting patients 592–4
  disguising medication in 269–70

driving, opioids and 740
droplet transmission 121
  extra precautions **128**
drops per minute, calculation 359
drug administration 255–345
  covert 269–70
  defined 255
  delivery *see* infusion devices
  errors 267–8
  indications 255
  legal and professional context 256–61
  multiple choice questions 344–5, 1178
  in parenteral nutrition solutions
      586–7
  in practice 266–89
  procedure guidelines 290–337
  self- 268–9, 290–2
  single nurse 268
  verbal orders 267–8
  via enteral feeding tubes 598–600
  via infusion devices 346–74
drug intoxication, cardiopulmonary
      arrest 215–16
drug users, intravenous 159
drugs *see* medicines
dry lips 863, 870
dry mouth 855
  during oxygen therapy 954
  treatment 862, 869
dry skin 880, 881
dryers, electric air 91
drying
  hand 91, 104
  skin 881
dual diagnosis patients 1083
dura mater 756, 756
dural puncture, inadvertent 764, 774
Durogesic *see* fentanyl
Duthie Report (1988) 261
DVT *see* deep vein thrombosis
dying, care of *see* terminal care
dysphagia
  dietary advice **578**
  problem solving 601–4
  see also swallowing difficulties
dysphasia 697
dyspnoea 647
  exertional 647

paroxysmal nocturnal 647
dysuria, catheterized patients 486

ear care 883–4
ear drops, procedure guidelines 312–13
ear swabs 969, 969
eating
  assisted, procedure guidelines 592–4
  difficulties 601–4
ECG *see* electrocardiogram
elastic compression stockings, graduated
      see antiembolic stockings
elastomeric balloons, infusion devices
      364
elderly
  blood pressure measurement 630, 632
  discharge planning 244–5
  hypothermia 659
  pressure ulcers 1121
  skin changes 880
  thermoregulation 659
  venepuncture 1059
electric hand dryers 91
electro-larynx device 995
electrocardiogram (ECG) 616
  cardiopulmonary resuscitation 224,
      226
  examples *617*
electrolytes
  monitoring, during parenteral
      nutrition **588**
  parenteral nutrition solutions 586
  postoperative management 819
  unconscious patients 1049
electronic records 46
elemental feeds 581–2
elixirs 263
embolism
  air 335, 1028
  particle, intravenous procedures 336
  see also pulmonary embolism; venous
      thromboembolism
embolus *see* embolism
emollients 881
empathy 66
emphysema 636, 640, 652
  see also chronic obstructive
      pulmonary disease

Employment Rights Act 1996 1081
empyema 501
end-of-life care *see* terminal care
endotracheal intubation,
    cardiopulmonary resuscitation
    209, 224
endotracheal tube, drug administration
    via 216
enemas 264, 416–22
    contraindications 417
    evacuant 417–18
    indications 416–17
    problem solving 421–2
    procedure guidelines 418–21
    retention 418
energy
    requirements 572, **573**
    supplements 576
enteral feeding tubes 577–9
    blocked **584**
    drug administration via 598–600
    see also gastrostomy tubes;
        nasogastric tubes
enteral tube feeding 577–83
    complications 583, **584**
    equipment 580, **581**
    feeds 581–2
    home 583
    indications 567
    monitoring 582
    nasal care 884
    procedure guidelines 594–600
    termination 583
    unconscious patients 1047
enteric coated tablets 262–3, 294
enterococci 130–1, 150
    see also vancomycin-resistant
        enterococci
Enterococcus faecalis 150
Enterococcus faecium 130–1, 150
Entonox (nitrous oxide and oxygen)
    729
environment (health care)
    cleaning *see* cleaning, environmental
    cleanliness 95, 121
    Clostridium difficile reservoirs 153
    enterococcal survival 130–1, 150–1
    MRSA contamination 146–7

prevention of violence 1086
    as reservoir of infection 120
epidermal growth factor (EGF) **1101**,
    1119–20
epidermis 880
epidural abscess 764, 776
epidural analgesia 754–82
    acute pain 726–7
    advantages 754–5
    bolus injections 761
    catheter removal 771–2
    checking height of block 763
    chronic pain 740–1, 755
        exit site dressing change 769–70
        pain assessment 763
        post-insertion management
        768–9
        problem solving 776–8
    complications 763–4, 774–6
    continuous infusion 759–61
    contraindications 755–6
    defined 754
    drug-related side-effects 761–2,
        772–4
    drugs used 757–9
    indications 755
    monitoring 761, 768
    multiple choice questions 782,
        1182
    pain assessment 762–3, 768–9
    patient controlled (PCEA) 761
    problem solving 772–8
    procedure guidelines 765–72
    pump alarm 776
    pumps 363
    safety checks 765, **765**
epidural catheter
    disconnection 777
    insertion, procedure guidelines 765–7
    migration 764, 775, 777
    occlusion 777
    optimal position 760
    removal, procedure guidelines
        771–2
epidural haematoma 763–4, 775
epidural space 756–7
epileptic seizures 710
epinephrine *see* adrenaline

equipment
  as reservoirs of infection 121
  spread of infection via 91–2, 120
errors
  blood pressure measurement 626,
    629–30
  infusion 348–9, 367
  medication 267–8
  transfusion 1024, 1025, 1027, *1028*
  tympanic temperature measurement
    664
  see also incidents; spillages
erythema, intravenous infusion site
    331–3
erythrocytes *see* red blood cells
Escherichia coli, antibiotic resistant 143
Essence of Care benchmarks 131, 573,
    853, 878–9
essential oils 1120
ethambutol 838
ethical issues
  cardiopulmonary resuscitation 219
  unconscious patients 1049
ethnic minorities, blind or partially
    sighted 73
Eton scale 411
European Association of Palliative Care
    (EAPC) 724
European Medicines Evaluation Agency
    (EMEA) 256
European Pressure Ulcer Advisory Panel
    (EPUAP) 1122, 1123
European Society of Hypertension 627
European Union (EU), CE mark *see* CE
    mark
evaluating care 42
evidence
  grading 19–20
  levels 20, **20**
  sources 17–18
evidence-based practice 16–19, 1168
  defined 16
  implementation 21
excreta
  barrier-nursed patients 137
  see also faeces; urine
exercise
  constipation management 413

pain management 732
  respiration during 636, 647
expert nurse 12
expert opinion 18
expiration *638*, 639, *639*
expiratory reserve volume (ERV) *640*,
    641
exposure-prone procedures (EPP) 161,
    162
  see also invasive procedures
extravasation 330–1
exudate, wound 1113
  assessment 1115
  chronic excessive **1100**
eye(s)
  anatomy and physiology *827*,
    827–30, *830*
  artificial 834, 884
  irrigation 833, 847–9, *849*
  opening, Glasgow coma scale 694–5,
    695
  swabbing 839–40, 970
  toxic effects of systemic drugs 837–8
eye care 826–52, 884
  comatose patient 838, 849–50, 884,
    1048, 1051
  general principles 830–1
  indications 826
  insensitive eye 834
  multiple choice questions 891, 1183
  procedure guidelines 839–50
eye drops
  contact lenses and 832–3
  instillation 831–2, 843–4, *844*
  storage 262
eye medications 834–7
eye ointments
  contact lenses and 832–3
  instillation 832, 845–6, *846*
  storage 262
eye protection (goggles)
  barrier nursing 129–30, 137
  operating theatre 800
eyelid closure, comatose patients 849–50

face masks *see* masks
faecal incontinence 880
faecal (stool) softeners **414**, 415

faeces (stools) 404
  assessment 406, *407*, 412
  leakage, stomas 453
  produced by stomas 440
  source barrier nursing 133, 137
  specimen collection 973
  see also defecation
fainting 479, 1073
family
  collusive behaviour 71–2
  communication 54
  deceased patients 528, 529, 536
  discharge planning and 236, 251–2
  stoma patients 442
  viewing body after removal from
    ward 537
  see also visitors
fasting, preoperative 785
fat
  dietary supplements 576
  emulsion, parenteral nutrition
    solutions 585
fatigue, positioning and 895
feeding, procedure guidelines 592–4
feet *see* foot
feline spongiform encephalopathy 1034
female patients
  midstream specimen of urine 968, 975
  urinary catheterization 460–1, 466–7,
    475–9
  urinary catheters 463
fentanyl (Durogesic) 735–6
  epidural/intrathecal 727, 757–9
  intravenous 725–6
  oral transmucosal 735–6
  transdermal patches 735, **736**
ferritin, serum **589**
fever 659–60
  transfusion reactions 1026, 1028,
    1040
  see also pyrexia
fibre, dietary 412–13
fibrillation, heart 615–16
fibrin sheath, causing occlusion 330
fibroblast growth factor 2 (FGF-2)
  1101, 1120
fibroblasts 1101–2
fibrosing alveolitis 640

finger massage, abnormal scars 1137
finger pricking, blood glucose
    monitoring 678, 681
fires, oxygen safety 940
fistulas, catheterized patients 485
Flamazine (silver sulphadiazine) 1135
flaps, surgical
  donor site problems 1135–6
  observation chart *1133–4*
flashback, venepuncture 1068
flatus (wind), bowel stoma patients 440,
    443
flossing, tooth 869
flowmeters 941
fluconazole 859–60, 861
fluid balance
  postanaesthetic recovery 806, *807*
  postoperative management 819
  unconscious patients 1049
fluid deficit *see* dehydration
fluid intake
  after lumbar puncture 561
  catheterized patients 486
  constipation management 413
  daily requirements 572–3, **573**
  urostomy 444
fluid overload *see* circulatory overload
fluids
  dying patients 278
  in hypovolaemia 214
  intravenous, safe administration
    284–5
  subcutaneous infusion 277–8
  see also body fluids; infusion fluids
fluoride 860, 862
5-fluorouracil (5-FU)
  prevention of oral complications 864
  skin complications 880
  toxic effects on eye 837
flushing
  after i.v. drug administration 289,
    322, 326–7
  enteral feeding tubes 599, 600
  occluded vascular access devices
    330
foam wound dressings **1109**
foamsticks 858, 867, 870
folate, serum **589**

Foley (balloon) catheters **461**, 461–2, *462*
  balloon deflation problems 486
  balloon size 461–2
  suprapubic catheterization 470
  see also urinary catheterization
food
  benchmarks 573, **574–5**
  charts 568–9
  disguising medication in 269–70
  hygiene 122, **123**
  oral drug administration and 294
  stoma patients 443–4
  see also diet; meals; nutrition
food-borne infections 122
  hepatitis A 155
  vancomycin-resistant enterococci 150
food poisoning 122
foot
  care 883
  venepuncture 1056
footwear
  barrier nursing 130
  operating theatre staff 800
  protective 94–5
forceps 91, 92
forearm
  blood pressure measurement 630
  veins for venepuncture 1056, *1057*
fractures, pathological 895
fresh frozen plasma (FFP) **1021**
FreshAire 451
friction 1122
5-FU *see* 5-fluorouracil
full blood count **589**
fully weight bearing (FWB) 906
Functional Health Patterns, Gordon's **30**, 30–1, **33–4**
functional residual capacity (FRC) *640*, 642, 946
funeral directors 537
fungal infections
  feet 883
  oral 859–60, 861
  specimen collection 966
fusidic acid, topical **1107**

gag reflex 701, 708
gargling medication 311
gas and air (Entonox) 729
gaseous exchange 642–4, *643*, **644**, 935, *936*
gastric contents
  aspiration *see* aspiration, gastric contents
  pH, enterally-fed patients 577–9, 596
gastric distension, during CPAP 947
gastrointestinal function, unconscious patients 1047
gastrostomy 579–80
gastrostomy buttons 579–80
gastrostomy tubes 579
  percutaneous endoscopically placed (PEG) 579, 580
  radiologically inserted (RIG) 579, 580
GCS *see* Glasgow Coma Scale
Gel-X capsules 450
Gelclair 862
gene therapy specimens 964
general anaesthesia *see* anaesthesia
general sales list (GSL) medicines 256
genitourinary function, unconscious patients 1047
gingivitis 572
Glasgow Coma Scale (GCS) 226, 694–8, 1046
  form 696
  procedure guidelines 705–6
  scoring **695**
glaucoma 828
glomerular filtration 667, *668*
glomerular filtration rate (GFR) 671
gloves 94
  barrier nursing 130, 137
  clean non-sterile (examination)
    indications for use 94, 98, 130
    procedure guidelines 107–8, *109*
  disposal of used 108
  materials 94
  operating theatre staff 800
  sterile
    aseptic technique 91, 101
    indications for use 94, 98, 130
  venepuncture 1063

gloving, double 130, 800
glucagon 675
glucose
  administration 676
  blood 673–82
    indications for measuring
      674
    monitoring 678–80
    parenteral nutrition **588**
    procedure guidelines 680–2
    see also hyperglycaemia;
      hypoglycaemia
  parenteral nutrition solutions 585
  in urine 676
glucose polymers
  dietary supplements 576
  enteral feeds 581–2
glutamine 582
gluteus muscle injections *280*, 281
glycerine-based hydrogel sheet 1138
glycerol (glycerin) suppositories 415,
  423
glyceryl trinitrate, to aid venous access
  1061
glycopeptide-resistant enterococci
  (GRE) *see* vancomycin-resistant
  enterococci
goggles *see* eye protection
goitre 572
Gordon's Functional Health Patterns *30*,
  30–1, **33–4**
gowns
  aseptic technique 94, 98
  barrier nursing 128–9, 136, 139
  operating theatre staff 800
graduated elastic compression stockings
  see antiembolic stockings
graft-versus-host disease (GVHD),
    transfusion-associated
    (TA-GVHD) 1031–2
Graftskin 1119
Gram-negative bacteria, antibiotic
    resistant 143–4
Gram-positive bacteria, antibiotic
    resistant 144–51
granulation tissue 1102
granulocyte colony-stimulating factor
    (G-CSF) 863–4

granulocyte macrophage
    colony-stimulating factor
    (GM-CSF) 863–4
granulocytes, apheresed **1020**
gravity drip rate controllers 360
gravity flow infusions 359–60
group protocols 270–1
  see also patient group directions
growth factors
  abnormal scarring 1137
  oral mucositis 863–4
  wound healing **1101**, 1102–3,
    1119–20

haematocrit, blood glucose testing and
    679
haematoma
  after venepuncture 1072–3
  epidural 763–4, 775
haematopoietic stem cell transplantation
    see stem cell transplantation
haematuria, bladder irrigation 390
haemodilution, acute normovolaemic
    (ANH) 1015
haemoglobin
  concentration 572
  oxygen transport *643*, 644–5, *937*,
    937–8
haemolytic disease of the newborn
    (HDN) 1017
haemolytic transfusion reactions
    1026–7, 1031
haemopneumothorax 501
haemorrhage *see* bleeding/haemorrhage
haemostasis 1099
haemothorax 501, 503–4
haemovigilance 1013–14
hair care 882–3
hair loss 883
hair removal, preoperative 784
hairdryers 883
halitosis 855
hand(s)
  Clostridium difficile spread
    154
  cuts and abrasions 103
  drying 91, 104
  MRSA transmission 146

spread of infection 89, 120
veins for venepuncture 1056, *1057*, 1058
hand washing 88–91, 120–1
after glove removal 108, 130
areas frequently missed 89, *89*
barrier nursing 135
compliance with 89, 90, 120
equipment and facilities 102
methods 89–90
MRSA control 146
operating theatre 106, 800
by patients 131
procedure guidelines 102–6
surgical procedures 106
handling, manual *see* manual handling
handover 46
handrubs, alcoholic *see* alcoholic handrubs
Hazard Analysis Critical Control Points (HACCP) 122
Hazardous Waste (England and Wales) Regulations 2005 132
HCAI *see* health care-acquired infections
head and neck tumours
enteral tube feeding *577*, *579*, *580*
swallowing difficulties 601
head coverings 129, 800
head injury 694, 703
head lice 883
head tilt/chin lift manoeuvre 208, *208*, 209, 222
headache
after inadvertent dural puncture 774
post-lumbar puncture *557*, 561, 562
healing, wound *see* wound healing
health and safety, occupational
diathermy smoke 798
hepatitis B 161, 162, 163
intravenous drug administration 286–7
MRSA 146
venepuncture 1063–4
see also inoculation accidents; personal protective equipment; violence

Health and Safety at Work, etc. Act 1974 1080
Health and Safety Executive (HSE), patient group directions 271, *272*
Health and Safety (Consultation with Employees) Regulations 1996 1081
health care-acquired infections (HCAI) 84–7, 118–23
consequences to patients 85, 87, 119
costs 84, 85, 86, 118
defined 84
diagnosis 87
prevention *see* barrier nursing; infection control
reservoirs 120
risk assessment 118–19
risk factors 85, 87–8, 118
routes of spread 88, 120–3
sites 84–5, 118
sources 119–20
health care assistants 14, 878
hearing, testing 709
hearing aids 73, 74, *795*
hearing-impaired patients, communication with 73–4
heart
apical beat assessment 616–18
conduction system *615*
rhythm 614–16
heart rate 612–14
factors affecting 613, *614*
see also pulse
heat and moisture exchanger (HM 949–50, **950**, *951*, 993
heat therapy
to aid venous access 1061, 1C
pain management 732–3
heel supports, during surgery 7
hemiplegic shoulder pain, prev 919
heparin 771
hepatitis 154–68
viruses **155**
hepatitis A 154–7, **155**
procedure guidelines 157
vaccine 156–7

hepatitis B **155**, 159–68
  death 163, 168
  prevention of spread 161–3
  procedure guidelines **164–8**
  screening 161
  transfusion-related 160, 1033
  transmission 159–60, 161
  vaccine 162–3
hepatitis B e antigen (HBeAg) 160, 161
hepatitis B immunoglobulin (HBIg)
    161–2
hepatitis B surface antigen (HBsAg) 160,
    161
hepatitis C **155**, 1033
hepatitis D **155**
hepatitis E **155**
hepatitis G **155**
...es, oral 861
...man lines (skin-tunnelled catheters),
    parenteral nutrition 585
...sm
    ...fices 540
    ...g and personal hygiene 882
    ...ream 1064
    ...999
    ...an immunodeficiency virus

    ...ng 583
    ...y **241**, 945
    ...ition 591
    ...re
    ...2

    ...ctions *see* health
    ...fections
    ...ouncil 539
    ...virus (HIV)

    ...HLA)

    ...in (HNIg)

    ...rus

procedure guidelines 953–4
tracheostomy/laryngectomy patients
    993, 1005
humidifiers
  cold water 950, **950**, *951*
  water bath **950**, 950–2, *951*
humidity 948–9
humour, using 730
Hyalofill 1119
hyaluronidase, subcutaneous fluid
    infusions 278
hydration
  in dysphagia 602
  terminally ill patients 278
  see also fluid intake
hydrocolloid wound dressings **1110**
hydrocortisone 221
hydrofibre wound dressings **1111**
Hydroframe 450
hydrogel-coated catheters 465
hydrogel wound dressings **1110**, 1114
hydrogen peroxide **1107**
hydromorphone 736
hygiene
  bed bathing *see* bed bathing
  food 122, **123**
  hospital 95
  personal *see* personal hygiene
  see also cleaning
hyperbaric oxygen therapy 1118
hypercapnia 932, 952
hyperglycaemia 676–8, 677
  parenteral nutrition 590
hyperkalaemia 214–15, 1031
hyperlipidaemia, blood glucose testing
    and 679
hyperpyrexia **661**
  malignant 816
hypertension 623–4
  blood pressure measurement 631
  postoperative 814
hyperthermia 659–61, **660**
  postoperative 816
hyperthyroidism 664
hypertonic fluid contraction 353, **354**
hypertrophic scars 1136–8
hyperventilation 647
  central neurogenic **702**

hypodermoclysis 277–8
hypoglycaemia 590, 675–6
hypokalaemia 214–15
hypophosphataemia 590
hypotension 623
　　blood pressure measurement 631
　　epidural/intrathecal analgesia 762,
　　　　773
　　orthostatic 623
　　postoperative 814
hypothalamus, thermoregulation 656,
　　658, 660
hypothermia 659
　　cardiopulmonary arrest 214
　　postoperative 811, 816
　　transfusion-associated 1029
hypothyroidism 664
hypotonic fluid contraction 353, **354**
hypoventilation, postoperative 813
hypovolaemia, cardiopulmonary arrest
　　213–14
hypoxaemia 932
hypoxia 645, 934, 938
　　cardiopulmonary arrest 212–13
　　tracheal suctioning-related 999
　　wound healing and 1100, 1102, 1118
hypoxic drive 636, 952

ibuprofen 728
identification, patient 14
　　blood transfusions 1024, 1037, 1039
　　dead body 532
　　surgery 795, 802
ileal–anal pouch 433
ileal conduits 434
　　postoperative function 441
　　urine specimen collection 454
　　see also urostomy
ileal loops 434
ileostomy 433–4, *434*
　　indications 435–6
　　postoperative care 441–2
　　postoperative function 440–1
　　pouches *446*, 447
　　problem solving 453–4
　　see also stoma(s)
immobility
　　bed rest 895–6

unconscious patients 1046–7
　　see also mobilization
immunocompromised patients 87–8
　　blood cultures 967
　　infection control 88
　　infection risks 85
　　intramuscular injections 281–2
　　microbiological specimen collection
　　　　960
　　oral complications 855
　　sources of infection 119–20
　　Staphylococcus epidermidis infections
　　　　149
　　temperature monitoring 664
　　wound infections 1112
immunoglobulin
　　human normal (HNIg) 156
　　intravenous, *Clostridium difficile*
　　　　infection 153
impartiality 1169
incidents (accidents)
　　inoculation *see* inoculation accidents
　　transfusion reactions and events
　　　　1013–14
　　violent *see* violence
　　see also errors; spillages
incompatibilities, drug 286, 287
incongruence 61, 62
incontinence
　　skin care 880
　　vancomycin-resistant enterococci 150
　　see also urinary incontinence
Incorrect Blood Component Transfused
　　(IBCT) 1025, 1026–7, 1031–2
indemnity insurance 1170
independent prescribing 271
individuals, treating people as 1165
indomethacin 838
infection control
　　aseptic technique 83–116
　　education 87
　　extra precautions 127, **128**
　　microbiological specimens 962
　　operating theatre 800–1
　　principles 87–96
　　rationale 84–7
　　standard precautions 127, **127**
　　see also barrier nursing

Infection Control Standards Working
Party 86
infections
  antimicrobial-resistant organisms
    142–51
  blood borne *see* blood borne
    infections
  blood pressure monitoring 631
  central venous catheter-related
    967–8
  complicating spinal analgesia 764–5,
    778
  endogenous (self-) 119
  exogenous (cross-infection) 120
  health and safety at work *see under*
    health and safety, occupational
  health care (hospital)-acquired *see*
    health care-acquired infections
  intravenous infusion-related 332
  isolation of sources *see* source
    isolation
  lumbar puncture site 552
  notification 133
  pulse monitoring 618
  reservoirs 120–3
  routes of spread 120–3
  sources 119–20
  specimen collection for
    microbiological analysis 960
  surgical risk categories **86**
  temperature monitoring 665
  tracheal suctioning-related 999
  transfusion-transmitted 160,
    1014–15, 1032–4
  venepuncture site 1073
  wound *see* wound infections
  see also sepsis
infectious diseases
  barrier nursing *see* barrier nursing
  isolation of patients with *see* source
    isolation
  last offices 529, 534
  purpose-built wards 125
  see also specific diseases
infiltration 330–1, 334
inflammation, wound 1112–13
inflammatory phase, wound healing
  1099–101

inflammatory reactions, pulse
  monitoring 618
information provision 57–9
  breaking bad news 72
  colleagues 1167
  at discharge 251–2
  procedure guidelines 57–8
  source barrier nursing 133–4
  see also communication; patient
    education
infusion(s) 275–89
  complications **348**, 352–5, **354**
    groups at risk **347**
  containers, height 351
  defined 275
  epidural/intrathecal analgesics
    759–61, **760**
  monitoring 368
  parenteral 265
  process of delivery 347
  routes of administration 275–89
  see also intravenous infusions;
    subcutaneous infusions
infusion devices 346–74
  ambulatory 363–7
  battery-operated 364–5
  decision tree for selecting 357
  defined 346
  factors affecting flow rates 350–2
  gravity 359–60
  indications 346–7
  mechanical 364
  MHRA classification **356**, 356–7
  monitoring 368
  multiple choice questions 374, 1178
  paediatric patients 355
  problem solving 369–71
  procedure guidelines 368
  requirements 357–9
  safe use 349, **350**, 367
  selection criteria 346–7, 348–9
  user errors 348–9, 367
  winged *see* winged infusion devices
  see also infusion pumps
infusion flow rates
  calculations 285–6, 359
  factors affecting 350–2
  slowing/stopping 328–31

infusion fluids
    addition of drugs to 285–6, 287
    effects on flow rate 350–1
    visual inspection 285
infusion pumps 360–7
    accuracy of delivery 357–8
    alarm systems 358, 361, 369–70
    ambulatory 363–7
    battery-operated 364–5
    MHRA categories **356**, 356–7
    occlusion response and pressure
        358–9
    parenteral nutrition 587
    problem solving 369–71
    specialist 362–3
    syringe *see* syringe pumps
    user errors 348–9
    volume calculations 286
    volumetric 360–1
inhalational analgesia (Entonox) 729
inhalations 265–6
    procedure guidelines 310–11
inhalers 266
injections 265, 275–89
    defined 275
    direct intermittent intravenous *see*
        intravenous injections, direct
        intermittent
    equipment 297
    multidose preparations 265, 300–2,
        303
    procedure guidelines 297–307, *303*
    routes of administration 275–89
    single-dose preparations 265,
        298–300
inoculation accidents 1073
    hepatitis B transmission 159, 161
    management guidelines 165
    prevention 164, 287
insect-borne infections 122–3
inspiration 637–8, *638*, *639*
inspiratory capacity (IC) *640*, 642
inspiratory reserve volume (IRV) *640*,
    641
Institute of Jainology 541
instruments, sterile 92
insulin
    blood glucose regulation 675

continuous subcutaneous infusion 278
deficiency 676–7, *677*
intravenous infusion 677–8
subcutaneous injection 276
insulin-like growth factor 1 (IGF-1)
    1101
insurance, indemnity 1170
integrity, personal 1169
interferon-α 163
intermediate care 244
intermittent catheterization catheters
    461
intermittent pneumatic compression
    786, 799
intermittent self-catheterization (ISC)
    471–2
International Association for the Study
    of Pain (IASP) 714–15
International Council of Nursing,
    definition of nursing 3
International Normalized Ratio (INR),
    parenteral nutrition **588**
interpersonal aspects of care 4
interpreters 68, 74
interviews, assessment 32–4, **33–4**
intra-arterial drug administration 275
intra-articular drug administration
    275
intra-operative cell salvage (ICS)
    1015–16
intracranial pressure (ICP), raised 552,
    614
    tracheal suctioning-induced 999
    vital signs 703
intradermal drug administration 276
intramuscular injections 279–83
    needles 282
    opioid analgesics 727
    pain 282–3
    procedure guidelines 305–7
    sites 279–81, *280*
    skin preparation 281–2
    technique 282–3
    Z-track technique 281
intraoperative care 797–804
    diathermy 797–8
    infection control and asepsis 800–1
    laparoscopic surgery 801

intraoperative care (*cont.*)
  multiple choice questions 824–5,
    1182–3
  patient positioning 798–800
  procedure guidelines 802–4
  see also operating theatre
intrapleural drainage 497–524
  changing bottle 515–16
  definitions 497
  indications 497, 500–2
  maintenance 505–6, 512–14
  multiple choice questions 524, 1180
  pain control 506–7
  problem solving 520–2
  procedure guidelines 508–19
  suction 507, 511–12
  systems 503–4, *504*, *505*
intrapleural drains (chest drains) 497,
  498
  clamping 503
  dressings for insertion site 506
  insertion procedure 508–11
  insertion site 502
  removal 507–8, 516–19
  securing 503
  size 502
  stripping/milking 503, 513
intrapleural pressure 500
intrathecal analgesia 740–1, 754–82
  advantages 754–5
  bolus injections 761
  chronic pain 740–1, 755
    changing exit site dressing 769–70
    pain assessment 763
    post-insertion monitoring 768
    problem solving 776–8
  complications 763–5, 774–6
  continuous infusion 759–61, **760**
  contraindications 755–6
  defined 754
  drug-related side-effects 761–2, 772–4
  drugs used 757–9
  indications 755
  monitoring 761, 768
  multiple choice questions 782, 1182
  pain assessment 762–3, 768–9
  problem solving 772–8
  procedure guidelines 765–72
  pump alarm 776
intrathecal catheter

  disconnection 777
  insertion, procedure guidelines 765–7
  migration 764, 775, 777
  occlusion 777
  optimal position 760, **760**
intrathecal drug administration 276,
  551
intrathecal (subarachnoid) space 552–3,
  756, 756–7
intravenous access *see* venous access
intravenous bolus injections 288–9
  procedure guidelines 323–7
intravenous drug administration 273–4,
  283–9
  acute/postoperative pain 725–6
  asepsis/prevention of infection 284–5
  calculations 285–6
  in chronic pain 724
  drug compatibilities 286, 287
  methods 287–9
  patient comfort 287
  principles 284–7
  pros and cons 283–4
  safety 285
intravenous fluids, safe administration
  284–5
intravenous infusions
  administration sets 284–5, 288
  blood pressure monitoring 631
  continuous 287–8
    parenteral nutrition 586
    procedure guidelines 313–17
  drug calculations 285–6
  drug injections into 287, 288–9,
    323–7
  flow rates
    calculations 285–6
    factors affecting 350–2
    slowing/stopping 328–31
  intermittent 288
    procedure guidelines 317–22
  postanaesthetic recovery 811
  problem solving 328–36
  reducing risk of infection 284–5
intravenous injections, direct
  intermittent 288–9
  problem solving 328–36
  procedure guidelines 323–7
intravenous push 288–9
  procedure guidelines 323–7

invasive procedures
  aseptic technique 84
  hepatitis B 167
IQRA Trust 543
iron
  overload 1031
  serum **589**
irritation, intravenous infusions
  331–2
ischaemia, pressure-induced 1122
Islam
  last offices 543
  washing and personal hygiene
    881–2
isolation *see* protective isolation; source
  isolation
isolation rooms 125–6
  cleaning 134, 139–40, 141
  entering 136–7
  leaving 139
  preparation 135–6
  transporting patients in/out 141
isolators, barrier nursing 125
isotonic fluid expansion 352–3, **354**
  see also circulatory overload
ispaghula husk 414–15

Jackson's silver tracheostomy tube 988,
  988
Jain Centre 541
Jainism, last offices 540–1
jaundice, blood glucose testing 679
Jehovah's Witnesses
  blood transfusion 1024–5
  last offices 541
jejunostomy feeding tubes 580
  procedure guidelines 597–8
jewellery
  deceased patients 532
  nursing staff 90–1, 103
  surgical patients 794
joint protection, neurological patients
  919
Judaism, last offices 525, 541–2

Kapitex Tracoetwist fenestrated
  tracheostomy tube *990*, 990–1
keloids 1136–8
keratinocyte growth factor (KGF) **1101**,
  1102

ketones 676–7
kidneys 667–9, *668*
Klebsiella pneumoniae, antibiotic
  resistant 143
knee-jerk reflex 708
knowledge, updating 1168
Korotkoff's sounds *625*, *628*,
  628–9
Kussmaul's respiration 647

labelling
  blood pack *1035*
  medicines 261
  microbiological specimens 963
laboratory specimen collection *see*
  specimen collection
lacrimal apparatus 830, *831*
lactic acid 934
lactulose 415
lamivudine 163
language
  nursing 38–9
  patients speaking different 68
laparoscopic surgery 801
large intestine 404
larval therapy 1107–12
laryngectomy 982–1012
  communication methods 995
  general nursing care 997–8
  humidification 993, 1005
  multiple choice questions 1011–12,
    1184
  stoma 983–4, 998
    button 992, *992*
    suctioning via 998–1000,
      1002–4
  swallowing difficulties 995–6
  total *983*, 983–4
  tubes 991–2, *992*
  see also tracheostomy
laryngotomy 984
last offices 525–50
  critical care patients 533–5
  different religious faiths 538–44
  equipment 527–8
  multiple choice questions 550, 1180
  problem solving 536–7
  procedure guidelines 527–33
  radioactive patients 536–7
  see also death

latex
 allergy 94, 465
  assessment 786–7, **787**
  management 787–8
 gloves 94
 urinary catheters 465
laundry *see* linen/laundry
laxatives **414**, 414–16
 abuse 411
 bulking agents **414**, 414–15
 opioid-treated patients 735
 osmotic agents **414**, 415–16
 stimulant **414**, 416
 stool softeners **414**, 415
laying out *see* last offices
LBF barrier film 448
Leeds Assessment of Neuropathic
  Symptoms and Signs (LANSS)
  721
left bundle branch *615*
leg *see* lower limb
leg drainage bags 469
leg straps, catheterized patients 469
legal aspects
 controlled drugs 257, **258–9**
 violence 1080–1, 1088, 1089
Legionnaire's disease 121
lethal response 353
leucoagglutination 1030
leucocytes *see* white blood cells
levomepromazine 279
liability, vicarious 1170
lice, head 883
lidocaine (lignocaine)
 cardiopulmonary resuscitation 216,
  221
 gel, urinary catheterization 467
 oral care 862
lifestyle changes, constipation
  412–13
light source, eye care 831
lignocaine *see* lidocaine
limb
 movements, intraoperative 798–9
 selection for venepuncture 1059
 see also lower limb; upper limb
Limone 451
linctuses 263

linen/laundry
 source barrier nursing 132–3, 138
 viral hepatitis infection 157, 164
lip reading 73–4, 994
lipid emulsions, changing administration
  sets 285
lips, dry 863, 870
liquid paraffin 415
listening 61–2
lithotomy position 798
liver function tests **588**
Lloyd Davies position 799
 antiembolic stockings and 786, 799
local anaesthesia
 postoperative blocks 729
 postoperative care 806
 see also topical anaesthesia
local anaesthetic agents
 epidural/intrathecal 759, 760
 eye 832, 836
 side effects 762, 772–4
long-chain triglycerides (LCT) 576,
  581
long lines (peripherally inserted central
  catheters), parenteral nutrition
  585
loop of Henle 669
loperamide 408
lower limb
 amputees 924, 925
 blood pressure measurement 630
 veins for venepuncture 1056
lozenges 263
LP *see* lumbar puncture
lubricating gels, urinary catheterization
  466–7
lumbar puncture 551–66
 anatomy 552–4, *553*, *554*
 complications 557
 contraindications 552
 defined 551
 indications 551
 leakage from site 561, 562
 multiple choice questions 565–6,
  1180–1
 nurse's role 557
 problem solving 562
 procedure guidelines 558–61, *561*

lung
  compliance and elasticity 640–1
  defence mechanisms 645
  gaseous exchange 642–4, *643*, **644**
  infections, health care acquired 118
lung volumes 641–2
  measurement 639, *640*
lying position *see* side lying position;
      supine position
lymphocytes
  count, total 572
  in CSF 556
lymphoedema, blood pressure
      measurement 630

macrophages 1099–100, 1101,
      1102
maggots 1107–12
magnesium
  deficiency 572
  plasma **588**
magnesium salts, laxative 415–16
magnesium sulphate 217, 221
malabsorption 576, 582
malaria 1033
male patients
  facial shaving 886
  midstream specimen of urine 974
  penile sheaths 487–90
  urinary catheterization 460, 466,
      472–5
malignant hyperpyrexia 816
malnutrition
  assessment 568–72
  biochemical investigations 571–2
  poor wound healing 1105
  postoperative prevention 819
  refeeding syndrome 590, **590**
  screening 568
  venepuncture 1059
malnutrition universal screening tool
      (MUST) 568
malodour *see* odour
Management of Health and Safety at
      Work Regulations (MHSWR)
      1081
mandelic acid solutions 376, 379
manual handling 893

surgical patients 799–800
  see also positioning; transfers
masks
  aseptic technique 94
  barrier nursing 129, 137
  grading 129
  MRSA control 148
  operating theatre 800
  oxygen *see* oxygen masks
  ventilation, CPR 209
massage, abnormal scars 1137
Matron Charter 131
mattresses, pressure-relieving 1129–31,
      1130
McGill Pain Questionnaire (MPQ) 721
meals
  barrier nursing 137
  oral drug administration and 294
  see also feeding; food
mean arterial pressure (MAP) 624
mean cell volume **589**
meatus, urinary *see* urethral meatus
mechanical irritation, intravenous
      infusions 332
mechanical ventilation 947–8
median cubital vein 1056, *1057*
medical devices, CE mark 92
Medical Devices Agency (MDA) *see*
      Medicines and Health Care
      Products Regulatory Agency
medicinal products, defined 255
medicines
  addition to intravenous fluids/diluents
      286, 287, 288–9
  administration *see* drug
      administration
  combinations, subcutaneous infusions
      278
  compatibilities 286, 287
  containers 261–2
  defined 266
  disposal of unused 132, 260
  formulations 262–6
  general sales list (GSL) 256
  labelling 261
  legislation 256–61
  mixtures 262, 264
  off label 256–7

medicines (*cont.*)
patient's own 262, 268–9
pharmacy (P) 256
prescription only (POM) 256
reconstitution of powders 299–302, *303*
stability 262
stock control 262
storage 261–2
unlicensed 256–7
venepuncture and 1059–60
Medicines Act 1968 256, 270
Medicines and Health Care Products Regulatory Agency (MHRA) (formerly Medical Devices Agency) 256
blood transfusion practice 1013–14
classification of infusion devices **356,** 356–7
mercury sphygmomanometers 625
safe use of infusion devices 349, **350**
thermometers 663
medium-chain triglycerides (MCT) 576, 581
meningitis, complicating spinal analgesia 764–5
menstruation, surgical patients 793, 801
mental illness, and violence 1083
mercury
sphygmomanometers 625–6
thermometers 663
metabolic disorders, cardiopulmonary arrest 214–15
metacarpal veins 1056, *1057,* 1058
methadone 736–7
methicillin *see* meticillin
methotrexate 557, 837
meticillin-resistant *Staphylococcus aureus* (MRSA) 85, 143, 144–8
community care 148
epidemic (EMRSA) 144
eradication therapy 145
isolation of infected patients 124, 125
psychological effects 134
risk assessment 148
risk factors 145, 148
screening 145–6
transmission 146–8

meticillin-sensitive *Staphylococcus aureus* (MSSA) 144
metronidazole, topical **1107**
MHRA *see* Medicines and Health Care Products Regulatory Agency
microbiological specimen collection *see* specimen collection
microbore infusion sets 351
midstream specimen of urine (MSU) 968, 974–5
minerals
dietary requirements 573
parenteral nutrition solutions 586
serum levels 572
supplements 577
mini assessment **31**
mini-tracheostomy 984
minute ventilation (MV) 639
miotics 835, *836*
Misuse of Drugs Act 1971 257–61
mixtures of medicines 262, 264
mobility
nutritional status and 571
see also immobility
mobilization 901–12
amputees 924
from lying to sitting 902–3, *903*
patients on bed rest 896
positioning in chair 904
postoperative 818
from sitting to standing 905, *906*
walking 906–12
see also transfers
modified-release tablets 263
moisturizers 881
monocytes, in CSF 556
mood, in undernutrition 571
Morform sachet 450
Mormons, last offices 542
morphine
acute/postoperative pain 725–6, 727
breakthrough pain 734–5, 738
chronic pain 734–5
conversion to fentanyl **736**
safer practice guidance 260–1
motor blockade, epidural/intrathecal analgesia 762, 773
motor control 902

motor function, assessment 700–1, 707–8
motor response, Glasgow coma scale **695**, 697–8
mouth 853–4
  dry *see* dry mouth
  painful/sore **578**, 862
mouth care 853–76
  advances 863–5
  agents 858–60
  defined 853
  equipment 857–8
  frequency 857
  multiple choice questions 891–2, 1183
  oral problems 861–3
  problem solving 869–70
  procedure guidelines 866–9
  unconscious patients 1048, 1051
mouth-to-face mask ventilation 209
mouth-to-mouth ventilation 208–9, *210*
mouthwashes 859, 860, 862
movements, abnormal 701
  positioning neurological patients with 919–22, *921*
MRSA *see* meticillin-resistant *Staphylococcus aureus*
MSU (midstream specimen of urine) 968, 974–5
mucositis, oral *see* oral mucositis
mucous membranes
  hepatitis B exposure 159, 161
  mouth 854
multidisciplinary approach
  discharge planning 238–40, **239**, **241–3**, 247–9
  home enteral feeding 583
  nutritional support 591
mupirocin cream 145, **1107**
muscle
  atrophy, unconscious patients 1047
  co-ordination testing 700, 708
  weakness, assessment 707
muscle strength 700
  testing 707
  unconscious patients 1047
muscle tone
  defined 919

positioning patients with abnormal 919–22, *921*
  testing 700, 707
music, for pain management 730
Muslims
  last offices 543
  washing and personal hygiene 881–2
mycosis 966
mydriatics 835, *835*
myelography 551
myofibroblasts 1102

nail bed pressure, neurological assessment 698
nail brushes 104
nail varnish/polish 103
nails 103
  artificial 91, 103
  care 883, 887
nalidixic acid **674**
naloxone 221, 261, 813
name (wrist) bands 14
  see also identification, patient
nasal analgesia 737
nasal cannulae, oxygen via *941*, 941–2
  oxygen flow rates **942**
  problem solving 954–5
nasal care 883–4
nasal drops, procedure guidelines 311–12
nasoduodenal feeding 577–9
nasogastric feeding 577–9
nasogastric tubes
  checking position 577–9, 596–7
  enteral feeding 577–9
  insertion without an introducer 594–7
  see also enteral feeding tubes; Ryle's tube
nasojejunal feeding 577–9
National Cancer Institute Common Toxicity Criteria (NCI-CTC) 856, 857
National Collaborating Centre for Acute Care, parenteral nutrition 583, 585, 586, **587**, **588–9**, 590
National Council of Hindu Temples 540

National Health Service (NHS)
Continuing Healthcare 245
health care-acquired infections 118
isolation facilities 124
management of violence 1079–80,
1081
Security Management Service 1080,
1081
National Institute for Health and
Clinical Excellence (NICE) 16
on communication 55, 56, 68
pressure ulcer guidance 1122–3,
1129–31
violence guideline 1080, 1081–2,
1086, 1090–2
wound management guidance
1107–12
National Patient Safety Agency (NPSA)
14, 260–1, 577–9
National Prescribing Centre (NPC)
273
National Service Framework for Older
People
discharge planning 232, 244
self-administration of medicines 268
National Spiritual Assembly of the
Bahais of the United Kingdom
538
Naturcare 451
nausea and vomiting
dietary advice **578**
enterally fed patients **584**
opioid-induced 762, 774
postanaesthetic control 806, *807*, 815
source barrier nursing 133
nebulization 266
necrotic tissue, debridement 1106–12
needle sampling port, urinary catheter
system 480, *481*
needleless injection systems 320
needleless sampling port, urinary
catheter system 480
needles
disposal of used 1063–4
injections 297
intramuscular injections 282
removal from vein 1064, 1069
venepuncture 1061, **1062**

needlestick injuries *see* inoculation
accidents
needs, patient 37
negative pressure therapy *see* topical
negative pressure therapy
Negus's silver tracheostomy tube *988*,
989
nelaton catheters **461**, *462*, 471–2
neonates
haemolytic disease 1017
infusions 355, **356**
oxygen toxicity 838
thermoregulation 659
nephron *668*
nerve blocks 740–1
nerve growth factor (NGF) **1101**
nerve injuries, complicating
venepuncture 1071
neurological disorders
positioning 916–23
abnormal tone and movement
patterns 919–22, *921*
environmental aspects 922–3
joint protection 919
soft tissue changes and contractures
922
rehabilitation 923
spinal analgesia 756
swallowing difficulties 601, 603
violence and 1083
neurological observations (and
assessment) 692–713
after lumbar puncture 561, 562
consciousness 693–8
emergency 710
frequency 703–4, **704**
general points 704
indications 692
motor function 700–1
multiple choice questions 712–13,
1182
procedure guidelines 705–10
pupillary activity 698–700
sensory function 701
unconscious patients 1051
visual acuity/visual fields 704, **704**
vital signs 701–3
neuromuscular blockade, persistent 813

neuropathic pain 721, 734
neutropenia
    blood pressure monitoring 631
    health care-acquired infections 85,
        118
    sources of infection 119–20
    temperature monitoring 664
neutrophils 1099–100
NHS *see* National Health Service
The NHS Plan (2000), discharge
    planning 244
NICE *see* National Institute for Health
    and Clinical Excellence
nil by mouth, preoperative 785
nitrogen
    dietary requirements 572–3, **573**
    parenteral nutrition solutions 585
    partial pressure 934
nitrous oxide and oxygen 729
NMC *see* Nursing and Midwifery
    Council
Nodor S drops 451
non-invasive ventilation 947
non-steroidal anti-inflammatory drugs
    (NSAIDs) **724**, 728, 733
non-touch technique 83, 91
non-verbal communication 62–3
non-verbal cues 59, 61
noradrenaline 675
normal saline *see* sodium chloride, 0.9%
    solution
Norton scale 1123–4, **1124**
nose care 883–4
nose swab 970, *970*
Nosocomial Infection National
    Surveillance Service (NINSS) 86
nosocomial infections *see* health
    care-acquired infections
notification of infections 133
novice nurses 10
Novogel 1138
NSAIDs *see* non-steroidal
    anti-inflammatory drugs
nurse consultants 13
nurse practitioners 13
nurse prescribing 270–3
    evaluation **274**
nurses

blocking behaviour 67–8
    psychological support 67
nursing
    context 3–22
    defined 3
    language 38–9
    patients' perspective 3–12
    practice guidance/recommendations
        44–5
    requirements of organizations 12–16
Nursing and Midwifery Council (NMC)
    Code 5, 10, 1088, 1121, 1163–70
    consent guidance 6
    consultation on advanced practice 13
    dealing with violence guidance 1079
    drug administration guidance 267–8,
        269–70, 274, 275, 289
    nurse prescribing 271, 273
nursing assessment *see* assessment
nursing care *see* care
nursing diagnosis *see* diagnosis, nursing
nursing homes, discharge to 244–5
nursing models 29–30, 878
nutrients
    deficiencies 571
    intake, assessment 568–9
nutrition
    assessment of status 568–72
    benchmarks 573, **574–5**
    laryngectomy patients 995–6
    oral complications and 865
    screening 568
    subjective global assessment (SGA)
        568, 571
    wound healing and 1104–5
    see also diet; food; malnutrition
nutritional requirements **573**
    calculation 572–3
    causes of increased 568
nutritional support 567–610
    defined 567
    in dysphagia 603
    indications 567–8
    multidisciplinary team 591
    multiple choice questions 609–10,
        1181
    planning 573
    problem solving 601–4

nutritional support (*cont.*)
   procedure guidelines 591–600
   unconscious patients 1047
   see also dietary supplements; enteral
      tube feeding; parenteral nutrition
nystatin 859, 861

obesity, nutritional assessment 569
observations 611–91
   blood glucose 673–82
   blood pressure 620–34
   multiple choice questions 689–91,
      1181–2
   neurological *see* neurological
      observations
   peak flow 652–5
   pulse 611–19
   respiration 635–51
   temperature 656–66
   urinalysis 667–72
   see also vital signs
occupational health and safety *see*
      health and safety, occupational
occupational therapy, discharge
      planning 247
octreotide 408
oculocephalic reflex 701
odour
   oral (halitosis) 855
   stomas 444, 446, 454
   urine 669, **673**
oedema
   intravenous infusion/injection-related
      333–4
   nutritional assessment 569, 571
   see also lymphoedema
oesophageal speech 995
oesophageal tumours
   enteral tube feeding 577, 580
   swallowing difficulties 602
ointments 264
   eye *see* eye ointments
older people *see* elderly
oliguria, postoperative 816
Omaha nursing classification system
      41
omega-3 fatty acids 582
Omnopon 727

operating room (OR) *see* operating
      theatre
operating theatre 797–804
   hand washing 106, 800
   infection control and asepsis 800–1
   patient transfers 796
   procedure guidelines 802–4
   see also intraoperative care;
      postanaesthetic recovery room
opioid analgesics
   acute pain 725
   chronic pain 734–8
   driving and 740
   epidural/intrathecal 726–7, 757–9
   intramuscular injections 727
   intravenous 725–6
   mild to moderate pain 734
   moderate to severe pain 734–8
   nasal 737
   oral 727
   oral mucositis pain 862
   in renal failure 739
   side effects 735, 761–2, 772–4
   subcutaneous 727
   transdermal patches 735, 738
optic nerve 828
OR *see* operating theatre
Orabase paste 449
Orahesive powder 449
oral assessment **856**, 856–7
Oral Assessment Guide (OAG) 856
oral cavity *see* mouth
oral complications 854–5
   nutrition and 865
   prophylaxis and treatment 861–3
oral contraceptives 838
oral drug administration
   acute/postoperative pain 727
   chronic pain 724
   formulations 262–4
   procedure guidelines 292–6
oral hygiene *see* mouth care
oral infections 855, 861–2
oral mucosa 854
oral mucositis 854–5
   prevention 859, 860
   treatment 860, 862
Oral Mucositis Index (OMI) 856

oral temperature 661–2
Oramorph 727, 734
  see also morphine
orientation, evaluation of **695**, 697, 705
orthopnoea 647
Ostobon deodorant powder 451
Ostoclear sachets or spray 450
Ostofix tape 450
OstoSorb gel 450
outcomes, patient **40**, 40–1
overinfusion 348, 352–3
  complications **348**
  problem solving 334, 371
  see also circulatory overload
overshoes, barrier nursing 130
oxycodone
  acute/postoperative pain 727
  chronic pain 734, 737
oxygen
  consumption 938–9
  eye toxicity 838
  liquid 945
  pulmonary exchange 642–4, **644**, 935, *936*
  supply 941
  toxicity 952
  transportation *643*, 644–5, 934, 937–8
  uptake 934–5, **935**
  utilization 934, 938
  see also hypoxia
oxygen condensers (concentrators) 945
oxygen cylinders 940, 941, 945
oxygen masks
  fixed performance/high-flow (Venturi-type) 942–4, *944*, **944**
  problem solving 954–5
  simple semi-rigid plastic 942, **943**, *943*
  tracheostomy 944
oxygen partial pressure (PO_2) 934–5
  in blood (PaO_2) 644, 937, 938
oxygen saturation (SaO_2) 648, 937
  factors affecting *937*, 937–8
  measurement 939
  monitoring 648–9, 650–1, *651*
  PaO_2 and 938
oxygen therapy 940–5

delivery systems 941–5
equipment 941
hazards 952
home (domiciliary) **241**, 945
humidification 949, 1005
hyperbaric 1118
nasal cannulae catheters *941*, 941–2, **942**
nasal care 884
oral care 857
postanaesthetic recovery 808, 810, 813
problem solving 954–5
safety measures 940, 955
T-piece circuit 945
oxygenation
  adequacy, during respiratory therapy 954
  cellular 934
  positioning to maximize 913, *913*
  tissue 934
oxyhaemoglobin dissociation curve *937*, 937–8

paediatric patients
  blood pressure measurement 630
  enteral feeds 582
  infusion devices 355
  nutritional assessment 569
  nutritional requirements 573
  oral drug administration 295
  pulse measurement 619
  urinary catheters 461–2, 463
  venepuncture 1059
  see also neonates
pain
  acute *see* acute pain
  during bladder lavage/irrigation 392–3
  breakthrough 715, 738
  cancer *see* cancer pain
  chronic *see* chronic pain
  defined 714
  evoked 721
  incident 739
  intensity 716–17
  intramuscular injections 282–3
  intrapleural drainage 506

infusion site 335
6
ncture 562
neuropathic 721, 734
positioning and 895
postoperative *see* postoperative pain
skin graft donor sites 1135
spontaneous 721, 739
total, concept of 717
during venepuncture 1071
pain assessment 715–21
chronic/cancer pain 717, **718**, 722,
743–4
epidural/intrathecal analgesia 762–3,
768–9
multiple choice questions 752–3, 1182
procedure guidelines 741–4
RMH patient held pain chart 719–21,
722, 743–4
surgical patients 715–17, 741–2,
819–20
tools 718–21, 720, 722
pain management 721–41
acute pain 725–33
anaesthetic interventions 740–1
chronic pain 723, 723–4, 733–41
multiple choice questions 752–3, 1182
need for effective 721
non-pharmacological measures
729–33
postanaesthetic recovery 806, 807
postoperative pain 724–33, 820
preoperative preparation 741–2
principles 725
see also analgesia
painful stimuli, response to, Glasgow
Coma Scale 697–8
palifermin 864–5
Palladone 736
palliative care
nutritional assessment 569–70
urgent discharge home 236, 237–8
see also terminal care
palmar-plantar erythrodysesthesia
syndrome 880
palpation, veins 1059
panic attacks 69–70

paper towels 91, 104
dispensers 91, 102
disposal of used 104
paracetamol 728, 733
combination preparations 728
mouthwash 862
paraphimosis, catheterized patients 485
paraphrasing 64
parasites 1033
parasympathetic nervous system 613,
614
parenteral infusions 265
parenteral nutrition (PN) 583–91
changing administration sets 285, 586
choice of regimen 586
delivery and management 586–7
home 591
indications 567–8, 583
metabolic complications 587–90,
588–9
monitoring 587, **587**, **588–9**
route of administration 585
solutions 585–6
termination 590
Parsees, last offices 544
partial pressure (P) 934–5
partially sighted patients,
communication with 72–3
partially weight bearing (PWB) 906
particle embolism, intravenous
procedures 336
Passy Muir speaking valve 989
pastilles 263
patient-controlled analgesia (PCA) 726
epidural (PCEA) 761
postoperative pain 784
pumps 362–3
patient education
hepatitis A 157
hepatitis B carriers 163
as pain control measure 730
preoperative 741–2, 784
stomas 436–7, 439–40, 443
see also information provision
Patient-Generated Subjective Global
Assessment 571
patient group directions (PGD) 270–3
defined 271

flowchart 272
off label medicines 257
unlicensed medicines 257
patient hygiene *see* personal hygiene
patient problems 37
patients
  expectations 3–4
  identification *see* identification,
    patient
  involvement 18
  own drugs 262
  perspective of nursing 3–12
  positioning *see* positioning
  problems/needs 37
  providing information to *see*
    information provision
  safety 14–16
  self-administration of medicines
    268–9, 290–2
  as sources of evidence 18, 20
  tampering with infusion devices
    352
peak flow (peak expiratory flow rate,
    PEFR) 652–5
  factors affecting 652–4
  normal values 653
  procedure guidelines 654–5, 655
  timing of readings 652
PEG enteral feeding tubes 579,
    580
penile pain on erection, catheterized
    patients 485
penile sheaths 487–90
  procedure guidelines 488–90
penile swabs 971
Penrose drain, shortening 1147
percutaneously endoscopically placed
    gastrostomy (PEG) tubes 579,
    580
perianal area, hygiene/care 409, 882
perinatal transmission, viral hepatitis
    156, 160
perineal care 882
periodontitis 863
perioperative care 783–825
  defined 783
  multiple choice questions 824–5,
    1182–3

see also intraoperative care;
    postoperative care; preoperative
    care
peripheral resistance 620
peripheral vascular access devices
  occlusion 330
  parenteral nutrition 585
  venepuncture 1061, **1062**
peripherally inserted central catheters
    (PICCs), parenteral nutrition 585
peristalsis 404
personal hygiene 877–92
  aseptic technique 95–6
  barrier nursing 131–2
  bed bathing *see* bed bathing
  defined 877
  eye care 826–52
  hepatitis A 157
  mouth care 853–76
  multiple choice questions 891–2, 1183
  oxygen therapy and 955
  procedure guidelines 885–8
  skin care 879–82
  unconscious patients 1049
personal protective equipment (PPE)
    93–5
  barrier nursing 127–30, 136–7
  last offices 529
  operating theatre 800
  see also aprons, plastic; eye
    protection; gloves; protective
    clothing
*Personal Protective Equipment at Work
    Regulations* 93
pessaries, vaginal 264
  procedure guidelines 307–9
pest control 122–3
pethidine 727
PGD *see* patient group directions
pH
  blood 644
  gastric contents, enterally-fed patients
    577–9, 596
  urine *see under* urine
pharmacists, covert drug administration
    and 270
pharmacy (P) medicines 256
phase angle 570

phenazopyridine (pyridium) **674**
phlebitis
    intravenous infusion-related 331
    VIP scale *337*
phosphate
    enemas 417–18
    plasma **588**
physical activity *see* exercise
physical restraint 1087–8
physiotherapist 907
physiotherapy, patients on bed rest 896
pia mater 756, *756*
pilocarpine 864
pituitary gland tumours 828
planning
    care 39–41, **43–4**
    nutritional support 573
plantar reflexes 701
plasma
    cryo-depleted **1023**
    fresh frozen (FFP) **1021**
    oxygen transport 937
    proteins 571–2
Plasmodium falciparum 1033
plastic catheters 465
plastic surgery wounds 1131–6
    assessment 1132
    associated problems 1132–6
platelet derived growth factor (PDGF)
        1101, **1101**, 1119–20
platelets
    transfusion **1020**
    wound healing 1099
pleura 498–9, *499*
pleural effusion 500–1
    drainage 501, 502, 503–4
pleural space 499–500
pleurisy 639
plugholes, hand basin 103, 105
plugs, colostomy 440, 447
pneumatic compression, intermittent
        787, 799
pneumococcus *(Streptococcus
        pneumoniae)* 149
pneumonia
    health care acquired 118
    prevention, unconscious patients 1050
    see also respiratory tract infections

pneumothorax 497, 500, 520, 639
    intrapleural drainage 502, 503–4, 507
    spontaneous 500
    tension 215, 500, 520
point-of-care testing (POCT) 678–9
poisoning, cardiopulmonary arrest
        215–16
police 1087
polydipsia 676
polymorphonuclear leucocytes
        1099–100
polytetrafluoroethylene (PTFE)-coated
        catheters 465
polyurethane tubes, enteral feeding 579
polyuria 676
polyvinylchloride (PVC)
    catheters 465
    tubes, enteral feeding 579
Portex cuffed tracheostomy tube *985*,
        985–6
positioning 893–931
    amputees 923–5
    assisting patients to move 901–12
    in bed 896–901, *899*, *901*
    in cardiorespiratory compromise
        915–16
    defined 893
    eye care 830
    infusion flow rate and 351
    intraoperative 798–800
    intrapleural drain insertion 509
    lumbar puncture 558, *561*
    medical considerations 895–6
    multiple choice questions 930–1, 1183
    in neurological impairment 916–23
    postoperative period 817
    pressure ulcer prevention 1129
    principles 894–5
    pulse rate and 612–13
    unconscious patients 1050–1
    see also manual handling
post-mortem examination 531, 534, 536
postanaesthetic recovery 804–16
    assessment for discharge 805–6, *807*
    defined 804
    local and regional anaesthesia 806
    problem solving 812–16
    procedure guidelines 808–12

postanaesthetic recovery room 805
  equipment 805, 808
  handover to 804
posterior popliteal artery, blood pressure
  measurement 630
postoperative care 804–20
  blood pressure measurement 631
  multiple choice questions 824–5,
    1182–3
  plastic surgery 1132–6, *1133–4*
  procedure guidelines 817–20
  pulse monitoring 618
  respiratory monitoring 648
  stomas 441–2
  temperature monitoring 664
  total laryngectomy 997–8
  tracheostomy 996–7
  see also postanaesthetic recovery
postoperative complications
  prevention on ward 817–20
  recovery room 805, 812–16
Postoperative Observation and Pain
  Assessment Chart 719–21, *720*
postoperative pain
  assessment 715–17, *720*, 819–20
  epidural analgesia 755, 761, 763
  management 724–33, 817, 820
  need for effective control 721
  patient education and 741–2, 784
  postanaesthetic recovery 815
  see also acute pain
postural alignment 902
potassium chloride 221
powder, reconstitution for injection
  299–302, *303*
preadmission clinics, discharge planning
  232, 246–7
prealbumin 572
precordial thump 206, 222
prednisolone enema 418
pregnancy
  preoperative checks 793
  see also perinatal transmission
premedication 796
preoperative autologous donation (PAD)
  1015
preoperative care 783–96
  defined 783

fasting 785
latex allergy 786–8
multiple choice questions 824–5,
  1182–3
objectives 783–4
patient education and pain control
  741–2, 784
procedure guidelines 793–6
skin preparation 784
stoma creation 436–9
thromboprophylaxis 785–6,
  788–92
prescribing
  independent 271
  nurse 270–3, **274**
  supplementary 273
prescription only medicines (POM)
  256
prescriptions
  controlled drugs 257, **259**
  drug administration without 267
pressure
  effects on tissues 1121–2
  treatment, abnormal scars 1137
pressure area care 1129
  positioning and 895
  unconscious patients 1051
  see also skin care
pressure-relieving devices 1129–31,
  1130
  during surgery 799
pressure ulcers (sores) 1120–31
  aetiology 1121–2
  assessment tools 1123–4
  defined 1120–1
  grades 1123
  identifying at-risk patients 1122–3
  prevalence 1121
  treatment and prevention 1129
  unconscious patients 1048
  undernourished patients 571
primary health care team, discharge
  planning 234, **241–3**
prion diseases 1034
Prisma 1119, 1120
privacy 877
probenecid **674**
probiotics 153

procedures
  consent to 6–9, **8**
  invasive *see* invasive procedures
  providing information on 57–9
professional boundaries, maintaining 1166
professional reputation, upholding 1169
proficient nurses 11
proflavin cream **1107**
Promogran 1119, 1120
proprioception, testing 709
prostaglandins 660
prostatic surgery, bladder irrigation after 376–7, 381
proteases 1119, 1120
protective clothing 93–5
  intravenous drug administration 286
  source barrier nursing 127–30
  see also personal protective equipment
protective isolation 117, 124
protein, dietary
  requirements 572–3, **573**
  supplements 576
proteins
  CSF 556
  plasma 571–2
Proteus mirabilis
  antibiotic resistant 143
  catheter encrustation and 378–9
protozoa 966
pruritus, opioid-induced 762, 774
pseudomembranous colitis 152, 153
Pseudomonas (aeruginosa) 1135
  antibiotic resistant 143–4
  urine of catheterized patients 379
psychological disorders 69–70
psychological implications
  source isolation 119, 133–4
  stoma surgery 444–5
psychological interventions, pain management 729–31
psychological support 60, 69–70
  after violent incidents 1089
  communication issues 55, 56
  for nursing staff 67
psychosocial factors
  acute pain 715
  chronic pain 717, **718**

pulmonary embolism (PE)
  cardiopulmonary arrest 215
  postoperative care 818
  prophylaxis *see* thromboprophylaxis
  risk factors 785, 788–9
  signs 792
pulmonary oedema, re-expansion 501
pulse 611–19
  amplitude 616
  assessing gross irregularity 616–18
  defined 611
  indications 611
  neurological patients 703, 707
  palpation sites 611, *612*
  paradoxical 616
  postanaesthetic recovery 810
  postoperative monitoring 817
  procedure guidelines 618–19, *619*
  rate 612–14, **613**, *614*
  rhythm 614–16
pulse oximetry 648–9, 939
  postanaesthetic recovery 808
  procedure guidelines 650–1, *651*
pulseless electrical activity (PEA) 205, 213, 216–17
pupils, examination 698–700, **699**, 706
purgatives 414
Purkinje fibres *615*
pus, specimen collection 962
pyrexia 659–61, 665
  grades **661**
  intravenous procedure-related 335
  time for recording 663
  see also fever

quality assurance, point-of-care testing (POCT) 678–9
quality improvement 15
questioning 63–4
questions, open and closed 63–4

radial artery, pulse 611, *619*
radioactive contamination, deceased patients 536–7
radiologically inserted gastrostomy (RIG) tubes 579, 580
radiotherapy
  for cancer pain management 739–40

oral complications 854–5
skin reactions 880
tracheostomy and 986
randomized controlled trials (RCTs) 19,
20, **20**
Rastafarians, last offices 543
RCN *see* Royal College of Nursing
reagent sticks (dipsticks), urine 671–2,
672, **674**
reconstitution, powders for injection
299–302, *303*
reconstructive surgery *see* plastic surgery
records *see* documentation
recovery
postanaesthetic *see* postanaesthetic
recovery
postoperative 817–20
recovery position 208, *209*
rectal drug administration 422–5
procedure guidelines **424–5**
see also enemas; suppositories
rectal drug preparations 264
rectal examination, digital (DRE)
412
rectal swabs 971
rectal temperature 662
rectum 404
rectus femoris injections *280*, 281
rectus sheath, stoma siting 439, *439*
red blood cells
in CSF 556
frozen **1019**
in SAGM **1019**
for transfusion **1019**
washed **1019**
Redivac drainage system, dressing
1143–4
refeeding syndrome 590, **590**
reference nutrient intake (RNI) 573
referrals, discharge planning 247–9
reflecting back 64
reflexes 700–1, 708
primitive developmental 918
Reform Synagogues of Great Britain 542
refrigeration, food **123**
refusals
respect for 59
to take medication 269–70

regional anaesthesia, postoperative care
806, 812
regional nerve blocks 740–1
rehabilitation
neurological patients 923
see also mobilization
relatives *see* family
relaxation techniques, pain control 730,
731
religious practices
last offices 526–7, 538–44
personal hygiene 877, 881–2
renal clearance 671
renal function
opioid analgesia and 739
parenteral nutrition **588**, 590
tests 671
renin 622
Reporting of Injuries, Diseases and
Dangerous Occurrences
Regulations 1995 1081
research evidence 17–18, 20
residential care homes
discharge to 244–5
MRSA control 148
residual volume *640*, 641
resistance
airway 641
to blood flow 620, *621*
respiration 635–51
control 636, *637*
defined 635
depth 647
external 933
gas transport *643*, 644–5,
933
history taking **646**
internal (cellular) 635, *643*, 645,
933
pattern 647–8, 702, **702**
physiology 933–9
see also breathing
respiratory assessment 939–40
respiratory capacities 642
respiratory centre 636
respiratory depression
opioid-induced 761, 772
postoperative 813

respiratory disease
  lung compliance 640
  non-invasive ventilation 947
  see also asthma; chronic obstructive
    pulmonary disease
respiratory effort, signs **646**
respiratory failure 932
  CPAP 945, 946
  type 1 (hypoxaemic) 932
  type 2 (hypercapnic) 932
respiratory observations 645–51, **646**
  epidural/intrathecal analgesia 768
  indications 635
  neurological **702**, 702–3, 706
  postanaesthetic recovery 806, *807*,
    810
  postoperative 817
  procedure guidelines 650–1, *651*
respiratory problems
  positioning in 915–16
  unconscious patients 1047–8
respiratory pump failure 932
respiratory rate **645**, 645–7
  indications for assessing 635
  neurological patients 703
  normal 645, **645**
respiratory secretions
  eating difficulties 603
  humidification and 949
  during oxygen therapy 954
  positioning to maximize drainage 916
  suctioning via
    tracheostomy/laryngectomy
    998–1000, 1002–4
  tracheostomy/laryngectomy patients
    996–7, 998, 1006
  see also sputum
respiratory system 635, 933
respiratory therapy 932–59
  CPAP 945–7
  defined 932
  equipment 941
  humidification 948–52
  indications 932–3
  mechanical ventilation 947–8
  multiple choice questions 958–9,
    1183–4
  non-invasive ventilation 947

problem solving 954–5
  procedure guidelines 953–4
respiratory tract infections
  tracheostomy patients 1007
  viral 965
rest, in pain management 732
restraint, physical 1087–8
resuscitation
  cardiopulmonary *see*
    cardiopulmonary resuscitation
  do not attempt (DNAR) 219–20
  equipment 218, 221
  training 218–19
resuscitation committee 218
Resuscitation Council UK (RCUK)
  218–19
Resuscitation Training Officer (RTO)
  218
reticular activating system (RAS) 693,
  693
retinol binding protein 572
rhesus (Rh) blood group system
  1017
rhesus (Rh) incompatibility 1017
rifampicin **674**, 838
RIG enteral feeding tubes 579, *580*
right bundle branch *615*
rigors 660
Riker scale 1045
rings
  nursing staff 90–1, 103
  surgical patients 794
risk, defined 15
risk assessment
  health care-acquired infections
    118–19
  MRSA infection 148
  pressure ulcers 1123–4
  violence 1084–5
risk management 15–16, 1167
rituals
  last offices 526–7
  nursing 16
Roberts catheters 464, *464*
role development 12–13
roller clamps 351
Royal College of Nursing (RCN)
  Advanced Practice Programme 13

do not attempt resuscitation guidance 219–20
pressure ulcer guidance 1131
on violence 1079
Royal National Institute of the Blind (RNIB) 73
Royal National Institute of the Deaf (RNID) 74
Rusch speaking valve 989, *989*
Ryle's tube, insertion 594–7

SABRE reporting system 1013–14
safety
  occupational *see* health and safety, occupational
  patient 14–16
Safety Representatives and Safety Committees Regulations 1977 1081
salicylates 647, **674**
saline, normal *see* sodium chloride, 0.9% solution
saliva 854
  artificial 860, 868
  autologous 863
  reduced flow 855, 862
salivary gland dysfunction 855
Salmonella food poisoning 122
Saltair No-roma 451
Saltair solution 449
Salts cohesive seals 449
SARS (severe acute respiratory syndrome) 129
satiety, early **578**
scars 1103, 1136–8
  hypertrophic and keloid 1136–8
  management of abnormal 1137–8
schizophrenia, and violence 1083
sciatica, intraoperative positioning and 798
The Scope of Professional Practice (UKCC 1992) 12–13
scopolamine 838
Scotts catheters **461**
scrapie 1034
screw clamps 351
scrub nurse 804
SecuPlast 450

security, stored medicines 261
sedation
  critically ill patients 1045
  opioid-induced 761–2, 773
segmentation, intestinal 403–4
seizures 710
self-catheterization, intermittent 471–2
semi-permeable films, wound management **1111**
senna 416
sensory function, assessment 701, 709
sepsis
  central venous catheter-related 967–8
  intravenous infusion-associated 331
  transfusion-associated 1030
  see also infections
septic shock 144, 664
septicaemia 335
septicaemic shock 631
Serious Adverse Blood Reactions and Events (SABRE) reporting system 1013–14
Serious Hazards of Transfusion (SHOT) scheme 1025
serological testing 965–6
seromas, flap donor site 1136
severe acute respiratory syndrome (SARS) 129
Sevredol 727, 734
  see also morphine
sexual dysfunction, stoma patients 444–5
sexual transmission, viral hepatitis 156, 159
sharps disposal 132, 1063–4
  see also inoculation accidents
shaving
  facial, male patients 886
  surgical site 784
Shaw's silver laryngectomy tube 991, 992
shearing 1122
Shiley laryngectomy tube 991, 992
Shiley tracheostomy tubes 986–8, *987*
  cuffed 986, *987*
  cuffed fenestrated *987*, 988
  cuffless 986, *987*
  fenestrated 986–8, *987*

shivering 659, 660
  postoperative 811, 816
shock
  blood glucose testing 679
  septic 144, 664
  septicaemic 631
  venepuncture in 1059
short bowel syndrome 591
SHOT (Serious Hazards of Transfusion)
      scheme 1025
shoulder, positioning in hemiplegia 919
showering 95–6, 131–2, 881
  preoperative 794
  see also bathing
shroud 527, 532
side lying position 900–1, *901*
  neurological patients 921, *921*
  sitting up from 902–3, *903*
Sikh Educational and Cultural
      Association 544
Sikh Missionary Society 544
Sikhism
  last offices 543–4
  personal hygiene 882
Silastic laryngectomy tube 992, *992*
silicone catheters 465
silicone elastomer-coated catheters 465
silicone gel sheeting, hypertrophic and
      keloid scars 1137
silicone tubes, enteral feeding 579
silver alloy-coated catheters 466
silver dressings 1135
silver sulphadiazine 1135
silver toxicity 466
Sims (Graseby) Medical MS16A syringe
      driver 366–7
Sims (Graseby) Medical MS26 syringe
      driver 366, 366–7
Single Assessment Process 240–4
single
  rooms
    availability in NHS hospitals 124
    source isolation 125–6
sinoatrial (SA) node 615, *615*
sinus rhythm 615
sip feeds 575–6
siphonage 355, 362
sitting position
  amputees 924

  in bed 898–9, *899*
  in chair 904
  moving from lying to 902–3, *903*
  standing from 905, *906*
skills
  Benner's model of acquisition 10, 13
  updating 1168
skin 879–80
  ageing 880
  assessment 880
  bio-engineered substitutes 1119
  dry 880, 881
  non-intact
    aseptic technique 103
    hepatitis B exposure 159, 161, 165
  radiation reactions 880
  soreness, stoma site 453
  temperature 657
skin barrier products
  stoma care 448–9
  wound management **1111**
skin care 879–82
  diarrhoea 409
  multiple choice questions 891, 1183
  oxygen therapy 954
  stoma patients 447
  subcutaneous infusion sites 279
  unconscious patients 1048
  see also pressure area care
skin cleaning *see* skin preparation
skin closure strips, adhesive **1139**
skin grafts 1131–2
  donor site problems 1132–5
  recipient site problems 1135–6
skin infections, lumbar puncture site 552
skin preparation (cleaning)
  intramuscular injections 281–2
  preoperative 784
  venepuncture 1061–3, 1067, *1070*
skin-tunnelled catheters, parenteral
      nutrition 585
skinfold thickness 570
Skinsafe non-sting protective film 448
small intestine 403–4
smell *see* odour
soap
  bactericidal 90, 105–6, 120–1
  dispensers 102, 104

hand washing 89–90, 103–4, 120–1
patient skin care 881
perineal/perianal area 882
social interaction, during procedures 4
social services, discharge planning 234,
   239, 247
sodium bicarbonate
   cardiopulmonary resuscitation 217,
      221
   mouthrinse 865
sodium chloride, 0.9% solution (normal
      saline)
   bladder washout 376, 379
   device flushing 289, 322, 326–7,
      330
   as drug diluent 278
   eye irrigation 833
   mouth care 859
   wound cleaning 1106, **1107**
sodium citrate enema 418
sodium fluoride mouthwash 862
Soft Seal products 450
soft tissue changes, neurological patients
      922
SOLER acronym 62
solution R *see* citric acid 6% solution
sore mouth **578**, 862
   see also oral mucositis
source isolation 117, 123–4, 124–41
   Clostridium difficile infection 154
   cohort nursing 117, 126, 147
   defined 124
   discharge from 141
   facilities required 125–6
   general principles 126–34
   hepatitis A 158
   indications 124
   MRSA-infected patients 147
   procedure guidelines 135–41
   psychological effects 119, 133–4
   rooms *see* isolation rooms
   standard and extra precautions 127,
      127, 128
   strict 117
spacer devices 266
spasticity
   defined 919
   patient positioning 920–1, *921*

speaking valves 989, 989–90
   problems 996
specimen collection 960–81
   blood *see* blood sampling
   body fluids 973–6
   defined 960
   documentation 962–3
   indications 960
   multiple choice questions 980–1,
      1184
   procedure guidelines 969–76
   swabs 969–72
   types of investigation 964–6
   urine *see* urine specimen collection
specimens
   hepatitis B-infected 167
   storage 963
   transport containers 961–2,
      963–4
   transportation 963–4
spectacles 795
speech and language therapists (SLT)
      601, 602, 603
speech deficits 62–3, 697
speed shock 336, 353–5
sphygmomanometers 624–7
   aneroid 626
   components 627
   mercury 625–6
   non-invasive automated 626–7
   postanaesthetic recovery 808
   servicing 630
   using *625*, 629, 632–4
SPIKES model 72
spillages
   blood 1074
   hepatitis B-positive material 165
   microbiological specimens 963
   source barrier nursing 138
spinal anaesthesia/analgesia 551
   postoperative care 812
   see also epidural analgesia; intrathecal
      analgesia
spinal cord 552–4, *756*, 756–7
spinal nerves *757*
spinal stability, positioning and 895
spirometry 639, *640*
spring coil piston syringes 364

sputum
  assessment **646**
  collection 973–4
  infected, tracheostomy patients 1007
  retention, positioning 916
  see also respiratory secretions
staff
  allocation to infected patients 134
  health and safety *see* health and
    safety, occupational
  training *see* training
  violence against *see* violence
standard precautions 127, **128**
  see also universal precautions
standing, assistance with 905, *906*
staphylococci, coagulase-negative 149
Staphylococcus aureus 144
  coagulase-positive 144–8
  glycopeptide intermediate (GISA)
    144–5
  meticillin-resistant *see*
    meticillin-resistant
    Staphylococcus aureus
  meticillin-sensitive (MSSA) 144
  on nurses' uniforms 127
  vancomycin intermediate (VISA)
    144–5
  vancomycin resistant (VRSA) 144–5
Staphylococcus epidermidis, antibiotic
    resistance 143, 149
staples **1139**
  removal 1141–3
stem cell transplantation (SCT)
  blood groups in 1017–18
  cryopreserved cells 1018
  see also bone marrow transplantation
Stenotrophomonas maltophila,
    antibiotic resistant 143
sterculia 414–15
sterile supplies, aseptic technique 92
sternal rub, neurological assessment 698
steroids *see* corticosteroids
stethoscope
  apical heart beat assessment 616–18
  blood pressure measurement 628–9,
    632–4, *634*
  postanaesthetic recovery 808
stock control, medicines 262

stockings, graduated elastic compression
    see antiembolic stockings
stoma(s) 432–59
  bridges or rods 433–4, *434*
  cleaning solutions 447
  defined 432
  deodorants 451
  diarrhoea management 406, 440
  diet 443–4
  discharge plans 443
  fear of malodour 444, 446
  indications 435–6
  management systems 445–7
  sexual function and 444–5
  siting 438–9, *439*
  types 432–4
  see also colostomy; gastrostomy; ileal
    conduits; ileostomy;
    laryngectomy; urostomy
stoma appliances 445–7
  obtaining supplies 443
  plug systems 447
  postoperative period 441–2
  pouches 445–7, *446*
  procedure guidelines 451–3
  skin barriers 448–9
stoma care 432–59
  accessories 447–51
  indications 432
  multiple choice questions 458–9,
    1179
  postoperative 441–2
  preoperative 436–9
  problem solving 453–4
  procedure guidelines 451–3
stoma nurse/therapist, postoperative
    care 440
Stomahesive products 448, 449
stomatitis 854, 870
  prevention 865
  see also oral mucositis
stool softeners **414**, 415
stools *see* faeces
storage
  controlled drugs **258**
  medicines 261–2
  microbiological specimens 963
  patients' own medicines 262, 269

Streptococcus pneumoniae 149
stress
  hormones 675
  response to surgery 721
  violence and 1083
  see also psychological implications
stroke
  joint protection 919
  positioning 918, 922–3
stroke volume 613
subarachnoid (intrathecal) space 552–3,
    756, 756–7
subcutaneous infusions 277–9
  choice of sites 279
  drugs 278
  fluids (hypodermoclysis) 277–8
  infusion devices 366
  site care 279
subcutaneous injections 276–7
  procedure guidelines 304–5
  sites 277
subcutaneous layer 879
subcutaneous route of administration
    276–9
  acute/postoperative pain management
    727
  chronic pain management 724
subjective global assessment (SGA) 568,
    571
sublingual tablets 263, 294
substance abuse, and violence 1083
Suby G *see* citric acid 3.23% and
    magnesium oxide solution
sucralfate 860, 862
suction
  intrapleural drainage 507, 511–12
  postanaesthetic recovery 808, 809
  tracheal *see* tracheal suctioning
sudden cardiac death 205
summarizing 65–6
supervision, drug administration 268
supine position
  in bed 897–8
  neurological patients 918, 921, *921*
  sitting up from 902–3, *903*
supplementary prescribing 273
supportive care *see* psychological
    support

suppositories 264, 422–5
  administration 423
  contraindications 422–3
  defined 422
  indications 422
  types available 423
supraorbital pressure, neurological
    assessment 698
suprapubic catheterization
    470–1
surfaces, antibacterial 131
surgery 783–825
  for cancer pain management
    739–40
  hypothermia risk 659
  infection risk categories **86**
  poor technique **1100**
  stress response to 721
  see also intraoperative care;
      postoperative care; preoperative
      care
surgical instruments, sterile 92
surgical wounds
  changing dressings 1140–1
  exposure to water 92, 95–6
  infection risk categories **86**
  infections 86
  plastic surgery 1131–6
  postanaesthetic recovery 811
  postoperative care 818
  see also wound drains
suspensions, drug 264
sustained-release tablets 263
sutures
  chest drains 503
  removal 1141–3
  wound closure **1139**
swabs 962, 969–72
  ear 969, *969*
  eye 839–40, 970
  nose 970, *970*
  penile 971
  rectal 971
  throat 971, *972*
  vaginal 972
  wound 972
swallow reflex 701
swallowing, normal *604*

swallowing difficulties 601–4
  laryngectomy patients 995–6
  problem solving 601–4
  tracheostomy patients 601, 603,
    995
  see also dysphagia
Swedish nose *see* heat and moisture
    exchanger
symmetrical tonic neck reflex 918
sympathetic nervous system 613, *614*
syphilis, CSF testing 556
syringe drivers 365–7
  problem solving 369–71
  procedure guidelines 368
syringe pumps 361–2
  alarm systems 358, 361
  ambulatory 365
  anaesthesia 363
  patient-controlled analgesia 362
  pros and cons 361–2
  siphonage 355, 362
  user errors 349
syringes, oral drug administration 295
syrups 264
systemic inflammatory response
    syndrome (SIRS) 1030
systolic blood pressure 622
  measurement 629, 634

T-piece circuit 945
tablets 262–3
  administration guidelines 292–5
  crushing or breaking 263, 294, 599,
    600
  storage 262
  via enteral feeding tube 599
tachycardia 613–14
  junctional *617*
  postoperative 815
  transfusion reactions 1026
tachypnoea 646–7
tamoxifen, toxic effects on eye 838
tamponade, cardiac 215
tampons, during surgery 793, 801
tapeworms 973
taps, for hand washing 91, 102, 121
taste changes 863
team working 1167

tears 830, *831*
  artificial 837
TED stockings *see* antiembolic stockings
TEDS *see* antiembolic stockings
teeth, loose 795, 1050
Teflon coated catheters 465
temperature
  body 656–66
    conditions requiring monitoring
      664–5
    defined 656
    indications for measuring 656
    neurological patients 703, 707
    oxygen transport and 644
    postanaesthetic recovery 811
    postoperative monitoring 817
    procedure guidelines 666
    recording sites 661–3
    regulation 656–9, *658*
    time for recording 663
    transfusion reactions 1026, 1040
    see also fever; pyrexia
  core 656, *657*
  food safety and **123**
  inspired gases 948–9
  skin *657*
  venepuncture and 1060
  wound **1100**, 1106
tendon reflexes 708
terminal care
  communication problems 56
  hydration 278
  unconscious patients 1045
  urgent discharge home 236, *237–8*
  see also death
theatre, operating *see* operating theatre
therapeutic relationships, trusting 729
thermometers 663–4, *665*
thermoregulation 656–9, *658*
thiamine deficiency 571
thinking, critical 27–8
threadworms 971
three-way taps, infection risk 284
throat swabs 971, *972*
thrombocytes *see* platelets
thromboembolic deterrent stockings *see*
    antiembolic stockings
thromboprophylaxis

patients on bed rest 896
surgical patients 785–6, 788–92
see also antiembolic stockings
thrombosis
intravenous infusion-related 334
see also deep vein thrombosis; venous
thromboembolism
thyrotoxic crisis 664
tidal volume (TV) 639, 641
Tieman-tipped catheters 464, *464*
Tilley's forceps 997
TIME principles, wound management
1104, 1106–15
tissue adhesive **1139**
tissue integrity, impaired
aetiology 1121–2
respiratory therapy 947, 954
unconscious patients 1048
see also pressure ulcers
tissue necrosis, debridement 1106–12
tissue oxygenation 934
TNP *see* topical negative pressure
therapy
Todd's paralysis 710
toilets, barrier-nursed patients 137
tone *see* muscle tone
tonic labyrinthine reflex 918
tonic neck reflex
asymmetrical 918
symmetrical 918
toothbrushes 857–8
toothbrushing 858, 867–8, 870
topical anaesthesia
eye drops 832
urinary catheterization 466–7
topical applications of drugs, procedure
guidelines 309–10
topical negative pressure therapy (TNP)
1118
procedure guidelines 1147–50
topical preparations 264–5
topical wound treatment dressings
1119–20
total lung capacity (TLC) *640*, 642
touch, without consent 6–7
tourniquets
to aid venepuncture 1060, 1066, 1067
for venepuncture site bleeding 1064

towels, paper *see* paper towels
toxic shock syndrome 801
toxicity, cardiopulmonary arrest 215–16
trace elements, parenteral nutrition
solutions 586
tracheal dilators 996
tracheal suctioning (via tracheostomy)
998–1000
catheters 1000, *1000*
indications 999
procedure guidelines 1002–4
tracheo-oesophageal puncture 995–6,
997
tracheostomy 982–1012
communication methods 993–4
defined 982
dressing changes 997, 1001
emergency 984
general nursing care 996–7
humidification 950, 993, 1005
indications 982
mini 984
multiple choice questions 1011–12,
1184
oxygen masks 944
percutaneous 984
permanent *983*, 983–4
problem solving 1006–7
procedure guidelines 1001–5
resuscitation 1000
suctioning via 998–1000, 1002–4
surgical 984
swallowing problems 601, 603, 995
temporary 982, *983*
see also laryngectomy
tracheostomy tubes 984–92, 996
changing 996–7
changing difficulties 1006–7
decannulation plug *990*, 991
dislodgement 1006
Jackson's silver 988, *988*
Kapitex Tracoetwist fenestrated *990*,
990–1
laryngectomy tubes 991–2, *992*
Negus's silver *988*, 989
occlusion 1006
Portex cuffed *985*, 985–6
Shiley 986–8, *987*

tracheostomy tubes (*cont.*)
  speaking valve 989, 989–90
  stoma button 992, 992
  total laryngectomy 997–8
trachphone 993, *994*
training
  blood glucose monitoring 679–80
  cardiopulmonary resuscitation
    218–19
  communication 67
  infusion device use 349
  violence prevention/management
    1086, 1087
tramadol 728, 734
transcutaneous electrical nerve
    stimulation (TENS) 732
transdermal patches 265
transfers
  interhospital, MRSA-infected patients
    148
  to/from operating table 799–800, 803
  to/from operating theatre 796
  see also manual handling;
    mobilization
transforming growth factor-β (TGF-β)
    864, **1101**, 1120
transfusion 1013–44
  appropriate use 1018
  blood and blood products used
    1019–23
  blood pack labelling *1035*
  care during 1024
  defined 1013
  incompatible 1017
  indications 1018, **1019–23**
  Jehovah's Witnesses 1024–5
  multiple choice questions 1043–4,
    1184–5
  observations during 618, 665, 1024,
    1038
  pre-administration checks 1027,
    1028, 1036–7
  problem solving 1039–40
  procedure 1036–9
  procedure guidelines 1036–9
  process 1024
  safety and quality of practice
    1013–14

transfusion-associated circulatory
    overload (TACO) 1028
transfusion-associated graft-versus-host
    disease (TA-GVHD) 1031–2
transfusion reactions 1025–34
  Blood Safety and Quality Regulations
    1013–14
  delayed 1030–2
  immediate 1026–30
  infectious complications 160,
    1014–15, 1032–4
  major 1026, **1027**
  management 1025–6, **1027**, 1040
  minor 1025–6
  monitoring for 1038
transfusion-related acute lung injury
    (TRALI) 1030
transmissible spongiform
    encephalopathies (TSEs) 1034
transmission based precautions *see*
    source isolation
transplant co-ordinators 537
transplant donors 537
transportation
  discharge planning 250
  hepatitis B-infected patients 167
  infected patients 141
  microbiological specimens 963–4
  MRSA-infected patients 148
trapezium squeeze, neurological
    assessment 698
trauma
  cardiopulmonary arrest 206, 215
  epidural analgesia 755
  tracheal suctioning 999
  urethral mucosal, catheterized
    patients 484
Trendelenburg position, during surgery
    799
tricyclic antidepressants **724**
triglycerides 576, 581
trusting therapeutic relationships,
    creating 729
tuberculosis (TB), last offices 534
tubing, infusion administration sets 351
tubular reabsorption 668, *668*
tubular secretion *668*, 669
tunica adventitia 1058

tunica intima 1058
tunica media 1058
tympanic membrane thermometers 661,
    663–4, *665*
    procedure guidelines 666

ulcerative colitis 434
unconscious patients 1045–54
    defined 1045
    ethical issues 1049
    eye care 838, 849–50, 884, 1048,
        1051
    multiple choice questions 1054,
        1185
    physiological changes 1046–9
    procedure guidelines 1049–51
    see also consciousness
underinfusion 353, **354**
    complications **348**
    problem solving 371
undertakers 537
uniforms, nurses 93, 127
Union of Liberal and Progressive
        Synagogues 542
universal precautions
    operating theatre 800
    see also standard precautions
upper limb
    amputees 923, 925
    veins for venepuncture 1056–8, *1057*
urea, plasma **588**, 590
urease-secreting micro-organisms 378
ureterostomy 435
urethral catheterization *see* urinary
        catheterization
urethral meatus
    cleaning
        catheterized patients 468
        midstream specimen of urine 968,
            974, 975
    crusting, catheterized patients 485
urethral mucosal trauma/irritation,
        catheterized patients 484
urinalysis 667–72
    dipstick (reagent) tests 671–2, *672*
    drugs affecting results **674**
    indications 667
    procedure guidelines 671–2, *672*

urinary catheter-associated infections
        377–8, 467, 487
    bladder lavage 377
    management 483
    multiple choice questions 397, 1178–9
    sites of entry 467, *468*
    specimen collection 968
urinary catheterization 460–96
    anaesthetic lubricating gel 466–7
    defined 460
    drainage bags *see* urine drainage bags
    indications 460–1
    intermittent self- 471–2
    leg straps 469
    meatal cleaning 468
    multiple choice questions 495–6, 1180
    postanaesthetic recovery 806
    problem solving 483–7
    procedure guidelines 472–9
    suprapubic 470–1
    unconscious patients 1047, 1051
    urine specimen collection 479–80, *481*
urinary catheters 461–6
    bags *see* urine drainage bags
    balloon size 461–2
    biofilm formation 377–8
    bladder irrigation 381, *382*
    encrustations and blockages
        378–80
    leakage around 392
    length 463
    maintenance solutions 375–97
        clinically-based studies 379–80
        defined 375
        indications 375–6
        patient assessment 380–1
        problem solving 392–3
        procedure guidelines 385–7
    materials 464–6
    removal 482–3
    size 463
    suprapubic 470
    three-way 381, *382*, **461**, *462*
    tip design 464, *464*
    types **461**, *462*
    valves 469–70
urinary diversion 434–5
    see also ileal conduits; urostomy

urinary incontinence 880
penile sheaths 487–90
see also incontinence
urinary retention
catheterized patients 487
epidural/intrathecal analgesia 762,
774
urinary tract infections (UTIs) 669
catheter-associated *see* urinary
catheter-associated infections
dipstick tests 671
health care-associated 118
observations 669, **673**
predisposing factors 670
urine 667–71
colour 669, **673**
formation 667–9, *668*
leakage
around catheters 486
urinary stomas 453
observations 669–71, **673**
pH 669
catheter encrustation and 379, 381
smell 669, **673**
source barrier nursing 133, 137
urine drainage bags 468–9
body-worn 469
changing 467
emptying 481–2
leg 469
positioning 467
urine output/production
impaired
catheterized patients 484, 485
postoperative 816
urostomy 441
urine specimen collection 968
catheter (CSU) 479–80, *481*
ileal conduit or urostomy 454
midstream (MSU) 968, 974–5
procedure guidelines 974–6
twenty-four hour 671, 975–6
urostomy 434, *435*
fluid intake 444
indications 436
postoperative care 441–2
postoperative function 441
pouches *446*, 447

problem solving 453–4
urine specimen collection 454
see also stoma(s)
urticaria, transfusion-induced 1030

vaccines, storage 262
vacs system *see* topical negative pressure
therapy
vacuum blood collection systems 1063
procedure guidelines 1065, 1068–9
vacuum drainage system
changing 1144–5
removal 1145–6
VADs *see* vascular access devices
vaginal medicines 264
administration, procedure guidelines
307–9
vaginal swabs 972
Valsalva manoeuvre, chest drain
removal 507, 517
valves, venous 1058
vancomycin-resistant enterococci (VRE)
142, 143, 150–1
barrier nursing 127, 132
environmental survival 150–1
vascular access devices (VADs)
blood pressure measurement and 630
central *see* central venous access
devices
direct intermittent injections 288–9,
323–7
infusion flow rates 352
occlusion 330
parenteral nutrition 585
vascular endothelial growth factor
(VEGF) **1101**, 1103
vasovagal reaction 479, 1073
vastus lateralis injections *280*, 281
vector-borne infections 122–3
veins
anatomy and physiology 1056–8
injuries, intravenous infusions 329
missed 1074
palpation 1059, *1070*
selection for venepuncture 1058–60
tapping 1061
for venepuncture 1056–8, *1057*
visual inspection 1058–9

venepuncture 1055–78
  choice of device 1061, **1062**
  choice of vein 1058–60
  defined 1055
  improving venous access 1060–1
  indications 1055
  multiple choice questions 1077–8,
    1185
  problem solving 1071–5
  procedure guidelines 1065–70,
    1070–1
  removal of device 1064
  safety of practitioner 1063–4
  skin preparation 1061–3
venipuncture *see* venepuncture
venous access
  cardiopulmonary resuscitation 216,
    225
  limited, problem solving 1072
  methods for improving 1060–1
  parenteral nutrition 585
  see also central venous access devices;
    vascular access devices
venous pressure, infusion flow and 358
venous spasm
  effect on flow rate 351
  during intravenous infusions 329
  during venepuncture 1060, 1075
venous thromboembolism (VTE)
  cardiopulmonary arrest 215
  postoperative care 818
  prophylaxis *see* thromboprophylaxis
  risk factors 785, 788–9
  unconscious patients 1048
  see also deep vein thrombosis;
    pulmonary embolism
venous valves 1058
ventilated patients
  enteral feeds 582
  humidification of inspired gases 950
  positioning 914, *915*
  tracheal suctioning 999
ventilation 637–41
  Ambu bag and mask 209, 223
  mechanical 947–8
  minute (MV) 639
  mouth-to-face mask 209
  mouth-to-mouth 208–9, *210*

non-invasive 947
  pulmonary 933
ventilation/perfusion *(V/Q)* ratio
  effect of CPAP 946
  positioning and 914, *915*
ventilation systems *see* air conditioning
    and ventilation systems
ventilators, positive pressure 948
ventricular fibrillation (VF) 616, *617*
  cardiopulmonary resuscitation 205,
    216, 217
ventricular tachycardia (VT), pulseless
    205, 216, 217
ventrogluteal intramuscular injections
    280, 281
Venturi-type oxygen masks 942–4, *944*
verbal communication 62
verbal orders, drug administration
    267–8
verbal response, Glasgow coma scale
    695, 695–7
vicarious liability 1170
vigilance 14–15
violence 1079–96
  defined 1079
  intervention and management
    1087–8, 1092
  legislation 1080–1
  multiple choice questions 1096,
    1185–6
  policy formation 1081
  post-incident review 1088–9, 1092
  prediction 1081–4, 1090–1
  prevalence 1079–80
  prevention 1085–6, 1091
  procedure guidelines 1090–2
  risk assessment 1084–5
viral infections
  oral 861
  specimen collection 965
  transfusion-transmitted 1032–3
  see also specific infections
viscosity, blood 620
visitors
  source isolation facilities 129, 133–4
  see also family
visual acuity testing 704, 709
visual field defects 704, **704**, 828

visual fields *829*
visual pathways 828, *829*
visually impaired patients,
    communication with 72–3
vital capacity (VC) *640*, 642
vital signs
    epidural/intrathecal analgesia in
        chronic setting 768
    neurological assessment 701–3, 706–7
    postanaesthetic recovery 810–11
    unconscious patients 1050
    see also blood pressure; observations;
        pulse; respiratory observations;
        temperature
vitamin A 1105
vitamin B_{12}, serum **589**
vitamin C (ascorbic acid) **674**, 679,
    1102, 1105
vitamin D deficiency 571
vitamins
    dietary requirements 573
    parenteral nutrition solutions 586
    serum levels 572
    supplements 577
vitreous humour 828
volumetric infusion pumps 360–1
    ambulatory 365
vomiting *see* nausea and vomiting
VRE *see* vancomycin-resistant
    enterococci

walking 906–12
    assistance, procedure guidelines 912
    using elbow crutches **909–10**
    using sticks **907–8**
    using walking frame **911–12**
walking aids 906, **907–12**
walking frame **911–12**
walking sticks **907–8**
wards
    cleaning *see* cleaning, environmental
    purpose built infectious disease 125
    see also single rooms
waste
    domestic 132
    hepatitis B-infected patients 164
    source barrier nursing 132, 135, 138
    venepuncture 1063–4, 1070

The Watch Tower Bible and Tract
    Society 541
watches, removal 90–1, 103
water
    balloon catheters 463
    exposure of wounds to 92, 95–6
    eye irrigation 833
    flushing enteral feeding tubes 599, 600
    hand washing 89–90, 103, 105, 121
    wound cleaning 1106, **1107**
water baths, blood warming 1029
water vapour 935, 948
Waterlow scale 1124, *1125–6*
weighing, procedure guidelines 591–2
weight, body *see* body weight
weight bearing
    fully (FWB) 906
    partially (PWB) 906
wheezing **646**
whistle-tipped catheters 464, *464*
white blood cells
    in CSF 556
    for transfusion **1020**
white coats, doctors' 129
WHO *see* World Health Organization
winged infusion devices 1061, **1062**
WISECARE project 35
women *see* female patients
World Health Organization (WHO)
    analgesic ladder 723, *723*, 733–8
    Mucositis Scale 856, 857
wound(s)
    acute 1098, 1101–2
        changing dressings 1140–1
    assessment 1115, *1116–17*
    bacterial colonization 1112
    chronic 1098, 1101
    classification 1097–8
    cleaning 1106, **1107**, 1141
    closure methods 1138, **1139**
    contraction 1103
    debridement 1106–12
    defined 1097
    exudate *see* exudate, wound
    improving blood flow to 1105
    inflammation and infection 1112–13
    moisture balance 1113, 1114
    re-epithelialization 1102

surgical *see* surgical wounds
swabs 972
wound bed preparation (WBP) 1103,
    1104
wound drains
    dressing, procedure guidelines 1143–4
    removal, procedure guidelines 1145–6
    shortening, procedure guidelines 1147
wound dressings **1108–11**
    changing, procedure guidelines
        1140–1
    closed drainage systems (Redivac)
        1143–4
    dry and wet 1114
    moisture balance control 1113, 1114
    occlusive 1114
    principles of use 1113–15
    promoting autolytic debridement
        1107
    slipping, skin graft donor sites 1135
    topical treatments 1119–20
    see also dressings
wound healing 1098–113
    assessment 1115
    edge non-advancement 1115
    factors affecting **1100**, 1103–5
    by first intention 1098
    growth factors **1101**, 1102–3,
        1119–20
    haemostasis 1099
    inflammatory phase 1099–101
    maturation phase 1103
    nutrition and 1104–5
    phases 1098–103
    poor 571

proliferative phase 1101–3
promoting good 1105–13
by secondary intention 1098
by tertiary intention 1098
wound infections 1112–13
    health care acquired 118
    skin graft donor sites 1135
wound management 1097–162
    bio-engineered skin substitutes
        1119
    complementary therapies 1120
    hepatitis B infection 166–7
    hyperbaric oxygen therapy 1118
    moisture balance 1113, 1114
    multiple choice questions 1161–2,
        1186
    pressure ulcers 1129
    procedure guidelines 1140–50
    TIME principles **1104**, 1106–15
    topical negative pressure therapy
        (TNP) 1118, 1147–50
    topical treatment dressings 1119–20
wrist bands 14
    see also identification, patient

xerostomia (dry mouth) 855, 862, 869

Yeates vacuum drainage system, removal
    1145–6

Z-track technique, intramuscular
    injections 281
zinc 1105
Zoroastrian Trust Funds of Europe 544
Zoroastrianism, last offices 544